Comprehensive Textbook of Perioperative Transesophageal Echocardiography

SECOND EDITION

EDITED BY

Robert M. Savage, MD, FACC

Head, Perioperative Echocardiography
Department of Cardiothoracic Anesthesia, Anesthesia Institute
Co-director Intraoperative Echocardiography
Department of Cardiovascular Medicine
Cleveland Clinic
Cleveland, Ohio

Solomon Aronson, MD, FACC, FCCP, FAHA, FASE

Professor of Anesthesiology
Executive Vice Chair
Department of Anesthesiology
Duke University Medical Center
Durham, North Carolina

Stanton K. Shernan, MD, FAHA, FASE

Associate Professor of Anaesthesia
Director of Cardiac Anesthesia
Brigham and Women's Hospital
Harvard Medical School
Boston, Massachusetts

ASSOCIATE EDITOR

Andrew Shaw, MB, FRCA, FCCM

Associate Professor
Department of Anesthesiology
Duke University Medical Center
Durham, North Carolina

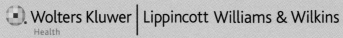
Wolters Kluwer | Lippincott Williams & Wilkins
Health

Philadelphia • Baltimore • New York • London
Buenos Aires • Hong Kong • Sydney • Tokyo

Acquisitions Editor: Brian Brown
Product Manager: Nicole Dernoski
Production Manager: Alicia Jackson
Senior Manufacturing Manager: Benjamin Rivera
Marketing Manager: Angela Panetta
Design Coordinator: Stephen Druding
Production Service: SPi Technologies

Second Edition

Printed in China

Library of Congress Cataloging-in-Publication Data
Comprehensive textbook of perioperative transesophageal echocardiography / edited by Robert M. Savage, Solomon Aronson, Stanton K. Shernan ; associate editor, Andrew Shaw. —2nd ed.
   p. ; cm.
  Includes bibliographical references and index.
  ISBN 978-1-60547-246-1 (hardback : alk. paper)
  1. Transesophageal echocardiography. 2. Heart—Surgery 3. Intraoperative monitoring.
I. Savage, Robert M., 1950–
  [DNLM: 1. Echocardiography, Transesophageal—methods. 2. Intraoperative Care.
WG 141.5.E2 C737 2011]
  RD52.T73C665 2011
  616.1'207543—dc22

                                         2010025181

To purchase additional copies of this book, call our customer service department at (800) 638-3030 or fax orders to (301) 223-2320. International customers should call (301) 223-2300.

Visit Lippincott Williams & Wilkins on the Internet: at LWW.com. Lippincott Williams & Wilkins customer service representatives are available from 8:30 am to 6 pm, EST.

                                      10 9 8 7 6 5 4 3 2 1

CCS0810

Dedication

This work is dedicated to Cheri, my wife and best friend, and our two amazing daughters (Lanier and Virginia). They make life an exciting adventure worth every second.

Robert M. Savage, MD

I would like to thank all my instructors, colleagues, and students over the years for teaching me that knowledge is endless and my family Leena, Rebecca, and Benjamin for helping me understand that each moment is precious. I dedicate this book to my Mother—Ethel Barbara Aronson—who is forever missed.

Solomon Aronson, MD

I would like to dedicate this book to my family Audrey, Ethan, and Mina for their precious support, patience, and love; to my parents Sidney and Phyllis Shernan for their guidance and encouragement to pursue a passion for learning and excellence; and finally to all my mentors, colleagues, and students over the years who have generously given me their extraordinary wisdom.

Stanton K. Shernan, MD

CONTENTS

CONTRIBUTORS

Nicolas Aeschlimann, MD
Department of Anesthesiology
Duke University Medical Center
Durham, North Carolina

Andrej A. Alfirevic, MD
Codirector
Perioperative Echocardiography
Department of Cardiothoracic Anesthesia
Anesthesia Institute
Cleveland Clinic
Cleveland, Ohio

Solomon Aronson, MD, FACC, FCCP, FAHA, FASE
Professor of Anesthesiology
Executive Vice Chair
Department of Anesthesiology
Duke University Medical Center
Durham, North Carolina

Edwin G. Avery, IV, MD, CPI
Assistant Professor of Anesthesiology
Division of Cardiac Anesthesia
Massachusetts General Hospital Heart Center
Harvard Medical School
Boston, Massachusetts

Atilio Barbeito, MD
Assistant Professor
Department of Anesthesiology
Duke University Medical Center
Staff Anesthesiologist
Anesthesiology Service
Durham VA Medical Center
Durham, North Carolina

Shahar Bar-Yosef, MD
Assistant Professor
Anesthesiology and Critical Care Medicine
Duke University
Staff Anesthesiologist
Department of Anesthesia
VA Medical Center
Durham, North Carolina

Erik A.K. Beyer, MD
Surgical Director
Atrial Fibrillation Center
Division of Cardiac Surgery
Methodist DeBakey Heart & Vascular Center
Houston, Texas

Bruce Bollen, MD
Missoula Anesthesiology PC
St. Patrick Hospital and Health Sciences Center
Missoula, Montana

Bernard E. Bulwer, MD
Noninvasive Cardiovascular Research
Cardiovascular Division
Brigham and Women's Hospital
Harvard Medical School
Boston, Massachusetts

Michael K. Cahalan, MD
Professor and Chair
Department of Anesthesiology
University of Utah School of Medicine
Salt Lake City, Utah

Michelle Capdeville, MD
Fellowship Program Director
Department of Cardiothoracic Anesthesia
Cleveland Clinic
Cleveland, Ohio

Jose Diaz-Gomez, MD
Department of Cardiothoracic Anesthesia
Anesthesia Institute
Heart and Vascular Institute
Cleveland Clinic
Cleveland, Ohio

Carlos Duran, MD
President/CEO
International Heart Institute of Montana
Missoula, Montana

Michael Essandoh, MD
Fellow
Department of Cardiothoracic Anesthesia
Cleveland Clinic
Cleveland, Ohio

Elyse Foster, MD, FACC, FAHA
Professor of Clinical Medicine & Anesthesia
Araxe Vilensky Endowed Chair in Cardiology
Director, Adult Non-Invasive Cardiology Laboratories
Director, Adult Congenital Heart Disease Service
University of California
California, San Francisco

A. Marc Gillinov, MD
The Judith Dion Pyle Chair in Heart Valve Research
Department of Thoracic and Cardiovascular Surgery
Cleveland Clinic
Cleveland, Ohio

Kathryn Glas, MD, FASE, MBA
Associate Professor
Anesthesiology
Department of Anesthesiology
Emory University School of Medicine
Atlanta, Georgia

Donald D. Glower, MD
Professor Division of Thoracic and Cardiovascular Surgery
Department of Surgery
Duke University Medical Center
Durham, North Carolina

Gonzalo Gonzalez-Stawinski, MD
Staff Surgeon
Department of Thoracic and Cardiovascular Surgery
Cleveland Clinic
Cleveland, Ohio

Ankur R. Gosalia, MD
Assistant Professor
Department of Anesthesiology
Western Pennsylvania Hospital
Pittsburgh, Pennsylvania

Alina M. Grigore, MD, MHS, FASE
Associate Professor of Anesthesiology
Department of Anesthesiology
University of Maryland School of Medicine
Director, Division of Cardiothoracic and Vascular
    Anesthesiology
Department of Anesthesiology
University of Maryland Medical Center
Baltimore, Maryland

Lori B. Heller, MD
Staff Attending
Swedish Covenant Hospital
Seattle, Washington

Jordan K.C. Hudson, MD, FRCPC
Assistant Professor
Department of Anesthesiology
The Ottawa Hospital, Civic Campus
Ottawa, Ontario

Christopher C. C. Hudson, FRCPC
Assistant Professor
Department of Anesthesiology
Division of Cardiac Anesthesiology and Critical Care Medicine
University of Ottawa Heart Institute
Ottawa, Ontario

G. Chad Hughes, MD
Director
Thoracic Aorta Program
Assistant Professor
Division of Thoracic and Cardiovascular Surgery
Department of Surgery
Duke University Medical Center
Durham, North Carolina

Jason N. Katz, MD
Assistant Professor of Medicine
Cardiology and Critical Care Medicine
UNC Center for Heart and Vascular Care
The University of North Carolina at Chapel Hill
Chapel Hill, North Carolina

Kyungrok Kim, MD
Fellow
Department of Cardiothoracic Anesthesia
Cleveland Clinic
Cleveland, Ohio

Colleen Gorman Koch, MD, MS, MBA
Vice-Chair, Research
Department of Cardiothoracic Anesthesia
Cleveland Clinic
Cleveland, Ohio

Ryan Lauer, MD
Assistant Professor
Department of Anesthesiology
Division of Cardiovascular Anesthesia
Loma Linda Medical Center
Loma Linda, Cailifornia

Teng C. Lee, MD
Department of Surgery
Division of Thoracic and Cardiovascular Surgery
Duke University Medical Center
Durham, North Carolina

Michael G. Licina, MD
Vice-Chairman, Operations
Department of Cardiothoracic Anesthesia
Cleveland Clinic
Cleveland, Ohio

Bruce W. Lytle, MD
CEO, Heart & Vascular Institute
Department of Thoracic and Cardiovascular Surgery
Cleveland Clinic
Cleveland, Ohio

G. Burkhard Mackensen, MD, PhD, FASE
Associate Professor of Anesthesiology
Division of Cardiothoracic Anesthesia and Critical Care
    Medicine
Department of Anesthesiology
Duke University Medical Center
Durham, North Carolina

Brenda M. MacKnight, MD
Department of Anesthesiology
Western Pennsylvania Hospital
Pittsburgh, Pennsylvania

Feroze Mahmood, MD
Director
Vascular Anesthesia and Perioperative Echocardiography
Beth Israel Deaconess Medical Center
Assistant Professor of Anesthesia
Harvard Medical School
Boston, Massachusetts

Carlo E. Marcucci, MD
Director of Cardiothoracic Anesthesia
Department of Anesthesia
University Hospital of Lausanne
Lausanne, Switzerland

Jonathan B. Mark, MD
Professor and Vice Chairman
Department of Anesthesiology
Duke University
Chief, Anesthesiology Service
Veterans Affairs Medical Center
Durham, North Carolina

Andrew Maslow, MD
Associate Professor
Department of Anesthesiology
Warren Alpert School of Medicine
Brown Medical School
Providence, Rhode Island

Joseph P. Mathew, MD
Director
Cardiac Anesthesia
Department of Anesthesiology
Duke University
Durham, North Carolina

Tomislav Mihaljevic, MD
Donna and Ken Lewis Endowed Chair in Cardiothoracic
    Surgery
Department of Thoracic and Cardiovascular Surgery
Cleveland Clinic
Cleveland, Ohio

Carmelo Milano, MD
Director
Cardiac Transplant
Assistant Professor
Division of Thoracic and Cardiovascular Surgery
Department of Surgery
Duke University Medical Center
Durham, North Carolina

K. Annette Mizuguchi, MD, PhD
Department of Anesthesiology
Perioperative and Pain Medicine
Brigham and Women's Hospital
Harvard Medical School
Boston, Massachusetts

Alina Nicoara, MD
Assistant Professor of Anesthesiology
Department of Anesthesiology
Duke University Medical Center
Durham, North Carolina

Albert Perrino, Jr, MD
Professor
Yale University School of Medicine
New Haven, Connecticut

Juan C. Plana, MD
Assistant Professor of Medicine
Department of Cardiology
Director
Cardiac Imaging
The University of Texas MD Anderson Cancer Center
Houston, Texas

Mihai V. Podgoreanu, MD
Associate Professor of Anesthesiology
Department of Anesthesiology
Duke University Medical Center
Durham, North Carolina

David T. Porembka, FCCM, FCCP
Professor of Anesthesia with Tenure
Professor of Surgery
Professor of Cardiology (Internal Medicine)
University of Cincinnati Academic Health Center
Anesthesiologist
Department of Anesthesiology
University Hospital
Cincinnati, Ohio

Scott T. Reeves, MD, MBA, FACC, FASE
John E. Mahaffey Endowed Professor and Chairman
Anesthesia and Perioperative Medicine
Medical University of South Carolina
Charleston, South Carolina

James Richardson, MD
Assistant Professor
Anesthesiology
Department of Anesthesiology
Emory University School of Medicine
Atlanta, Georgia

Kathryn Rouine-Rapp, MD
Professor of Anesthesia and Perioperative Care
University of California
California, San Francisco

Isobel Russell, MD, PhD, FACC
Professor of Anesthesia University of California
California, San Francisco

Joseph Sabik, MD
Chair
Thoracic and Cardiovascular Surgery
Cleveland Clinic
Cleveland, Ohio

Robert M. Savage, MD, FACC
Head, Perioperative Echocardiography
Department of Cardiothoracic Anesthesia
Codirector Intraoperative Echocardiography
Department of Cardiovascular Medicine
Cleveland Clinic
Cleveland, Ohio

Rebecca A. Schroeder, MD
Associate Professor
Department of Anesthesiology
Duke University
Durham, North Carolina

Carl Schwartz, MD
Assistant Professor
Department of Anesthesiology
Warren Alpert School of Medicine
Brown Medical School
Providence, Rhode Island

Jack S. Shanewise, MD
Professor of Anesthesiology
Chief Division of Cardiothoracic Anesthesia
Department of Anesthesiology
Columbia University Medical Center
New York City, New York

Andrew D. Shaw, MB, FRCA, FCCM
Associate Professor
Department of Anesthesiology
Duke University Medical Center
Durham, North Carolina

Stanton K. Shernan, MD, FAHA, FASE
Associate Professor of Anesthesia
Department of Anesthesiology
Perioperative and Pain Medicine
Director of Cardiac Anesthesia
Brigham and Women's Hospital
Harvard Medical School
Boston, Massachusetts

Joyce J. Shin, MD
Staff
Department of Cardiothoracic Anesthesia
Cleveland Clinic
Cleveland, Ohio

Douglas C. Shook, MD
Program Director, Cardiothoracic Anesthesiology
Fellowship, Department of Anesthesiology
Perioperative and Pain Medicine
Brigham and Women's Hospital
Harvard Medical School
Boston, Massachusetts

Linda Shore-Lesserson, MD, FASE
Chief
Cardiothoracic Anesthesiology
Montefiore Medical Center
Bronx, New York

Saket Singh, MD
Department of Anesthesiology
Western Pennsylvania Hospital
Pittsburgh, Pennsylvania

Nikolaos J. Skubas, MD, FASE, DSc
Associate Professor of Anesthesiology
Department of Anesthesiology
Weill Cornell Medical College
Associate Attending
Department of Anesthesiology
New York-Presbyterian Weill Cornell Medical Center
New York, New York

Nicholas G. Smedira, MD
Staff Surgeon
Department of Thoracic and Cardiovascular Surgery
Cleveland Clinic
Cleveland, Ohio

Edward G. Soltesz, MD, MPH
Staff Surgeon
Department of Thoracic and Cardiovascular
    Surgery
Cleveland Clinic
Cleveland, Ohio

William J. Stewart, MD, FACC, FASE
Co-director of Intraoperative Echocardiography
Department of Cardiovascular Medicine
Cleveland Clinic
Cleveland, Ohio

Christopher F. Sulzer, MD
Staff Anesthesiologist
Director of Cardiac Anesthesia
Department of Anesthesiology
University Hospital of Lausanne (CHUV)
Lausanne, Switzerland

Lars G. Svensson, MD
Staff Surgeon
Director of the Aorta Center
Director of the Marfan Syndrome and Connective
    Tissue Disorder Clinic
Department of Thoracic and Cardiovascular
    Surgery
Cleveland Clinic
Cleveland, Ohio

Madhav Swaminathan, MD, FASE, FAHA
Associate Professor of Anesthesiology
Division of Cardiothoracic Anesthesia and
    Critical Care Medicine
Department of Anesthesiology
Duke University Medical Center
Durham, North Carolina

Dilip R. Thakar, MD
Professor
Department of Anesthesiology and Pain
    Medicine
MD Anderson Cancer Center
Houston, Texas

James D. Thomas, MD
Department of Cardiovascular Medicine
Heart & Vascular Institute
Cleveland Clinic
Cleveland, Ohio

Christopher A. Thunberg, MD
Instructor
Department of Anesthesiology
Mayo Clinic College of Medicine
Senior Associate Consultant
Department of Anesthesiology
Mayo Clinic Hospital
Phoenix, Arizona

Daniel M. Thys, MD
Chairman Emeritus
Department of Anesthesiology
St. Luke's-Roosevelt Hospital Center
Professor Emeritus
Department of Anesthesiology
College of Physicians & Surgeons
Columbia University
New York, New York

Christopher A. Troianos, MD
Chairman and Program Director
Department of Anesthesiology
Western Pennsylvania Hospital
Pittsburgh, Pennsylvania

E. Murat Tuzcu, MD, FACC, FAHA
Vice-Chairman
Department of Cardiovascular Medicine
Heart & Vascular Institute
Cleveland Clinic
Cleveland, Ohio

Rosemary N. Uzomba, MD
Department of Anesthesiology
Western Pennsylvania Hospital
Pittsburgh, Pennsylvania

Daniel P. Vezina, MD, MSc, FRCPC
Associate Professor
Department of Anesthesiology
University of Utah School of Medicine
Salt Lake City, Utah

Patrick L. Whitlow, MD
Department of Cardiovascular Medicine
Heart & Vascular Institute
Cleveland Clinic
Cleveland, Ohio

Dominik Wiktor, MD
Lerner Research institute
Cleveland Clinic
University Hospitals
Case Western University
Cleveland, Ohio

Matthew L. Williams, MD
Fellow
Division of Thoracic and Cardiovascular
   Surgery
Department of Surgery Duke University
   Medical Center
Durham, North Carolina

FOREWORD

It is a pleasure to be asked to contribute in a small way to the *Comprehensive Textbook of Perioperative Transesophageal Echocardiography*. This text is one that Drs. Savage, Aronson, and Shernan should be justifiably proud. The transition from the first edition's focus on intraoperative transesophageal echocardiography (TEE) to the second edition's focus on perioperative transesophageal echocardiography is indicative of the progression of not only the imaging technique, but also the subspecialty of cardiac anesthesiology and perioperative medicine. Knowing that many of our trainees develop skills in TEE that contribute each and every day to improved patient outcomes, it should be real satisfaction for these editors and their contributors to know that their work is truly changing the specialty and patient care.

These editors have been persistent in advancing perioperative imaging to the benefit of patients. As Calvin Coolidge once said,

> Nothing in the world can take the place of persistence. Talent will not; nothing is more common than unsuccessful men with talent. Genius will not; unrewarded genius is almost a proverb. Education will not; the world is full of educated derelicts. Persistence and determination alone are unstoppable.

The persistence of these authors and editors in bringing this work forward is remarkable since time for creativity is increasingly being challenged in our academic medicine environments. As those of us involved in academic medicine know, it is this outlet for creativity that drew many of us into our academic careers, and I laud Bob, Sol, and Stan for their willingness to stay persistent and creative. What we are increasingly seeing is that patients benefit from those with skills in TEE, who apply their TEE skills along the continuum of perioperative. I find the organization of this second edition to be well thought out and the progression from basic material up through decision making is well-designed. So very often the "tools of our trade" are discussed in some detail, but the progression from the "basics" into decision making is left out of so many other texts.

Again, I thank the three editors and all their contributors for staying focused and persistent on what we all entered medicine to do—help the patient.

David L. Brown, MD
Chairman, Anesthesiology Institute
Cleveland Clinic

PREFACE

In 1972, Johnson and Holmes first demonstrated the usefulness of epicardial M-Mode echocardiography in assessing the effectiveness of open mitral commissurotomy leading to a limited expansion of intraoperative applications of ultrasound. The introduction of intraoperative transesophageal echocardiography in the early 1980's served as a catalyst leading to its accelerated clinical use and development of innovative technologies. Current state-of-the-art probes and consoles provide high resolution, multiplane 2-D, and real time 3-D imaging enabling detailed structural and flow evaluation that has contributed to improved perioperative clinical decision-making and clinical outcomes.

Over the last few decades, the utility of perioperative echocardiography for monitoring cardiac performance and diagnosing pathology has become increasingly evident. Peri-operative echocardiography is now considered an essential part of modern cardiac surgery and is becoming increasingly common in non cardiac anesthesia care for high risk patients as well. Its clinical applications are well recognized and numerous, including assessment of left ventricular (LV) and right ventricular (RV) function, assessment of preload, measurement of cardiac output, detection of myocardial ischemia, assessment of valvular function, detection and assessment of various congenital heart diseases, and evaluation of aortic atheromatous disease. These applications have significantly improved provider knowledge and therefore patient care. The essential information provided by perioperative echocardiography for hemodynamic management and diagnostic assessment has further accelerated its widespread use. It can be performed using transesophageal, epicardial, epiaortic, and transthoracic approaches. It is preformed preoperatively, intraoperatively, and postoperatively to diagnose pathology, assess treatment, and validate success or failure of actions directed to manage physiology. The invaluable use of echocardiography has also been identified in the cardiac catheterization and electrophysiology laboratories with direct, real time guidance of less invasive percutaneous cardiovascular procedures. An advanced understanding of perioperative TEE skills is expected from physicians supporting perioperative patient care including cardiovascular surgery or percutaneous interventions and non-cardiac surgery. As the 1990s saw the widespread adaptation of perioperative TEE into clinical practice, there was a growing interest in developing interdisciplinary guidelines for its use. This resulted in the publication of collaborative standards for perioperative echocardiography as endorsed by societies representing the cardiovascular disciplines. These standards are based on literature reviews and expert, multidisciplinary opinions of task force members from the Society of Cardiovascular Anesthesiologists, American Society of Anesthesiologists, and American Society of Echocardiography in addition to representations from other national and international cardiovascular associations. The interdisciplinary cooperation in this area is a testament to the clinical importance of this tool. Among cardiologists, cardiac surgeons, and cardiac anesthesiologists, perioperative echocardiography remains the most widely recognized monitoring and diagnostic tool used in guiding the perioperative decision-making process.

Like its predecessor, our second edition of the *Comprehensive Textbook of Perioperative Transesophageal Echocardiography* has been structured to permit gradual progression for the novice into the more advanced applications of ultrasound. It consists of 40 chapters presented in 3 sections covering "Basic Perioperative Echocardiography", "Echocardiography in the Critical Care Setting", and "Advanced Applications of Perioperative Echocardiography". For more experienced echocardiographers, their foundation will be reinforced thereby expanding the likelihood of their confidently performing advanced and complex diagnostic assessments in emergencies. Comprehensive tables of reference measurements of cardiovascular structures, hemodynamic formulas, and severity assessment criteria are included in an expanded appendix with perforated inner margins to encourage their lamination and posting in front-line clinical settings. This textbook represents the cumulative experience of leading cardiovascular surgeons, cardiologists, and anesthesiologists who have advanced the transformation of a once novel tool to its current widespread clinical application. It is our sincere hope that the second edition of the *Comprehensive Textbook of Perioperative Transesophageal Echocardiography* will serve as the ultimate resource for understanding the fundamental principles, clinical applications, and technological advances encompassing perioperative echocardiography. Furthermore, we believe this textbook reflects the extraordinary enthusiasm that will encourage the adoption of this invaluable technology as we seek to enhance the quality and value of care provided to our patients.

Robert M. Savage, MD
Solomon Aronson, MD
Stanton K. Shernan, MD

ACKNOWLEDGMENTS

The editors are indebted to the outstanding group of authors who have participated in our second edition of the *Comprehensive Textbook of Perioperative Transesophageal Echocardiography*. Some of the unsung heroes on our team included our associate editor, Dr. Andrew Shaw, along with colleagues Dr. Andrej Alfirevic and Dr. Anand Mehta. A special note of thanks is due to Dr. Bill Stewart who has provided unwavering support for our joint intraoperative imaging program with a shared vision for one standard of excellence. The success of our first edition was due, in large part, to the superb medical illustration and graphic design provided by Beth Halasz (medical illustrator), Mark Sabo (3D graphic designer) and their Director, Ann Paladino. We are especially grateful to our professional team from Wolters Kluwer/Lippincott Williams & Wilkins including Nicole Dernoski (Senior Product Manager), G. Biju Kumar (Project Manager), and Brian Brown (Senior Acquisitions Editor). They have consistently provided valuable insight, enthusiastic encouragement, and an unwavering commitment for impacting the care of our patients. Lastly, we wish to thank our colleagues, fellows, and members of the cardiovascular teams at the Cleveland Clinic, Duke, and Brigham & Women's Hospital for their support and participation. This monumental undertaking would not have been possible without their support and daily contributions to our understanding of perioperative imaging and its value in directing patient care. Lastly, we are indebted, beyond recompense, to our spouses and families for their long suffering patience in tolerating absences and vacations crowded by stacks of manuscripts, portable hard drives, and deadlines.

Robert M. Savage, MD
Solomon Aronson, MD
Stanton K. Shernan, MD

Basic Perioperative Echocardiography

CHAPTER 1

Physics of Echocardiography

Bernard E. Bulwer ■ Stanton K. Shernan ■ James D. Thomas

INTRODUCTION

Echocardiography, or cardiac ultrasonography, uses reflected ultrasound waves (echoes) from the heart and great vessels to generate information on cardiovascular structure and function. Optimal acquisition, display, and interpretation of echocardiographic data require an understanding of the physical principles of sound and the mechanisms underlying ultrasound generation, transmission, reflection, and reconstruction. Echocardiography, like other cardiac imaging techniques, has its strengths and weaknesses (1,2). Understanding these is a prerequisite for optimal utilization of this technology in clinical practice (Fig. 1.1).

ECHOCARDIOGRAPHY AND THE PROPERTIES OF ULTRASOUND

Echocardiographic images are produced by processing received ultrasound echoes reflected from the heart and great vessels (3–5). *Sound* is a mechanical vibration or wave of particles within a physical medium (such as air, fluids, or tissues) that is transmitted to particles in its path—causing them to vibrate (back and forth) at the frequency of the source. *Ultrasound* likewise propagates as longitudinal waves that cause tissues in its path to resonate, thereby propagating as microscopic cycles of compression and decompression (6). As waves propagate, differential interactions with the tissues they encounter, for example, reflection, refraction, diffraction, and attenuation, can be detected and translated into clinically useful graphical data. Ultrasound waves can be graphically depicted as a sine wave to illustrate important concepts pertinent to echocardiography (Fig. 1.2).

The sound spectrum can be classified as infrasonic (subsonic), audible, and ultrasonic. Audible sound (at frequencies below 20,000 cycles/s [20×10^3 Hertz, Hz] in adults) stimulates the auditory apparatus, thereby producing the sensation of hearing. Ultrasound, with frequencies greater than 15 to 20 kHz (15×10^3–20×10^3 cycles/s), is inaudible. The principal advantages of using ultrasound for diagnostic imaging are that (i) ultrasound can

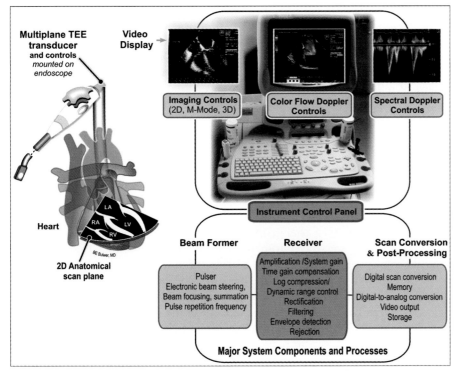

Figure 1.1. Overview of the Processes and Display Options in Transesophageal echocardiography (TEE). Optimal utilization of the technology in clinical practice requires an understanding of the principles that underlie the generation, transmission, interactions, reception, processing, and display of cardiac ultrasound data. **Left:** Schema showing perspectives of a multiplane TEE transducer mounted on a drivable endoscope along with the cardiac scan plane. **Right:** A composite summary of the instrument control panel, system components, major processes, and echocardiographic image displays.

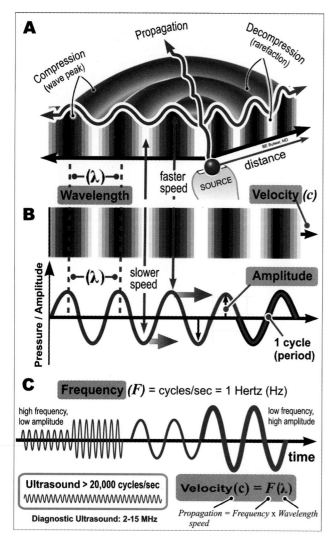

Figure 1.2. The Basic Properties of Ultrasound Waves. Ultrasound wavelength, amplitude, frequency, and propagation velocity all influence optimal image acquisition and interpretation (see text).

be directed as a beam, (ii) it obeys the laws of reflection and refraction, and (iii) it is differentially reflected from cardiac structures. A major disadvantage of ultrasound is that it propagates poorly through a gaseous medium. As a result, cardiac ultrasound in general and transthoracic echocardiography in particular require "windows" to avoid the air-filled lung. Diagnostic medical ultrasonography uses transducers with center frequencies ranging from 2 million Hz to 15 million Hz, or 2 to 15 megahertz (MHz), with newer applications like intravascular ultrasound employing frequencies exceeding 40 MHz (7).

Where the particles in a medium are most compressed, i.e., at the crest or maximal height of the sound wave, there is maximal acoustic pressure and intensity (Fig. 1.2). This maximal height is the wave *amplitude* (A) and is analogous to the loudness of sound expressed in decibels (dB). It is the changes in amplitude or brightness of the received ultrasound waves (echoes) that are harnessed

to produce grayscale or B-mode (brightness-modulated) images (Fig. 1.3) (8). The processed echoes can be displayed in real time using (i) a one-dimensional (1D; "ice-pick") format over time as in M-mode echocardiography, (ii) a two-dimensional (2D) or cross-sectional anatomical format, or (iii) a three-dimensional (3D) anatomical format (Fig. 1.4) (6,8). Wave amplitude can be measured in Pascals (Pa), but the decibel (logarithmic) scale is preferred as the amplitude and intensity of the transmitted ultrasound pulse may be a millionfold greater than that of the reflected echo. The decibel logarithmic scale (dB) compresses this very large and difficult-to-display range, for example, from 1,000,000:1 to 1,000:1, into a narrow and easily displayed logarithmic range, for example, from 60 to 30 dB. The decibel scale, therefore, facilitates the display of low-amplitude (weak) signals alongside high-amplitude (strong) signals. This compression of amplitudes of the received echoes using the dB scale is important in processing echo signals because amplitude measurements are the basis of B-mode echocardiography and its various display formats—whether M-mode, 2D, or 3D (Figs. 1.3 and 1.4; see "Ultrasound Interactions and the Challenges to Signal Processing") (6,9,10). The acoustic *intensity* of the ultrasound wave (or beam) is the acoustic power measured in watts (W) per squared meter (m²) of tissue. This concept is represented as Intensity (I) = Power (W)/beam area (m²). Intensity is proportional to the amplitude of the ultrasound wave squared: $I \sim A^2$. Higher ultrasound wave amplitudes generate greater intensities and hence carry a greater risk of tissue injury. Based on the relationship $I \sim A^2$, a doubling of the pressure amplitude would quadruple its intensity. This principle is harnessed in lithotripsy, where high-intensity ultrasound waves are used to fragment renal calculi. Echocardiography, on the other hand, uses low-intensity ultrasound waves that have not been shown to cause injury in routine clinical practice (5,11,12).

Wavelength (λ) is the length of one cycle or spatial oscillation, like the distance between two peaks or troughs (Fig. 1.2). The number of wavelengths per unit time is the *frequency* of the wave (F) and is commonly expressed as cycles per second or *hertz*. The product of the *wavelength* (λ) and the *frequency* (F) is equal to the *propagation velocity* (c) of the wave and is expressed by the formula: $c = F \times \lambda$. The propagation velocity of sound waves in human soft tissues averages 1,540 m/s (1.54×10^3 m/s or 1.54 mm/μs) (9,10). Wavelength is directly proportional to propagation velocity. The frequency of ultrasound in tissues is constant, and it corresponds to the transducer frequency. However, a change in velocity occurs whenever ultrasound waves travel from one tissue interface to another, like when moving from the heart to the lung. Therefore, at such an interface (i.e., the pericardial-pleural interface) where velocity changes, the wavelength must also change to accommodate the new velocity in the second tissue (6,13). Sound travels much faster in muscle (c = ~1,570 m/s) compared to air (c = ~330 m/s). Wavelength is inversely related to the frequency of the sound wave and may be calculated as

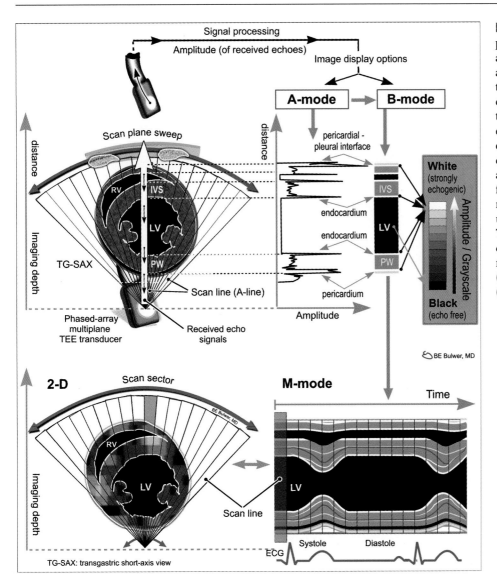

Figure 1.3. Schema showing scan plane anatomy (transgastric short-axis view, TG-SAX), scan lines, and received echoes returning to the transducer from various depths (**upper left**). Processing the amplitudes of the received echo signals reflected from various depths can be graphically depicted on an oscilloscope as an amplitude-modulated (A-mode) format or alternatively as a brightness-modulated (B-mode) display using gray scale (**upper right**). The same B-mode data can be displayed over time in 1D as a motion mode (M-mode) format (**lower right**), or as a 2D format (**lower left**).

$$\lambda = c\,/\,F = \frac{1.54 \times 10^{3} \text{ m/s}}{F(\text{MHz})}$$

$$= 1.54 \,/\, F(\text{m})$$

Accordingly, a 1.5 MHz and a 15 MHz transducer wave will have wavelengths of approximately 1.0 and 0.1 mm, respectively. Wavelength determines the ability to distinguish two points or structures as separate. This ability to resolve or visualize image detail is called the spatial resolution (see Chapter 3: Optimizing Two-Dimensional Echocardiographic Imaging) (9,10). The higher the frequency of the transmitted ultrasound wave (hence the shorter the wavelength), the better will be the axial resolution (along the path of the ultrasound beam). Additionally, the depth of penetration or range of the ultrasound wave is directly proportional to its wavelength. The longer the wavelength, the greater the tissue penetration and hence better imaging of deeper structures like the cardiac

apex on transesophageal echocardiography (TEE). This deeper penetration comes, however, at the expense of image resolution (12). The converse is also true; higher frequency ultrasound, for example, the 5 or 7.5 MHz transducers used in TEE, provides better image resolution due to their shorter wavelengths. However, this improved image resolution is observed only with near-field structures like the aortic and mitral valves on TEE. Deeper structures like the cardiac apex are suboptimally visualized due to less tissue penetration, or greater attenuation, of high-frequency, short-wavelength ultrasound.

THE PIEZOELECTRIC EFFECT AND ULTRASOUND

The stage for ultrasonography was set back in 1880, when Pierre and Jacques Curie noted that quartz and other crystals could generate electrical surface charges when subjected to mechanical stress. This ability to generate

Figure 1.4. Brightness-Modulated (B-mode) Grayscale Display Options. **Upper panel, from left to right:** Schema showing imaging of cardiac anatomy, where the amplitudes of the received echoes (scan line data) can be optionally displayed as M-mode (a 1D motion-mode format over time), or as a 2D scan sector. Both image display options are based on gray scale or brightness-modulation (B-mode). **Lower panel, from left to right:** Real-time imaging of cardiac anatomy (parasternal long axis views): The amplitudes of the received echoes can be processed into B-mode data that can be displayed using a 1D (M-mode), 2D (cross-sectional anatomy), or 3D anatomy formats.

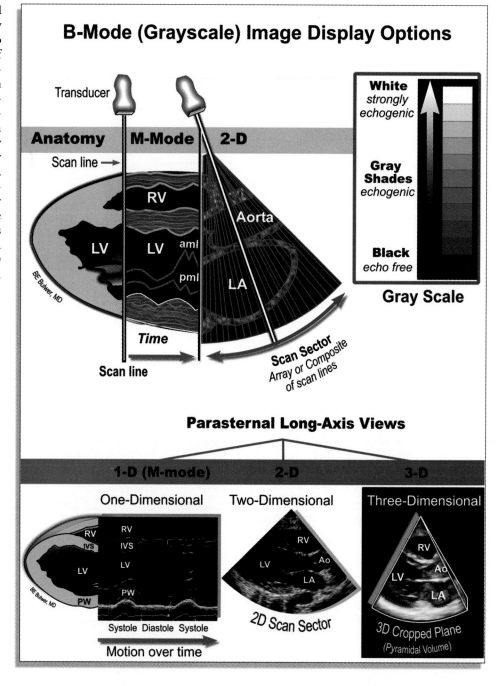

electricity following application of mechanical stress on crystals is known as the pressure-electric effect or "direct" *piezoelectric effect*. A year later, the Curies also observed the reverse of this principle—that when such crystals are exposed to electricity, they vibrate in a predictable fashion (6,9,14). This is the basis of ultrasonography: that electrical charges applied to piezoelectric (PZE) elements generate an ultrasound beam (*"transmit"* mode), and the converse—that ultrasound echoes impacting PZE elements generate electrical signals (*"receive"* mode) (Figs. 1.5 and 1.6).

Molecules within PZE materials used in ultrasound transducers, for example, lead-zirconate-titanate (PZT),

are highly charged dipoles. At rest, the dipoles are in equilibrium with zero net charge. However, when an electrical charge is placed across the PZE element, these dipoles undergo realignment, triggering PZE element vibrations at its natural *resonant frequency* (Fig. 1.6). Such vibrations are transmitted toward their target in the form of ultrasound waves. Following a brief period measured in microseconds, echoes arising from imaged structures impact the PZE element. When this occurs, the mechanical energy of the echoes induces an electric signal by mechanical realignment of the molecular dipoles (Fig. 1.6). These electrical signals are then elaborately processed and displayed as the ultrasound image (6,9,10).

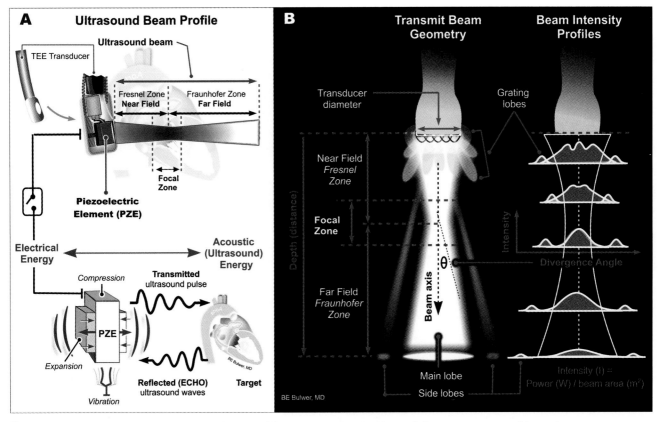

Figure 1.5. A: The PZE element and the ultrasound beam generation. **B:** Transmit beam geometry and intensity profiles.

ULTRASOUND TRANSDUCERS: THE BASICS

Ultrasound transducers vary widely in design and capabilities, depending on the clinical application. Standard transducer components include the PZE element, matching layer or faceplate, acoustic lens, electrodes, and backing material enclosed within the transducer housing (10,15). A motorized multiplane *phased array* transducer mounted on a flexible endoscope is used in TEE (Fig. 1.7). The PZE elements are the acoustic center of the transducer. Modern ultrasound transducers contain arrangements or "arrays" of PZE elements, which may

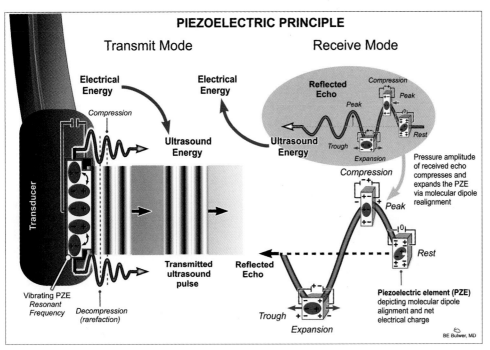

Figure 1.6. The transducer PZE element: transmission and reception modes. **Left panel:** During transmit mode, electrical excitation of the transducer PZE elements converts electrical energy into acoustic energy. The result is transmission of the ultrasound pulse. **Right panel:** During receive mode the reverse occurs when the reflected ultrasound (received echoes) impact the PZE element. Here acoustic energy is converted into electrical energy.

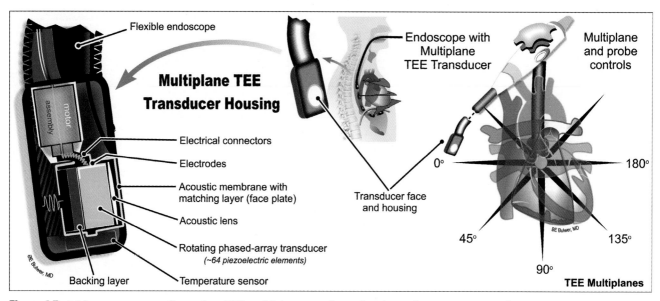

Figure 1.7. Major components of a modern TEE multiplane transducer showing endoscope mount and orientation of the standard TEE examination multiplanes.

be linear (linear array), curved (curved or curvilinear array), annular (annular array), or a rectangular matrix (matrix array) where the PZE elements are arranged in rows, typically 3 to 7. Phased-array transducers typically utilize very thin (~0.3 wavelength thick) PZE elements, in arrays of 64, 128, or 256 individual elements, compared to around 3,000 in modern 3D matrix-array transducers (Fig. 1.8) (16). Phased array refers to operational capacity, not the physical PZE element arrangement. *Phasing* describes the capacity to phase or control the timing of PZE element excitation. This is the basis of electronic steering and focusing of the ultrasound beam, which previously required bulky steering components (Figs. 1.9 and 1.10).

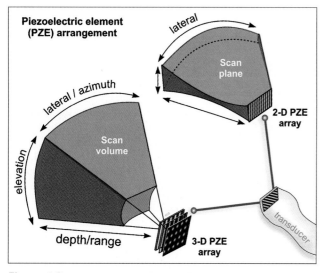

Figure 1.8. Basic outline of PZE element arrangements and geometrical scan planes in a 2D phased array and a 3D matrix-array transducer.

Phased array operation facilitates the scanning of a wide field of view (FOV) despite being confined to a small "footprint," for example, the intercostal "windows" or the confines or the esophageal lumen. The basis of the FOV or image scan sector, therefore, is the ability of phased-array transducers to pivot or "sweep" through the anatomical scan plane, thereby acquiring a wide FOV despite transducer footprint limitations (Figs. 1.3, 1.4, and 1.9) (9,10,15).

Transducer PZE elements are electronically interconnected via various circuits within the *beam former*, including transmit/receive switches, digital time-delays, preamplifiers, analog-to-digital converters, dynamic receive focusing, signal summation, and time gain compensation (TGC) circuits (see Fig. 3.3). Selective excitation times of individual PZE elements facilitate dynamic beam focusing and steering during transmission; selective delays of received echo signals permit focusing on reception (Fig. 1.11) (9,15). When PZE elements within an array are excited, they generate multiple spherical ultrasound "wavelets" that interfere constructively to produce a compound planar wave front (Huygens' principle; Fig. 1.12) (9,10). Unlike linear array transducers where only a portion of the PZE elements contribute to beam formation during each pulse-echo sequence (transmission-reception cycle), *all* PZE elements produce the beam that interrogates every scan line (typically >100) within the fan-shaped scan sector (Fig. 1.13). This transmission-reception cycle is repeated as the beam is swept across the anatomical scan sector (see Figs. 1.3, 1.4, 1.9, and 1.14). Electrical excitation of each PZE element initiates a cycle of contraction and expansion (vibrations), resulting in the generation of ultrasound pulses (Figs. 1.5 and 1.6). The length of these vibrations is limited by *damping*. The

Phased Array Transducer, Electronic Beam Steering, and Generation of Scan Sector

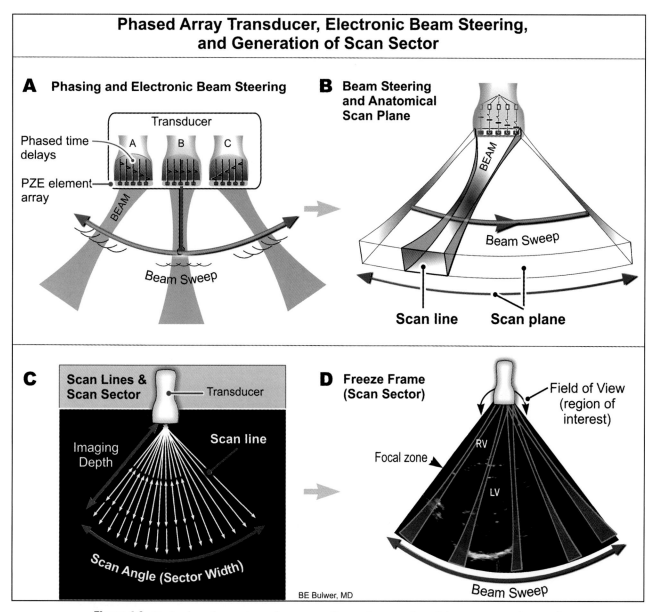

Figure 1.9. Basic phased array transducer operation and generation of the scan sector (see text).

damping block or *backing material* is juxtaposed to the back of the PZE element and absorbs those vibrations that do not contribute to beam formation (Fig. 1.7). More importantly, the damping element mechanically dampens or limits ("ring down") PZE element vibrations, thereby shortening the *pulse duration* and *spatial pulse length*—an important determinant of image quality (axial resolution) (Fig. 1.6; see Figs. 1.15 and 3.4 to 3.7). Imaging pulses are typically two or three wavelengths long, compared to the longer pulse lengths (5–25 cycles) used in Doppler echocardiography (6,9,13).

A recent innovation has been the use of specially crafted broadband PZE elements. This facilitates multifrequency, multi-Hertz transducer operation during "transmit" mode (9,17,18). Another is the ability to transmit at one frequency and receive at another frequency—a requirement for *harmonic imaging*. This has significantly improved image quality (see "Tissue Harmonic Imaging"). Although the same PZE element functions as both a transducer and a receiver of ultrasound (except in the continuous-wave [CW] Doppler operation where these functions are separate), it spends >> 99% of the time in "receive" mode, i.e., receiving multiple echoes that arise from the initial pulse (3–5). Modern transducers are highly sensitive and can detect echoes of magnitude less than 1% that of the transmitted pulse (7,8). The transducer *electrodes* are serially connected to the PZE elements. The *matching layer* or *face plate* is a thin, but crucial, component that interfaces with the PZE element on one side and the skin or esophagus on the other (Fig. 1.7). Without the matching layer, the large difference in acoustic impedance between the PZE and the skin (or esophagus) would result in a major loss

Figure 1.10. Focused and unfocused ultrasound beam mechanisms. **Left panel:** Generation of an unfocused ultrasound beam that results from simultaneous excitation of the PZE elements. **Middle and right panels:** The ultrasound beam can be focused, with resultant improved image quality, by *phasing* or controlled timing of PZE element excitation, either using an external lens, or by digital beam focusing.

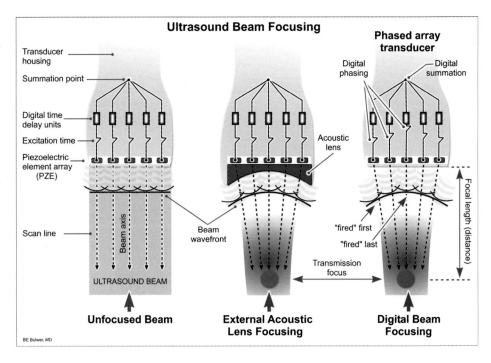

of acoustic energy on both transmission and reception. An ideal matching layer is designed with an impedance gradient that matches one surface to the other, thereby optimizing ultrasound energy transfer. The use of *coupling gel* between the matching layer and the skin (or esophagus) eliminates air pockets that would otherwise greatly diminish ultrasound transmission. A convergent *acoustic lens*, usually made of polystyrene or epoxy resin, enhances the

focus of the ultrasound beam. A *temperature sensor* at the probe tip warns of potential thermal injury from possible overheating resulting from PZE element vibrations. Such sensors would automatically shut down transducer operations should a preset temperature threshold be exceeded. The case and insulator surrounding the transducer are a plastic or metal housing that offers protection from electrical noise and potential electrical shock to the patient.

Figure 1.11. Ultrasound beam focusing on transmission and reception. **Left panel:** Transit Focusing. Phased excitation of individual PZE elements by the introduction of variable digital time delays is used to focus and steer the ultrasound beam during transmission. **Right panel:** During reception, introducing selective time delays into the received echo signals that differentially impact the PZE elements is necessary to align (or put *in phase*) these signals that are then summed up (electronic beam summation) to form the net or averaged signal.

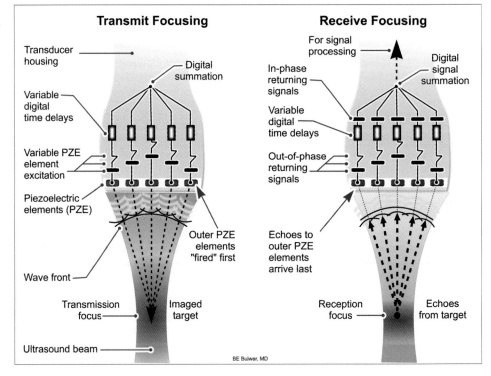

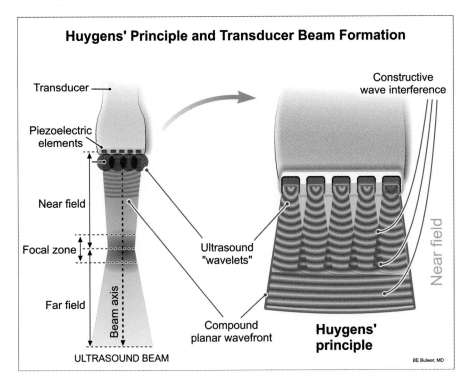

Figure 1.12. Formation of the ultrasound beam wavefront (Huygens' principle). Excitation of the piezoelectric elements triggers transmission of spherical ultrasound wavelets from the transducer face. These tiny wavelets merge to form a near parallel compound planar wavefront (Huygens' principle). This narrow 3D ultrasound beam is slightly convergent in the near field, becoming more focused in the focal zone, before diverging in the far field.

ULTRASOUND BEAM GEOMETRY

The ultrasound beam, analogous to that of a flashlight, is a directed stream of ultrasound waves (pulses) along the beam axis (Fig. 1.5). It remains largely confined to a predictable 3D space with axial, lateral, and elevational ("slice-thickness")

dimensions (Figs. 1.5 and 1.9; see Fig. 3.4) (6,9,15). With phased array transducers, the beam is dynamic, being swept through the anatomical scan plane to generate the scan sector (Figs. 1.3 and 1.9). Anatomical structures lying within the ultrasound beam path are both targets of the transmitted ultrasound pulse as well as the source of the received

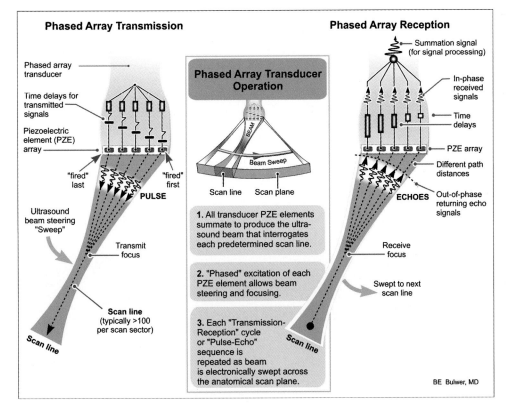

Figure 1.13. Phased array transducer operation. Phased array transducer operation. **Left and right panels:** Simultaneous transmission and reception of ultrasound signals occur, although for clarity, they are displayed separately. **Left panel:** During phased array transmission, all transducer PZE elements are excited and summate to form the ultrasound beam or scan line. **Right panel:** During reception, the returning echoes (arising from that same scan line) are time-shifted, phase-adjusted, and summated.

Figure 1.14. Pulse-echo operation. Diagnostic ultrasound imaging is based on the *pulse-echo operation*. Here, the *predictable relationship between time and distance* serves as the basis for constructing ultrasound images. The return-trip times (in microseconds) for the transmitted ultrasound pulse to return (1), and translation of these times into anatomical distances (2), which are then mapped to create the composite anatomical B-mode image display (3), are the basic steps involved in the pulse-echo technique.

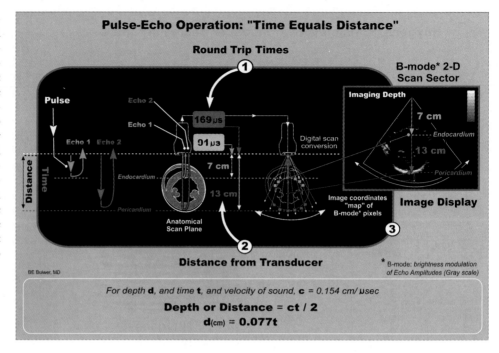

echoes. Therefore the transmitted beam, as well as its received echoes, comprises the ultrasound beam—making the ultrasound beam a "two-way street" (Figs. 1.9, 1.11, and 1.13, see Fig. 1.22). The transducer design elements, including transducer size (diameter), frequency, aperture, and focusing mechanisms, are important determinants of the ultrasound beam configuration and image quality. As stipulated by Huygens' principle, emitted spherical wavelets of ultrasound pulses transmitted from each PZE element interfere or merge to form a nearly parallel beam wave front

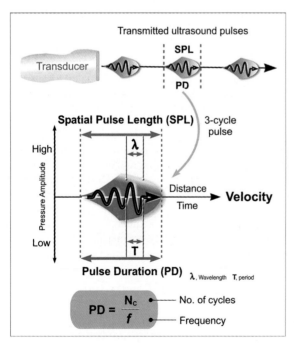

Figure 1.15. Pulse geometry: pulse duration and spatial pulse length.

(Fig. 1.13). When unfocused, the ultrasound beam travels initially in a columnar geometrical pattern in its *near field* or *Fresnel zone* and then diverges in the *far field* or *Fraunhofer zone* (Figs. 1.5 and 1.10).

The properties of ultrasound waves were discussed earlier (Fig. 1.2). These same fundamental properties apply to the ultrasound beam. The length of the near field—the beam region that provides superior image resolution as compared to the far field—is largely determined by transducer diameter and transducer frequency (Fig. 1.5; see Fig. 3.9). As both increase, the near-field length increases—a desirable result in ultrasound imaging (Fig. 1.13) (6,9,11). Based on the relationship, *ultrasound velocity, c = Fλ*, where both transducer frequency (F) and ultrasound velocity in soft tissues average 1.54×10^3 m/s, the wavelength λ becomes a useful variable for calculating near-field length. Hence, near-field length is directly proportional to transducer diameter (D), but inversely related to the wavelength (λ), and is represented by the equation: Near-field length = $D^2/4\lambda$ (see Fig. 3.9). For example, a 5 MHz transducer with a 5-mm diameter

$$\lambda = c/F = \frac{1.54 \times 10^3 \text{ m/s}}{F \text{ (MHz)}} = 0.3 \text{ mm}$$

$$= \frac{1.54 \times 10^3 \text{ m/s}}{5 \text{ (MHz)}} = 0.3 \text{ mm}$$

Nearfield length = $D^2/4\lambda$
= 25 mm^2/4 × 0.3 mm = 20.8 cm.

Distal to the near field, the beam diverges into the far field. The far field's dimensions, in direct contrast with those of the near field, are directly proportional to the transducer diameter and are inversely related to the wavelength. The *angle of divergence*, θ, approximately equals arc sin (1.22λ/D) or sin θ = 1.22λ/D (Fig. 1.5) (3,4,7). Lateral resolution is heavily influenced by the geometry of the far field. The less beam divergence (i.e., the smaller the divergence angle, θ), the better will be the lateral resolution of structures imaged in the far field (see Figs. 3.8 and 3.9). Theoretically, the best way to achieve optimal lateral resolution is by using a large diameter–high-frequency/short-wavelength transducer. However, a trade-off exists between resolution and tissue penetration (see Fig. 3.6). High-frequency transducers could theoretically deliver improved lateral resolution in the far field. However, high-frequency beams suffer greater attenuation with increasing depth, and hence diminished tissue penetration. A phenomenon associated with transducer beams is the unwanted transmission of acoustic *side lobes* (Fig. 1.5). These are additional low-intensity acoustic beams that stray from the main beam path. They result from radial vibrations of the PZE element, as contrasted with the longitudinal PZE element vibrations that generate the main beam (6,9,12). Side lobes image structures outside the main beam path, i.e., structures that lie outside the anatomical scan plane. Echoes received from such structures can be mapped into the final image, thereby displaying side lobe artifacts that misrepresent the true anatomy. Apodization, a technique for optimizing the geometry of the main ultrasound beam, effectively minimizes side lobe and *grating lobe* formation and the genesis of related artifacts. Grating lobes, so-called due to the grating-like arrangement of multiple PZE elements, are multiple low-intensity accessory beams that appear near the transducer face (Fig. 1.5) (9,10).

When focused, either electronically or via the use of a curved acoustic lens, the near-field geometry converges with the result being a shorter *focal distance*, i.e., the distance from the transducer to the narrowest beam width (Fig. 1.10). Electronic beam focusing is achieved by manipulating the PZE element electronic activation sequence (Fig. 1.11) (9,10,15).

PULSE-ECHO OPERATION: TIME EQUALS DISTANCE

Diagnostic ultrasound imaging, with the exception of the CW Doppler technique, is based on the *pulse-echo method* of operation. Pulse-echo ultrasound systems—whether A-mode, B-mode, pulsed-wave (PW) Doppler, color flow Doppler, or tissue Doppler echocardiography—acquire anatomical images, or assess velocities, by transmitting short pulses of ultrasound into the body and analyzing echoes reflected from anatomical structures in its path (Fig. 1.3) (6,9). Analysis of the *round-trip times* and *amplitudes* of the received echoes is the basis of anatomical imaging. Analysis of the *frequency change* or *shifts* between the transmitted and received echoes to determine blood flow velocities is the basis of Doppler echocardiography. This section describes

the pulse-echo method in anatomical imaging. The pulsed-echo technique in Doppler imaging is discussed separately (see "Pulsed Doppler Echocardiography").

A *predictable relationship between time and distance* is the basis for constructing ultrasound images (Fig. 1.14). The time it takes for the reflected wave to return to the transducer is indicative of the distance, or how deep structures lie with respect to the transducer. This is how the structure of an ultrasound image takes shape—by calculating the times taken for its echoes to return and translating these times (and their amplitudes) into a composite anatomical B-mode image map of the heart (Figs. 1.3 and 1.14) (6,9,10). As ultrasound travels at near constant speeds in soft tissues, the round-trip travel time is used to calculate the distances. When an ultrasound pulse is generated, it travels at an average velocity of 0.154 cm/μs. As depicted in Figure 1.14, the ultrasound pulse encounters and is reflected from two structures—one at 7 cm (the endocardium) and the other at 13 cm (the pericardium). The incident pulse first reaches the reflecting surface located 7 cm away from the transducer. Its echo travels 7 cm back to the transducer, with a total round-trip distance of 14 cm. The second pulse (actually the nonreflected or transmitted portion of the same pulse) has to travel farther to the reflecting surface located 13 cm away and back, a journey totaling 26 cm. The first ultrasound pulse takes 91 μs, and the second 169 μs, to complete the return journey. The basis of the determining and assigning depth or distance of a structure from the transducer, i.e., its spatial anatomical location, is the time it takes for its echoes to return. These distances are collectively mapped according to spatial coordinates or "addresses" for each echo and are collated to construct a composite ultrasound image (see "Scan conversion and storage in computer memory" in Chapter 3). If the round-trip time is t ms, then the depth or distance (d) cm of a returning echo will be approximately: d (cm) = 0.077t (μs)—considering the average velocity of ultrasound in soft tissues as 0.154 cm/μs and with d being 1/2 the round-trip distance (5–7). An important limitation of ultrasound is that for unambiguous visualization of structures, a second ultrasound pulse cannot be emitted until echoes have returned from the deepest structures of interest. This is the pulse repetition frequency (PRF) in kHz, and is approximately 77,000/d (cm); PRF typically ranges from 1,000 to 5,000 pulses/s (1–5 kHz).

INTERACTION OF ULTRASOUND WITH TISSUES

Reflection: The Central Principle

The ultrasound beam, like light, obeys the laws of reflection and refraction. When ultrasound encounters tissues in its path, for example, the skin → subcutaneous tissue → chest wall → pleura → lung → pericardium →

myocardium → endocardium → blood → heart valves (as in transthoracic echocardiography), it interacts differentially with each tissue boundary (Figs. 1.16 and 1.17). The ultrasound wave may be reflected, scattered, refracted, diffracted, and attenuated to varying extents as it traverses these tissues. *Reflection* is the basis of all ultrasonic imaging. Only those reflected ultrasound waves (echoes) that are received by the transducer contribute to image formation. The strongest reflections, i.e., echoes with the largest amplitudes, arise principally at tissue interfaces (boundaries) (Fig. 1.16) (5,6,9,13).

The extent to which the wave is reflected depends on (i) the *angle* of the incident ultrasound beam relative to the target—whether perpendicular or oblique, (ii) the "*smoothness*" or *size* of the target reflector relative to the *wavelength* of the incident ultrasound beam, whether *specular* (mirror-like) or *nonspecular*, and (iii) the difference in *acoustic* impedance, which is the degree to which

different tissues impede ultrasound transmission (Figs. 1.16 and 1.17).

Specular and Nonspecular Reflection

When the incident beam travels perpendicular to a *specular* tissue boundary or interface, for example, the pericardium, endocardium, or pleura—one where surface irregularities are smaller than the wavelength of the incident beam—most is reflected directly back along its incident path (Figs. 1.16 and 1.17). The remainder of the beam is transmitted into deeper tissues in the same direction as the incident beam. Specular reflections produce the strongest echoes, i.e., echoes with the largest amplitude spikes on A-mode, and appear as highly *echoreflective* (hyperechoic or "*echobright*") structures on B-mode (Figs. 1.3, 1.16, and 1.17). Therefore, on B-mode echocardiography, images are optimally visualized when

Figure 1.16. Tabular summary of ultrasound interactions with tissues. The strengths or amplitudes of the returning echoes directly influence the appearance of the ultrasound image display (compare Fig. 1.17). Three major interactions between the incident ultrasound and the target structures determine the *degree of reflection*—and hence the amplitudes of the received echoes. They are: (i) the angle of incidence between the transmitted ultrasound pulse and the target structure or reflector, (ii) the "smoothness" or relative size of the reflector compared to the incident ultrasound wavelength, and (iii) the difference in acoustic impedance encountered at tissue boundaries. The transmitted remnant of the original pulse is subject to further reflection, scattering, refraction, diffraction, and absorption. The net effect is attenuation with distance traveled.

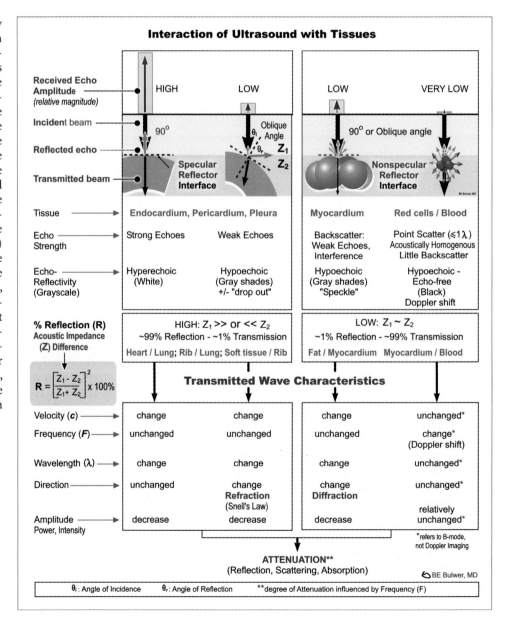

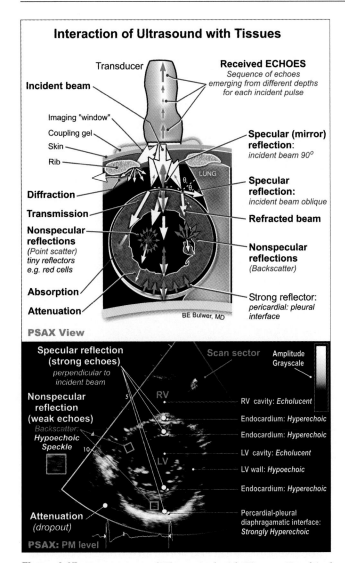

Figure 1.17. Interactions of Ultrasound with Tissues. Graphical depiction of various interactions on transthoracic echocardiography (parasternal short-axis [PSAX] views) at the mid-left ventricle (LV) or papillary muscle (PM) level (**Above**), with corresponding B-mode appearance (**Below**).

To accommodate the velocity change, and since frequency remains unchanged, the transmitted wave must bend or *refract* (Figs. 1.16 and 1.17). However, because the velocity of ultrasound does not change markedly in tissues, *refraction* does not cause major distortions of echocardiographic image quality but can cause refraction artifacts. The refractive property of ultrasound waves can be harnessed in acoustic lenses to focus the ultrasound beam.

When tissue interface irregularities are larger than the incident beam wavelength—or conceptually rough or *nonspecular*—the beam is acoustically scattered in multiple directions, typically in a cone-like spread (*cone angle*) about the reflection axis (Figs. 1.16 and 1.17). The echoes they produce are called *backscatter*. Although most backscatter never directly return to the transducer, they generate useful echo patterns that manifest as inhomogeneous granular "speckles" that serve as tissue "signatures," especially within the myocardium. These speckles are not images of actual structures but are artifacts resulting from constructive and destructive interference of the backscattered echoes (Fig. 1.18). As myocardial regions exhibit their own "signature" speckle patterns, these patterns can be tracked through the cardiac cycle. This is the basis of *speckle tracking* echocardiography—a new technique to assess regional myocardial motion and deformation (Fig. 1.19).

When the ultrasound beam strikes tiny structures like the red blood cells with spatial dimensions ≤ one wavelength, the incident ultrasound wave is scattered in all directions (Figs. 1.16 and 1.17). These *point scatterers* (or Rayleigh-Tyndall scatterers) result in tiny spherical wavelets that are much weaker than echoes arising from nonspecular and specular reflectors. The received backscatter is the summation of multiple points of scatter from the total red cell mass (within the sample volume) due to constructive interference. As these aggregate echoes are still comparatively very tiny, they produce little or no backscatter on pulse-echo imaging (B-mode echocardiography). For this reason, unclotted blood, as well as serous effusions, appears black or echolucent ("echofree") on the grayscale image display (8,9). With pulse-echo Doppler imaging, which utilizes longer pulses (10–25 cycles long compared to the 2- or 3- cycle pulses used in B-mode

the structures of interest are oriented perpendicular to the ultrasound beam. The converse applies in Doppler echocardiography (discussed later) where parallel alignment of beam and blood flow provides optimal velocity measurements. This poses challenges in *duplex* scanning, where real-time B-mode images are simultaneously acquired and displayed with pulsed Doppler or color flow Doppler information. Here, excellent B-mode images may be displayed, but the Doppler recordings may be suboptimal, and vice versa (9,11).

When the incident beam impacts the tissue interface at an oblique angle, a portion is reflected at an angle (θ) equivalent to and away from the incident beam (Figs. 1.16 and 1.17). The transmitted portion of the beam now traverses a tissue with a different acoustic impedance or mismatch. This mismatch triggers a change in velocity (as well as wavelength) of the transmitted beam.

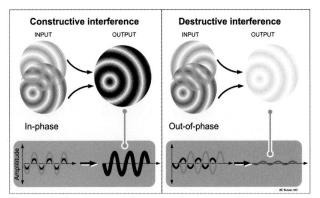

Figure 1.18. Ultrasound wave-wave interactions. **Left:** constructive or additive, **right:** destructive interference.

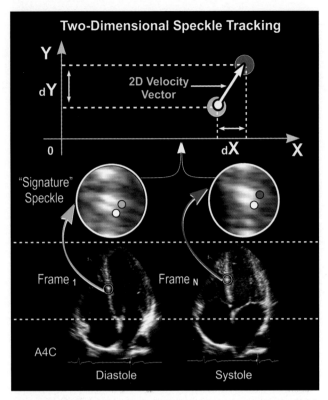

Figure 1.19. Speckle Tracking. B-mode "speckles" can be tracked during the cardiac cycle to provide clinically useful measures of cardiac motion and deformation. Such B-mode speckle tracking parameters are comparatively unaffected by the insonation angle limitations seen with corresponding Doppler-derived measures.

echocardiography), it is the change or *shift in frequency* of the received echoes that is transformed into blood flow velocity and direction (see "Doppler Echocardiography").

Acoustic Impedance

A major determinant of the fraction of ultrasound reflected is the acoustic impedance of tissues. *Acoustic impedance* is that property of tissues that resists or impedes the propagation of ultrasound (5,6–9). Quantitatively, the acoustic impedance (Z) is the product of the tissue density (ρ, in kg/m³) and the velocity of sound (v, in m/s) within that tissue:

$$Z = \rho \times v$$

The fraction of ultrasound reflected, or the *reflection coefficient*, depends on the difference in the acoustic impedance between two tissues: the greater the difference, the greater the reflection (Fig. 1.16). The reflection coefficient (R) is defined as

$$R = \left[\frac{Z_1 - Z_2}{Z_1 + Z_2}\right]^2 \times 100\%$$

where Z_1 is the acoustic impedance of the tissue proximal to the reflective interface, and Z_2 is that of the tissue distal to the reflective interface. The unit of acoustic impedance is measured in kg/m²/s or rayl (from Rayleigh; 1 *rayl* = 1 kg/m²/s).

As ultrasound passes through an acoustically homogeneous medium, for example, blood or a serous pericardial effusion, it travels in a linear fashion, i.e., with its velocity and direction unchanged. Such tissues are excellent transmitters of ultrasound. They produce few reflections on B-mode imaging and therefore appear echo-free (black) (Fig. 1.17). They have a *low reflection coefficient*, with a negligible fraction of the incident ultrasound reflected. However, when ultrasound encounters an interface between two tissues with a large difference in acoustic impedance, for example, the heart-lung interface, nonlinear sound propagation occurs. Most of the incident wave is reflected (>>99%), thereby producing very strong (hyperechoic or "echo bright") echoes (Figs. 1.12 and 1.13).

Air, a comparatively sparse medium, has a very low acoustic impedance ($\sim$0.0004 × 10⁶ *rayls* (kg/m²/s). Ultrasound travels very poorly in air because air reflects almost all the incident ultrasound beam. This leads to difficulty in visualizing an air-filled lung and the aortic arch and great vessels on TEE due to the presence of the interposing air-filled, left main-stem bronchus. Despite this anatomical challenge, an experienced sonographer can perform certain maneuvers to minimize its impact. For example, the aortic arch and great vessels can be seen in more than 90% of patients using an appropriate probe-tip flexion and multiplane angle rotation (5). Alternatively, an epiaortic surface probe can be utilized to improve the quality of ascending aorta and aortic arch images. Loss of the TEE probe tip-tissue contact interface is also a significant source of compromised image quality when imaging from the transgastric depth. However, ultrasound image quality can be improved at this depth by removing gastric air with orogastric suctioning and using a generous amount of ultrasound coupling gel immediately prior to TEE probe insertion. This eliminates air pockets between the probe tip and the gastroesophageal interface. The acoustic properties of air also explain (i) why strong echoes arise from heart/lung interface (Figs. 1.16 and 1.17), (ii) why the application of acoustic coupling gel to the skin is essential (to displace air pockets) in transthoracic examination studies, and (iii) the rationale for "bubble" (agitated saline contrast) studies.

Denser tissues like blood (Z = $\sim$1.67 × 10⁶ kg/m²/s) and bone (Z = $\sim$4–7 × 10⁶ kg/m²/s) are good transmitters of ultrasound. However, because the trabecular architecture of bone acts as multiple reflective surfaces, this greatly attenuates the ultrasound beam, thereby producing echo "dropout" or shadowing artifacts. Calcified and metallic structures like prosthetic valves strongly reflect ultrasound, leading to poor visualization distally due to acoustic shadowing.

Attenuation

The amplitude and intensity of the ultrasound beam invariably decrease with imaging depth (Fig. 1.5). This loss of signal strength occurs due to reflection, scattering, and absorption of ultrasound energy (Figs. 1.16 and 1.17). Absorption occurs when ultrasound wave energy is converted into another energy form, such as heat, because of mechanical friction. Absorption is frequency dependent—the higher the beam frequency, the greater the absorption, and hence the poorer the tissue penetration. A doubling of the beam frequency halves its intensity. Hence, a 7.5 MHz TEE transducer (in the mid-esophageal position) will suboptimally visualize the cardiac apex due to poor tissue penetration that is in turn due to marked attenuation. In soft tissues, absorption is the primary cause of attenuation. With the air-filled trachea, or with large bronchi, calcified structures, and prosthetic valves, reflection is the primary cause. Attenuation degrades image quality and results in dropout artifacts. The *attenuation coefficient* of ultrasound (in dB/cm) is the log relative energy intensity loss per centimeter that the ultrasound beam travels. The attenuation coefficient is roughly proportional to the beam frequency and is nearly constant in soft tissues, averaging between 0.5 and 1.0 dB/cm/MHz (Fig. 1.20). The *half-power distance, half-amplitude value,* and *half-value layer* are measures describing the degree to which the initial power, intensity, or amplitude of the ultrasound beam is attenuated by one half (6,9,12).

Ultrasound Interactions and the Challenges to Signal Processing

The fate of the generated ultrasound beam—reflection, refraction, scattering, and attenuation—poses challenges to processing of the raw echo to construct the B-mode image display (5–10,13). Signals received by the transducer are generated from a broad range of very weak echoes within signal strengths that vary by many 1,000-folds. These signals contain phase as well as amplitude information. Therefore, processing this raw echo signal into echocardigraphic images involves a number of critical steps (see Fig. 3.3), including

1. *Amplification* using *system gain* or *coarse gain* prior to processing: to provide a general increase in amplitude of the very low amplitude radiofrequency echo signals. This process is operator controlled.
2. *Differential amplification* using *time-gain* or *depth-gain compensation (TGC/DGC)*: to compensate or differentially amplify those late-retuning echoes that arise from greater depths and which, as a result, suffer greater attenuation (Fig. 1.21; see Fig. 3.12). Sliding controls on the instrument panel permit real-time differential TGC adjustment.

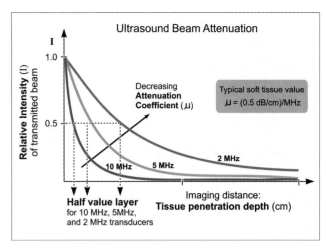

Figure 1.20. Ultrasound Beam Attenuation. Graphical overview showing the relationship between ultrasound beam intensity, transducer frequency, and distance (imaging depth). The half-value layer, the distances it takes for beam intensity to be reduced by one half, is a commonly used measure of transducer beam attenuation.

3. *Logarithmic compression/dynamic range control*: to reduce an unwieldy broad range of echo amplitudes into a more practical display scale that permits visualization of the weakest as well as the strongest echoes, i.e., those ranging from threshold to saturation (Fig. 1.21).
4. *Filtering* using a *low-pass spatial filter/noise smoothing*: to remove unwanted noise and high-frequency echoes, hence improving the *signal-to-noise ratio*.
5. *Digital scan conversion*: to digitally convert the received echoes signals into 2D B-mode pixelated images in preparation for display (see Chapter 3).

In addition to the amplitude and timing of the received echoes to construct the B-mode anatomical display, changes in frequency of echoes reflected from blood and moving structures are the basis of hemodynamic Doppler and tissue Doppler echocardiography. Accurate recording of Doppler data poses additional challenges which are discussed under the corresponding headings.

IMAGE DISPLAY FORMATS

A-Mode Versus B-mode; B-mode Display Formats

Echocardiographic image displays utilize the pulse-echo method described earlier to calculate distances and to create a structural image map of the heart. The interaction of ultrasound with tissues determines the echoreflectivity or appearance of each picture element (pixel) within the digital image and is based on the amplitude of the received echoes. Historically, there were two basic display modalities: (i) Amplitude-modulated or A-mode display and (ii) brightness-modulated or B-mode

Figure 1.21. Scan Line Processing. Because the exponential attenuation in signal strength varies up to a millionfold with imaging depth, it is necessary to logarithmically compress the signal to make its decay linear. Differential amplification is then applied, based on depth (time-gain compensation) to flatten out the background signal and allow the true ultrasound reflections to emerge.

Scan-Line Processing

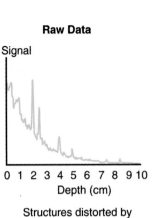

Raw Data

Structures distorted by
attenuation and
1,000,000-fold variation
in signal strength

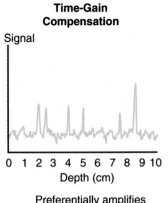

**Time-Gain
Compensation**

Preferentially amplifies
deeper signals to adjust
for attenuation

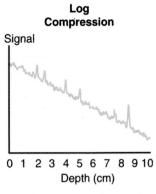

**Log
Compression**

Compresses signal so it
can be displayed to the
viewer. Adjusted by
"Dynamic Range"

displays (Figs. 1.3 and 1.4). On the A-mode display format, A-mode spikes showing the relative amplitudes of echoes arising from structures at different depths were displayed on an oscilloscope (Fig. 1.3). A-mode oscilloscopic displays are no longer used in echocardiography as cardiac structures were identified only along a fixed beam direction and therefore not suited for assessment of moving structures. Furthermore, such displays were very difficult to interpret and were superseded by B-mode displays. On B-mode echocardiography, the amplitudes of the received echoes are displayed according to their degree of brightness on grayscale. B-mode echoes can be displayed as a 1D anatomical format over time—as with M- or motion mode, or as 2D or 3D anatomic images in real time—as with 2D or 3D echocardiography (Fig. 1.4) (6,15). Although largely superseded by subsequent developments, M-mode displays remain useful for precise timing of cardiac events because of its superior temporal resolution afforded by high sampling rates. This averages 1,000 to 2,000 scan lines/s compared to frame rates of 30 to 60 frames/s with 2D echocardiography (5–10,13).

2D ECHOCARDIOGRAPHY: TRANSDUCER OPERATION, FRAMES, AND FRAME RATE

In 2D echocardiography, image frames are created from rapid and repetitive sweeps along multiple scan lines across a fan-shaped arc or sector scan (Figs. 1.3 and 1.9). This sweep or swivel angle is typically ±45 degrees. Each transducer PZE element within the phased array transducer will sequentially phase or transmit a short (2–3 cycle) pulse of ultrasound and will then wait microseconds for its echoes reflected from different depths to return. This cycle of transmission and reception is represented by a single scan line (Figs. 1.3, 1.6, and 1.9) Scan line signals are received and processed in real time

before the beam is electronically steered across the anatomical scan plane (Figs. 1.3, 1.9, and 1.13). Based on the pulse-echo principle, echoes must first return to the transducer from the deepest structures before the transmitted beam proceeds to create the next scan line. How long the transducer takes before sweeping to the next scan line depends on the length of the scan line, i.e., the maximum depth or distance from the transducer. Each sweep of the ultrasound beam across the anatomical scan plane, when processed and displayed, is called a *frame* (Figs. 1.3 and 1.9). Acquiring, processing, and displaying frames at rates exceeding 30 times/s produce real-time, dynamic images of the heart (9–11). The time required to process each frame depends upon the number of scan lines per frame *(line density)* (see Fig. 3.10). The finite speed of ultrasound in tissues imposes limits on the maximum number of pulses that can be transmitted each second. Therefore considering (i) the finite speed of sound (1,540 m/s), (ii) the impact of imaging depth, and (iii) the scan line density on processing and display times, there is a fundamental limit on frame rates in 2D echocardiography. The number of scan lines per frame multiplied by the number of frames per second cannot exceed the finite limits of ultrasound and the PRF (see Fig. 3.10). Higher frame rates can be achieved, however, by (i) imaging at shorter distances (shallow depths), (ii) employing fewer scan lines (lower scan line density), and (iii) narrowing the scan sector angle or width. This problem is compounded in color flow Doppler imaging due to the additional demands to simultaneously analyze and process blood velocities along scan lines. Therefore, a trade-off must occur between imaging depth, frame rate, and image quality (resolution). Recently, *parallel processing* of multiple (rather than single) scan lines simultaneously, rather than sequentially, has resulted in a marked increase in 2D and color flow Doppler frame rates (Fig. 1.22; Table 1.1). Parallel processing is

	Serial (Hz)	Parallel (Hz)
TABLE 1.1 **Echocardiographic Frame Rates Serial Versus Parallel Processing**		
M-mode	200	400
2D	30–40	120–400
Color Doppler	10–15	40–120
Tissue Doppler	7–12	30–90
Spectral Doppler	50–200	50–400

achieved by employing multiple digital beam formers in parallel that can simultaneously process multiple scan lines per each transmitted pulse. The resulting time savings is exploited to increase frame rate, improve lateral resolution, and flow velocity assessment, especially during the color flow Doppler examination (9,10,15).

TISSUE HARMONIC IMAGING

Tissue harmonic imaging is an ultrasound imaging technique that has significantly improved suboptimal or "technically difficult" studies by delivering better spatial

resolution and fewer artifacts (Fig. 1.23) (9). As the transmitted ultrasound wave moves deeper into tissues, the typical linear sinusoidal propagation pattern becomes increasingly distorted or nonlinear. In wave terms, this means that the wave peak or crest, the region of maximal acoustic pressure, moves faster than its trough. The result is a saw-tooth-shaped wave propagation pattern that resembles the movement of a caterpillar (19–21). This occurs because the transmitted wave causes the imaged tissue itself to vibrate—akin to a conductor leading a choir. These microscopic tissue vibrations, in chorus with the first harmonic or fundamental frequency, inject additional acoustic energy ("the choir") in multiples of the transmitted (first harmonic) frequency ("the conductor"). Therefore, it is these tissue-generated harmonics, for example, second-, third-, and fourth-order harmonics, that are added to the first harmonic or fundamental frequency, thereby distorting it. Echoes derived from these distorted waves exhibit these same harmonic frequencies, and it is the second harmonics that are selectively processed in tissue harmonic imaging to generate the image display (9,15,16).

Second-order harmonic echoes arise from the central regions of the ultrasound beam and from deeper structures near the focal zone. This confers upon harmonic echoes three principal advantages that are exploited to

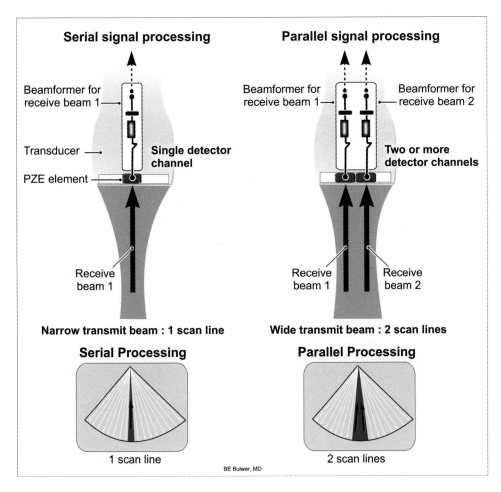

Figure 1.22. Serial Versus Parallel Processing. By simultaneously processing multiple scan lines, it is possible to increase frame rate dramatically compared to the limitations of single scan line processing. **Left panel:** Schema showing serial processing of a single scan line or beam received per transmitted pulse. Such processing is hostage to the finite acoustic propagation velocity in tissues. **Right panel:** Parallel processing techniques facilitate a two- or multifold increase in processing times by simultaneous acquisition and processing of B-mode image lines.

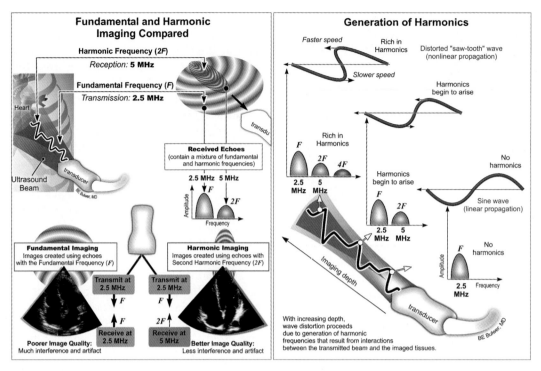

Figure 1.23. **Left panel:** Fundamental and harmonic imaging compared. In fundamental imaging, images are created using echoes with frequencies equal to that of the transmitted ultrasound. Harmonic imaging employs echoes arising from deeper tissues with frequencies twice that of the transmitted ultrasound. **Right panel:** Echoes with harmonic frequencies, unlike their fundamental counterparts, propagate nonlinearly and possess key properties that enhance image quality (see text).

improve ultrasound image quality: First, being confined to the central portions of the beam means that second harmonic echoes are not plagued by acoustic "noise" and artifacts (e.g., diffraction, side lobe, and reverberation artifacts) commonly seen with echoes near the beam periphery. Secondly, these less bulky (spatially smaller with lower amplitude) harmonic echoes encounter less interference from structures like the ribs (Fig. 1.23). Combined with the need to travel only a one-way journey from their origins to the transducer, they suffer comparatively less attenuation and their received signals are relatively large despite their higher frequencies. Thirdly, the focal zone and central regions of the ultrasound beam have the strongest intensities (amplitudes). This is a prerequisite for generating harmonics. Low-intensity beam regions, such as side grating lobes and side lobes (Fig. 1.5), produce low-amplitude echoes that are devoid of harmonics, and therefore eliminated from harmonic image creation (9,10,15,16).

Although tissue harmonic imaging has led to significant improvements in transthoracic image quality, especially with endocardial border delineation in "technically difficult" studies, this marked advantage has less significance in TEE. By virtue of the close proximity to the heart and the avoidance of the chest wall, TEE has benefitted from the superior image resolution wrought by the use of high-frequency transducers. Harmonic imaging has a downside. Its lower signal-to-noise ratio removes some of the speckle "noise" associated with echoes having the fundamental frequency (Figs. 1.18 and 1.19). Therefore,

tissue harmonic imaging may result in some loss of myocardial "speckle" and the associated imaging benefits of speckle tracking echocardiography (22,23).

CONTRAST ECHOCARDIOGRAPHY

The use of ultrasound contrast agents has contributed greatly to the diagnostic quality of echocardiographic studies. Contrast echocardiography is a highly specialized field and relies on the physical properties of the contrast agent and its interactions and behavior when exposed to ultrasound (Fig. 1.24) (24–27). Gas-containing contrast agents are distributed within the heart and circulation. They intensely reflect ultrasound, providing a marked increase in echoreflectivity far beyond that of normal body tissues and fluids. Therefore, ultrasound contrast agents are widely used to enhance visualization and assessment of cardiac structure, blood flow hemodynamics, and myocardial perfusion imaging. An ideal ultrasound contrast agent should (i) be nontoxic, (ii) distribute readily into the microcirculation, and (iii) be highly echoreflective with stable harmonics, and susceptible to rapid bubble disruption when subjected to clinically safe ultrasound beam intensities (24).

Contrast agents employed in echocardiography may be simply air agitated in saline ("bubble study"), or engineered microspheres typically 3 to 6 μm in diameter (slightly smaller than red blood cells with diameters

6–8 μm). These microspheres contain an insoluble gas, for example, nitrogen or perfluorocarbons trapped within an outer shell. This construction enables the highly echoreflective gas to maintain stability until its delivery to the desired target. Encapsulation of the gas leads to marked signal enhancement, not only due to markedly increased point scatter (because of the large acoustic impedance difference between the microbubble and the surrounding tissues), but also from bubble resonance (harmonics), and bubble rupture that can occur (Figs. 1.24 and 1.25). The degree to which these interactions occur depends on the acoustic intensity/power or mechanical index (MI, or peak negative acoustic pressure) of the transmitted ultrasound beam. Therefore, in addition to standard B-mode imaging, there are "contrast-specific" imaging modes when using contrast agents. These include high- and low-power (high-MI and low-MI) techniques, Doppler harmonic imaging and special Doppler modes, for example, phase correlation techniques. Image acquisition modes used in contrast imaging may be continuous or triggered or involve bubble destruction-detection sequences.

Myocardial contrast echocardiography (MCE) is a diagnostic technique that utilizes an ultrasound contrast agent and adapted ultrasound systems to enhance imaging quality. Early MCE techniques used contrast solutions containing relatively large bubbles (~16 μm) that were injected into the venous circulation to demonstrate gross anatomic abnormalities. Newer contrast agents are smaller (averaging 2.5–3 μm) with more stable microbubbles that behave as intravascular tracers (28,29). When contrast is used to image intracardiac shunts, right heart valvular incompetence, and/or pericardial effusions, hand-agitated saline (or blood or both) is often used. These microbubbles, however, are unstable. When new contrast agents are injected intravenously, they cross into the pulmonary circulation and enhance left-sided structures. In addition to left-sided valvular incompetence, they are valuable for enhancing endocardial borders and thereby facilitate regional wall motion assessment. Despite the improved resolution delivered by higher frequency TEE transducers, approximately 5% to 10% of the time, adequate wall motion abnormality interpretation is still not possible

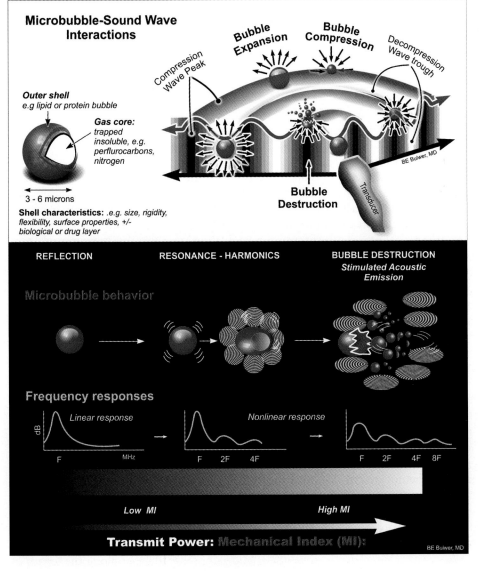

Figure 1.24. Above: Microbubble-Sound Wave Interactions. Microbubbles are gas-containing contrast agents that greatly reflect ultrasound, thereby markedly enhancing image quality. When exposed to an ultrasound field, microbubbles undergo cycles of compression and expansion. **Below:** Such microbubble behavior is further exploited in ultrasonography, as increasing the transmit power (or *mechanical index*) leads to generation of addition bubble harmonics due increasing bubble resonance or bubble destruction.

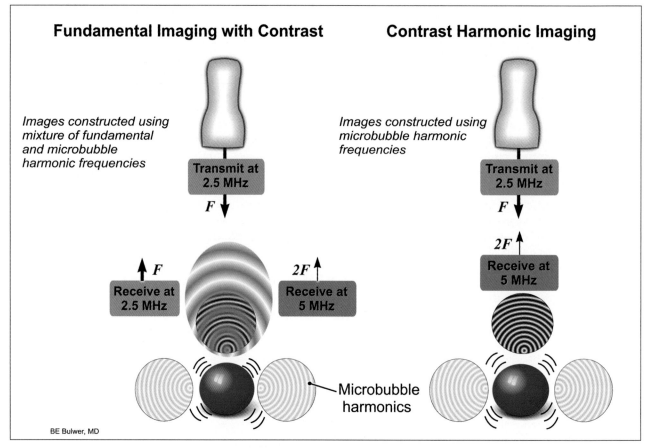

Figure 1.25. Fundamental imaging with contrast and contrast harmonic imaging compared (see text).

during surgical imaging. In 70% of cases, the intraoperative use of contrast with TEE enables visualization of regions that were missed when not using contrast (30). MCE also enhances Doppler interrogation when there is suboptimal visualization of the spectral Doppler time-velocity display (or envelope). Since ultrasound contrast agents behave as surrogate RBCs, they greatly improve Doppler signals. Direct, real-time interpretation of cardioplegic distribution and myocardial function reserve are applications of contrast agents combined with stress echocardiography. This has enabled both sonographer and surgeon to assess the adequacy of myocardial protection and surgical revascularization (31,32).

DOPPLER ECHOCARDIOGRAPHY

The most important addition to anatomical B-mode echocardiography is Doppler echocardiography (12,33, 34). This has made possible the noninvasive assessment of physiologic, hemodynamic, and mechanical measures of cardiac function. Blood flow velocity, direction, and flow patterns are the major applications of hemodynamic Doppler echocardiography. Newer Doppler measures, for example, myocardial tissue Doppler imaging (TDI), tissue velocity imaging, and myocardial deformation imaging, have significantly improved the assessment of systolic and diastolic function.

Blood Flow Hemodynamics, Flow Velocity Profiles, and Doppler Echocardiography

Blood flow through the heart and blood vessels is not uniform. A range or spectrum of velocities within cardiac chambers and blood vessels exists at each instant during the cardiac cycle (34–38). This spectrum, at each instant, can be analyzed and displayed on spectral Doppler echocardiography (Fig. 1.26). Several factors influence blood flow velocity profiles. These include cardiac chamber geometry, phase of the cardiac cycle, blood vessel diameter, vessel length, wall characteristics, flow rate, blood viscosity, and frictional forces. The range of velocities may become broadened or dispersed where blood vessels narrow or constrict, and where heart valves become stenosed or regurgitant. Complex flow patterns occur where blood vessels bifurcate and near valve orifices. Normal blood flow through the heart is mostly *laminar* or streamlined but can become *turbulent* or disorganized in the presence of valvular pathology and prosthetic heart valves. Laminar flow within cardiac chambers and great arteries typically exhibits an initial flat or *plug flow* profile during the initial systolic cardiac upstroke, becoming *skewed or blunted parabolic* as the flow proceeds, and *parabolic* in long straight vessels like the descending thoracic and abdominal aortae (Figs. 1.27 and 1.28).

In laminar flow, concentric laminae (streamlines) or isovelocities glide smoothly together along the length of

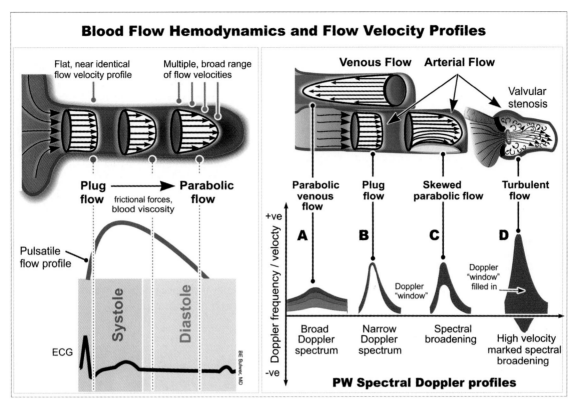

Figure 1.26. Simplified depiction of blood flow velocity profiles in a large blood vessel or cardiac chamber during the cardiac cycle (**left**), Flow velocity profiles in various blood vessels and their corresponding spectral Doppler appearance (**right**) (see text).

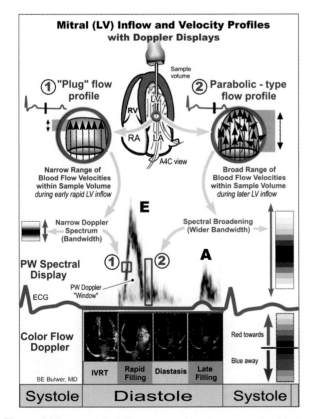

Figure 1.27. Simplified illustration showing transmitral inflow velocity profile with corresponding color flow Doppler and pulsed Doppler spectra as viewed on transthoracic echocardiography—apical 4-chamber (A4C) view (see text).

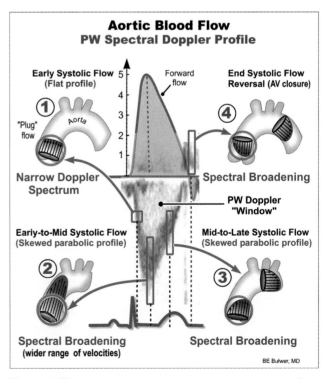

Figure 1.28. Simplified illustration showing aortic outflow velocity profiles with corresponding pulsed Doppler spectra as viewed on transthoracic echocardiography—apical 5-chamber view (see text).

blood vessels. Laminar flow with a parabolic flow profile displays the highest (maximum) velocities at the axial center of tubular blood vessels. Velocities are lowest, approaching zero adjacent to the vessel wall. The concentration of red blood cells, the main source of backscattered Doppler signals, mirrors the velocity profile and is evident on the intensity of the spectral Doppler display. With plug flow, the flat velocity profile indicates that almost all blood cells (across the vessel lumen) are flowing at the same velocity. This is represented by a narrow range or band of velocities on the time-velocity spectral Doppler display, a reflection of the near uniform flow velocities across the vessel lumen (Figs. 1.27 and 1.28). This is typical of early systolic flow. Turbulent flow is disorganized blood flow that exhibits the widest range of flow velocities—both positive and negative—due to vortex formation and multidirectional currents (Fig. 1.26). Turbulent flow is typically seen with obstructive and regurgitant valvular lesions, prosthetic heart valves, shunts, and arteriovenous fistulae (35–38).

The Doppler Principle and Doppler Frequency Shift

Doppler echocardiography is based on the principle that there is change in frequency of the received echoes reflected from flowing red blood cells compared to the interrogating

transducer frequency—akin to the change in pitch (frequency) when you listen to a moving siren (Fig. 1.29) (33,39). The change in frequency (pitch) can provide measurable information about blood flow velocity and direction. When the target (blood) is moving toward the transducer, the frequency of the received echoes compared to that of the transmitted ultrasound wave is shifted upward. If blood is moving away from the transducer, the frequency is shifted downward (Figs. 1.28 and 1.30). In hemodynamic Doppler echocardiography, this *shift in frequency* of the received echoes (f_R) compared to that of the transmitted ultrasound wave (f_T), is used to derive (i) blood flow velocity, (ii) blood direction, and (iii) blood flow characteristics (Figs. 1.30 and 1.31). This *Doppler frequency shift*, or simply the *Doppler shift*, is defined as the received frequency minus the transmitted frequency (Fig. 1.31) (9,40).

For sound reflected from moving blood cells, the shift in frequency is proportional to blood cell velocities relative to the speed of sound in blood. Therefore, if blood were

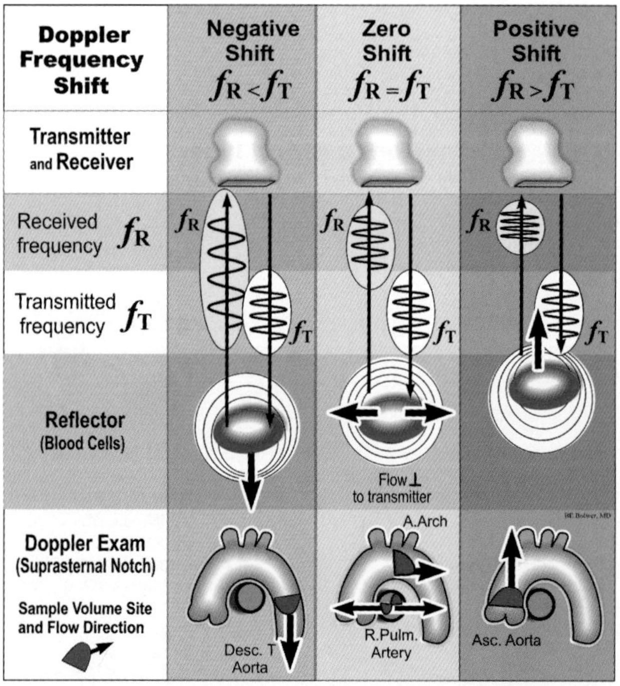

Figure 1.29. The Doppler principle as applied to normal blood flow dynamics within the thoracic aorta (suprasternal notch view on transthoracic echocardiography). The Doppler frequency shift, sometimes called the Doppler frequency or Doppler shift, is a change or shift in frequency of the received echoes compared to the frequency of the transmitted ultrasound wave. Note the impact of flow direction on the frequency of the received echoes (*shown in yellow*) (see text).

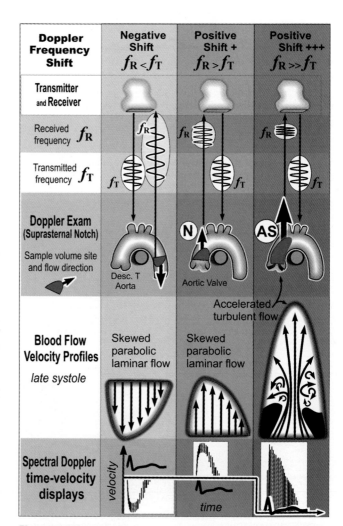

Figure 1.30. Simplified schema of the Doppler examination of flow velocities within the thoracic aorta as viewed from the suprasternal notch window (compare Figs. 1.26 and 1.29). Note flow direction, the associated Doppler frequency shifts, and their corresponding time-velocity spectral Doppler displays (see text).

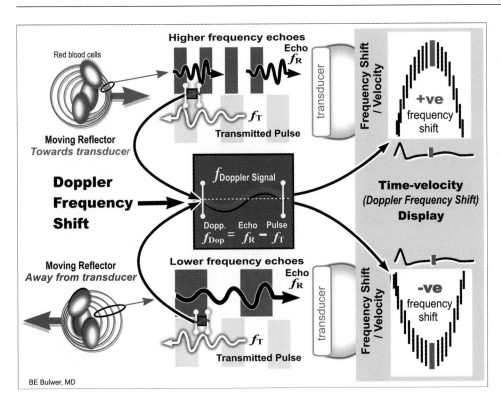

Figure 1.31. The Doppler Frequency Shift. **Upper panel:** Echoes reflected from blood moving toward the transducer exhibit higher frequencies compared to the transmitted Doppler ultrasound pulses. This difference in frequency is the *Doppler frequency shift*. It is a wave with its own frequency (**center**); it carries valuable information on blood flow velocity and direction that can be graphically displayed over time (**right panel**). Flow moving away from the transducer demonstrates a negative shift in frequency (**lower panel**), and is displayed accordingly.

moving at 1% the speed of sound, there would be a 1% shift in the frequency of that sound. With Doppler ultrasonography, there are actually *two* Doppler shifts: one when the sound is first received by moving blood cells and a second when sound is reflected back to the transducer. Therefore, blood moving at 1% of the speed of sound will shift the frequency by 2 (41).

The Doppler frequency shift is proportional only to the blood velocity component that is directed straight (parallel or at 0 degrees) to the transducer (Fig. 1.32). This velocity component that is parallel to the interrogating ultrasound beam equates to v cos θ, where v is the blood flow velocity being interrogated and θ is the angle between the beam and the interrogated blood vessel. The smaller the beam-vessel (or Doppler) angle, i.e., the more parallel the alignment, the bigger will be the Doppler shift. The mathematical relationship between the change in frequency of the reflected signal and the velocity of the red cell is:

$$V = \frac{f_r - f_t \times c}{\cos \theta \times 2\, f_t}$$

where Doppler frequency shift, $\Delta f = f_r - f_r$ (Fig. 1.32), θ = the angle of incidence between the transducer and

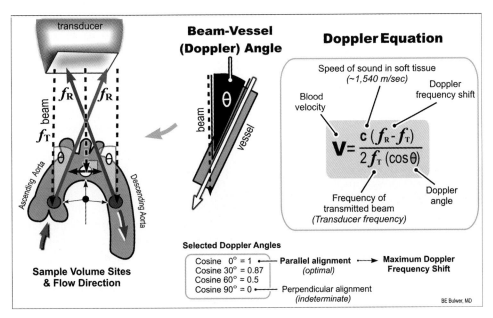

Figure 1.32. The Doppler angle and the Doppler equation. **Left panel:** The alignment of the ultrasound beam relative to that of blood flow can markedly affect the accuracy of flow velocity measurements. Optimal transducer beam alignment is parallel to blood flow, i.e., at a Doppler angle of zero (0) degrees where the cosine equals 1 (**middle panel**). The Doppler equation (**right panel**) describes the mathematical relationship between the measured Doppler frequency shift and target blood flow velocity, adjusted for the Doppler angle.

the velocity vector. As the angle θ approaches 90 degrees, the cos θ becomes zero. Whereas at an angle θ of 0 degree, the cos θ = 1. c is the velocity of sound in tissue (1,540 m/s), constant. f_t is the frequency of the transmitted signal. This is the transducer frequency. 2 represents the round-trip travel to and then travel from the reflector. f_r is the reflected signal frequency.

The cosine relationship of the relative blood flow velocity to the true blood flow velocity imposes an error in measurement with increasing Doppler angles. The larger the Doppler angle, the greater is the error estimate of the actual blood flow velocity. The best Doppler measurements or the most accurate measured blood flow velocities, therefore, are made with the Doppler beam aligned parallel to the targeted blood flow. This contrasts with B-mode echocardiography where the greatest reflections, and hence the best images, are acquired when the transducer beam is aligned perpendicular to the region of interest (Figs. 1.16 and 1.17). This is the *first paradox* of Doppler echocardiography. This is noteworthy because during 2D-guided placement of the Doppler sample volume, the best Doppler signals are often obtained when the 2D images appear suboptimal.

Optimal resolution of 2D (B-mode) images is obtained using high-frequency transducers. In contrast, higher blood flow velocities can be measured from the same Doppler frequency shifts when using low-frequency transducers (<2 MHz). This is the *second paradox* of Doppler echocardiography (12,39).

CONTINUOUS-WAVE DOPPLER ECHOCARDIOGRAPHY

During CW Doppler echocardiography, ultrasound is continually transmitted from a dedicated PZE element and continually received by another (9,40,42). The CW Doppler sample volume conforms to the area of overlap between the transmitted and received beams (Fig. 1.33). The returning echoes that impact the receiving PZE element include stronger (high-amplitude–low-frequency) echoes that emerge from slow-moving structures like the ventricular and vessel walls, as well as weaker (low-amplitude–high-frequency) echoes backscattered from fast-moving red blood cells. These received echoes induce a "raw" multifrequency electrical signal from which the desired Doppler signal—the Doppler frequency shift—must be extracted, processed, analyzed, and visualized on a time-velocity spectral Doppler display (Figs. 1.31 and 1.33). To extract the desired Doppler frequency shift, the received echoes sequentially undergo

1. *Amplification* in the receiver using nonlinear or logarithmic amplification.
2. *Demodulation* in the mixer/multiplier-demodulator to extract the low-frequency (kHz-range) Doppler shift

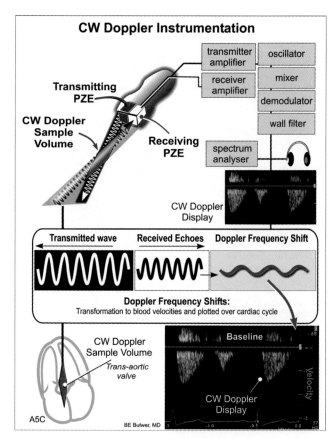

Figure 1.33. CW Doppler instrumentation (see text).

from the high frequency (MHz-range) ultrasound echoes by employing a "low-pass" (high velocity reject) filter that discards the high-frequency signals.

3. *Phased-sensitive demodulation* using a *quadrature detection* technique to determine the velocity direction—whether toward or away from the transducer.
4. The output Doppler signal is again filtered, this time using a "high-pass" (low velocity reject) or "wall" filter to reduce or eliminate high-amplitude, low-velocity "wall thump" echoes that arise from vessel walls, tissues, and transducer movements.
5. The "pure" Doppler frequency shift is then processed using a *digital Fourier spectral analysis* program called the *fast Fourier transform (FFT)*. This computational program prismatically resolves the composite multifrequency Doppler signal into its frequency spectrum (bandwidth), and corresponding intensities, to create the visual time-velocity spectral Doppler display (Fig. 1.33; see Fig. 1.37 and "Graphical Display of Doppler Frequency Spectra") (14–17).
6. The Doppler-shifted frequencies are in the low-frequency (kHz)/audible range, permitting audio output through a speaker or headphone. This property is harnessed in transthoracic studies where the sounds/tones of the Doppler signals serve as a guide to optimal Doppler placement when using a nonimaging (Pedoff) CW Doppler probe (9,33,42–44).

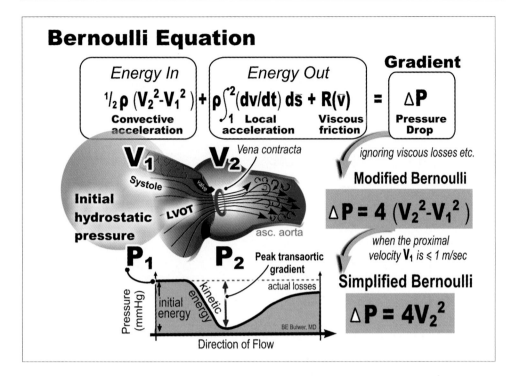

Bernoulli Equation

Energy In

$$\tfrac{1}{2}\rho\,(V_2{}^2\text{-}V_1{}^2)$$

Convective acceleration

Energy Out

$$\rho\int_1^2 (dv/dt)\,d\bar{s} + R(\bar{v})$$

Local acceleration   Viscous friction

Gradient

$$\Delta P$$

Pressure Drop

=

V$_1$ **V$_2$** Vena contracta

Systole   valve

Initial hydrostatic pressure   LVOT   asc. aorta

P$_1$ **P$_2$**   Peak transaortic gradient

ignoring viscous losses etc.

Modified Bernoulli

$$\Delta P = 4\,(V_2{}^2\text{-}V_1{}^2)$$

when the proximal velocity **V$_1$** is ⩽ 1 m/sec

Simplified Bernoulli

$$\Delta P = 4V_2{}^2$$

Pressure (mmHg)

initial energy   kinetic energy   actual losses

BE Bulwer, MD

Direction of Flow

Figure 1.34. The Bernoulli Equation. By accounting for the balance between potential energy and kinetic energy, it is possible to quantify the pressure drop across a stenotic valve. The equation serves as the basis for calculating pressure gradients ("driving pressure") across a narrowed orifice. The Bernoulli principle broadly states that as velocities increase, the pressure must decrease. This assumes the conservation of energy. However, in reality some energy is lost through heat, turbulent friction, and vortex formation. **ρ**-mass density of blood; **v**-velocity; **P**-pressure.

CW Doppler can measure high blood flow velocities in excess of 7 m/s as can occur across stenotic valves. However, it lacks the capacity to precisely identify the depth where this maximum velocity originates. This lack of depth specificity is also called *range ambiguity*. This technical drawback, as well as the large size of the CW Doppler sample volume, result in the inclusion of unwanted signals that arise from slower moving structures like the myocardium and blood vessel walls. A high-pass wall filter is employed to discard this high-amplitude-low velocity clutter. The most common clinical application of CW Doppler is the *Bernoulli equation* to quantify pressure drop across a stenotic valve or vessel (9,35,37). The fundamental principle of the Bernoulli equation is the law of conservation of energy—that the total fluid energy along a streamlined flow is constant. This means that any increase in velocity must be accompanied by a decrease in pressure. Therefore, an increase in kinetic energy as blood accelerates through a stenotic orifice must be accompanied by a concomitant fall in potential energy, represented by a pressure drop and accelerated flow across that stenosis. For a sufficiently abrupt and severe stenosis, with pressure drop (or pressure gradient) measured in mm Hg and velocity in meters per second, the pressure drop Δp can be described simply as $\Delta p = 4v^2$ (Fig. 1.34).

PULSED DOPPLER ECHOCARDIOGRAPHY

Pulsed Doppler or PW Doppler imaging involves operator-directed Doppler interrogation of blood flow velocities at specified depths (33,39). This *depth or range specificity* of the PW Doppler examination contrasts with the indiscriminate depth sampling of the CW Doppler examination. With PW Doppler, the same PZE element acts as both receiver and transmitter of ultrasound (Fig. 1.35). The transducer emits an ultrasound pulse (with spatial pulse length of 5–25 cycles) that targets a specified depth within a comparatively small sample volume. Based on the pulse-echo principle described earlier—where "time equals distance" (see Fig. 1.14)—an electronic time window or receiver "gate" opens only to, and analyzes only those echoes that return during a specified time window (that equates to that specified distance or depth). It is only those echoes received during this time "gate" that contain the desired Doppler frequency shifts corresponding to flow velocities found within the sample volume at the specified depth. These select echoes are then (i) extracted, (ii) filtered, (iii) sampled, and (iv) transformed into the time-velocity PW Doppler spectral display using processes in common with those described above for CW Doppler signal processing (43,44).

Following transmission of a pulse, the PZE element must wait (in "listening mode") for the specified echoes, reflected from the selected depth, to return before transmitting another pulse (see "Pulse-Echo Ultrasonography: Time Equals Distance"). The time for this return trip equals 2*d*, where *d* is the distance between transmitter and the specified depth (Figs. 1.14 and 1.36). This complete cycle of transmitting, waiting, and receiving is called the PRF; it is defined as the number of pulses per second (Fig. 1.36). The time between the pulses is the *pulse repetition period* (PRP); it is the reciprocal of the PRF, i.e., PRP = 1/PRF (PRP = pulse duration + listening time). Each time the receiver gate opens, i.e., once per PRP, the Doppler signal is *sampled* (Fig. 1.35).

Figure 1.35. Pulsed (PW) Doppler Instrumentation. The "range specificity" advantage afforded by PW Doppler interrogation of blood flow requires an elaborate design to receive and analyze only those echoes (and their Doppler shifts) that arise at specified depth. Once during each pulse-echo cycle (i.e., once per the PRP), the receiver gate opens only to those selected echoes. Range delay regulates the time delay, and the duration of time that the receiver gate opens is regulated by the length delay. Received Doppler signals are sampled in the sample-and-hold unit that "reconstructs" the Doppler signal prior to derivation of blood velocities by the fast Fourier transformation. The pulse Doppler operation, compared with continuous-wave Doppler (see Fig. 1.33), involves a more elaborate circuitry. Based on the gating requirements, as well as the limitations of ultrasound, the pulsed Doppler technique is subject to a Nyquist limit—or a maximum measurable velocity. When such velocity is exceeded, aliasing, or erroneous frequency estimation results (see Fig. 1.37).

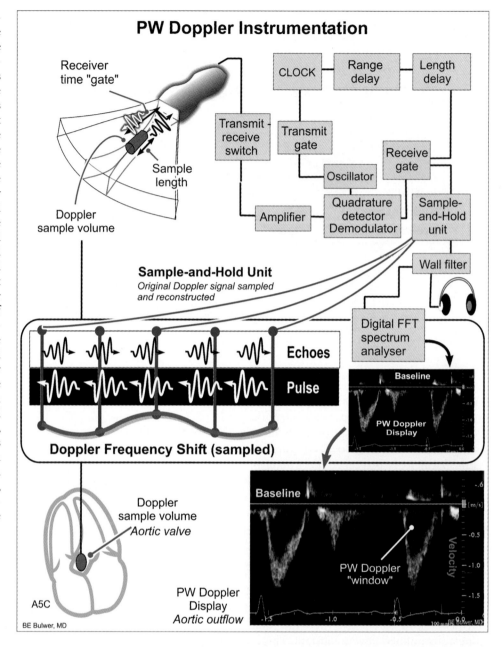

The *sampling rate* or *sampling frequency*, therefore, equals the pulse repetition frequency (sampling rate = PRF). The PRF is depth dependent since the speed of sound is finite and since echoes from greater depths need more time to return to the transducer before the next pulse transmission. As a result, the maximum PRF, and hence the maximum sampling rate, is depth dependent. This is a major limitation of PW Doppler interrogation of blood flow velocities (9,10,45). (see "2D Echocardiography: Transducer Operation, Frames, and Frame Rate"). The *duty factor* is the percentage or fraction of "work time" that the transducer element is transmitting pulses. With CW Doppler interrogation, the duty factor = 1% or 100%. With PW Doppler imaging, the *duty factor* = pulse duration/PRP × 100% (Fig. 1.36). The average PW transducer transmits only during a tiny fraction of the cycle, <<1%, with "listening mode" >>99%. A duty factor of 0.002%

or 0.2% is typical. Therefore, the greater the depth of interrogation, the lower (slower) is the PRF, the longer must be the waiting period (PRP), the lower the duty factor, and hence the lower the maximum measurable velocity. In other words, the deeper you image, the longer you wait, the more you listen, the less work you do, and the less capacity you have to measure high-velocity blood flows when using PW Doppler (9,10,45).

This round-trip distance, 2(d), requires a delay (T_d, time gate) between transmission and reception and is expressed as $T_d = 2d/c$, where c is the velocity of ultrasound in soft tissues (4). As the depth of interrogation increases, or if blood flow velocities are too high, the rate of sampling (PRF) becomes too slow to accurately measure and reconstruct the Doppler frequency shift. According to Shannon's wave sampling rule or theorem—also called the Nyquist criterion for analyzing frequencies—you must sample a

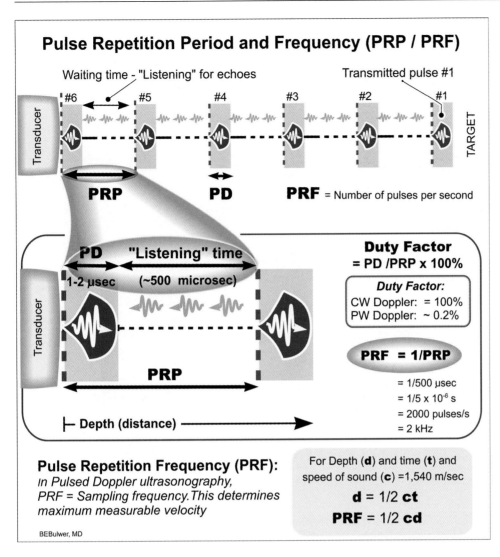

Pulse Repetition Period and Frequency (PRP / PRF)

Waiting time - "Listening" for echoes

Transmitted pulse #1

#6   #5   #4   #3   #2   #1

Transducer

TARGET

PRP   **PD**   **PRF** = Number of pulses per second

PD "Listening" time
1-2 µsec (~500 microsec)

Duty Factor
= PD /PRP x 100%

Duty Factor:
CW Doppler: = 100%
PW Doppler: ~ 0.2%

PRF = 1/PRP

= 1/500 µsec
= 1/5 x 10^{-6} s
= 2000 pulses/s
= 2 kHz

Transducer

PRP

├─ **Depth (distance)** ──────────────►

Pulse Repetition Frequency (PRF):
In Pulsed Doppler ultrasonography,
PRF = Sampling frequency. This determines
maximum measurable velocity

For Depth (**d**) and time (**t**) and
speed of sound (**c**) =1,540 m/sec

d = 1/2 ct
PRF = 1/2 cd

BEBulwer, MD

Figure 1.36. Upper panel: Schema showing six sequential ultrasound along with two important time intervals: pulse duration (PD) and pulse repetition period (PRP). In pulsed ultrasonography, following transmission of a single ultrasound pulse, the transducer must wait and listen for the return of echoes from the deepest structures—before transmitting another pulse. Violation of this principle leads to range ambiguity. The complete cycle of transmitting, waiting, and receiving is called the pulsed repetition frequency (PRF), and this PRF determines the maximum measurable velocity. **Lower panel:** The ratio of PD to the PRP is the duty factor. For a structure or sample volume located 10 cm from the transducer, the ultrasound round-trip time takes about 130 µs (µs; sound velocity in tissue is ~1540 m/s). To accurately interrogate such a sample volume 130 µs is needed to accurately acquire data from this depth (see text).

wave at least twice (*2f*) during its cycle in order to faithfully reproduce it (Fig. 1.37) (9,10,33). Therefore when analyzing the Doppler frequency shift (which is itself a wave, Fig. 1.31), you must sample it at least twice per cycle to faithfully reproduce it—and hence the velocity it represents. As the sampling frequency equals the PRF, and as two samples (hence two PRFs) per Doppler shift cycle are required for its accurate reconstruction, the maximum measureable Doppler frequency shift (blood flow velocity) is one half the sampling rate, i.e., 1/2 PRF. At Doppler frequency shifts greater than 1/2 the PRF, which happens with high-velocity flows and with flows interrogated at greater depths, the PRF or the sampling frequency is exceeded. This means that the sampling frequency is now too slow—it cannot keep up and faithfully reconstruct the Doppler frequency signal (Fig. 1.37). The result is an unfaithful or aliased reconstruction of the true Doppler signal. Therefore, an ambiguous or *aliased* signal is seen whenever the *Nyquist frequency*, akin to a "speed limit" (*Nyquist limit*), is exceeded. The Nyquist limit = PRF/2 (9,10,12).

The Nyquist limit, therefore, is the maximum measurable Doppler frequency shift (maximum measurable blood velocity) that can be accurately measured. At Doppler frequency shifts (velocities) greater than the

Nyquist limit, aliasing, a major form of PW Doppler display artifact, occurs (Fig. 1.37). An aliased PW Doppler signal "wraps around" the baseline of the time-velocity spectral display and appears to come from the opposite direction (Fig. 1.37). With color flow Doppler imaging, a PW Doppler-based technique, the wrap around appears as an unexpected color change—from blue to red or red to blue (see "Color flow Doppler Imaging," Figs. 1.44 and 1.50). The visual illusion of wagon wheels spinning in reverse in old Western movies results from the same principle. Here, the old movie cameras ("sampling rate") were too slow to accurately capture the comparatively fast-moving wagon wheels. More aliasing is seen with (i) high-velocity flows (as occurs downstream from a stenotic valve or vessel), (ii) lower PRFs (deep gating), and (iii) when using higher frequency transducers. Therefore, aliasing is less with slower blood velocities, higher PRF (shallow gating), and with lower frequency transducers (9,10,12).

These considerations explain the fundamental differences and the increased technical demands of the PW Doppler operation compared to the more straightforward CW Doppler technique. PW Doppler instrumentation requires a *sample and hold* unit where samples or snippets of the demodulated Doppler signals (from the receiver

Figure 1.37. Sampling Frequency, the Nyquist Limit, and Aliasing in Pulsed (PW) Doppler Operation. The time between the pulses is the PRP; it is the reciprocal of the PRF, i.e., PRP = 1/PRF (PRP = pulse duration + listening time). Each time the receiver gate opens, i.e., once per PRP, the Doppler signal is sampled (Fig. 1.35). The sampling rate or sampling frequency, therefore, equals the PRF (sampling rate = PRF). Shannon's wave sampling theorem (Nyquist criterion) for analyzing wave frequencies stipulates that you must sample a wave at least twice 2× during each cycle, or at twice its frequency (2F), in order to faithfully "recreate" it. Therefore, the maximum measurable Doppler frequency shift, i.e., the maximum measurable blood flow velocity, equals one half of the sampling rate, i.e., 1/2 PRF.

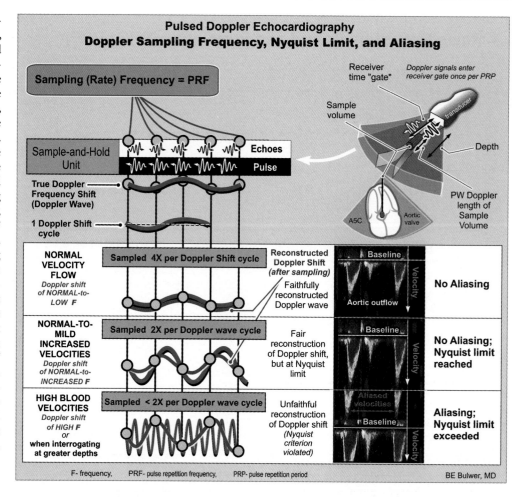

gate) are analyzed (Figs. 1.35 and 1.37). PW Doppler is useful to determine blood flows at precise locations. However, the receiving circuitry is turned on ("gated") only for a brief interval, corresponding to the specific depth of interest. This process is repeated at each instant during the cardiac cycle, allowing the processing and display of a series of Doppler-shifted signals using *fast Fourier transformation*. This yields the specific velocity profile in the sample volume at teach instant during the cardiac cycle (Figs. 1.26 to 1.30; see "Graphical Display of Doppler Frequency Spectra" and Fig. 1.38).

High PRF Mode and Multigate Doppler

Newer cardiac ultrasound platforms are equipped with the capacity for "high PRF mode" or "extended range/depth" Doppler measurements (9,10,42). As discussed above, the Nyquist limit equals PRF/2. Therefore, the PRF determines the maximum measurable velocity (Nyquist limit) without aliasing. The rationale for using "high PRF mode" Doppler is that if, for example, you succeed in doubling the PRF, you can effectively double the maximum velocity that you could measure with ordinary PW Doppler alone. The solution lies in gating the instrument to simultaneously receive two echoes: one—the echo expected from a specified depth (range) as per normal pulsed Doppler operation, and two—the echo from twice this depth that arose

from a previous pulse. Therefore, if you set the sample volume at half the depth of the region of interest, and you then measure the velocity after two consecutive pulses, you have then effectively doubled the PRF and the maximum measurable velocity. This principle can be exploited further by gating the instrument to simultaneously receive echoes from regions at depths multiples (e.g., 2×, 3×, 4×) that of primary sample volume depth, thereby doubling, tripling, or quadrupling the PRF and the maximal measurable velocity (without aliasing) all during a single listening gate. The downside is the potential for range ambiguity or image artifact appearance at multiples or fractions of the true depth (46). Multigate PW Doppler techniques simultaneously process multiple Doppler signals from multiple closely spaced sample volumes using multiple parallel receiver gates with time delays. Together, they can provide an instantaneous blood flow velocity profile across a valve or blood vessel. The use of multiple receiver gates is a principle used in color flow Doppler mapping.

GRAPHICAL DISPLAY OF DOPPLER FREQUENCY SPECTRA

To generate the spectral Doppler display, the raw echo signals must be demodulated and filtered. Like a prism that separates light into the colors of the spectrum or

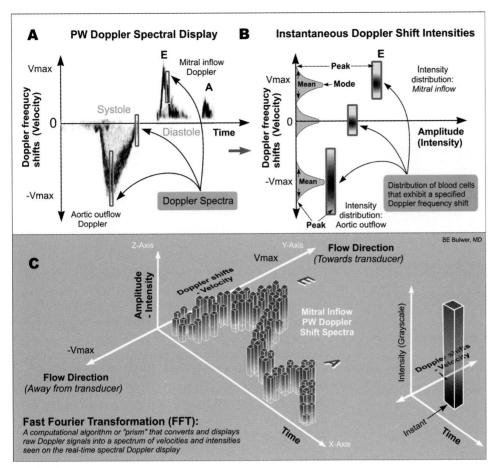

Figure 1.38. Graphical display of Doppler frequency spectra and the FFT. The time-velocity spectral Doppler display conveys much information about blood flow characteristics (**A**) (see Figs. 1.26 to 1.31, 1.39, and 1.40). To generate such information, the raw Doppler data is subjected to a computational algorithm—the *fast Fourier transformation*. This transforms the raw Doppler data into spectral bands of Doppler frequency shifts—representing blood flow velocities and intensities found within the sample volume at each instant during the cardiac cycle (**B** and **C**). (see text).

the cochlea that separates sounds into different frequency tones, so is the *fast Fourier transformation* that converts the raw Doppler shift signal into its spectrum of frequencies and intensities that correspond to flow velocities found within the sample volume (Fig. 1.38) (43,44). The fast Fourier transformation is a computational algorithm that transforms the raw Doppler frequency shift waveform into its spectral band of Doppler frequency shifts and intensities over time—*the time-velocity spectral Doppler display*. The Doppler frequency shifts in each vertical spectral band corresponds to the range of velocities present within the sample volume at each instant in time (during the cardiac cycle). The largest Doppler shifts correspond to peak velocities, and the smallest Doppler shifts correspond to the lowest velocities at each instant in time. A series of such spectral bands are analyzed, plotted, and displayed in real time as the time-velocity spectral Doppler display, or alternatively called the Doppler velocity profile or Doppler envelope.

The time-velocity spectral Doppler display reveals (Figs. 1.26 to 1.31)

1. The spectral band or range of Doppler frequency shifts that are present within the sample at each instant during the cardiac cycle. These correspond to the *range of blood flow velocities* and *flow characteristics*, for example, plug versus parabolic or turbulent flow patterns.

A number of clinically useful Doppler-derived parameters can easily be measured using automated calculations, for example, peak or maximal velocity, average or mean velocity, the velocity-time integral, pressure half time, and deceleration time.

2. Positive, negative, or no Doppler frequency shift: These indicate the *presence and/or direction of blood flow* with respect to the transducer.

3. The amplitude of each Doppler frequency shift is a measure of the intensity or brightness of the Doppler display. This corresponds to the percentage of blood cells exhibiting each Doppler shift (43,44).

With PW Doppler, *laminar plug flow* exhibits a narrow band or range of Doppler frequency shifts. This is displayed as a narrow spectral band with a spectral "window" (Figs. 1.26, 1.27, 1.31, 1.35, 1.39, and 1.40). The spectral band broadens as *laminar parabolic flow* ensues. With *turbulent flows*, the wide range of velocities encountered appear as broad spectral bands of Doppler frequency shifts (*spectral broadening*) with the resultant "filled-in" spectral window. Absence of a Doppler "window" typically appears on the CW Doppler display (Fig. 1.26 and 1.33). This reflects the wide range of velocities found within this much larger sample volume. The spectral Doppler examination is typically done with 2D and color flow Doppler serving as a guide for optimal sample volume placement (Fig. 1.40) (43,44).

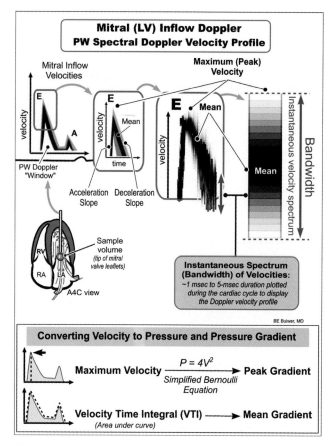

Figure 1.39. The Pulsed (PW) Spectral Doppler Display Illustrating the Bandwidth (spectrum) of Frequencies Encountered Within Each Sample Volume. A4C, apical 4-chamber view on transthoracic echocardiography. Velocities can be converted to intracardiac pressures and pressure gradients by applying the Bernoulli equation.

TISSUE DOPPLER ECHOCARDIOGRAPHY

Just as optimal hemodynamic Doppler assessment requires a basic understanding of blood flow characteristics, optimal tissue Doppler assessment also requires some insight into basic cardiac mechanics (24,47). Cardiac form and function are implied in the helical myofiber arrangement and electromechanical design (48,49). Cardiac motion is complex and includes global translation and rotation in addition to regional 3D deformation. The normal heart deforms—shortens, thickens, and twists—during systole, with active reversal of these regional movements during diastole (Fig. 1.41) (50). Such motion can be assessed using TDI, a PW Doppler-based technique, and TDI-derived measures of regional myocardial function (47–50).

With hemodynamic Doppler imaging, low-amplitude–high-frequency Doppler signals received from normal intracardiac flow averaging 100 to 150 cm/s must be separated from high-amplitude–low-frequency Doppler signals received from slower moving (10–15 cm/s) ventricular walls and other cardiac structures. This is achieved using a high-pass filter (51). With TDI, the reverse is executed, and the Doppler signals arising from sampled myocardial segments are separated from blood flow signals by low-pass filtering or by increasing the system gain. The Doppler shift signal is analyzed using an *autocorrelation* method. Numerous TDI display formats are used, for example, the longitudinal spectral TDI at the mitral annulus, color-coded 2D TDI, color-coded TDI M-mode, average velocity curves, and proprietary parametric displays (Fig. 1.42). TDI and TDI-derived measures of cardiac motion and deformation, for example, longitudinal velocities, strain

Figure 1.40. Annotated PW Doppler freeze frame. The time-velocity spectral Doppler display conveys much information about blood flow characteristics (see Figs. 1.26 to 1.31, 1.39, and 1.40). To generate such information, the raw Doppler data is subjected to a computational algorithm—the *fast Fourier transformation*. This transforms the raw Doppler data into spectral bands of Doppler frequency shifts—representing blood flow velocities and intensities found within the sample volume at each instant during the cardiac cycle.

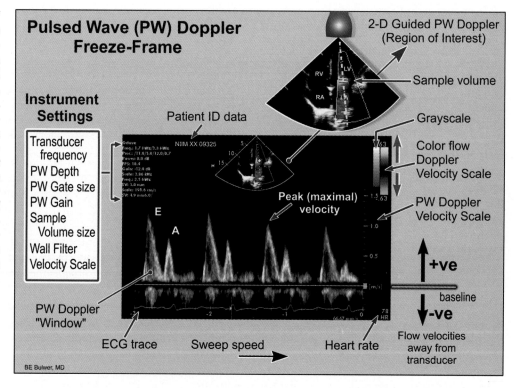

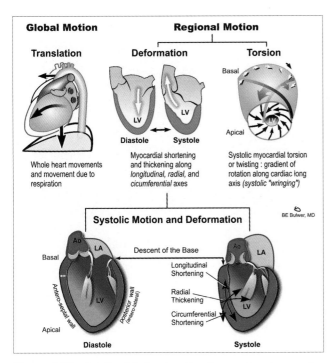

Figure 1.41. Cardiac Mechanics. Cardiac motion is complex and includes translational as well as myocardial motion and deformation. TDI and TDI-derived measures can assess aspects of cardiac motion and deformation but are limited by Doppler angle dependence. Speckle tracking echocardiography can over come this and can better assess myocardial torsion—an important functional parameter of clinical importance.

and strain-rate, have found increasing applications in the assessment of systolic and diastolic functions (23,52,53). TDI imaging is beset by the same angle dependency of spectral Doppler techniques, and this largely restricts its utility to the assessment of longitudinal motion and deformation (47).

COLOR FLOW DOPPLER ECHOCARDIOGRAPHY

One of the great advances in echocardiography was the advent of color flow Doppler imaging (or mapping) in the 1980s (54,55). This PW Doppler-based technique is a visually intuitive, spatially correct real-time display of (i) blood flow velocities, (iii) blood flow direction, and (iii) blood flow pattern—all superimposed on B-mode images, whether M-mode, 2D, or 3D displays.

The technique simultaneously interrogates multiple sample volumes, using multiple receiver "gates" per scan line. There are literally hundreds of gates represented in each color scan sector. However, unlike the 2D B-mode display where there is a 1:1 relationship between the acoustic scan line and the display scan line (see Fig. 1.3), each color flow Doppler-2D display represents a *packet* (variously termed a *burst, pulse train,* or *ensemble*) of acoustic scan lines. Each *packet size,* comprising four to eight acoustic scan lines from which the Doppler frequency shifts (velocities), are simultaneously analyzed, are encoded in color: *red* indicating flow toward the transducer and *blue* indicating flow away from the transducer (Fig. 1.43). This arrangement of four to eight acoustic scan lines, represented visually as 1 display scan line, is to facilitate optimal visual assessment of the color-coded velocities. However, processing and displaying this enormous amount of data in real-time impose huge computational demands. Because color flow mapping is an expanded application of the PW Doppler principle, it is subject to PW Doppler limitations such as aliasing. Indeed, the much increased computational demands cause aliasing to occur at even lower velocities than with PW Doppler, even at normal intracardiac flow rates. As with PW Doppler, if the highest Doppler shift frequency exceeds one-half of the PRF (PRF/2) for that particular depth, aliasing of the color signal will occur. This appears as an immediate change or color inversion from light blue to light yellow when blood flow velocities exceed the established maximal measurable

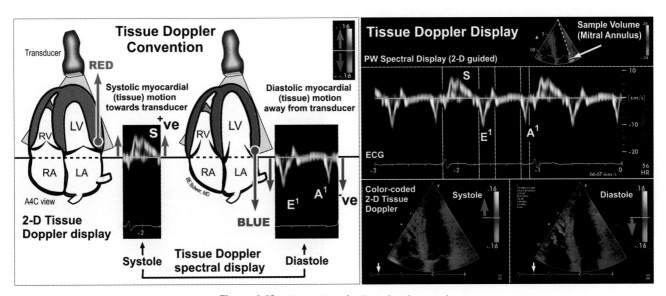

Figure 1.42. Tissue Doppler Imaging (see text).

Figure 1.43. Color flow Doppler velocity scales. Three color flow Doppler display options. By convention, flow (mean velocities) toward the transducer are color-coded red, and flow away from the transducer are color-coded blue. No measureable flow is displayed as black. Lighter shades denote higher mean flow velocities. Variance maps introduce a third color, usually green, to display the wider variations found in turbulent flows.

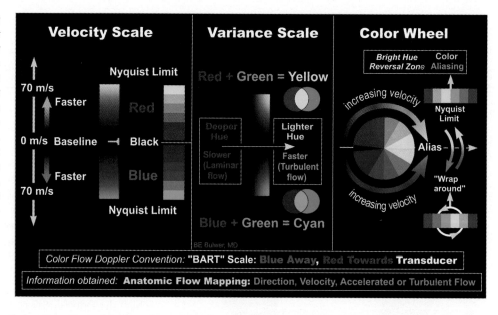

velocity (Fig. 1.43, see Fig. 1.50) (54,55). Optimization of color Doppler mapping and increasing the Nyquist limit, i.e., the maximal measurable velocity without aliasing, can be achieved by

1. Optimizing the Doppler angle (parallel transducer beam-flow direction)
2. Reducing the depth (distance) of color scan sector or region of interest, thereby increasing the PRF
3. Narrowing the color scan sector width, which effectively reduces the number of scan lines
4. Reducing the scan line density
5. Reducing the density of ultrasound bursts (smaller packet size)
6. Shifting the velocity scale/PRF to suit flow conditions

The color scan sector represents color-encoded velocities of blood present within that sector. It uses a fundamentally different method of signal processing than the fast Fourier transformation used with PW and CW Doppler. This is because of the enormous amount of data that must be processed by color flow mapping. As shown in Figure 1.44, a brief burst of ultrasound is emitted, but then the entire returning sound train for the whole sector of interest is received, amplified, and stored in memory. Then a second pulse is emitted and likewise is stored in digital memory. Using a mathematical method called *autocorrelation*, the wave fronts in pulses 1 and 2 are compared to each other. In regions where blood flow is moving toward the transducer ("red" flow), the waves of pulse 2 tend to be shifted forward relative to the signal in pulse 1. When blood is going away from the transducer, the pulse 2 signal lags a bit behind pulse 1 ("blue" flow). This permits the equipment to determine velocity along the length of the scan line. If only two pulses were emitted, then about all that could be determined from the autocorrelation method would be whether the blood was moving toward or away from the transducer. Instead, multiple pulses are emitted and all are compared with each other, generating a family of velocity estimates as shown in Figure 1.45. These

velocity estimates have a characteristic (i) *phase* (the angle around the circle, proportional to the velocity), (ii) *amplitude* (the strength of the signal), and (iii) *variance* (the degree of scatter between successive estimations related to turbulence). By averaging these together, it is possible to obtain a more precise estimate of velocity for every point along the scan line (54–56).

With color flow mapping, as with 2D echocardiography, there is a trade-off between temporal resolution and the accuracy of the information in the image. If the packet size is increased, the velocity accuracy is increased but the temporal or real-time resolution is decreased. Most packet sizes are between 3 and 20 pulses but are typically 8. If there are too few packets, the velocity determinations will be inaccurate. If there are too many packets, the frame rate will be low. The same is true for the line density (the number of scan lines per frame). *Velocity mode* display of color flow Doppler mapping represents the average of the packet velocities along a scan line. The *variance mode* of color flow Doppler mapping is a continuation of the velocity mode. However, packet velocities are averaged, and then the variability between the individual velocity

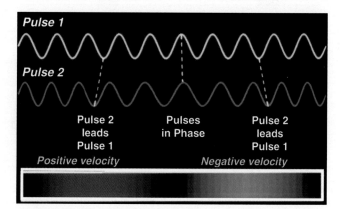

Figure 1.44. Color Doppler processing by autocorrelation. By comparing the phase shift in successive pulses of ultrasound, it is possible to determine the velocity all along the sector of interest.

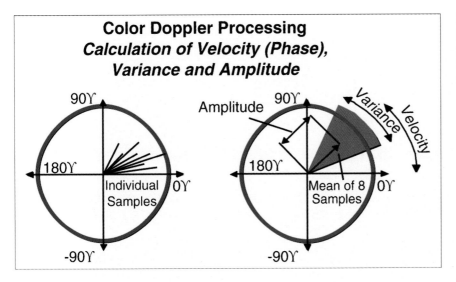

Figure 1.45. Color Doppler processing. By averaging the phase and amplitude of multiple color Doppler pulses together, it is possible to obtain a more precise estimate of color flow velocity (see text).

estimates in the packet is examined. If the packet contains a broad band of velocities, then another color is introduced into the color map (Fig. 1.43). These colors are typically green or yellow. If the range of these velocities is small, then only a small amount of variance color is introduced (Fig. 1.43). If the range is large, then a large amount of variance color is introduced (55,57).

Instrumentation Factors in Color Flow Doppler Imaging

One of the most important applications of color Doppler echocardiography is the assessment of valvular regurgitation. The size of the regurgitant jet, as visualized by color Doppler, is an important method for characterizing the severity of regurgitation. Consequently, an understanding of the principles of ultrasound and instrumentation impacting the color jet area is essential. First, one must consider the physical parameter that best determines jet size—jet momentum—given by the product of flow rate through the regurgitant orifice and the driving velocity. Thus, for

the same amount of flow going through a valve, a high-pressure jet will appear larger than a low-pressure jet ("billiard ball effect"). This also explains why blood pressure should be measured during the echocardiographic examination. There also is the important issue of jet constraint and distortion by adjacent walls. As shown in Figure 1.46, an eccentrically directed wall jet tends to flatten out along the wall and appears considerably smaller than an equal sized central jet, by a factor of more than half (Coanda effect) (58). Finally, there are a host of instrumentation factors that can impact the appearance of the jet. Figure 1.47 shows the impact of color gain on a mitral regurgitant jet as visualized on TEE. As gain is increased, the jet appears larger, and ultimately (at gain = 56) there is extraneous coloration of the B-mode image (tissue), indicating excessive color gain setting. In general, the color Doppler gain should be increased until color pixels just begin to appear within the B-mode image (tissue) and then reduced slightly to eliminate these. Output power has a similar impact on jet size and should generally be set at levels that are well within the Food and Drug Administration (FDA)

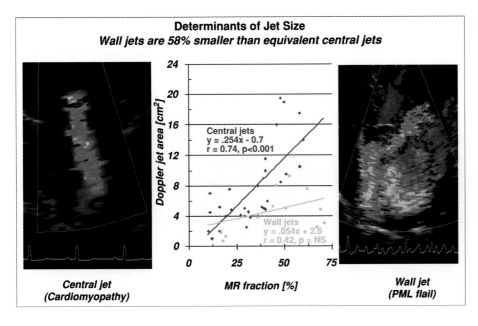

Central jet (Cardiomyopathy)

Wall jet (PML flail)

Figure 1.46. Impact of Wall Impingement on Jet Size. Jets that are directed eccentrically against a chamber wall are less than half the size of centrally directed jets (see text).

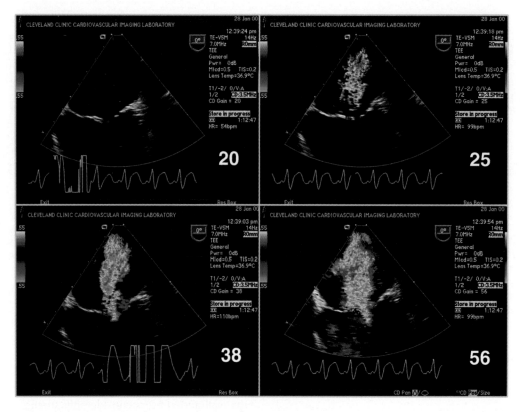

Figure 1.47. Impact of Color Gain on Jet Size. By highlighting weaker Doppler signals, color gain (and the corresponding transmission parameter, output power) critically impacts jet size.

standards for output power. Figure 1.48 demonstrates the impact of PRF or scale on the size of the color Doppler jet. For color flow Doppler, there are a finite number of velocity "bins" that are represented on the display, typically about 16 forward and 16 backward. Therefore, the lowest velocity that is visible is approximately 1/16 of the maximal velocity (14). Because the PRF and the transducer frequency determine the maximal measurable velocity, reducing PRF can make the color jet appear larger by encoding lower velocities within the jet. When the color velocity scale is set at the maximum value (69 cm/s), the instrument displays all velocities greater than about 4 cm/s. Reducing the scale to 39 now encodes velocities greater than 2 cm/s, with a

larger jet, while reducing it still further to 17 cm/s encodes velocities greater than 1 cm/s. These adjustments make jet sizes appear larger.

Transducer frequency has a dual effect on the size of the regurgitant jet. The primary effect of increasing transducer frequency is to encode lower velocities within the jet, making the jet appear larger. However, higher frequency ultrasound is attenuated more by intervening tissue, so this may make the jet appear smaller. Typically, the frequency effect dominates in TEE, where there is little attenuation, whereas the attenuation effect is dominant in transthoracic echocardiography (Fig. 1.49). There are other ways of influencing the color flow Doppler

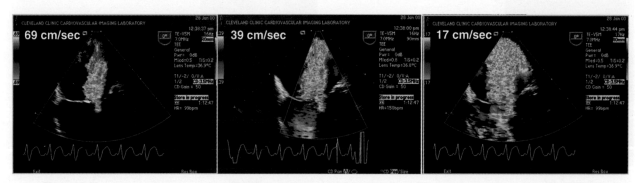

Figure 1.48. Impact of Color Scale on Jet Size (Velocity Effect). Reducing the PRF lowers the minimal velocity displayed by color Doppler, thus making jets appear larger.

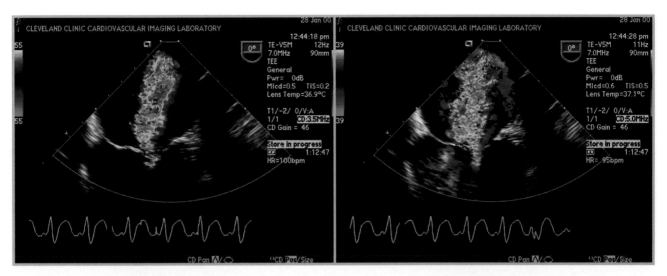

Frequency = 3.5 MHz
Nyquist Limit = 55 cm/sec
Vmin ⊕3.5 cm/sec

Frequency = 5 MHz
Nyquist Limit = 39 cm/sec
Vmin ⊕2.5 cm/sec

Figure 1.49. Impact of Transducer Frequency on Jet Size. Increasing the transducer frequency lowers the minimal velocity displayed by color Doppler, thus making jets appear larger.

display, but the recommendation is for each laboratory to establish internal standards in conformity with the appropriate instrument settings guidelines. The aim is to foster consistency in the assessment and interpretation of regurgitant jets (54–58).

CW, PW, AND COLOR FLOW DOPPLER COMPARED

The three most commonly used hemodynamic Doppler modalities are summarized in Table 1.2 and Figure 1.50.

TABLE 1.2	**Doppler Echocardiography Techniques Compared**		
	CW Doppler	**PW Doppler**	**Color Flow Doppler**
Sample volume	Large (measured in cm)	Small (2–5 mm)	Large (adjustable color scan sector)
Velocities measured	A Spectrum: maximum-to-minimum (hence the term "spectral" Doppler)	A Spectrum: maximum-to-minimum (hence the term "spectral" Doppler)	Mean velocity (each color pixel or voxel codes for mean velocity and flow direction on "BART" scale)
Display format	Time-velocity spectral graph	Time-velocity spectral graph	Color-coded velocity pixels (2D) and voxels (3D) superimposed on B-mode image
Spectrum of blood flow velocities detected and displayed	Wide; spectral broadening (no "window" seen on time-velocity graphical display)	Narrow; spectral window (but spectral broadening seen with turbulent flows)	Wide; wide spectrum of velocities displayed as color mosaic—green color added to conventional "BART" scale
Detection of high blood flow velocities	No aliasing; accurate assessment	Aliasing; inaccurate assessment with high flow velocities	Color aliasing (even with normal intracardiac flows)
Aliasing artifact and display	No aliasing; no Nyquist velocity limit; peak velocities on the correct side of baseline	Aliasing; Nyquist limit; aliased velocities appear on opposite side of baseline	Aliasing; color aliasing appears as color inversion on BART scale (e.g., light blue-light light yellow and vice versa)
Depth resolution/ range ambiguity	Range ambiguity	Range resolution (single gate)	Range resolution (multiple gates)

BART, *Blue Away, Red Towards.*

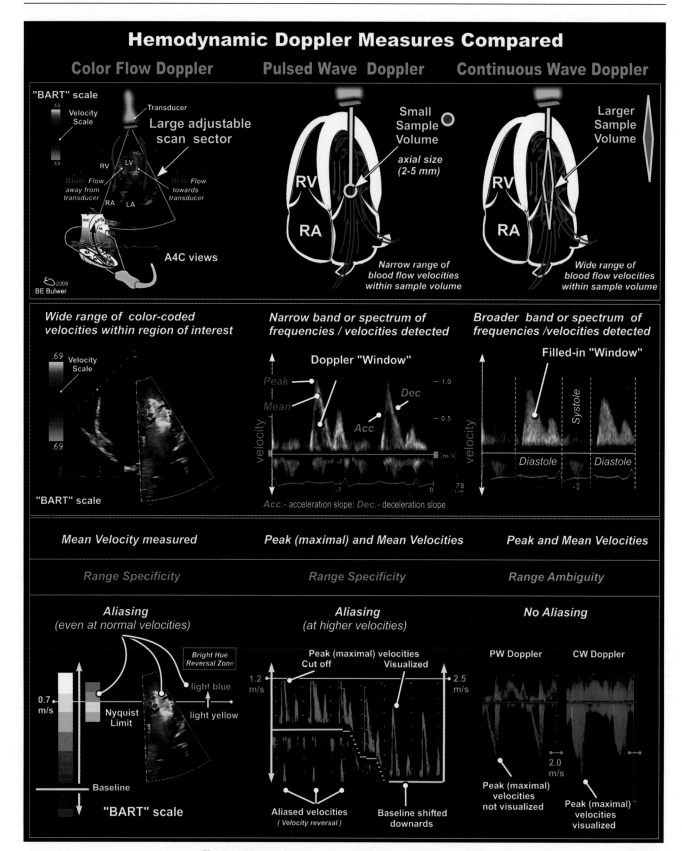

Figure 1.50. Hemodynamic Doppler measures compared.

CONCLUSIONS

Echocardiography or cardiac ultrasonography is the most widely used and versatile cardiac imaging modality with established utility in the diagnosis and management of patients with suspected or established cardiovascular disease. Optimal use of this technology requires a working understanding of the basic physical principles that influence ultrasound generation, transmission, interactions, image processing, and display. Ultrasound—sound with inaudible frequencies beyond 20,000 Hz—has physical properties that can be harnessed to provide clinically useful information about cardiac structure and function. Image reconstruction and display of cardiac structures depend on the pulse-echo method; this converts the times between ultrasound wave transmission and the reception of its echoes into anatomical depths or distances. The amplitudes of the received echoes determine their grayscale brightness, and these B-mode images are optionally displayed using M-mode, 2D, or 3D formats. Additional developments, like parallel processing, tissue harmonic imaging, and contrast echocardiography, have improved the quality of B-mode imaging.

Doppler echocardiography, especially spectral Doppler, color flow Doppler, and TDI, has delivered clinically important data on cardiac hemodynamics and mechanics. It is based on the principle that the shifts in the frequency of the received echoes compared to the emitted ultrasound beam can be used to derive blood flow and tissue velocities. All ultrasound imaging modalities harness the strengths, but are subject to the intrinsic weaknesses of ultrasound. Understanding these should foster, not just improved ultrasound image acquisition and interpretation, but also optimal cardiovascular assessment in the clinical setting.

KEY POINTS

- Ultrasound propagates as longitudinal waves that cause tissues to resonate, thereby propagating as cycles of compression and decompression. As waves propagate, differential interactions occur with the tissues they encounter, including reflection, refraction, diffraction, and attenuation. These can be detected and translated into graphical data.
- The product of the wavelength (λ) and the frequency (F) is equal to the propagation velocity (c) of the wave and is expressed by the formula: $c = F \times \lambda$. Wavelength is directly proportional to propagation velocity. The frequency of ultrasound in tissues is constant and corresponds to the transducer frequency. However, a change in velocity occurs whenever ultrasound waves travel from one tissue interface to another.

- The higher the frequency of the transmitted ultrasound wave, the better the axial resolution. The longer the wavelength, the greater the tissue penetration.
- Modern ultrasound transducers contain arrangements or arrays of PZE elements, which may be linear (linear array), curved (curved or curvilinear array), annular (annular array), or a rectangular matrix (matrix array).
- The ultrasound beam is largely confined to a predictable 3D space with axial, lateral, and elevational dimensions. The length of the near field is largely determined by transducer diameter and transducer frequency. As both increase, the near-field length increases. Optimal lateral resolution is achieved with a large-diameter–high-frequency/short-wavelength transducer.
- The most accurately measured Doppler blood flow velocities are made with the Doppler beam aligned parallel to the targeted blood flow. This contrasts with 2D echocardiography where the greatest reflections and hence the best images are acquired when the transducer beam is aligned perpendicular to the region of interest. This is the first paradox of Doppler echocardiography. In addition, optimal resolution of 2D images is obtained with high-frequency transducers. In contrast, higher blood flow velocities can be measured from the same Doppler frequency shifts when using low-frequency transducers (<2 MHz). This is the second paradox of Doppler echocardiography.
- Pulsed Doppler echocardiography interrogates blood flow velocities at a specified depth but is susceptible to aliasing. With CW Doppler echocardiography, ultrasound is continually transmitted from a dedicated PZE element and continually received by another. Although CW lacks range specificity unlike PW, it is not susceptible to aliasing.

REFERENCES

1. Bulwer BE, Rivero J, Solomon SD. Basic principles of echocardiography and tomographic anatomy. In: Solomon SD, Braunwald E, eds. *Atlas of Echocardiography*. New York: Current Science/Springer Science, 2008:1–24.
2. Bulwer BE, Shamshad F, Solomon SD. Clinical utility of echocardiography. In: Solomon SD, ed., Bulwer BE, Assc. ed. *Essential Echocardiography. A Practical Casebook with DVD*. Totowa, NJ: Humana Press, 2007:71–86.
3. Edler I, Hertz CH. The use of ultrasonic reflectoscope for the continuous recording of the movements of heart walls. 1954. *Clin Physiol Funct Imaging* 2004;24(3):118–136.
4. Edler I, Lindström K. The history of echocardiography. *Ultrasound Med Biol* 2004;30(12):1565–1644.

5. Geiser EA. Echocardiography: physics and instrumentation. In: Skorton DJ, Schelbert HR, Wolf GL, Brundage BH, eds. *Marcus Cardiac Imaging: a Companion to Braunwald's Heart Disease.* 2nd ed. Philadelphia: WB Saunders, 1996:273–295.

6. Weyman A. Physical principles of ultrasound. In: Weyman A, ed. *Principles and Practice of Echocardiography.* 2nd ed. Philadelphia: Lea & Febiger, 1994:3–28.

7. Jensen JA. Medical ultrasound imaging. *Prog Biophys Mol Biol* 2007;93(1–3):153–165.

8. Orihashi K, et al. Principle of transesophageal echocardiography and modes. In: Oka Y, Goldiner PL, eds. *Transesophageal Echocardiography.* Philadelphia: J. B. Lippincott Co., 1992:9–27.

9. Bushberg JT, Siebert JA, Leidholdt EM Jr, et al. *The Essential Physics of Medical Imaging.* 2nd ed. Philadelphia: Lippincott Williams & Wilkins, 2002:469–553.

10. Kremkau F. *Diagnostic Ultrasound: Principles and Instruments.* 7th ed. Philadelphia: W.B. Saunders Company, 2002.

11. Feigenbaum H. Physics and instrumentation. In: Feigenbaum H, ed. *Echocardiography.* 6th ed. Baltimore: Williams & Wilkins, 2004:11–45.

12. Otto C. Principles of echocardiographic image acquisition and Doppler analysis. In: Otto C, ed. *Textbook of Clinical Echocardiography.* 2nd ed. Philadelphia, W.B. Saunders Company, 2004:1–28.

13. Dowsett DJ, Johnston RE, Kenny PA. Principles of ultrasound. In: Dowsett DJ, Johnston RE, Kenny PA, eds. *The Physics of Diagnostic Imaging.* 2nd. ed. London: Arnold Publishers Ltd, 2006:511–529.

14. Thomas JD. Principles of imaging. In: Fozzard HA, Haber E, Jennings RB, Katz AM, eds. *The Heart and Cardiovascular System.*, 2nd ed. New York: Raven Press, 1996:625–668.

15. Whittingham TA. Medical diagnostic applications and sources. *Prog Biophys Mol Biol.* 2007;93(1–3):84–110.

16. Houck RC, Cooke JE, Gill EA. Live 3D echocardiography: a replacement for traditional 2D echocardiography? *Am J Roengenol* 2006;187(4):1092–1106.

17. Wells PN. Ultrasound imaging. *Phys Med Biol* 2006;51(13): R83–R98.

18. Hung J, Lang R, Flachskampf F, et al. 3D echocardiography: a review of the current status and future directions. *J Am Soc Echocardiogr* 2007;20(3):213–233.

19. Prior DL, Jaber WA, Homa DA, et al. Impact of tissue harmonic imaging on the assessment of rheumatic mitral stenosis. *Am J Cardiol* 2000;86(5):573–576, A10.

20. Rubin DN, Yazbek N, Garcia MJ, et al. Qualitative and quantitative effects of harmonic echocardiographic imaging on endocardial edge definition and side-lobe artifacts. *J Am Soc Echocardiogr* 2000;13(11):1012–1018.

21. Desser TS, Jeffrey RB. Tissue harmonic imaging techniques: physical principles and clinical applications. *Semin Ultrasound CT MR* 2001;22(1):1–10.

22. Marwick TH. Measurement of strain and strain rate by echocardiography: ready for prime time? *J Am Coll Cardiol* 2006;47:1313–1327.

23. Kirkpatrick JN, Vannan MA, Narula J, et al. Echocardiography in heart failure: applications, utility, and new horizons. *J Am Coll Cardiol* 2007;50:381–396.

24. McCulloch M, Gresser C, Moos S, et al. Ultrasound contrast physics: a series on contrast echocardiography, article 3. *J Am Soc Echocardiogr* 2000;13(10):959–967.

25. Kaufmann BA, Wei K, Lindner JR. Contrast echocardiography. *Curr Probl Cardiol* 2007;32(2):51–96.

26. Raisinghani A, DeMaria AN. Physical principles of microbubble ultrasound contrast agents. *Am J Cardiol* 2002;18;90(10A):3J–7J.

27. Amyot R, Morales MA, Rovai D. Contrast echocardiography for myocardial perfusion imaging using intravenous agents: progress and promises. *Eur J Echocardiogr* 2000;1(4):233–243.

28. Rubin DN, Thomas JD. New imaging technology: measurement of myocardial perfusion by contrast echocardiography. *Coron Artery Dis* 2000;11(3):221–226.

29. Pasquet A, Greenberg N, Brunken R, et al. Effect of color coding and subtraction on the accuracy of contrast echocardiography. *Internat J Cardiol* 1999;70(3):223–231.

30. Erb JM, Shanewise JS. Intraoperative contrast echocardiography with intravenous optison does not cause hemodynamic changes during cardiac surgery. *J Am Soc Echocardiogr* 2000;14(6):595–600.

31. Aronson S, Savage R, Lytle B, et al. Identifying the etiology of left ventricular dysfunction during coronary bypass surgery: the role of myocardial contrast echocardiography. *J Cardiovasc Thorac Anes* 1998;12:512–518.

32. Aronson S, Jacobsohn E, Savage R, et al. The influence of collateral flow on distribution of cardioplegia in patients with an occluded right coronary artery. *Anesthesiology* 1998;89:1099–1107.

33. Hatle L, Angelsen B. *Doppler Ultrasound in Cardiology: Physical Principles and Clinical Applications.* 2nd ed. Philadelphia: Lea & Febiger, 1985.

34. Spencer MP. *Cardiac Doppler Diagnosis.* Vol. II. Dordrecht: Martinus Nijhoff Publishers, 1986.

35. Hatle L, Angelsen B. Physics of blood flow. In: Hatle L, Angelsen B, eds. *Doppler Ultrasound in Cardiology: Physical Principles and Clinical Applications.* 2nd ed. Philadelphia: Lea & Febiger, 1985:8–31.

36. Weyman A. Principles of flow. In: Weyman A, ed. *Principles and Practice of Echocardiography.* 2nd ed. Philadelphia: Lea & Febiger, 1994:184–200.

37. O'Rourke MF, Nichols WW. The nature of flow in a liquid. In: O'Rourke MF, Nichols WW, eds. *McDonald's Blood Flow in Arteries.* 5th ed. New York: Oxford University Press, 2005:11–48.

38. O'Rourke MF, Nichols WW. Ultrasonic blood flow and velocimetry. In: O'Rourke MF, Nichols WW, eds. *McDonald's Blood Flow in Arteries.* 5th ed. New York: Oxford University Press, 2005:149–163.

39. Weyman A. Principles of Doppler flow measurement. In: Weyman A, ed. *Principles and Practice of Echocardiography.* 2nd ed. Philadelphia: Lea & Febiger, 1994:143–162.

40. Kremkau F. *Doppler Ultrasound: Principles and Instruments.* 7th ed. Philadelphia: W.B. Saunders Company, 1990.

41. Thomas JD, Licina MG, Savage RM. Physics of echocardiography. In: Savage RN, Aronson SA, eds. *Comprehensive Textbook of Intraoperative Transesophageal Echocardiography.* Philadelphia: Lippincott Williams & Wilkins, 2005:3–22.

42. Weyman A. Doppler instrumentation. In: Weyman A, ed. *Principles and Practice of Echocardiography.* 2nd ed. Philadelphia: Lea & Febiger, 1994:163–183.

43. Weyman A. Doppler signal processing. In: Weyman A, ed. *Principles and Practice of Echocardiography.* 2nd ed. Philadelphia: Lea & Febiger, 1994:201–217.

44. Hatle L, Angelsen B. Blood velocity measurements using the Doppler effect of backscattered ultrasound. In: Hatle L, Angelsen B, eds. *Doppler Ultrasound in Cardiology: Physical Principles and Clinical Applications.* 2nd ed. Philadelphia: Lea & Febiger, 1985:32–73.

45. Dowsett DJ, Johnston RE, Kenny PA. Principles of ultrasound. In: Dowsett DJ, Johnston RE, Kenny PA, eds. *Ultrasound Imaging*. 2nd. ed. London: Arnold Publishers Ltd, 2006:530–558.

46. Giesler M, Goller V, Pfob A, et al. Influence of pulse repetition frequency and high pass filter on color Doppler maps of converging flow in vitro. *Int J Cardiac Imaging* 1996;12(4): 257–261.

47. Thomas JD, Popovic ZB. Assessment of left ventricular function by cardiac ultrasound. *J Am Coll Cardiol* 2006;48:2012–2025.

48. Buckberg GD, Weisfeldt ML, Ballester M, et al. Left ventricular form and function: scientific priorities and strategic planning for development of new views of disease. *Circulation* 2004;110:e333–e336.

49. Torrent-Guasp F, Ballester M, Buckberg GD, et al. Spatial orientation of the ventricular muscle band: physiologic contribution and surgical implications. *J Thorac Cardiovasc Surg* 2001;122(2):389–392.

50. Sengupta PP, Korinek J, Belohlavek M, et al. Left ventricular structure and function: basic science for cardiac imaging. *J Am Coll Cardiol* 2006;48:1988–2001.

51. Desco M, Antoranz JC. Technical principles of Doppler tissue imaging. In: *Doppler Tissue Imaging Echocardiography*. Madrid: McGraw-Hill, 1998: 7–22.

52. Teske AJ, De Boeck BW, Melman PG, et al. Echocardiographic quantification of myocardial function using tissue deformation imaging, a guide to image acquisition and analysis using tissue Doppler and speckle tracking. *Cardiovasc Ultrasound* 2007;5:27.

53. Pislaru C, Abraham TP, Belohlavek M. Strain and strain rate echocardiography. *Curr Opin Cardiol* 2002;17:443–454.

54. Kisslo J, Adams DB, Belkin RN. *Doppler Color-Flow Imaging*. New York: Churchill Livingstone, 1988.

55. Weyman A. Principles of color flow mapping. In: Weyman A, ed. *Principles and Practice of Echocardiography*. 2nd ed. Philadelphia: Lea & Febiger, 1994:218–233.

56. Lee R. Physical principles of flow mapping in cardiology. In: *Textbook of Color Doppler Echocardiography*. Philadelphia: Lea & Febiger, 1989:18–49.

57. Aggarwal KK, Philpot EF, Nanda NC. Understanding different types of color Doppler systems. In: *Textbook of Color Doppler Echocardiography*. Philadelphia: Lea & Febiger, 1989:74–98.

58. Chao K, Moises V, Shandas R, et al. Influence of the Coanda effect on color Doppler jet area and color encoding. In vitro studies using color Doppler flow mapping. *Circulation* 1992;85(1):333–341.

QUESTIONS

1. As a diagnostic imaging technique, which of the following properties of ultrasound imaging is most limiting?
   A. Ultrasound can be directed as a beam
   B. Ultrasound is differentially reflected from cardiac structures
   C. Ultrasound obeys the laws of reflection and refraction
   D. Ultrasound propagates poorly through a gaseous medium

2. The acoustic properties of air are least likely to explain which of the following?
   A. Improved surface ultrasound imaging by applying acoustic coupling gel
   B. Difficulty in visualizing the aortic arch and great vessels with TEE
   C. Poor TEE imaging of the ventricular apex from mid-esophageal depths
   D. Strong echoes arising from heart/lung interface
   E. The rationale for "bubble" contrast studies.

3. Improved temporal resolution can most easily be achieved with which of the following maneuvers?
   A. Imaging at shallower depths
   B. Increasing scan line density
   C. Lowering the transducer frequency
   D. Widening the scan sector angle

4. Optimal color Doppler mapping can best be achieved by which of the following?
   A. Aligning the Doppler angle parallel to transducer beam-flow direction
   B. Decreasing the PRF
   C. Increasing the depth of color scan sector
   D. Increasing the scan line density
   E. Widening the color scan sector width

5. Compared to hemodynamic Doppler imaging, optimal tissue imaging is by which of the following?
   A. Adjusting the system for a higher amplitude, lower frequency signal
   B. Decreasing system gain
   C. Increasing the scale
   D. Using a high-pass filter

CHAPTER 2

Imaging Artifacts and Pitfalls

Lori B. Heller ■ Solomon Aronson ■ Linda Shore-Lesserson

An *artifact* can be defined as any structure in an ultrasound image that does not have a corresponding anatomic tissue structure. Artifacts are a common occurrence in an ultrasound display because they are often the result of the physical properties of ultrasound itself. Recognizing artifacts is essential to proper ultrasound interpretation, because not identifying an artifact as such may lead to unwarranted clinical intervention or concern. Similarly, pitfalls may also cause improper diagnoses. *Pitfalls* are normal anatomic structures that are often erroneously interpreted as pathologic. This chapter discusses the detection and avoidance of artifacts, as well as the identification of common echocardiographic pitfalls.

ARTIFACTS

Artifacts may be classified into four main categories: missing structures, degraded images, falsely perceived objects, and structures with a misregistered location.

MISSING STRUCTURES

The absence of an object or area that should be projected on the ultrasound display is considered an artifact. *Missing structures* occur for several reasons and can be related to the resolution of the ultrasound image. *Resolution* is defined as the ability to distinguish between two distinct structures that are in close proximity. Lateral resolution, or the ability to distinguish between two objects in a horizontal plane, is related to the bandwidth of the ultrasound beam. If two structures are closer together than the width of the lateral resolution, they will appear as a single image; in essence, the display is missing images. The best lateral resolution occurs at the focal zone, where the near field meets the far field and where the beam width is the narrowest (Fig. 2.1). Longitudinal, or axial, resolution is the ability to distinguish between two structures in the longitudinal plane. Longitudinal resolution is determined by the spatial pulse length. Because the smallest resolvable distance between two reflectors is one wavelength, higher frequency (and therefore shorter wavelength) transducers have greater axial resolution (1). It follows, then, that lower frequency transducers are less able to distinguish two separate objects in the vertical plane.

Acoustic shadowing may also create missing images. It occurs when the ultrasound beam reaches a strong reflector. This reflector decreases the beam intensity to distal structures, essentially blocking the beam to that area. Therefore, any image that lies deep to the strongly reflecting item cannot be seen. It places a shadow (or anechoic) area distal to the original structure. This commonly occurs with high-density structures, such as prosthetic valves, and heavily calcified objects (2). When shadowing occurs, an alternate acoustic window is required to view the objects or areas of interest (Fig. 2.2).

DEGRADED IMAGES

An image of imperfect or poor quality is referred to as a degraded image and is often due to artifact phenomena. *Reverberations* are a type of image degradation. They are secondary reflections that occur along the path of a sound pulse and are a result of the ultrasound "bouncing"

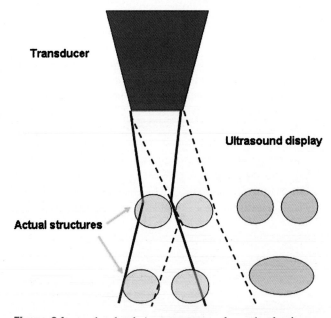

Figure 2.1. As the depth increases away from the focal zone, lateral resolution is decreased. Even as the scan line moves laterally, noted by the dotted lines, the two separate objects seen in the far field are unable to be viewed as distinct entities.

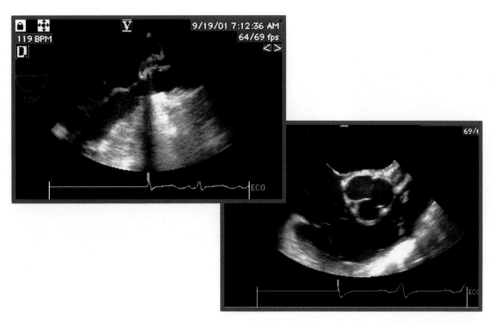

Figure 2.2. Shadowing. **Left:** Long-axis view of the left ventricle and the left ventricular outflow tract (LVOT) demonstrating shadowing through the center of the image. This resulted from a suture line of a bioprosthetic valve. **Right:** To image the aortic annulus in its entirety, a change in imaging plane from 120 to 30 degrees was required.

in between the structure and another reflecting surface. Reverberations appear as parallel yet irregular lines extending from the object away from the transducer. They occur when the near side of the object, a second object, or the transducer itself functions as another reflecting surface. When the transducer functions as this additional reflector, an image is displayed as expected after the ultrasonic beam is returned to the transducer. However, this same beam is then sent back to the object, is reflected back again to the transducer, strikes the transducer face, and is reflected back to the target (Fig. 2.3). These repeated journeys traveled by the same beam produce additional signals that are interpreted as the same object at twice the distance from the primary target. This can occur multiple times, and the result is multiple images displayed on the screen in a straight line from the object away from the transducer. Therefore, a reverberation is two or more equally spaced echo signals at increasing depths, twice the distance as the original signal. Reverberations generally occur with strong, superficial reflectors, such as calcified structures and metallic objects (3). A common site for this is in the descending thoracic aorta and is known as a linear reverberation. More commonly, reverberations are merged together and appear as a solid line directed away from the transducer. This is called *comet tail* or *ring down* (Fig. 2.4).

Enhancement is another type of image degradation and is the reciprocal of acoustic shadowing. If a structure is a weak reflector or if the medium through which the ultrasound travels has a lower attenuation rate than soft tissue, the beam is attenuated less than normal. The echoes below the weak reflector are then enhanced and these structures appear to be brighter than normal or hyperechoic (Fig. 2.5). This can be adjusted in the vertical plane by decreasing the time-gain compensation on the console.

Noise can also degrade the quality of an image. Noise has many etiologies, including excessive gain and other

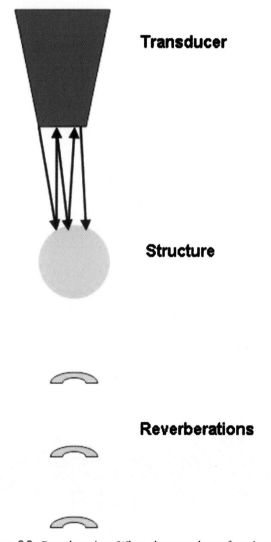

Figure 2.3. Reverberation. When the transducer functions as an alternate reflecting source, reverberations appear as parallel yet irregular lines away from the structure.

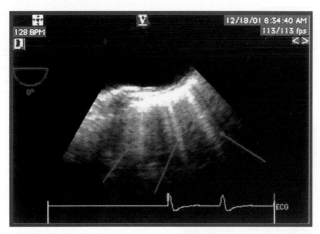

Figure 2.4. Reverberation. Merged reverberations form a single line away from the transducer and are called *ring down* or *comet tail.*

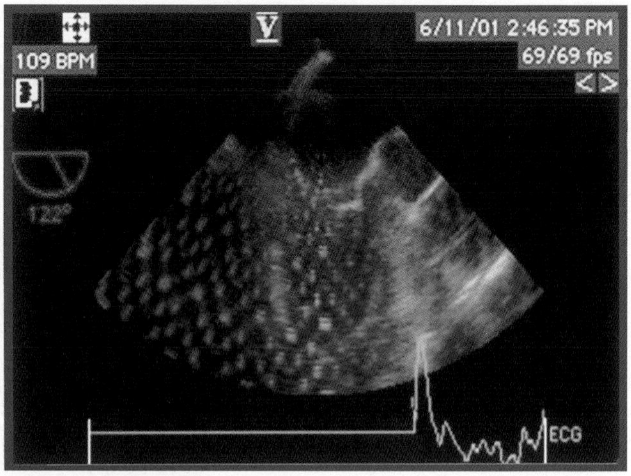

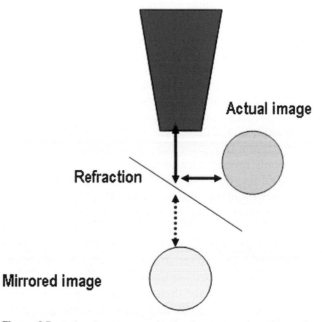

Figure 2.6. Noise. Artifact from the electrocautery degrades this midesophageal, long-axis view.

changes in settings, but in the operating room arena, it is most commonly from electrical interference such as electrocautery. Noise appears as very small amplitude echoes on the scan. It is most likely to affect low-level echolucent areas rather than bright echogenic areas (Fig. 2.6).

FALSELY PERCEIVED OBJECTS

Falsely perceived objects may occur as a result of *refraction.* Refracted ultrasound waves are beams that have been deflected from their original uniform path and occur as a result of the waves passing through a medium with a different acoustic impedance. The transducer assumes the reflected signal originated from the initial scan line and the image is displayed as such (Fig. 2.7). Objects may therefore appear laterally or otherwise displaced from their true position, and a side-by-side double image is created. A mirror image can also be created as a result of the ultrasound wave bouncing in between the near and the far side of the structure before returning to the transducer, similar to a reverberation. This mirrored image is always located on a straight line between the transducer and the artifact and is always deeper than the true reflector. A common place of occurrence for this is the descending aorta and is often referred to as a double-barrel aorta (3) (Fig. 2.8). Falsely perceived objects due to refraction and mirror images can often be overcome by altering the scanning angle.

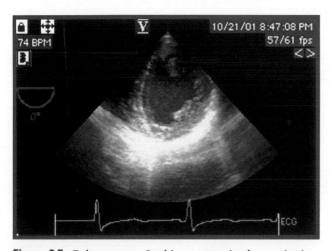

Figure 2.5. Enhancement. In this transgastric, short-axis view, enhancement is seen along the anterior wall and anterior pericardium. This can be improved by adjusting the time-gain compensation or vertical gain.

Figure 2.7. Refraction. As a result of a change in acoustic impedance of the tissue, some of the sound waves are refracted from their original courses. A false mirror image is then placed distal to the actual object.

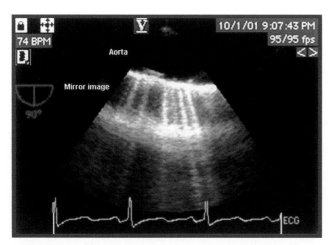

Figure 2.8. Double-Barrel Aorta. A mirror image is created in the descending thoracic aorta. This is a common artifact.

MISREGISTERED LOCATIONS

Although the main ultrasound beam is central, multiple beams are projected out from the transducer at various angles to the central beam (Fig. 2.9). These beams are referred to as *side lobes* and can result in images being placed in the wrong location on the displayed image.

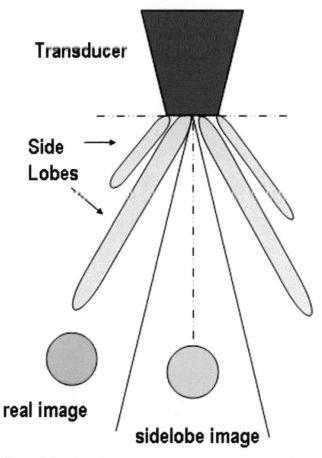

Figure 2.9. Side Lobes. Extraneous beams are projected from the transducer. Information is relayed as though the objects are in the path of the main ultrasound beam.

Generally, the energy in these extraneous beams is much lower than that of the main beam, and therefore no effect or image is produced. However, if these beams, or side lobes, reach a strong specular reflector, the reflected energy will be high and will be added to the reflected energy of the main beam. Side-lobe artifacts usually become apparent when they do not conflict with real, more intense echoes. An enlarged cardiac chamber often provides this setting. If the emitted echo beam is rapidly oscillating, then multiple side-lobe artifacts may be displayed as a curved line at the level of the true object with the brightest area corresponding to the original structure (Fig. 2.10) (1). In the ascending aorta, a side-lobe artifact may create the appearance of a false dissection (Fig. 2.11) (although more commonly, false dissections in the ascending aorta are a reverberation artifact related to the posterior left atrial wall) (4). Identification is accomplished by recognition of the fact that the side-lobe artifacts cross anatomic walls and cavities without regard for natural borders and always have a common radius from the transducer. They may disappear with adjustment of the depth or angle of the transducer.

Beam-width artifacts occur when superimpositions of structures within the beam profile are merged into a single tomographic image (5). A common beam-width artifact can sometimes appear as a right atrial mass (6).

Range ambiguity can also result in the display of structures in false locations and occurs with a high pulse-repetition frequency (PRF). With a high PRF, a second Doppler pulse is sent out before the first Doppler signal along the same scan line is received. Therefore, the machine is unable to recognize the returning signal as originating from the first, second, or even a subsequent pulse. This results in deep structures appearing closer to the transducer than their true locations. When an unexpected object is observed in a cardiac chamber, it is often due to range ambiguity. This can be differentiated from a real structure by changing the depth setting of the image (and therefore the PRF) (Fig. 2.12) (7).

Pitfalls

Pitfalls are normal structures that are often erroneously interpreted as pathologic. It is important for an echocardiographer to review and become familiar with these entities in order to avoid advocating unnecessary clinical intervention. These structures can be organized according to the cardiac chambers and are reviewed here in order of the right atrium, right ventricle, left atrium, left ventricle, aortic valve, and pericardium.

Right Atrium

In the right atrium, the *eustachian valve* is often visualized. It is an embryologic remnant of the right valve of the sinus venosus and serves to divert the blood flow from the inferior vena cava (IVC) through the foramen ovale into the

Figure 2.10. Side Lobes. The oscillation of the transducer may cause the side-lobe artifact to appear curved.

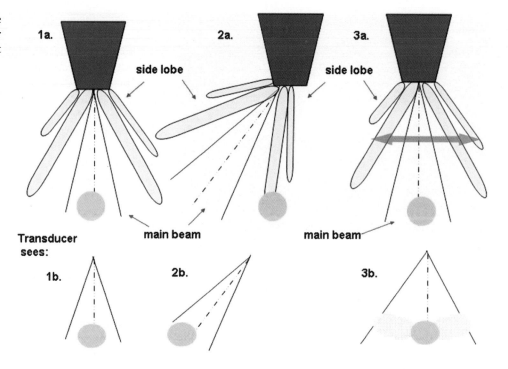

left atrium in utero. It is a thin, elongated structure located at the junction of the IVC and the right atrium and is seen in approximately 57% of individuals (8). It can be quite large and extend all the way to the fossa ovalis; however, it does not cross the tricuspid valve and enter into the right ventricle (8–10). It can often be seen in multiple views of the right atrium, including the four-chamber and bicaval views. While the eustachian valve has long been considered to be of no physiological consequence, a recent study found a strong correlation between persistent eustachian valve and patent foramen ovale, thus predisposing these patients to increased risk of paradoxical emboli (10). In addition, the eustachian valve can be a source of infective endocarditis (11) and has been mistaken for intracardiac tumor or thrombus (12).

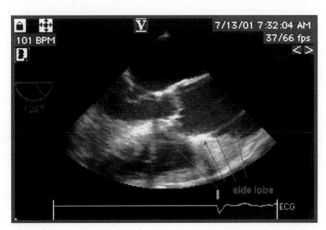

Figure 2.11. Side Lobe. Side lobes can create the appearance of an ascending aortic flap or false dissection.

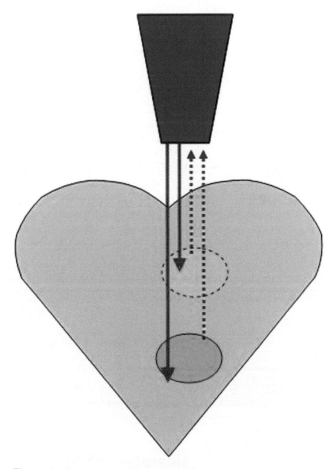

Figure 2.12. Range Ambiguity. When there is range ambiguity, it is not clear which pulse is being received back by the transducer. As a result, some objects can be placed falsely close to the transducer.

Another right atrial structure most likely derived from the sinus venosus is the *Chiari's network*. It is a thin, mobile, web-like structure that can be seen in 2% of patients undergoing transesophageal echocardiography. While this structure is benign, there is a high likelihood of an associated patent foramen ovale (83% vs. 28%) with a high degree of right-to-left shunting (13). In one study of 1,400 patients, Chiari's network was found more frequently in patients with unexplained arterial embolic events than in those being evaluated for other reasons. Atrial septal aneurysms, which are also associated with patent foramen ovale, occur at a higher frequency in patients with Chiari's network (24%) (13).

The *crista terminalis* is a muscular ridge that extends anteriorly from the superior vena cava (SVC) to the IVC and divides the trabeculated portion of the right atrium from the posterior smooth-walled sinus venarum segment. It is formed by the junction of the sinus venosus and the primitive right atrium and can be confused with a thrombus or tumor. It is best seen in the bicaval view (Fig. 2.13).

Lipomatous hypertrophy of the interatrial septum also occurs in normal individuals. Adipose tissue will infiltrate the interatrial septum, giving the septum a dumbbell appearance because the lipomatous infiltration spares the fossa ovalis (Fig. 2.14).

Right Ventricle

Trabeculations are part of the normal ventricular chamber musculature and are seen as muscle bundles on the endocardial surface. While located on both sides of the heart, they are often more frequently visualized on the right. Right ventricular hypertrophy may accentuate trabeculations. The *moderator band* is the most prominent muscular ridge in the right ventricle. It appears as a linear structure in the apical third of the right ventricle extending from the free wall to the septum (Fig. 2.15). The moderator

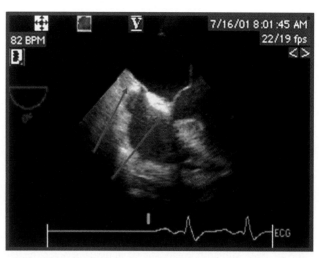

Figure 2.14. Lipomatous Hypertrophy of the Interarterial Septum. The fatty infiltration of the atrial septum spares the fossa ovalis and gives it a dumbbell-shaped appearance.

band corresponds to part of the electrical conduction system, housing some Purkinje fibers. It sometimes can be confused with thrombus.

Left Atrium

There is a distinct raphé between the left superior pulmonary vein and the left atrial appendage (LAA). This area extends into the left atrium and often has the appearance of a ridge or crest of tissue. It is normal atrial tissue, but its appearance, when imaged at certain angles, can look like a mass protruding into the body of the atrium. Historically, this has resulted in unnecessary anticoagulation in patients suspected of having an atrial clot. For this reason, it is often referred to as the "Coumadin ridge." A two-chamber image (midesophageal at 90 degrees) usually provides the view required to visualize this raphé (Fig. 2.16).

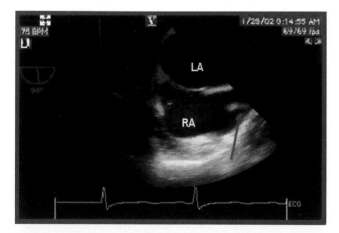

Figure 2.13. Crista Terminalis. This structure, seen in the bicaval view, divides the trabeculated anterior wall of the right atrium from the smooth-walled posterior portion. It can sometimes be confused with thrombus.

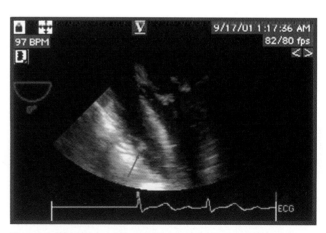

Figure 2.15. Moderator Band. The most prominent muscular bundle in the right ventricle. It extends from the RV free wall to the septum.

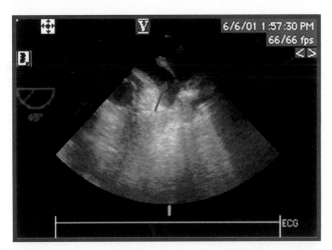

Figure 2.16. Coumadin Ridge. The atrial tissue between the left upper pulmonary vein and the atrial appendage can be mistaken for an atrial thrombus.

Left Atrioventricular Groove

The left atrioventricular (AV) groove is a very common location for the occurrence of pitfalls. Many normal structures lie with the left AV groove and can be normal in appearance yet confused with abnormal structures. These structures can also become pathologic and can present as abnormal structures, other than what they truly are. The normal structures that occur in the left AV groove include the mitral annulus, coronary sinus, lipomatous tissue, the circumflex coronary artery, and the descending thoracic aorta. Mitral annular calcification can appear as a shadow or a usual structure obscuring the normal view of the left AV groove. A dilated coronary sinus (as a result of persistent left SVC) will distend the AV groove and cause it to be abnormal in its anatomic relations with other structures. Enlarged lymph nodes can cause the fatty tissue in the AV groove to appear pathologic, and hiatal hernias can also distort this structure. An aneurysm of the circumflex coronary artery of the descending thoracic aorta can present as an abnormal mass in the left AV groove (14); furthermore, an echogenic AV groove can sometimes be mistaken for an LAA thrombus (15,16). Sometimes true cardiac pathology can mimic atrial appendage thrombus as well. A case of a pedunculated, multilobulated cardiac papillary fibroelastoma is reported to have been surgically removed from the LAA when cardiac thrombus was the presumed diagnosis (17).

Left Ventricle

The left ventricular papillary muscles are much more prominent on transesophageal echocardiography than the right ventricular papillary muscles. The papillary muscles identify the midventricular level. Rarely, one of the papillary muscles may be bifid, can give the appearance of a

third papillary muscle, and can sometimes be confused with a left ventricular mass. If rupture of the papillary muscle occurs as a complication of acute myocardial infarction, the entire muscle or a portion of the muscle can be seen as a prolapsing mass in the left atrium during systole.

The left ventricle is characterized as having a smooth endocardial surface but may occasionally have trabeculations, usually finer than those seen in the right ventricle. Similar to the moderator band on the right, the left ventricle may have a prominent band in the apical third of the chamber and is referred to as a *false tendon* (Fig. 2.17). This structure is thought to represent false chordae tendineae and is not pathologically significant (10).

Aortic Valve

Some normal variants of the aortic valve can be confused with valvular vegetations. The *nodules of Arantius* are the normal leaflet thickening seen at the central portion of the leaflets of the aortic valve. These nodules tend to enlarge with age. *Lambl's excrescences* are small mobile densities consisting of connective tissue. They protrude out linearly from the coaptation point of the aortic valve and on the aortic side and can be up to 5 mm in length. These also increase in prevalence with increasing age. They can sometimes be confused with vegetations; however, repeat examinations revealing unchanged densities and the lack of a clinical correlation often assist in ruling out the diagnosis of endocarditis. There is no evidence that Lambl's excrescences are associated with strokes (18). This is in contrast to papillary fibroelastomas, previously referred to as giant Lambl's excrescences, which are lobulated masses on the valve leaflet. These tumors can be found on either side of the valve and range in size from a few millimeters to 4 cm. Unlike Lambl's excrescences, they are associated with embolic events and often warrant excision.

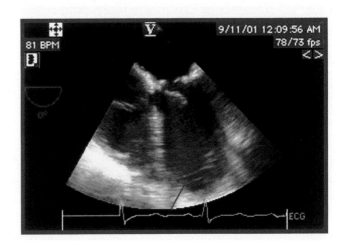

Figure 2.17. False Tendon. A prominent band seen in the apical third of the left ventricle. It is thought to represent a false chordae.

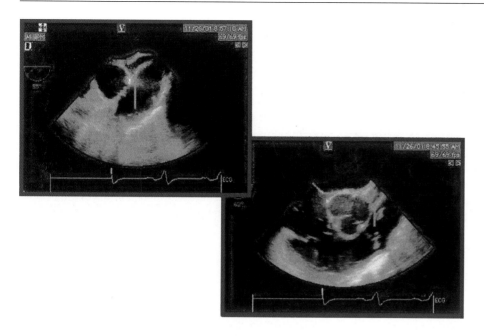

Figure 2.18. Transverse Sinus. This echo-free space between the posterior descending aorta and the LAA is the reflection of the pericardium. It indicates a pericardial effusion. Fibrinous material can collect in the space (**right**).

In the four-chamber view with anterior flexion at the level of the aortic valve, only the right and noncoronary cusps are visualized. The left coronary cusp is imaged on end and may appear to be a valvular vegetation as it moves in and out of the imaging plane. Confirmation of the nonpathologic nature of this structure can be achieved by imaging this area from a different angle, thus transecting the valve in a plane more parallel to its axis (19). This ideal plane is usually at 30 degrees but will vary in different individuals.

TABLE 2.1	**Transesophageal Imaging Pitfalls**	
Right atrium	Eustachian valve	Embryologic remnant. Thin, elongated structure located at the junction of the IVC and the RA.
	Chiari network	Embryologic remnant. Thin, web-like structure located in lower third of RA.
	Crista terminalis	Muscular ridge that extends from the SVC to the IVC.
	Lipomatous hypertrophy of the interatrial septum	Fatty infiltration of the interatrial septum (IAS).
	Pacing wires/catheters	Also seen in other chambers. Cause of multiple artifacts and extraneous echoes.
Right ventricle	Moderator band	Prominent muscular trabeculation in apical third of chamber.
	Papillary muscles	Chordal attachment of tricuspid valve.
Left atrium	Persistent left superior vena cava	Echo-free space between left upper pulmonary vein (LUPV) and LAA. Suspected with dilated coronary sinus (CS); confirmed with injection of agitated saline into upper extremity.
	Coumadin ridge	Atrial tissue between LUPV and LAA. Can have Q-tip–like appearance.
	Interatrial septal aneurysm	Bulging fossa ovalis >1.5 cm. Associated with patent foramen ovale (PFO).
Left ventricle	Papillary muscles	Chordal attachment of mitral valve.
	False tendon	Band in apical third of chamber. Thought to represent false chordae tendineae.
Aortic valve	Nodules of Arantius	Thickening at central coaptation point of leaflets.
	Lambl's excrescences	Fibroelastic densities that protrude from the leaflets toward the ventricular side.
Pericardium	Transverse sinus	Pericardial reflection between posterior descending aorta and left atrium. Most notable when pericardial fluid is present.

Aorta

The innominate vein is a common structure seen anterior to the transverse aorta in the upper esophageal long-axis view of the aortic arch. The innominate vein can be quite large and distended. Its size usually varies with respiration. A long-axis view of the vein as it lies directly anterior to the aorta can appear as an aortic dissection. Differentiation of this structure is accomplished by demonstration of its venous flow pattern by color or spectral Doppler.

A hematoma in the wall of the aorta can mimic an intimal flap. Oscillation or flutter of the suspected intimal flap independent of the aortic wall can help prevent the false-positive diagnosis of aortic dissection (20).

Pericardium

When a pericardial effusion occurs, the echo-free space between the pericardium and the myocardium becomes more apparent. Sometimes this space may mimic an abscess or false chamber. The transverse sinus is an example of such a space. It is the pericardial reflection between the posterior wall of the ascending aorta and the anterior wall of the left atrium. The transverse sinus can be seen in the short- and long-axis views of the aortic valve (Fig. 2.18). Depending on the plane of the echo, the atrial appendage or epicardial fat may be seen floating in the space, giving the illusion of an intracardiac mass (19,21).

When chronic pericardial disease occurs, fibrinous material can be seen in the sac (Fig. 2.18). If the stranding has a more nodular appearance, the presence of a malignant effusion with metastases must be considered.

CONCLUSION

Recognizing imaging artifacts and mastering the diagnosis of common echocardiograph pitfalls are essential parts of echocardiography. Many artifacts are based on the physical properties of ultrasound itself and require at least a basic understanding of these concepts. While the pitfalls of ultrasound imaging require some amount of memorization or recall of true anatomy, many artifacts can be distinguished from true structures by noting their characteristics or by altering the imaging settings.

KEY POINTS

- Artifacts are any structure in a display that does not have a corresponding anatomic tissue structure.
- Artifacts can be classified as missing structures, degraded images, falsely perceived objects, and structures in the wrong location.
- Artifacts occur as a result of limitations in detail resolution, the properties of ultrasound itself, or equipment malfunction.
- Resolution is the ability to distinguish between two distinct structures. Decreased resolution can result in missing structures.
- Two common artifacts are acoustic shadowing and reverberation.
- Acoustic shadowing occurs when a strong reflector blocks the interpretation of the ultrasound images below it. An alternate window that images the structure more proximally or from a different angle is required to see these structures.
- Reverberations are equally spaced image artifacts that appear at increasing depths from the strong reflector being imaged.
- Pitfalls are errors in the interpretation of normal structures. It is important to be able to identify these normal structures or variants to prevent unnecessary clinical intervention.

REFERENCES

1. Feigenbaum H. *Echocardiography*. 5th ed. Feigenbaum H, ed. Philadelphia: Lea and Febiger, 1993.
2. Bach DS. Transesophageal echocardiographic (TEE) evaluation of prosthetic valves. *Cardiol Clin* 2000;18(4):751–771.
3. Kremkau FW, Taylor KJW. Artifacts in ultrasound imaging. *J Ultrasound Med* 1986;5:227–237.
4. Flachskampf FA, Daniel WG. Transesophageal echocardiography. Aortic dissection. *Cardiol Clin* 2000;18(4):807–817.
5. Otto CM. Principles of echocardiographic image acquisition and Doppler analysis. In: *Textbook of Clinical Echocardiography*. 3rd ed. Philadelphia: Saunders, 2004:12–13.
6. Chen MS, Sun JP, Asher CR. A right atrial mass and pseudomass. *Echocardiography* 2005;5:441–444.
7. Losi MA, Betocchi S, Briguori C, et al. Determinants of aortic artifacts during transesophageal echocardiography of the ascending aorta. *Am Heart J* 1999;137(5):967–972.
8. Limacher MC. Echocardiographic anatomy of the eustachian valve. *Am J Cardiol* 1986;57(4):363–365.
9. Otto CM. Transthoracic views, normal anatomy and flow patterns. In: *Textbook of Clinical Echocardiography*. 3rd ed. Philadelphia: Saunders, 2004:39–40.
10. Schuchlenz HW, Saurer G, Weihs W, et al. Persisting eustachian valve in adults: relation to patent foramen ovale and cerebrovascular accidents. *J Am Soc Echocardiogr* 2004;17(3):231–233.
11. San Roman JA, Vilacosta I, Sarria C, et al. Eustacian valve endocarditis: is it worth searching for? *Am Heart J* 2001;142(6):1037–1040.
12. Carson W, Chiu SS. Image in cardiovascular medicine: eustachian valve mimicking intracardiac mass. *Circulation* 1998;97:2188.
13. Schneider B, Hofmann T, Justen MH, et al. Chiari's network: normal anatomic variant or risk factor for arterial embolic events? *J Am Coll Cardiol* 1995;26(1):203–210.

14. Zuber M, Oechslin E, Jenni R. Echogenic structures in the left atrioventricular groove: diagnostic pitfalls. *J Am Soc Echocardiogr* 1998;11:381–386.
15. Schneider B, Stöllberger C, Schneider B. Diagnosis of left atrial appendage thrombi by multiplane transesophageal echocardiography: interlaboratory comparative study. *Circ J* 2007;71:122–125.
16. Kurisu K, Hisahara M, Ando Y. Missing left atrial thrombus: dislodgement or artifact? *Ann Thorac Surg* 2008;86:1011–1012.
17. Barcena J, Geroge JC, Grommes C, et al. Cardiac papillary fibroelastoma mimicking left atrial appendage thrombus. *J Am Soc Echocardiogr* 2008;21:1177.
18. Goldman JH, Foster E. Transesophageal echocardiographic (TEE) evaluation of intracardiac and pericardial masses. *Cardiol Clin* 2000;18(4):849–860.
19. Shively B. Transesophageal echocardiographic (TEE) evaluation of the aortic valve, left ventricular outflow tract, and pulmonic valve. *Cardiol Clin* 2000;18(4):711–729.
20. Alter P, Herzum M, Maisch B. Echocardiographic findings mimicking type A aortic dissection. *Herz* 2006;31:153–155.
21. Aronson S, Ruo W, Sand M. Inverted left atrial appendage appearing as a left atrial mass with TEE during cardiac surgery. *Anesthesiology* 1992;76:1054–1055.

QUESTIONS

1. Increasing frequency
   A. creates more reverberations
   B. improves resolution
   C. increases penetration
   D. causes shadowing
2. Which of the following can cause structures to be displayed in a false location?
   A. Acoustic shadowing
   B. Noise
   C. Refraction
   D. Reverberation
3. Range ambiguity results in structures being placed in the wrong location. The actual location can be determined by
   A. changing the omniplane
   B. harmonic imaging
   C. decreasing the gain
   D. changing the depth setting
4. Which of the following is an embryologic remnant that has no pathologic significance?
   A. Eustachian valve
   B. Moderator band
   C. Transverse sinus
   D. Lambl's excrescence

CHAPTER 3

Optimizing Two-Dimensional Echocardiographic Imaging

Bernard E. Bulwer ■ Stanton K. Shernan

INTRODUCTION

Optimal interpretation of echocardiographic images is contingent on optimal image acquisition, display, and storage. This requires a sound understanding of practical ultrasound physics, instrument control settings, individual patient characteristics, and their collective impact on the technical and diagnostic qualities of echocardiographic data (Figs. 3.1 and 3.2) (1). Accurate perioperative assessment and appropriate surgical decision making rely on the optimal integration of these important technical influences. Knowledge and experience with the critical details of the acquired echocardiographic data will permit optimal echocardiographic assessment, minimization of artifacts, and avoidance of important pitfalls. Distinguishing pathology from artifact will avoid delivery of inaccurate or erroneous information, injudicious therapeutic intervention, and their attendant impact on patient outcomes (2). This chapter reviews important concepts for optimizing the acquisition, processing, and display of real-time, two-dimensional (2D) echocardiographic images. Optimization of spectral Doppler and color flow Doppler imaging are discussed in Chapter 1.

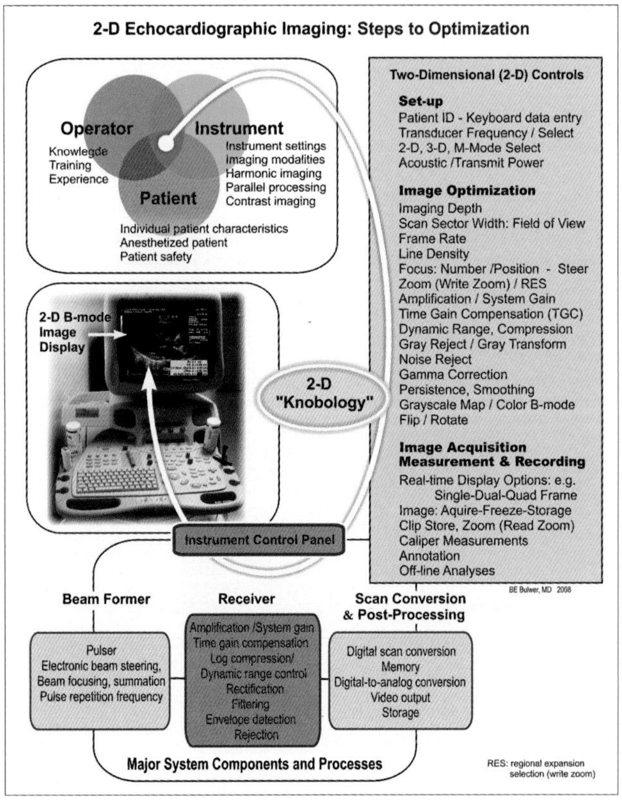

THE IMPACT OF ULTRASOUND INSTRUMENTATION ON IMAGE GENERATION AND DISPLAY

The conversion of reflected ultrasound signals into real-time, 2D echocardiographic images is a complex process, involving numerous electronic and digital manipulations (3–5). The basic technological requirements for diagnostic medical ultrasound imaging include instrumentation capable of beam generation, reception of the returning echoes, signal processing, and image display (Fig. 3.3). Optimizing the generation of cardiac images requires an appreciation for the contributions of each essential component of this elaborate circuitry.

Figure 3.1. Steps to image optimization in 2D echocardiography.

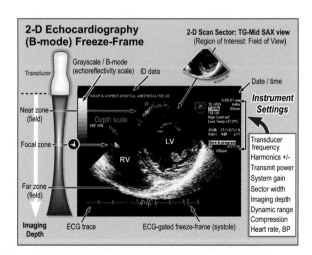

Figure 3.2. 2D B-mode image depicting annotations and instrument settings.

MASTER SYNCHRONIZER (CLOCK)

"Timing is everything" in cardiac ultrasonography. Intricate *timing systems* lie at the heart of transducer phased array operation, ultrasound beam generation, transmission, reception, electronic beam steering and transmit/receive focusing, pulse repetition frequency, signal processing, and multiple user controls. The *master clock* or *synchronizer* (Fig. 3.3) coordinates the elapsed time intervals between electronic signal emission from the transmitter (that results in the generation of the pulsed ultrasound beam from the transducer), and the electronic conversion of the received echo signal (see Figs. 1.3, 1.6, and 1.14). These time intervals are important for correlating the signal amplitude to the depth of the tissue interfaces. The received echo amplitude ultimately determines *pixel* (picture element) brightness or grayscale, while the time for the sound to return determines the image depth. The *synchronizer* also assists with the introduction of any special amplification based on elapsed time (6). Decreasing the voltage amplitude produced by the transmitter (power) results in a decrease in the amplitude of the ultrasound pulse produced by the transducer and a decrease in the corresponding amplitude of the returning signal.

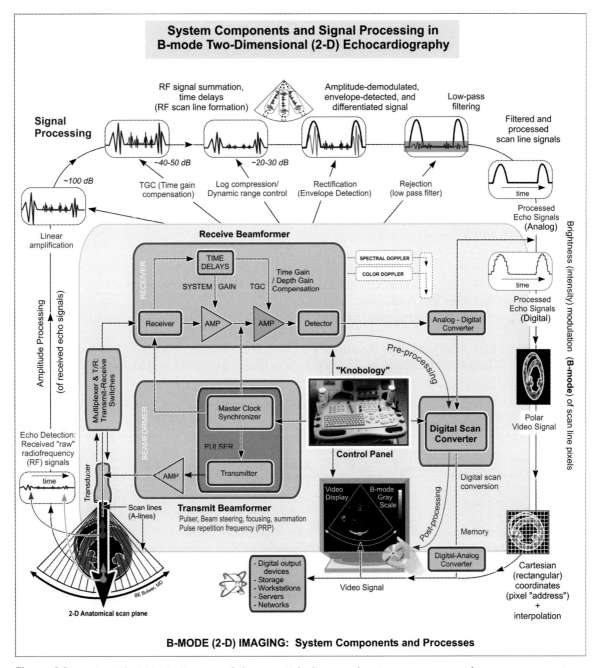

Figure 3.3. A simplified block diagram of the essential ultrasound system components that are necessary to generate, transmit, receive, process, and display 2D echocardiographic images. AMP, amplifier; TGC, time-gain compensation; VCR, videocassette recorder.

TRANSDUCERS AND SPATIAL RESOLUTION

The transducer serves as an electroacoustic conversion device composed of multiple piezoelectric crystals that are capable of generating, transmitting, and receiving ultrasound waves (see Figs. 1.5–1.7). In response to an alternating electrical current from the transmitter, the crystal alternately compresses and expands, thereby generating an imaging pulse 2 to 3 cycles in length (see Fig. 1.6). Conversely, when a returning ultrasound signal (echo) contacts a piezoelectric crystal, an electric current is generated that is eventually amplified and processed before being displayed on the monitor for interpretation. A transducer's *fundamental resonance frequency* is inversely proportional to the thickness of the piezoelectric material. The pulse of ultrasound, however, is actually composed of a range of frequencies called the *frequency bandwidth* (Fig. 3.4).

In generating an ultrasound image, the piezoelectric crystals of the transducer emit a short burst of ultrasound, which is followed by a passive period of "listening" for returning echoes. Ideally, all echoes from one pulse must be received before the next pulse is emitted. Emission of a pulse prior to the reception of all echoes from greater depths would result in range ambiguity. The number of times the crystal is pulsed or electrically stimulated per second is coordinated through the synchronizer and is called the *pulse repetition frequency* (PRF) (see Fig. 1.36). The *pulse repetition period* (PRP) is the amount of time required to transmit a pulsed ultrasound wave plus the time devoted to listening. The PRF is limited by the maximum sampling depth and the velocity of ultrasound in the medium. Because the velocity of ultrasound is nearly constant for most interacting tissues, the PRF will increase if the depth of interest is decreased.

The *pulse duration* (PD) is the product of the number of cycles within a burst or packet of ultrasound (N_c) and its duration (Fig. 3.4). The PD can also be calculated using transducer frequency:

$$PD = \frac{N_c}{f}$$

The spatial geometry of the ultrasound pulses that constitute the ultrasound beam impacts ultrasound image quality or resolution in three dimensions in space. The *spatial resolution* of the beam is described using three parameters: *axial* (depth), *lateral*, and *elevational* (slice thickness) resolution (Fig. 3.4). The ability to distinguish (separately) two points in space in the axial dimension (in the directing of the main ultrasound beam axis) is the *axial resolution*. *Lateral* (side-to-side) *resolution* refers to image detail in a direction perpendicular, with *elevational resolution* along the beam thickness. Of the three different types of spatial resolution, *axial* is the most precise. *Lateral* resolution is dependent on the width of the generated beam. Narrow beams have better lateral resolution. Far distances from the transducer lead to a wider beam width. This wider beam width decreases the lateral resolution. Thus, there will be image blurring at greater depths of field.

The length of the pulse (*spatial pulse length*) and PD directly affect *axial resolution*, which is the ability to distinguish two structures that are close to each other along the direction of beam propagation as two separate structures (Fig. 3.5). One way for the sonographer to optimize axial resolution is to increase the transducer frequency, which decreases the wavelength and therefore shortens the PD. It is important to remember, however, that increasing the ultrasound frequency decreases the depth of penetration and may compromise far-field imaging (Fig. 3.6) (1). The PD can also be shortened by using transducers with broad frequency *bandwidths*, which include a greater mixture of high and low frequencies compared to narrow

Figure 3.4. Pulse Geometry and Spatial Resolution Parameters. **Left panel:** Schema depicting the geometry of a three-cycle ultrasound pulse and concept of pulse duration. **Center:** Spatial resolution parameters of the ultrasound beam oriented along the axial, lateral, and slice thickness (elevational) planes. **Right panel:** The concept of transducer bandwidth and its relationship to damping, spatial pulse length, and frequency spectrum.

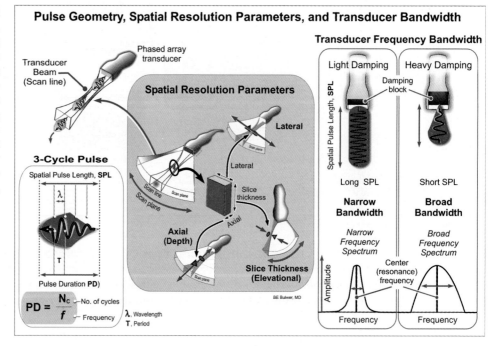

bandwidths (Fig. 3.4). Consequently, broad bandwidth transducer pulses are more likely to preserve higher frequencies as ultrasound waves penetrate through tissues; they have a greater sensitivity than narrow frequency bandwidth transducers (6). Finally, the use of damping material in the construction of transducers minimizes piezoelectric crystal ringing and vibration, thereby producing a shorter PD (Fig. 3.4). Thus, axial resolution can be improved by assuring a short PD through the use of an appropriately dampened transducer with a high-frequency and broader frequency bandwidth (Fig. 3.7).

Ultrasound beam geometry is also an important factor for determining image quality and is dependent upon several factors. For a *nonfocused transducer*, the near field is columnar shaped and nondivergent. The length of the near field, also known as the *Fresnel zone*, is determined by the diameter of the transducer face aperture (D) and the wavelength (λ) according to the equation:

$$\text{Near field length} = D^2/4\,\lambda$$

The beam begins to diverge beyond the focal point into the far field known as the *Fraunhofer zone*. Objects are generally better imaged when they are in the Fresnel zone,

especially within the focal zone, because the beam is comprised of more parallel waves, and reflecting surfaces in the zone tend to be more perpendicular (7). *Lateral resolution* is one of the most significant variables in determining ultrasound image quality. It tends to deteriorate in the far-field region because of beam divergence. Lateral resolution describes the ability of a transducer to resolve two objects that are adjacent to each other and perpendicular to the beam axis (Fig. 3.8). Lateral resolution also refers to the ability of the beam to detect single small objects across the width of the beam (6). In general, lateral resolution is optimal when the ultrasound beam width is narrow. Lateral resolution can therefore be improved by increasing the frequency (shortening the wavelength), although at the expense of tissue penetration (Fig. 3.9). Increasing the transducer aperture diameter can also improve lateral resolution by lengthening the near-field depth at the expense of a wider proximal near field. Furthermore, unlike transthoracic probes, the size of the transducer is limited by esophageal diameter. Increasing the ultrasound signal amplitude (intensity) increases the detection of echoes at the beam margins, thus effectively increasing beam width and decreasing lateral resolution (7,8).

Focusing the transducer improves lateral resolution by concentrating ultrasound energy into a narrower beam. (Fig. 3.9). Focal depth can be altered by adding an acoustic lens or mirror (*external focusing*), making the surface of the piezoelectric crystal concave (*internal focusing*), or via direct manipulation by the sonographer through the use of electronic focusing methods (6). With increasing degrees of focusing, the beam width narrows at the focal point, thus optimizing image quality by increasing the beam intensity. Focusing, however, limits the near-field depth because the beam diverges rapidly beyond the focal zone.

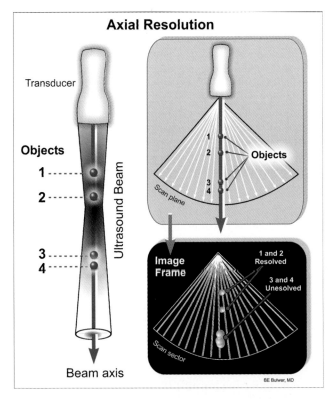

Figure 3.5. Axial resolution refers to the minimum distance between two structures oriented parallel to the ultrasound beam axis that permits visualization of the structures as separate, distinct reflectors on the monitor screen. The structures (*objects 1 and 2*) closest to the transducer are spaced far enough apart to be distinguished as separate reflectors. The two distant structures (*objects 3 and 4*) are too closely spaced along the direction of the ultrasound beam to be resolved and, therefore, appear merged on the image display.

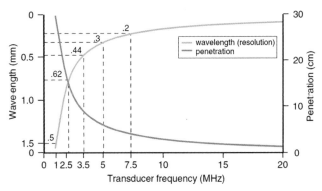

Figure 3.6. Graph of transducer frequency (horizontal axis) versus wavelength (*red line*) and penetration (*blue line*) of the ultrasound signal in soft tissue. Although higher frequency (shorter wavelength) transducers offer improved axial, lateral, and temporal resolution, the depth of penetration is greater with lower frequency (longer wavelengths) transducers. mm, millimeters; cm, centimeters; MHz, megahertz (From Otto C. Principles of echocardiographic image acquisition and Doppler analysis. In: Otto C, ed. *Textbook of Clinical Echocardiography.*, 2nd ed. Philadelphia: W.B. Saunders Company, 2000, with permission).

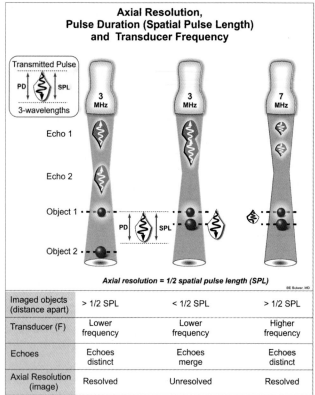

Axial Resolution, Pulse Duration (Spatial Pulse Length) and Transducer Frequency

Imaged objects (distance apart)	> 1/2 SPL	< 1/2 SPL	> 1/2 SPL
Transducer (F)	Lower frequency	Lower frequency	Higher frequency
Echoes	Echoes distinct	Echoes merge	Echoes distinct
Axial Resolution (image)	Resolved	Unresolved	Resolved

PD - pulse duration(microseconds)

Figure 3.7. Axial Resolution and Pulse Duration (Spatial Pulse Length), and Transducer Frequency. **A:** The two reflectors (Objects 1 and 2) are far enough apart to permit resolution by the separately returning echo pulses. **B:** The two reflectors (Objects 1 and 2) are too close to prevent the returning echo pulses from merging. **C:** Increasing the transducer frequency from 3 to 7 MHz shortens the pulse duration and spatial pulse length, thus permitting resolution by preventing merging of the returning echo pulses (*spheres*). Note: axial resolution = 1/2 spatial pulse length.

Temporal Resolution and Real-Time Imaging

In addition to axial and lateral resolution, *temporal resolution* is also an important consideration for real-time, 2D ultrasound imaging. Temporal resolution refers to the ability to display rapidly moving structures and distinguish closely spaced events in time. Temporal resolution is related to the time required to generate one complete frame and is therefore directly related to the *frame rate*. Each frame is composed of multiple scan lines, which determine the scan-line density of the image (Fig. 3.10; see "2D Echocardiography: Transducer Operation, Frames, and Frame Rate" in Chapter 1). Each scan line must be traversed twice (round trip) by the ultrasound pulse before the next pulse can be emitted.

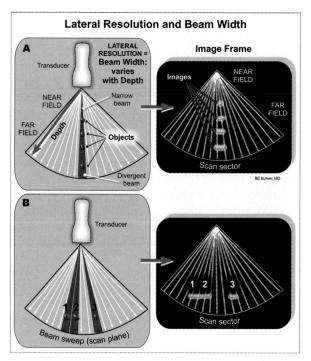

Figure 3.8. Lateral Resolution and Beam Width. Lateral resolution refers to the ability to resolve two adjacent structures that are oriented perpendicular to the beam axis as separate entities. Lateral resolution also refers to the ability of the beam to detect single small objects across the width of the beam. **A:** A single object (*sphere*) smaller than the ultrasound beam width will be imaged as long as it remains within the beam. Consequently, the size of the object will lengthen proportionally with the width of a diverging beam. **B:** If two structures are separated from each other by a distance perpendicular to the axis of the ultrasound beam that is greater than the beam width (*spheres 2 and 3*), they can be resolved. Conversely, if this distance between two structures is shorter than the beam width (*spheres 1 and 2*), the structures will not be resolved and the ultrasound image will merge. Therefore, a small beam width provides optimal lateral resolution.

Lateral resolution is an important variable in determining ultrasound image quality and is ultimately influenced by transducer size, shape, frequency, and focusing.

The PRF, which is dependent upon the speed of sound in tissue and the depth, is therefore limited by the transmit time for the signal to reach the designated target and back (8).

The frame rate and temporal resolution are affected by how quickly the pulse can interrogate each scan line. Assuming that the velocity of ultrasound in tissues is 1,540 m/s, the round-trip time for traversing each individual scan line is 13 μs/cm. The time (T_{line}) required to scan a single line of length (D) can therefore be calculated from the following formula (9):

$$T_{line} = 13 \text{ μs/cm} \times D \text{ (cm)}$$

The time required to scan a frame (T_{frame}) consisting of a given number of scan lines (N), can also be calculated:

$$T_{frame} = NT_{line}$$

Lateral Resolution and Ultrasound Beam Geometry

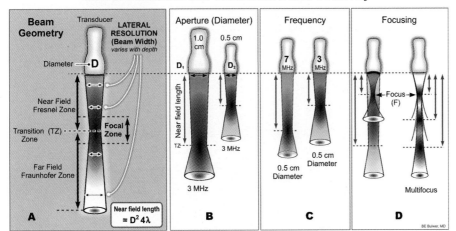

Figure 3.9. Lateral Resolution and Ultrasound Beam Geometry. **A:** An unfocused ultrasound beam is composed of a near field, which ends at the transition zone (TZ) before diverging into the far field. Lateral resolution is optimal in the near field where the ultrasound beam remains narrow. **B:** Increasing the diameter of the transducer aperture (D1 > D2) produces a longer near field. **C:** Increasing the transducer frequency (7 vs. 3 MHz) produces a longer near-field length at the expense of decreased penetration. **D:** A focused transducer produces a focal point (F) that is closer to the transducer thus creating a narrower and shorter near field.

The maximum frame rate (FR_{max}) can then be calculated from the reciprocal of T_{frame}:

$$FR_{max} = 1/T_{frame}$$

$$FR_{max} = \frac{77,000/s}{N \times D \; (cm)}$$

Therefore, assuming preservation of scan-line density and spatial resolution, the temporal resolution and frame rate can be improved only by reducing *depth* or *scan angle* (sector width) (Figs. 3.10 and 3.11). Alternatively, for a given depth and sector width, using a higher frequency transducer with decreased tissue penetration will also permit an increased frame rate and improved temporal resolution. Temporal resolution is dependent upon depth, scan angle, scan-line density, and the transducer frequency. The major determinants of image resolution are summarized in Table 3.1.

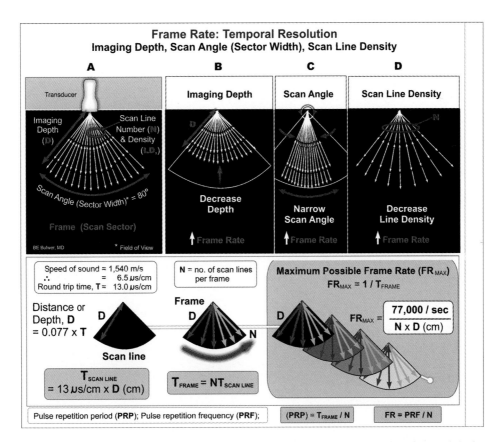

Figure 3.10. Temporal Resolution, Depth, and Scan Angle. For a given scan-line density (**A**), the frame rate and temporal resolution can be improved by decreasing depth (**B**), narrowing the scan angle (**C**), or decreasing scan line density (**D**).

Figure 3.11. The effect of changing depth on temporal and spatial resolution. Decreasing the scan depth (**A:** 180 mm; **B:** 120 mm; **C:** 80 mm; **D:** 40 mm) allows for a balance of improved temporal resolution (maximum frame rate) by decreasing the time required to scan all the lines within the sector while maintaining or improving spatial resolution. mm, millimeter.

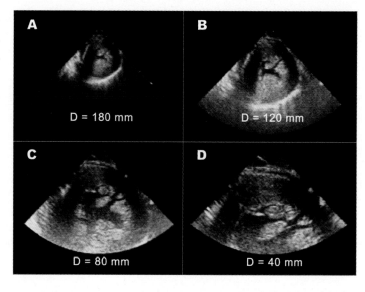

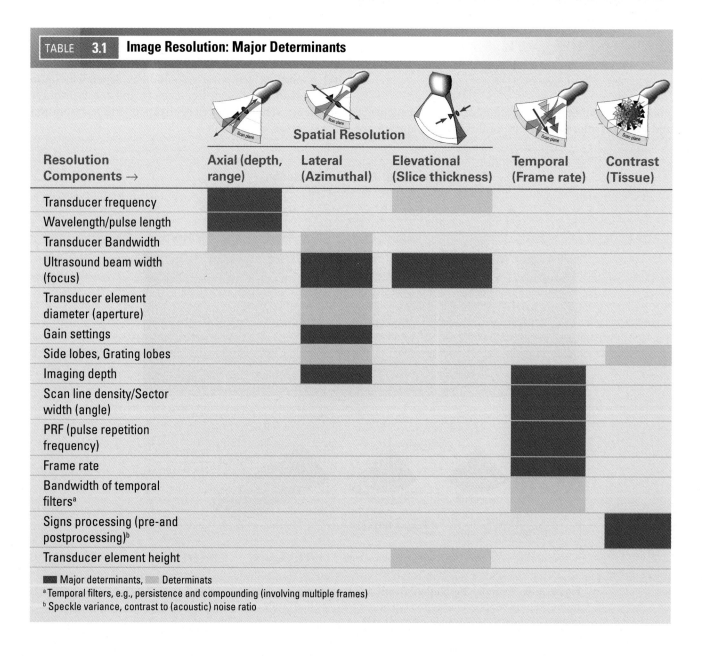

| TABLE 3.1 | Image Resolution: Major Determinants | | | | |

| | Spatial Resolution | | | | |
Resolution Components →	Axial (depth, range)	Lateral (Azimuthal)	Elevational (Slice thickness)	Temporal (Frame rate)	Contrast (Tissue)
Transducer frequency	Major		Determinant		
Wavelength/pulse length	Major				
Transducer Bandwidth	Determinant	Determinant			
Ultrasound beam width (focus)		Major	Major		
Transducer element diameter (aperture)		Major			
Gain settings		Major			
Side lobes, Grating lobes		Major			Determinant
Imaging depth		Major		Major	
Scan line density/Sector width (angle)				Major	
PRF (pulse repetition frequency)				Major	
Frame rate				Major	
Bandwidth of temporal filters[a]				Determinant	
Signs processing (pre-and postprocessing)[b]					Major
Transducer element height			Determinant		

■ Major determinants, ▨ Determinats
[a] Temporal filters, e.g., persistence and compounding (involving multiple frames)
[b] Speckle variance, contrast to (acoustic) noise ratio

AMPLIFICATION AND TIME-GAIN COMPENSATION

Signal processing can be initiated once the returning echoes are received by the transducer and converted back into an electrical form called the *radiofrequency signal*. *Amplifiers* increase the small voltage amplitudes received from the transducer to allow further signal processing (Fig. 3.3). The *system gain* control determines the amplification of the returning signal and is similar to the volume control on an audio system. Increasing the gain can compensate for signal loss due to attenuation; however, excessive gain can cause saturation and interfere with lateral resolution (7). This is an important matter in the operating room where, because of high ambient lighting, excessive gain settings are commonly used. *Time-gain compensation* (TGC) provides selective depth-dependent amplification, by increasing receiver gain with increasing echo arrival time (Fig. 3.12). Consequently, amplification can be progressively increased from the near to far field to compensate for attenuation-associated decreases in the signal amplitude of echoes returning from distant structures. Alternatively, *lateral gain compensation* allows for compensation of nonuniformities in image brightness caused by different amounts of attenuation along individual scan lines from side to side within the scan sector (9).

PREPROCESSING

Signal processing involves numerous complex manipulations of the electrical signal prior to its display. *Preprocessing* refers to modifications of the signal that determine the specific numeric values assigned to the echo intensities. Because preprocessing occurs prior to storage in the computer memory, these functions cannot typically be performed on "frozen" images (Fig. 3.3). Preprocessing begins with *signal amplification* and includes other complex manipulations such as *filtering, demodulation,* and *differentiation*. Initial signal preprocessing involves filtering the noise from returning echoes by eliminating frequencies outside the desired echo bandwidth. The signal can be further processed through *detection* or *demodulation*, which converts echo voltages from radio frequency form to video form, thereby displaying only the

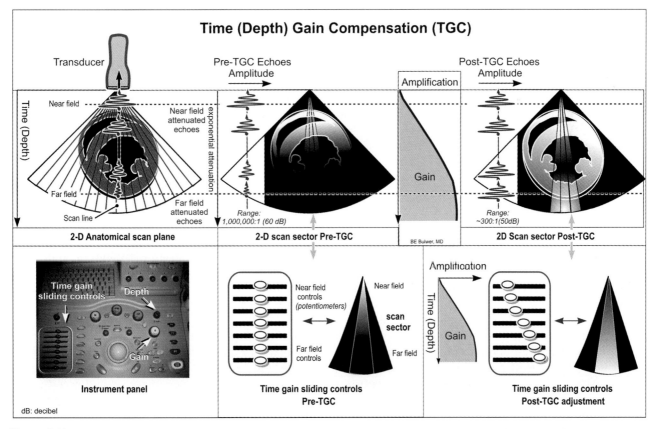

Figure 3.12. TGC provides selective depth-dependent amplification by increasing receiver gain with increasing echo arrival time. Increasing the amplitude of signals arriving from reflectors at greater depths compensates for attenuation associated with greater traveling distances. When TGC is optimally increased from the near to far field, echoes from similar reflectors are displayed with uniform brightness regardless of their depth in the image scan.

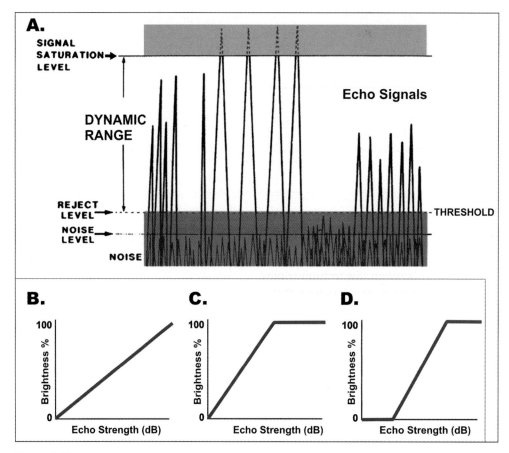

Figure 3.13. Displayed Dynamic Range (DR) and Compression. **A:** The displayed DR includes the ultrasound signal range measured in decibels that remains after excessively strong signals falling beyond the saturation level are eliminated along with weak signals below the reject and noise levels (Adapted from Thys M, Hillel Z. How it works: basic concepts in echocardiography. In: Bruijn N, Clements F, eds. *Intraoperative Use of Echocardiography*. Philadelphia: JB Lippincott, 1991, with permission). **B–D:** The effect of compression on narrowing the displayed DR: (**B**) fully displayed DR; (**C**) narrowing the DR by compressing stronger ultrasound signals to white (100% brightness); (**D**) narrowing the DR by compressing both weaker ultrasound signals to black (0%) and stronger ultrasound signals to white (100%), respectively.

positive components of the signal (10). Differentiating the signal accentuates the leading edge, shortening the signal duration and making the width of the echo less gain sensitive (7). Edge enhancement is responsible for improved resolution and easier quantitative measurements during M-mode scanning, although it is not commonly utilized for 2D imaging (11).

Dynamic-range manipulation is also a preprocessing option within limited control of the sonographer. *Dynamic range* (DR) refers to the range of useful ultrasound signals that can be identified and used by a given component of the ultrasound system (9). The displayed DR includes the range of ultrasound signals remaining after excessively strong signals falling beyond the saturation level are eliminated along with weak signals below the reject and noise levels (Fig. 3.13). A compromise must still exist, however, between the desire to maintain a wide DR for optimal grayscale recording, and the advantage that a narrow range offers in facilitating the discrimination between true image signals and noise (11). Although

a broad DR may increase the detection of weaker signals, this may occur at the expense of noise amplification. The displayed DR can be controlled by the operator by adjusting the *compression*. Logarithmic compression of the linear scale, representing the breadth of echo intensities, can be altered to reassign the values of some weak echo amplitudes to zero (black) or some of the strongest to maximum (white) (Fig. 3.13) (10). Increasing compression generally reduces the DR to produce a higher contrast image.

Additional preprocessing functions may be introduced later in image processing, yet still prior to actual memory storage. For example, increasing the *persistence* provides a smoother image of a slower moving structure by averaging and updating sequential frames. Although temporal resolution may be compromised by the requirement for increased sampling time, the image quality of slower moving structures improves because of less variation in signal levels from regions of comparable strength echoes (12). Persistence should be kept to a minimum to preserve temporal resolution when visualizing cardiac structures, which tend to be moving relatively rapidly. Increasing persistence also reduces the grainy appearance in the image associated with *speckle*, which represents the constructive and destructive interference patterns of scattered (nonspecular) reflections. Speckle is further reduced by *spatial compounding*, which averages frames obtained from scan lines directed at multiple angles, thereby increasing the probability that specular echoes will be produced from a perpendicular angle of incidence (10).

The numeric value of a given pixel can also be altered by employing preprocessing modifications that take into consideration the values of pixels in the near vicinity. *Spatial processing* and *smoothing* (12) are used to calculate the value of a particular pixel by averaging the values of surrounding pixels. Although this technique may improve the display of an image in which there is minimal change in echo density, the averaging of adjacent pixels may compromise some spatial detail (10,11). *Edge enhancement* utilizes a convolution or filtering process that alters the magnitude or number of weighting factors to change signal levels across an interface in order to detect subtle changes in echo density (12). Finally, *write zoom* or *regional expansion selection* (RES) is a preprocessing magnification technique applied during data collection that actually increases the number of pixels within the expanded region thus improving spatial resolution at the expense of a smaller field of view (FOV) (Fig. 3.14).

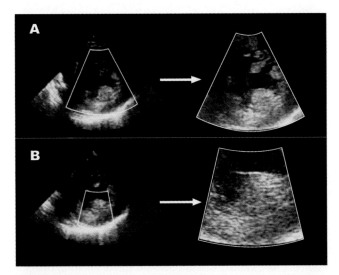

Figure 3.14. Write zoom or RES is a preprocessing function that permits magnification while improving spatial resolution. **A:** The area of interest is first selected by positioning a box (*outlined quadrangular box*) within the image scan. Activating the write zoom function (®) provides magnification and improved spatial resolution of the outlined area. **B:** Decreasing the size of the initial outlined quadrangular box results in further magnification and spatial resolution at the expense of a smaller FOV.

ANALOG-TO-DIGITAL CONVERTERS

In *analog* form, voltage amplitudes are continuously variable and proportional to the echo amplitude. However, in modern echocardiography, analog 2D echocardiography data are difficult to integrate with other echo modalities like color flow Doppler. *Digitized signals* are more stable, flexible, and facilitate quantitative manipulation, processing, and analysis of received echoes, for example quantification and automated interpretation—feats not easily achievable using analog data. Therefore, modern echocardiography systems employ *analog-to-digital converters* (ADC) that convert analog signals (polar acquisition format) to digitized format (checkerboard matrix/rectangular grid with Cartesian [x,y] coordinates) by assigning it discrete numeric values (Fig. 3.15). Analog-to-digital conversion can occur at a variety of sites along the circuit, but moving this process closer to the front end enables greater flexibility and increased accuracy of beam steering and dynamic focusing. For example, some array instruments employ digital beam formers that digitize raw ultrasound signals from each transducer element before they are combined into a single reflector along each scan line (9). Indeed, modern instruments maintain digital processing throughout the circuit—the result being optimal signal processing and analysis of the acquired echo data (13).

Digital signals are temporarily stored in random access memory (RAM) as a series of "bits" (*binary digit*), which can only exist in either a 1 or 0 ("on" or "off") state. Further precision is acquired by using the binary system to generate large numbers from individual bits known as bytes (8-bit with a maximum decimal count of 256), or words (16-bit word of 2^{16} decimals; or 32-bit word and 64-bit word—the current industry standard) (Table 3.2). Thus, in the binary system, 8-bit resolution corresponds to a precision of one part in 2^8 or 256 levels (10,13). More permanent computer memory and faster computer systems store digital echo signals using larger word sizes (32- and 64-bit)—measured as megabytes (MB; 10^6), gigabytes (GB; 10^9), or terabytes (TB; 10^{12}) (14,15).

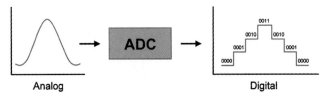

Figure 3.15. The ADC converts an analog signal to a digitized format by assigning it discrete numeric values, using a binary number system. Digital signals offer some advantages over their analog counterparts, including longer-term stability of the displayed image and facilitation of quantitative manipulation, processing, and analysis of received echoes.

TABLE 3.2	Digital Storage Capacity: Bits, Bytes, and Binary Numbers				
Levels	Number of Bits (Bit = Binary Digit)	Power of Two	Bytes 1 Byte (Binary Digit) = 8 Bits	Units	Note
1	2	2^1		Bit	0 or 1
2	4	2^2		Bits	
3	8	2^3		Bits	
4	16	2^4		Bits	Hexadecimal
5	32	2^5		Bits	
6	64	2^6		Bits	
7	128	2^7		Bits	
8	256	2^8	1 byte	Byte	1 character
9	512	2^9		Byte	
10	1,024	$1,024^1\ (2^{10})$	1 Kilobyte (KB)	Bytes	1 page
20	1,048,576	$1,024^2\ (2^{20})$	Megabyte (MB)	bytes	1 book
30	1,073,741,824	$1,024^3\ (2^{30})$	Gigabyte (GB)	Bytes	Encyclopedia
40	1,099,511,627,776	$1,024^4\ (2^{40})$	Terabyte (TB)	Byte	

Graphic "bits": 1-bit image: monochrome; 8-bit image: 256 colors or grayscales; 24- or 32-bit image: graphic supports true color.

SCAN CONVERSION AND STORAGE IN COMPUTER MEMORY

The initial ultrasound sector scan is represented by approximately 100 scan lines containing thousands of digitized coordinates. The scan converter locates each series of echoes corresponding to the scan line representing pulses from the transducer (Fig. 3.3). *Digital scan conversion* converts information obtained within these radial sector scan lines into a rectangular, checkerboard matrix (Cartesian coordinates) of picture elements or pixels (usually 512 × 512) suitable for storage in memory and eventual video display (16). During the construction of an ultrasound image, the echo signals are oriented into corresponding pixel locations or addresses (Cartesian [x,y] coordinates, which are determined from the echo delay time and transducer beam coordinates (Fig. 3.16)). Each pixel is assigned the digitized value representing the echo intensity of the ultrasound signal returning from a specific anatomic site. In the B (brightness)-mode image display format, the greater the number of gray levels or colors (bits per pixel), the better is the image resolution and the greater data size per pixel. A trade-off exits between image quality and processing, transmission, and display speed (17). The combination of a binary storage system and multiple layered matrices allows up to 1,024 shades of gray to be stored for a 10-bit system, far exceeding the 32 to 64 shades of gray that a monitor can display for each pixel, and the 50 to 100 shades of gray that can be differentiated by human vision (1×).

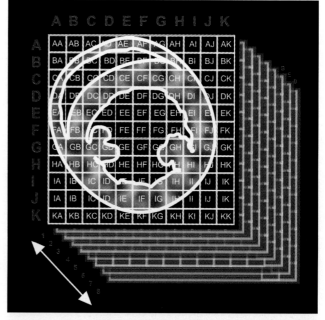

Figure 3.16. Scan conversion involves the orientation of echo signals into corresponding pixel locations (AA, AB, AC, etc.) on a matrix. The pixel locations are determined from the echo delay time and transducer beam coordinates. Each pixel is assigned a discrete digitized value representing the echo intensity of the ultrasound signal returning from a specific anatomic site. The combination of a binary storage system and multiple layered matrices (at least *8–10 layers*) allows for a greater number of gray shades.

POSTPROCESSING

Following scan conversion and storage in memory, the signal can be further modified. In contrast to preprocessing, *postprocessing* refers to image processing performed after data are retrieved from system memory (Fig. 3.3). Postprocessing primarily determines the particular shade of gray assigned to a pixel depending on the signal amplitude versus brightness level relationship selected by the operator (Fig. 3.17). Furthermore, because the range of echo amplitudes in stored memory far exceeds the number of brightness levels that can be displayed on the monitor, a range of pixel values may be assigned to a single brightness level. The translation of the range of pixel values stored in RAM to brightness levels is called *grayscale mapping*. The assignment of a particular grayscale map only affects the brightness of the displayed pixel and not its original stored value. Consequently, in comparison to preprocessing, a postprocessing function can generally be performed on a frozen image. Black-and-white inversion reverses the grayscale assignments, such that white represents low-echo intensity and black represents high-echo intensity.

B color is another postprocessing function that represents echo intensity in various colors rather than shades of gray (Fig. 3.18). B color may improve contrast resolution by facilitating the ability to distinguish subtle differences in echo intensity between adjacent tissues (10). *Read zoom* is a postprocessing magnification function. In comparison to write zoom, the spatial resolution is not improved during read zoom magnification because the number of pixels representing the original scanned area remains the same.

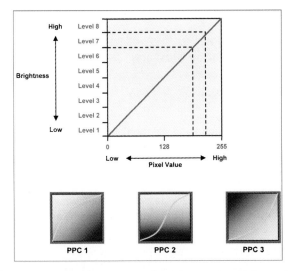

Figure 3.17. Postprocessing (grayscale mapping) determines the range of pixel values assigned to a particular brightness level (**top**). This linear relationship can be further altered (**bottom**) by selecting one of several postprocessing curves (PPC) that suppress gray levels at either end of the spectrum of pixel values (PPC₁, PPC₂, PPC₃). The assignment of a particular grayscale map only affects the brightness of the displayed pixel and not its original stored value.

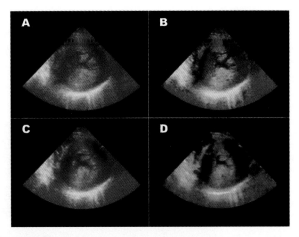

Figure 3.18. B color is a postprocessing function that represents echo intensity in various colors rather than shades of gray. A variety of B color maps can be selected (**A–D**).

IMAGE DISPLAY, RECORDING, AND STORAGE

Following final postprocessing modification of the signal, a *digital-to-analog converter* converts the digitized data stored as discrete numbers in memory, back into analog format as continuously variable voltages that control the brightness of the monitor for display (Fig. 3.3). A typical television monitor uses an interlaced scan-line system in which each video frame is composed of two fields. One field contains the even-numbered, horizontal scan lines (*raster lines*) while the other includes the odd raster lines. Consequently, an interlaced scan-line system provides 60 video fields/s, resulting in a 30 Hz frame rate. In contrast, a noninterlaced computer monitor provides improved temporal resolution with frame rates of at least 75 to 80 Hz (Fig. 3.19). The brightness and contrast controls of the computer monitor should also be adjusted accordingly (Fig. 3.20). In addition, it may be necessary to diminish the brightness of the ambient lighting in order to optimize the visualization of ultrasound images.

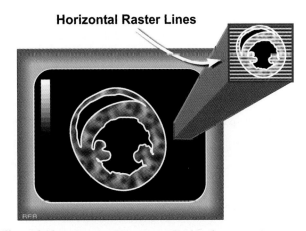

Figure 3.19. Ultrasound images are displayed on a monitor screen as a composition of horizontal raster lines (525 lines/frame).

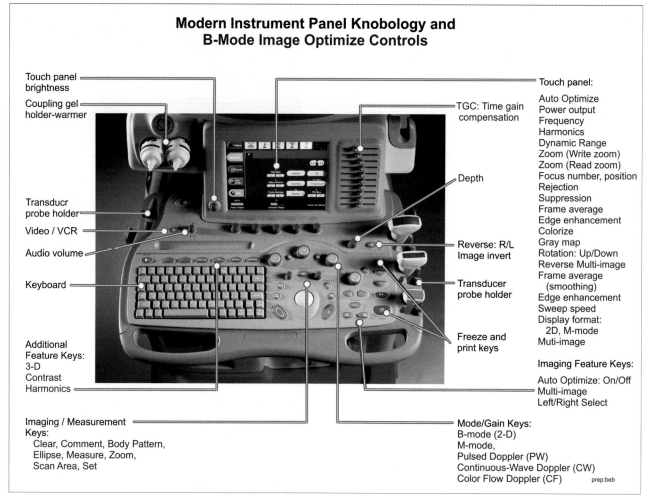

Figure 3.20. Ultrasound console and digital instrument panel of a modern ultrasound machine. See B-mode Echocardiography: Selected Knobology Optimization Glossary.

B-mode Echocardiography: Selected Knobology Optimization Glossary	
2D	Two-dimensional echocardiography; commonly referred to as "B-mode"
3D	Three-dimensional echocardiography
Acoustic power	Transmit power; acoustic energy output of the ultrasound beam per unit time (in watts, W); control feature that adjusts the amount of energy delivered to the patient; use high-power default setting to optimize image quality (better signal-to-noise ratio); acoustic output indices: mechanical index (MI) and thermal index (TI) typically displayed on image frame.
Amplitude	Ultrasound wave height above baseline; a basic physical characteristic of sound waves that is used in processing B-mode or grayscale images; ultrasound beam energy, intensity, and power are closely related
Annotation keys	Function keys to enter labels or measurements on the B-mode image display
Archiving	Transferring echo images to storage media, e.g., CDs, DVDs, flash drives
Artifact	Imaging artifact; false representations of the imaged tissue; can result from operator, instrument settings, and patient factors
B-color	See Color B-mode
B-mode	Brightness modulation of amplitudes of the received echo signals using grayscale; display formats include M-mode, 2D, and 3D options

(continued)

Calipers	Function tools for measurements, typically activated by pointing device
Cine loop /Playback	For review of recently acquired images within system memory before applying freeze or save functions
Coded excitation	Technique for improving far-field image resolution and penetration
Color B-mode	B-mode contrast-enhancing technique using various color options
Colorize	See Color B-mode
Compression	Postprocessing setting which, in conjunction with log compression (dynamic range control, which is a preprocessing function), improves or softens the appearance of B-mode images
Depth	Distance from the transducer; adjust as needed to visualize specified region of interest; depth scale visible on scan sector; frame rate decreased with greater imaging depth due to finite speed of ultrasound
Depth gain	Depth gain compensation (DGC), see Time-gain compensation (TGC)
Dynamic range/log compression	Range of echo intensities ranging from threshold (smallest) to saturation (largest) that can be displayed on the B-mode ultrasound image; increasing the dynamic range increases the number of gray shades (improved contrast resolution); decreasing the dynamic range decreases number of gray shades (decreased contrast resolution—image appears more black and white)
Edge enhancement	Selective enhancement of the grayscale pixel differences to improve tissue definition
Field of View	FOV; region of interest (ROI) or scan sector width; pie-shaped image with scan sector swivel or sweep angle ± 45 degrees (typical range 15–90 degrees); see Scan sector; Sector width
Focal zone	See Focus
Focus	Narrowest region of the ultrasound beam that exhibits the best spatial resolution; also called focal zone, focal spot, focal point
Focus, dynamic	Technique for adjusting the focus of an ultrasound beam
Focus number and position	For increasing the number of transmit focal zones or moving the position of the focal zone
FOV	See Field of view; Scan sector width
Frame	Digital memory of cardiac ultrasound display (typical display is composed of 512 × 512 pixels). Still-frame or freeze-frame of B-mode video display; display scan sector
Frame average	Temporal filter for averaging frames to display an aesthetically smoother image.
Frame rate	The rate or frequency at which the ultrasound equipment can process and display image frames in real time (frames/sec); ~30 frame/s processing power needed to display flicker-free images in real time. To increase frame rate: narrow scan sector, decrease imaging depth, and decrease line density
Freeze	Freeze-frame; still-frame of video image display
Freeze-frame	See Freeze; still-frame
Frequency	See Transducer Frequency; Pulse Repetition Frequency (PRF); Multifrequency
Gain	System gain; used to amplify weak echoes and improve image contrast; avoid excessive gain (especially in the operating theatre setting)
Gray map	see Grayscale map
Grayscale map	Scale displayed with B-mode (grayscale) images that indicate echo strength or intensity; structures that produce echoes with the highest intensities appear white (echoreflective, "echobright"); structures that produce few or no echoes appear black (echolucent or "echo free"); the human eye can discern 16–32 intermediate shades of gray out of a potentially displayable 256 shades of gray
Harmonic imaging	A technique to improve image quality; selectively uses echoes with harmonic frequencies echoes to create the image; it can reduce artifact and improve image quality
Harmonics	See Harmonic imaging
Image	Reconstruction of the anatomical scan plane to form the scan sector display (image frame) by processing the received echo signals

(continued)

B-mode Echocardiography: Selected Knobology Optimization Glossary (*Continued*)

Image optimization	Includes: Presets, transducer frequency, imaging depth, focal points, gain/TGC, auto-optimize functions
Imaging artifact	See Artifact
Keyboard	Input device for entering patient data, annotations, and other entries
Line density	Scan line density; adjust to optimize B-Mode frame rates or spatial resolution; the number of scan lines within scan sector; frame rate and temporal resolution decreased with increased line density due to finite speed of ultrasound
Log compression	Preprocessing function that compresses the amplitudes of received echo signals using a logarithmic scale—this facilitates improved image display
Mechanical index (MI)	Acoustic output measure to describe the nonthermal and biosafety effects of ultrasound, e.g., cavitation, microbubble rupture; compares two parameters: peak rarefactional pressure and center frequency of the transmitted ultrasound
M-mode	Time-motion mode (T-M Mode); one-dimensional echocardiography over time with time on the x-axis and depth on the y-axis
Multifrequency	Feature that allows multi-Hertz transducer operation
Multi-Hertz	See Multifrequency
Operator	Instrument operator, sonographer
Optimization	See Image Optimization
Persistence	Postprocessing feature that averages acquired image frames to smoothen the appearance of the moving heart (video image); if persistence is set too high, heart appears to be in slow motion
Postprocessing	Image manipulation following digital scan conversion; inputs following image freeze or save
Preprocessing	Inputs and manipulations prior to digital scan conversion; entries prior to image freeze or save
Probe	Transducer housing, but commonly called the transducer
PRF	See Pulse-repetition frequency
Pulse repetition frequency	Pulse rate or PRF; the number or separate pulses that are sent out every second by the transducer; the pulse-echo operation requires that the transducer must wait for the echoes ("round trip") before transmitting another imaging pulse; PRF typically ranges from 1,000 to 5,000 pulses/s (1–5 kHz); PRF and hence improved frame rates are possible when imaging at shallow depths
Read zoom	A postprocessing function that allows simple image magnification of an operator-defined region of interest within a stored image (no change in image resolution compared to "write zoom")
Region of interest (ROI)	Anatomical area of interest within the ultrasound imaging plane
Rejection	Selection of amplification and processing threshold; removal of unwanted "noise"
RES	regional expansion selection (see Write zoom)
Resolution	Imaging detail; the ability to display image detail without blurring; axial, lateral, slice-thickness, temporal, and contrast resolution
Scan line density	See Line density
Scan plane	Anatomical scan plane within range of transducer beam
Scan sector	Pie-shaped image frame of anatomical scan plane produced by phased array transducers
Sector scan	See Scan sector
Sector size	See Sector width; Field of view (FOV); scan angle plus image depth
Sector width	pie-shaped image with scan sector sweep angle ± 45 degrees; a wide scan sector (with increased line density) results in lower frame rates and temporal resolution
Smoothing	Image smoothing or softening; a postprocessing function
Spatial compounding	Technique for improving image quality by combining or averaging ultrasound images acquired from multiple insonation angles into a single image

(*continued*)

Suppression	Removal of unwanted low-level echoes or acoustic "noise"
Sweep speed	To change speed at which the timeline is swept
Thermal index (TI)	Standard measure to describe ratio of transmitted acoustic power to power required to raise the tissue temperature by 1°C (tissue assumed to have attenuation of 0.3 dB/cm/MHz along the beam axis); there thermal index for soft tissue (TIS) as well as bone (TIB)
TGC	See Time-gain compensation
Time-gain compensation	TGC; compensates for beam attenuation (loss of acoustic energy with increasing imaging depth); depth-dependent amplification of echoes using sliding controls on display panel (apply based on appearance of image display); also called depth gain compensation (DGC), time varied gain, or variable swept gain
Trace	Measurement tool for tracing selected region of interest, e.g., circumferences and cross-sectional areas
Trackball/joystick	Pointing device or computer mouse for controlling multiple operations of the ultrasound system, e.g., position, scroll, measurements, and analyses
Transducer	The probe housing the piezoelectric elements; phased array transducers permit a wide range of view despite confinement to a small transducer "foot print," e.g., the intercostal spaces or the esophageal lumen
Transducer frequency	A fundamental characteristic of the ultrasound beam (measured in megaHertz, MHz); for transthoracic and transesophageal echocardiography, typical values range 2–5 MHz and 5–7.5 MHz, respectively; modern transducers are capable of multiHertz operation
Transmit power	See Acoustic power
Write zoom	A preprocessing function to allow image magnification of operator-defined region of interest within an active image; improved image resolution achieved by re-scanning of selected region (with increase in line density and pixels compared to "read zoom"); RES: regional expansion selection
Zoom	See Read zoom, Write zoom

Resolution, the ability to distinguish two point targets as separate entities, is better preserved by recording and storing ultrasound images on an optical disk in comparison to video tape, which requires further compression of the data.

CONCLUSIONS

Optimizing the 2D echocardiographic examination requires knowledge and experience in the principles involved in ultrasound instrumentation, image acquisition, and display. Echocardiographic images are constructed by complex series of manipulations of the received echo signals. Many of these manipulations are within the control of the echocardiographer. Optimal signal processing, amplification, time-gain compensation, logarithmic compression and display DR control, filtering, digital scan conversion, and analog-to-digital conversion are important intermediate steps that directly impact the quality of the echograph display. Transducer design and ultrasound beam characteristics directly influence image resolution. Axial, lateral, and temporal resolution must be optimized to limit the interference associated with artifacts. Postprocessing and data storage are also useful—not just for optimizing work flow,

but also because of the increased availability of off-line analyses in the modern echocardiography laboratory. Ultimately, accurate interpretation and diagnosis of cardiac anatomy, physiology pathology on echocardiography requires a practical understanding of the multiple variables that influence optimal 2D image acquisition and display.

KEY POINTS

- *Signal processing* of the received echoes require important intermediate steps prior to image display: amplification, time-gain compensation, logarithmic compression, dynamic range control, filtering, digital scan conversion, and analog-to-digital conversion.
- *Axial resolution* refers to the minimum distance between two structures oriented parallel to the ultrasound beam axis that permits visualization of the structures as separate, distinct reflectors on the monitor screen.
- *Axial resolution* of 2D echocardiographic images is optimized by shortening the pulse duration through the use of high-frequency transducers with broad frequency bandwidths and appropriate damping.

- *Lateral resolution* refers to the ability to resolve two adjacent structures that are oriented perpendicular to the beam axis as separate entities. Lateral resolution also refers to the ability of the beam to detect single small objects across the width of the beam.
- *Lateral resolution* of 2D echocardiographic images is optimized by avoiding the use of excessive transmit power or gain, and using a focused high-frequency transducer and large aperture diameter.
- *Temporal resolution* for 2D echocardiographic imaging can be optimized while maintaining line density by minimizing depth, reducing the sector angle, and using high-frequency transducers.
- *Preprocessing* refers to modifications of the signal that determine the specific numeric values assigned to the echo intensities prior to storage in the computer memory.
- *Postprocessing* (grayscale mapping) determines the range of pixel values assigned to a particular brightness level after retrieval from computer memory and only affects the brightness of the displayed pixel rather than its original stored value.
- The *analog-to-digital converter* converts an analog signal to a digitized format by assigning it discrete numeric values, using a binary number system.

REFERENCES

1. Otto C. Principles of echocardiographic image acquisition and Doppler analysis. In: Otto C, ed. *Textbook of Clinical Echocardiography*. 2nd ed. Philadelphia: W.B. Saunders Company, 2004:1–28.
2. Zagebski J. Physics of diagnostic ultrasound. In: Zagebski J, ed. *Essentials of Ultrasound Physics*. St. Louis: Mosby, 1996:1–19.
3. Dowsett DJ, Johnston RE, Kenny PA. The principles of ultrasound. In: Dowsett DJ, Johnston RE, Kenny PA, eds. *The Physics of Diagnostic Imaging*. 2nd ed. London: Arnold Publishers Ltd, 2006:511–529.
4. Weyman A. Physical principles of ultrasound. In: Weyman A, ed. *Principles and Practice of Echocardiography*. 2nd ed. Philadelphia: Lea & Febiger, 1994:3–28.
5. Geiser EA. Echocardiography: physics and instrumentation. In: Skorton DJ, Schelbert HR, Wolf GL, Brundage BH, eds. *Marcus Cardiac Imaging: a Companion to Braunwald's Heart Disease*. 2nd ed. Philadelphia: W.B. Saunders, 1996:273–295.
6. Hedrick W, Hykes D, Starchman D. Basic ultrasound instrumentation. In: Hedrick W, Hykes D, Starchman D, eds. *Ultrasound Physics and Instrumentation*. 3rd ed. St. Louis: Mosby, 1995:31–70.
7. Bushberg JT, Siebert JA, Leidholdt EM Jr, et al. *The Essential Physics of Medical Imaging*. 2nd ed. Philadelphia: Lippincott Williams & Wilkins, 2002:469–553.
8. Feigenbaum H. Instrumentation. In: Feigenbaum H, ed. *Echocardiography*. 5th ed. Baltimore: Williams & Wilkins, 1993:1–67.
9. Zagebski J. Pulse-echo ultrasound instrumentation. In: Zagebski J, ed. *Essentials of Ultrasound Physics*. St. Louis: Mosby, 1996:46–68.
10. Kremkau F. Imaging instruments. In: Kremkau F, ed. *Diagnostic Ultrasound: Principles and Instruments*. 7th ed. Philadelphia: W.B. Saunders Company, 2002:101–166.
11. Thys M, Hillel Z. How it works: basic concepts in echocardiography. In: Bruijn N, Clements F, eds. *Intraoperative Use of Echocardiography*. Philadelphia: JB Lippincott, 1991: 13–44.
12. Hedrick W, Hykes D, Starchman D. Digital signal and image processing. In: Hedrick W, Hykes D, Starchman D, eds. *Ultrasound Physics and Instrumentation*. 3rd ed. St. Louis: Mosby, 1995:208–238.
13. Thomas J. Digital image processing. In: Weyman A, ed. *Principles and Practice of Echocardiography*. 2nd ed. Philadelphia: Lea & Febiger, 1994:56–74.
14. Dowsett DJ, Johnston RE, Kenny PA. Computers in radiology. In: Dowsett DJ, Johnston RE, Kenny PA, eds. *The Physics of Diagnostic Imaging*. 2nd ed. London: Arnold Publishers Ltd, 2006:276–277.
15. Dowsett DJ, Johnston RE, Kenny PA. The digital image. In: Dowsett DJ, Johnston RE, Kenny PA, eds. *The Physics of Diagnostic Imaging*. 2nd ed. London: Arnold Publishers Ltd, 2006:313–318.
16. Zagebski J. Image storage and display. In: Zagebski J, ed. *Essentials of Ultrasound Physics*. St. Louis: Mosby, 1996:69–86.
17. Bansal S, Ehler D, Vacek JL. Digital echocardiography: its role in modern medical practice. *Chest* 2001;119(1):271–276.

QUESTIONS

1. Axial resolution can be optimized by employing which one of the following characteristics of an ultrasound transducer?
   A. Decreased damping
   B. Lower frequency
   C. Decreasing the focal depth
   D. Wider bandwidth
2. Lateral resolution can be optimized by employing which one of the following variables?
   A. Lower transducer frequency
   B. Narrower transducer aperture diameter
   C. Focused transducer
   D. Increased power
3. Temporal resolution can be improved by which one of the following variables?
   A. Decreasing depth
   B. Increasing scan angle
   C. Decreasing transducer frequency
   D. Increasing scan-line density

CHAPTER 4

Surgical Anatomy of the Heart

Bruce Bollen ▪ Carlos Duran ▪ Andrej A. Alfirevic ▪ Robert M. Savage

A familiarity with cardiovascular anatomy is fundamental to understanding the standard imaging planes commonly utilized in daily clinical applications of ultrasound in the perioperative environment. This is especially true for intraoperative transesophageal and epicardial echocardiography where anatomic localization of pathology is required to answer specific surgical questions. In addition, pathologic processes, such as endocarditis, dilatation of cardiac chambers and vascular structures, and congenital abnormalities, may result in distortion of normal relational anatomy, making it challenging even for experienced echocardiographers to recognize the structural anatomy of the heart. Understanding the three-dimensional anatomic relation of the cardiac fibrous skeleton, cardiac chambers, valves, and vascular structures provides a greater ability to recognize resulting distortions of normal anatomy. It will be the purpose of this discussion to introduce the novice echocardiographer to basic cardiac anatomy, yet challenge the experienced echocardiographer to develop a greater understanding of cardiac anatomy in relation to their practice.

FIBROUS SKELETON OF THE HEART

The fibrous skeleton of the heart is formed by the U-shaped cords of the aortic annulus and their extensions forming the right trigone, left trigone, and a smaller fibrous structure from the right aortic coronary cusp to the root of the pulmonary artery (1) (Fig 4.1). This "skeleton" plays a primary function of supporting the heart within the pericardium. A continuum of fibrous tissue extends from the fibrous skeleton providing attachments for the atriums, ventricles, and valve leaflets.

Three U-shaped cords of the aortic annulus join to each other at the commissures of the aortic valve, forming a scalloped fibrous crown-like skeleton of the aortic valve. The right fibrous trigone extends from the base of the noncoronary cusp (NCC) and is more substantial than the left fibrous trigone. The left fibrous trigone extends from the base of the left coronary cusp (LCC). A scalloped area is formed between the right and left trigones and the annular attachment of the left and NCC. This is called the *intertrigonal space* and has no proper skeletal structure. A broad membranous curtain, extending from the aortic annulus to the mitral annulus, covers this space.

This broad membrane is often referred to as the aortic curtain and the space as the mitral aortic interstitial fibrosis or intervascular space. This membrane merges with the anterior third of the mitral annulus, becoming the middle portion of the anterior leaflet of the mitral valve.

From the left and right fibrous trigones, a fibrous tissue continuum extends around the left and right atrioventricular (AV) orifices, forming the annuli fibrosi of the mitral and tricuspid annuli. The mitral annulus is the transition area where the left atrium, mitral valve leaflets, and left ventricle (LV) come together. The mitral valve leaflets form a membranous curtain attaching to the mitral annulus. The anterior circumferential portion of the mitral annulus associated with the left trigone, intertrigonal

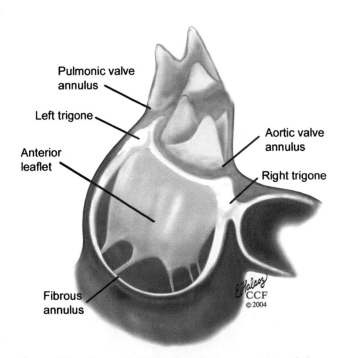

Figure 4.1. Fibrous skeleton of the heart consisting of three U-shaped cords of the aortic annulus, the right and left trigones, and the fibrous structure from right coronary cusp (RCC) to the root of the pulmonary artery. Extensions from skeleton include the aortic curtain, mitral and tricuspid annulus, and anterior leaflet of the mitral and pulmonic valves.

space, and right trigone area is the attachment point of the anterior leaflet of the mitral valve. This anterior portion of the mitral annulus has minimal shape change during the cardiac cycle and is less prone to dilation because of its rigid structure. Its margins are defined surgically by two dimples raised at the border of the right and left trigones when lifting the anterior leaflet.

The annuli fibrosi of the mitral annulus becomes thinner and poorly defined as it extends posteriorly from the left and right trigones. This portion of the annulus is poorly supported and is prone to dilation in pathologic states. The posterior leaflet of the mitral valve attaches to this portion of the annulus. Dilation of the annular attachment of the posterior leaflet creates increased tension on the middle scallop of the posterior leaflet, explaining the 60% occurrence of chordal tears in the middle scallop of the posterior leaflet (2).

From the base of the annular cord of the NCC, a membrane extends becoming continuous with the interventricular septum. Its downward extension forms the membranous septum. This relationship is important in understanding the anatomy of the left ventricular outflow tract (LVOT).

CARDIAC VENTRICLES

The right ventricle (RV) has two openings—the tricuspid and pulmonic valves—separated by a band of myocardium, the crista supraventricularis. The LV has a common opening at its base shared by the aortic root and the mitral valve (Fig. 4.2). Although sharing a common opening in the LV, the aortic and mitral valves are set at an angle to each other (Fig. 4.3)(6). The LVOT is defined anteriorly by the membranous and the muscular portions of the interventricular septum (3,4). The superior part of the membranous septum is directly continuous with the right wall of the aortic root. The membranous septum is beneath

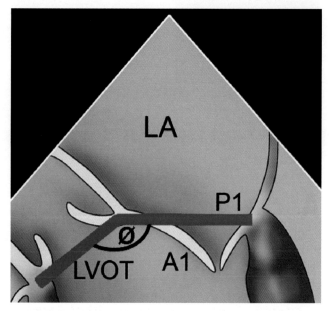

Figure 4.3. The aortic and mitral valves share a common opening in the LV and are set at an angle to each other.

the NCC. The posterior portion of the LVOT is defined by the anterior leaflet of the mitral valve.

To facilitate reporting of left ventricular function, the ventricle is divided into segments. Various segmental classifications have been utilized. The Society of Cardiovascular Anesthesiologists (SCA) and the American Society of Echocardiography (ASE) have developed a 16-segment model of the LV based on the recommendations of the Subcommittee on Quantification of the ASE Standards Committee. This model divides the LV into three levels: basal, mid, and apical. The basal and mid levels are each divided circumferentially into six segments and the apical level into four segments (Figs. 4.4 and 4.5) (5).

TRICUSPID VALVE

The tricuspid valve of the RV has three leaflets. Its orifice viewed from the RV is triangular with anterior, posterior, and septal sides. The tricuspid annulus is relatively indistinct especially in the septal region. The tricuspid valve has three leaflets: anterior, posterior, and septal. The anterior leaflet, the largest of the three, is semicircular to quadrangular in shape. Chordae attaching to the anterior leaflet arise from the anterior and medial papillary muscles (PPMs). The posterior leaflet is usually the smallest. The leaflet has several indentations or clefts that give it a scalloped appearance. Its chordae arise from the posterior and anterior PPMs. The septal leaflet is primarily attached to the septum, the remainder attaching to the posterior wall of the RV (Fig. 4.6). Part of its basal attachment is to

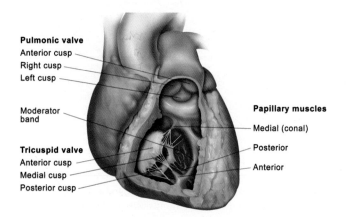

Figure 4.2. Diagram showing that the tricuspid and pulmonary valves occupy separate openings within the RV. Reproduced with permission from Jonathan B. Mark.

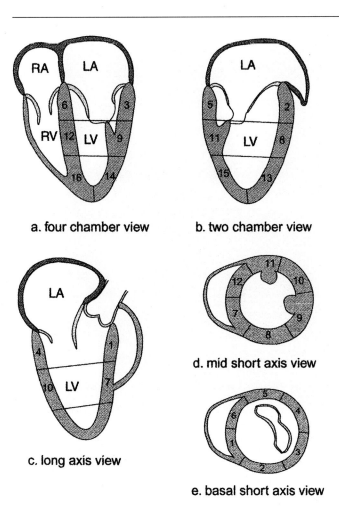

Basal Segments	Mid Segments	Apical Segments
1=Basal Anteroseptal Anterior	7=Mid Anteroseptal	13=Apical
2=Basal Anterior	8=Mid Anterior	14=Apical Lateral
3=Basal Lateral	9=Mid Lateral	15=Apical Inferior
4=Basal Posterior	10=Mid Posterior	16=Apical Septal
5=Basal Inferior	11=Mid Inferior	

a. four chamber view

b. two chamber view

c. long axis view

d. mid short axis view

e. basal short axis view

Figure 4.4. Sixteen-Segment Model of the LV. **A:** Four-chamber views show the three inferoseptal and three ante-rolateral segments. **B:** Two-chamber views show the anterior and three inferior segments. **C:** Long-axis views show the two anteroseptal and two inferolateral segments. **D:** Mid short-axis views show all six segments at the mid level. **E:** Basal short-axis views show all six segments at the basal level.

the posterior wall of the RV but most of its attachment is to the septal wall. Its chordae arise from the posterior and septal PPMs.

Silver et al. (8) defined three commissures: anteroseptal commissure, anteroposterior commissure, and posteroseptal commissures. These commissures define the margins of the leaflets of the tricuspid valve. The antero-septal commissure is defined by a deep indentation in the membranous interventricular septum where the anterior and septal walls of the RV join. The anteropos-terior commissure is defined by fan-shaped chorda at the acute margin of the RV and the anterior PPM point-ing to the commissure. The posteroseptal commissure is defined by attaching fan-shaped chordae, the most medially placed posterior PPM, and a fold of tissue on the septal leaflet.

The basal attachments of the leaflets to the annulus are at different levels in the heart. The posterior leaflet and the posteroseptal half of the septal leaflet are roughly hor-izontal and about 15 mm lower than the highest part of

the valve's attachment, which occurs at the anteroseptal commissure near the midpoint of the membranous interventricular septum.

The chordae of the tricuspid valve originate from PPMs or directly from the muscle of the posterior or septal walls of the RV. Silver et al. (8) defined chordae as being rough zone, fan shaped, basal, free edge, and deep chordae.

PULMONIC VALVE

The pulmonic annulus is not part of the fibrous skel-eton as is the aortic annulus. It is attached to the base of the aorta by a flimsy fibrous extension of the aortic root called the *tendon of conus*. The rest of the pulmonic valve has muscular attachments to the RV and interventricular septum (Fig. 4.7). The pulmonic valve normally has three cusps with a nodule at the midpoint of each free edge. The pocket behind the cusp is the sinus.

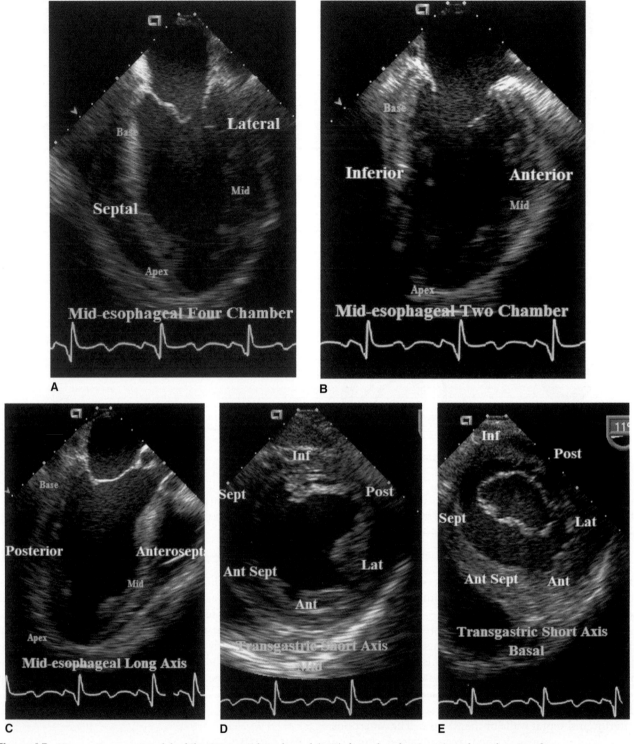

Figure 4.5. Sixteen-Segment Model of the LV. **A:** Midesophageal (ME) four-chamber imaging plane showing the three inferoseptal and three anterolateral segments. **B:** ME two-chamber showing the three anterior and three inferior segments. **C:** ME long-axis views showing the two anteroseptal and two posterior segments. **D:** Transgastric mid short-axis views showing all six segments. **E:** Transgastric two-chamber view showing anterior and inferior segments at base, mid, and apical levels.

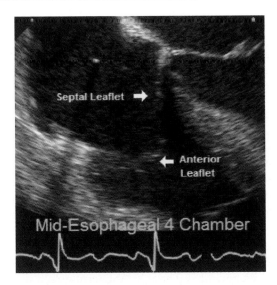

Figure 4.6. ME four-chamber, two-dimensional image plane with focus on tricuspid valve.

MITRAL VALVE APPARATUS

The mitral valve apparatus is an anatomical term describing structures of the LV associated with mitral valve function (Fig. 4.8). These structures consist of the fibrous skeleton of the heart (Fig. 4.1), the mitral annulus, mitral leaflets, mitral chordae, and the PPM-ventricular wall complex. This anatomic description oversimplifies the complex mechanical interaction of

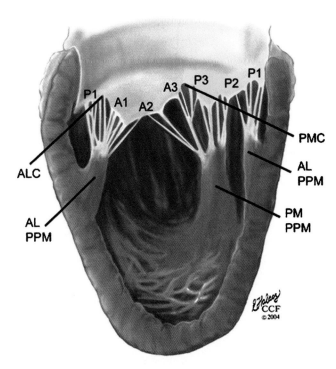

Figure 4.8. The valve apparatus consisting of the mitral valve leaflets, chordae, PPMs, free wall of the LV and the mitral annulus.

the heart, which makes the left ventricular chamber functional.

The important role of TEE in mitral valve repair makes it imperative that the echocardiographer understands mitral valve anatomy. This understanding of anatomy is then used to define the mitral valve anatomy visualized by multiplane TEE imaging of the mitral valve. The echocardiographer must be able to communicate important anatomic/pathological findings to the surgeon performing a mitral valve repair. In addition to the anatomical terms for portions of the mitral valve, there are two surgical nomenclatures used: the Carpentier terminology (adopted by ASE/SCA) (5,7) and the Duran terminology (8,9). Ideally, the echocardiographer should be familiar with all of these terminologies (Fig. 4.9). Intraoperative echocardiographic identification of the different

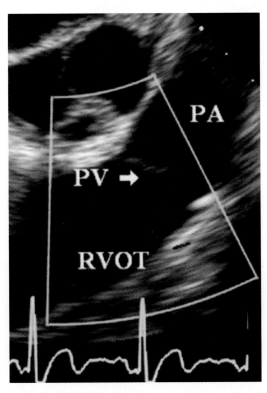

Figure 4.7. ME RV inflow-outflow two-dimensional imaging plane with focus on pulmonic valve.

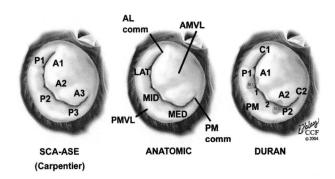

Figure 4.9. Comparison of SCA/ASE terminology with the anatomic nomenclature and Duran terminology.

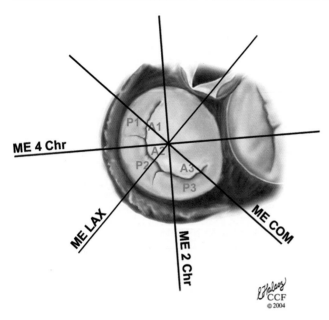

Figure 4.10. Standard imaging planes and mitral valve anatomy. Imaging planes depicted above: ME four chamber (ME 4Chr), ME commissural (ME COM), ME two chamber (ME 2Chr), ME long axis (ME LAX).

segments of the anterior and posterior mitral valve leaflets (PMVL) is dependent on understanding this terminology and their relation to the standard imaging planes (Figs. 4.10 and 4.11).

MITRAL VALVE LEAFLETS: CARPENTIER-SCA TERMINOLOGY

The Carpentier terminology is solely a terminology of the mitral leaflets and does not involve naming chordae or PPMs (7). The lateral scallop of the posterior leaflet is named P1, middle scallop named P2, and medial scallop named P3. The anterior leaflet is divided into A1, A2, and A3 based upon the portion of the anterior leaflet making contact with P1, P2, and P3 during systole (Figs. 4.9, 4.10, 4.12, and 4.13). The SCA/ASE terminology does not in fact define chordal attachment to the leaflets. However, it is important for the echocardiographer to understand the orientation of chordae as related to this terminology. For this purpose, their attachments are explained and related to the Carpentier terminology (Figs. 4.12, and 4.13). The chordae tendineae are fibrous strings radiating

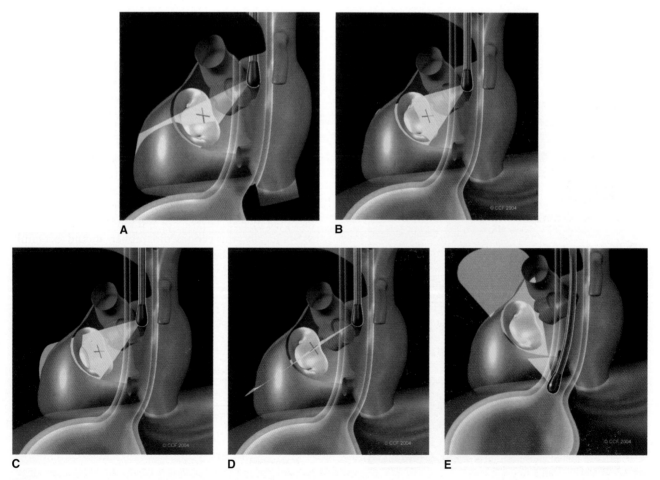

Figure 4.11. Three-dimensional illustration of relationship between TEE and mitral valve apparatus in imaging planes commonly used for three-dimensional evaluation of mitral valve.

ASE/SCA Terminology
(per Carpentier)

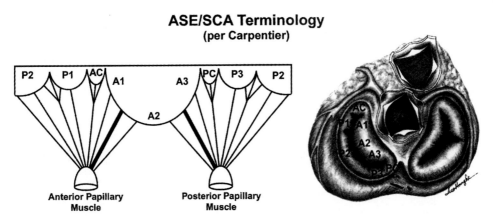

Figure 4.12. Chordal Relationships—ASE/SCA Terminology. Anterior leaflet divided into A1, A2, and A3. Posterior leaflet divided into P1 (anterolateral scallop), P2 (middle scallop), and P3 (posteromedial scallop). Commissural clefts not named anterior or posterior. Chordae arising from the anterior PPM attach to A1, AC, and P1, and the lateral half of P2 and A2. Chordae arising from the posterior PPM attach to A3, PC, and P3, and the medial half of P2 and A2.

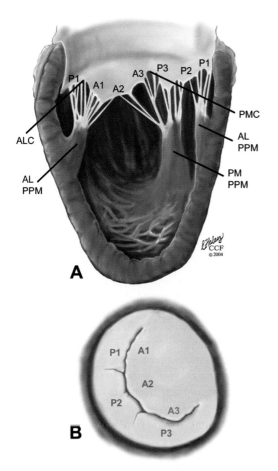

Figure 4.13. Chordal Relationships—ASE/SCA Terminology. The anterior mitral valve leaflet (AMVL) is shown in *tan*. The PMVL is shown in *blue*. Chordae arising from the anterior PPM attach to A1-P1, and the lateral half of P2 and A2. Chordae arising from the posterior PPM attach to A3-P3 and the medial half of P2 and A2. Depicted above: Anterior leaflet divided into A1, A2, and A3. Posterior leaflet divided into P1 (anterolateral scallop), P2 (middle scallop), and P3 (posteromedial scallop). ALC, PMC, posteromedial PPM (PM PPM), anterolateral PPM (AL PPM).

from the left ventricular PPMs or the ventricular free wall (posterior leaflet only) and attaching to the mitral leaflets in an organized manner (10). Chordae from the PPMs radiate upward attaching to the corresponding halves of the anterior and posterior leaflets. Chordae arising from the anterior PPM attach to A1, P1, (AC), and the lateral half of P2 and A2. Chordae arising from the posterior PPM attach to A3, P3, (PC), and the medial half of P2, and A2 (Figs. 4.12 and 4.13). This relation aids in defining the portion of the mitral valve that is echocardiographically visualized.

There are two chordae attaching to the ventricular surface of the anterior leaflet that are by far the thickest and largest of the chordae to the mitral valve. They have been called strut or stay chordae. One arises from the anterior PPM and attaches to the mid A1/A2 area of the anterior leaflet; the other arises from the posterior PPM and attaches to the mid A2/A3 portion of the anterior leaflet (Fig. 4.13).

MITRAL VALVE APPARATUS—DURAN TERMINOLOGY

The Duran mitral valve nomenclature is based on dividing the structures of the mitral valve into what is seen by the surgeon observing the valve through a left atriotomy.

The structures of the mitral apparatus in this orientation are defined as being anterior (A) or posterior (P) and being left or right, as viewed by this surgical view. Left-sided structures are noted by the numeral 1 and right-sided by the numeral 2. The chordae tendineae are named by the area of the leaflet into which they are inserted, independent of whether they are inserted into the free edge or the ventricular surface. Chordae tendineae are defined by the location of attaching to the anterior leaflet based upon the area of attachment

Duran Terminology

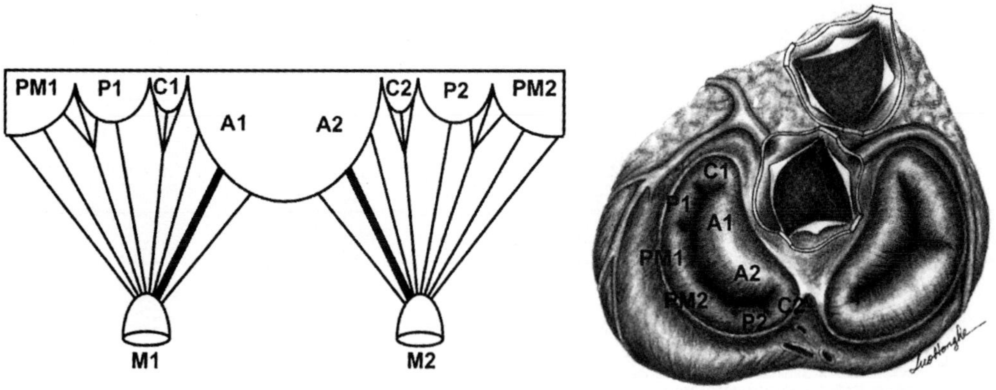

Figure 4.14. Duran Terminology. Diagram of the mitral valve apparatus. Anterior leaflet is divided into A1 and A2. Posterior leaflet is divided into P1, PM, and P2. PM is further divided into PM1 and PM2. Anterior PPM M1 and posterior PPM M2. Commissural scallops are labeled as C1 and C2. Observe that all leaflets with a numerical 1 are held by chordae arising from M1 and those leaflets with a numerical 2 are held by chordae arising from M2. Darkened chordae from M1 to A1 and M2 to A2 represent strut or stay chordae.

and right and left orientation to their related strut (stay) chords. The PPMs are defined as M1 (anterior PPM) and M2 (posterior PPM) (11). A curtain of fibroelastic tissue extends from the mitral annulus forming the mitral valve leaflets (12–14). The combined surface area of the mitral leaflets is twice that of the mitral orifice, permitting large areas of coaptation. The free edge of this curtain has multiple indentations. These indentations do not extend to the annulus. The commissural area between the anterior and posterior leaflets is in fact a small leaflet and is delineated by the attachment of the commissural fan chordae. These chordal attachments define the commissural area attaching to the commissural scallops, which have variable size but great importance for the function of the mitral valve. Duran defines the commissural scallops as left (C1) and right (C2), as seen by the surgeon through an atriotomy (Fig. 4.14) (8).

The anterior leaflet is semicircular in shape. The base-to-apical height of the anterior leaflet is almost twice as great as the posterior leaflet. The annular attachment of the anterior leaflet runs along approximately 30% of the annular circumference. Duran defines the anterior leaflet as A, and divides it into left (A1) and right (A2) halves, as seen by the surgeon through a left atriotomy. The posterior leaflet is attached to the mitral annulus along the free wall of the LV. It extends from the anterior commissure (C1) attachment of the LV free wall to the junction of the posterior LV and the muscular ventricular septum (C2). The posterior leaflet attachments involve about 70% of the mitral annulus. Small indentations in the posterior leaflet most commonly give it a three-scallop appearance: a larger middle scallop (PM), lateral scallop (P1), and smaller medial scallop (P2) on either side of PM. PM is further divided into a left half (PM1) and right half (PM2), as viewed by the surgeon through an atriotomy

(Fig. 4.14). The echocardiographer performing TEE is able to measure the height of the anterior leaflet and the three scallops of the posterior leaflet. Anatomic measurements of normal heights of these leaflets are given in Tables 4.1 and 4.2 (12).

The chordae tendineae are fibrous strings radiating from the left ventricular PPMs or the ventricular free wall (posterior leaflet only) and attaching to the mitral leaflets in an organized manner (11). Chordae from the PPM radiate upward attaching to the corresponding halves of the anterior and posterior leaflets. Chordae arising from M1 (anterior PPM) attach to A1, C1, P1, and PM1. Chordae arising from M2 (posterior PPM) attach to A2, C2, P2, and PM2. This relation aids in defining the portion of the mitral valve visualized echocardiographically. The majority of chordae branch either soon after leaving the PPM or before insertion into the leaflet. There are also cross-connections between chordae as they radiate to the valve leaflets. Lam defined three orders of chordae (12). First-order chordae attach on the free margin of the leaflet. Second-order chordae insert anywhere from a few to several millimeters back from the free edge. Third-order chordae travel from the ventricular wall and insert into the base of the posterior leaflet only (Fig. 4.15). Chordal morphology may also be identified on the basis of how they attached to the mitral leaflet. Lam classified chordae into rough zone, cleft, basal, and commissural chordae (13). Understanding this different chordal morphology is helpful to the surgeon in defining the scallops of the mitral valve. There are two chordae attaching to the ventricular surface of the anterior leaflet that is by far the thickest and largest of the chordae to the mitral valve. They have been called "strut" or "stay chordae." One arises from M1 and attaches to A1 of the anterior leaflet; one arises from M2 and attaches to the A2 portion of the anterior leaflet.

| TABLE 4.1 | **Height and Spread of the Anterolateral and PMCs of the Mitral Valve** |

Commissural Area (cm)	Present Study Male (26)	Female (24)	Commissure	Rusted, Scheifley, and Edwards (1952) Male (25)	Female (25)	Junctional Tissue	Cheichi and Lees (1956) Male (60)	Female (45)
	Anterolateral			*Anterior*			*Anterior*	
Height	0.8 (0.5–1.3)	0.7 (0.5–1.0)	Height (cm)	0.8 (0.5–1.3)	0.7 (0.4–1.1)	Height (cm)	0.8 (0.6–1.2)	0.7 (0.6–1.1)
Spread	1.2 (0.6–1.9)	0.9 (0.3–1.5)	—	—	—	Breadth (cm)	1.7 (0.7–2.4)	1.5 (0.7–2.1)
	Posteromedial			*Posterior*			*Posterior*	
Height	0.8 (0.6–1.2)	0.8 (0.4–1.1)	Height (cm)	0.8 (0.5–1.3)	0.7 (0.3–1.0)	Height (cm)	0.7 (0.5–0.9)	0.6 (0.4–0.8)
Spread	1.8 (1.2–2.6)	1.5 (0.9–2.2)	—	—	—	Breadth (cm)	1.3 (0.7–1.8)	1.2 (0.7–1.6)

Note: Measurements of the commissures given by Rusted, Scheifley, and Edwards (Anatomic Features of the Normal Mitral Valve and Associated Structures. *Circulation* 1952; 6[6I]: 825–831) and of the junctional tissues given by Cheichi MA, Lee WM, Thompson R (Functional anatomy of the normal mitral valve. *Journal of thoracic surgery* 1956) are added for comparison.

The PPMs are large trabeculae carnae originating from the junction of the middle and apical third of the left ventricular wall in a plane posterior to the intercommissural plane in diastole. Rusted et al. (16), suggested the nomenclature anterior (anterolateral) and posterior (posterolateral) based upon the consistent relationship that each PPM bears with its respective commissural area (C1, C2). According to Duran's surgical classification, the anterior PPM is termed M1 and the posterior termed M2. The anterior PPM (M1) is located on the anterior-lateral free wall of the LV. The posterior PPM (M2) originates at the junction of the posterior left ventricular free wall and the muscular ventricular septum (8). They extend into the upper third of the ventricular cavity below the

| TABLE 4.2 | **Height and Width of the Anterior and Posterior leaflets of the Mitral Valve, Comparing the Data of Rusted, Scheifley, and Edwards (1952) and of Cheichi and Lees (1956)** |

Height and Width (cm)	Present Study Male (26)	Female (24)	Rusted, Scheifley, and Edwards (1952) Male (25)	Female (25)	Cheichi and Lees (1956) Male (60)	Female (25)
	Anterior Cusp		*Anterior Cusp*		*Aortic Leaflet*	
Height	2.4 (2.0–3.0)	2.2 (1.8–3.5)	2.3 (1.6–2.9)	2.1 (1.6–2.5)	2.1 (1.9–3.2)	2.2 (1.8–2.7)
Width	3.6 (2.5–4.8)	2.9 (1.8–4.2)	—	—	3.7 (2.5–4.5)	3.3 (2.4–4.2)
	Posterior Leaflet		*Posterior Cusp*		*Ventricular Leaflet*	
	Middle Scallop					
Height	1.4 (0.9–2.0)	1.2 (0.7–1.8)	1.3 (0.8–1.8)	1.2 (0.7–2.4)	1.4 (1.8–2.5)	1.2 (0.8–2.4)
Width	2.3 (1.3–3.8)	1.8 (0.6–2.6)	—	—	3.3 (2.5–4.1)	3.0 (2.3–3.6)
	Anterolateral Commissural Scallop				*Anterior Leaflet Accessory*	
Height	1.1 (0.9–2.0)	1.0 (0.8–1.4)	—	—	1.1 (0.8–1.8)	1.0 (0.7–1.3)
Width	1.6 (0.9–4.0)	1.4 (0.9–2.0)	—	—	1.5 (1.1–1.8)	1.2 (1.0–1.6)
	Posteromedial Commissural Scallop				*Posterior Accessory Leaflet*	
Height	1.0 (0.6–1.7)	0.8 (0.5–1.1)	—	—	0.9 (0.6–1.2)	0.9 (0.7–1.0)
Width	1.5 (0.9–3.1)	1.1 (0.5–2.2)	—	—	1.1 (0.8–1.5)	0.8 (0.7–1.2)

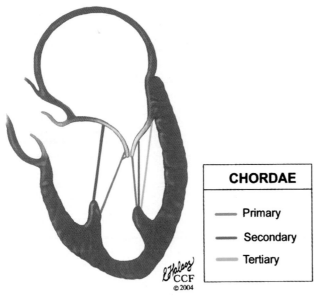

Figure 4.15. There are Three Orders of Chordae. Primary chordae attach on the free margin of the leaflet. Secondary chordae insert anywhere from a few to several millimeters back from the free edge. Tertiary chordae travel from the PPM and ventricular wall and insert into the base of the posterior leaflet only.

commissural tissue (C1, C2) of the LV. The PPMs most commonly have one head but may have double, triple, or multiple heads. The M1 PPM is more commonly supplied by two separate arteries: the first obtuse marginal arising from the left circumflex and the first diagonal arising from the left anterior descending (LAD) artery (15–17). A single artery, usually from the right coronary artery or the third obtuse marginal of the left circumflex, most commonly perfuses the M2 PPM. The greater incidence of M2 PPM dysfunction or rupture in myocardial ischemia has been associated with the single artery supply to it versus the common dual supply to the M1 PPM. The PPMs do not function in isolation from the left ventricular wall and chordae/leaflets to which they attach. The whole mitral valve apparatus interaction is important for proper ventricular function.

AORTIC ROOT

The aortic root is the portion of the ventricular outflow that supports the leaflets of the aortic valve. The superior boundary of the aortic root is the sinotubular junction, and the inferior boundary is the plane defined by the bases of the aortic semilunar valves attaching to the crown-shaped aortic annulus. Within these boundaries, the aortic root is composed of the aortic valve leaflets, the sinuses of Valsalva, and the interleaflet triangles (Fig. 4.16) (16).

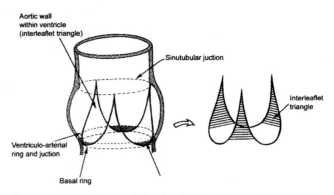

Figure 4.16. Diagram of the Aortic Root. **Inset:** The coronet-like arrangement of the valvar attachments.

There are three functional semilunar leaflets of the normal aortic valve. Each leaflet has

1. A functional hinge point where it attaches to the aortic root
2. A body of the semilunar valve
3. A coaptation surface of the leaflet with a thickened central nodule (nodule of Arantii)

The hinge point of the aortic leaflets attaches to the aortic root in a semilunar fashion along the crown-shaped aortic annulus (annulus fibrosus). The superior apex of each leaflet, attaching to the annulus fibrosus, attaches to the sinotubular junction. The bases of the aortic leaflets attach to the annulus at or below the anatomic ventricular

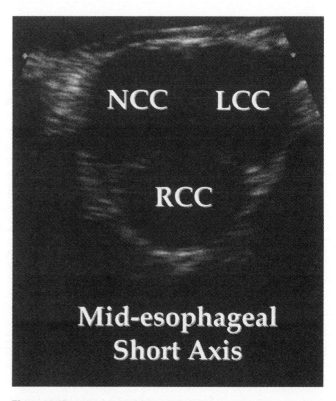

Figure 4.17. ME aortic valve short-axis imaging plane demonstrating the three coronary cusps: RCC, NCC, and LCC.

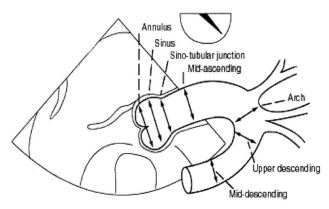

Figure 4.18. Schematic representation of the ME long-axis imaging plane demonstrating the aortic root. Measurements are taken at the annulus (hinge point of the aortic valve), sinus of Valsalva, sinotubular junction, and ascending aorta.

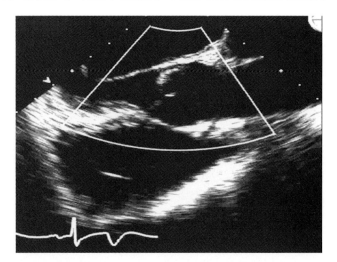

Figure 4.19. The ME aortic valve long-axis imaging plane demonstrating the aortic root. It includes the annulus (*1*), aortic valve leaflets (*2*), coronary sinuses (*3*), sinotubular junction (*4*), and ascending aorta (*5*).

arterial junction. The three cusps are referred to as right coronary, left coronary, and NCCs based on the coronary ostium associated with the cusp (Fig. 4.17).

The cusps are of similar but not equal sizes. Corresponding with each cusp of the aortic valve, the aortic root is expanded forming the three sinuses of Valsalva. The sinuses of Valsalva are defined inferiorly by the attachments of the aortic valve leaflets and superiorly by the sinotubular junction (Figs. 4.18 to 4.20). The sinotubular junction is thicker than the adjacent sinuses and is circular, defining the beginning of the aorta proper. The thickness and circular nature of the sinotubular junction play an important role in supporting the aortic valve leaflets. Dilation of the sinotubular junction can cause aortic insufficiency and may be a contraindication for placing a stentless aortic valve. The interleaflet triangles are the portion of the aortic root between the attachments of the aortic valve leaflets along the annulus fibrosus and the plane defined by the three bases of the aortic annulus (18). These interleaflet triangles, although part of the

aortic root, are exposed to left ventricular pressures in that they lay below the basal attachment of the aortic leaflets. Understanding the anatomic relationships of the aortic root to other cardiac structures is critical when evaluating abnormal cardiac shunts and fistulas (Table 4.3). Measurement of the diameter of the annular base of the aortic valve, sinus of Valsalva, sinotubular junction, and ascending aorta provides important data for surgical decision making (Figs. 4.18, 4.19, and 4.20) (18).

CORONARY ANATOMY

The left main and right coronary arteries (RCA) supplying the heart arise from ostia in the left sinus of Valsalva and right sinus of Valsalva, respectively. The left main coronary artery then divides into the LAD coronary artery and the circumflex coronary artery. At the base of the heart, the RCA and circumflex artery form a circle around the heart in the AV groove. A long-axis

TABLE 4.3	Relationship of Various Portions of the Aortic Root to Surrounding Structures
Portion of aortic root	Related structure
Noncoronary sinus	Left and right atriums, transverse sinus
Right coronary sinus	Right atrium, free pericardial space
Left coronary sinus	Left atrium, free pericardium
Noncoronary/right coronary interleaflet triangle (membranous septum)	Right atrium, conduction system, septal leaflet of tricuspid valve, RV
Right/left coronary interleaflet triangle	Potential space between aorta and pulmonary trunk or infundibulum
Left/noncoronary interleaflet triangle (subaortic curtain)	Left atrium, makes up large portion of the aortic leaflet of the mitral valve

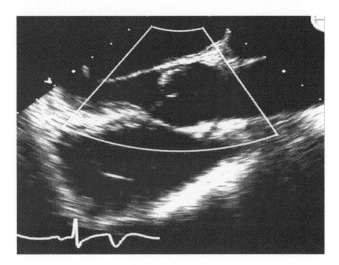

Figure 4.20. Schematic representation of four levels of aortic root where measurements are taken.

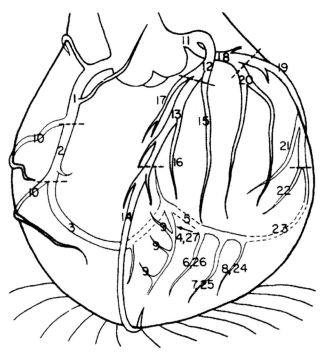

Figure 4.21. Diagram of the anatomic segments of the coronary arteries for use in locating lesions in individual patients. Proximal, mid, and distal portions of the right coronary artery (*1, 2, 3*). Posterior descending coronary artery, which as the dotted segments proximal to it indicate, may arise from the right (*4*) or left (*27*) system (*4, 27*). Right posterolateral segment (*5*), an extension of the right coronary artery in association with right dominant systems (*6, 7, 8*). From it come several inferior surface (marginal) branches, called right posterolateral arteries, to the back of the LV. Left dominant systems have a comparable left posterolateral segment, leading to the posterior descending artery (*9*). Acute marginal branches of the coronary artery (*10*). Left main coronary artery (*11*). Proximal, mid, and distal portions of the LAD coronary artery (*12, 13, 14*). First and second diagonal branches (*15, 16*). The first diagonal may originate almost from the bifurcation of the left main coronary artery and was formerly called a ramus intermedius. Additional diagonal branches may be present. First septal branch of the anterior descending artery (*17*). The proximal and distal portions of the left circumflex coronary artery (*18, 19*). The first, second, and third obtuse marginal branches of the circumflex artery, the first is usually the largest vessel (*20, 21, 22*). An extension of the circumflex artery, called the left AV artery, present only in patients with a left dominant system (*23*). In such patients, this vessel gives off further inferior surface ("marginal") branches to the back of the LV, now called left posterolateral arteries (*24, 25, 26*), before terminating in the left posterior descending coronary artery (*27*). (From the National heart, Lung, and Blood Institute Coronary Artery Surgery Study (CASS), and the American Heart Association, Inc., with permission.)

loop is formed by the LAD and the posterior descending coronary artery (Fig. 4.21) (19). The posterior descending artery originates as a termination of the right coronary and/or circumflex coronary artery. The term *dominance* in regard to the coronary circulation defines which of these two vessels terminate to form the posterior descending artery (PDA). A right dominant circulation is one in which the PDA is formed as a termination of the RCA. A left dominant coronary circulation is one where the PDA is formed as a branch of the circumflex coronary artery. Right dominance occurs in 85% of hearts, whereas left dominance occurs in about 10% to 15% of hearts. Vessels may be codominant, if the right coronary gives rise only to the posterior descending artery and the circumflex to vessels supplying the posterior LV. The left main coronary artery originates from an ostium in the left sinus of Valsalva. The left main coronary artery bifurcates into the LAD artery and the circumflex coronary artery. Occasionally, an additional branch comes off that parallels the diagonal arteries of the LAD artery. Such a branch off the left main is called the *ramus intermedius.*

The LAD coronary artery originates from the left main and travels along the anterior interventricular sulcus to the apex of the heart. In most cases, the artery extends to the posterior aspect of the heart communicating with the posterior descending artery. The LAD sends large septal perforating arteries perpendicularly into the interventricular septum. Diagonal branches of the LAD course obliquely between the LAD and circumflex artery supplying the left ventricular free wall anteriorly and laterally. The LAD supplies a few small branches to the right ventricular free wall. The left circumflex coronary artery originates from the left main coronary artery and then travels along the left atrial ventricular groove on the left, coursing posteriorly, and supplies the posterior segment of the LV. Obtuse marginal branches of the

circumflex anterior supply the obtuse margin of the LV. In left dominant circulation, the circumflex provides left posterolateral (marginal) arteries to the inferior portion of the LV.

The right coronary originates from an ostium in the right sinus of Valsalva. Traveling in the right AV

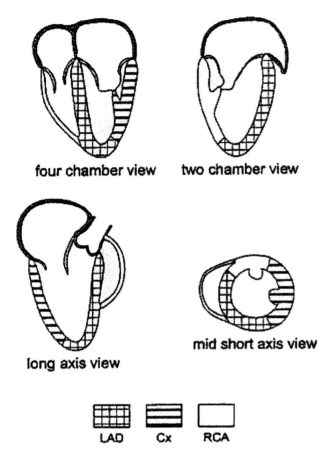

Figure 4.22. Typical regions of myocardium perfused by each of the major coronary arteries to the LV. Other patterns occur as a result of normal anatomic variations or coronary disease with collateral flow. LAD, left anterior descending; cx, circumflex; RCA, right coronary artery.

The circumflex artery supplies the basal, mid, and apical lateral segments and the basal and mid posterior segments. In hearts that have a left dominant circulation, the circumflex gives rise to the posterior descending artery supplying both the inferior wall, the inferior third of the septum, and the AV node. In addition, it provides blood supply to the posteromedial PPM and portions of the posterior fascicle of the left bundle. The proximal left circumflex supplies the sinoatrial node in 65% of hearts.

The RCA in right dominant circulations provides basal, mid, and apical inferior segments of the LV (Fig. 4.22). In addition, in right dominant systems (85% of patients), the RCA provides blood supply for the inferior one third of the septum and is the origin of the AV node artery.

CONCLUSION

It has been the purpose of this discussion to familiarize the echocardiographer with the cardiovascular anatomy, which is essential for utilizing ultrasound in the perioperative management of patients. We have reviewed cardiac structure from the fibrous skeleton to a detailed examination of the cardiac valves. This discussion will serve as the basis for a fuller understanding of three-dimensional cardiac structure and enable a more capable provision of the critical information that will guide the management of the patient's clinical course.

groove, the RCA gives off branches to the anterior right ventricular free wall. Traveling in the region of the acute margin of the RV, the RCA gives off acute marginal branches, which course to the apex of the heart. In right dominant circulations, the RCA courses posteriorly, terminating by bifurcating into the posterior descending and right posterolateral segment artery. The posterior descending artery travels in the posterior interventricular sulcus, giving rise to septal, right ventricular, and left ventricular branches. The right posterolateral segment artery gives rise to marginal branches supplying the inferior surface of the LV.

The general areas of the left ventricular wall supplied by the coronary arteries have been summarized in the standard ASE/SCA Guidelines for Performing Intraoperative TEE according to the standardized 16 segmental views (Fig. 4.22) (5). The LAD supplies the basal, mid, and apical septal segments; basal and mid anteroseptal segments; basal, mid, and apical anterior segments. The LAD provides blood to the anterior two thirds of the septum. The LAD supplies conduction tissue, including the bundle of His, the right bundle branch, and the anterior fascicle of the left bundle.

KEY POINTS

- The fibrous skeleton of the heart is formed by the U-shaped cords of the aortic annulus forming the right and left trigones. From the left and right trigones, a fibrous tissue continuum extends around the left and right AV orifices, forming the annuli fibrosi of the mitral and tricuspid annuli. The mitral annuli fibrosi thins posteriorly, permitting pathologic annular dilatation and increased tension on the middle scallop of the PMVL.
- The SCA and ASE have jointly developed a 16-segment model of the LV based on the recommendations of the Subcommittee on Quantification of the ASE Standards Committee, which divides the LV into three levels (basal, mid, and apical). The base and mid levels are divided into six segments and the apex into four.
- The three leaflets of the tricuspid valve are the anterior, posterior, and septal. The anterior leaflet is usually the largest leaflet and the posterior leaflet the smallest. The valve has three commissures: anteroseptal commissure, anteroposterior commissure, and posteroseptal commissure.

■ The pulmonic annulus and valve are attached to the base of the aorta by a fibrous extension of the aortic root called the *tendon of conus*.

■ The mitral valve apparatus consists of the fibrous skeleton of the heart, the mitral annulus, mitral leaflets, mitral chordae, and the PPM-ventricular wall complex. There are three nomenclatures used to describe the apparatus: anatomic terminology, SCA/ASE (Carpentier) terminology, and Duran terminology.

■ The aortic root is comprised of the aortic annulus, valve leaflets, sinuses of Valsalva, and sinotubular junction. Pathologic distortion of any of these components may result in aortic-valve dysfunction.

■ The aortic valve has three coronary cusps (right, left, and noncoronary) with corresponding expanded sinuses inferiorly defined by attachment of the leaflet and the sinotubular junction.

■ The heart is supplied by three coronary arteries: the LAD, the circumflex (LCx), and the right coronary artery (RCA). The LAD supplies the anterior two thirds of the interventricular septum, anterolateral free wall of the LV, and the infranodal conduction system (Bundle of His, right bundle branch, and left anterior fascicle). The LCx supplies the posterior and inferior (7% of patients) wall of the LV and portions of the posterior fascicle of the left bundle branch (LBB). It also supplies the posteromedial PPM. The RCA supplies the RV and the inferior LV (in 85% of patients) in addition to the AV node. Myocardial ischemia produces regional wall-motion abnormalities and dysrhythmias that may be predicted on the basis of coronary circulation.

REFERENCES

1. Zimmerman J, Bailey CP. The surgical significance of the fibrous skeleton of the heart. *J Thorac Cardiovasc Surg* 1962;44: 701–712.
2. Kunzelman KS, Reimink MS, Cochran RP. Annular dilation increases stress in the mitral valve and delays coaptation: a finite element computer model. *Cardiovasc Surg* 1997;5(4):427–434.
3. Lee KS, Stewart WJ, Lever HM, et al. Mechanism of outflow tract obstruction causing failed mitral valve repair. *Circulation* 1993;88(Pt 2):24–29.
4. Mihaileanu S, Mariono JP, Chauvaud S, et al. Left ventricular outflow obstruction after mitral repair (Carpentier's technique): proposed mechanism of disease. *Circulation* 1988;78(Suppl. 1):I-78–I-84.
5. Maslov AD, Regan MM, Haering JM, et al. Echocardiographic predictors of left ventricular outflow tract obstruction and systolic anterior motion of the mitral valve after mitral valve reconstruction for myxomatous disease. *J Am Coll Cardiol* 1999;34:2096–2104.
6. Walmsley R, Watson H. The outflow tract of the left ventricle. *Br Heart J* 1966;28:435–447.
7. Shanewise JS, Cheung AT, Aronson S, et al. ASE/SCA for performing a comprehensive multiplane transesophageal echocardiography council for intraoperative echocardiography and the Society of Cardiovascular Anesthesiologist task force for certification in perioperative transesophageal echocardiography. *J Am Soc Echocardiogr* 1999;12:884–900.
8. Silver MD, Lam JHC, Ranganathan N, et al. Morphology of the human tricuspid valve. *Circulation* 1971;43:33–48.
9. Carpentier AF, Lessana A, Relland JYM, et al. The "physio-ring": an advanced concept in mitral valve annuloplasty. *Ann Thorac Surg* 1995;60:1177–1186.
10. Kumar N, Kumar M, Duran CMG. A revised terminology for recording surgical findings of the mitral valve. *J Heart Valve Dis* 1995;4:70–75.
11. Bollen BA, Lou HH, Oury JH, et al. A systematic approach to intraoperative transesophageal echocardiographic evaluation of the mitral valve with anatomic correlation. *J Cardiothorac Vasc Anesth* 2000;14(3):330–338.
12. Lam JHC, Ranganathan N, Wigle ED, et al. Morphology of the human mitral valve. II. The valve leaflets. *Circulation* 1970;41:459–467.
13. Lam JHC, Ranganathan N, Wigle ED, et al. Morphology of the human heart valve. I. Chordae tendineae: a new classification. *Circulation* 1970;41:449–458.
14. DePlessis LA, Marchand P. The anatomy of the mitral valve and its associated structures. *Thorax* 1964;19:221–227.
15. Silverman ME, Hurst JW. The mitral complex. Interaction of the anatomy, physiology, and pathology of the mitral annulus, mitral valve leaflets, chordae tendineae, and papillary muscles. *Am Heart J* 1968;3:399–418.
16. Rusted IE, Schiefly CH, Edwards JE. Studies of the mitral valve. I. Anatomical features of the normal mitral valve and associated structures. *Circulation* 1952;6:825–831.
17. Voci P, Bilotta F, Caretta Q, et al. Papillary muscle perfusion pattern: a hypothesis for ischemic papillary muscle dysfunction. *Circulation* 1995;91:1714–1718.
18. Kirkland JW, Barratt-Boyes BG. *Cardiac Surgery*. New York: John Wiley and Sons, 1986:19.
19. Principal Investigators of CASS and Their Associates. The National Heart, Lung, and Blood Institute Coronary Artery Surgery Study (CASS). *Circulation* 1981;62(Suppl. 1):793–802.

QUESTIONS

1. The right fibrous trigone is adjacent to which anatomic structure?
   A. Middle scallop of the PMVL
   B. Aortic valve left coronary cusp (LCC)
   C. Posteromedial commissure (PMC)
   D. The medial base of the anterior mitral valve leaflet (AMVL)

2. Which of the following best characterizes the shape of the mitral annulus during systole?
   A. Saddle-shaped circle
   B. Planar-shaped circle
   C. Saddle-shaped ellipse
   D. Circular-shaped ellipse

3. The thinnest portion of the annulus fibrosa is located adjacent to
   A. Middle base of AMVL
   B. Anterolateral commissure (ALC)
   C. Posteromedial commissure
   D. Middle base of PMVL

4. The SCA and ASE standard nomenclature divides the apex into how many segments?
   A. One
   B. Three
   C. Four
   D. Six

5. Strut or stay chordae are thicker and originate from the anterior and posterior muscles and attach to which of the following segments of the mitral valve?
   A. Edge of the AMVL
   B. Midportion of the AMVL
   C. Lateral base of the PMVL
   D. Middle edge of the PMVL

CHAPTER 5

Comprehensive and Abbreviated Intraoperative TEE Examination

Jack S. Shanewise ■ Joyce J. Shin ■ Daniel P. Vezina ■ Michael K. Cahalan

Since its first use assessing cardiac function in the operating room over 20 years ago (1–3), transesophageal echocardiography (TEE) has come to play a critical role in the anesthetic management of patients undergoing surgery that involves the heart and great vessels. It is used as a diagnostic tool during cardiac surgery as well as a monitor of cardiac function, and many studies have shown that it has a significant impact on both the surgical care and anesthetic management these patients receive (4–7). This chapter reviews an approach to performing a comprehensive intraoperative TEE examination using a multiplane probe.

There are several good reasons to complete a comprehensive TEE examination whenever possible. One important aspect of learning TEE is to become familiar with normal and abnormal anatomy of the heart and great vessels as imaged with echocardiography. The more complete examinations performed, the more exposure there is to normal and abnormal pathology. Complete examinations also maximize exposure to the various TEE views, allowing one to become familiar with these more quickly. Performing and recording a comprehensive TEE examination at the beginning of an operation establishes a set of baseline findings. Should unexpected problems arise later in the case, this baseline record can be reviewed to determine whether subsequently noted findings are new or were preexisting. Finally, there is a small but important percentage of patients in which the comprehensive TEE examination reveals an unexpected incidental finding, which often can have an important impact on the care a patient receives. There may be situations in which the patient is unstable and a complete examination cannot be performed; in such situations, the main purpose of the TEE examination should be accomplished first so that the important issue for the case is addressed. Then, the remainder of the comprehensive examination may be completed as the situation allows.

PREVENTION OF TEE COMPLICATIONS

Although generally a very safe procedure when performed in appropriately selected patients with proper technique, TEE can, on rare occasions, result in serious complications (8,9). Therefore, every comprehensive TEE examination begins with a search for contraindications to the procedure (Table 5.1). Symptomatic esophageal stricture, esophageal diverticulum, recent esophageal surgery, and esophageal tumor are generally considered absolute contraindications to TEE. Assessment before the procedure includes a review of the medical record and an interview with the patient whenever possible. Specific questions are asked regarding the presence of dysphagia, hematemesis, and a history of esophageal disease. When a history of esophageal disease or symptoms is discovered, the relative risk of performing TEE must be balanced against the potential benefit of the procedure. The decision to proceed despite such symptoms should be documented in the medical record with an acknowledgement of the increased risk, including informed consent from the patient. Evaluation by a gastroenterologist with esophagoscopy can be helpful in assessing the risk of performing TEE.

Excessive force must never be used to insert or manipulate the probe within the esophagus. Perforation of the pharynx by TEE probe insertion and perforation of the esophagus from TEE examination have been reported (10,11) and may be more likely in elderly women, possibly due to more delicate tissue and smaller body size. Less catastrophic complications of TEE include dental and oropharyngeal trauma, mucosal injuries causing GI bleeding, and laryngeal dysfunction, possibly increasing

TABLE 5.1 Contraindications for TEE
I Absolute
Recent esophageal or gastric surgery
Symptomatic esophageal stricture
Esophageal diverticulum
Esophageal tumor or abscess
II Relative
History of mediastinal radiation
Symptomatic hiatal hernia
Coagulopathy
Unexplained upper gastrointestinal (UGI) bleed
Esophageal varices
Cervical spine disease

the risk of aspiration postoperatively (12,13). One case report also documented the displacement of an esophageal stethoscope into the stomach occurring during a TEE examination. The dislodged device was retrieved several weeks later using endoscopy (14).

INTRAOPERATIVE TEE INDICATIONS

There are three categories of indications for intraoperative TEE described by the ASA/SCA Practice Guidelines (15). Category one indications are supported by the strongest evidence in the literature and expert opinion and include hemodynamic instability and valve repair surgery. Category two indications are supported by weaker evidence in the literature and expert consensus. These include patients at risk for myocardial ischemia during surgery and operations to remove cardiac tumors. Category three indications have little scientific evidence or expert support for their use and include monitoring for emboli during orthopedic procedures and intraoperative assessment of graft patency. In judging whether intraoperative TEE is indicated in a particular situation, three factors must be considered. First are patient characteristics—specifically the presence and nature of cardiovascular disease and risk factors for complication due to TEE. Second, the surgical procedure and the role that TEE could play in facilitating its accomplishment must be considered. Finally, the availability of appropriate echocardiographic equipment and expertise in the institution where the procedure is to be formed must be considered.

OPTIMIZING IMAGE QUALITY

The settings of the echocardiography system have an important impact on the quality of the images obtained. One of the challenges of learning TEE is to know when the image has been optimized, even if it is of poor quality, and when further efforts to improve it are a waste of time. There is a fair amount of variation in the quality of echo images from patient to patient. The depth of the image is adjusted so that the entire structure of interest is included and centered in the image. General image gain and dynamic range (compression) are adjusted so that the blood in the chambers is nearly black but distinct from the gray scales of the soft tissues. Time gain controls are adjusted so that there is a uniform level of overall brightness from the near field to the far field of the image. Most TEE probes can provide images on several frequencies. Higher frequencies have better resolution but less penetration than lower frequencies, so the highest frequency with adequate penetration to provide a clear image of the structure being examined is selected. Color flow Doppler (CFD) is adjusted by increasing the gain until background noise appears in the color sector, and then decreasing it until the noise is just no longer visible. The size and position of the color sector are set

to be as small as possible but still including the entire area of interest. This helps increase the frame rate or temporal resolution of the image.

COMPREHENSIVE TEE EXAMINATION

The American Society of Echocardiography (ASE) and the Society of Cardiovascular Anesthesiologists (SCA) jointly published guidelines for performing a comprehensive intraoperative TEE examination (16,17). The guidelines describe 20 views of the heart and great vessels that include all four chambers and valves of the heart as well as the thoracic aorta and the pulmonary artery (PA) (Fig. 5.1). The order in which these views are acquired during a TEE examination may vary from person to person. The following is a description of an approach to performing a comprehensive intraoperative TEE. It is merely one example of many equally valid ways to proceed. It is usually most efficient to complete all of the midesophageal (ME) views first, proceed to the trans-gastric (TG) views, and then finish up with an examination of the thoracic aorta.

General Considerations

The process of examining cardiac structures with TEE begins with moving the transducer into the desired location, and then pointing the imaging plane in the proper direction by manipulating the probe to obtain the desired image. This is accomplished primarily by watching the image develop as the probe is manipulated rather than by relying on the depth markers of the probe or the multiplane angle icon on the screen. These markers and orientation guides can provide a general indication of the transducer location and imaging plane orientation, but final development of the image is always based on the appearance of the structures displayed in the image. There is individual variation in the anatomic relationship of the esophagus to the heart, and this relationship must be taken into consideration when performing a TEE examination. In some patients, the esophagus is lateral to the heart, while in others, it is more directly posterior to the left atrium (LA). The up-down and left-right orientation of the TEE image can be adjusted on the machine as desired. Figure 5.2 shows the image orientation recommended in the ASE/SCA guidelines.

TEE produces a two-dimensional image or cross section through the structure being examined, which exists in three dimensions in space. In order to examine each structure in its entirety, it is necessary to move the imaging plane through the three-dimensional extent of the structure by manipulating the probe. This is done for the more horizontal imaging planes (multiplane angles close to 0 and 180 degrees) by advancing and withdrawing the probe within the esophagus and for the more vertical imaging planes (multiplane angles close to 90 degrees) by turning the probe to the patient's left and right. The imaging

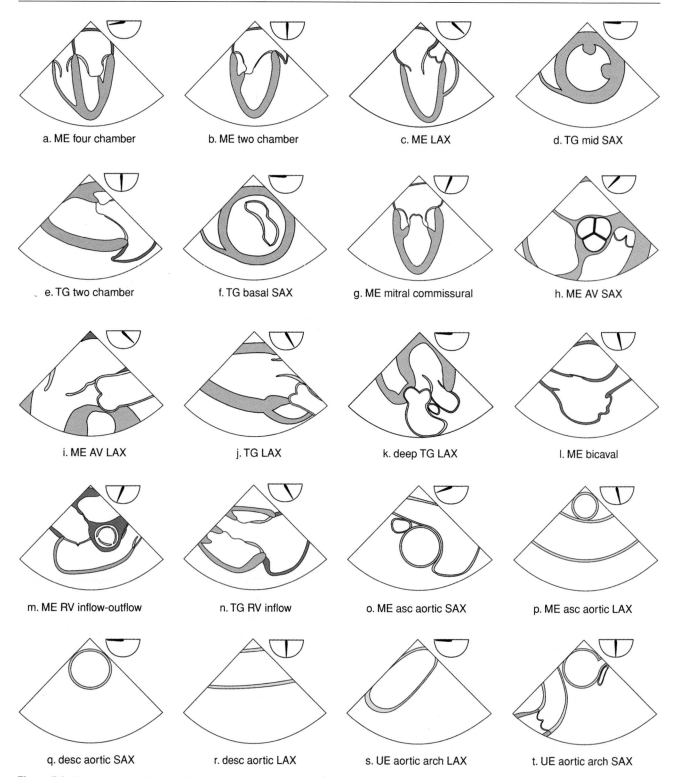

a. ME four chamber

b. ME two chamber

c. ME LAX

d. TG mid SAX

e. TG two chamber

f. TG basal SAX

g. ME mitral commissural

h. ME AV SAX

i. ME AV LAX

j. TG LAX

k. deep TG LAX

l. ME bicaval

m. ME RV inflow-outflow

n. TG RV inflow

o. ME asc aortic SAX

p. ME asc aortic LAX

q. desc aortic SAX

r. desc aortic LAX

s. UE aortic arch LAX

t. UE aortic arch SAX

Figure 5.1. Twenty Cross-Sectional Views Comprising the Recommended Comprehensive TEE Examination. Approximate multiplane angle is indicated by the icon adjacent to each view. ME, midesophageal; TG, transgastric; UE, upperesophageal; SAX, short axis; LAX, long axis; AV, aortic valve; RV, right ventricle; asc, ascending; desc, descending.

plane can also be moved through a structure by increasing or decreasing the multiplane angle while holding the probe still with the structure in the centerline of the image. It is best to focus attention on one structure at a time, following the same sequence in each study. The preferred sequence of the examination will vary from person to person, but if followed routinely it will ensure that each structure is checked on each examination. Each structure should be examined with multiple imaging planes and from more than one transducer position if possible.

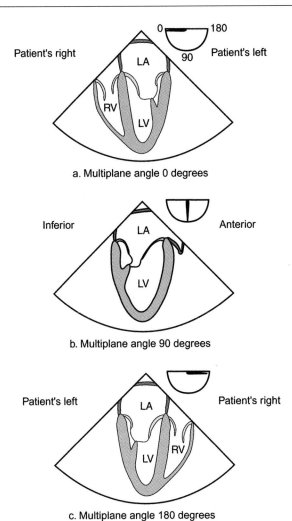

Figure 5.2. Conventions of Image Display Followed in the Guidelines. Transducer location and the near field (vertex) of the image sector are at the top of the display screen and far field at the bottom. **A:** Image orientation at multiplane angle 0 degrees. **B:** Image orientation at multiplane angle 90 degrees. **C:** Image orientation at multiplane angle 180 degrees. LA, left atrium; LV, left ventricle; RV, right ventricle.

TEE Probe Insertion

The TEE probe is inserted into the esophagus after induction of general anesthesia and tracheal intubation when used during surgery. An orogastric tube is inserted into the stomach prior to inserting the probe and suction applied to remove air or fluid that may be present in the stomach and esophagus. After the orogastric tube is removed, the TEE probe is inserted gently into the midline of the posterior pharynx while the mandible is displaced anteriorly with a jaw lift or thrust in order to lift the tongue and the glottis off the posterior pharynx. Gentle attempts to insert the probe blindly may be tried. However, if after a few attempts the probe does not pass into the esophagus, a laryngoscope is used to displace the mandible anteriorly and provide visualization that the probe is in the midline. Excessive force must never

be used, and on rare occasions the TEE probe simply will not pass into the esophagus, and the procedure must be abandoned.

TEE Probe Manipulation

After the TEE probe is inserted, it is manipulated to develop and acquire a series of images of the heart and great vessels. The following terminology is used in the ASE/SCA guidelines to describe the manipulation of the probe (Fig. 5.3). These terms are made assuming that the imaging plane is directed anteriorly from the esophagus through the heart in a patient in the standard supine anatomic position. Rotating the anterior aspect of the probe within the esophagus toward the patient's right is called "turning to the right," and rotating it toward the left is called "turning to the left." Pushing the tip of the probe more distal into the esophagus or the stomach is called "advancing the transducer," and pulling the tip more proximally is called "withdrawing." Flexing the tip of the probe with the large control wheel anteriorly is called "anteflexing," and flexing it posteriorly "retroflexing." Flexing the tip of the probe with the small control wheel to the patient's right is called "flexing to the right," and flexing it in the opposite direction is called "flexing

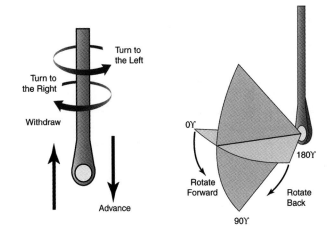

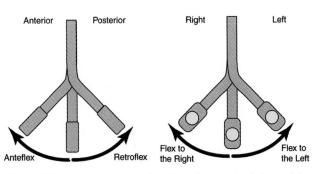

Figure 5.3. Terminology used to describe manipulation of the probe and transducer during image acquisition.

to the left." Finally, increasing the transducer multiplane angle from 0 degrees toward 180 degrees is called "rotating forward," and decreasing in the opposite direction toward 0 degrees is called "rotating back."

Left Atrium and Pulmonary Veins

The comprehensive TEE examination is started by locating the transducer at the ME level posterior to the LA. The LA is then examined from top to bottom with the multiplane angle at 0 degrees (horizontal plane) by advancing the probe until the plane passes through the floor of the LA and then withdrawing until the dome of the atrium is reached. The multiplane angle is then increased to about 90 degrees and the probe turned to the left. Near the lateral and superior aspect of the LA, the base of the left atrial appendage (LAA) is seen opening into the atrium. The LAA is examined carefully for thrombus by increasing and decreasing the multiplane angle while holding the LAA on the centerline of the image. Turning the probe to the left and withdrawing slightly identifies the left upper pulmonary vein (LUPV), which enters the LA from an anterior to posterior direction just lateral to the LAA. Pulsed wave Doppler is used to examine the LUPV flow velocity profile by placing the sample volume at least 1 cm within the vein. Advancing 1 to 2 cm and turning slightly further to the left will identify the left lower pulmonary vein (LLPV). In some patients, the LUPV and LLPV enter the LA as a single vessel. Adjusting the multiplane angle up and down will often open up the veins in the image. The right upper pulmonary vein (RUPV) is next examined by turning the probe to the right at the level of the LAA beyond the interatrial septum (IAS). Like the LUPV, the RUPV can be seen to enter the superior aspect of the LA in an anterior to posterior direction. The right lower pulmonary vein (RLPV) is then seen by turning the probe slightly to the right and advancing 1 to 2 cm.

Mitral Valve Midesophageal Views

Attention is now turned to the mitral valve (MV), which is examined with several ME views. The MV apparatus includes the anterior and posterior leaflets, annulus, chordae tendinae, papillary muscles, and left ventricle (LV) walls. The two leaflets meet at the anterolateral and posteromedial commissures, each of which is related to a corresponding papillary muscle with a similar name. The posterior leaflet anatomically consists of three scallops: lateral (P1), middle (P2), and medial (P3). For descriptive purposes, the anterior leaflet is divided into thirds: lateral third (A1), middle third (A2), and medial third (A3) (Fig. 5.4).

The first step in developing the ME views of the MV is to position the transducer posterior to the midlevel of the LA and direct the imaging plane through the middle of the mitral annulus parallel to the transmitral flow. Retroflexion of the probe tip is often necessary to achieve this

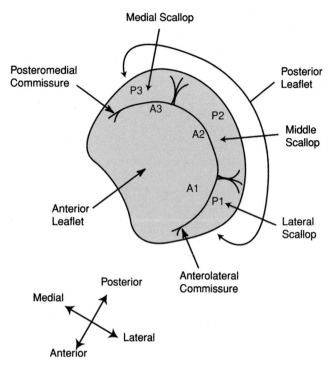

Figure 5.4. Mitral Valve Anatomy. A1, lateral third of the anterior leaflet; A2, middle third of the anterior leaflet; A3, medial third of the anterior leaflet; P1, lateral scallop of the posterior leaflet; P2, middle scallop of the posterior leaflet; P3, medial scallop of the posterior leaflet.

because the MV annulus is located inferior to the base of the heart in many patients. The multiplane angle is then increased just until the aortic valve (AV) disappears to develop the ME four-chamber view (Fig. 5.1A), usually around 10 to 20 degrees. In this view, the posterior mitral leaflet is to the right of the image display, and the anterior mitral leaflet is to the left. Because the ME four-chamber view transects the MV obliquely, it is difficult to be sure exactly which portion of the anterior and posterior leaflets is seen in a particular image. A transition in the image occurs as the multiplane angle is increased to about 60 to 80 degrees. Beyond the transition point, the anterior leaflet is to the right of the display and the posterior leaflet is to the left. At this transition angle, the imaging plane intersects both commissures of the MV simultaneously, forming the ME mitral commissural view (Fig. 5.1G). In this view, the middle third of the anterior leaflet (A2) is seen in the middle between portions of the posterior leaflet on each side; the lateral scallop (P1) to the right of the display, and the medial scallop (P3) to the left. From the ME mitral commissural view, turning the probe to the right moves the plane toward the medial or right side of the MV through the base of the anterior leaflet, and turning the probe to the left moves the plane toward the lateral side through the posterior leaflet. Next, the multiplane angle is rotated forward to between 120 and 160 degrees until the left ventricular outflow tract (LVOT), AV, and proximal ascending aorta line up in the image to develop the

ME LAX view (Fig. 5.1C). The ME LAX view, like the ME mitral commissural view, is oriented to the anatomy of the MV and is useful for identifying regions of the leaflets. In this view, the anterior mitral leaflet (middle third, A2) is to the right of the display and the posterior mitral leaflet (middle scallop, P2) is to the left. With proper orientation of the imaging plane through the center of the mitral annulus, the entire MV can be examined from the ME window without moving the probe by rotating forward from 0 to 180 degrees. CFD is applied to the ME views of the MV to detect flow disturbances such as mitral regurgitation or mitral stenosis. This is easily accomplished by rotating the multiplane angle backward from the ME LAX view through the mitral commissural and four-chamber views. The transmitral inflow velocity profile is examined with pulsed wave Doppler in the ME four-chamber view or ME LAX view by placing the sample volume between the open tips of the mitral leaflets. This is useful for assessing mitral stenosis and diastolic function of the LV.

Aortic Valve Midesophageal Views

Following examination of the MV with ME views, attention is turned to the AV, which is a semilunar valve located close to the center of the heart and with three cusps. The ME AV short-axis (SAX) view (Fig. 5.1H) is developed from the ME window by advancing or withdrawing the probe until the AV comes into view, and then turning the probe until the AV is centered in the display. The image depth is adjusted to between 10 and 12 cm until the AV is at the midlevel of the display. The multiplane angle is then rotated forward until a symmetrical image of all three cusps of the AV is seen, approximately 30 to 60 degrees. The cusp adjacent to the atrial septum is the noncoronary cusp, the cusp farthest from the probe is the right coronary cusp, and the remaining is the left coronary cusp. The imaging plane is moved superiorly through the sinuses of Valsalva by withdrawing and anteflexing the probe slightly to bring the right and left coronary ostia and then the sinotubular junction into view. The probe is then advanced by moving the imaging plane through and then under the AV annulus, showing a SAX view of the LVOT. CFD is applied to the midesophageal AV SAX view to detect flow disturbances such as aortic regurgitation and aortic stenosis.

The midesophageal AV LAX view (Fig. 5.1I) is developed by rotating the multiplane angle forward to 120–160 degrees while keeping the AV in the center of the display until the LVOT, AV, and proximal ascending aorta line up in the image. The proximal ascending aorta appears toward the right of the display and the LVOT to the left. The right coronary cusp is always toward the bottom of the display, but the cusp that appears posteriorly in this view may be the left or the noncoronary cusp depending on exactly how the imaging plane passes through the valve. This view is similar to the ME LAX view in that it shows where both left-sided valves come together but has

less depth to include only the AV. The midesophageal AV LAX view is the best view for measuring the size of the aortic root. The diameters of the AV annulus, sinuses of Valsalva, sinotubular junction, and proximal ascending aorta may be measured, adjusting the probe from side to side to maximize the internal diameter of these structures. The diameter of the AV annulus is measured during systole where the AV cusps attach to the ventricle and is normally between 1.8 and 2.5 cm. CFD is applied to the midesophageal AV LAX view to detect flow abnormalities through the LVOT, AV, and proximal ascending aorta. It is particularly useful for detecting and quantifying the severity of aortic regurgitation.

Left Ventricle Midesophageal Views

Following examination of the MV and AV with the ME views, attention is turned to the LV. Figure 5.5 illustrates the segmental model recommended in the guidelines for describing regional wall motion abnormalities as modified to comply with standards adopted by the American Heart Association in 2002 (18). Currently in clinical practice, analysis of LV regional function is based on a qualitative visual assessment of the motion and thickening of a segment during systole. The recommended qualitative grading scale for wall motion is 1 = normal (>30% thickening), 2 = mildly hypokinetic (10%–30% thickening), 3 = severely hypokinetic (<10% thickening), 4 = akinetic (does not thicken), and 5 = dyskinetic (moves paradoxically and thins during systole). The apex (apical cap, segment 17) does not include endocardium and is not usually assigned a wall motion score. All 17 segments can be examined by obtaining the three ME views of the LV. To obtain these, the transducer is again positioned behind the midlevel of the LA and the imaging plane aimed through the center of the mitral annulus and the apex of the LV. The apex is usually somewhat more inferior than the MV annulus, so the tip of the probe may need to be retroflexed to direct the imaging plane through the apex. Excessive force should never be applied, and in some patients, it may not be possible to align the imaging plane in this manner. The depth of the image is increased to include the entire apex, usually to 16 cm. Rotating the multiplane angle forward from 0 degrees to between 10 and 20 degrees until the diameter of the tricuspid annulus is maximized and the AV is no longer in view develops the ME four-chamber view (Fig. 5.1A), which shows the basal, mid, and apical segments in the anterolateral wall and the inferoseptal wall. Rotating the multiplane angle forward until the right atrium (RA) and right ventricle (RV) disappear, usually about 80 to 100 degrees, develops the ME two-chamber view (Fig. 5.1B), which shows the basal, mid, and apical segments in the inferior wall and the anterior wall. Finally, by rotating the multiplane angle forward until the LVOT, AV, and the proximal ascending aorta come into view and are aligned, usually between 120 and 160 degrees, the ME LAX view (Fig. 5.1C) is developed.

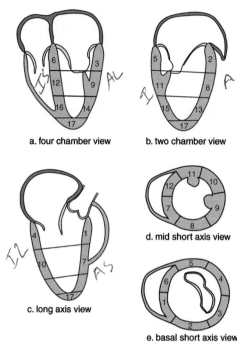

a. four chamber view   b. two chamber view

c. long axis view

d. mid short axis view

e. basal short axis view

Basal Segments	Mid Segments	Apical Segments
1= Basal Anteroseptal	7= Mid Anteroseptal	13= Apical Anterior
2= Basal Anterior	8= Mid Anterior	14= Apical Lateral
3= Basal Anterolateral	9= Mid Anterolateral	15= Apical Inferior
4= Basal Inferolateral	10= Mid Inferolateral	16= Apical Septal
5= Basal Inferior	11= Mid Inferior	17= Apex (Apical Cap)
6= Basal Inferoseptal	12= Mid Inferoseptal	

Figure 5.5. Seventeen-Segment Model of the Left Ventricle. **A:** Four-chamber view shows the three inferoseptal and three anterolateral segments and the apex (apical cap). **B:** Two-chamber view shows the three anterior and three inferior segments and the apex (apical cap). **C:** LAX view shows the two anteroseptal and two inferolateral segments and the apex (apical cap). **D:** Mid-SAX views show all six segments at the midlevel. **E:** Basal SAX views show all six segments at the basal level.

This view shows the basal and midanteroseptal segments and the basal and midinferolateral segments. As with the MV, the entire LV can be examined by simply rotating forward from 0 to 180 degrees without moving the probe, if the imaging plane is properly oriented through the center of the mitral annulus and the LV apex.

Right Heart Midesophageal Views

Following examination of the LV, attention is directed to the RV. Examination of the RV begins with the ME four-chamber view. From there, the probe is turned to the right until the tricuspid valve (TV) is in the center of the display. The image depth is adjusted to include the tricuspid annulus and RV apex. In this view, the apical portion of the anterior RV free wall is to the right of the display and the basal anterior free wall to the left. Next, the ME RV inflow-outflow view (Fig. 5.1M) is obtained by increasing the multiplane angle to between 60 and 90 degrees while keeping the TV visible until the right

ventricular outflow tract (RVOT), pulmonic valve (PV), and main PA come into view and are aligned. This view shows the RVOT to the right side of the display and the inferior (diaphragmatic) portion of the RV free wall to the left. The TV apparatus includes three leaflets (anterior, posterior, and septal), namely, annulus, chordae tendinae, papillary muscles, and RV walls and is examined with the views used to examine the RV. In the ME four-chamber view, the TV is seen with the septal leaflet to the right of the display and the posterior or anterior leaflet to the left, depending on the exact orientation of the imaging plane. The probe is advanced and withdrawn to move the imaging plane through the tricuspid annulus from its inferior to superior extent. Next, the multiplane angle is rotated forward keeping the tricuspid annulus in the center of the display to develop the ME RV inflow-outflow view. In this view, the anterior leaflet of the TV is to the right side of the display and the posterior leaflet to the left. CFD is applied to these views to detect flow abnormalities of the TV. The PV is seen to the right of the display in LAX in the ME RV inflow-outflow view. The PV is a trileaflet, semilunar valve, like the AV. Its leaflets, however, are more difficult to image with TEE because they are thinner and farther from the esophagus. Views of the PV are repeated with CFD to detect regurgitation or stenosis.

Examination of the RA begins with the ME four-chamber view, which allows direct comparison of its size to the LA. The probe is turned to the right to bring the RA into the center of the display and the depth of the image adjusted to maximize the size of the RA in the display. The probe is then advanced and withdrawn to show the atrium in its entire inferior to superior extent. The superior vena cava (SVC) and inferior vena cava (IVC) are examined from the ME four-chamber view by withdrawing or advancing the probe from their junctions with the RA to their more proximal portions. The coronary sinus is shown next by identifying it along the posterior surface of the heart in the atrioventricular groove as it empties into the RA at the most inferior and posterior extent of the atrial septum adjacent to the septal leaflet of the TV. A LAX of the coronary sinus may be developed from the ME four-chamber view by slightly advancing or retroflexing the probe to move the imaging plane through the floor of the LA.

Increasing the multiplane transducer angle forward until the IVC in the left side of the display and the SVC appears in the right side (usually between 80 and 110 degrees) develops the ME bicaval view (Fig. 5.1L). The right atrial appendage, extending superiorly from the anterior aspect of the RA, is seen in this view (Fig. 5.1L). The right atrial appendage, extending from the anterior, superior aspect of the RA, is also seen in this view. The imaging of the RA is completed by turning the probe to the left and the right through the lateral to the medial extent of the atrium.

The IAS is shown through its entire medial-lateral extent with the ME bicaval view by turning the probe to the right and left. The IAS has a thin region centrally called the "fossa ovalis" and thicker regions called the "limbus," anteriorly and posteriorly. To detect interatrial shunts, CFD is applied to the IAS. Low velocity flow through an atrial septal defect or a patent foramen ovale (PFO) may be more easily detected if the scale (Nyquist limit) of the CFD is decreased to about 30 cm/s. Another way to detect right to left interatrial shunting is to inject agitated saline into the RA as positive airway pressure is released. The appearance of contrast in the LA in less than five cardiac cycles indicates the presence of an interatrial shunt.

Left Ventricle Transgastric Views

The TG views of the LV are developed by advancing the probe into the stomach and anteflexing the tip until the heart comes into view. At a multiplane angle of 0 degrees, the SAX view of the LV will be seen, and the probe is then turned as needed to the left or right to center the LV in the display. The depth of the image is set to include the entire LV, usually 12 cm. Next, to facilitate final positioning of the probe the multiplane angle is increased to 90 degrees to show a view of the LV with the apex to the left and the mitral annulus to the right of the display. The probe is advanced or withdrawn as needed to position the transducer at the midpapillary level and the anteflexion of the probe adjusted until the LAX of the LV is horizontal in the display. The multiplane angle is decreased to between 0 and 20 degrees until the circular symmetry of the chamber is maximized to obtain the TG mid-SAX view (Fig. 5.1D). This view is the most popular view for monitoring LV function because it simultaneously shows regions of the LV supplied by the right, circumflex, and left anterior descending coronary arteries. It can be used to measure LV chamber size and wall thickness at end diastole. Normal LV wall thickness is less than 1.2 cm and LV SAX diameter less than 5.5 cm. Calculation of fractional area change as an index of LV systolic function may be performed in this view by measuring the end diastolic and end systolic areas of the chamber. Rotating the multiplane angle forward to approximately 90 degrees until the apex and the mitral annulus come into view develops the TG two-chamber view (Fig. 5.1E). The length of the displayed LV image is maximized by turning the probe as needed to the left or right. This view displays the basal and mid segments of the inferior and anterior walls. The apex of the LV is often not visible in the TG two-chamber view. It is useful for examining the chordae tendinae, which are perpendicular to the ultrasound beam in this view. The chordae to the anterolateral papillary muscle are at the bottom of the display and those to the posteromedial papillary muscle are at the top.

Mitral Valve Transgastric Views

Withdrawing the probe from the TG mid-SAX view until the MV appears develops the TG basal SAX view (Fig. 5.1F), which shows all six basal segments of the LV. The TG basal SAX view shows a SAX view of the MV. Advancing the transducer slightly deeper into the stomach with more anteflexion in order to align the imaging plane as parallel as possible to the mitral annulus may improve the SAX view of the MV. If the cross section obtained is not perfectly parallel to the annulus, which is often the case, the probe may be withdrawn to image the posteromedial commissure and then advanced to image the anterolateral commissure. In these views of the MV, the anterolateral commissure is in the far field to the right of the display, the posteromedial commissure in the near field to the left. The anterior leaflet is to the left of the display and the posterior leaflet to the right. These views of the MV are very useful for localizing leaflet abnormalities. CFD applied to the TG basal SAX view can be used to determine the location of a regurgitant orifice in patients with MR.

Right Heart Transgastric Views

In the TG mid-SAX view, the RV is seen to the left side of the display from the LV. The TG RV inflow view (Fig. 5.1N) is developed by turning the probe to the right to center RV cavity in the display and then rotating the multiplane angle forward to between 100 and 120 degrees until the apex of the RV appears in the left side of the display. This view provides good views of the inferior (diaphragmatic) portion of the RV free wall, located in the near field. In some patients, images of the RVOT and PV can be developed from the TG RV inflow view by decreasing the multiplane angle toward 0 degrees and anteflexing the probe. The TV is also seen in the TG RV inflow view with the RA to the right of the display and the RV to the left, and CFD is applied to detect flow abnormalities. It also usually shows the best images of the tricuspid chordae tendinae because they are perpendicular to the ultrasound. A SAX view of the TV can be developed by withdrawing the probe slightly toward the base of the heart until the tricuspid annulus is centered in the display and decreasing the multiplane angle to about 30 degrees. In this view, the posterior leaflet of the TV is in the near field to the left, the anterior leaflet is in the far field to the left and the septal leaflet to the right side of the display. CFD is applied to these views to detect flow disturbances.

Aortic Valve Transgastric Views

The primary use of the two TG views of the AV is to make Doppler measurements of the flow through the LVOT and AV. ME views cannot be used for this purpose because this flow is perpendicular to the Doppler beam from the ME window. Transgastric views of the AV also provide images of the ventricular aspect of the valve in some patients. The TG LAX view (Fig. 5.1J) is obtained from the TG mid-SAX view by rotating the multiplane angle forward to 90–120 degrees until the AV comes into view in the far field to the right side of the display. Turning the probe slightly to the right may help to bring the AV and LVOT into view in some cases.

To develop the deep TG view of the AV, the probe is advanced deep into the stomach from the TG mid-SAX view and positioned adjacent to the LV apex. The probe is then anteflexed until the imaging plane is oriented toward the base of the heart producing the deep TG LAX view (Fig. 5.1K). Deep in the stomach the exact position of the probe and transducer is more difficult to determine and control, but some trial and error turning, flexing, withdrawing, advancing, and rotating of the probe develop this view in most patients. The AV is located at the bottom of the display in the far field in the deep TG LAX view, with the LV outflow directed away from the transducer. Doppler quantification of flow velocities through the LVOT and the AV is usually possible with one or the other of these views in most patients, but detailed images of the valve anatomy are difficult to obtain because it is so far from the transducer. Flow velocity through the AV is measured by aiming the continuous wave Doppler beam through the LVOT across the valve. Normal peak AV flow velocity is less than 1.5 m/s. Positioning the pulsed wave Doppler sample volume just proximal to the AV in the center of the LVOT allows the blood flow velocity in the LVOT to be measured. Normal peak LVOT flow velocity is less than 1.2 m/s. Using CFD to image the flow through the LVOT and AV may facilitate directing the Doppler beam through the area of maximum flow.

TEE EXAMINATION OF THE THORACIC AORTA

After finishing the TG views of the heart, the thoracic aorta is examined. The probe is withdrawn to the level of the diaphragm and turned to the patient's left at 0 degrees multiplane angle until the distal descending thoracic aorta is seen developing the descending aorta SAX view (Fig. 5.1Q). The descending thoracic aorta is examined from the diaphragm to the arch by withdrawing the probe to the aortic arch. At the level of the diaphragm, the esophagus is located anterior to the aorta. It winds around within the thorax until at the level of the distal arch it is posterior to the aorta, so as the probe is withdrawn, it is turned to the right (anteriorly) keeping the descending aorta centered in the image. It is difficult to maintain contact between the transducer and the aorta within the stomach, so the mid and distal abdominal aorta are difficult to see with TEE. The multiplane angle is rotated forward to 90 degrees to obtain the descending aorta LAX view (Fig. 5.1R), and the probe is withdrawn and advanced to examine the entire descending thoracic aorta.

It is difficult to determine anterior and posterior or right to left orientations related to the descending thoracic aorta in the TEE images because of the lack of internal anatomic landmarks and the variable relationship between it and the esophagus. One approach describing lesion locations is to record probe depth from the incisors. The presence of an adjacent structure, such as the LA or the base of the LV, may also be used to determine the level of the descending aorta being shown.

Next, the probe is withdrawn to the upper esophageal window about 20 to 25 cm from the incisors at 0 degrees multiplane angle to develop the upper esophageal aortic arch LAX view (Fig. 5.1S). The probe is turned to the right (anterior) as it is withdrawn to keep the aorta in view because the midaortic arch lies anterior to the esophagus. The distal arch is to the right of the display and the proximal arch to the left. Withdrawing the transducer above the upper esophageal aortic arch LAX view produces images of the left carotid artery and proximal left subclavian artery in some individuals. Because the trachea often lies between the proximal aorta and the esophagus, the right brachiocephalic artery is more difficult to image. The left brachiocephalic vein is also often seen anterior to the arch in these views.

Next, the upper esophageal aortic arch SAX view (Fig. 5.1T) is developed by increasing the multiplane forward to 90 degrees. With this view, the probe is turned to the right (anteriorly) to image the arch more proximally and to the left (posteriorly) to image distally. In many patients, images of the main PA and the PV can be obtained in the left side of the display by turning the probe back and forth until these structures are seen. Retroflexing the probe will often improve this view of the PV. If the PA and the PV are seen in this view, blood flow velocities through each of these structures can be measured using Doppler echocardiography. The origin of the branches of the aortic arch is often seen to the right of the display.

Finally, the comprehensive TEE examination is completed by advancing the probe to a depth of about 30 cm from the incisors placing the transducer at the level of the right PA to image the proximal and midascending aorta. The ascending aorta is positioned in the center of the image and the multiplane angle adjusted until the vessel is a circle, usually between 0 and 60 degrees, developing the ME ascending aortic SAX view (Fig. 5.1O). The probe is advanced and withdrawn to see different portions of the ascending aorta. The ME ascending aortic LAX view (Fig. 5.1P) is then developed by increasing the multiplane angle until the anterior and posterior walls of the aorta appear as two parallel, curved lines, usually between 100 and 150 degrees. The inside diameter of the ascending aorta at the sinotubular junction and the midlevel may be measured from these LAX and SAX images.

This completes the acquisition of the images for the comprehensive intraoperative TEE examination. Another abbreviated examination is usually performed immediately after cardiopulmonary bypass to check the results of the surgery and again after the chest is closed. It is important that the results of the TEE examination be reported to the surgeon and other subsequent caregivers, such as the ICU team. It is best to speak directly with the surgeon to avoid any confusion about what was and was not seen on the TEE examination. The findings should also be documented in the medical record.

ABBREVIATED TEE EXAMINATION

Because of time constraints and relatively narrow diagnostic goals, anesthesiologists often perform a more limited intraoperative examination than described in the ASE/SCA's task force recommendation for a comprehensive TEE examination (see previous section) (16,17). However, even when time is critical, the examination performed should allow at least the basic applications of TEE as outlined in the 1996 guidelines for perioperative TEE: to detect markedly abnormal ventricular filling or function, extensive myocardial ischemia or infarction, large air embolism, severe valvular dysfunction, large cardiac masses or thrombi, large pericardial effusions, and major lesions of the great vessels (15). A minimum of eight different cross sections, drawn from the 20 cross sections delineated in the comprehensive examination, are required to meet these diagnostic goals. Four of the cross sections are imaged in both two-dimensional and color Doppler to assess valvular function. The next paragraph will describe the probe manipulations required to achieve these cross sections. The reader should review Figure 5.1 to understand the terms used in this description (16).

Probe Manipulations and Examination Sequence

After the TEE probe is introduced safely into the esophagus, it is advanced to the ME level (28–32 cm measured at the upper incisors), and the AV is imaged in the SAX by turning the probe, adjusting its depth in the esophagus, and rotating the multiplane transducer to 25–45 degrees until the three cusps of the valve are seen as approximately equal in size and shape (Fig. 5.1H). Image depth is set to 10–12 cm as required to position the AV in the center of the video screen. This cross section is ideal for detection of aortic stenosis. The videotape is activated at this point and kept running throughout the rest of the examination. Videotape is very inexpensive relative to the cost of a missed diagnosis. Next, the probe is turned slightly to position the AV in the center of the video screen, and then the multiplane angle is rotated forward to 110–130 degrees to bring the LAX of the AV in view (Fig. 5.1I). This cross section is best for detection of ascending aortic abnormalities including type I aortic dissection. Color Doppler is used for assessment of AV competence. For detection of valvular stenosis and regurgitation, the maximum possible Nyquist limit is used (ideally above 50 cm/s). Next, the color Doppler is discontinued and the probe is turned rightward until the ME bicaval cross section comes into view (Fig. 5.1L). This cross section is seen best usually at a multiplane angle between 90 and 110 degrees and is ideal for assessing caval abnormalities, as well as compression of the RA from anteriorly located masses or effusions and the LA from posteriorly located masses

or effusions. In addition, the bicaval cross section may reveal collections of air located anteriorly in the left or RA, as well as the structure of the IAS including the foramen ovale. Next, the multiplane angle is rotated back to 60–80 degrees and the probe is turned leftward, just past the AV, to bring the ME RV inflow and outflow cross section into view (Fig. 5.1M). Usually, an image depth of 12 to 14 cm is required to position the RV outflow track in the center of the video screen. This cross section reveals the contractile function of the RV, the outflow tract, as well as the pulmonary valve function with the application of color Doppler. Next, the transducer is rotated back to 0 degrees, the probe advanced 4 to 6 mm into the esophagus, and gently retroflexed until all four cardiac chambers are visualized (ME four-chamber) (Fig. 5.1A). Often, rotating the transducer 10 to 15 degrees will enhance the view of the tricuspid annulus. Usually, an image depth of 14 to 16 cm is required to include the LV apex in the sector scan. In two-dimensional imaging, the free wall of the RV and the anterolateral and inferoseptal wall segments are evaluated for contractile function. With color Doppler, both the MV and TV are assessed. Stenotic and regurgitant lesions can be diagnosed accurately. During this assessment, the image depth is decreased to 10–12 cm to afford a magnified view of the valves and maximization of the Nyquist limits (above 50 cm/s). Next, color Doppler is discontinued, the LV is positioned in the center of the screen, and the multiplane angle is rotated forward to 90 degrees to bring into view the ME two-chamber cross section (Fig. 5.1B). The image depth is returned to 14–16 cm. This cross section is best for revealing the function of the basal and apical segments of the anterior and inferior LV walls as well as anterior and inferior pericardial collections. When air emboli collect in the LV, they can be seen best usually in this view as very echogenic areas, located along the anterior apical endocardial surface. Then, the transducer is rotated forward to 135 degrees to reveal the ME LAX cross section that is best for assessment of the anteroseptal and inferolateral wall segments for contractile LV function (Fig. 5.1C). Together, the ME four-chamber, two-chamber, and LAX cross sections reveal all 17 segments of the LV (Fig. 5.5). However, the next and last of the basic cross sections provide a second look at the mid-ventricular segments as well as other benefits. To achieve this cross section, the transducer is rotated back to 0 degrees, the LV is centered in the screen and the probe advanced 4 to 6 cm into the stomach. Then, it is flexed gently anteriorly to reveal the TG SAX cross section (Fig. 5.1D). This cross section is ideal for monitoring LV filling and contractile function. All major coronary arteries supplying the myocardium are viewed in this cross section. Moreover, changes in preload cause greater changes in the LV SAX than in the LAX dimension, and movement of the probe from this cross section is readily apparent because the papillary muscles provide prominent landmarks. Since this cross section is used to judge filling and ejection, image depth is consistently set to 12 cm so that the size and function of the heart are judged easily relative to previously examined hearts.

Limitations

The abbreviated examination has significant limitations that must be appreciated. Clearly, it is an insufficient examination for the quantitative evaluation of hemodynamics, comprehensive valvular assessment, detection of flawed cardiac repairs, and other advanced TEE applications. Advanced applications of perioperative TEE should not be provided based on the abbreviated examination alone. Instead, the abbreviated examination is viewed best as serving two needs: first, as an emergency tool for the very rapid detection of life-threatening cardiac problems not diagnosed readily with other less invasive perioperative techniques; and second, as the minimum examination of basic perioperative TEE practitioners, who recognize the limitations of this examination and seek appropriate consultation when advanced TEE applications are required (19).

TEE AND NONCARDIAC SURGERY

Perioperative TEE Indications for Noncardiac Surgery

As previously outlined by the ASA practice guidelines, the category I indications (support by the strongest evidence or expert opinion) of TEE in noncardiac surgical circumstances are acute, persistent, and life-threatening hemodynamic disturbances. The use of TEE for monitoring myocardial ischemia or infarction is supported by

weaker evidence and expert consensus (i.e., a category II indication).

Basic Perioperative TEE Examination for Noncardiac Surgery

Currently, there are 20 cross-sectional views comprising the recommended comprehensive TEE examination (Fig. 5.1). Of these, seven cross-sectional views can be utilized to perform a basic TEE examination for noncardiac surgery (Table 5.2).

As with any TEE examination, assessment of the patient must be made prior to TEE probe insertion. Contraindications for TEE should be actively sought and if any concerns are detected, these should be discussed with the patient followed by documenting in the medical record with an acknowledgement of the increased risk, including informed consent from the patient. The Task Force on Perioperative TEE recommends two levels of training: basic and advanced. These refer to specialized training that extends beyond the minimum exposure to TEE that occurs during normal anesthesia residency training. Anesthesiologists with basic training are able to use TEE for indications that lie within the customary practice of anesthesiology. Those with advanced training are, in addition to the above, able to exploit the full diagnostic potential of perioperative TEE.

With basic training emphasizing monitoring rather than making specific diagnoses, when an anesthesiologist with basic training encounters TEE findings that require intraoperative cardiac surgical intervention or postoperative medical/surgical management, except in an emergency, consultation with a physician with advanced skills in perioperative TEE must be sought in a timely manner. Basic and advanced proficiency levels relative to specific conditions are discussed in the ASA/SCA Practice Guidelines and summarized in Table 5.3.

TABLE 5.2	Seven Cross-Sectional Views for the Basic Perioperative TEE Examination for Noncardiac Surgery	
Cross-sectional views	**Examinations**	
ME four chamber	LV, RV, LA, RA, MV (+CFD), TV (+CFD), IAS (+CFD)	
ME two chamber	LV, LA, LAA, MV (+CFD), PV inflow velocity profile	
ME LAX	LV, LA, MV (+CFD), AV (+CFD), mitral inflow velocity profile	
TG mid SAX	LV, RV	
ME RV inflow-outflow	RV, RA, TV (+CFD), PV (+CFD), AV (+CFD), TR velocity profile	
Desc aortic SAX	Descending aorta from diaphragm to arch, left pleural space	
UE aortic arch LAX	Aortic arch	

AV, aortic valve; CFD, color flow doppler; Desc, Descending; IAS, interatrial septum; LA, left atrium; LAX, long axis; LV, left ventricle; ME, midesophageal; MV, mitral valve; PV, pulmonic valve; SAX, short axis; RA, right atrium; RV, right ventricle; TG, transgastric; TV, tricuspid valve; UE, upperesophageal.

TABLE 5.3	**Basic and Advanced Proficiency Levels Discussed Relative to Specific Conditions**	
	Basic Proficiency	**Advanced Proficiency**
Wall motion, myocardial ischemia, and coronary artery disease	1. Able to use TEE to detect unequivocal changes in segmental wall thickening and motion (i.e., from normal wall motion to akinesis). 2. Able to distinguish these changes in segmental wall thickening and motion from artifacts (i.e., translational motion of the heart, changing cross section, image dropout, abnormal ventricular activation).	Advanced training required to be able to evaluate or quantify subtle changes in segmental wall motion and thickening associated with myocardial ischemia and infarction.
Hemodynamic function	1. Able to make qualitative assessments of hemodynamic status. 2. Have a cognitive understanding of more sophisticated TEE techniques for quantifying hemodynamic function.	Able to make quantitative hemodynamic assessments.
Valvular surgery	1. Have an understanding of the anatomy and function of native and prosthetic valves, the hemodynamic changes that occur in valvular disease, and the echocardiographic tools (i.e., CWD) that are available for valve assessment. 2. Able to obtain multiple views of all valves, recognize gross valvular dysfunction on two-dimensional echocardiography and appreciate the color patterns of antegrade and retrograde flow on color Doppler examinations. 3. Able to detect air embolic during valve surgery.	Advanced training required to obtain quantitative echocardiographic measurements of valve function (i.e., jet area, flow velocity pattern, effective valve orifice area).
Congenital heart surgery	1. Have an understanding of how TEE is used during congenital heart surgery.	When repair of congenital heart defects will be dictated by the results of intraoperative TEE assessment, TEE should be performed by, or in timely consultation with, a physician with advanced pediatric TEE training in complex congenital heart disease.
Cardiomyopathy, cardiac aneurysms, endocarditis, foreign bodies, intracardiac thrombi, pulmonary emboli, traumatic cardiac injuries, thoracic aortic aneurysms and dissections, traumatic thoracic aortic disruption, and pericarditis		TEE should be performed by, or in timely consultation with, a physician with advanced TEE training.

(continued)

TABLE 5.3	Basic and Advanced Proficiency Levels Discussed Relative to Specific Conditions (*Continued*)	
	Basic Proficiency	**Advanced Proficiency**
Cardiac tumors	1. Able to detect large, unequivocal cardiac masses.	The use of TEE to accurately detect smaller or ill-defined masses, especially to distinguish potential masses from normal intracardiac structures, identify associated lesions, inspect IVC, and rule out iatrogenic valve injury during resection of intracardiac masses, should be performed by, or in timely consultation with, a physician with advanced TEE training.
Air emboli	1. Have an understanding of the physiologic effects of air emboli. 2. Technically capable of detecting air emboli intraoperatively, especially during upright neurosurgical procedures.	The use of intraoperative TEE to accurately detect PFO should be performed by, or in timely consultation with, a physician with advanced TEE training.
Pericardial effusion and tamponade	1. Able to detect large pericardial effusions.	Advanced training required to detect and assess hemodynamically significant effusions.
Transplant surgery	1. Able to evaluate hemodynamic disturbances (see "Hemodynamic function"). 2. Able to detect entrapped air (see "Air emboli") during transplant operations.	Advanced training required to evaluate the surgical results of transplant surgery (i.e., integrity of anastomoses).
MCS, defibrillators and catheter placement	1. Able to evaluate accurately the mechanism of hemodynamic disturbances in patients receiving MCS.	Advanced training required to monitor placement and function mechanical circulatory assistance devices.
Nonoperative CCM		Advanced training required if TEE indicated other than determining the cause of hemodynamic disturbances.

CCM, critical care medicine; CWD, continuous wave Doppler; HOCM, hypertrophic obstructive cardiomyopathy; IVC, inferior vena cava; MCS, mechanical circulatory support; PFO, patent foramen ovale; TEE, transesophageal echocardiography.

KEY POINTS

- The comprehensive perioperative TEE examination recommended by the SCA/ASE guidelines consists of 20 views.
- Develop a consistent, systematic approach to performing the comprehensive examination.
- Performing a comprehensive TEE examination whenever possible rapidly increases knowledge and skill, provides a baseline for later comparison, and is more likely to detect previously undiagnosed abnormalities.
- Screen for esophageal disease *before* inserting the TEE probe.
- *Never* apply excessive force when inserting or manipulating the TEE probe.

- Adjust image depth, overall gain, dynamic compression, time delay gain, focus, and frequency to optimize two-dimensional image quality.
- Determine the location of the TEE transducer in relation to the heart, then the orientation of the imaging as it passes through the heart.
- The imaging plane can be moved through the structure being examined by advancing and withdrawing the probe, turning (rotating) the probe to left and right, or increasing and decreasing the multiplane angle.
- The centerline of the image stays the same if the probe is not moved as the multiplane angle is changed.
- Examine each structure with multiple views.
- An abbreviated examination of eight views can achieve the basic applications of perioperative TEE more rapidly than the comprehensive.

REFERENCES

1. Matsumoto M, Oka Y, Strom J, et al. Application of transesophageal echocardiography to continuous intraoperative monitoring of left ventricular performance. *Am J Cardiol* 1980;46(1):95–105.

2. Cahalan MK, Kremer P, Schiller NB, et al. Intraoperative monitoring with two-dimensional transesophageal echocardiography. *Anesthesiology* 1982;57(3):A153.

3. Dubroff JM, Clark MB, Wong CY, et al. Left ventricular ejection fraction during cardiac surgery: a two-dimensional echocardiographic study. *Circulation* 1983;68(1):95–103.

4. Stevenson JG, Sorensen GK, Gartman DM, et al. Transesophageal echocardiography during repair of congenital cardiac defects: identification of residual problems necessitating reoperation. *J Am Soc Echocardiogr* 1993;6(4):356–365.

5. Hartman GS, Yao FS, Bruefach M III, et al. Severity of aortic atheromatous disease diagnosed by transesophageal echocardiography predicts stroke and other outcomes associated with coronary artery surgery: a prospective study. *Anesth Analg* 1996;83(4):701–708.

6. Sheikh KH, Bengtson JR, Rankin JS, et al. Intraoperative transesophageal Doppler color flow imaging used to guide patient selection and operative treatment of ischemic mitral regurgitation. *Circulation* 1991;84(2):594–604.

7. Grigg LE, Wigle ED, Williams WG, et al. Transesophageal Doppler echocardiography in obstructive hypertrophic cardiomyopathy: clarification of pathophysiology and importance in intraoperative decision making. *J Am Coll Cardiol* 1992;20(1):42–52.

8. Daniel WG, Erbel R, Kasper W, et al. Safety of transesophageal echocardiography. A multicenter survey of 10,419 examinations. *Circulation* 1991;83(3):817–821.

9. Kallmeyer IJ, Collard CD, Fox JA, et al. The safety of intraoperative transesophageal echocardiography: a case series of 7200 cardiac surgical patients. *Anesth Analg* 2001;92(5):1126–1130.

10. Spahn DR, Schmid S, Carrel T, et al. Hypopharynx perforation by a transesophageal echocardiography probe. *Anesthesiology* 1995;82(2):581–583.

11. Brinkman WT, Shanewise JS, Clements SD, et al. Transesophageal echocardiography: not an innocuous procedure. *Ann Thorac Surg* 2001;72(5):1725–1726.

12. Hogue CW Jr, Lappas GD, Creswell LL, et al. Swallowing dysfunction after cardiac operations. Associated adverse outcomes and risk factors including intraoperative transesophageal echocardiography. *J Thorac Cardio Surg* 1995;110(2):517–522.

13. Rousou JA, Tighe DA, Garb JL, et al. Risk of dysphagia after transesophageal echocardiography during cardiac operations. *Ann Thorac Surg* 2000:69(2):486–489; discussion 489–490.

14. Humphrey LS. Esophageal stethoscope loss complicating echocardiography. *J Cardiothoracic Anesth* 1988;2:356.

15. Practice guidelines for perioperative transesophageal echocardiography. A report by the American Society of Anesthesiologists and the Society of Cardiovascular Anesthesiologists Task Force on Transesophageal Echocardiography. *Anesthesiology* 1196;84(4):986–1006.

16. Shanewise JS, Cheung AT, Aronson S, et al. ASE/SCA guidelines for performing a comprehensive intraoperative multiplane transesophageal echocardiography examination: recommendations of the American Society of Echocardiography Council for Intraoperative Echocardiography and the Society of Cardiovascular Anesthesiologists Task Force for Certification in Perioperative Transesophageal Echocardiography. *Anesth Analg* 1999;89(4):870–884.

17. Shanewise JS, Cheung AT, Aronson S, et al. ASE/SCA guidelines for performing a comprehensive intraoperative multiplane transesophageal echocardiography examination: recommendations of the American Society of Echocardiography Council for Intraoperative Echocardiography and the Society of Cardiovascular Anesthesiologists Task Force for Certification in Perioperative Transesophageal Echocardiography. *J Am Soc Echocardiogr* 1999;12(10):884–900.

18. Cerqueira MD, Weissman NJ, Dilsizian V, et al. Standardized myocardial segmentation and nomenclature for tomographic imaging of the heart: a statement for healthcare professionals from the Cardiac Imaging Committee of the Council on Clinical Cardiology of the American Heart Association. [Review] [11 refs] [Consensus Development Conference. Journal Article. Review] *Circulation* 2002;105(4):539–542.

19. Miller JP, Lambert AS, Shapiro WA, et al. The adequacy of basic intraoperative transesophageal echocardiography performed by experienced anesthesiologists. *Anesth Analg* 2001;92:1103–1110.

QUESTIONS

1. What is the major use of the deep transgastric (TG) long-axis (LAX) view?
   A. Measure velocities in the left ventricular outflow tract (LVOT) and aortic valve (AV)
   B. Obtain detailed two-dimensional images of the AV
   C. Assess global left ventricular (LV) function
   D. Measure the size of the LVOT
   E. Examine the mitral chordae tendinae

2. The basal posterior segment of the LV is in which of the following transesophageal echocardiography (TEE) views?
   A. Midesophageal (ME) four-chamber
   B. ME two-chamber
   C. TG two-chamber
   D. TG mid short-axis (SAX)
   E. TG basal SAX

3. Which two ME TEE views are aligned with the anatomy of the mitral valve?
   A. Four-chamber and two-chamber
   B. Two-chamber and LAX
   C. Mitral commissural and LAX
   D. Four-chamber and mitral commissural
   E. Two-chamber and mitral commissural

4. What is the minimum number of views needed to achieve the basic perioperative TEE applications described in the 1996 guidelines?
   A. 6
   B. 8
   C. 10
   D. 15
   E. 20

CHAPTER 6

Updated Indications for Intraoperative TEE

Scott T. Reeves ∎ Daniel M. Thys

In the United States, intraoperative echocardiography (IOE) has become integral to the care of many cardiac surgical patients (1). In a 2001 survey of active members of the Society of Cardiovascular Anesthesiologists (SCA) residing in the United States or Puerto Rico, Morewood et al. (2) documented that 94% of respondents practice at institutions that use IOE. Furthermore, 72% of anesthesiologists working at such institutions responded that they personally employed transesophageal echocardiography (TEE) during anesthetic care.

IOE is widely used because it is thought to provide information that significantly influences clinical management and improves patient outcome. Although there is limited scientific evidence to substantiate such perception, several recent case series have documented the usefulness of IOE in adult cardiac surgery (3–9). Investigators have usually examined whether IOE yielded new information and how frequently the new information had an impact on anesthetic or surgical management. In adult cardiac surgery, the total number of patients included in these reports was 11,444 (Table 6.1). The incidence of new information ranged from 12.8% to 38.6%, while the impact on treatment ranged from 9.7% to 48.8%. In 1996, a task force of the American Society of Anesthesiologists/Society of Cardiovascular Anesthesiologists (ASA/SCA) published practice guidelines for perioperative TEE (10). In 2000, Couture et al. (4) prospectively evaluated the relative impact of each ASA

category–based TEE indication in 851 cardiac surgical patients. The nature of the clinical impact included modification of medical therapy (53%), modification of planned surgical intervention (30%), and confirmation of a diagnosis (30%). Couture concluded that the ASA practice guidelines were useful in demonstrating a greater impact of TEE on clinical management for category I versus category II patients.

As in adult cardiac surgery, the use of IOE has become routine in many pediatric cardiac surgery centers. While epicardial echocardiography was used most commonly in the early years, the use of TEE has increased with the development of smaller TEE probes. Several recent studies have documented the utility of intraoperative TEE, particularly for the detection of residual defects after cardiopulmonary bypass (CPB) in pediatric cardiac surgery (10–15). These reviews reported on a total of 2,589 cases. The detection of significant residual defects after CPB ranged from 4.4% to 14.4% (Table 6.2).

Because of their retrospective nature, most of these reports do not withstand rigorous scientific scrutiny. Nonetheless, they confirm the clinical opinion that IOE provides new information on cardiac pathology in a significant number of patients and that the new information results in frequent management changes. Most physicians who care for cardiac surgical patients believe these benefits to be real and have adopted the technique in their clinical practice.

TABLE 6.1 The Usefulness of IOE in Adult Cardiac Surgery		
Number of Patients	New Information	Change in Management
3,245 (3)	15%	14%
851 (4)	—	14.6%
203 (5)	12.8%	10.8%
5,016 (6)	22.9%	—
238 (7)	38.6%	9.7%
1,891 (8)	—	48.8%

TABLE 6.2 The Usefulness of IOE in Pediatric Cardiac Surgery	
Number of Patients	Residual Defects
86 (9)	12.8%
200 (10)	10.5%
667 (11)	6.6%
1,000 (12)	4.4%
532 (13)	8%
104 (14)	14.4%

PRACTICE GUIDELINES

As previously discussed, a task force of the ASA/SCA published practice guidelines for perioperative TEE in 1996 (10). A new ASA/SCA Task Force on Perioperative TEE is currently working on revising the initial guidelines (17). Practice guidelines are recommendations that may be adopted, modified, or rejected according to clinical needs and constraints and are not intended to replace local institutional policies. The purposes of the new guidelines are to assist the physician in determining the appropriate application of TEE and to improve outcomes of surgical patients by defining the utility of perioperative TEE based on the strength of supporting evidence. The revised evidence-based guidelines focus only on the application of TEE in surgical patients and potential surgical patients in the setting of cardiac surgery, noncardiac surgery, and postoperative critical care.

The most recent task force developed the proposed practice guidelines by means of a seven step process.

1. The Task Force on Perioperative TEE was composed of leading cardiothoracic anesthesiologists and intraoperative cardiologists who reached consensus on the criteria for evidence.
2. Original published research studies from peer-reviewed journals relevant to TEE were reviewed and evaluated.
3. Expert consultants were asked to (a) participate in opinion surveys on the effectiveness of TEE imaging and (b) review and comment on a draft of the guidelines developed by the Task Force.
4. Opinions about the guideline recommendations were solicited from a sample of active members of the ASA who personally perform TEE as part of their practice.
5. The Task Force held an open forum at the SCA 2008 annual meeting to solicit input on its draft recommendations.
6. The consultants were surveyed to assess their opinions on the feasibility of implementing the guidelines.
7. All available information was used to build consensus within the Task Force to finalize the guidelines.

Evidence for the guidelines was obtained from two sources: scientific and opinion-based evidence. The scientific evidence was divided into four categories and included supportive literature, suggestive literature, equivocal literature, and insufficient evidence from the literature. The opinion-based evidence was divided into expert, membership, and informal opinion. A complete summary of the guideline can be found at the ASA Web site (www.asahq.org) under practice guidelines.

From the cumulative data obtained above, five specific recommendations were made. A summary of the recommendations follows:

1. **Cardiac and Thoracic Aortic Surgery:** For adult patients without contraindications, TEE should be considered in all open heart (e.g., valvular procedures) and thoracic aortic surgical procedures, and should be considered in CABG surgeries as well, to (a) confirm and refine the preoperative diagnosis, (b) detect new or unsuspected pathology, (c) adjust the anesthetic and surgical plan accordingly, and (d) assess results of the surgical intervention. In small children, the use of TEE should be considered on a case-by-case basis because of risks unique to these patients (e.g., bronchial obstruction).
2. **Catheter-Based Intracardiac Procedures:** For patients undergoing transcatheter intracardiac procedures, TEE may be used.
3. **Noncardiac surgery:** TEE may be used when the nature of the planned surgery or the patient's known or suspected cardiovascular pathology might result in severe hemodynamic, pulmonary, or neurologic compromise. If equipment and expertise are available, TEE should be used when unexplained life-threatening circulatory instability persists despite corrective therapy.
4. **Critical care:** TEE should be used when diagnostic information that is expected to alter management cannot be obtained by TTE or other modalities in a timely manner.
5. **Contraindications for the use of TEE:** TEE may be used for patients with oral, esophageal, or gastric disease, if the expected benefit outweighs the potential risk, and provided the appropriate precautions are applied. These precautions may include considering other imaging modalities (e.g., epicardial echocardiography), obtaining a gastroenterology consultation, using a smaller probe, limiting the examination, avoiding unnecessary probe manipulation, and employing the most experienced operator.

In 1997, the American Heart Association (AHA) and American College of Cardiology (ACC) published guidelines for the clinical application of echocardiography (18). In 2000, the AHA/ACC Task Force was reconvened to update the guidelines that were published in 2006 (19). The Task Force also decided to include a new section on IOE. In the preparation of the intraoperative section, a literature search was conducted that identified an additional 118 articles related to the intraoperative use of echocardiography.

The AHA/ACC guidelines utilize the following classification system for indications.

Class I: Conditions for which there is evidence and/or general agreement that a given procedure or treatment is useful and effective.
Class II: Conditions for which there is conflicting evidence and/or a divergence of opinion about the usefulness/efficacy of a procedure or treatment.
   IIa: Weight of evidence/opinion is in favor of usefulness/efficacy.
   IIb: Usefulness/efficacy is less well established by evidence/opinion.
Class III: Conditions for which there is evidence and/or general agreement that the procedure/treatment is not useful/effective and in some cases may be harmful.

In addition, the weight of the evidence in support of the recommendation was determined as follows:

Level of Evidence A: Data derived from multiple randomized trials.

Level of Evidence B: Data derived from a single randomized trial or nonrandomized studies.

Level of Evidence C: Only consensus opinion of expert, case studies, or standard of care.

The 2006 AHA/ACC guidelines had three Class I and one Class II specific recommendations regarding intraoperative assessment.

Class I

1. Intraoperative TEE is recommended for valve repair surgery. (Level of Evidence: B.)
2. Intraoperative TEE is recommended for valve replacement surgery with a stentless xenograft, homograft, or autograft valve. (Level of Evidence: B.)
3. Intraoperative TEE is recommended for valve surgery for infective endocarditis. (Level of Evidence: B.)

Class IIa

Intraoperative TEE is reasonable for all patients undergoing cardiac valve surgery. (Level of Evidence: C.)

INDICATIONS FOR SPECIFIC LESIONS OR PROCEDURES

Mitral Valve Repair

Two studies from Japan have confirmed the usefulness of intraoperative TEE for the assessment of residual regurgitation after mitral valve repair (20,21). Kawano et al. (20) observed that 5 out of 34 patients had 1+ regurgitation on postoperative ventriculography. Four of these patients demonstrated a maximal mosaic area greater than 2 cm^2 on color flow Doppler by TEE immediately after CPB. All four patients developed rapidly progressing mitral regurgitation (MR) in the postoperative period. In a study by Saiki et al. (21), 40 out of 42 patients with no or trivial MR (mosaic area ≤ 2 cm^2) also had no or trivial MR early and late postoperatively. The other two patients in whom moderate MR was detected intraoperatively by TEE, evolved to moderate regurgitation three months later.

Aklog et al. (22) have recently examined the role of intraoperative TEE in the evaluation of ischemic MR. They studied 136 patients with a preoperative diagnosis of moderate ischemic MR, without leaflet prolapse or pathology, who underwent isolated coronary artery bypass grafting (CABG). They observed that IOE downgraded MR in 89% of patients and that CABG alone leaves many patients with significant residual MR. A reduction in MR severity when assessed by IOE was also reported by Grewal et al. (23). They studied 43 patients with moderate to severe MR and observed that MR improved by at least one grade in 51% of patients when assessed under general anesthesia.

The AHA/ACC guideline document assigned intraoperative TEE a Class I indication for valve repair surgery (18). In summary, TEE examination prior to CPB allows for the evaluation of the mechanism of valvular dysfunction and hence facilitates surgical planning. Post-CPB intraoperative TEE allows for the immediate assessment of the repair. This post-CPB evaluation should assess for residual MR, systolic anterior motion of the leaflets, and restriction of leaflet opening indicating possible stenosis. It is critical that the IOE examination occurs under similar loading conditions to the patients baseline status.

Valve Replacement

Nowrangi et al. (24) reviewed the impact of intraoperative TEE in patients undergoing aortic valve replacement (AVR) for aortic stenosis (AS). They reviewed the clinical data of 383 patients and observed that 54 patients had mitral valve replacement (MVR) at the time of the AVR. In six patients, MVR was not planned but was performed on the basis of the IOE findings. In 25 patients, MVR was cancelled because of the IOE findings, while the surgical plan was altered in an additional 18 patients.

The clinical impact and cost-saving implications of routine IOE were studied prospectively in 300 patients by Ionescu et al. (25). In two patients undergoing AVR, significant MR detected by IOE resulted in MVR and in one patient undergoing MVR, aortic regurgitation resulted in AVR. The authors calculated that the extension of an existing TEE service to routine IOE resulted in savings of $109 per patient per year in 2001.

Morehead et al. (26) have studied the significance of paravalvular jets detected by IOE after valve replacement. In 27 patients, multiple jets were detected after valve replacement. They were more common and larger in the mitral position and after insertion of mechanical valves. Reversal of anticoagulation with protamine reduced the incidence and size of the jets in all patients.

The outcome of mild periprosthetic regurgitation identified by IOE was also studied by O'Rourke et al. (27). Of 608 patients undergoing isolated AVR or MVR, 113 were found to have trivial or mild periprosthetic regurgitation at surgery. While the observation was benign in most patients, four patients were found to have progression of the regurgitation by late transthoracic echocardiographic examination.

The AHA/ACC guidelines recommend intraoperative TEE for valve replacement surgery with a stentless xenograft, homograft, or autograft valve (Class I) and consider reasonable for all patients undergoing cardiac valve surgery (Class IIa) (19). TEE is important to detect paravalvular regurgitation or abnormal leaflet motion post valve implantation. In addition, for both mitral valve repair and replacement surgery, it is important to evaluate the left ventricle (LV) for possible left circumflex coronary artery injury and the aortic valve for a suture-related injury to an aortic cusp.

Coronary Artery Surgery

Bergquist et al. (28) studied how TEE guides clinical decision making in myocardial revascularization. For the 584 intraoperative interventions that were recorded, TEE was the single most important guiding factor in 98 instances (17%). TEE was the single most important monitor influencing fluid administration; antiischemic therapy; and vasotrope, inotrope, vasodilator, or antiarrhythmic administration. In two patients, critical surgical interventions were made solely on the basis of TEE. During high-risk CABG, Savage et al. (29) observed that in 33% of patients at least one major surgical management alteration was initiated on the basis of TEE, while in 51% of patients, at least one major anesthetic/hemodynamic change was initiated by a TEE finding. Arruda et al. (30) evaluated the role of power Doppler imaging to assess the patency of CABG anastomosis. In 11 out of 12 patients, the flow in the left anterior descending coronary artery could be visualized before and after the anastomosis. In one patient, the graft was revised because of worsened flow after CPB.

Gurbuz et al. (31) recently found that intraoperative TEE frequently modified the strategy in off-pump coronary artery bypass surgery (OPCAB). They prospectively evaluated 744 patients scheduled for OPCAB surgery and found that intraoperative TEE resulted in a major or minor modification in operative strategy in 16% or 10% of patients, respectively. Major modifications included graft revisions, no touch technique due to ascending aorta atherosclerosis or intraoperative balloon pump insertion.

Previously Undetected Aortic Stenosis or Mitral Regurgitation During CABG

Elderly patients frequently require CABG and AVR secondary to AS. Occasionally, a patient may present for CABG with AS diagnosed during the intraoperative TEE examination. Indications for AVR are the same as if the patient was diagnosed preoperatively. If the AS is moderate or severe, AVR is indicated. Controversy exist if the degree of AS appears to be mild. Optimization of TEE windows is necessary to assure that the maximum mean and peak transvalvular pressure gradients are being obtained. Epicardial echocardiography and direct surgical transduction of LV and aortic pressures may also add in the decision making (19).

Undiagnosed MR in a patient undergoing CABG surgery is more controversial. A comprehensive examination of the mitral valve is necessary to determine the mechanism of the MR. Significant MR with a structural abnormality such as a prolapsed or flailed segment warrants repair or replacement. Patients with moderate or mild MR during surgery are more difficult to evaluate due to the hemodynamic effects of anesthesia, which typically lessen the degree of regurgitation. It is therefore reasonable to perform MV repair in patients with newly diagnosed moderate MR detected on the intraoperative TEE examination (19).

Minimally Invasive Cardiac Surgery

With the growing interest in minimally invasive cardiac surgery, the role of IOE in these procedures has been evaluated. Applebaum et al. (32) reported that TEE facilitated the placement of intravascular catheters during port-access surgery, thereby avoiding the use of fluoroscopy. Fluoroscopy was only helpful as an aide to TEE for placement of the coronary sinus catheter. Falk et al. (33) observed that TEE was particularly useful for monitoring the placement and positioning of the endoaortic clamp that is used in these procedures. Similar benefits were reported by Schulze et al. (34).

In minimally invasive valve surgery, Secknus et al. (35) noted intracardiac air in all patients. New LV dysfunction was more common in patients with extensive air by IOE. Second CPB runs were required in 6% of patients. Kort et al. (36) examined the role of IOE in 153 patients undergoing minimally invasive AVR. Postbypass mild AI was observed in two patients. On follow-up, moderate regurgitation was observed in 4 patients, mild-to-moderate in 2, and mild in 18 patients. The regurgitation was paravalvular in eight of these patients.

In patients undergoing CABG without CPB, Moises et al. (37) detected 31 new regional wall motion abnormalities (RWMA) during 48 coronary artery clampings. At the time of chest closure, 16 segments had partial recovery and 5 of these had not recovered. Seven days later, the RWMA persisted in the 5 without recovery and in 2 with partial recovery. These patients had more complicated postoperative courses.

Aortic Atheromatous Disease

The relationship between the severity of aortic atheromatous disease and postoperative dysfunction has been established previously. Choudhary et al. (38) documented severe atheromatous disease in 12 out of 126 patients undergoing CABG. Protruding atheromas were significantly more common in patients over 60 years of age. Out of four patients with grade V atheromas, two developed right hemiplegia postoperatively. To determine the optimal method to detect ascending aortic atheromas intraoperatively, manual palpation, TEE, and epiaortic scanning were compared in 100 patients (39). Age, greater than 70 years, and hypertension were significant risk factors for severe ascending atheromas. Epiaortic scanning was found superior to both manual palpation and TEE. In order to advance the recognition of intraoperative epiaortic scanning, the ASE and SCA jointly published guidelines for the performance of a comprehensive intraoperative epiaortic ultrasonographic examination in 2007 (40).

NEW APPLICATIONS

Three-Dimensional Echocardiography

With the development of three-dimensional (3D) echocardiography, several investigators have explored its incremental value for the intraoperative detection of valvular lesions (9,41–43). In many instances, 3D-echocardiography provided complementary morphologic information that explained the mechanisms of abnormalities seen with conventional two-dimensional (2D) echocardiography. 3D echocardiography also allowed direct visualization and planimetry of regurgitant orifice areas and measurement of regurgitant volumes. Vogel et al. (44) used 3D-echocardiography to image congenital cardiac lesions as they would be visualized by a surgeon. This approach yielded additional information in the diagnosis of supravalvular mitral membranes, doubly committed subarterial ventricular septal defects, and subaortic stenoses caused by restrictive ventricular septal defects in double inlet LVs. Muller et al. (45) also demonstrated in a series of 74 patients that 3D image reconstruction was more sensitive in detecting mitral valve bileaflet and commissural defects in patients with Carpentier type II mitral valve lesions than TEE alone. More recently, Grewal et al. (46) demonstrated, in 42 consecutive patients undergoing MV repair for MR, that real-time intraoperative 3D TEE imaging was superior to 2D TEE imaging in the diagnosis of P1, A2, A3, and bileaflet disease (P < 0.05).

Intraoperative Stress Echo

Intraoperative dobutamine stress echocardiography has been utilized to detect inducible demand ischemia in patients with severe coronary artery disease and to predict functional changes after myocardial revascularization (47,48). In 75 out of 80 anesthetized patients with severe coronary artery disease scheduled for noncardiac surgery, inducible ischemia was detected after a standard dobutamine-atropine stress protocol. None of the patients suffered significant complications. The diagnostic value of intraoperative dobutamine stress echocardiography in this patient population remains to be determined. In CABG surgery, changes in myocardial function after low-dose dobutamine were highly predictive for early and late changes in myocardial function from baseline function. When improvement in function was noted after dobutamine, the odds ratios for early and late improvement were 20.7 and 34.6, respectively.

COMPLICATIONS

Intraoperative TEE is not without risks. Hogue et al. (49) studied independent predictors of swallowing dysfunction after cardiac surgery. In addition to age and length of intubation after surgery, intraoperative use of TEE was a highly significant (P < 0.003) predictor of swallowing dysfunction. In another study of 838 consecutive cardiac surgical patients, significant factors causing postoperative dysphagia were studied by multiple logistic regression (50). After controlling for other significant factors such as stroke, LV ejection fraction, intubation time, and duration of operation, the patients with intraoperative TEE had 7.8 times greater odds of dysphagia than those without.

In a recent review of 7,200 adult cardiac surgical patients, Kallmeyer et al. reported on the safety of intraoperative TEE (51). They observed no mortality and a morbidity of only 0.2%. Most complications were related to probe insertion or manipulation that resulted in oropharyngeal, esophageal, or gastric trauma. In seven patients, diagnostic esophagogastroduodenoscopy (EGD) was indicated because of postoperative odynophagia. Acute upper gastrointestinal bleeding occurred in two patients. In one of these patients, EGD revealed several linear esophageal tears while in the other only erythema and diffuse oozing were observed. Esophageal perforation occurred in one elderly female patient. The patient suffered from dyspnea 2 days after the surgical procedure. The perforation resulted in a hydropneumothorax and required surgical repair. One esophageal perforation was also reported by Schmidlin et al. (8) in a series of 2,296 intraoperative TEE examinations. Finally, Lennon et al. investigated the incidence of intraoperative TEE-related gastrointestinal complications in 516 cardiac surgical patients. This group found that compared to a group of 343 cardiac surgical patients in whom intraoperative TEE was not performed, patients in whom intraoperative TEE was performed had a higher overall incidence of major gastrointestinal complication (1.2% vs. 0.29%), including 2 patients with an early (<24 hours) presentation and 4 patients with a later (>24 hours) presentation (52).

Greene et al. (53) evaluated the safety of TEE in pediatric cardiac surgery by performing an endoscopic examination of the esophagus following TEE. In 50 patients undergoing repair of congenital cardiac surgery, the endoscopic examination was performed after removal of the TEE probe. In 32 patients, mild mucosal injury was observed, but none resulted in long-term feeding or swallowing difficulties.

Despite its overwhelming popularity, the TEE approach as described above has some limitations. The recommendations of the ASE and SCA Task Force guidelines for training in perioperative echocardiography include epicardial and epiaortic imaging as core components of advanced training (54). Guidelines for performing a comprehensive epicardial and epiaortic examination were recently published (40,55). Hence in patients where a TEE probe is difficult or impossible to advance into the esophagus or in patients with gastroesophageal pathology, epicardial and epiaortic ultrasound are viable alternatives (56,57).

9. Sugeng L, Shernan SK, Weinert L, et al. Real-time three-dimensional transesophageal echocardiography in valve disease: comparison with surgical findings and evaluation of prosthetic valves. *J Am Soc Echocardiogr* 2008;21(12):1347–1354.
10. Practice Guidelines for perioperative transesophageal echocardiography. A report by the American Society of Anesthesiologists and the Society of Cardiovascular Anesthesiologists Task Force on transesophageal echocardiography. *Anesthesiology* 1996;84:986–1006.
11. Rosenfeld HM, Gentles TL, Wernovsky G, et al. Utility of intraoperative transesophageal echocardiography in the assessment of residual cardiac defects. *Pediatr Cardiol* 1998;19:346–351.
12. Sheil ML, Baines DB. Intraoperative transesophageal echocardiography for pediatric cardiac surgery by an audit of 200 cases. *Anaesth Intensive Care* 1999;27:591–595.
13. Stevenson JG. Role of intraoperative transesophageal echocardiography during repair of congenital cardiac defects. *Acta Paediatr Suppl* 1995;410:23–33.
14. Ungerleider RM, Kisslo JA, Greeley WJ, et al. Intraoperative echocardiography during congenital heart operations: experience from 1,000 cases. *Ann Thorac Surg* 1995;60(6 Suppl.): S539–S542.
15. Sloth E, Pedersen J, Olsen KH, et al. Transesophageal echocardiographic monitoring during paediatric cardiac surgery: obtainable information and feasibility in 532 children. *Paediatr Anaesth* 2001;11:657–662.
16. Durongpisitkul K, Soongswang J, Sriyoschati S, et al. Utility of intraoperative transesophageal echocardiogram in congenital heart disease. *J Med Assoc Thai* 2000;83(Suppl. 2):S46–S53.
17. Practice Guidelines for perioperative transesophageal echocardiography. A report by the American Society of Anesthesiologists and the Society of Cardiovascular Anesthesiologists Task Force on transesophageal echocardiography. *Anesthesiology* 2010; 12:1084–1096.
18. Cheitlin MD, Alpert JS, Armstrong WF, et al. ACC/AHA guidelines for the clinical application of echocardiography. *Circulation* 1997;95:1686–1744.
19. Bonow RO, Carabello BA, Chatterjee K, et al. ACC/AHA 2006 Guidelines for the management of patients with valvular heart disease. *JACC* 2006;48:e1–e148.
20. Kawano H, Mizoguchi T, Ayoagi S. Intraoperative transesophageal echocardiography for evaluation of mitral valve repair. *J Heart Valve Dis* 1999;8:287–293.
21. Saiki Y, Kasegawa H, Kawase M, et al. Intraoperative TEE during mitral valve repair: does it predict early and late postoperative mitral valve dysfunction? *Ann Thorac Surg* 1998;66: 1277–1281.
22. Aklog L, Filsoufi F, Flores KQ, et al. Does coronary artery bypass grafting alone correct moderate ischemic mitral regurgitation? *Circulation* 2001;104(Suppl. 1):I68–I75.
23. Grewal KS, Malkowski MJ, Piracha AR, et al. Effect of general anesthesia on the severity of mitral regurgitation by transesophageal echocardiography. *Am J Cardiol* 2000;85(2):199–203.
24. Nowrangi SK, Connolly HM, Freeman WK, et al. Impact of intraoperative transesophageal echocardiography among patients undergoing aortic valve replacement for aortic stenosis. *J Am Soc Echocardiogr* 2001;14:863–866.
25. Ionescu AA, West RR, Proudman C, et al. Prospective study of routine perioperative transesophageal echocardiography for elective valve replacement: clinical impact and cost-saving implications. *J Am Soc Echocardiogr* 2001;14:659–667.

KEY POINTS

■ Although intraoperative TEE is widely utilized during cardiac surgery because it is perceived to be useful, scientific evidence demonstrating its usefulness is limited.

■ Practice guidelines developed by professional organizations classify indications for perioperative TEE on the basis of the strength of supporting evidence or expert opinion that the technology improves outcomes.

■ In the ACC/AHA guidelines for perioperative echocardiography, new Class I indications include the evaluation of complex valve replacements and the placement of intracardiac devices.

■ In the ACC/AHA guidelines for perioperative echocardiography, new Class IIb indications include the evaluation of regional myocardial function during off-pump CABG, intraoperative dobutamine stress testing, and assessment of residual duct flow after interruption of patent ductus arteriosus.

■ While the incidence of complications after perioperative TEE is low, probe insertion and manipulation may result in oropharyngeal, esophageal, or gastric trauma. In these patients, epicardial and epiaortic ultrasound are appropriate alternatives.

REFERENCES

1. Thys DM. Echocardiography and anesthesiology: successes and challenges. *Anesthesiology* 2001;95:1313–1314.
2. Morewood GH, Gallagher ME, Gaughan JP, et al. Current practice patterns for adult perioperative transesophageal echocardiography in the United States. [See comment.] [Journal Article] *Anesthesiology* 2001;95(6):1507–1512.
3. Click RL, Abel MD, Schaff HV. Intraoperative transesophageal echocardiography: 5-year prospective review of impact on surgical management. *Mayo Clin Proc* 2000;75:241–247.
4. Couture P, Denault AY, McKenty S, et al. Impact of routine use of intraoperative transesophageal echocardiography during cardiac surgery. *Can J Anaesth* 2000;47:20–26.
5. Michel-Cherqui M, Ceddaha A, Liu N, et al. Assessment of systematic use of intraoperative transesophageal echocardiography during cardiac surgery in adults: a prospective study of 203 patients. *J Cardiothorac Vasc Anesth* 2000;14:45–50.
6. Mishra M, Chauhan R, Sharma KK, et al. Real-time intraoperative transesophageal echocardiography—how useful? Experience of 5,016 cases. *J Cardiothorac Vasc Anesth* 1998;12(6): 625–632.
7. Sutton DC, Kluger R. Intraoperative transesophageal echocardiography: impact on adult cardiac surgery. *Anaesth Intensive Care* 1998;26:287–293.
8. Schmidlin D, Bettex D, Bernard E, et al. Transesophageal echocardiography in cardiac and vascular surgery: implications and observer variability. *Br J Anaesth* 2001;86(4):497–505.

26. Morehead AJ, Firstenberg MS, Shiota T, et al. Intraoperative echocardiographic detection of regurgitant jets after valve replacement. *Ann Thorac Surg* 2000;69(1):135–139.

27. O'Rourke DJ, Palac RT, Malenka DJ, et al. Outcome of mild periprosthetic regurgitation detected by intraoperative transesophageal echocardiography. *J Am Coll Cardiol* 2001;38:163–166.

28. Bergquist BD, Bellows WH, Leung JM. Transesophageal echocardiography in myocardial revascularization. Influence on intraoperative decision making. *Anesth Analg* 1996;82:1139–1145.

29. Savage RM, Lytle BW, Aronson S, et al. Intraoperative echocardiography is indicated in high-risk coronary artery bypass grafting. *Ann Thorac Surg* 1997;64:368–373.

30. Arruda AM, Dearani JA, Click RL, et al. Intraoperative application of power Doppler imaging: visualization of myocardial perfusion after anastomosis of left internal thoracic artery to left anterior descending coronary artery. *J Am Soc Echocardiogr* 1999;12(8):650–654.

31. Gurbuz AT, Hecht ML, Arslan AH. Intraoperative transesophageal echocardiography modifies strategy in off-pump coronary artery bypass grafting. *Ann Thorac Surg* 2007;83:1035–1040.

32. Applebaum RM, Cutler WM, Bhardwaj N, et al. Utility of transesophageal echocardiography during port-access minimally invasive cardiac surgery. *Am J Cardiol* 1998;82:183–188.

33. Falk V, Walther T, Diegeler A, et al. Echocardiographic monitoring of minimally invasive mitral valve surgery using an endoartic clamp. *J Heart Valve Dis* 1996;5:630–637.

34. Schulze CJ, Wildhirt SM, Boehm DH, et al. Continuous transesophageal echocardiographic (TEE) monitoring during port-access cardiac surgery. *Heart Surg Forum* 1999;2:54–59.

35. Secknus MA, Asher CR, Scalia GM, et al. Intraoperative transesophageal echocardiography in minimally invasive cardiac valve surgery. *J Am Soc Echocardiogr* 1999;12:231–236.

36. Kort S, Applebaum RM, Grossi EA, et al. Minimally invasive aortic valve replacement: echocardiographic and clinical results. *Am Heart J* 2001;142:391–392.

37. Moises VA, Mesquita CB, Campos O, et al. Importance of intraoperative transesophageal echocardiography during coronary artery surgery without cardiopulmonary bypass. *J Am Soc Echocardiogr* 1998;11:1139–1144.

38. Choudhary SK, Bhan A, Sharma R, et al. Aortic atherosclerosis and perioperative stroke in patients undergoing coronary artery bypass: role of intraoperative transesophageal echocardiography. *Int J Cardiol* 1997;67:31–38.

39. Sylivris S, Calafiore P, Matalanis G, et al. The intraoperative assessment of ascending aortic atheroma: epiaortic imaging is superior to both transesophageal echocardiography and direct palpation. *J Cardiothorac Vasc Anesth* 1997;11:704–707.

40. Glas KM, Swaminathan M, Reeves ST, et al. Guidelines for the performance of a comprehensive intraoperative epiaortic ultrasonographic examination: recommendations of the American Society of Echocardiography and the Society of Cardiovascular Anesthesiologists *J Am Soc Echocardiogr* 2007;20:1227–1235.

41. Abraham TP, Warner JG, Jr, Kon ND, et al. Feasibility, accuracy, and incremental value of intraoperative three-dimensional transesophageal echocardiography in valve surgery. *Am J Cardiol* 1997;80(12):1577–1582.

42. Breburda CS, Griffin BP, Pu M, et al. Three-dimensional echocardiographic planimetry of maximal regurgitant orifice area in myxomatous mitral regurgitation: intraoperative comparison of proximal flow convergence. *J Am Coll Cardiol* 1998;32(2):432–4437.

43. De Simone R, Glombitza G, Vahl CF, et al. Three-dimensional color Doppler for assessing mitral regurgitation during valvuloplasty. *Eur J Cardiothorac Surg* 1999;15(2):127–133.

44. Vogel M, Ho SY, Lincoln C, et al. Three-dimensional echocardiography can simulate intraoperative visualization of congenitally malformed hearts. *Ann Thorac Surg* 1995;60(5):1282–1288.

45. Muller S, Muller L, Laufer G. comparison of three-dimensional imaging to transesophageal echocardiography for preoperative evaluation in mitral valve prolapsed. *Am J Cardiol* 2006;98:243–248.

46. Grewal J, Mankad S, Freeman WK, et al. Real-time three-dimensional transesophageal echocardiography in the intraoperative assessment of mitral valve disease. *J Am Soc Echocardiogr* 2009;22:34–41.

47. Seeberger MD, Skarvan K, Buser P, et al. Dobutamine stress echocardiography to detect inducible demand ischemia in anesthetized patients with coronary artery disease. *Anesthesiology* 1998;88(5):1233–1239.

48. Aronson S, Dupont F, Savage R, et al. Changes in regional myocardial function after coronary artery bypass graft surgery are predicted by intraoperative low-dose dobutamine echocardiography. *Anesthesiology* 2000;93(3):685–692.

49. Hogue CW Jr, Lappas GD, Creswell LL, et al. Swallowing dysfunction after cardiac operations. Associated adverse outcomes and risk factors including intraoperative transesophageal echocardiography. *J Thorac Cardiovasc Surg* 1995;110(2):517–522.

50. Rousou JA, Tighe DA, Garb JL, et al. Risk of dysphagia after transesophageal echocardiography during cardiac operations. *Ann Thorac Surg* 2000;69(2):486–489.

51. Kallmeyer IJ, Collard CD, Fox JA, et al. The safety of intraoperative transesophageal echocardiography: A case series of 7,200 cardiac surgical patients. *Anesth Analg* 2001;92:1126–1130.

52. Lennon MJ, Gibbs NM, Weightman WM, et al. Transesophageal echocardiography-related gastrointestinal complications in cardiac surgical patients. *J Cardiothorac Vasc Anesth* 2005;19:141–145.

53. Greene MA, Alexander JA, Knauf DG, et al. Endoscopic evaluation of the esophagus in infants and children immediately following intraoperative use of transesophageal echocardiography. *Chest* 1999;116:1247–1250.

54. Cahalan MK, Abel M, Goldman M, et al. American Society of Echocardiography and Society of Cardiovascular Anesthesiologists task force guidelines for training in perioperative echocardiography. *Anesth Analg* 2002;94:1384–1388.

55. Reeves ST, Shernan S, Glas K, et al. Guidelines for Performing a Comprehensive Epicardial Echocardiography Examination: Recommendations of the American Society of Echocardiography Council for Intraoperative Echocardiography. *J Am Soc Echocardiogr* 2007;20:427–437.

56. Eltzschig HK, Rosenberger P, Löffler M, et al. Impact of intraoperative transesophageal echocardiography on surgical decisions in 12,566 patients undergoing cardiac surgery. *Ann Thorac Surg* 2008;85(3):845–852.

57. Rosenberger P, Shernan SK, Löffler M, et al. The influence of epiaortic ultrasonography on intraoperative surgical management in 6051 cardiac surgical patients. *Ann Thorac Surg* 2008;85(2):548–553.

QUESTIONS

1. Practice guidelines for perioperative echocardiography
   A. define the allowed usage of echocardiography
   B. are based on proven indications only
   C. refer to clinical problems rather than to individual patients
   D. determine the level of reimbursement for the procedure

2. In the AHA/ACC/ASE guidelines, the meaning of a Class I indication is that TEE
   A. should be used whenever the condition is present
   B. is useful and effective
   C. is not associated with harmful effects
   D. will guarantee reimbursement for the procedure

3. In minimally invasive cardiac surgery, IOE has been found useful for all of the following *except*

   A. placement of intracardiac and intravascular catheters
   B. assessment of post-CPB valvular function
   C. assessment of regional wall motion during coronary artery clamping
   D. evaluation of intracardiac air after valvular surgery
   E. prediction of long-term outcome after coronary artery bypass surgery

4. In cardiac surgical patients, the reported morbidity after intraoperative TEE is approximately
   A. 1 per 10,000 patients
   B. 1 per 5,000 patients
   C. 1 per 1,000 patients
   D. 1 per 500 patients
   E. 1 per 100 patients

Organization of an Intraoperative Echocardiographic Service: Personnel, Equipment, Maintenance, Safety, Infection, Economics, and Continuous Quality Improvement

Saket Singh ■ Joseph P. Mathew ■ Christopher A. Troianos

Since the mid-1980s, transesophageal echocardiography (TEE) has been used with increasing frequency in both cardiac and noncardiac operating rooms. Intraoperative TEE services are provided at nearly all of the institutions in North America where cardiac anesthesiologists practice (1,2). Echocardiography provides the operating room clinician with real-time information about cardiac function, anatomy, hemodynamics and has shown to improve outcomes in high-risk surgical patients (3). The recent introduction of three-dimensional (3D) echocardiography has shown great potential, enabling the echocardiographer to generate far more detailed imaging of anatomic structures, and enabling navigation of medical instruments based on stereoscopic images. Cardiac anesthesiologists have become partners in the surgical decision making, given their in-depth knowledge of pathophysiology, cardiac surgical anatomy, and surgical approaches. TEE has proven utility in liver transplantation, plays an essential role in percutaneous valve placement, robotic, and other noncardiac surgeries. The expanded role of TEE benefits patient care but entails risks, liability, costs, and additional training (4).

Developing an intraoperative TEE service requires considerable investment in equipment and training of personnel. Close collaborative relationships among anesthesiologists, cardiologists, and TEE support staff are necessary in order to assure safe patient care. The purchase and maintenance of TEE probes and machines incur significant expense and require dedicated space for probe sterilization and storage. This chapter reviews several essential components involved in the organization of a successful intraoperative TEE service.

PERSONNEL

Although cardiologists have traditionally performed and interpreted echocardiographic studies outside of the operating room setting, anesthesiologists have assumed an integral role in the development of intraoperative echocardiography (IOE) since the introduction of monoplane TEE probes into clinical practice nearly 30 years ago. Anesthesiologists quickly recognized the utility of TEE as an accurate and sensitive monitor of left ventricular filling and global and regional systolic function. The development of advanced Doppler imaging techniques greatly enhanced the monitoring and diagnostic capabilities of the clinician caring for the high-risk surgical patient while 3D TEE has enabled excellent visualization of shape, spatial orientation, and navigation of various intracardiac catheters, stents, and atrial septal defect occluders (5).

In North America, cardiovascular anesthesiologists or cardiologists perform the majority of intraoperative TEE studies. Poterack et al. conducted a survey of anesthesiology training programs in 1992 to determine who uses TEE in the operating room. Fifty-four percent of respondents reported that the anesthesiologist was primarily responsible for interpretation of TEE data, whereas the remaining respondents reported that the cardiologist is responsible. Ninety-one percent of academic institutions reported routine use of intraoperative TEE (6). Members of the cardiovascular section of the Canadian Anesthesiologists' Society received a survey in 2000 (2). Nearly all respondents (91%) noted that their hospital offered intraoperative TEE services as follows: 13% reported that cardiologists provided the service, 35% by anesthesiologists only, and 52% by both. A survey of the Society of Cardiovascular Anesthesiologists (SCA) in the United States yielded similar results (1). Fifty-two percent of respondents noted that an anesthesiologist performed intraoperative TEE examinations, 18% reported that a cardiologist performed the studies, and 29% reported that either physician could be involved. A majority of anesthesiologists (66%) noted that a cardiologist assisted with interpretation of the TEE only upon request (51%) or not at all (15%). One third of respondents reported that a cardiologist was involved in data interpretation when specific surgical procedures were performed (e.g., valve surgery). In 2007, Wax et al. conducted a survey of anesthesiologists performing liver transplant (LT) at high volume centers to investigate the utilization of TEE, training, and credentialing. Among 217 anesthesiologists who responded, 86% performed TEE in some or all LT cases. Most users performed a limited scope examination, although some performed a comprehensive TEE exam. Only 12% of users were board certified to perform TEE and only one center reported a policy regarding credentialing requirements for TEE (7). Bettex et al. analyzed 865 routine TEE examinations in patients younger than 17 years of age who were undergoing surgery for congenital heart disease (median age 36 months). TEE made a diagnostic impact in 18.5% of cases and led to surgical alterations of management in 12.7% of cases; this included need for repeat bypass run in 7.3%. Their observation indicated that a regular team of cardiac anesthesiologists, appropriately trained in TEE, competently performed the service (8).

The cognitive and technical skills of anesthesiologists using TEE may vary due to differences in training and clinical experience. In 1996, a Task Force on Practice Guidelines for Transesophageal Echocardiography established by the American Society of Anesthesiologists (ASA) and the SCA recognized two levels of training in perioperative TEE: basic and advanced (9). Anesthesiologists with basic training "should be able to use TEE for indications that lie within the customary practice of anesthesiology." This includes assessment of ventricular function, hemodynamics, and cardiovascular collapse. Anesthesiologists with advanced training should be able to utilize the full diagnostic potential of TEE. The training or experience requirement calls for either completion of 12 months of cardiothoracic anesthesiology fellowship or 24 months experience in the perioperative care of patients with cardiovascular disease, respectively. Advanced training should take place in a training program specifically designed to accomplish comprehensive training in perioperative echocardiography (9). Both accredited and nonaccredited programs offer fellowship training. Clinicians with basic training must recognize their limitations and obtain assistance from expert echocardiographers when needed. When presented with complex diagnostic decisions in the operating room, even anesthesiologists with advanced training may require the assistance of a cardiologist. Training objectives include specific cognitive and technical skills required for the basic and advanced levels (Table 7.1) (10). Most importantly, these training guidelines published jointly by the American Society of Echocardiography and the SCA recommend that 150 TEE examinations be completed under appropriate supervision with at least 50 of them personally performed, interpreted, and reported by the trainee as part of "basic" training. Advanced training requires 300 complete examinations performed under appropriate supervision, with at least 150 of these personally performed, interpreted, and reported by the trainee (Table 7.2).

Both task forces have noted that proficiency in TEE could be gradually obtained "on the job" through practice and repetition for physicians unable to participate in a formal training program. However, the same cognitive and technical skills outlined in Table 7.1 are required of these physicians. Physicians who complete their core residency training before July 1, 2009 will forever be able to follow the Practice Experience Pathway to certification in Perioperative TEE; anesthesiologists could begin to master the essential cognitive and technical skills by studying standard texts and training videos and by attending TEE workshops and training sessions. In addition, the Task Force recommended that anesthesiologists seeking basic training via this pathway should have at least 20 hours of continuing medical education (CME) devoted to echocardiography while physicians seeking advanced training should have at least 50. Physician should document the experience in detail and be able to demonstrate its equivalence in depth, diversity, and case numbers to match the desired training levels. Letters or certificates from the director of the perioperative echocardiography training program document competence (10). The National Board of Echocardiography (NBE), Inc. administers examinations that provide a means for which physicians can demonstrate their knowledge of echocardiography, based on an objective standard. The title of "Testamur" designates successfully passing of the written examination, while "Diplomate" designates board certification in echocardiography. The certification is valid for 10 years after the physician successfully passed the Examination of Special Competence. NBE also offers a Recertification Examination that is similar in format but designed specifically for those who have previously passed the exam. The purpose of the Recertification Examination is to promote continued excellence in the performance and interpretation of cardiac ultrasound, in conjunction with ongoing CME in the field. Applicants who seek recertification must have performed and interpreted at least 50 perioperative transesophageal echocardiograms per year during 2 of the last 3 years and obtained at least 15 hours of AMA Category I CME devoted to echocardiography (10,11). The ASA Committee on Outreach Education formed a workgroup to develop a strategic plan regarding basic perioperative echocardiography during its 2006 Annual Meeting. The workgroup organizes workshops on Basic Perioperative Echocardiography. The attendees have the ability to obtain a "Certificate of Completion" at the conclusion of these workshops. Though credentialing is a local hospital process, such "Certificate of Completion" may serve as a starting point for some physicians seeking hospital credentials in basic nondiagnostic TEE. The ASA and the NBE may offer a Certificate in Basic Perioperative Echocardiography in the near future. Regardless of certification level, a collaborative relationship with an expert in TEE is strongly encouraged. The expert in TEE should be immediately available so that essential intraoperative findings are not overlooked or missed. Although the presence of the expert

TABLE 7.1	Recommended Training Objectives for Basic and Advanced Perioperative Echocardiography

Basic Training

Cognitive Skills

1. Knowledge of the physical principles of echocardiographic image formation and blood velocity measurement
2. Knowledge of the operation of ultrasonographs including all controls that affect the quality of data displayed
3. Knowledge of the equipment handling, infection control, and electrical safety associated with the techniques of perioperative echocardiography
4. Knowledge of the indications, contraindications, and potential complications for perioperative echocardiography
5. Knowledge of the appropriate alternative diagnostic techniques
6. Knowledge of the normal tomographic anatomy as revealed by perioperative echocardiographic techniques
7. Knowledge of commonly encountered blood flow velocity profiles as measured by Doppler echocardiography
8. Knowledge of the echocardiographic manifestations of native valvular lesions and dysfunction
9. Knowledge of the echocardiographic manifestations of cardiac masses, thrombi, cardiomyopathies, pericardial effusions, and lesions of the great vessels
10. Detailed knowledge of the echocardiographic presentations of myocardial ischemia and infarction
11. Detailed knowledge of the echocardiographic presentations of normal and abnormal ventricular function
12. Detailed knowledge of the echocardiographic presentations of air embolization

Technical Skills

1. Ability to operate ultrasonographs, including the primary controls affecting the quality of the displayed data
2. Ability to insert a TEE probe safely in the anesthetized, tracheally intubated patient
3. Ability to perform a comprehensive TEE examination and to differentiate normal from markedly abnormal cardiac structures and function
4. Ability to recognize marked changes in segmental ventricular contraction indicative of myocardial ischemia or infarction
5. Ability to recognize marked changes in global ventricular filling and ejection
6. Ability to recognize air embolization
7. Ability to recognize gross valvular lesions and dysfunction
8. Ability to recognize large intracardiac masses and thrombi
9. Ability to detect large pericardial effusions
10. Ability to recognize common echocardiographic artifacts
11. Ability to communicate echocardiographic results effectively to health care professionals, the medical record, and patients
12. Ability to recognize complications of perioperative echocardiography

Advanced Training

Cognitive Skills

1. All the cognitive skills defined under basic training
2. Detailed knowledge of the principles and methodologies of qualitative and quantitative echocardiography
3. Detailed knowledge of native and prosthetic valvular function including valvular lesions and dysfunction
4. Knowledge of congenital heart disease (if congenital practice is planned, then this knowledge must be detailed)
5. Detailed knowledge of all other diseases of the heart and great vessels that is relevant in the perioperative period (if pediatric practice is planned, then this knowledge may be more general than detailed)
6. Detailed knowledge of the techniques, advantages, disadvantages, and potential complications of commonly used cardiac surgical procedures for treatment of acquired and congenital heart disease
7. Detailed knowledge of other diagnostic methods appropriate for correlation with perioperative echocardiography

(*continued*)

Advanced Training (*Continued*)

Technical Skills

1. All the technical skills defined under basic training

2. Ability to acquire or direct the acquisition of all necessary echocardiographic data, including epicardial and epiaortic imaging

3. Ability to recognize subtle changes in segmental ventricular contraction indicative of myocardial ischemia or infarction

4. Ability to quantify systolic and diastolic ventricular function and to estimate other relevant hemodynamic parameters

5. Ability to quantify normal and abnormal native and prosthetic valvular function

6. Ability to assess the appropriateness of cardiac surgical plans

7. Ability to identify inadequacies in cardiac surgical interventions and the underlying reasons for the inadequacies

8. Ability to aid in clinical decision making in the operating room

Reproduced with permission from Cahalan MK, Abel M, Goldman M, et al. American Society of Echocardiography and Society of Cardiovascular Anesthesiologists task force guidelines for training in perioperative echocardiography. Anesth Analg 2002;94:1384–1388.

echocardiographer would be required less frequently as the expertise of the anesthesiologist increases, a collaborative relationship with the primary echocardiographers in the hospital (cardiologist, radiologist) may be essential for the long-term viability of an intraoperative service. The conduct of a comprehensive examination should not compromise patient safety. Anesthesiologists should anticipate and seek additional support especially during percutaneous valve placements, coronary sinus catheter placements, and while providing offsite services.

Qualified TEE support personnel are an important component of the intraoperative TEE team. Support personnel may be responsible for the daily maintenance of the TEE probes to include visual inspection of the probe for defects, cleaning and disinfection following each use, and regular testing for leakage currents. Support staff may improve efficiency in the operating room by entering patient data before each examination and retrieving and storing data (either digital or videotape) when studies are completed. In smaller centers, TEE equipment is often shared among anesthesiologists, cardiologists, and intensivists. The TEE support personnel can assist in transporting and coordinating the use of TEE machines and probes.

EQUIPMENT AND MAINTENANCE

The cost of purchasing and maintaining an intraoperative echocardiographic system can be considerable. Basic equipment needed for a TEE service includes an ultrasound machine, a TEE probe, a process for cleaning and disinfecting probes, a leakage current tester, a holder for storing the probes between uses, tools to archive data, report and bill generation capacities, and a service contract. A dedicated machine and probe is not necessarily required in every operating room, but hospitals must carefully evaluate how they will provide intraoperative TEE services before investing in new or additional equipment. Smaller services share a single TEE system among

TABLE 7.2	The American Society of Echocardiography and the SCA Guidelines for Training in Perioperative Echocardiography (2002)		
	Basic	**Advance**	**Director**
Echocardiographic examinations	150	300	450
Minimum Intraoperative TEE examinations	50	150	300
Total duration of training	NS	NS	NS
Total CME hours	20	50	NS
Perioperative TEE examinations	NS	NS	NS
MOC:CME hours	NS	NS	NS
MOC: number of TEE per year	50	50	50

physicians in the echocardiography lab, the operating room, and the ICU (6). Centers caring for a larger volume of high-risk surgical patients may use more than one probe with each ultrasound machine (e.g., four probes are used with two ultrasound machines), which necessitates that the ultrasound machine be transported between operating rooms as needed. Larger cardiac centers in the United States provide TEE services for most patients undergoing cardiac surgery (1) and often devote a single echocardiography system to each cardiac operating room. Interest and utilization of real-time 3D TEE are increasing as published appraisals appear in the medical literature. 3D echocardiography provides improved accuracy and reproducibility over two-dimensional (2D) methods for LV volume and function calculation and the derivation of mitral valve area in patients with mitral stenosis (12). Live 3D is not gated, does not require an ECG, and is not affected by extra cardiac movement. 3D reconstruction is gated and more time consuming as one has to wait for reconstruction, and then determine if the image is optimal. 3D reconstruction, however, enables the user to utilize cropping function and view the structures in any imaginable plane within a heart. In practice, both types of 3D acquisition are used during an examination. Four-dimensional (4D) is equivalent to 3D in motion; all live 3D used in the heart is 4D because of the obvious need to show motion. A recent study in the *Journal of the American College of Cardiology* suggested that live 3D echocardiography permits faster image acquisition and delivers superior images of certain cardiac structures as compared with either real-time transthoracic echocardiography (TTE) or reconstructed 3D TEE imaging technology (13). There are various options available for adding 3D capabilities to old 2D TEE machines with a software upgrade. Most major imaging companies are in the process of developing real-time 3D TEE systems, but currently only one manufacturer has the commercially available technology with a matrix array transducer (13). It should be noted that a traditional 2D TEE costs approximately 20% less than live 3D system. Another benefit of the matrix array 3D transducer is the superior 2D image quality.

The addition of echocardiographic equipment to an operating room requires planning and organization to avoid cluttering and interference with patient care. One such example is depicted in Figure 7.1, where a Skytron boom with an S video and data port was placed above the typical location of the echocardiography machine within the operating room. The S video connection allows TEE images to be displayed throughout the room on multiple video monitors while data port connection enables rapid transfer of acquired images to a permanent offsite storage hard drive. A further benefit of this configuration is that it allows for the review and comparison of all perioperative studies.

Storage devices specifically designed for TEE probes are recommended because of the significant risk of mechanical damage in the operating room. Draping an unprotected TEE probe over an anesthesia cart or ultrasound machine

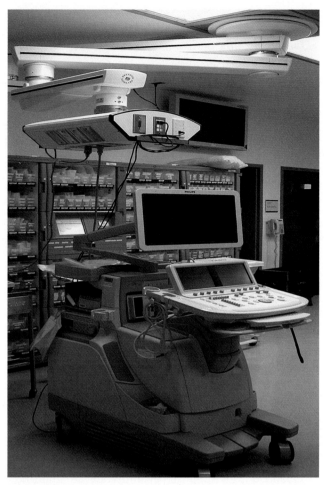

Figure 7.1. TEE machine connected to a Skytron boom via S video and data port.

is strongly discouraged. The possibility of intraoperative damage is enhanced by the fact that a variety of personnel handle the probe. Dropping the probe or striking it against a hard surface can damage the transducer elements and acoustic lens, the connector, or the control housing. Tears and abrasions on the probe can occur as it is advanced and withdrawn against a patient's teeth. After each examination, the probe should be carefully inspected for cracks, abrasions, and perforations. Physical defects in the housing of the probe can expose the patient to infective or electrical hazards. Larger defects can traumatize the esophagus during probe manipulation. In addition, procedures and chemicals that are used for cleaning and sterilization can damage TEE probes (Table 7.3). The electrical safety of the TEE system may be compromised with mechanical damage to the probe. The entire probe and cable should therefore be inspected before each use for defects in the housing and the probe should never be used for patient care if obvious defects are present. Since visual inspection may not detect small cracks or perforations, a leakage current test should be performed according to the recommendations of the manufacturer (some require testing following every use of the probe) (Fig. 7.2). Commercially available devices measure the electrical impedance of the

TABLE 7.3	Procedures and Chemicals That Damage TEE Probes

Procedures That Damage Probes

Autoclaving

Immersion in chlorine bleach or alcohol

Immersion of the control handle in any liquid

Dry heat sterilization

Ultraviolet sterilization

Gas sterilization

Prolonged immersion (several hours) in disinfecting solution

Chemicals That Damage Probes

Iodine

Mineral oil

Acetone

Spray aerosol anesthetics (if applied directly to the probe)

Adapted from Sequoia Ultrasound System: User and Reference Manuals. *Mountain View, CA: Accuson Corp., 2000–2001.*

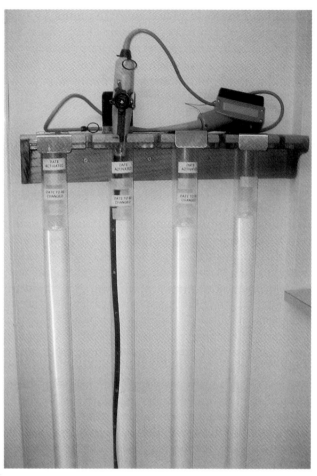

Figure 7.3. Example of a wall-mounted rack designed to protect TEE probes during storage.

system and provide a warning signal if leakage currents exceed recommended standards (approximately 50 μA) (14). The leakage current test is most often performed immediately prior to the disinfection process.

Proper storage of the probe will reduce the risk of mechanical damage. For storage between patient examinations, the probe should be maintained in a straight rather than flexed position to minimize tension on the cable connections. Commercial wall-mounted racks that protect the transducer in a straight plastic tube can be used in the operating room and cleaning room (Fig. 7.3). The probes should not be exposed to direct sunlight during disinfection or storage. Specialized probe holders that stabilize the control housing while the probe is inserted in a patient have been described (Fig. 7.4) (15). A probe holder can

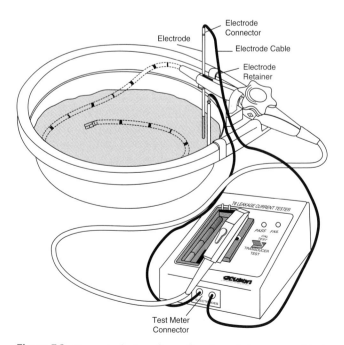

Figure 7.2. Proper technique for performing a leakage current test.

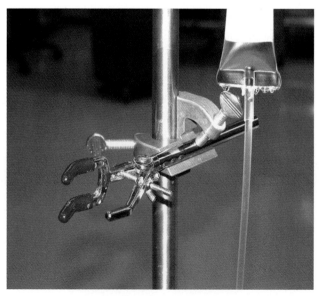

Figure 7.4. Holder for TEE probe.

prevent dropping or mishandling of the control housing, as well as prevent kinking or twisting of cables. During transportation to different sites in the hospital, the probe should be placed in a carrying case, or a protective device should be placed over the transducer elements in the tip of the probe.

SAFETY

Denault et al. reported on the perioperative use of TEE by anesthesiologists and its impact in noncardiac surgery and in the ICU. TEE altered therapy in 60% for indications classified as Category I ASA guidelines. The most frequent reason for changing management was a modification in medical therapy in 45% of these cases (16). This clearly illustrates the benefits of TEE, but the potential for cause serious complications must also be appreciated. Fortunately, serious complications associated with the use of TEE are rare (Table 7.4). Patients should be informed of a 1% risk of minor complications and 0.01% risk of major complications. TEE requires informed consent, which should be obtained in a manner compatible with hospital policies (17). With the exception of life-threatening emergencies, an echocardiographic procedure should not be performed without a written request. The request should clearly state the reasons for the study, the query to be answered and become part of patient's permanent medical record (18,19). The largest safety study reviewed data from 10,419 TEE procedures performed in awake patients. Morbidity occurred in 0.18% of examinations: and mortality in 0.0098% (20). The safety of intraoperative TEE

was examined in a case series of 7,200 cardiac surgical patients (21). No deaths related to intraoperative TEE were reported in this retrospective study. Morbidity occurred in 14 patients (0.2%); severe odynophagia accounted for half of these complications. In two other large series, morbidity was reported in 0.47% of 1,500 ambulatory adult patients and 0% of 5,016 cardiac surgical patients (22,23). The safety of TEE appears comparable with upper gastrointestinal (UGI) endoscopy (24). The live 3D TEE probe is 1 mm wider in diameter than 2D probes; although this should not lead to any higher rate of morbidity, no studies are currently available.

Complications Related to the Gastrointestinal System

Several types of trauma to the esophagus and stomach can occur during TEE examinations. Esophageal perforation is a rare but potentially lethal complication. Only one case of esophageal perforation was reported following 7,200 intraoperative studies (21). Brinkman et al. (25) described three patients who sustained intrathoracic esophageal perforations over a 2-year period at a large academic center. This form of trauma may present initially as subcutaneous emphysema, substernal chest pain, hemorrhage, or the appearance of the TEE probe in the surgical field (21,25). Mortality has been reported following esophageal perforation by the TEE probe (26). Trauma to the GI system may also produce significant hemorrhage. Injury consistent with a Mallory-Weiss tear has been observed in patients with UGI bleeding following the removal of the TEE probe (21,27). Lennon et al. conducted a retrospective database audit of 859 patients who underwent cardiac surgery at a single institution in Australia. The patients were identified by cross-referencing cardiac surgery and endoscopy databases. A major GI complication was defined as a perforation of the esophagus or stomach or upper GI bleeding, requiring transfusion, endoscopic, or surgical intervention. Early presentation was defined as less than 24 hours; late presentation was defined as greater than 24 hours. Five hundred sixteen patients had cardiac surgery with TEE (group 1), and 343 patients had cardiac surgery without TEE (group 2). Six patients were identified: 1.2% (95% confidence interval [CI], CI, 0.5%–2.5%) in group 1 who had a major upper GI complication consistent with TEE injury. Two patients, 0.38% (95% CI, 0.05%–1.40%), presented early, and four patients, 0.76% (95% CI, 0.21%–1.98%), presented late. One patient in group 2 developed a major upper GI complication, 0.29% (95% CI, 0.01%–1.6%). They concluded that the incidence of major GI complications attributed to TEE, in this group of cardiac surgical patients, was higher than previously reported. Late presentation was more common than early presentation. Previous studies, that have not included late presentations, may have underestimated the true incidence of major GI complications related to TEE (28). Factors most commonly associated with esophageal injuries are listed in Table 7.5 (29–31).

TABLE 7.4	Complications of Intraoperative TEE

Complications Related to the GI System

Esophageal perforation

Esophageal bleeding

Dysphagia

Odynophagia

Thermal injury

Transient bacteremia

Lip and dental trauma

Complications Related to Compression of Adjacent Structures

Tracheal compression

Displacement of the endotracheal tube

Vocal cord paralysis

Cardiac arrhythmias

Hypertension or hypotension

Splenic injury

TABLE 7.5	Risk Factors Most Commonly Associated with Esophageal Injury
Small patient size	
Prolonged procedure	
Cardiomegaly	
Cardiopulmonary bypass and low cardiac output	
Advanced age	
Zenker's diverticulum	
Long-term steroid use	
Radiation therapy	
Candida esophagitis	
Schatzki ring	
Poor preoperative cardiac function requiring inotropic support	

TABLE 7.6	Risk Factors for Dysphagia in Pediatric Patients
Age <3 y	
Preoperative patient acuity status	
Longer intubation times(more than 7 days)	
Operation of left-sided obstructive lesions	

An association between intraoperative TEE and postoperative swallowing dysfunction has been noted in cardiac surgical patients. In a study of 869 patients undergoing cardiac operations, swallowing dysfunction was identified in 34 subjects (32). Multivariate logistic regression analysis identified intraoperative use of TEE as an independent predictor of this complication. Patients with an impaired swallowing reflex were more likely to develop postoperative aspiration and pneumonia. In a second study of 838 consecutive cardiac surgical patients, TEE use was also significantly related to the development of postoperative dysphagia (33); patients monitored with TEE were 7.8 times as likely to experience dysphagia as those who did not have TEE. In contrast to these studies, two small prospective clinical trials demonstrated no association between intraoperative TEE and postoperative dysphagia in adults (34,35). In a prospective study of 50 pediatric patients, Kohr et al. reported an 18% incidence of dysphagia after open heart surgery with TEE. The incidence of vocal cord paralysis was noted to be 8%, and adverse events related to aspiration occurred in 4%. Resolution of dysphagia ranged from 13 to 150 days in this cohort of patients. They suggest vigilance in monitoring for signs of preoperative and postoperative dysphagia, with prompt referral to a speech therapist. These steps can

substantially reduce patient morbidity, length of hospital stay, and requirement for prolonged nasogastric tube use (36). The most common causes for dysphagia are listed in Table 7.6. Anesthesiologists, involved with congenital heart disease cases, should familiarize themselves with the report published by the Task Force of Pediatric Council of the American Society of Echocardiography, providing guidelines and indications for performance of TEE in the patient with acquired or congenital heart disease (37).

Several mechanisms may contribute to esophageal and gastric injuries during TEE examinations. The majority of injuries are likely the result of direct trauma produced by the probe. Although data are limited, some investigators recommend against blind placement of probes. The pyriform sinus mucosa is extremely thin and fragile, especially in the lateral portion. Only a small muscle layer separates it from the carotid sheath. In a study by Aviv et al. (38), no perforations were reported in the study group, but some hypopharyngeal hematomas and lacerations were found; none required intervention. Extensive manipulation of the probe tip to obtain required images may damage normal tissue. In an animal model, however, no mucosal injury was produced following prolonged and sustained contact of a probe with the esophagus (39). Direct trauma is more likely to occur in the setting of extensive gastric or esophageal pathology. In 2006, Augoustides et al. reported perforation of the esophagus despite routine placement of the TEE probe. The likely mechanism was esophageal compression from severe left atrial enlargement. A diagnosis of esophageal perforation should be considered if there are signs of pleural effusion, and confirmed by fluid analysis for particulate matter, low Ph, and an elevated level of salivary amylase (40). A summary of the UGI injuries reported in the literature is provided in Tables 7.7–7.9.

| TABLE 7.7 | Reported Pharyngeal Injuries Associated with TEE |

Author	Indication for TEE	Risk Factor	Clinical Presentation	Time to Presentation	Therapy	Length of Stay	Outcome
Spahn et al. (1995)	75-year-old female, CABG	Severe dysphagia	TEE probe visualized in mediastinum	Intraoperative	Primary repair	49 days	Survival

Modified with permission from Augoustides JG, Hosalkar HH, Milas BL, et al. Upper gastrointestinal injuries related to perioperative transesophageal echocardiography: index case, literature review, classification proposal, and call for a registry. J Cardiothorac Vasc Anesth 2006;20(3):379–384.

TABLE 7.8	Reported Esophageal Injuries Associated with Perioperative TEE						
Author	Indications For TEE	Risk Factor	Clinical Presentation	Time to Presentation	Therapy	Length of Stay	Outcome
Brinkman et al. (2001)	85-year-old female, CABG	None	Pleural effusion	2 d	Primary repair	40 d	Survival
Lecharny et al. (2002)	37-year-old male, valve replacement	Cardiomegaly with esophageal compression	Septic shock	7 d	No definitive therapy as patient demised	Unspecified	Fatal
Ghafoor et al. (2004)	71-year-old male, CABG	Schatzki ring Candida esophagitis	Intraoperative blood on TEE probe	Intraoperative CABG postponed	Conservative management	Unspecified	Survival
Nana et al. (2003)	70-year-old female, CABG	None	Pleural effusion with fever	2 d	Esophageal stent	17 d	Survival
Kharach et al. (1996)	66-year-old male, possible mitral disease	Chronic gastritis mesenteric ischemia	Abdominal pain pneumomediastinum	1 d	Esophagectomy	Unspecified	Fatal
Brinkman et al. 2001	80-year-old female, AVR with CABG	Long-term steroid use	Pleural effusion Pneumothorax	20 d	T tube esophageal drainage	11 wk	Survival
Zalunardo et al. (2002)	72-year-old female, acute M.I.	Esophageal ischemia	Pleural effusion	8 d	Esophageal stent	2 mon	Survival
Fujii et al. (2003)	62-year-old male, CABG	Thermal transfer	Nasogastric blood Mallory Weiss tear	1 d	Conservative	Unspecified	Survival
Massey et al. (2000)	59-year-old female, mitral and tricuspid surgery	Cardiomegaly with esophageal compression	Pleural effusion	5 d	Esophagectomy, gastrostomy, mediastinal drainage	Unspecified	Fatal
MacGregor et al. (2004)	2 females >70 y old, CABG and carotid endarterectomy AVR and ascending aortic arch replacement	Biatrial enlargement	Coffee ground emesis: endoscopy showed tear at gastroesophageal junction	3 d	EGD injection of epinephrine with blood transfusion	9 d	Survival
			Right pleural effusion	6 d	Primary repair	Prolonged	Survival
Han et al. (2003)	62-year-old male, valve replacement	TEE probe compression, nonpulsatile CPB flow; atrial enlargement	Septic shock	12 d	Operative repair	Prolonged	Survival
DeVries et al.	59-year-old female, mitral and tricuspid valve surgery	Giant left atrium	Septic shock	5 d	Operative repair	9 d	Fatal

Modified with permission from Augoustides JG, Hosalkar HH, Milas BL, et al. Upper gastrointestinal injuries related to perioperative transesophageal echocardiography: index case, literature review, classification proposal, and call for a registry. J Cardiothorac Vasc Anesth 2006;20(3):379–384.

TABLE 7.9	Reported Gastric Injuries Associated with TEE						
Author	Indications for TEE	Risk Factors	Clinical Presentations	Time to Presentation	Therapy	Length of Stay	Outcome
Latham et al. (1995)	65-year-old male, aortic valve replacement	Smoking; Attempted apical 4 chamber view	Blood from orogastric tube	Immediately postoperative	Conservative blood transfusion	Unspecified	Survival
Kihara et al. (1999)	CABG		Blood from nasogastric tube	Immediately postoperative	Conservative, endoscopic		
Lennon et al. (2005)	6 cases CABG+/− valve	Possible operator inexperience	Abdominal pain, hematemesis; Free air on imaging three tears; one ulcer, two perforations	Immediate or delayed	Conservative; Endoscopic; Surgical with laparotomy	Unspecified	Survival

Modified with permission from Augoustides JG, Hosalkar HH, Milas BL, et al. Upper gastrointestinal injuries related to perioperative transesophageal echocardiography: index case, literature review, classification proposal, and call for a registry. J Cardiothorac Vasc Anesth 2006;20(3):379–384.

Since all ultrasound transducers generate heat, thermal injury may be produced at the site where the transducer contacts tissue. Theoretically, the risk of thermal injury would be increased during prolonged use or when a significant temperature gradient existed between the transducer tip and the esophagus (during hypothermic cardiopulmonary bypass). Heat-sensing thermistors are now incorporated into the tips of transducers such that when a temperature limit is reached, transmitting power is automatically switched off. Transducers should be inactivated when not in use to reduce the potential for thermal injury. Trauma to the tissue of the esophagus may also occur due to buckling or doubling over of the tip of the TEE probe. This complication can be caused by improper insertion techniques or by excessive mobility in the tip of the probe due to stretching and elongation of the steering cables. The possibility of transducer buckling should be considered whenever difficulty is encountered while withdrawing the probe or adjusting the control knobs. Probe doubling over has been successfully treated by advancing the transducer into the stomach and straightening the tip (41). There are some options available if difficulty is encountered in introducing the probe into the esophagus. Reverse Sellick maneuver involves lifting the cricoid cartilage forward while the head is kept in neutral position, "lateral neck pressure" where external medially directed pressure can be applied to the ipsilateral neck by multiple fingers at the lateral border of the thyrohyoid membrane. These techniques have been used and reported in literature to be very useful in adults and children during difficult TEE placement while avoiding instrumentation. There are also reports of the successful use of Glidescope (42), when faced with difficulty placing the probe and the use of temporary esophageal overtube for diverticular disease (43). If difficulties with probe insertion are encountered, alternative imaging modalities such as epicardial echocardiography should be considered. Resistance to manipulation after "successful" insertion should alert the operator to possible false passage formation. In such cases, an esophageal endoscopy is recommended for evaluation of the esophagus and prompt initiation of appropriate management for potentially fatal complications (20).

Complications Related to Compression of Adjacent Structures

Several types of airway-related complications have been reported in the literature. Direct compression of the trachea or the tracheal tube by the TEE probe has been described in infants and small children. In a series of 1,650 pediatric TEE examinations, airway obstruction occurred in 14 patients (44). However, a prospective study in pediatric patients demonstrated no changes in pulmonary function variables or gas exchange when a pediatric biplane probe was used (45). Airway obstruction associated with intraoperative TEE has been reported in adult patients with aortic pseudoaneurysms and aortic dissections (46,47). Acute hypoxemia, secondary to TEE-induced malposition of the tracheal tube, can occur in the operating room. Extensive manipulation of the probe may result in advancement of the oral tracheal tube into the right main stem bronchus or inadvertent tracheal extubation (48). There are also reports of edema of the tongue due to the TEE probe that typically resolves on the first post-operative day (49). Sriram et al. reported tongue necrosis and cleft after approximately 8.3 hours of probe contact, presumably from compression of glossal blood vessels. When edema of the tongue is noted, an attempt should be made to reposition any transoral device. ENT could be consulted and if actual necrosis is noted, early debridement is indicated (50).

Hemodynamic changes during TEE probe placement are common. Hypertension and tachycardia are frequently observed during passage of the probe and following laryngoscopy-assisted placement. These events are usually brief and self-limited. Hemodynamically significant supraventricular and ventricular arrhythmias have been reported, but significant arrhythmias occur in less than 0.5% of TEE examinations performed in awake patients (20,51). The incidence of dysrhythmias is reduced when probe insertion and manipulation occur in anesthetized patients (9,21). Pharmacologic interventions are rarely required to treat cardiovascular disturbances since removing the probe can terminate the majority of hemodynamic events.

Vocal cord paralysis is a rare complication of intraoperative TEE. Transient unilateral vocal cord paralysis has been reported in two patients undergoing neurosurgical procedures in the upright position with neck flexion (52,53), with compression of the recurrent laryngeal by the probe being the most likely cause of this injury. Recurrent laryngeal nerve palsy has also been observed in 1.9% to 6.9% of cardiovascular surgical patients in the early postoperative period (54,55). Although an association between intraoperative TEE use and recurrent laryngeal nerve injury in cardiac surgical patients has been suggested (56), a prospective study demonstrated that the incidence of recurrent laryngeal nerve palsy was not significantly different in cardiac surgical patients monitored with or without TEE (49). Other factors appear to be responsible for this complication, including surgical manipulation and the duration of cardiopulmonary bypass and tracheal intubation.

Contraindications

TEE examinations should be avoided or performed with great caution in patients with significant esophageal or gastric pathology (Table 7.10). Flexion and extension of the cervical spine are often required during passage of the probe into the esophagus, creating the potential for injury to the spinal cord or esophagus in patients with significant atlantoaxial disease or cervical arthritis. A careful patient examination for any signs or symptoms related to the GI system should be conducted prior to each TEE examination. Clinicians should be aware of any history of dysphagia, odynophagia, UGI bleeding, esophageal or gastric surgery, mediastinal radiation, or esophageal strictures, tumors, varices, or diverticula. Absolute contraindications to the use of TEE include patient refusal, esophageal strictures, webs, rings, esophageal perforation, obstructing esophageal neoplasms, and cervical spine instability. Physicians must weigh the risks and benefits of IOE in patients with relative contraindications to TEE.

Infection

Bacteremia and Endocarditis

Transient bacteremia may occur during any GI instrumentation. The incidence of bacteremia during UGI endoscopy without biopsy averages approximately 4% (57). Insertion and manipulation of a TEE probe could induce mild trauma to mucosa and allow the introduction of bacteria from the oral cavity and esophagus into the bloodstream. However, the risk of bacteremia during TEE examinations appears low. Several prospective studies have demonstrated that positive blood cultures are obtained in only 0% to 4.2% of patients during and following TEE probe placement (58–60).

In susceptible patients, transient bacteremia can result in bacterial endocarditis. In an analysis of 41 studies of upper endoscopy-induced bacteremia, only two possible cases of endocarditis were noted (57). In both of these patients, factors other than the procedure may have contributed to the development of endocarditis. No cases of endocarditis were reported in the ten studies examining the incidence of bacteremia after TEE (58). A review of the literature reveals only one case report describing a temporal relationship between TEE and endocarditis (61), but a clear cause-and-effect relationship could not be clearly demonstrated.

Infective endocarditis prophylaxis is not necessary for nondental procedures that do not penetrate the mucosa, such as TEE, diagnostic bronchoscopy, esophagogastroscopy, or colonoscopy, in the absence of active infection.

TABLE 7.10	Contraindications to TEE Probe Placement
Absolute Contraindications	
Patient refusal	
Esophageal strictures, webs, or rings	
Esophageal perforation	
Obstructing esophageal neoplasm	
Cervical spine instability	
Relative Contraindications	
Esophageal diverticulum	
Large hiatal hernia	
Recent esophageal or gastric surgery	
Esophageal varices	
History of dysphagia or odynophagia	
Cervical arthritis	
History of radiation to the mediastinum	
Deformities of the oral pharynx	
Severe coagulopathy	

However, in high-risk patients with infections of the GI or GU tract, it is reasonable to administer antibiotic therapy to prevent wound infection or sepsis (62). Thus, there appears to be little scientific evidence to justify endocarditis prophylaxis for TEE in the perioperative setting.

Cleaning and Disinfection of TEE Probes

Bacterial and viral cross-infection between patients has been documented following upper endoscopy (63). A risk of transmission of infective agents between patients also exists with the TEE probe. At the present time, no formal guidelines have been published that describe recommended techniques for sterilization of the TEE probe. When cleaning the TEE probe, most echocardiographers have adopted guidelines established by gastroenterologists for the disinfection of endoscopes (64).

A space outside of the operating room should be dedicated to the cleaning of the probe immediately following each use. This area must be well ventilated and temperature controlled. Heavy-duty gloves and protective eyewear will protect personnel handling the probe from the caustic effects of glutaraldehyde-based solutions. A sink for washing the probe and a container for holding glutaraldehyde disinfectant solution are the minimal requirements for this area. Figure 7.5 illustrates a workstation for cleaning and disinfection of probes. The establishment of dedicated storage areas for contaminated and clean probes will reduce the risk of transducer damage.

The first step in the decontamination of TEE probes is precleaning. Precleaning is the process of mechanically or chemically removing material from the surface of the probe (14). A variety of precleaning methods can be used to remove blood or other organic matter from the probe. Scrubbing the probe with soap and water or isopropyl alcohol will remove most adherent secretions. Several commercially prepared enzymatic precleaning solutions are also available.

Following precleaning, the probe can be either manually or automatically disinfected (Fig. 7.5). The automated disinfectors are less labor intensive compared to the manual process of disinfection and rinsing. The probe is placed in the machine, which occupies little space and is programmed by following the prompts on the display; this takes less than 1 minute. Once the cycle starts, it requires no manual input and takes 15 minutes to complete. Upon completion of the cycle, the probe is disinfected, rinsed, and ready to use. The glutaraldehyde is disposed off by the machine, and a log receipt is printed. Manual cleaning is performed by immediately placing the probe in a disinfecting solution. Only glutaraldehyde-based solutions, approved by the FDA and the manufacturer of the probe, should be used. The probe is immersed in the solution only up to the last depth mark since damage to the system will occur if the control handle is submerged in any liquids. The duration of the manual disinfecting process should be at least 20 minutes to eliminate bacterial and viral contaminants. After removal from the solution, the probe is rinsed in water and allowed to dry for at least 20 to 30 minutes so that residual glutaraldehyde evaporates. It is highly recommended that a logbook be maintained specifying details like patient name, date, time, and name of the person disinfecting the probe. Standards for inspection, cleansing, and disinfection of TEE probes are recommended for each echocardiographic laboratory.

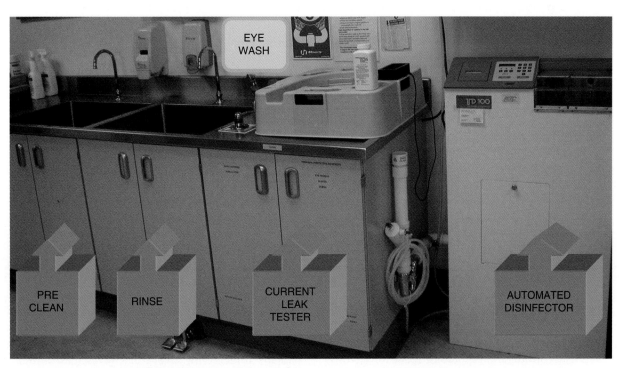

Figure 7.5. Organization of sterilization and disinfection equipment.

Manufacturers' specifications for disinfection soaking time should be followed. Damage to the probe encasement can also occur with use of a wrong disinfectant or excessive immersion time in the recommended disinfectant (14). Probes are covered by warranty but commonly occurring events, such as damage caused by Cidex immersion, dropping, and bite damage, are excluded.

ECONOMICS OF AN INTRAOPERATIVE ECHO SERVICE

The economic considerations that are important for providing IOE services include (i) capital, personnel, and service costs, (ii) improved patient care and outcomes leading to fewer operative complications, (iii) proper billing and documentation, (iv) generation of patient reports and archival of patient studies, and (v) costs associated with credentialing and attaining/maintaining certification. It is important that physicians and institutions understand the practical and financial implications of this service from the cost, patient benefit, and reimbursement perspectives (65).

Capital Equipment Costs

The initial costs related to initiating a new intraoperative echo service include the capital purchase of equipment and training of personnel. An ultrasound system capable of providing the essential services costs between $150,000 and $250,000, depending on the features, software packages, number and type of probes, training, and the purchase of an ongoing service contract. A multiplane TEE transducer will cost between $20,000 and $50,000, depending on the vendor, 3D capabilities, and whether the probe is new or refurbished. 3D TEE imaging is becoming increasingly available so that physicians and hospitals, considering a purchase, should strongly consider systems capable of producing 3D imaging.

A complete IOE service should also provide epicardial and epiaortic imaging, which requires additional probes that are compatible with the same intraoperative system. These surface probes are also used for transthoracic echocardiography and for imaging the internal jugular or subclavian veins to provide ultrasound-guided central venous cannulation (66). The higher frequency probes (7 MHz) are used for pediatric transthoracic echocardiography while lower frequency probes (2 or 3 MHz) are used for adult transthoracic echocardiography. 3D echocardiography is also possible with certain transthoracic probes. A complete system for perioperative echocardiography thus includes a wide variety of probes, which must be compatible with one or more ultrasound machines.

An IOE service may operate independently or in association with an echocardiography service outside the operating room. If an IOE is to operate independently of other services, consideration should be made for securing storage space for digital media, patient reports, viewing stations, and cleaning and storage areas. Maintenance costs include service contracts for upgrades, repair and maintenance of the echocardiographic system, cleaning and storage, report generation, a quality improvement program, and digital media storage.

Training Personnel

A new IOE service requires one or several competent physician echocardiographers. The costs associated with training or hiring physicians depend on the particular service model at each institution. A few options are possible to fulfill this need. An anesthesiologist or cardiologist may already be on staff who possesses appropriate training, experience, and proficiency in performing IOE. Such a scenario enables the service to commence without significant "start-up" costs in personnel training. If an experienced echocardiographer is not on staff, costs will be incurred for recruiting a new cardiovascular anesthesiologist or cardiologist with appropriate training and expertise. One experienced echocardiographer can provide "on the job" training to others using a mentoring approach (67). This is probably the most cost-effective manner to train anesthesiologists and is a particularly attractive option in private practice settings. Another approach is for an individual anesthesiologist to spend a dedicated period of time in a more formal educational program (68), such as during a cardiovascular anesthesia fellowship. Taking the time away from an established practice setting, whether academic or private practice, is costly and may not be practical in all situations. Savage et al. (68) have described their 1-year educational program for IOE, which focuses on acquiring the necessary cognitive and technical skills to proficiently perform IOE.

Patient Benefit

IOE is used to evaluate cardiac function, volume status, pathologic lesions, and corrective surgical repairs. The monetary benefit varies, depending on the particular indication for TEE. Use of IOE to assess valvular pathology and to evaluate a surgical repair allows for immediate detection of a pathologic defect during the initial surgical procedure, reducing the likelihood of repeat cardiac surgery. Potential savings per patient from a TEE-detected defect not requiring further intervention has been estimated between $30,000 and $70,000 per patient at one institution (69). Use of IOE to assess congenital heart disease and evaluate the corrective repair allows for immediate detection of inadequate surgical repair. A discussion on the cost-effectiveness of intraoperative TEE reported that TEE was instrumental in diagnosing inadequate surgical repair in 20% of pediatric cardiac patients, saving between $30,000 and $70,000 per patient in which intraoperative echo altered the surgical plan (69). In a study of high-risk patients undergoing myocardial revascularization, IOE was responsible for alterations in surgical management in

TABLE 7.11	Monetary Benefit of IOE
Type of Surgery	**Monetary Benefit per Case**
Congenital	$875
Valve repair	$750
CABG	$100–$500
Valve	$125

33% and alterations in anesthetic management in 51% of patients (70). The monetary benefit for ischemia monitoring with IOE is unclear.

A cost-benefit analysis by Benson and Cahalan (71) accounted for the incidence of problems detected by TEE in various types of cardiac surgery and the cost associated with not discovering the problem intraoperatively. Their analysis revealed a monetary benefit to TEE use as presented in Table 7.11.

TEE Report and Billing

The ability to effectively communicate the TEE examination results to other health care professionals and the medical record is an essential component of performing intraoperative TEE (72). Many third party insurers require a complete interpretation and report to be generated by the echocardiographer for payment of professional services. The best way to insure a complete examination and report is to perform the comprehensive multiplane TEE examination in a routinely consistent manner and to document the results of the examination on a standardized reporting form. The SCA Web site (www.scahq.org) provides a sample reporting form for intraoperative echo. Key components of this form are a brief patient history that indicates the planned surgical procedure, operation performed, requesting physician, indication for TEE (e.g., evaluate valve repair), probe placement procedure, echocardiographic services performed, and pertinent TEE findings.

Billing for TEE

Reimbursement for intraoperative TEE is dependent on third party payer contracts, whether the echocardiographer is a cardiologist or anesthesiologist, and the geographical region. Many third party payers have adopted the following Center of Medicare Services policy that defines reimbursable indications for intraoperative TEE:

The interpretation of TEE during surgery is covered only when the surgeon or other physician has requested echocardiography for a specific diagnostic reason (e.g., determination of proper valve placement, assessment of the adequacy of valvuloplasty or revascularization, placement of shunts or other devices, assessment of vascular integrity, or detection of intravascular air). To be a covered service, TEE must include

a complete interpretation/report by the performing physician. When TEE is used for monitoring during a surgical procedure, the placement of the probe (93313) is covered. Coverage for evaluation, however, is not allowed for monitoring, technical trouble shooting, or any other purpose that does not meet the medical necessity criteria for the diagnostic test.

The key points for reimbursement of IOE services should include

1. **Documentation that the surgeon or other physician is requesting echocardiography for a specific diagnostic reason.** The medical record should indicate this request either by an order in the medical record, the operative consent form, progress notes, or at the very least within the dictated echocardiography report. It is a good practice for the patient report to indicate the medical necessity for performing the TEE and the physician who requested the IOE service. It should also be clear whether the IOE was performed for diagnostic, monitoring, or research purposes.
2. **A complete interpretation and report are generated by the echocardiographer.** Best practices include submission of a copy of the completed, signed TEE report with the billing sheet.
3. **When TEE is used for monitoring, only placement of the probe is covered.** There is no reimbursement for diagnosis when intraoperative TEE is used only for monitoring.

Billing Codes for Intraoperative TEE

The Relative Value Guide (RVG) published by the ASA includes a "Statement on Transesophageal Echocardiography" that pertains to billing codes for intraoperative TEE. The most commonly used billing codes include

93312—Echocardiography, transesophageal, real time with image documentation (2D) (with or without M-mode recording); including probe placement, image acquisition, interpretation, and report. This service involves placement of the transesophageal probe, obtaining the appropriate images and views, and critical analysis of the data. Patients with increased risks of hemodynamic disturbances may require probe insertion and interpretation of the echocardiogram. This includes, but is not limited to, histories of congestive heart failure, severe ischemic heart disease, valvular disease, aortic aneurysm, major trauma, and burns. It may also be indicated in certain procedures that involve great shifts in the patient's volume status. Such procedures may include vascular surgery, cardiac surgery, liver resection/transplantation, extensive tumor resections, and radical orthopedic surgery. The use of TEE may also be indicated when central venous access is contraindicated or difficult, and it is not possible to adequately assess blood loss and replacement, impairment of venous return, and right and left heart function without the TEE.

93313—Echocardiography, transesophageal, real time with image documentation (2D) (with or without M-mode recording); placement of transesophageal probe only. Although the procedure is generally safe, the proper insertion of the probe requires skill and judgment. There are a few inherent risks to placement of the probe, including pharyngeal and/or laryngeal trauma, dental injuries, esophageal trauma, bleeding, arrhythmias, respiratory distress, and hemodynamic effects. There have even been case reports of perioperative death attributed to TEE probe placement.

93314—Echocardiography, transesophageal, real time with image documentation (2D) (with or without M-mode recording); image acquisition, interpretation, and report only. This code is used when one physician inserts the probe and another physician interprets the images. Physicians who obtain and interpret cardiac images and provide a report but who did not place the TEE probe should use this code to report their service.

93315—TEE for congenital cardiac anomalies, including probe placement, image acquisition, interpretation, and report. This service involves placement of the transesophageal probe, obtaining the appropriate images and views, and critical analysis of the data in patients with congenital cardiac anomalies. This includes, but is not limited to, congenital valve problems, such as bicuspid aortic valve, septal defects, including patent foramen ovale, and more complicated congenital heart defects. This includes, but is not limited to, all the indications listed for code 93312 but in patients with congenital cardiac anomalies.

93316—Placement of transesophageal probe only (for congenital cardiac anomalies). This is the equivalent of code 93313 but in patients with congenital cardiac anomalies.

93317—Image acquisition, interpretation, and report only (for congenital cardiac anomalies). This is the equivalent of code 93314 but in patients with congenital cardiac anomalies.

93318—Echocardiography, transesophageal (TEE) for monitoring purposes, including probe placement, real-time 2D image acquisition and interpretation leading to ongoing (continuous) assessment of (dynamically changing) cardiac pumping function and to therapeutic measures on an immediate time basis. This code is used when the patient's condition, as described under 93312, requires repetitive evaluation of cardiac function in order to guide ongoing management.

93320—Doppler echocardiography, pulsed wave and/or continuous wave with spectral display. This code is used to evaluate blood velocity and flow patterns through various cardiac and vascular structures. Stenotic lesions generally lead to increased blood velocity proportional to the degree of stenosis, thereby providing a method to assess the severity of stenosis.

Velocity measurements are also used to calculate the area of stenotic valves and regurgitant orifices. This code may be submitted along with code 93312 or 93315.

93325—Doppler color flow velocity mapping. This code is used to evaluate the direction and character of blood flow through various cardiac and vascular structures. This code may be submitted along with code 93312 or 93315.

Use of Modifiers

If the TEE is performed for diagnostic purposes by the same anesthesiologist who is providing the anesthesia service, modifier 59 should be appended to the TEE code to note that it is distinct and independent from the anesthesia service. If the anesthesiologist does not own the TEE equipment, s/he reports only the professional component of the TEE service and should append modifier 26 (Professional Component) to the TEE code.

Bundling Issues

TEE is a special diagnostic tool, which may be used by properly trained physicians (i.e., anesthesiologists, cardiologists) to benefit patient care. Perioperative use of TEE should be separately reported and paid for the following reasons:

1. TEE is a special tool and not a standard intraoperative technique. It provides unique information that no other diagnostic procedure can provide. TEE permits ongoing assessment of cardiovascular function and immediate treatment of abnormalities related to surgical interventions, anesthesia effects, and changing patient conditions.

2. Intraoperative TEE is a relatively new diagnostic tool, which has not been factored in any of the current base unit values for anesthesia care reimbursement. The ASA-RVG unit values for anesthesia services do not include the special information TEE provides or the increased risk and work of the echocardiographer.

3. Because medical conditions that indicate the use of TEE exist in patients undergoing a great variety of operations, the unit values of specific anesthesia services do not reflect the use of the TEE.

4. A TEE examination is a service extending beyond the scope of standard perioperative anesthesia care. This is obvious when the service is requested by the surgeon or other physician but is also true if the anesthesiologist believes the TEE to be clinically indicated in a given patient.

5. Any physicians using TEE should be specifically credentialed by their institution to do so.

6. Anesthesiologists using TEE provide information equivalent to that provided by any consulting physician (e.g., cardiologist) using echocardiography for a given indication. This is not part of, but rather in addition to, the anesthesia service being provided.

TEE BILLING FORM

Date of Service: _____

Physician requesting service: _____

Physician Echocardiographer: _____

PROCEDURE CODES (check all procedures performed)

[ ] 93312-26: Echocardiography, transesophageal, real time with image documentation (2D) (with or without M-mode recording) including probe placement, image acquisition, interpretation & report

    [ ] 93313-26 TEE probe placement only [ ] 93314: Interpretation/report only

[ ] 93315-26 Echocardiography, transesophageal, real time with image documentation (2D) including probe placement, image acquisition, interpretation & report (as 93312) **for congenital anomalies**

    [ ] 93316-26 TEE probe placement only [ ] 93317: Interpretation/report only for congenital anomalies

[ ] 93318-26: **TEE used for monitoring purposes only**

[ ] 93320-26: Doppler echocardiography, pulsed wave and/or continuous wave with spectral display

[ ] 93325-26: Doppler color flow velocity mapping

ICD-9 CODES (Check all that identify the diagnostic indication for TEE)

LEFT VENTRICLE

[ ] Cardiomegaly	429.3
[ ] Functional disturbance following cardiac surgery	429.4
[ ] Fluid overload	276.6
[ ] Hypertrophic obstructive cardiomyopathy	425.1
[ ] Alcoholic cardiomyopathy	425.5
[ ] Other cardiomyopathy	425.4
[ ] Ventricular septal defect	745.4
[ ] Left ventricular aneurysm	414.10
[ ] Acquired cardiac septal defect	429.71

MITRAL VALVE

[ ] Rheumatic mitral stenosis	394.0
[ ] Rheumatic mitral regurgitation	394.1
[ ] Rheumatic mitral stenosis with regurgitation	394.2
[ ] Mitral regurgitation – non rheumatic	424.0
[ ] Ruptured chordae tendinae	429.5
[ ] Ruptured papillary muscle	429.6
[ ] Other papillary muscle disorders	429.81

AORTIC VALVE

[ ] Rheumatic aortic stenosis	395.0
[ ] Rheumatic aortic insufficiency	395.1
[ ] Rheumatic aortic stenosis with insufficiency	395.2
[ ] Other aortic valve disease with AS or AI	424.1
[ ] Congenital stenosis of aortic valve	746.3
[ ] Congenital insufficiency of aortic valve	746.4

COMBINED AORTIC/MITRAL VALVE DISEASE

[ ] Mitral stenosis with aortic stenosis	396.0
[ ] Mitral stenosis with aortic insufficiency	396.1
[ ] Mitral insufficiency with aortic stenosis	396.2
[ ] Mitral insufficiency with aortic insufficiency	396.3
[ ] MS and/or MI with AS and/or AI	396.8

TRICUSPID VALVE

[ ] Rheumatic disease, stenosis or regurgitation	397.0
[ ] Other, stenosis or regurgitation	424.2

PULMONIC VALVE

[ ] Rheumatic diseases of the pulmonic valve	397.1
[ ] Pulmonary valve disorder, non-rheumatic	424.3

ENDOCARDITIS (any valve)

[ ] Bacterial	421.0
[ ] Endocarditis, not specified as bacterial	424.90

AORTA

[ ] Atherosclerosis	440.0
[ ] Dissection of thoraic aorta	441.01
Thoracic aneurysm: [ ] ruptured 441.1 [ ] unruptured 441.2	
[ ] Injury to thoracic aorta	901.0

HYPOTENSION

[ ] Septicemia	038.9
[ ] Volume depletion	276.5
[ ] Cardiogenic shock	785.51
[ ] Traumatic shock	958.4
[ ] Postoperative shock	998.0
[ ] Shock, unspecified	785.50
Hypotension: [ ] specified 458.8 [ ] unspecified	458.9

TUMORS

[ ] Benign neoplasm of the heart	212.7
[ ] Neoplasms of unspecified nature	239.8

CONGENITAL

[ ] Ostium secundum ASD or patent foramen ovale	745.5
[ ] Ostium primum	745.61
[ ] Partial anomalous pulmonary venous connection	747.42
[ ] Patent ductus arteriosus	747.0

MISCELLANEOUS

[ ] Air embolism	999.1
[ ] Iatrogenic pulmonary embolism	415.11
[ ] Other pulmonary embolism	415.19
[ ] Atrial fibrillation	427.31
[ ] Atrial flutter	427.32

Figure 7.6. TEE billing form.

Diagnosis Codes

Equally important for billing is to indicate the appropriate ICD-9 code that identifies the pathologic lesion for which the echocardiogram is performed. Common ICD-9 codes that qualify for reimbursement are listed in the CMS Report Policy of each particular Local Carrier Determination. Any diagnosis not listed is not covered for reimbursement. Claims submitted without a covered ICD-9 code are denied for reasons of failing to justify medical necessity. A typical billing sheet that includes both commonly used CPT and ICD-9 codes is provided in Figure 7.6.

Credentialing

Many third party carrier policies include a statement similar to that of the CMS policy, which states, "**Physicians who perform, supervise, and/or interpret the studies must be capable of demonstrating training and experience specific to the study performed or interpreted and maintain documentation for post payment audit.**" At the very least, the institution in which the TEE is performed should credential the physician echocardiographer. Further demonstration of qualifications may be accomplished on the successful completion of either of two examinations administered by the NBE: the "**Perioperative Transesophageal Echocardiography Certification Examination**" or "**An Examination of Special Competence in Echocardiography.**" Board certification is also available through NBE after requisite training in perioperative echocardiography (10). CMS Policy does not specifically state that the physician echocardiographer should pass one of these examinations. However, physicians may use the successful completions of these exams combined with clinical experience to demonstrate training and expertise worthy of reimbursement or credentialing within their hospital.

ASSESSING QUALITY IN AN INTRAOPERATIVE TEE SERVICE

In the last two decades, the use of TEE in the operating room has seen significant technological advances, which have permitted the anesthesiologist to perform a comprehensive examination on every patient but have also heightened the complexity of the procedure. Diagnostic interpretations of these TEE examinations may vary widely, particularly when the anesthesiologist performing the examination is responsible for the anesthetic management of the patient (73). The clinical experience of the examiner conducting a test may also have a favorable or perhaps even a detrimental effect on outcome (74). In recent years, the goal of improving quality in health care has gained national prominence, triggered in large part by a publication on medical errors from the Institute of Medicine (IOM) (75). This report galvanized the public and the private sector and the medical profession into a collaborative effort at building a safer health care system.

A centerpiece of that strategy has been the assessment and improvement of quality in health care delivery.

Any dialogue on CQI first merits a definition of the word "quality." The IOM has defined quality as "the degree to which health services for individuals and populations increase the likelihood of desired health outcomes and are consistent with current professional knowledge" (76). Continuous quality improvement (CQI) is a management methodology adapted by health care providers from business and industry that is designed to identify and analyze problems in health care delivery. More importantly, once a problem is identified, CQI encourages the development, testing, and implementation of solutions without assigning blame. The essential elements of CQI include an "orientation towards customers and systems (processes), a commitment to understanding and minimizing process variations, and the development of teams that can broaden vision and implement solutions" (77). CQI in perioperative echocardiography is a continual process characterized by three assumptions about quality: (a) technological advancements in echocardiography may redefine quality and therefore the ensuing recommendations, (b) assessments of quality often require comparisons, and (c) quality is enhanced by repetitive practice (78).

In 2006, the American Society of Echocardiography and the SCA developed a series of recommendations for CQI in perioperative echocardiography (79). Prior to establishing the principles of CQI, this document outlined the components of a "high quality" perioperative echocardiography service, which included (a) equipment and recording, (b) the request for echocardiographic services, (c) patient interactions, (d) the role of the physician and sonographer, (e) performance and interpretation time, and (f) the role of a comprehensive versus limited examination. To begin with, an ultrasound machine with multiplane imaging and full diagnostic capabilities (2D, Doppler, and M-mode) is required to provide a comprehensive perioperative echocardiographic examination. Additionally, a system for permanently recording data onto a media format that allows for offline review or analysis is needed, and ideally, this would be an all-digital capture, storage, and review process that incorporates the Digital Imaging and Communications in Medicine (DICOM) format, high-speed networking, and permanent storage with built-in redundancy. The second component of a perioperative service is the request for echocardiographic services, which must be documented on the surgical schedule, anesthesia record, or permanent medical record. Furthermore, the indications for performing perioperative echocardiography should be documented clearly, either in the anesthesia record or on the report of echocardiographic findings. With regard to patient interactions, the echocardiographer is expected to discern relative or absolute contraindications to examination, review risk and benefits of the procedure, document informed consent, either separately or as part of the general anesthetic consent, and use the clinical history in conjunction with echocardiographic data to guide perioperative management decisions.

The cardiac sonographer in the echocardiography laboratory plays a well-respected and integral role in acquiring comprehensive echocardiographic examinations by applying independent judgment and problem-solving skills. He or she has specific training in obtaining accurate images and integrating diagnostic information during the performance of the examination. In the perioperative environment, a sonographer may assist the physician in manipulation of the controls on the ultrasonography system; however, the physician must always be present to insert the TEE probe, perform a perioperative TEE examination, interpret the echocardiographic data, and assist the surgeon by providing information pertinent to surgical decisions.

The time needed to complete a comprehensive perioperative examination will vary depending on the complexity of the case. No minimal time has been established to perform a comprehensive evaluation; however, initial study time may last 10 to 45 minutes, including time for discussion between cardiologists, surgeons, and anesthesiologists. Additional time may be needed for important Doppler calculations and complementary evaluations. It is also recognized that the entire duration of an intraoperative examination may total several hours, as repeated sequential examinations are conducted to assess acute hemodynamic changes or the adequacy of surgical repair. Echocardiographic data that will influence the surgical plan should be interpreted and reported to the surgeon in an ongoing and timely manner. A verbal report must be provided throughout and in particular, at the completion of the initial examination to both the surgical and anesthesia care teams. A written or electronic description of the findings should be left in an obvious location within the operating room upon completion, so that it is available for immediate reference. Furthermore, a written or electronic report outlining key findings should be included in the medical record by the end of the procedure. Official reports of all the intraoperative data may be generated after completion of the surgical procedure and should be consistent with the real-time interpretation provided to the surgeon. Such a report should be legible, placed in the patient's medical record within 24 hours of surgery, and include (i) a description of the echocardiographic procedure, (ii) indications for the procedure, and (iii) important findings.

Although a comprehensive examination is always recommended, a limited or focused study may be occasionally indicated. Typically, these patients have had a recent comprehensive examination with no expected interval change other than in the area being reexamined. A limited intraoperative TEE examination may also be warranted following a request to determine the etiology of acute hemodynamic compromise such as during an intraoperative cardiac arrest. Although not all components of the comprehensive examination may be needed in every patient, the practitioner should attempt to acquire all 20 of the recommended views (80) accompanied by appropriate Doppler and hemodynamic data in the event they are needed for remote consultation.

Six fundamental principles guide the formation of an intraoperative CQI process (16). To begin with, physicians who perform and interpret intraoperative echocardiographic studies must have adequate primary training. Guidelines for basic and advanced training have been published and discussed earlier in this chapter (9,10). A certifying examination in perioperative TEE has also been developed and administered with higher overall examination performance associated with longer than 3 months of training and performance and interpretation of at least six examinations a week (81). Beyond primary training and testing, the process of CQI must require that those who perform intraoperative studies maintain a case volume sufficient to maintain their skills and competency. Upon completion of the primary training requirements, a minimum of 50 examinations per year, with at least 25 personally performed, is required to remain proficient in performing perioperative echocardiography. In addition, CME in perioperative echocardiography is essential to keep pace with technical advances, refinements in established techniques, and application of new methods. Physicians practicing perioperative echocardiography should obtain a minimum of 15 hours every 3 years of Category I CME credits in echocardiography.

Third, CQI requires periodic impartial review of study performance and interpretation by those at a higher training level. This includes caseload review, performance review, record keeping review, and documentation of proper equipment performance. In addition to the caseload requirements for training at the basic and advanced level, a minimum of 25 intraoperative TEE studies per month should be performed by a perioperative echocardiographic service. A minimum of five cases for each echocardiographer in a service should also be subjected to review every 12 months in order to assess the documentation of the indications for the procedure and patient consent, appropriate use of ultrasound system technology and controls, the adequacy and presentation of the imaging planes, and concurrence between the recorded images and the written report. In a similar fashion, an interpretation review should be conducted every year on five of the cases for each physician in the service. Here the focus is not on the performance variables but rather on whether the examination has been accurately interpreted. The two interpretations should be compared and any differences discussed with the primary physician. A final component of the periodic review process is that of equipment review. All electrical systems should be checked for current leakage according to industry standards. TEE probes should be checked for leakage at a minimum of every 3 months. Regular preventive maintenance service should be conducted according to manufacturer's recommendations. In the intraoperative environment, it is critical that echocardiographic equipment such as the TEE probes be cleaned according to institutional guidelines. In addition, the ultrasound system and electrocardiographic cables should be wiped carefully with an antiseptic solution after each patient use.

Fourth, CQI requires formal continuing education at local, regional, and national levels to maintain competence in a rapidly changing field. In addition to the CME requirements outlined earlier, every perioperative echocardiographic service should conduct a service conference lasting between 30 and 60 minutes at least once a month. This conference should cover a wide assortment of echocardiographic topics and may range in format from case reviews to formal didactic presentations. Fifth, continuing performance, competence, and education must be documented and submitted to a hospital or departmental quality assurance committee. Finally, CQI requires a yearly utilization review of echocardiographic services. Utilization review should aim to determine if the study was indicated, if the appropriate views were obtained, if the question at hand was answered, and if the study was interpreted and the report distributed in a timely fashion.

Research into the importance of training and CQI processes for perioperative TEE is limited but a few studies merit discussion. Stevenson has reported on the outcome of congenital cardiac surgery when TEE was performed by physicians who met training guidelines and compared it to those who did not meet the criteria (73). In his study, 219 patients undergoing repair of congenital cardiac defects were included in the study where, in the first year of the study, physicians who met ASE guidelines for pediatric TEE performed intraoperative TEE. In the second year of the study, physicians who performed the examinations did not meet the guidelines for training. Despite similar mortality rates for both groups, physicians who did not meet training guidelines had lower rates of adequacy of TEE studies, detection of residual cardiac lesions, and use of TEE in returning to cardiopulmonary bypass for additional surgery. Stevenson concluded that patient outcome is better when physicians who meet published guidelines perform intraoperative TEE and a physician other than the physician providing intraoperative care for the patient should perform the echocardiography examination. In an accompanying editorial, Fyfe further argued that "the conflicting responsibilities of serving as both the intraoperative anesthesiologist and the echocardiographer" might preclude performing either task well (82).

In response, Mathew et al. (83) assessed the quality of intraoperative TEE examinations performed by 10 cardiac anesthesiologists participating in a CQI program at a university hospital. The anesthesiologists first interpreted 154 comprehensive TEE examinations from adult patients undergoing cardiac surgery shortly after the examinations were completed in the operating room. A second interpretation of these examinations was then conducted off-line by two primary echocardiographers (a radiologist and cardiologist), and interrater agreement between the three raters was measured using the kappa coefficient (κ) and percent agreement. Between anesthesiologist and

radiologist, the agreement was 83% (κ: 0.58), between anesthesiologist and cardiologist 80% (κ: 0.57), and between radiologist and cardiologist 82% (κ: 0.60). This study demonstrated that an anesthesiologist responsible for the anesthetic management of an adult cardiac patient could in fact function as an intraoperative echocardiographer. Furthermore, the performance and interpretation of the TEE examinations can be conducted at a level comparable to that provided by "experts" evaluating the TEE examinations removed from the demands of the operating room (i.e., off-line). Thus, the anesthesiologist and intraoperative echocardiographer need not be mutually exclusive.

Although it appears that the anesthesiologist may be able to simultaneously serve as an echocardiographer, the need for adequate training cannot be minimized. The study by Mathew et al. (83) did reveal that, when compared to the "expert," anesthesiologists with more than 5 years of experience had higher levels of agreement than those with less than 5 years of experience. For instance, using bias analysis, they demonstrated that anesthesiologists as a group underestimated fractional area change (FAC) when compared to the off-line assessment of the expert. Much of this underestimation was related to the experience of the user. Similarly, Bergquist et al. (84), in a study evaluating real-time intraoperative interpretation, showed that anesthesiologists can estimate FAC in real time to within ±10% of off-line values in only 75% of all cases but to within ±20% in 93% of all cases.

Finally, although a CQI process may appear cumbersome, it is a process that can function well in the intraoperative environment. Miller et al. (85) reported on a process of providing educational aids and regular TEE performance feedback to eight cardiac anesthesiologists conducting 135 intraoperative TEE studies. The process of education and feedback increased the ability to record a basic TEE examination from 42% to 81%. Furthermore, 79% of the images were interpreted accurately while 15% were not evaluated and only 6% were incorrectly interpreted when compared to the consensus interpretation of up to three experts.

In summary, the demands of the perioperative environment dictate that a CQI process be implemented as soon as the service is established. A CQI process always seeks to identify problems and fix them without assigning blame. Once problems have been fixed, new ones are identified and the cycle repeats itself endlessly. It is vital that assessments of quality not be directed simply at meeting training requirements or passing tests. Quality is not equivalent to accreditation or certification—it is not examinations, tests, or numbers and it is not determined by the user but by the consumer (patient, surgeon, referring cardiologist). Aside from being a mandate of various accreditation agencies, CQI is a process that will aid perioperative echocardiographers in improving the delivery of care to patients. CQI in the perioperative environment is feasible but must move from the periphery to the core of the echocardiography service.

KEY POINTS

■ Physicians performing intraoperative TEE should establish a collaborative relationship with a colleague who has advanced training in TEE.

■ Alternative methods like epicardial echocardiography should be considered if TEE cannot be performed.

■ The TEE probe should be carefully inspected for any cracks or perforations after each examination.

■ The risks of an electrical injury to a patient will be reduced if a leakage current test is performed after each use of the probe.

■ Patients should be evaluated for any signs or symptoms of esophageal or gastric disease during the preoperative history and physical examination. The risks and benefits of TEE must be carefully weighed in patients with relative contraindications to TEE.

■ Routine antibiotic prophylaxis to prevent endocarditis is not required prior to TEE except in high-risk patients.

■ TEE probes must be disinfected for at least 20 minutes in a glutaraldehyde-based solution to eliminate bacterial and viral contaminants.

■ A thorough and complete understanding of the economics of an intraoperative TEE service is important for identifying patient benefit and justifying acquisition of necessary equipment and personnel.

■ Proper billing practices require adequate documentation of medical necessity for performing IOE services, use of correct CPT procedural codes, and accurate ICD diagnostic codes.

■ A CQI process must be implemented as soon as an IOE service is established.

■ A CQI process always seeks to identify problems and fix them without assigning blame.

REFERENCES

1. Morewood GH, Gallagher ME, Gaughan JIP, et al. Current practice patterns for adult perioperative transesophageal echocardiography in the United States. *Anesthesiology* 2001; 95:1507–1512.

2. Lambert AS, Mazer CD, Duke PC. Survey of the members of the cardiovascular section of the Canadian Anesthesiologists' Society on the use of perioperative transesophageal echocardiography—a brief report. *Can J Anaesth* 2002;49:294–296.

3. Shapira Y, Vaturi M, Weisenberg DE, et al. Impact of intraoperative transesophageal echocardiography in patients undergoing valve replacement. *Ann Thorac Surg* 2004;78:579–583.

4. Kneeshaw JD. Transoesophageal echocardiography (TOE) in the operating room. *Br J Anaesth* 2006;97:77–84.

5. Handke M, Heinrichs G, Moser U, et al. Transesophageal real-time three-dimensional echocardiography methods and initial in vitro and human in vivo studies. *J Am Coll Cardiol* 2006;48(10):2070–2076.

6. Poterack KA. Who uses transesophageal echocardiography in the operating room? *Anesth Analg* 1995;80:454–458.

7. Wax DB, Torres A, Scher C, et al. Transesophageal echocardiography utilization in high-volume liver transplantation centers in the United States. *J Cardiothor Vasc Anesth* 2008;22(6):811–813.

8. Bettex DA, Schmidlin D, Bernath MA, et al. Intraoperative transesophageal echocardiography in pediatric congenital cardiac surgery: a two-center observational study. *Anesth Analg* 2003;97:1275–1282.

9. Practice guidelines for perioperative transesophageal echocardiography. A report by the American Society of Anesthesiologists and the Society of Cardiovascular Anesthesiologists Task Force on Transesophageal Echocardiography. *Anesthesiology* 1996;84:986–1006.

10. Cahalan MK, Abel M, Goldman M, et al; American Society of Echocardiography and Society of Cardiovascular Anesthesiologists task force guidelines for training in perioperative echocardiography. American Society of Echocardiography; Society of Cardiovascular Anesthesiologists. *Anesth Analg* 2002;94(6):1384–1388.

11. National Board of Echocardiography, Inc: Board certification in perioperative transesophageal Echocardiography. Available at http://echoboards.org/certification /pte/reqs.html-4

12. Hung J, Lang R, Flachskampf F, et al. 3D echocardiography: a review of the current status and future directions. *J Am Soc Echocardiogr* 2007;20(3):213–233.

13. Sugeng L, Shernan SK, Salgo IS, et al. Live 3-dimensional transesophageal echocardiography: initial experience using the fully-sampled matrix array probe. *J Am Coll Cardiol* 2008; 52:446–449.

14. Sequoia Ultrasound System: User and Reference Manuals. Mountain View, CA: Accuson Corp., 2000–2001.

15. Taillefer J, Couture P, Sheridan P, et al. A comprehensive strategy to avoid transesophageal echocardiography probe damage. *Can J Anaesth* 2002;49:500–502.

16. Denault AY, Couture P, McKenty S, et al. Perioperative use of transesophageal echocardiography by anesthesiologists: impact in noncardiac surgery and in the intensive care unit. *Can J Anaesth* 2002;49(3):287–293.

17. Sanfilippo AJ, Bewick D, Chan KL, et al. Guidelines for the provision of echocardiography in Canada: recommendations of a joint Canadian Cardiovascular Society/Canadian Society of Echocardiography Consensus Panel. *Can J Cardiol* 2005;21:763–780.

18. European Association of Echocardiography recommendations for standardization of performance, digital storage and reporting of echocardiographic studies. *Eur J Echocardiogr* 2008;9:438–448.

19. Douglas PS, Khandheria, B, Stainback RF, et al. ACCF/ASE/ACEP/ASNC/SCAI/SCCT/SCMR 2007 appropriateness criteria for transthoracic and transesophageal echocardiography, *J Am Coll Cardiol* 2007;50(2):187–204.

20. Daniel WG, Erbel R, Kasper W, et al. Safety of transesophageal echocardiography. A multicenter survey of 10,419 examinations. *Circulation* 1991;83:817–821.

21. Kallmeyer IJ, Collard CD, Fox JA, et al. The safety of intraoperative transesophageal echocardiography: a case series of 7,200 cardiac surgical patients. *Anesth Analg* 2001;92:1126–1230.

22. Chan KL, Cohen GI, Sochowski RA, et al. Complications of transesophageal echocardiography in ambulatory adult patients: analysis of 1,500 consecutive examinations. *J Am Soc Echocardiogr* 1991;4:577–582.

23. Mishra M, Chauhan R, Sharma KK, et al. Real-time intraoperative transesophageal echocardiography—how useful? Experience of 5,016 cases. *J Cardiothorac Vasc Anesth* 1998;12:625–632.

24. Silvis SE, Nebel O, Rogers G, et al. Endoscopic complications. Results of the 1974 American Society for Gastrointestinal Endoscopy Survey. *JAMA* 1976;235:928–930.

25. Brinkman WT, Shanewise JS, Clements SD, et al. Transesophageal echocardiography: not an innocuous procedure. *Ann Thorac Surg* 2001;72:1725–1726.

26. Massey SR, Pitsis A, Mehta D, et al. Esophageal perforation following perioperative transesophageal echocardiography. *Br J Anaesth* 2000;84:643–646.

27. St-Pierre J, Fortier LP, Couture P, et al. Massive gastrointestinal hemorrhage after transesophageal echocardiography probe insertion. *Can J Anaesth* 1998;45:1196–1199.

28. Lennon MJ, Gibbs NM, Weightman WM, et al. Transesophageal echocardiography-related gastrointestinal complications in cardiac surgical patients. *J Cardiothor Vasc Anesth* 2005;19(2): 141–145.

29. Spahn DR, Schmid S, Carrel T, et al. Hypopharynx perforation by a transesophageal echocardiography probe. *Anesthesiology* 1995;82:581–583.

30. Han YY, Cheng YJ, Liao WW, et al. Delayed diagnosis of esophageal perforation following intraoperative transesophageal echocardiography during valvular replacement—A case report. *Acta Anaesthesiol Scan* 2003;41(2):81–84.

31. Muir AD, White J, McGuigan JA, et al. Treatment and outcomes of esophageal perforation in a tertiary referral center. *Eur J Cardiothoracic Surg* 2003;23:799–804.

32. Hogue CW, Jr, Lappas GD, Creswell LL, et al. Swallowing dysfunction after cardiac operations. Associated adverse outcomes and risk factors including intraoperative transesophageal echocardiography. *J Thorac Cardiovasc Surg* 1995;110:517–22.

33. Rousou JA, Tighe DA, Garb JL, et al. Risk of dysphagia after transesophageal echocardiography during cardiac operations. *Ann Thorac Surg* 2000;69:486–489; discussion 489–490.

34. Messina AG, Paranicas M, Fiamengo S, et al. Risk of dysphagia after transesophageal echocardiography. *Am J Cardiol* 1991;67:313–314.

35. Hulyalkar AR, Ayd JD. Low risk of gastroesophageal injury associated with transesophageal echocardiography during cardiac surgery. *J Cardiothorac Vasc Anesth* 1993;7:175–177.

36. Kohr LM, Dargan M, Hague A, et al. The incidence of dysphagia in pediatric patients after open heart procedures with transesophageal echocardiography. *Ann Thorac Surg* 2003;76:1450–1456.

37. Ayres NA, Fyfe DA, Stevensone GL, et al. Indications and guidelines for performance of transesophageal echocardiography in the patient with pediatric acquired or congenital heart disease: a report from the Task Force of the Pediatric Council of the American Society of Echocardiography. *J Am Soc Echocardiogr* 2005;18(1):91–98.

38. Aviv JE, Di Tullio MR, Homma S, et al. Hypopharyngeal perforation near–miss during transesophageal echocardiography. *Laryngoscope* 2004;114:821–826.

39. O'Shea JIP, Southern JE, D'Ambra MN, et al. Effects of prolonged transesophageal echocardiographic imaging and probe manipulation on the esophagus an echocardiographic-pathologic study. *J Am Coll Cardiol* 1991;17:1426–1429.

40. Augoustides JG, Hosalkar HH, Milas BL, et al. Upper gastrointestinal injuries related to perioperative transesophageal echocardiography: index case, literature review, classification proposal, and call for a registry. *J Cardiothorac Vasc Anesth* 2006;20(3):379–384.

41. Kronzon I, Cziner DG, Katz ES, et al. Buckling of the tip of the transesophageal echocardiography probe: a potentially dangerous technical malfunction. *J Am Soc Echocardiogr* 1992;5:176–177.

42. Hirabayaski Y. GlideScope-assisted insertion of a transesophageal echocardiography probe. *J Cardiothorac Vasc Anesth* 2007;21(4):628.

43. Willens HJ, Lamet M, Migikovsky B, et al. A technique for performing transesophageal echocardiography safely in patients with Zenker's diverticulum. *J Am Soc Echocardiogr* 1994;7(5):534–537.

44. Stevenson JG. Incidence of complications in pediatric transesophageal echocardiography: experience in 1650 cases. *J Am Soc Echocardiogr* 1999;12:527–532.

45. Andropoulos DB, Ayres NA, Stayer SA, et al. The effect of transesophageal echocardiography on ventilation in small infants undergoing cardiac surgery. *Anesth Analg* 2000;90:47–49.

46. Arima H, Sobue K, Tanaka S, et al. Airway obstruction associated with transesophageal echocardiography in a patient with a giant aortic pseudoaneurysm. *Anesth Analg* 2002;95: 558–560.

47. Nakao S, Eguchi T, Ikeda S, et al. Airway obstruction by a transesophageal echocardiography probe in an adult patient with a dissecting aneurysm of the ascending aorta and arch. *J Cardiothorac Vasc Anesth* 2000;14:186–187.

48. Ziegeler S, Pulido MA, Hirsch D. Acute oxygen desaturation and right heart dysfunction secondary to transesophageal echocardiography-induced malpositioning of the endotracheal tube. *Anesth Analg* 2002;95:255–256.

49. Yanamoto H, Fujimura N, Namiki A. Swelling of tongue afvter intraoperative monitoring by transesophageal echocardiography. *Masui* 2001;50:1250–1252.

50. Sriram S, Khorasani A, Mbekeani K. Tongue necrosis and cleft after prolonged transesophageal echocardiography probe placement. *Anesthesiology* 2006;105:635.

51. Khanderia BK, Tajik AJ, Freeman WK. Transesophageal echocardiographic examination: technique, training, and safety. In: Freeman WK, ed. *Transesophageal Echocardiography*. Boston, MA: Little Brown, 1994:599.

52. Gussenhoven EJ, Taams MA, Roelandt JR, et al. Transesophageal two-dimensional echocardiography: its role in solving clinical problems. *J Am Coll Cardiol* 1986;8:975–979.

53. Cucchiara RF, Nugent M, Seward JIB, et al. Air embolism in upright neurosurgical patients: detection and localization by two-dimensional transesophageal echocardiography. *Anesthesiology* 1984;60:353–355.

54. Shafei H, el-Kholy A, Azmy S, et al. Vocal cord dysfunction after cardiac surgery: an overlooked complication. *Eur J Cardiothorac Surg* 1997;11:564–566.

55. Kawahito S, Kitahata H, Kimura H, et al. Recurrent laryngeal nerve palsy after cardiovascular surgery: relationship to the placement of a transesophageal echocardiographic probe. *J Cardiothorac Vasc Anesth* 1999;13:528–531.

56. Shintani H, Nakano S, Matsuda H, et al. Efficacy of transesophageal echocardiography as a perioperative monitor in patients undergoing cardiovascular surgery. Analysis of 149 consecutive studies. *J Cardiovasc Surg (Torino)* 1990;31:564–570.

57. Botoman VA, Surawicz CM. Bacteremia with gastrointestinal endoscopic procedures. *Gastrointest Endosc* 1986;32: 342–346.

58. Mentec H, Vignon P, Terre S, et al. Frequency of bacteremia associated with transesophageal echocardiography in intensive care unit patients: a prospective study of 139 patients. *Crit Care Med* 1995;23:1194–1199.

59. Voller H, Spielberg C, Schroder K, et al. Frequency of positive blood cultures during transesophageal echocardiography. *Am J Cardiol* 1991;68:1538–1540.

60. Shyu KG, Hwang JJ, Lin SC, et al. Prospective study of blood culture during transesophageal echocardiography. *Am Heart J* 1992;124:1541–1544.

61. Foster E, Kusumoto FM, Sobol SM, et al. Streptococcal endocarditis temporally related to transesophageal echocardiography. *J Am Soc Echocardiogr* 1990;3:424–427.

62. Practice Guideline: Focused Update ACC/AHA 2008 Guideline Update on Valvular Heart Disease: Focused Update on Infective Endocarditis. *J Am Coll Cardiol* 2008;52:676–685.

63. Birnie GG, Quigley EM, Clements GB, et al. Endoscopic transmission of hepatitis B virus. *Gut* 1983;24:171–174.

64. Banerjee S, Shen B, Nelson BD. Infection control during GI endoscopy. Prepared by: ASGE Standards of Practice Committee. *Gastrointest Endosc* May 2008; 67(6): 781–790.

65. Shanewise JS. Development and costs of an intraoperative echocardiography service. *Semin Cardiothorac Vasc Anesth* 1999;3:235–241.

66. Troianos CA, Savino JS. Internal jugular vein cannulation guided by echocardiography. *Anesthesiology* 1991;74:787–789.

67. Cahalan MK, Foster E. Training in transesophageal echocardiography: in the lab or on the job? *Anesth Analg* 1995;81:217–218.

68. Savage RM, Licina MG, Koch CG, et al. Educational program for intraoperative transesophageal echocardiography. *Anesth Analg* 1995;81:399–403.

69. Murphy PM. Pro: intraoperative transesophageal echocardiography is a cost-effective strategy for cardiac surgical procedures. *J Cardiothorac Vasc Anesth* 1997; 11:246–249.

70. Savage RM, Lytle BW, Aronson S, et al. Intraoperative echocardiography is indicated in high-risk coronary artery bypass grafting. *Ann Thorac Surg* 1997; 64:368–374.

71. Benson MJ, Cahalan, MK. Cost-benefit analysis of TEE in cardiac surgery. *Echocardiography* 1995;12:171–183.

72. Pearlman AS, Gardin JM, Martin RP, et al. Guidelines for physician training in transesophageal echocardiography: Recommendations of the American Society of Echocardiography Committee for physician training in echocardiography. *Am Soc Echocardiogr* 1992;5:187–194.

73. Stevenson JG. Adherence to physician training guidelines for pediatric transesophageal echocardiography affects the outcome of patients undergoing repair of congenital cardiac defects. *J Am Soc Echocardiogr* 1999;12(3):165–172.

74. Jollis JG, Peterson ED, DeLong ER, et al. The relation between the volume of coronary angioplasty procedures at hospitals treating Medicare beneficiaries and short-term mortality. *N Engl J Med.* 1994;331(24):1625–1629.

75. Kohn LT, Corrigan J, Donaldson MS. To err is human: building a safer health system. Washington, DC: National Academy Press, 2000.

76. Institute of Medicine (U.S.). Division of Health Care Services., Lohr KN, Institute of Medicine (U.S.). Committee to Design a Strategy for Quality Review and Assurance in Medicare., United States. Health Care Financing Administration. *Medicare: A Strategy for Quality Assurance.* Washington, DC: National Academy Press, 1990.

77. Applegate KE. Continuous quality improvement for radiologists. *Acad Radiol* 2004;11(2):155–161.

78. Kisslo J, Byrd B, Geiser E, et al. Recommendations for continuous quality improvement in echocardiography. *J Am Soc Echocardiogr* 1995;8:S1–S28.

79. Mathew JP, Glas K, Troianos CA, et al. American Society of Echocardiography/Society of Cardiovascular Anesthesiologists recommendations and guidelines for continuous quality improvement in perioperative echocardiography. *J Am Soc Echocardiogr* 2006;19(11):1303–1313.

80. Shanewise JS, Cheung AT, Aronson S, et al. ASE/SCA guidelines for performing a comprehensive intraoperative multiplane transesophageal echocardiography examination: recommendations of the American Society of Echocardiography Council for Intraoperative Echocardiography and the Society of Cardiovascular Anesthesiologists Task Force for Certification in Perioperative Transesophageal Echocardiography. *J Am Soc Echocardiogr* 1999;12(10):884–900.

81. Aronson S, Thys DM. Training and certification in perioperative transesophageal echocardiography: a historical perspective. *Anesth Analg* 2001;93(6):1422–1427.

82. Fyfe D. Transesophageal echocardiography guidelines: return to bypass or to bypass the guidelines? *J Am Soc Echocardiogr* 1999;12(5):343–344.

83. Mathew JP, Fontes ML, Garwood S, et al. Transesophageal echocardiography interpretation: a comparative analysis between cardiac anesthesiologists and primary echocardiographers. *Anesth Analg* 2002;94(2):302–309.

84. Bergquist BD, Leung JM, Bellows WH. Transesophageal echocardiography in myocardial revascularization: I. Accuracy of intraoperative real-time interpretation. *Anesth Analg* 1996;82(6):1132–1138.

85. Miller JP, Lambert AS, Shapiro WA, et al. The adequacy of basic intraoperative transesophageal echocardiography performed by experienced anesthesiologists. *Anesth Analg* 2001;92(5): 1103–1110.

QUESTIONS

1. Which of the following is an absolute contraindication to the placement of a TEE probe?
   A. Esophageal varices
   B. Esophageal strictures
   C. Cervical arthritis
   D. History of mediastinal radiation

2. All of the following statements about complications related to intraoperative TEE are true *except*
   A. Compression of the membranous portion of the trachea by the TEE probe can produce airway obstruction.
   B. The ultrasound transducer should be inactivated when not in use to reduce the risk of thermal injury.
   C. Failure to provide antibiotic prophylaxis prior to a TEE examination increases the risk of bacterial endocarditis.
   D. Compression of the recurrent laryngeal nerve by the TEE probe may result in transient vocal cord paralysis.

3. The minimal recommended time required to effectively disinfect a TEE probe in a glutaraldeyde-based solution is
   A. 10 minutes
   B. 15 minutes
   C. 20 minutes
   D. 30 minutes

CHAPTER 8

Organizing Education and Training in Perioperative Transesophageal Echocardiography

Andrej A. Alfirevic ■ Robert M. Savage

INTRODUCTION

A perioperative transesophageal echocardiography (TEE) is used for either initial diagnosis of cardiovascular disease or to confirm and monitor previously documented state. According to the survey of active members of the Society of Cardiothoracic Anesthesiologists (SCA), TEE was a routine diagnostic modality tool used in 90% of valvular surgeries as well as 41% of coronary artery bypass surgeries (1). In addition to the wide spread indication for TEE use in the cardiac operating rooms, the intraoperative hemodynamic disturbances unresponsive to therapy represent an indication for TEE use during noncardiac surgeries as well. Along with the increased clinical application, the use of TEE is responsible for the improvement in patients' outcome in both cardiac and noncardiac surgical arena (2). Therefore, proper organization of the educational training program, which yields competent echocardiographers, is of great importance. The need to establish strong perioperative echocardiographic training programs comes from the wide spread use of TEE in large academic institutions and smaller clinical practice groups. The wide spread use of TEE is also followed by the increased involvement of cardiac and general anesthesiologists in providing perioperative TEE service. Initial burden of performing intraoperative TEE was carried on by cardiologists, but more recently, Morewood et al. (1) presented the survey, which showed that 81% of anesthesiologists practiced in institutions where they carried some or all responsibility for TEE studies performed.

HISTORY OF TRAINING IN TEE

The initial recommendation of the American Society of Echocardiography (ASE) specified three levels of training and was primarily based on the experience of cardiologists performing perioperative echocardiographic studies (2,3). Based on the prior recommendations for training in transthoracic echocardiography, the ASE Committee for Physician Training in Echocardiography published the guidelines for training in TEE (4). These guidelines were directed at training for TEE in both the operative and nonoperative settings. Growing use and interest for obtaining proper certification in perioperative echocardiography have prompted the making of practice guidelines directed toward the anesthesia practitioners.

A multidisciplinary task force of the American Society of Anesthesiologists (ASA) and SCA published guidelines for perioperative TEE, which defined two levels (basic and advanced) of training (5). The guideline was a result of collaborative work between the anesthesiologists and cardiologists in facilitating the training in perioperative TEE and enhancing the quality improvement of individual studies performed. The same goals were reemphasized in the ASE and SCA Task Force guidelines for training in perioperative echocardiography (6). As a result of the multidisciplinary approach, the training guidelines in basic and advanced perioperative echocardiography are similar to the training guidelines for level 1 and level 2 in general echocardiography except for greater number of personally performed cases as well as longer duration of training specified for general echocardiography training (7). The difference is justified by more specific orientation of the perioperative echocardiography toward surgical practice. The essential components of basic training include "independent work, supervised activities, and assessment programs" (6,7). In addition to previously mentioned basic training components, the emphasis of the advanced training lies in the comprehensiveness (6,7). The 1996 ASA and SCA guidelines delineated goals and objectives for cognitive and technical skills required for performing the intraoperative TEE (see Tables 8.1 and 8.2) (5). These guidelines were slightly redefined in 2002, with the addition of epicardial and epiaortic imaging (6). In addition to delineating cognitive and technical objectives, the guideline also recommends necessary number of examinations and methodology for performing a comprehensive intraoperative multiplane TEE examination needed to fulfill the requirements of certification (see Table 8.3) (8). The SCA Task Force for Certification endorsed the standard of nomenclature for 20 cross-sectional TEE views comprising the comprehensive perioperative examination (8).

The perioperative TEE rotation for CTA fellows at the Department of Cardiothoracic Anesthesia (CTA)

| TABLE 8.1 | Basic Competencies |

Cognitive Skills	Technical Skills
1. Knowledge of the physical principles of echocardiographic image formation and blood velocity measurement	1. Ability to operate ultrasonographs including the primary controls affecting the quality of the displayed data
2. Knowledge of the operation of ultrasound platform including all controls that affect the quality of data displayed	2. Ability to insert a TEE probe safely in the anesthetized, tracheally intubated patient
3. Knowledge of the equipment handling, infection control, and electrical safety associated with the techniques of perioperative echocardiography	3. Ability to perform a comprehensive TEE examination and differentiate normal from markedly abnormal cardiac structures and function
4. Knowledge of the indications, contraindications, and potential complications for perioperative echocardiography	4. Ability to recognize marked changes in segmental ventricular contraction indicative of myocardial ischemia or infarction.
5. Knowledge of the appropriate alternative diagnostic techniques	5. Ability to recognize marked changes in global ventricular filling and ejection
6. Knowledge of the normal tomographic anatomy, as revealed by perioperative echocardiographic techniques	6. Ability to recognize air embolization
7. Knowledge of commonly encountered blood flow velocity profiles, as measured by Doppler echocardiography	7. Ability to recognize gross valvular lesions and dysfunction
8. Knowledge of the echocardiographic manifestations of native valvular lesions and dysfunction	8. Ability to recognize large intracardiac masses and thrombi
9. Knowledge of the echocardiographic manifestations of cardiac masses, thrombi, cardiomyopathies, pericardial effusions, and lesions of the great vessels	9. Ability to detect large pericardial effusions
10. Detailed knowledge of the echocardiographic presentations of myocardial ischemia and infarction	10. Ability to recognize common echocardiographic artifacts
11. Detailed knowledge of the echocardiographic presentations of normal and abnormal ventricular functions	11. Ability to communicate echocardiographic results effectively to health care professionals and in the medical record
12. Detailed knowledge of the echocardiographic presentations of air embolization	12. Ability to recognize complications of perioperative echocardiography

at The Cleveland Clinic consists of four 2-week blocks spread throughout the educational year, with emphasis on preparation for the clinical practice of Cardiovascular Anesthesia as well as successful completion of the National Board of Echocardiography Perioperative TEE Certifying Examination (PTEeXAM). The goals and objectives of the rotation are a modification of the ASE/SCA Task Force Guidelines for Training in Perioperative Echocardiography (5). This guideline divides the required cognitive and technical competencies of the individual echocardiographer into the basic and advanced categories. Therefore, CTA fellows are evaluated according to basic category at the finish of their second block and to the advanced category at the end of their fourth block.

In order to emphasize staged ASE/SCA Task Force goals and objectives, the rotation is set up into the basic and advanced stages.

1. *BASIC perioperative TEE* includes CTA fellows' *Blocks I and II.* The goals of the rotation include the fulfillment of the cognitive and technical skills items listed as a part of the basic competency requirement (Table 8.1). The educational focus during this stage is on the introduction to perioperative echocardiography and basic imaging acquisition. At the end of the block/module, echocardiographer in training must be able to perform the basic echocardiographic examination, without assistance, which will be evaluated by CTA staff credentialed in advanced perioperative TEE.

TABLE 8.2	Advanced Competencies*

Cognitive Skills	Technical Skills
1. All the cognitive skills defined under basic training	1. All the technical skills defined under basic training
2. Detailed knowledge of the principles and methodologies of qualitative and quantitative echocardiography	2. Ability to acquire or direct the acquisition of all necessary echocardiographic data, including epicardial and epiaortic imaging
3. Detailed knowledge of native and prosthetic valvular function, including valvular lesions and dysfunction	3. Ability to recognize subtle changes in segmental ventricular contraction indicative of myocardial ischemia or infarction
4. Knowledge of congenital heart disease (If pediatric or adult congenital practice is planned, then this knowledge must be detailed.)	4. Ability to quantify systolic and diastolic ventricular functions and to estimate other relevant hemodynamic parameters
5. Detailed knowledge of all other diseases of the heart and great vessels that is relevant in the perioperative period (If pediatric practice is planned, then this knowledge may be more general than detailed.)	5. Ability to quantify normal and abnormal native and prosthetic valvular functions
6. Detailed knowledge of the techniques, advantages, disadvantages, and potential complications of commonly used cardiac surgical procedures for treatment of acquired and congenital heart diseases	6. Ability to assess the appropriateness of cardiac surgical plans
7. Detailed knowledge of other diagnostic methods appropriate for correlation with perioperative echocardiography	7. Ability to identify inadequacies in cardiac surgical interventions and the underlying reasons for the inadequacies
	8. Ability to aid in clinical decision making in the operating room

*Adapted from Cahalan MK, et al. American Society of Echocardiography and Society of Cardiovascular Anesthesiologists Task Force Guidelines for Training in Perioperative Echocardiography. J Am Soc Echocardiogr 2002;15:647–652.

TABLE 8.3	Numbers of Examinations for Basic and Advance Perioperative Echocardiography

	Basic[a]	Advanced[a]
Minimum number of examinations[b]	150	300
Minimum number personally performed[c]	50	150

[a] Totals for basic training may be counted toward advanced training, provided the basic training was completed in an advanced training environment.
[b] Complete echocardiographic examinations interpreted and reported by the trainee under appropriate supervision. May include transthoracic studies recorded by qualified individuals other than the trainee.
[c] Comprehensive intraoperative TEE examinations personally performed, interpreted, and reported by the trainee under appropriate supervision. Adapted from Cahalan MK, et al. American Society of Echocardiography and Society of Cardiovascular Anesthesiologists Task Force Guidelines for Training in Perioperative Echocardiography. J Am Soc Echocardiogr 2002;15:647–652; Quinones, et al. ACC ACC/AHA Clinical competence statement on echocardiography: a report of the American College of Cardiology/American Heart Association/American College of Physicians—American Society of Internal Medicine Task Force on Clinical Competence. J Am Coll Cardiol 2003;41(4): 687–708.

2. *ADVANCED perioperative TEE* includes CTA fellows' *Blocks III and IV.* The goals of the rotation include the fulfillment of the cognitive and technical skill items listed as a part of the advanced competency requirement (Table 8.2). The educational focus is on developing the capabilities to utilize full diagnostic capabilities of TEE and competence in performing the advanced comprehensive perioperative TEE examination. At the end of each block, the echocardiographer-in-training should be able to independently perform the comprehensive echocardiographic examination. Their performance will be evaluated by a CTA staff credentialed in advanced perioperative TEE.

DEPARTMENT OF CARDIOTHORACIC ANESTHESIA: ADVANCED PERIOPERATIVE TEE TRAINING

CTA fellows receive a total of 8 weeks of dedicated Perioperative TEE training divided into four 2-week Periop TEE Modules designed to provide the trainee with the cognitive and technical skills required to be an advanced independent echocardiographer. The daily curriculum of the rotation (Table 8.4) includes (a) hands-on

TABLE 8.4	CTA Perioperative TEE Curriculum			
	Module 1	**Module 2**	**Module 3**	**Module 4**
Practical skills	Platform setup Perform supervised basic exam TEE study entry	Perform supervised advanced exam Interpretation of advanced exam Record TEE study	Performance, interpretation, recording, and presentation of findings under supervision Incorporation of TEE exam into patient management and surgical decisions	Similar to Module 3, with greater independence under supervision Perform epicardial study
Technical skills	Basic competencies	Advanced competencies	Advanced competencies	Transthoracic experience and epicardial echo
Cognitive skills	Basic competencies	Advanced competencies	Participate in echo curriculum lectures	Submit case presentation for publication
Hands-on studies[a] Module/clinical care	20/25	40/50	60/75	80/100
Studies reviewed[b]	40	80	120	160

[a] Performed, interpreted, and recorded under credentialed supervision.
[b] Independently interpreted and reviewed under credentialed supervision.

performance studies, (b) independent interpretation of preassigned TEE studies for group review, (c) daily reading assignments, and (d) a daily Periop TEE Quiz reviewed with the attending staff. The textbook and the quizzes are designated for the specific module and differ for the basic and advanced modules, respectively. Performing, interpreting, and writing the final report of the intraoperative TEE studies supervised by the attending Staff and daily review of studies previously interpreted by trainees enable the individual trainee to develop their technical imaging skills as well as ability to recognize and evaluate a full spectrum of perioperative cardiovascular pathophysiology. In addition to studies performed during their Periop TEE Modules, Fellows perform a complete TEE examination on all of their assigned surgical patients requiring TEE assessment. A monthly log of cases personally performed and interpreted/review is provided for every Fellow to follow their progress. In the daily review sessions, Fellows also provide a more detailed presentation of the most interesting "Case of the Day," which is then added to the departmental teaching library. A comprehensive lecture series supplements the daily curriculum in addition to quarterly interdisciplinary anatomic "wet-lab" workshops and clinical case conferences. A yearly "Review of Perioperative TEE" workshop is provided for all current and former trainees to keep them current and assess their perioperative imaging skills.

KEY POINTS

- Intraoperative TEE is performed by anesthesiologists ≥80% of time.
- Proper organization of the educational training program is necessary for the success.
- Perioperative TEE training is divided into two levels (basic and advanced) by the ASA and the Society of Cardiovascular Anesthesiologists (SCA).
- Essential components of basic training include independent work, supervised activities, and assessment programs as well as comprehensive examination.
- The SCA Task Force for Certification endorsed the standard of nomenclature for 20 cross-sectional TEE views comprising the comprehensive perioperative examination.

REFERENCES

1. Morewood GH, Gallagher ME, Gaughan JP, et al. Current practice patterns for adult perioperative transesophageal echocardiography in the United States. *Anesthesiology* 2001;95:1507–1512.
2. Pearlman AS, Gardin JM, Martin RP, et al. Guidelines for optimal physician training in echocardiography: recommendations of the American Society of Echocardiography Committee for Physician Training in Echocardiography. *Am J Cardiol* 1987;60:158–163.

3. Stewart WJ, Aurigemma GP, Bierman FZ, et al. Guidelines for training in adult cardiovascular medicine: Core Cardiology Training Symposium (COCATS). Task force 4: training in echocardiography. *J Am Coll Cardiol* 1995;25:16–19.

4. Pearlman AS, Gardin JM, Martin RP, et al. Guidelines for physician training in transesophageal echocardiography: recommendations of the American Society of Echocardiography Committee for Physician Training in Echocardiography. *J Am Soc Echocardiogr* 1992;5:187–194.

5. Practice guidelines for perioperative transesophageal echocardiography. A report by the American Society of Anesthesiologists and the Society of Cardiovascular Anesthesiologists Task Force on Transesophageal Echocardiography. *Anesthesiology* 1996;84:986–1006.

6. Cahalan MK, et al. American Society of Echocardiography and Society of Cardiovascular Anesthesiologists Task Force Guidelines for Training in Perioperative Echocardiography. *J Am Soc Echocardiogr* 2002;15:647–652.

7. Quinones, et al. ACC ACC/AHA Clinical competence statement on echocardiography: a report of the American College of Cardiology/American Heart Association/American College of Physicians—American Society of Internal Medicine Task Force on Clinical Competence. *J Am Coll Cardiol* 2003;41(4):687–708.

8. Shanewise JS, Cheung AT, Aronson S, et al. ASE/SCA guidelines for performing a comprehensive intraoperative multiplane transesophageal echocardiography examination: recommendations of the American Society of Echocardiography Council for Intraoperative Echocardiography and the Society of Cardiovascular Anesthesiologists Task Force for Certification in Perioperative Transesophageal Echocardiography. *Anesth Analg* 1999;89:870–884.

QUESTIONS

1. What are the components of the echocardiographic training?
   A. Independent performance of the study
   B. Supervision
   C. Assessment of the performed study
   D. Performance of the comprehensive exam
   E. All of the above

2. Which competency belongs to the advanced technical skills group?
   A. Ability to recognize large intracardiac masses and thrombi
   B. Ability to recognize intracardiac air
   C. Ability to recognize common echocardiographic artifacts
   D. Ability to quantify normal and abnormal native and prosthetic valvular functions

3. Which competency belongs to the advanced cognitive skills group?
   A. Knowledge of the operation of ultrasound platform
   B. Knowledge of the indications, contraindications, and potential complications for perioperative echocardiography
   C. Knowledge of congenital heart disease
   D. Knowledge of commonly encountered blood flow velocity profiles as measured by Doppler echocardiography

4. How many images are required per the ASE/SCA definition of the comprehensive echocardiographic examination?
   A. 12
   B. 15
   C. 18
   D. 20

5. What determines NBE Diplomat status?
   A. Passing the NBE perioperative echocardiographic examination
   B. Independently reviewed 300 studies
   C. Independently performed 150 studies
   D. Passing ABA Oral Boards
   E. All of the above

CHAPTER 9

Assessment of Global Ventricular Function

Carlo E. Marcucci ■ Ryan Lauer ■ Solomon Aronson

Left ventricular (LV) systolic function is a powerful predictor of clinical outcome for a wide range of cardiovascular diseases including ischemic cardiac disease, cardiomyopathy, and valvular heart disease. Data from the CASS registry indicate that LV function, determined by ejection fraction (EF), is more important for predicting survival than the number of diseased vessels (1). Echocardiography provides both a quantitative and a qualitative measure of systolic function by estimating global and regional ventricular functions and by measuring ventricular volumes and EF. A multitude of techniques have been developed to overcome the fundamental shortcoming of two-dimensional (2D) echocardiography. The estimation of the volume and function of a three-dimensional (3D) structure with a 2D technique necessitates geometrical assumptions and possible erroneous extrapolation. The advent of live 3D echocardiography largely overcomes these problems and allows for more accurate quantification of LV volumes and EF.

NORMAL ANATOMY AND PHYSIOLOGY OF THE LEFT VENTRICLE

The left ventricle is a thick-walled, bullet-shaped chamber with an average LV wall thickness of 10.9 ± 2.0 mm and an average mass of 92 ± 16 g/m^2. In cross section, the left ventricle has a nearly circular configuration that increases in area from base to apex. It is obliquely positioned in the chest with its apex pointing left, slightly anteriorly and inferiorly. It shares a triangular-shaped interventricular septum with the right ventricle in the anteromedial portion. The remainder of the LV wall, called the free wall, is not in contact with any other chamber. Two papillary muscles originate from the ventricular free wall, one anterolateral and one inferomedial, onto which the chordae of the mitral valve are inserted.

PHASES OF VENTRICULAR SYSTOLE

During the cardiac cycle, systole starts with mitral valve closure and ends with aortic valve closure. On an electrocardiogram, onset of systole is identified at the peak of the QRS complex and end of systole after repolarization at the end of the T wave. Systole also can be determined

by events in the left ventricle (Fig. 9.1). Mitral valve closure marks the beginning of systole and is followed by an isovolumic contraction period. During this period, ventricular pressure rises rapidly while volume stays constant. As ventricular pressure exceeds aortic pressure, the aortic valve opens. The ejection phase follows, marked by acceleration and deceleration. During the first half of the ejection phase when LV pressure exceeds aortic pressure, blood rushes from the left ventricle into the aorta. Then in the deceleration phase of systole, when aortic pressure exceeds ventricular pressure, the forward flow of blood at a progressively slower velocity is reflected by the downward slope of the velocity tracing. After aortic valve closure, during the isovolumic relaxation phase, the myocardium relaxes and pressure returns to baseline. Consequently, intraventricular pressure drops below atrial pressure and diastolic filling begins with opening of the mitral valve.

LEFT VENTRICULAR SYSTOLIC FUNCTION

Ventricular systolic function is described by both load-independent and load-dependent indices of myocardial performance. Load-dependent variables vary with changes in preload and afterload. Therefore, estimates of contractility require measurement of ventricular ejection performance during different loading conditions. Examples of load-dependent measures are fractionals shortening, fractionals area change, and estimation of EF using different geometric models. The clinical evaluation of ventricular function often relies on evaluating preload, afterload, cardiac output (CO), EF, end-systolic volumes, and dimensions. Load-independent measures of ventricular contractility are systolic elastance and preload recruitable stroke work (Fig. 9.1). Echocardiographic modalities designed for evaluating contractility independent of load include the systolic index of contractility, pressure-area relationships, and strain rate (SR) imaging. During systole, the ventricular myocardium rotates or twists around the longitudinal axis. The direction of rotation at the valvular level (base) is opposite to the apical level. Looking from the apex upward to the base (the transthoracic long-axis view), the rotation at the base is clockwise and at the apex counterclockwise. This counterdirectional rotation results in ventricular torsion. Rotation or twist is quantified in angular degrees, and torsion is calculated as

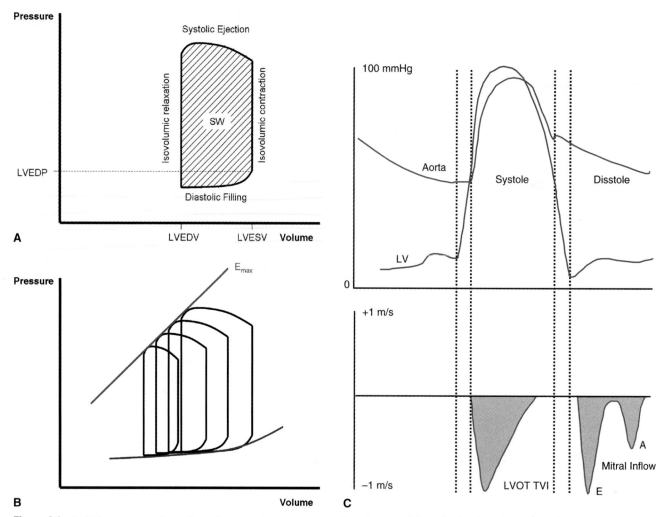

Figure 9.1. **A.** LV pressure-volume loop. Isovolumic contraction: after closure of the mitral valve, the ventricular myocardium contracts without a reduction in intraventricular volume. Systolic ejection: when intraventricular pressure exceeds pressure in the aorta, the aortic valve opens and ejection occurs. Isovolumic relaxation: after closure of the aortic valve, myocardial relaxation produces an intraventricular pressure drop without change in volume until pressure drops beneath left atrial pressure. Diastolic filling begins with the opening of the mitral valve and continues until the onset of isovolumic contraction. **B.** By abruptly reducing preload (caval occlusion), variable pressure-volume loops can be recorded. The slope connecting the maximal generated pressure under the various loading condition represents myocardial elastance (E_{max}). Plotting the Stroke work of every loop against the EDV generates a linear curve, the slope of which is the preload recruitable stroke work (PRSW). Both E_{max} and PRSW are load-independent measures of ventricular contractility. **C.** The ventricular cycle and the corresponding Doppler flow velocity profiles in the LV outflow tract and the mitral inflow tract. LV stroke work is defined as the area within the pressure-volume loop. LVEDP, left ventricular end diastolic pressure; LVEDV, left ventricular end diastolic volume; LVESV, left ventricular end systolic volume; SW, stroke work.

the difference between basal and apical rotation. Speckle tracking is the only echocardiographic modality that allows for the measurement of twist and torsion.

TWO-DIMENSIONAL EXAMINATION OF THE LEFT VENTRICLE

In 2D echocardiography, the left ventricle, a 3D object, is studied in real time by manipulating the transesophageal echocardiographic (TEE) probe to produce multiple imaging planes. To reproduce and compare measurements, standardized views have been developed based on internal and external references of the ventricle. The imaging planes used to describe and quantitate global LV function include midesophageal four-chamber view (ME 4C) (Fig. 9.2), the midesophageal two-chamber view (ME 2C) (Fig. 9.3), midesophageal long-axis view (ME LAX) (Fig. 9.4), transgastric short-axis view (TG SAX) (Fig. 9.5), and transgastric long-axis view (TG LAX) (Fig. 9.6). During a TEE examination for global ventricular assessment, artifactual shortening of the LV long axis

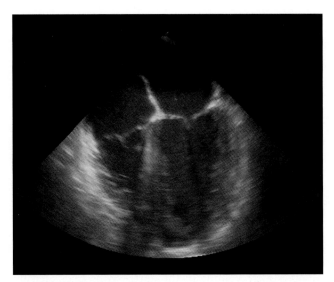

Figure 9.2. The ME 4C view.

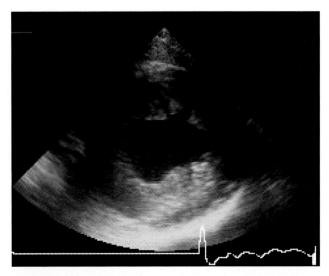

Figure 9.5. The TG SAX view.

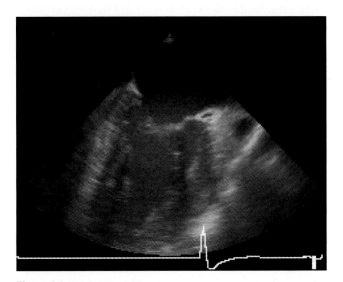

Figure 9.3. The ME 2C view.

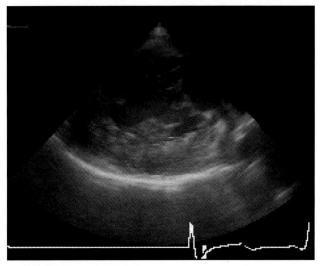

Figure 9.6. The TG LAX view.

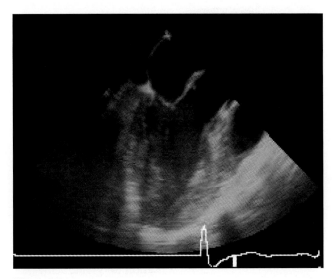

Figure 9.4. The ME LAX view.

should be avoided or the myocardium at the mid- to apical segments will appear falsely thickened. A foreshortened left ventricle in the four-chamber view may represent a more proximal segment of the anterior wall rather than the true LV apex. The four- and two-chamber views are used to measure mitral inflow velocity, and LV volume and area are used as surrogates for LV preload.

To obtain the four-chamber view, the TEE probe is inserted into the midesophagus approximately 20 cm, the omniplane is rotated to 10 to 20 degrees, and the probe is slightly retroflexed. From the four-chamber view, the long axis of the left ventricle is centered in the middle of the sector and the image plane is slowly rotated toward 90 degrees to obtain the two-chamber view. Again, slight angulation and manipulation of the probe are necessary to obtain the two-chamber view, which includes the full length of the left ventricle and avoids foreshortening.

The orthogonal axis of the two-chamber view may be used to calculate LV volumes and EF. The omniplane is rotated toward 120 degrees from the two-chamber view to obtain the long-axis view. This view may be used to study the aortic valve apparatus, the left ventricle, and the LV outflow tract.

From the midesophageal level, the probe is advanced into the stomach to obtain the transgastric midpapillary short-axis view. With the omniplane at 0 degrees, the tip is anteflexed to bring the short axis into view. The short-axis midpapillary plane is preferred intraoperatively because it provides information regarding volume, contractility, ventricular dimensions, and thickness. The short axis of the left ventricle can be imaged at many levels; however, only two imaging planes are consistently reproducible from good internal references: the transgastric midpapillary short-axis view through the body of the papillary muscles and the transgastric basal short-axis view through the mitral valve. Intraoperatively, the transgastric midpapillary view reveals changes in volume status that are reflected in the end-diastolic cavity size. Change in fractional area and fractional shortening, surrogates of EF, can be calculated with this view. Distributions of the three coronary arteries are represented in this view, making it particularly useful for monitoring new regional wall motion abnormalities.

To obtain the transgastric two-chamber view of the left ventricle, start at the transgastric midpapillary short-axis view, center the left ventricle in the middle of the imaging, and rotate the omniplane out to 90 degrees. In this view, the inferior wall is at the top of the sector and the anterior wall is at the bottom, directly opposite the inferior wall. This view allows for the evaluation of the subvalvular apparatus of the mitral valve, the papillary muscles, and the entire anterior and inferior walls of the left ventricle, although the apical segments often drop out of the imaging sector in TEE.

EJECTION PHASE INDICES OF LEFT VENTRICULAR PERFORMANCE

LV global systolic performance is commonly expressed in terms of CO or EF. Before the development of 3D echocardiography, these volumetric variables could be derived form flow velocity profiles and 2D measurements. All of these techniques, however, are based on the assumption that cardiac cavities and outflow tracts have regular shapes and contract homogenously.

CO and stroke volume (SV) can be derived using Doppler velocities and estimations of surface area. Using simple 2D grayscale imaging, EF can be approximated by fractional shortening, fractional area change (FAC), and Simpson's method.

All these indices are very sensitive to changes in preload and afterload.

CARDIAC OUTPUT

CO is calculated from the equation CO = SV × HR, where SV is stroke volume and HR is heart rate. SV is defined as the difference between the end-diastolic and end-systolic volume in the left ventricle. Since volume is a 3D parameter, calculation of SV with 2D echo requires measuring a cross-sectional area (CSA) and the flow through that area with Doppler flow measurement using the equation below:

$$SV = CSA \times VTI$$

where SV is stroke volume, CSA is the cross-sectional area, and VTI is the velocity time integral.

During systole, the left ventricle ejects a given amount of blood (SV) into the cylindrically shaped aorta, which occupies a set volume in the aorta. SV is calculated by measuring the area and height of this blood column in the aorta. The CSA at the base of this column is derived by measuring the diameter (D) of the base of the aorta and applying the formula for the area of a circle: πr^2 or $\pi(D/2)^2$. The height of the column is obtained with Doppler to measure the flow through the aorta during systole. The area under the Doppler systolic flow velocity curve or the VTI represents the height of the cylinder. Thus, the volume of the cylinder or SV is the product of the CSA and VTI (Fig. 9.7).

Using this method to derive volume from area and flow measurements, we make several assumptions. First, the area measured for the calculation of SV is constant during the entire period of systole. Second, a small error in diameter measurement quadruples the error in the calculation for the CSA. Third, flow across the area of interest is assumed to be laminar such that the recorded flow represents the average flow and distance of flow in that region. In the presence of aortic valve disease, SV measurement in the ascending aorta will be inaccurate because flow distal to

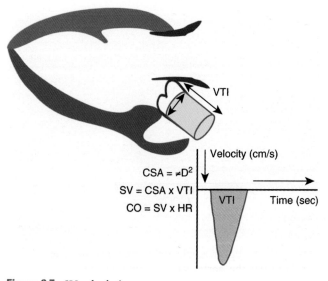

Figure 9.7. SV calculation.

the valve is not laminar. Fourth, the Doppler beam angle of incidence is assumed to be parallel to the direction of blood flow in that area. Finally, the area and flow measurements must be made at the same anatomic site. Several investigators have looked into the optimal site for measurements of the Doppler flow velocity. Muhiudeen et al. (2) looked at the pulmonary artery as a site for CO measurement. They measured the CSA and pulsed-wave Doppler signal of the pulmonary artery systolic flow. The result correlated modestly with CO measured by the thermodilution method (r = 0.65). Pulmonary systolic flow detected only intraoperative increases in CO greater than 15% (sensitivity, 71%; specificity, 82%), not decreases (sensitivity, 54%; specificity, 90%). Darmon et al. (3) used the TG LAX to obtain a spectral envelope with the continuous wave beam placed in the path from the LV outflow tract to the ascending aorta (3). The angle between the Doppler beam and the aortic valve plane was 7 ± 5 degrees with a range of 0 to 18 degrees. For the CSA, they used the time-averaged shape of the aortic valve aperture, measured in the upper esophageal view at 30 degrees. They obtained the TEE frame where the aortic valve cusp tips were as close to a straight triangle as possible, thus equating this structure to an equilateral triangle. The length of each side of the aortic valve (S) was measured, and the three values were averaged before calculation of the area of the aortic valve orifice in systole.

$$AVA = 0.5 \times \cos 30° \times S^2$$

$$AVA = 0.433 \times S^2$$

When the triangular model was used to calculate aortic valve area (AVA), Doppler-derived cardiac output (DCO) correlated tightly with thermodilution results for cardiac output (r = 0.93) (Fig. 9.8).

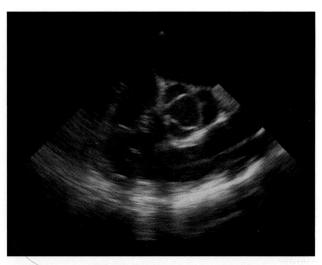

Figure 9.9. The upper esophageal aortic valve short-axis view demonstrating the aortic valve near peak systole resembling the shape of a circle.

This same group also substantiated the circular model to describe the aortic valve based on the observation that at maximal valve aperture, near peak systole, the aortic valve orifice appears nearly circular (Fig. 9.9). The aortic valve diameter (D) was measured in the longitudinal view, at the hinge points using the inner leaflet surface to inner leaflet surface method (Fig. 9.10). The aortic valve orifice area was then calculated using the equation:

$$AVA = p \times \left(\frac{D}{2}\right)^2$$

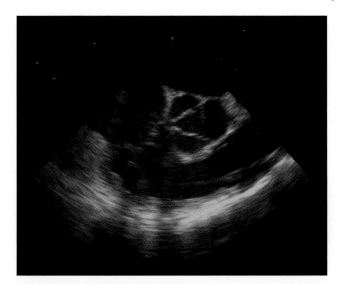

Figure 9.8. The upper esophageal aortic valve short-axis view demonstrating the aortic valve resembling the shape of an equilateral triangle.

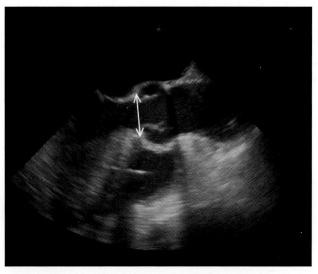

Figure 9.10. The ME LAX view demonstrating the aortic valve diameter (D) at the hinge points using the inner leaflet surface to inner leaflet surface method.

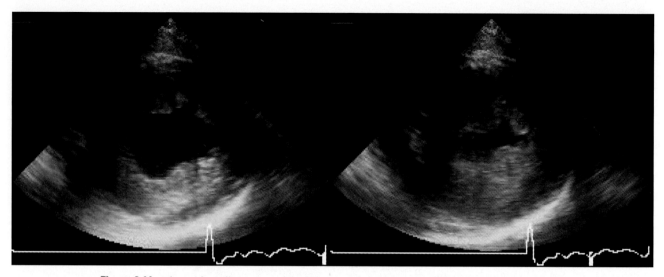

Figure 9.11. The midpapillary view of the left ventricle at end-diastole (**A**) and end-systole (**B**).

The TG LAX was used to obtain the Doppler spectral envelope with the continuous wave beam placed in the path from the LV outflow tract to the ascending aorta. CO based on this circular model has a correlation coefficient of 0.88 when compared to the thermodilution method (3).

In an intraoperative study, Perrino et al. (4) used the triangular aortic valve method to calculate CO with high reproducibility. In 32 of 33 patients (97%), they were able to image the LV outflow tract in the TG LAX and calculate CO with a correlation of r = 0.98 for intrasubject changes in CO. Serial changes in CO >1 L/min were tracked correctly in 97% of the cases. The magnitude of change in CO was underestimated by 14% with DCO when compared to the thermodilution method (4). Thus, DCO predicted the direction of change with high correlation; in a dynamic setting, it can underestimate the magnitude of the change.

FRACTIONAL SHORTENING

Fractional shortening (FS) is a 1D approximation of EF calculated as

$$FS = (LVEDd) - (LVESd)/LVEDd \times 100\%$$

where LVEDd is left ventricular end-diastolic diameter and LVESd is end-systolic diameter. The ventricular diameters are measured in the transgastric midpapillary short-axis view using M-mode. In the absence of regional wall motion abnormalities (RWMAs), it provides a rough idea of global ventricular function. For transthoracic imaging, a FS of 30% is considered the lower limit of normal ventricular function (5).

FRACTIONAL AREA CHANGE

FAC is measured in the transgastric midpapillary view. The equation is as follows:

$$FAC\% = \left[\frac{(LVEDA - LVESA)}{LVEDA} \right] \times 100\%$$

where FAC is the fractional area change, LVEDA is the area at end-diastole, and LVESA is the area at end-systole. To calculate the area, the endocardial surface is traced, without considering the papillary muscles. This index of systolic performance is heavily preload and afterload dependent. Intraoperatively, FAC is routinely used as a surrogate for EF. Several studies with intraoperative TEE, using the midpapillary short-axis view to calculate EF, have demonstrated a close correlation between EF based on FAC and radionuclide angiography and scintigraphy (r = 0.96 and 0.82, respectively) (Fig. 9.11) (6,7). FS and FAC measure the percent of change in a single or two myocardial dimensions as an estimate of LV contractile performance. RWMAs outside the scanned area will lead to important overestimation of global ventricular function. Conversely, RMWAs in the scanning plane may underestimate global function, if the remainder of the myocardium contracts normally.

EJECTION FRACTION

EF is calculated by the following formula:

$$EF\% = \left[\frac{(EDV0 - ESV)}{EDV} \right] \times 100\%$$

where EDV, volume at end-diastole; ESV, volume at end systole. The American Society of Echocardiography

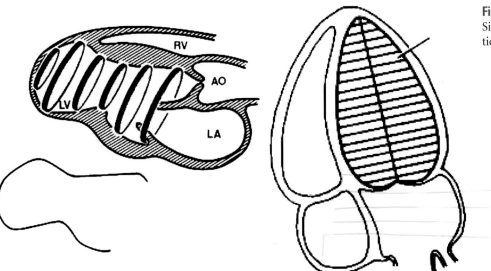

Figure 9.12. Illustration of the Simpson's method for calculation of LV volumes.

recommends using the modified Simpson's method to derive the ventricular volumes. The Simpson's method uses two orthogonal imaging planes to derive volume and makes no geometric assumptions about the ventricle. This method uses the four- and two-chamber views to derive LV end-diastolic volume (LVEDV), left ventricular end systolic volume, and LVEF. The endocardial borders of the selected planes are traced out manually or detected automatically. Then, the length of the left ventricle is divided into 20 cylinders of different diameters but equal thickness. This "method of discs" requires that the volumes of the cylinders are calculated and summed to estimate the ventricular volume. Most new models of echocardiography machines calculate the EDV, ESV, and EF automatically after the echocardiographer identifies the four-chamber plane and traces out the endocardium (Fig. 9.12).

However, the limitations of the method must be recognized. First, endocardial definition is affected by the physics of ultrasound and by anatomic limitations. For example, the lateral wall in the ME 4C is often difficult to visualize and trace because of the anatomic position of the endocardial-ventricular interface in this imaging plane. The border is parallel to the echo beam and therefore appears "blurred" as a result of poor lateral resolution. Signal attenuation by calcium deposits on the mitral annulus can create "drop out" of the echo signal distal to the deposits, further complicating endocardial detection of the ventricular walls. The numerous trabeculations in the left ventricle, most notably its apex, may sometimes be falsely identified as the endocardial border. Therefore, the endocardium identified by echocardiography is often different than the endocardium identified by angiography, in which the contrast material fills the trabeculations and distinguishes them from the true endocardium. With ultrasound contrast, the true endocardial border is easily revealed. Although popular in transthoracic echocardiography, the use of contrast agents has not been

reported in TEE. Second, this method is further limited by the fact that the measurements of end-diastolic area (EDA) and end-systolic area (ESA) in the two orthogonal scanning planes cannot be performed during the same cardiac cycle. Variations in preload or afterload while repositioning the probe will lead to errors in the calculated volumes.

CALCULATING PRELOAD AND AFTERLOAD

Preload

Echocardiography provides several ways to qualitatively and semiqualitatively assess preload as defined by the volume in the ventricle at the end of diastole. Because echocardiography images the heart in a 2D perspective, calculations derived from a single 2D imaging plane provide information regarding area. To derive volume, more than one imaging plane is often necessary. Volumetric calculations must be based on geometric assumptions about the shape of the left ventricle. Geometric models vary from the simple ellipsoid shape to the complex cylinder-cone shape and the cylinder - truncated cone - cone shape in which two or more geometric shapes are used to describe the left ventricle (Fig 9.13). The accuracy of any model depends on the number of imaging planes used. The area-length method is based on the ellipsoid shape as a model of the left ventricle. Measurement of the LV length is obtained from the ME 4C, and the area calculated from the 2D area is measured in the same view. In clinical conditions such as dilated cardiomyopathy or LV aneurysms, the ventricle does not resemble geometrical shapes; therefore, the equations used to calculate the ventricular volume based on the ellipsoid shape do not apply.

Because of the differences in scanning planes, the validation studies done with TTE cannot be directly applied

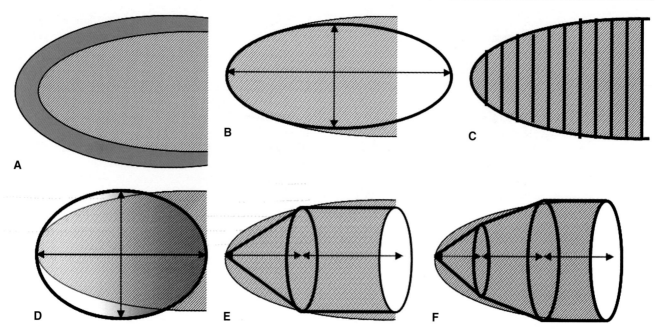

Figure 9.13. Geometric models for the calculation of LV volumes. **A.** Normal LV shape. **B.** Simple ellipsoid shape **C.** Simpson's method of discs. **D.** Area-length method. **E.** Cylinder-cone model. **F.** Cylinder-truncated cone-cone model.

to TEE. Smith et al. (8) compared LV volumes and EF, derived from transesophageal short-axis and four-chamber images, with similar variables obtained from ventriculography. They tested the three commonly used algorithms (Simpson's method, the area-length method, and the diameter-length method) for predicting volumes using TEE and validated those against ventricular angiography. The modified Simpson's method correlated best with angiography; the area-length method had the next highest correlation. Diastolic and systolic volumes were underestimated with all methods when compared with values assessed with angiography. Measurements of LV length by TEE were smaller for systole and diastole when compared to measurements by ventriculography. The underestimation of ventricular length, possibly because of foreshortening in the four-chamber view, is a major factor contributing to the smaller volumes obtained by TEE. Compared to TTE, TEE may be more accurate in estimating ventricular volumes due to the superior detection of the endocardial border.

When Clements et al. (6) evaluated ventricular area as a surrogate for volume, they used the transgastric mid-papillary short-axis view to measure ESA, EDA and from that calculated FAC. Approximately 87% of the SV is derived from the fiber shortening in the short axis. The level of the midpapillary is ideal for measurement since the papillary muscles provide reproducible internal reference. Clements et al. validated their measurements with simultaneous radionucleotide imaging and found a correlation of r = 0.86 with TEE EDA. TEE ESA also correlated with radionuclide ESA (r = 0.92), as did the FAC (r = 0.96).

This validation study by Clements et al. supports the use of the LV EDA as a surrogate for preload. In patients with normal or abnormal LV function and graded hypovolemia, acute blood loss caused directional changes in LV EDA. 2D TEE detected a change in LV EDA with as little as a 2.5% estimated blood volume deficit (~1.75 mL/kg). The mean change in LV EDA was 0.3 cm²/1% estimated blood-volume deficit (9). Reich et al. (10) manipulated blood volumes in pediatric patients following sternal closure after repair of congenital heart lesions and recorded images of the midpapillary short axis during these interventions. Mild reductions in blood volume were identified with high sensitivity (80%–95%) and specificity (80%).

The EDA is measured by acquiring the midpapillary short-axis view and scrolling to the end of diastole as defined by the image frame corresponding to the peak of the QRS complex. Without an ECG for reference, the image on which the LV cavity is largest is selected. Next, with planimetry the borders of the endocardium are traced, using the leading-edge-to-leading-edge method and including the papillary muscles in the measurement. After the cavity is traced out, the software package on most machines will automatically give a calculated area and circumference. If the body surface area of the patient is known, the EDA index will be calculated; less than 5.5 cm²/m² defines hypovolemia.

In summary, 2D TEE can be used to measure LV volumes. Although the absolute volumes calculated underestimate those derived from angiography, detecting change in volume and the direction of change is more important than calculation of absolute volume.

The experienced echocardiographer can detect changes in preload by visual inspection of the left ventricle at end-diastole and end-systole. With decreases in preload, there is a linear decrease in LV EDA and LV ESA. End-systolic cavity obliteration or "kissing ventricle" is a potentially useful "alarm" for hypovolemia. Obliteration can also reflect an increased inotropic state and decreased systemic vascular resistance. Leung and Levine (11) found that although end-systolic cavity obliteration detected by TEE is frequently associated with decreased LV preload, 10% of the time it reflects only an increase in EF. End-systolic cavity obliteration is very sensitive in predicting decreases in ESA (100%), but the specificity for predicting decrease in preload is low (10%–30%).

AFTERLOAD

Afterload is the force that acts to resist myocardial shortening during systole. At the level of the arterial system, it is defined in terms of systemic vascular resistance. Alternatively, afterload is the stress imposed on the ventricular wall during systole. The use of wall stress to measure myocardial function is based on the principle of equilibrium. The forces acting within the wall must exactly balance the forces acting on the wall. The stress forces acting on the wall are expressed as dynes/cm^2. LV wall stress depends on chamber size, myocardial thickness, interventricular pressure, and to some extent configuration. There are three types of ventricular wall stress: circumferential, meridional, and radial (Fig. 9.14). In the ellipsoid model, the forces act on the left ventricle in orthogonal planes. Peak ventricular wall stress occurs during the first third of systole; at the end-systole, ventricular wall stress is about half of the peak value.

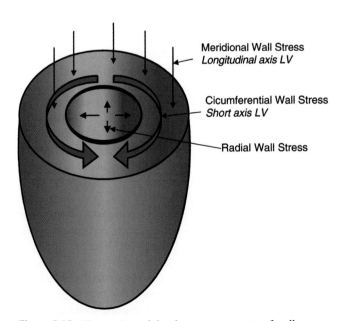

Figure 9.14. Illustration of the three components of wall stress.

Echocardiography can be used to noninvasively measure meridional and circumferential wall stress. Meridional stress acts on the long axis of the LV; the circumferential stress acts on the short axis of the LV. The shape of the ventricle, which changes throughout the cardiac cycle, affects wall stress. In patients with heart failure, the shape of the left ventricle is spherical. In a spherical model, meridional stress equals circumferential stress. The normal left ventricle resembles the ellipsoid model in which circumferential stress at the end of systole is 2.57 times higher than meridional stress (5). In a dilated failing heart, the left ventricle gradually begins to resemble a sphere, and the meridional and circumferential stress gradually equalize.

Meridional wall stress can be measured with 2D echocardiography using the method that has been validated with angiography (12).

$$\sigma_m (dynes/cm^2) = \frac{1.35 \times P(LVID)}{4h\,(1+h/LVID)}$$

σ_m = end-systolic meridional wall stress
P = pressure in the LV at the end of systole
LVID = LV internal diameter
h = end-systolic posterior wall thickness

1.35 is the factor to convert the blood pressure from millimeters of mercury to dynes/cm^2.

Reichek et al. (13) used the same equation but substituted systolic blood pressure for LV pressure. When they simultaneously measured pressure using a noninvasive blood pressure cuff and an invasive LV micromanometer catheter, they found that the two pressures strongly correlated (r = 0.89). Transthoracic echocardiography using M-mode was used to measure the thickness (h) of the posterior wall. End-systolic stress derived from a noninvasive blood pressure cuff correlated extremely well with stress measured invasively (r = 0.97). The mean value of meridional stress calculated from their study was 64.8 ± 19.5 × 10^3 dynes/cm^2.

Meridional wall stress can also be calculated using 2D echocardiography recordings with the formula:

$$\sigma_m (dynes/cm^2) = 1.33 \times \frac{BP_{syst}(A_m)}{A_c} \times 10^3$$

A_c = LV cavity area in the short-axis view
A_m = myocardial area
BP_{syst} = systolic blood pressure

The value for meridional wall stress was slightly higher (86 ± 16 × 10^3 dynes/cm^2) compared to that found with the M-mode (5).

Ventricular wall stress varies throughout the cardiac cycle; end-systolic wall stress indicates afterload. Given the complexity of the calculation, this approach has not been widely adopted clinically. Furthermore, most of the validation studies were done using TTE. In general, measurements of wall stress to estimate overall ventricular function are most useful in the situation of ventricular pressure or volume predominant states such as hypertension, or with valvular lesions such as stenosis or regurgitation.

SYSTOLIC INDEX OF CONTRACTILITY (dP/dt)

Although ejection phase indices of LV performance are easy to obtain, their load dependency may confound the accurate assessment of LV systolic function. The maximal rate of pressure increase during the isovolumic phase of ventricular systole dP/dt$_{(max)}$ is sensitive to changes in contractility, insensitive to changes in afterload and wall motion abnormalities, and only mildly affected by changes in preload. Continuous wave Doppler is used to determine the velocity of the mitral regurgitation jet. From that, the rate of pressure increase or dP/dt$_{(mean)}$ is determined (14). This method requires that one has a mitral regurgitant jet. Since the method gives the mean dP/dt, the value often underestimates the peak dP/dt. To obtain the dP/dt, the continuous wave velocity profile of the mitral regurgitant jet is optimized. Then, the time it takes for the mitral regurgitant velocity to rise from 1 to 3 m/s is measured (Fig. 9.15). Using the simplified Bernoulli equation, the velocities are converted into pressures.

$$P = 4V^2 = 4(1)^2 = 4 \text{ mm Hg}$$

$$P = 4V^2 = 4(3)^2 = 36 \text{ mm Hg}$$

$$dP/dt = 4(3)^2 - 4(1)^2 / \Delta t \text{ (ms)}$$

$$\frac{dP}{dt} = \frac{(36-4) \times 1,000}{\Delta t \text{ (second)}}$$

$$\frac{dP}{dt} = \frac{32,000 \text{ mm Hg}}{\Delta t \text{ (second)}}$$

A dP/dt value greater than 1,200 mm Hg/s or a time of ≤27 ms is considered normal and dP/dt value less than 1,000 mm Hg/s or a time of ≥32 ms is considered abnormal. In one study, dP/dt and −dP/dt indices were

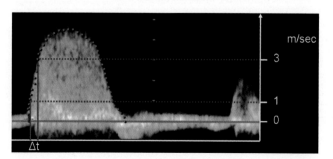

Figure 9.15. Systolic index of contractility (dP/dt). A continuous Doppler trace of a regurgitant mitral jet is obtained and the time (Δt) from 1 to 3 m/s is measured. Systolic index of contractility is calculated as dP/dt = 32,000 mm Hg/dt.

determined prospectively in 56 patients with chronic congestive heart failure and low EF < 50% to predict event-free survival (15).

Unlike ejection phase indices described above, pressure volume relationships describe the contractile state of the myocardium. The slope of the pressure volume loops or the end-systolic elastance is a load-independent indicator of preload-recruitable stroke work and, therefore, reflects true contractility. Using automated border detection algorithms, continuous measurement of the LV area as a surrogate for LV volume is possible. Combined with intraventricular hi-fidelity catheters, pressure area loops can be constructed. Gorcsan et al. (16) coupled continuous area measurements, obtained with TEE, with continuous pressure data measured at the level of the left ventricle in 13 patients undergoing coronary artery bypass grafts. They found that stroke force derived from pressure area loops closely correlated with changes in estimates of stroke work from pressure volume loops for individual patients before bypass (mean correlation r = 0.99 ± 0.03) and after bypass (mean correlation r = 0.96 ± 0.05). Pressure estimates of end-systolic elastance, maximal elastance, and preload-recruitable stroke force decreased from before to after cardiopulmonary bypass. The load-dependent measures of LV function, such as SV, CO, and FAC, were unchanged after surgery in these patients (Figs. 9.12–9.14).

TISSUE DOPPLER IMAGING

Although contractility independent of different LV loading conditions can be measured using 2D TEE, this method has not been widely adopted because it is cumbersome. Tissue Doppler imaging provides quantitative measurement of global as well as segmental LV function. Tissue Doppler technology is based on the same principles as color flow Doppler mapping.

With advances in Doppler technology, the high velocity and low amplitudes that are characteristic of blood flow can be filtered out to display the high-amplitude, low-velocity signals that are characteristic of cardiac tissue. Cardiac structures move in a velocity range of 0.06 to 0.24 m/s, approximately ten times slower than myocardial blood flow. Tissue Doppler displays the velocity of the myocardium through the cardiac cycle, with movement toward the transducer depicted as a positive deflection and movement away from the transducer depicted as a negative deflection. Four distinct velocities are typically seen on the wave form obtained by TEE (Fig. 9.16). The first negative velocity (S1 velocity) is associated with isovolumic contraction. The next negative deflection is the systolic shortening velocity; the peak systolic velocity is S2. These velocities are depicted as negative because as the ventricle contracts there is a net movement toward the apex and away from the transducer. The two velocities in diastole, the E and A velocities, correspond to the Doppler mitral inflow E and A velocities. These are depicted as

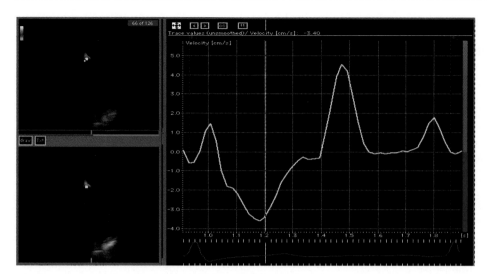

Figure 9.16. Tissue Doppler velocity tracing with sample site placed at the septal mitral annulus. On the right is the corresponding tissue velocity profile through one cardiac cycle. See text for explanation of the four velocities depicted above.

positive velocities because in diastole the myocardium moves toward the transducer. The Em is the peak early diastolic myocardial relaxation velocity, and Am is the late diastolic velocity associated with atrial contraction.

Myocardial velocity imaging is angle dependent and limited by some of the same variables that limit conventional Doppler echocardiography. The myocardial velocity measured at the site of interest is the sum of all the velocities in that area. In other words, this velocity does not differentiate between the three components that affect the motion of the heart: radial contraction, longitudinal shortening, and rotation. A translational motion of the heart within the thorax can generate a velocity measurable by tissue Doppler imaging. Tissue Doppler imaging does not discriminate between actively contracting myocardium and a "tethered" myocardium. Thus, an akinetic segment may demonstrate a velocity, if it is being pulled along by an adjacent contracting segment of myocardium. These limitations explain the poor reproducibility of this technique.

Despite these limitations, however, tissue Doppler imaging can be used to measure global ventricular function. The descent of the mitral annulus from the base to the apex is a well-described feature of normal LV function. Earlier studies using M-mode and 2D echocardiography have demonstrated the importance of the longitudinal vector of contraction to global LV function. Gulati et al. (17) used tissue Doppler M-mode to evaluate the velocity of mitral annular descent. The average peak mitral annular descent velocity correlated linearly with LVEF (r = 0.86) using radionuclide ventriculograms as the standard of reference. They derived an equation for predicting EF from average peak mitral annular descent velocity.

$$LVEF = 8.2 \times (average\ peak\ mitral\ annular\ velocity) + 3\%$$

When the average peak mitral annular velocity at six sites (septal, lateral, inferior, anterior, posterior, and anteroseptal annulus) was greater than 5.4 cm/s, the velocity was 88%

sensitive and 97% specific for EF > 50%. A velocity greater than 5.4 cm/sec at a single annular site predicted an LVEF > 50% with an 89% sensitivity and 85% specificity. Clinically, this has potential value of rapidly estimating global LV function in cases where endocardial border definition is suboptimal for tracing, although, one must keep in mind a significant limitation to this method—preload dependency. In an intraoperative TEE study, it has been demonstrated that significant changes in peak mitral annular velocity with changes in preload (18).

The concept of myocardial strain was introduced in the 1970s to facilitate the understanding of elastic stiffness of myocardial tissue. With strain and SR imaging, regional myocardial contractile movement can be measured independent of traction and tethering effects from other regions.

Strain is a dimensionless quantity that represents the percentage change of length from a resting state to one achieved following the application of a force (stress). In general terms, strain, ε, means relative deformation, and SR means rate of deformation. If an object has an initial length L_0 that after a certain time changes to L, strain is defined as

$$\varepsilon = \frac{(L - L_0)}{L_0}$$

And SR is calculated as

$$SR = \frac{\varepsilon}{\Delta t}$$

When a myocardial segment shortens, L_0 is larger than L, and strain is negative. When a segment lengthens, strain is positive (Fig. 9.17).

Strain occurs simultaneously in all three dimensions, longitudinal or meridional, transmural or radial, and circumferential as force is applied to a segment of myocardium. Since myocardial tissue is incompressible and the volume

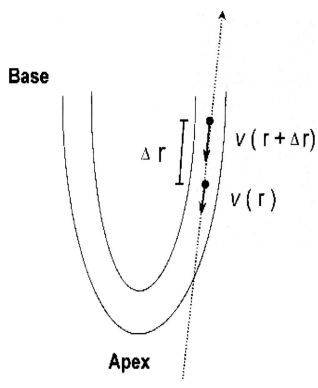

Figure 9.17. Schematic of how SR of tissue segment (Δr) is estimated from tissue velocity (v). *Dashed line* indicates orientation of ultrasound beam. Distance along beam is denoted by r. SR is calculated by subtracting $v(r + \Delta r)$ from $v(r)$ over distance (Δr) between these two points. When velocities are equal, SR is zero and there is no compression or expansion. If $v(r + \Delta r) > (r)$, SR is negative and there is compression. When $v(r)$ exceeds $v(r + \Delta r)$, SR is positive, indicating expansion. (From Urheim S, Edvardsen T, Torp H, et al. Myocardial strain by Doppler echocardiography. Validation of a new method to quantify regional myocardial function. *Circulation* 2000;102(10):1158–1164.)

must remain constant, shortening from base to apex combined with circumferential shortening must be balanced by transmural thickening. Therefore, longitudinal and circumferential myocardial deformation measured by strain is simultaneously and inversely related to radial strain.

Figure 9.18. Illustration of systolic shortening mitral annulus moving toward the apex and away from the transducer (**A**). Diastolic expansion with mitral annulus moving toward the transducer (**B**).

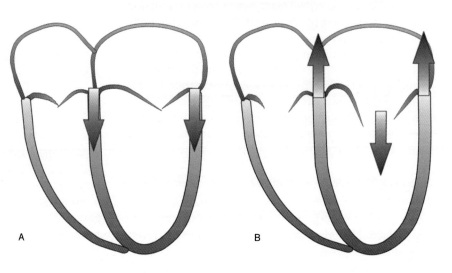

The myocardial base descends toward the apex during systole and reverts during diastole (Fig. 9.18). The apex is nearly stationary, moving only a few millimeters in the same direction as the base. As the base moves toward the relatively stationary apex, the tissue velocities decrease from base to apex. Therefore, measuring the velocity gradient subtracts its translational component because this motion would affect both sampling points equally.

The instantaneous change in length (dL) in a small time increment (dt) is related to the velocities (v_1 and v_2) of the end points of the object:

$$dL = (v_2 - v_1)dt$$

By dividing the equation above by L, we see that the instantaneous change in length per unit length equals the velocity gradient (i.e., SR) times the time increment:

$$\frac{dL}{L} = \frac{(v_2 - v_1)dt}{L}$$

Because it is not feasible to track the end points of the object, the velocity gradient SR is estimated from two points with a fixed distance:

$$\frac{dL}{L} \approx \frac{(v_r - v_{(r+\Delta r)})dt}{\Delta r} = SR\,dt$$

Finally, by integrating this equation from time t_0 to t, we arrive at the following relation between SR and strain:

$$\text{Log}\,\frac{L}{L_0} = \int_{t_0}^{t} SR\,dt$$

where log denotes the natural logarithm and L_0 and L denote the object length at times t_0 and t, respectively. This gives the equation:

$$\varepsilon = \exp\left(\int_{t_0}^{t} SR\,dt\right) - 1$$

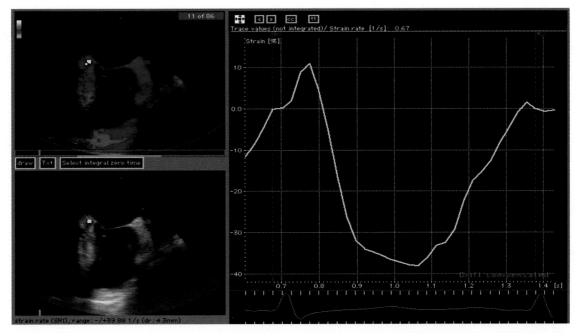

Figure 9.19. Myocardial strain by Doppler. Negative strain denotes myocardial shortening (compression) while positive strain (expansion) denotes myocardial lengthening. Also during the integration procedure, the random noise is cancelled out and a relatively smooth signal is obtained.

Velocity gradients (SRs) in the direction of the ultrasonic beam can be estimated from the spatial variation in Doppler shift frequency of the received signal. For calculation of strain, (Eq. 5) SR is integrated throughout each cardiac cycle, starting at peak R wave on the ECG. Because SR equals velocity (m/s) divided by distance (m), the units for SR is 1/s, and strain, which is the time integral (with units $1/s \times s$), is reported as a fraction or percentage of end-diastolic dimension (19).

Myocardial strain and SR imaging is a potentially powerful tool since it allows for quantification of segmental myocardial function that is independent of the tethering effect and potentially independent of loading conditions (Figs. 9.19 and 9.20). Some data from animal studies

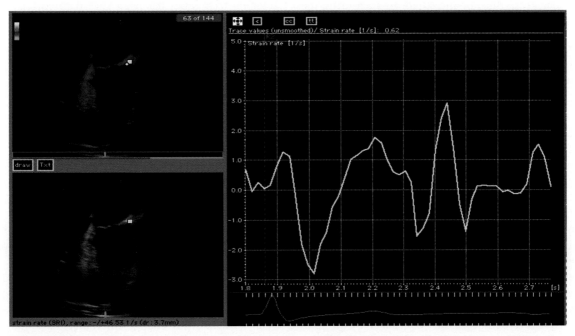

Figure 9.20. Myocardial SR by Doppler (1/s). Of note, SR signal has significant noise mainly from random noises in the velocity signal.

suggest that the peak systolic SR from the interventricular septum correlates reliably with invasively derived measures of ventricular function, such as, $dP/dt_{(max)}$ (20). It also eliminates the problem of preload dependency associated with mitral annular descent velocity. Another animal study shows that peak SR, this time during isovolumic contraction and relaxation, also correlates well with dP/dt regardless of loading conditions (21). The feasibility of using this technique by TEE in an intraoperative setting has been studied with good results (22).

SPECKLE TRACKING

One of the most important limitations of Doppler-based techniques for evaluating myocardial deformation and ventricular function is the angle dependency tissue motion with respect to the ultrasound beams. Particularly in TEE, it can be difficult to properly align the interrogating sound beam with the region of interest. 2D speckle tracking has the great advantage of measuring tissue velocities and deformation in an angle-independent fashion. This new technology is now routinely used in transthoracic echocardiography, but it has not been validated for TEE. Ultrasound reflectors that distort the sound wave in a relatively constant way are found within the myocardium. A consistent grayscale tone will be attributed to the pixels representing these reflectors throughout the cardiac cycle. Speckles are comprised of groups of 20 to 40 of these pixels. Each speckle will, thus, show a distinct grayscale pattern throughout the cardiac cycle (23). Using pattern recognition algorithms, the position of these speckles can be tracked from image to image in a digitally stored cineloop. The displacement of the speckle in both dimensions of the 2D image can, thus, be measured. By measuring the changing distance between different speckles throughout diastole and systole, myocardial shortening or strain can be calculated. Speckle tracking has, however, some limitations. The quality of speckle tracking depends highly on the spatial resolution of the image and on the frame rate of the cineloop. Myocardial deformation occurs in the three spatial dimensions, resulting in speckles moving out of the 2D scanning plane. The computer compensates for this out-of-plane motion by tracking new speckles as they move in while previous ones fade out of the scanning plane. Low frame rates will lead to undersampling, and speckles will move out of the search area too soon for the digital compensation. High frame rates will reduce this problem but may lead to inadequate tracking due to reduced spatial resolution. The optimal frame rate for adequate speckle tracking seems to be approximately 90 frames/s, which is considerably lower than Doppler-based techniques and may lead to inadequate detection of short lasting events, such as the isovolumetric phases of the cardiac cycle (24). Artifacts, like reverberations, can be mistaken by the software as myocardium resulting in falsely low strain calculations or drift. Drift occurs when, at the end of the cycle,

strain does not return to baseline. The computer software will correct the difference by drift compensation. Strong reflectors in the near field can cast an acoustic shadow and cause drop out, leading to the inability of the software to track the segments in the far field. Apart from the temporal, radial, and lateral resolution, accurate tracking also depends on the orientation of the myocardial fibers and the blood-tissue interface. In the transesophageal short-axis views in TEE, for example, the fiber orientation and the endocardial border of the septal and lateral walls are parallel to the ultrasound beam, frequently resulting in low resolution with inadequate tracking.

Visual control of the tracking process remains necessary to correct misinterpretation of artifacts by the software.

Although Speckle tracking can be performed on any 2D grayscale image, the images acquired in the harmonics mode allow superior endocardial border delineation. When obtaining images, special attention must be given to image quality and frame rate. For adequate timing of cardiac events, a constant HR in sinus rhythm and a clear ECG signal as well as aortic valve opening and closure times are necessary.

The software arbitrarily divides the LV myocardium into six segments that are color coded and displays velocity, displacement, strain and SR curves for the entire ventricle or for the individual segments (Fig. 9.21). The global ventricular strain values, in the longitudinal, radial, or circumferential dimension, are calculated as an average of all the strains measured over the entire myocardium in the respective directions. Compared to techniques calculating derived parameters representing global ventricular function, such as mitral annular velocity, this technique has the advantage of evaluating the entire visible myocardium in its calculation of global function. EF calculated using speckle tracking techniques has been shown to correlate closely with visual estimation and Simpson's method (r = 0.82) for TTE (25). And several studies reported the technique to have low interobserver and intraobserver variability (8.6%–11.8% and 5.2%–8.8% respectively) (26,27).

Global longitudinal strain has been proposed as a new index for LV systolic function with a high specificity and sensitivity for the diagnosis of myocardial infarction (28). Reductions in global longitudinal strain closely correlate to infarct size in chronic ischemic heart disease (29). And, speckle tracking has been shown to demonstrate early decreases in global longitudinal, radial, and circumferential strain in patients with subclinical hypertrophic cardiomyopathy (30).

Global diastolic SRs in the isovolumic relaxation phase correlate to diastolic function, as assessed by intraventricular pressure measurements (31).

By tracking angular displacement in the short-axis views, speckle tracking allows for the quantification of ventricular twist and torsion (32). This unique feature has been used to study changes in ventricular rotation and rotation rate in the elderly (33), in patients with essential hypertension (34), myocardial ischemia (35), ventricular

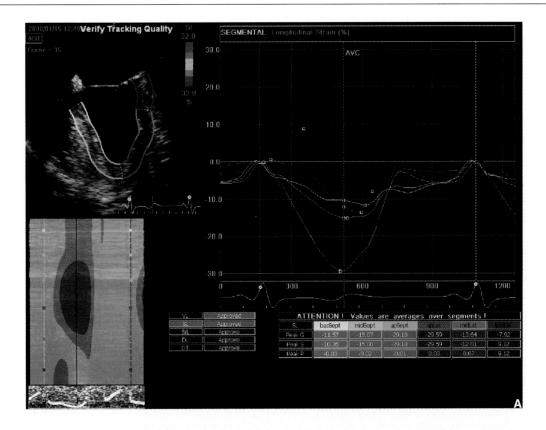

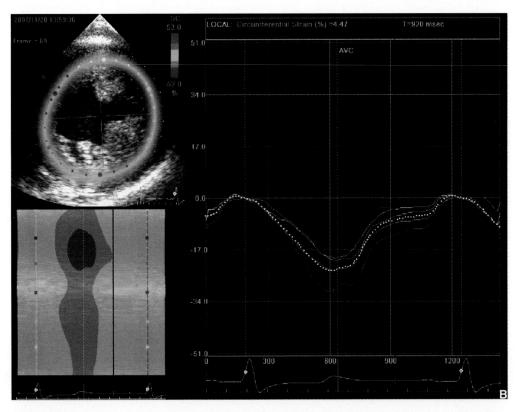

Figure 9.21. Ventricular Strain, SR, and Rotation Measured by Speckle Tracking. **A.** Color-coded regional longitudinal strain curves in the midesophageal four-chamber view. Note the positive strain (segmental lengthening) of the latero-basal segment in systole, indicating dyskinesia. **B.** Circumferential strain in transgastric midpapillary short-axis view. Segments are color coded; global circumferential strain is represented by the white dotted line.

(Continued)

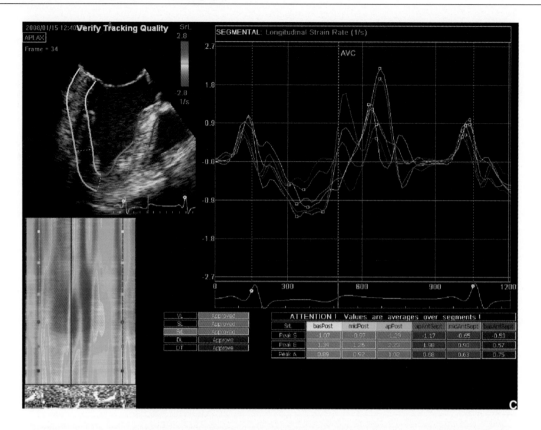

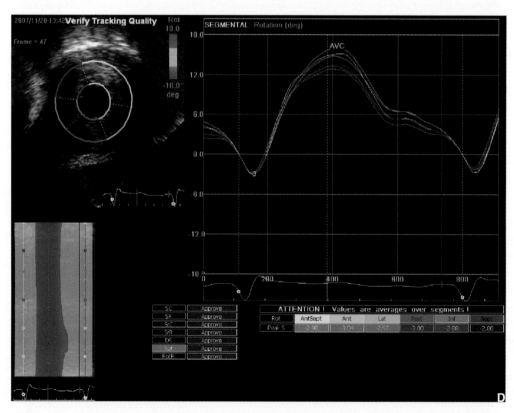

Figure 9.21. (*Continued*). **C.** Longitudinal SR in midesophageal long-axis view. Systolic and diastolic waves are preceded by biphasic undulations occurring during the isovolumic phases. **D.** LV apical rotation in the transgastric apical short-axis view. Systolic apical rotation occurs counterclockwise and is by convention positive; basal rotation is clockwise and negative. The software erroneously identifies the most negative point on the tracing as maximal apical rotation illustrating the need for visual verification of automated tracking.

hypertrophy (36), dilated cardiomyopathy (20), and chronic mitral regurgitation (37). In one study, the rate of early diastolic untwist has been shown to correlate to the degree of diastolic dysfunction, as defined by classic echocardiographic measures (38).

CALCULATING LEFT VENTRICULAR FILLING PRESSURE

Swan et al. (39) first described the clinical use of flow-directed balloon-tipped catheters to measure intracardiac pressures in man. Since that introduction, pulmonary artery occlusion pressure (PAOP) has been considered the standard for estimation of mean left atrial pressure and LV filling pressure. LV filling pressure or LV end-diastolic pressure (LVEDP) changes, however, with changes in LVEDV, the true indicator of LV preload. With the pulmonary artery catheter, LVEDP is used to estimate a volume index, the LVEDV. The error introduced by this approximation is clinically insignificant in conditions of low LV filling pressures. However, in critically ill patients, the PCWP grossly misrepresents the LVEDV. Echocardiography, on the other hand, provides an accurate diagnostic tool in any situation for the assessment of LV filling pressure and preload.

INTERATRIAL SEPTUM

The interatrial septum provides qualitative information regarding the filling pressure of the right and left ventricles. The atrial septum can be examined in the four-chamber view, the bicaval view, or the right ventricular inflow-outflow view. The directional movement of the interatrial septum and its curvature may reflect the pressure relations between the left and right atria. Normally due to higher left-sided pressures, the interatrial septum bulges toward the right atrium. During passive mechanical expiration, right atrial pressure transiently exceeds left atrial pressure, and the atrial septum momentarily bows toward the left atrium. This midsystolic atrial reversal occurs when the corresponding PAOP is ≤15 mm Hg. A rightward midsystolic bowing or absence of the leftward bowing of the interatrial septum indicates PAOP > 15 mm Hg, with a sensitivity of 89%, specificity of 95%, and a positive predictive value of 0.97 (40).

PULMONARY VEIN FLOW

At the midesophageal level, the TEE transducer is placed behind the left atrium allowing excellent visualization of the left upper pulmonary vein (LUPV) in the two-chamber view. With slight manipulation of the probe, the left lower and right pulmonary veins can be easily identified as well. Doppler interrogation of the LUPV in the two-chamber

view has several advantages. First, the LUPV can easily be visualized with the aid of color flow Doppler. Second, a long segment of the vein can be visualized enabling proper placement of the pulse wave cursor 1 to 2 cm into the vein. Lastly, the pulmonary vein visualized here parallels the direction of the Doppler beam, thus increasing the accuracy of the Doppler measurements.

Sampling too close to the left atrium leads to underestimation of atrial reversal velocity. An inadequate signal may be improved by increasing the sample volume size to 3 to 4 mm. Color flow Doppler may help find the pulmonary vein flow stream as it enters the atrium.

The normal velocity of the pulmonary vein flow consists of an antegrade systolic flow (PVS1) produced by the forward flow of blood into the atrium as the left atrial pressure decreases during relaxation (Fig. 9.22). Then, downward movement of the mitral annulus during LV ejection creates a second systolic peak (PVS2) with higher amplitude. In the presence of low left atrial pressure, the biphasic nature of the S wave becomes more prominent because of the temporal dissociation of atrial relaxation and mitral annular motion (41). With TEE, the biphasic systolic wave is commonly seen. The descent of the S wave corresponds with the V wave in the left atrial pressure tracing. The second large flow velocity is the diastolic wave (PVD) prompted by the antegrade flow of blood from the pulmonary veins into the left ventricle during early diastole. It coincides with the Y descent of the left atrial pressure tracing during early ventricular filling. During this phase, because the left atrium is an open conduit between the pulmonary veins and the left ventricle, the pulmonary veins reflect abnormalities in the compliance of the left ventricle. The D wave is followed by a retrograde velocity called the A wave, which coincides with atrial contraction during late diastole and represents flow from the atrium into the pulmonary vein during atrial contraction (Table 9.1).

Multiple factors can affect the pulmonary vein flow pattern. Sinus tachycardia may cause the systolic and

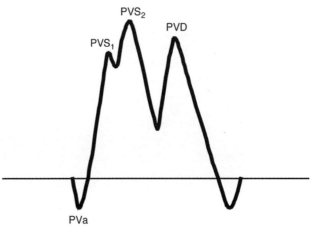

Figure 9.22. Illustration of the four components of the pulmonary vein Doppler flow velocities. See text for explanation.

TABLE 9.1	Determinants of Pulmonary Vein Flow Velocities
Velocity	**Determinants**
Early systole (PVS1)	LA relaxation
Late systole (PVS2)	RV output, LA compliance, mean LAP
Diastole (PVd)	LV relaxation
Atrial reversal (PVa)	LA contractility, LV compliance

diastolic waves to fuse. The peak systolic to diastolic filling ratio increases with sinus tachycardia because the diastolic filling period is shortened. In patients with atrial fibrillation, systolic forward flow is diminished or absent, and diastolic flow is the main contributor to left atrial filling. Mechanical ventilation may decrease systolic flow during inspiration because of elevated airway pressure and increase diastolic flow at the end of expiration (42). The position of the sample volume in the pulmonary vein affects the flow characteristics as well. The systolic phase decreases as the sample volume is moved closer to the orifice where the pulmonary vein empties into the left atrium. Atrial flow reversal may be detected at a site other than that used to obtain the maximal systolic and diastolic flow velocities. Motion artifact from prominent atrial contraction may make it difficult to detect reversal of atrial contraction because it is a low-velocity signal. The shape and size of the pulmonary flow velocity profile provide quantitative and qualitative information about LV preload. Normally, the S wave is equal to or slightly larger than the D wave. The degree

of systolic forward flow in the extraparenchymal pulmonary veins is determined by atrial relaxation, LV systolic function (suction effect), mitral regurgitation, and left atrial compliance and pressure. In situations of elevated left atrial pressure (LAP > 15), the S wave is blunted, reflecting that most forward flow into the LA occurs during diastole. Kuecherer et al. speculated that the decrease in left atrial compliance from increased LAP or left atrial volume or both best explains the shift in pulmonary venous flow (43). They used TEE Doppler to measure the pulmonary vein inflow velocity in 47 patients during cardiovascular surgery, excluding patients with mitral regurgitation. Fractional area shortening was the index of LV systolic function. They found that the systolic fraction, defined as systolic fraction = $TVI_{PVS}/(TVI_{PVS} + TVI_{PVD})$, correlated strongly with mean PAOP (r = −0.88) and LAP measured directly by an intra-atrial catheter (r = −0.78). In their study, systolic fraction less than 40% usually implied wedge pressure ≥ 20 mm Hg (Fig. 9.23).

Kinnaird et al. (44) reexamined the accuracy of pulmonary venous flow as a predictor of left atrial pressure. Unlike Kuecherer et al. (43), who used both direct LAP and PAOP measurements, Kinnaird used only direct LAP measurements. Measured PAOP consistently overestimated LAP. Kinnaird et al. reported that the deceleration time of the pulmonary vein during early diastole (DT_D) was more accurate than pulmonary wedge pressure in predicting LAP in cardiac surgical patients. A close correlation (r = −0.92) was found between LAP and pulmonary vein diastolic deceleration time. A DT_D of less than 175 ms had 100% sensitivity and 94% specificity for LAP > 17 mm Hg. A DT_D > 275ms predicted LAP of ≤6 mm Hg with 88% sensitivity and 95% specificity (44).

In summary, systolic flow pattern can be used as an "eyeball index" of LAP during cardiovascular surgery,

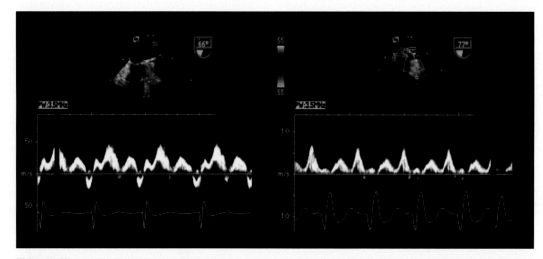

Figure 9.23. Illustration of low filling pressure (**left**), where the systolic waveform is greater than the diastolic waveform and the two components of systole, PVS1 and PVS2, are seen clearly. **Right:** Illustration of high left atrial pressure with LAP > 15 mm Hg showing the systolic component blunted and the diastolic waveform greater than the systolic waveform.

if patients do not have serious mitral regurgitation. The PVD deceleration time and the PVS to PVD velocity ratio are noninvasive tools for measuring LAP.

MITRAL INFLOW VELOCITIES AND TISSUE DOPPLER

Tissue Doppler imaging may also be used in conjunction with conventional Doppler techniques to estimate LV filling pressure. Mitral E wave velocity is directly influenced by LAP and inversely related changes in LV relaxation. Measures of E wave velocity via conventional Doppler correlate poorly with LAP because abnormal relaxation and high filling pressure often coexist in cardiac patients. Nagueh et al. (45) demonstrated that dividing the E wave blood flow velocity by the annulus tissue E velocity (Ea) provides an alternative method to correct the transmitral velocity for the influence of relaxation. They found that the E/Ea correlated well with PCWP (r = 0.87, p < 0.001) and derived a formula for predicting wedge pressure from the E/Ea ratio.

$$PCWP = 1.24 \left(\frac{E}{Ea} \right) + 1.9$$

In patients with sinus tachycardia with fused mitral inflow E and A waves, the E/Ea ratio correlated well with PCWP (r = 0.86, p < 0.001). As a general guideline, E/Ea > 10 predicts a mean PCWP > 15 mm Hg with a 92% sensitivity and 80% specificity.

Kim and Sohn (46) evaluated 200 patients prospectively to compare the ratio of E/Ea to that of invasive LV diastolic pressure measured before atrial contraction (pre-A wave). They found that the E/Ea ratio correlated well with pre-A wave pressure (r = 0.74, p < 0.001), and the correlation was not dependent on LV systolic function (EF ≥ 50%; r = 0.74 vs. EF < 50%; r = 0.70).

The slight discrepancy between the Nagueh and Kim studies may be explained by the following differences. Kim and Sohn used pre-A pressure to represent the LV filling pressure rather than PCWP. Second, the tissue velocity sample volume was placed on the septum in Kim and Sohn's study, whereas Nagueh et al. sampled the lateral mitral annulus. In both studies, an E/Ea ratio of ≥9 predicted an elevated LV filling pressure ≥12 mm Hg. Kim and Sohn also derived an equation for predicting LV pressure.

$$LV \text{ filling pressure} = E / Ea + 4$$

THREE-DIMENSIONAL EVALUATION OF GLOBAL VENTRICULAR PERFORMANCE

The increase of computational power and the miniaturization of ultrasound equipment have recently allowed for the development of real-time 3D echocardiography

(RT3DE), which allows for rapid, accurate, real-time assessment of cardiac volumes.

The matrix array ultrasound transducer has up to 3,000 ultrasound elements that fire nonsimultaneously to reproduce a real-time, pyramid-shaped, and 3D image of the interrogated region of the heart. Presently, the size of the imaged volume is not enough to contain the entire adult LV. Therefore, a series of four or more gated cycles need to be combined to recreate a full volume image of the ventricle, resulting in a maximum frame rate of 25 Hz (47).

Currently, RT3DE for TEE offers three different modalities: live 3D, 3D zoom, and full volume. The first and second provide an online, ungated 3D image of a portion of the heart while imaging of the entire LV cavity requires the summation of several gated cycles. Only the latter, gated view encompasses the whole left ventricle and can be used for the volumetric assessment of global LV function. For the acquisition of a high-quality full volume loop, all manipulation of the patient and surgical interference must be paused and the ventilation paused. The ultrasound machine acquires four to seven ECG-gated images that will be summed to create the full volume projection of the heart. The accuracy of the gating process can be verified by evaluating the superposition of different ECG tracings. Improper alignment of the images due to movement or artifacts will show up as "stitch lines" in the 3D image.

When a full volume 3D image is acquired, only the outer surface of the pyramid shape is displayed. The image can then be cropped in different planes to expose the structures within and to evaluate wall motion of the different segments.

Several semiautomated algorithms have been developed to calculate LV volumes (48). After identifying several landmarks, the endocardium is traced by an automated endocardial border detection algorithm, which can be visually inspected and manually corrected if needed. Based on this data, an endocardial cast and its displacement throughout the cardiac cycle are generated and displayed as the "jelly-bean image" (Fig. 9.24).

Ventricular volumes are numerically and graphically displayed as time-volume curves, and end-diastolic volume (EDV), end-systolic volume (ESV), and EF are calculated. The accuracy of the calculated volumes and EF depends on the number of elements in the transducer, the spatial and temporal resolution of the image, and the accuracy of the endocardial border delineation. The accuracy and reproducibility of RT3DE have been established in several studies. Global LV volume and EF measurements using RT3DE correlate highly with cardiac MRI (r = 0.98) with minimal bias (1.4 mL) and narrow limits of agreement (±20 mL) (49). In fact, the correlation with cardiac MRI is better for RT3DE than for single photon emission computed tomography and cardiac computed tomography, albeit with higher variability (50,51). The limited temporal and spatial resolution of the technology accounts for some of the reported underestimation and variability of LV volumes by RT3DE. As in 2D echocardiography, the interposition of the mitral valve apparatus between the transducer and the

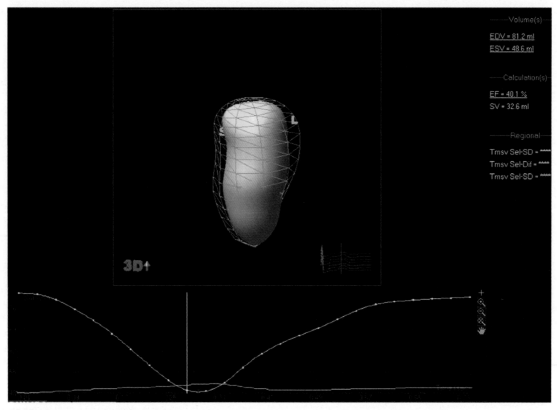

Figure 9.24. Real-time 3D cast of LV endocardium reconstructed out of 7 ECG gated cardiac cycles. The LV cavity is presented in the "jelly-bean" image as a cast of the endocardium at end-systole within a frame representing the end-diastolic dimensions. EDV, ESV, EF, and SV are automatically calculated and graphically displayed. The superposition of the ECG signals represents the gating process.

LV cavity can cause acoustic shadowing with signal drop out in the 3D projection. This will lead to inaccuracy of the automated endocardial detection and necessitates manual correction with extrapolation of visible ventricular walls.

Nevertheless, the interobserver and intraobserver variability is significantly lower for RT3DE than for 2D echocardiography (52). Its superiority to 2D echocardiographic imaging is largely due to the fact that no geometrical assumptions and no extrapolation of the endocardial border for the regions in between scanning planes are necessary.

KEY POINTS

Normal anatomy and physiology of the left ventricle
- Normal anatomy
- Phases of ventricular systole
- LV systolic function

2D examination of the left ventricle
- Midesophageal four-chamber view
- Midesophageal two-chamber view
- Midesophageal long-axis view
- Transgastric midpapillary short-axis view
- Transgastric two-chamber view

Ejection phase indices of LV performance
- CO
- Fractional shortening
- FAC
- EF

Calculating preload and afterload
- Preload
  - Area-length method
  - Modified Simpson's
  - LV EDA
- Afterload
  - End-systolic meridional wall stress

Load-independent indices of LV contraction
- Systolic index of contractility (dP/dt)
- Preload recruitable stroke work and elastance

Tissue Doppler imaging
- Tissue velocity imaging
- Tissue strain imaging

Speckle tracking

Calculating LV filling pressure
- Interatrial septum
- Pulmonary vein flow
- Mitral inflow velocities and tissue Doppler

3D evaluation of global ventricular performance

REFERENCES

1. Alderman EL, Bourassa MG, Cohen LS, et al. Ten-year follow-up of survival and myocardial infarction in the randomized Coronary Artery Surgery Study. *Circulation* 1990;82(5): 1629–1646.

2. Muhiudeen IA, Kuecherer HF, Lee E, et al. Intraoperative estimation of cardiac output by transesophageal pulsed Doppler echocardiography. *Anesthesiology* 1991;74(1):9–14.

3. Darmon PL, Hillel Z, Mogtader A, et al. Cardiac output by transesophageal echocardiography using continuous-wave Doppler across the aortic valve. *Anesthesiology* 1994;80(4): 796–805; discussion 25A.

4. Perrino AC Jr, Harris SN, Luther MA. Intraoperative determination of cardiac output using multiplane transesophageal echocardiography: a comparison to thermodilution. *Anesthesiology* 1998;89(2):350–357.

5. Douglas PS, Reichek N, Plappert T, et al. Comparison of echocardiographic methods for assessment of left ventricular shortening and wall stress. *J Am Coll Cardiol* 1987;9(4): 945–951.

6. Clements FM, Harpole DH, Quill T, et al. Estimation of left ventricular volume and ejection fraction by two-dimensional transoesophageal echocardiography: comparison of short axis imaging and simultaneous radionuclide angiography. *Br J Anaesth* 1990;64(3):331–336.

7. Urbanowicz JH, Shaaban MJ, Cohen NH, et al. Comparison of transesophageal echocardiographic and scintigraphic estimates of left ventricular end-diastolic volume index and ejection fraction in patients following coronary artery bypass grafting. *Anesthesiology* 1990;72(4):607–612.

8. Smith MD, MacPhail B, Harrison MR, et al. Value and limitations of transesophageal echocardiography in determination of left ventricular volumes and ejection fraction. *J Am Coll Cardiol* 1992;19(6):1213–1222.

9. Cheung AT, Savino JS, Weiss SJ, et al. Echocardiographic and hemodynamic indexes of left ventricular preload in patients with normal and abnormal ventricular function. *Anesthesiology* 1994;81(2):376–387.

10. Reich DL, Konstadt SN, Nejat M, et al. Intraoperative transesophageal echocardiography for the detection of cardiac preload changes induced by transfusion and phlebotomy in pediatric patients. *Anesthesiology* 1993;79(1):10–15.

11. Leung JM, Levine EH. Left ventricular end-systolic cavity obliteration as an estimate of intraoperative hypovolemia. *Anesthesiology* 1994;81(5):1102–1109.

12. Grossman W, Jones D, McLaurin LP. Wall stress and patterns of hypertrophy in the human left ventricle. *J Clin Invest* 1975;56(1):56–64.

13. Reichek N, Wilson J, St John Sutton M, et al. Noninvasive determination of left ventricular end-systolic stress: validation of the method and initial application. *Circulation* 1982;65(1):99–108.

14. Bargiggia GS, Bertucci C, Recusani F, et al. A new method for estimating left ventricular dP/dt by continuous wave Doppler-echocardiography. Validation studies at cardiac catheterization. *Circulation* 1989;80(5):1287–1292.

15. Kolias TJ, Aaronson KD, Armstrong WF. Doppler-derived dP/dt and -dP/dt predict survival in congestive heart failure. *J Am Coll Cardiol* 2000;36(5):1594–1599.

16. Gorcsan J III, Gasior TA, Mandarino WA, et al. Assessment of the immediate effects of cardiopulmonary bypass on left ventricular performance by on-line pressure-area relations. *Circulation* 1994;89(1):180–190.

17. Gulati VK, Katz WE, Follansbee WP, et al. Mitral annular descent velocity by tissue Doppler echocardiography as an index of global left ventricular function. *Am J Cardiol* 1996;77(11):979–984.

18. Toyoda T, Baba H, Akasaka T, et al. Assessment of regional myocardial strain by a novel automated tracking system from digital image files. *J Am Soc Echocardiogr* 2004;17(12):1234–1238.

19. Urheim S, Edvardsen T, Torp H, et al. Myocardial strain by Doppler echocardiography. Validation of a new method to quantify regional myocardial function. *Circulation* 2000;102(10): 1158–1164.

20. Popovic ZB, Grimm RA, Ahmad A, et al. Longitudinal rotation: an unrecognised motion pattern in patients with dilated cardiomyopathy. *Heart* 2008;94(3):e11.

21. Hashimoto I, Li X, Hejmadi Bhat A, et al. Myocardial strain rate is a superior method for evaluation of left ventricular subendocardial function compared with tissue Doppler imaging. *J Am Coll Cardiol* 2003;42(9):1574–1583.

22. Simmons LA, Weidemann F, Sutherland GR, et al. Doppler tissue velocity, strain, and strain rate imaging with transesophageal echocardiography in the operating room: a feasibility study. *J Am Soc Echocardiogr* 2002;15(8):768–776.

23. Leitman M, Lysyansky P, Sidenko S, et al. Two-dimensional strain-a novel software for real-time quantitative echocardiographic assessment of myocardial function. *J Am Soc Echocardiogr* 2004;17(10):1021–1029.

24. Teske AJ, De Boeck BW, Melman PG, et al. Echocardiographic quantification of myocardial function using tissue deformation imaging, a guide to image acquisition and analysis using tissue Doppler and speckle tracking. *Cardiovasc Ultrasound* 2007;5:27.

25. Perk G, Tunick PA, Kronzon I. Non-Doppler two-dimensional strain imaging by echocardiography—from technical considerations to clinical applications. *J Am Soc Echocardiogr* 2007;20(3): 234–243.

26. Amundsen BH, Helle-Valle T, Edvardsen T, et al. Noninvasive myocardial strain measurement by speckle tracking echocardiography: validation against sonomicrometry and tagged magnetic resonance imaging. *J Am Coll Cardiol* 2006;47(4):789–793.

27. Korinek J, Wang J, Sengupta PP, et al. Two-dimensional strain— a Doppler-independent ultrasound method for quantitation of regional deformation: validation in vitro and in vivo. *J Am Soc Echocardiogr* 2005;18(12):1247–1253.

28. Reisner SA, Lysyansky P, Agmon Y, et al. Global longitudinal strain: a novel index of left ventricular systolic function. *J Am Soc Echocardiogr* 2004;17(6):630–633.

29. Gjesdal O, Hopp E, Vartdal T, et al. Global longitudinal strain measured by two-dimensional speckle tracking echocardiography is closely related to myocardial infarct size in chronic ischaemic heart disease. *Clin Sci (Lond)* 2007;113(6):287–296.

30. Serri K, Reant P, Lafitte M, et al. Global and regional myocardial function quantification by two-dimensional strain: application in hypertrophic cardiomyopathy. *J Am Coll Cardiol* 2006;47(6):1175–1181.

31. Wang J, Khoury DS, Thohan V, et al. Global diastolic strain rate for the assessment of left ventricular relaxation and filling pressures. *Circulation* 2007;115(11):1376–1383.

32. Helle-Valle T, Crosby J, Edvardsen T, et al. New noninvasive method for assessment of left ventricular rotation: speckle tracking echocardiography. *Circulation* 2005;112(20):3149–3156.

33. Zhang L, Xie M, Fu M. Assessment of age-related changes in left ventricular twist by two-dimensional ultrasound speckle tracking imaging. *J Huazhong Univ Sci Technolog Med Sci* 2007;27(6):691–695.

34. Han W, Xie M, Wang X, Lu Q. Assessment of left ventricular global twist in essential hypertensive heart by speckle tracking imaging. *J Huazhong Univ Sci Technolog Med Sci* 2008;28(1):114–117.

35. Bansal M, Leano RL, Marwick TH. Clinical assessment of left ventricular systolic torsion: effects of myocardial infarction and ischemia. *J Am Soc Echocardiogr* 2008;21(8):887–894.

36. Takeuchi M, Borden WB, Nakai H, et al. Reduced and delayed untwisting of the left ventricle in patients with hypertension and left ventricular hypertrophy: a study using two-dimensional speckle tracking imaging. *Eur Heart J* 2007;28(22):2756–2762.

37. Borg AN, Harrison JL, Argyle RA, et al. Left ventricular torsion in primary chronic mitral regurgitation. *Heart* 2008;94(5):597–603.

38. Perry R, De Pasquale CG, Chew DP, et al. Assessment of early diastolic left ventricular function by two-dimensional echocardiographic speckle tracking. *Eur J Echocardiogr* 2008;9(6):791–795.

39. Swan HJ, Ganz W, Forrester J, et al. Catheterization of the heart in man with use of a flow-directed balloon-tipped catheter. *N Engl J Med* 1970;283(9):447–451.

40. Kusumoto FM, Muhiudeen IA, Kuecherer HF, et al. Response of the interatrial septum to transatrial pressure gradients and its potential for predicting pulmonary capillary wedge pressure: an intraoperative study using transesophageal echocardiography in patients during mechanical ventilation. *J Am Coll Cardiol* 1993;21(3):721–728.

41. Nishimura RA, Abel MD, Hatle LK, et al. Relation of pulmonary vein to mitral flow velocities by transesophageal Doppler echocardiography. Effect of different loading conditions. *Circulation* 1990;81(5):1488–1497.

42. Orihashi K, Goldiner PL, Oka Y. Intraoperative assessment of pulmonary vein flow. *Echocardiography* 1990;7(3):261–271.

43. Kuecherer HF, Muhiudeen IA, Kusumoto FM, et al. Estimation of mean left atrial pressure from transesophageal pulsed Doppler echocardiography of pulmonary venous flow. *Circulation* 1990;82(4):1127–1139.

44. Kinnaird TD, Thompson CR, Munt BI. The deceleration [correction of declaration] time of pulmonary venous diastolic flow is more accurate than the pulmonary artery occlusion pressure in predicting left atrial pressure. *J Am Coll Cardiol* 2001;37(8):2025–2030.

45. Nagueh SF, Middleton KJ, Kopelen HA, et al. Doppler tissue imaging: a noninvasive technique for evaluation of left ventricular relaxation and estimation of filling pressures. *J Am Coll Cardiol* 1997;30(6):1527–1533.

46. Kim YJ, Sohn DW. Mitral annulus velocity in the estimation of left ventricular filling pressure: prospective study in 200 patients. *J Am Soc Echocardiogr* 2000;13(11):980–985.

47. Picard MH, Popp RL, Weyman AE. Assessment of left ventricular function by echocardiography: a technique in evolution. *J Am Soc Echocardiogr* 2008;21(1):14–21.

48. Sugeng L, Weinert L, Lang RM. Left ventricular assessment using real time three dimensional echocardiography. *Heart* 2003;89(Suppl. 3):29–36.

49. Corsi C, Lang RM, Veronesi F, et al. Volumetric quantification of global and regional left ventricular function from real-time three-dimensional echocardiographic images. *Circulation* 2005;112(8):1161–1170.

50. Chan J, Jenkins C, Khafagi F, et al. What is the optimal clinical technique for measurement of left ventricular volume after myocardial infarction? A comparative study of 3-dimensional echocardiography, single photon emission computed tomography, and cardiac magnetic resonance imaging. *J Am Soc Echocardiogr* 2006;19(2):192–201.

51. Sugeng L, Mor-Avi V, Weinert L, et al. Quantitative assessment of left ventricular size and function: side-by-side comparison of real-time three-dimensional echocardiography and computed tomography with magnetic resonance reference. *Circulation* 2006;114(7):654–661.

52. Jenkins C, Bricknell K, Hanekom L, et al. Reproducibility and accuracy of echocardiographic measurements of left ventricular parameters using real-time three-dimensional echocardiography. *J Am Coll Cardiol* 2004;44(4):878–886.

QUESTIONS

1. All of the following indicate elevated LV filling volumes *except*
   A. Rightward bowing of the interatrial septum in midsystole.
   B. Blunting of the systolic component of the pulmonary vein flow velocity spectral display.
   C. Pulmonary vein flow systolic fraction less than 40%.
   D. E/Ea ratio more than 10.
   E. Leftward bowing of the interatrial septum in midsystole.

2. Comprehensive examination of LV systolic function includes all the following views *except*
   A. ME 2C view
   B. ME 4C view
   C. ME LAX view
   D. Transgastric midpapillary short-axis view
   E. The deep TG LAX view

3. All of the following statements regarding LV wall stress is true *except*
   A. Meridional wall stress can be calculated using noninvasive BP and myocardial area measured in M-mode.
   B. Meridional wall stress acts on the long axis of the left ventricle.
   C. Circumferential wall stress acts on the long axis of the left ventricle.
   D. In the normal ventricle, circumferential stress at the end of systole is 2.57 times higher than meridional stress.
   E. In the dilated ventricle, circumferential to radial wall stress ratio at the end of systole is 1.

4. Which of the following statements regarding pulmonary vein flow is false?

A. Tachycardia can cause the systolic and diastolic waveforms to fuse.

B. In patients with atrial fibrillation, diastolic flow is the main contributor to left atrial filling.

C. With low left atrial pressure, the biphasic nature of the systolic waveform becomes more prominent.

D. The pulmonary S wave corresponds to the Y descent of the left atrial filling pressure tracing.

5. All of the following statements regarding measurements of SV and CO are true *except*

A. CSA can be calculated by measuring the LV outflow tract diameter in the ME LAX view.

B. CSA can be calculated by measuring the length of each side of the aortic valve seen in the aortic valve short-axis view.

C. The TG LAX view can be used to obtain the spectral envelope for measuring the VTI used in the SV calculation.

D. The spectral envelope, used to measure the VTI, obtained from the pulmonary artery is equivalent to that from the aorta in the TG LAX view.

CHAPTER 10

Assessment of Right Ventricular Function

Shahar Bar-Yosef ■ Rebecca A. Schroeder ■ Atilio Barbeito ■ Jonathan B. Mark

INTRODUCTION

In the past, greater emphasis has been placed on indices of left ventricular (LV) function than right ventricular (RV) function. In fact, the RV was often viewed as a simple passive conduit contributing little to overall cardiac performance (1). Recent studies, however, have emphasized the prognostic significance of RV dysfunction in various perioperative settings, leading to a closer examination of the so-called "neglected ventricle" (2–4).

Several factors complicate the echocardiographic evaluation of the RV. It has a nongeometric complex shape that precludes characterization using simple formulae. As a result, wall segmentation is not standardized. Both a thin wall and extensive trabeculations interfere with endocardial tracing as well as with evaluating wall thickening. Also, systolic excursions are normally smaller than in the LV, again hindering distinction of normal from abnormal wall movement. And for standard midesophageal echocardiographic views, the RV is in the far field and has an oblique orientation. Consequently, assessment of RV size and function requires multiple echocardiographic views and techniques.

STRUCTURE AND FUNCTION OF THE RIGHT VENTRICLE

The RV is an asymmetric, complex chamber, which normally appears crescent shaped in short axis cross section. It is comprised of an inflow tract and an outflow tract; each has a separate embryologic origin (Fig. 10.1). The inflow tract begins at the tricuspid valve (TV) and is located posteroinferiorly. Trabeculae carneae or muscle bundles line most of the RV inflow chamber, making it difficult to delineate the endocardial border. The smooth-walled outflow tract, also known as the infundibulum, is positioned antero-superiorly and leads to the pulmonic valve and pulmonary artery (PA). An encircling muscular ring separates the inflow and outflow portions of the RV and is composed of four distinct muscular bands: the parietal band, supraventricular band (crista supraventricularis), septal band, and moderator band (5). Of these, the moderator band is of considerable importance to the echocardiographer. This structure appears as a prominent muscular trabeculation extending from the lower ventricular septum to the RV

free wall, and it must not be mistaken for an abnormal intracardiac mass or thrombus (Fig. 10.2).

The RV medial wall is formed by the interventricular septum that it shares with the LV. The lateral wall, also termed free wall, may be divided into basal, mid, and apical segments corresponding to the adjacent LV segments as seen in the midesophageal four-chamber view. The third wall of the RV is the inferior wall and is adjacent to the diaphragm. Papillary muscles (PM) arise from the RV walls and support the TV via chordae tendineae. These muscles are more variable in location and size compared to the mitral valve support structures.

The isovolumic phases of the cardiac cycle are shorter for the RV than for the LV. As a result, while onset of LV contraction normally occurs prior to the onset of RV contraction, RV ejection begins earlier, lasts longer, and has a reduced ejection velocity and a later peak compared with LV ejection. RV systolic contraction has three components: *longitudinal shortening* caused by the PM and longitudinal fibers in the free wall, increased rightward *septal curvature* caused by LV contraction, and a *bellows-like* movement of the RV lateral wall toward the interventricular septum caused by contraction of circular fibers in the RV free wall. Of these, the major contributor to RV ejection is the longitudinal shortening, especially in younger individuals (6).

One other factor that should be considered during qualitative assessment of RV systolic function is the effect

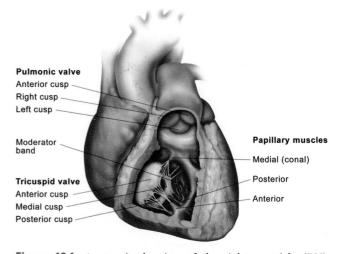

Figure 10.1. Anatomic drawing of the right ventricle (RV) major structures labeled.

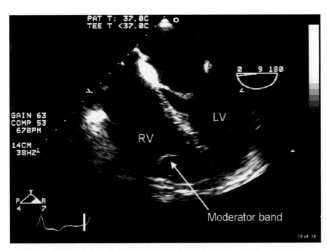

Figure 10.2. Midesophageal four-chamber view showing the moderator band inside the right ventricle (RV). LV = left ventricle.

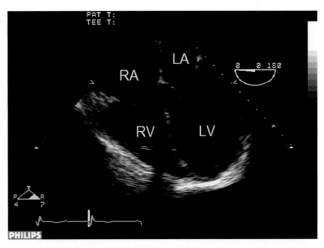

Figure 10.3. Midesophageal four-chamber view of the right ventricle (RV), left ventricle (LV), right atrium (RA) and left atrium (LA).

of afterload on RV performance. Because the thin-walled RV is a volume-pumping chamber, its ejection fraction is extremely sensitive to acute increases in PA pressure. In contrast, the thick-walled LV is a pressure-pumping chamber, and its ejection fraction, while influenced by the systemic arterial pressure, is generally less influenced by afterload. These hemodynamic factors must be considered for proper interpretation of RV systolic function.

TRANSESOPHAGEAL ECHOCARDIOGRAPHIC IMAGING OF THE RIGHT VENTRICLE

Because of its unique geometry, the RV requires multiple images for accurate structural and functional assessment. The most useful transesophageal echocardiography (TEE) scan planes for RV examination include the midesophageal four-chamber view, midesophageal RV inflow-outflow view, transgastric mid–short-axis view, and transgastric RV inflow view (7).

The *midesophageal four-chamber view* is the single most useful view for assessing overall RV anatomy and global function and allows evaluation of the apex, mid, and basal segments of this ventricle. In the four-chamber view, the RV appears triangular compared to the elliptical LV, and its length extends to only two thirds the length of the LV. As a result, the LV, not the RV, normally forms the cardiac apex (Fig. 10.3).

The *midesophageal RV inflow-outflow view* is sometimes termed the "wrap-around view," as the right atrium (RA), RV, and PA appear to encircle the aortic valve and left atrium, circumscribing a 180 to 270 degrees arc (Fig. 10.4). This view is particularly helpful for assessing motion of the diaphragmatic segment of the RV free wall and the RV infundibulum. It also often enables quantitative Doppler evaluation of a tricuspid regurgitation jet, because this jet is often parallel to the ultrasound beam in this scan plane.

The *transgastric mid–short-axis view* may be obtained in the horizontal scan plane with the TEE probe inserted approximately 35 to 40 cm from the incisors, with the tip anteflexed to achieve a true short-axis view. Slight clockwise (rightward) probe rotation will center the RV in the image screen. While this view is used most often to monitor LV function, it also allows assessment of the RV free wall and ventricular septum (Fig. 10.5). This view reveals the crescent-like shape of the RV seen in cross section.

Finally, the *transgastric RV inflow view* provides a long-axis view of the RV similar to the transgastric two-chamber view of the LV. To acquire this view, one begins with the transgastric mid–short-axis view of the RV and advances the multiplane angle to approximately 90 degrees or until the RA and RV are seen in long axis, with the RV inflow and TV centered in the image (Fig. 10.6). Alternatively, one develops the transgastric two-chamber view of the left

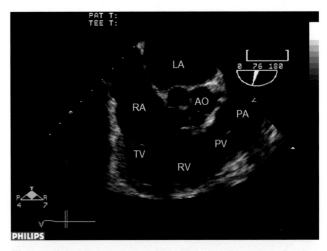

Figure 10.4. Midesophageal RV inflow-outflow view showing the right heart structures in the far field "wrapped" around the aorta (AO): right atrium (RA), tricuspid valve (TV), right ventricle (RV), pulmonary valve (PV), and pulmonary artery (PA). LA, left atrium.

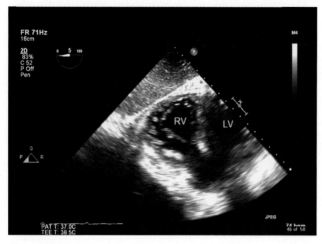

Figure 10.5. Transgastric mid–short axis view of the right ventricle (RV) with the tricuspid valve (TV) seen in cross section. LV, left ventricle.

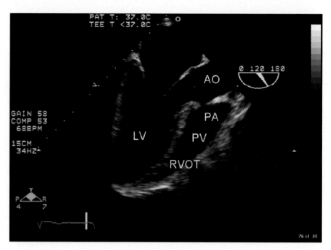

Figure 10.7. Midesophageal long-axis view of the left ventricle (LV) and aorta (AO) with the right ventricular outflow tract (RVOT), pulmonary valve (PV), and pulmonary artery (PA) visible on the right side.

atrium and ventricle and then rotates the probe clockwise (rightward) until the two right-sided chambers are displayed. In this view, the inferior or diaphragmatic aspect of the RV free wall can be seen in the near field while the anterior segments are in the far field.

Other TEE views may be used to supplement these four standard ones in patients who have abnormal RV anatomy and function. The *midesophageal long-axis view* includes a portion of the RVOT, and often, the pulmonic valve can be seen to the right of the aortic valve (Fig. 10.7). The *transgastric RV inflow-outflow view* provides an image with many of the same structures seen in the midesophageal RV inflow-outflow view, including the RA, RV, PA, and both tricuspid and pulmonic valves (Fig. 10.8). This view is acquired beginning with the transgastric mid–short-axis view, advancing the multiplane angle to approximately 110 to 140 degrees, and then rotating the TEE probe slightly clockwise (rightward). Finally, the *deep*

transgastric RV apical view provides an image similar to the deep transgastric long-axis view but focused instead on the RV, TV, and RA (Fig. 10.9). This view is acquired by slight clockwise (rightward) rotation of the probe from the deep transgastric long-axis view.

RIGHT VENTRICULAR HYPERTROPHY AND DILATATION

Evaluation of global RV function should include an assessment of the presence or absence of hypertrophy and/or dilatation. RV hypertrophy results from pressure overload of the ventricle, and common causes include pulmonic valve stenosis and pulmonary hypertension, either primary or secondary to other causes like LV failure or mitral stenosis. In addition to secondary hypertrophy that results from increased RV systolic pressures,

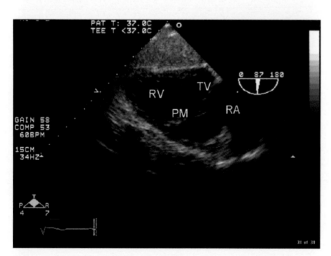

Figure 10.6. Transgastric RV inflow view showing the right ventricle (RV), tricuspid valve (TV), and right atrium (RA). One of the papillary muscles (PM) is seen as well.

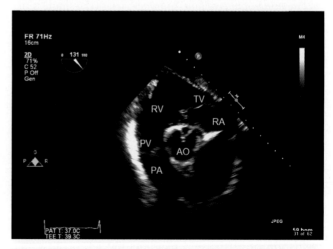

Figure 10.8. Transgastric RV inflow-outflow view with the right heart structures in the near field "wrapped" around the aorta (AO): right atrium (RA), tricuspid valve (TV), right ventricle (RV), pulmonary valve (PV), and pulmonary artery (PA).

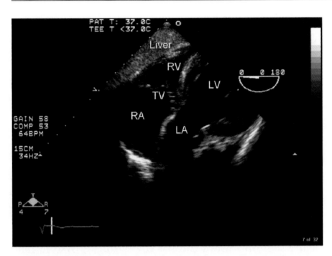

Figure 10.9. Deep transgastric view of the right ventricle (RV) with the tricuspid valve (TV) and right atrium (RA) visible. Also seen are the left ventricle (LV) and left atrium (LA).

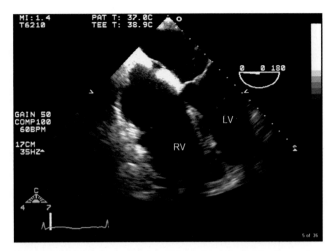

Figure 10.11. Dilation of the right ventricle (RV). Note that the RV makes the apex of the heart and is larger than the left ventricle (LV).

less common causes for increased RV free wall thickness include primary myocardial diseases such as amyloidosis and endocardial fibroelastosis (8).

RV free wall thickness is measured to determine the presence of hypertrophy. Normal RV free wall thickness is less than half that of the LV, and RV hypertrophy is diagnosed when RV wall thickness measured at end-diastole exceeds 5 mm (9,10). The diagnosis of mild RV hypertrophy is difficult and confounded by the trabeculations that give the endocardial surface of the chamber an uneven appearance. In patients with chronic cor pulmonale and severe pulmonary hypertension that raises PA pressures to systemic levels, RV wall thickness may exceed 10 mm (Fig. 10.10). Another clue to the presence of significant RV hypertrophy is the intracavitary trabecular pattern, which becomes more prominent, particularly at the apex.

RV dilatation occurs with RV volume overload and also often develops in patients with chronic RV pressure overload. An important clue to the presence of RV dilatation may be found through examination of the cardiac

apex. Normally the RV length extends to only two thirds the length of the LV. Therefore, in the midesophageal four-chamber view, the cardiac apex is formed by the LV (Fig. 10.3). When the RV rather than the LV forms the cardiac apex, the RV is dilated. The degree of RV enlargement is often categorized semiquantitatively by comparing the end-diastolic areas of the RV and LV in the midesophageal four-chamber view with the view adjusted to maximize the tricuspid annulus (often at 5–25 degrees multiplane angle rotation). The RV is generally no more than two thirds the size of the LV in this view. With moderate dilatation, RV area equals LV area, and with severe RV dilatation, the RV cross-sectional area exceeds that of the LV (Fig. 10.11). A final clue to the presence of RV enlargement is gleaned from its shape because as the RV dilates, its shape changes from triangular to spherical (9,10).

In addition to the semiquantitative evaluation described above, formal quantitative measurements of RV dimensions from the midesophageal four-chamber and inflow-outflow views can be made (Figs. 10.12 and 10.13) (11).

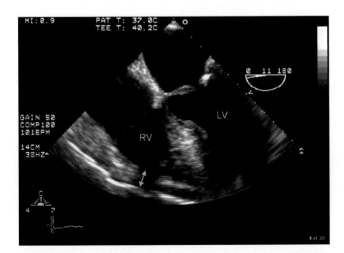

Figure 10.10. Severe hypertrophy of the right ventricle (RV). The *double headed arrow* shows the hypertrophied right ventricular wall width. LV, left ventricle.

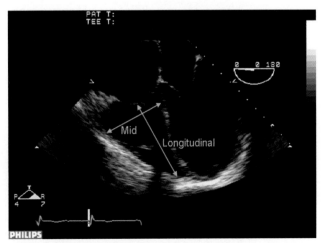

Figure 10.12. Measurements of the right ventricle (RV) in the midesophageal four-chamber view: Mid-short axis perpendicular to the long axis of the RV.

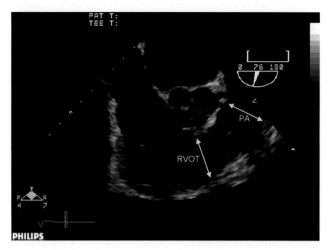

Figure 10.13. Measurements of the right ventricle in the midesophageal inflow-outflow view. Right ventricular outflow tract (RVOT) and pulmonary artery (PA) dimensions.

The views are oriented to maximize tricuspid annulus diameter and the chamber dimensions are measured at end-diastole. Normal and abnormal values are summarized in Table 10.1.

RIGHT VENTRICULAR OVERLOAD AND THE VENTRICULAR SEPTUM

Examination of the ventricular septum may help distinguish RV volume overload from RV pressure overload. Septal motion is determined primarily by the pattern of myocardial depolarization, the state of musculature contraction, and the pressure gradient between RV and LV. Normally, the LV contains the center of cardiac mass, and LV pressures exceed RV pressures throughout the cardiac cycle. Consequently, the ventricular septum functions primarily as part of the LV and maintains a convex curvature toward the RV during systole and diastole. As the RV becomes hypertrophied, the interventricular septum flattens, resulting in a D-shaped rather than a round LV cavity on transgastric short axis imaging. This septal shift is maximal at end-systole and early diastole, when intracavitary pressures in the RV peak (10,12,13). Other signs of chronic RV pressure overload include RV dilatation, tricuspid regurgitation from annular dilatation, and RV hypocontractility.

In contrast to pressure overload, RV volume overload results in septal flattening at end-diastole, at the time of maximal ventricular filling and distension (12). This leftward movement is then reversed during ventricular ejection as the RV empties, resulting in paradoxical motion of the septum toward the RV cavity during systole. The abnormal ventricular septal motion caused by RV volume overload should not be confused with the transient abnormality of septal motion that occurs during ventricular pacing. Owing to delayed activation of the LV during RV pacing, a characteristic septal "bounce" may be observed, which reflects the early systolic RV depolarization (14).

RIGHT VENTRICULAR SYSTOLIC FUNCTION— QUALITATIVE AND REGIONAL ASSESSMENT

Owing to difficulties in quantitative evaluation of global RV systolic function, most clinical assessment focuses on qualitative measures of chamber size, wall thickness, RV systolic wall excursion, and extent of systolic obliteration of the RV cavity. Assessment of regional RV function is also difficult because of the complexity of RV anatomy and the reduced systolic excursion of the RV compared to the LV walls. Mild degrees of RV hypocontractility are rarely reported, and it is recommended that RV dysfunction be diagnosed only when a wall segment is either akinetic or dyskinetic (7).

TABLE 10.1 Reference Measurements for RV Dimensions				
View	Normal	Mild	Moderate	Severe
Midesophageal four-chamber view				
Mid-ventricular	2.7–3.3	3.4–3.7	3.7–4.1	≥4.2
Longitudinal	7.1–7.9	8.0–8.5	8.6–9.1	≥9.2
Midesophageal inflow-outflow view				
RV outflow tract	2.5–2.9	3.0–3.2	3.3–3.5	≥3.6
Pulmonary artery	1.5–2.1	2.2–2.5	2.6–2.9	≥3.0

All values are in cm.
RV, right ventricle.
Adapted from Lang RM, Bierig M, Devereux RB, et al. Recommendations for chamber quantification: a report from the American Society of Echocardiography's Guidelines and Standards Committee and the Chamber Quantification Writing Group, developed in conjunction with the European Association of Echocardiography, a branch of the European Society of Cardiology. J Am Soc Echocardiogr 2005;18:1440–1463.

Regional RV function can be impaired when global function remains preserved. This is seen most often in patients with occlusion of the right coronary artery or one of its acute marginal branches. Because a small portion of the anterior RV free wall may be supplied by the conus branch of the left anterior descending artery, occlusion of this artery also may influence regional RV function (15). In addition to coronary occlusion, cardiac surgery is another common cause of RV dysfunction. The RV is particularly susceptible to ischemic injury during cardiac surgery for several reasons. Cardioplegia delivery may be inadequate for RV protection, particularly when retrograde cardioplegia is employed, and the anteriorly located RV is more prone to ambient warming from surgical lights (16). Furthermore, the anterior, nondependent location of the right coronary artery ostium and the proximal anastomotic site of a right coronary artery saphenous vein bypass graft make these favored sites for coronary air or atheromatous embolization.

Significant RV infarction is typically accompanied by LV inferior wall myocardial infarction because these portions of the myocardium share the right coronary artery as a common blood supply (17). Ancillary signs of RV infarction include RA enlargement, RV dilatation, tricuspid regurgitation, and paradoxical ventricular septal motion (18,19). If a patent foramen ovale is present, increases in RA pressure accompanying RV infarction may lead to hypoxemia from a right to left shunt.

A unique pattern of dynamic RVOT obstruction has been described in approximately 5% of patients undergoing cardiac surgery (20). It is characterized by end-systolic obliteration of the RV, especially its outflow portion and an associated significant pressure gradient (>25 mm Hg) across the RVOT. Possible risk factors for this condition include RV hypertrophy, hypovolemia, and increased adrenergic tone leading to infundibular hypercontractility. This condition, which is usually associated with hemodynamic instability, can be diagnosed easily with TEE.

RIGHT VENTRICULAR GLOBAL SYSTOLIC FUNCTION—QUANTITATIVE ECHOCARDIOGRAPHIC ASSESSMENT

Quantitative assessment of global RV function includes measurement of RV volume and ejection fraction. Because of the irregular shape of the RV, acquisition of multiple images may be necessary to fully define chamber size and shape. Additionally, the frequent occurrence of tricuspid regurgitation also confounds the interpretation of ejection indices. The simplest ejection phase index is the one-dimensional *shortening fraction*, which can be calculated in either the short or long axis (21). Based on planimetry measurements in the midesophageal four-chamber view, RV *fractional area change (FAC)* can be calculated as FAC = [(end-diastolic area − end systolic area)/end-diastolic area] × 100. Normal FAC values range between 32% and 60%, and this wide range of normal values further emphasizes the difficulty of quantifying RV dysfunction. The degree of RV dysfunction can be classified as mild (FAC 25%–31%), moderate (FAC 18%–24%), and severe dysfunction (FAC < 18%) (11). In patients undergoing coronary artery bypass surgery, RV FAC values less than 35% were associated with worse early and late postoperative outcome (2).

Another quantitative measure of RV function, *ejection fraction*, can be determined using summation of smaller geometric volumes (ellipsoid, prism, or pyramid) to model the RV (22–24). Alternatively, a modified Simpson's method can be used to calculate RV ejection fraction (25). Normal values for RV ejection fraction are 45% to 65%, slightly smaller values compared to normal LV ejection fraction. Finally, three-dimensional echocardiography can be used to obtain more accurate measurements of RV size (26,27). Given the complexity and potential inaccuracies in all of these methods, quantitative assessment of RV volume is rarely performed in clinical TEE practice.

Because the echocardiographic methods described above are often inaccurate or too cumbersome to use in the operating room, other means of quantifying RV function have been investigated. One method focuses on the unique pattern of RV systolic contraction. As mentioned above, the main contribution to RV systole is the contraction of longitudinal muscle fibers causing long-axis shortening and motion of the tricuspid annulus toward the RV apex. Because the septal attachment of the tricuspid annulus is relatively fixed, the majority of tricuspid annular motion occurs in its lateral aspect. This gives the motion of the tricuspid annulus a hinge-like appearance, moving more laterally than medially. This motion contrasts with that of the mitral annulus, which has a more symmetrical or piston-like appearance during systole. *Tricuspid annular plane systolic excursion (TAPSE)* describes this long-axis systolic excursion of the lateral aspect of the tricuspid annulus and has been validated as a useful additional measure of global RV systolic function. TAPSE can be measured either in the midesophageal four-chamber view (Fig. 10.14) or from the transgastric inflow-outflow view (Fig. 10.15). The latter view might be preferable because the axis of annular movement is more parallel to the ultrasound beam, enabling more accurate measurement of annular motion and annular velocity (see below) (28). Measurement of TAPSE can be expressed as an absolute value or as a shortening fraction. Normal TAPSE is 15 to 20 mm toward the cardiac apex, and this value is slightly greater than normal mitral annular plane systolic excursion (11). Using radionuclide RV ejection fraction as a reference method, TAPSE had a better correlation with global RV function than RV FAC (29,30). Decreased TAPSE is a poor prognostic factor in patients with acute myocardial infarction (31). Similarly, TAPSE less then 12 mm was associated with increased mortality after mitral valve repair surgery in patients with dilated cardiomyopathy (32). A note of caution is needed

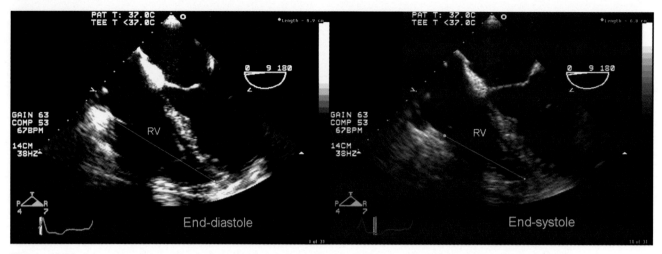

Figure 10.14. Measurement of Tricuspid Annular Plane Systolic Excursion (TAPSE) in the midesophageal four-chamber view. The TAPSE is the difference between the end-diastolic length (8.9 cm) and end-systolic value (6.8 cm).

in interpreting TAPSE as a measure of RV function alone, because some data suggest that TAPSE is also affected by LV function, independent of RV function (33).

An index of RV function closely related to TAPSE is the *tricuspid annular velocity*, which can be measured using tissue Doppler with the sample volume located on the lateral tricuspid leaflet attachment to the RV free wall (28).

Other spectral Doppler measurements are also valuable adjuncts for assessing RV function. In patients with tricuspid regurgitation, the acceleration of the regurgitant jet reflects the rate of increase in RV pressure during systole and can therefore be used as a measure of RV contractility. The index, called dP/dT, can be calculated by measuring the time interval between a jet velocity

of 1 m/s (corresponding to ventriculo-atrial pressure gradient of 4 mm Hg) and 3 m/s (corresponding to pressure gradient of 36 mm Hg). The dP/dT is calculated by dividing this pressure difference (36 − 4 = 32 mm Hg) by the time interval (seconds) between these points on the spectral Doppler envelope (Fig. 10.16). Normal values for RV dP/dT are above 1,100 mm Hg/s. Calculation of RV dP/dT using this method provides values similar to those derived from invasive cardiac catheterization and appear to be independent of RA pressure (34). Compared to ejection phase indices, dP/dT is more sensitive to preload changes and less sensitive to afterload changes (35).

Another ventricular performance index free of any geometrical assumptions is the *myocardial performance*

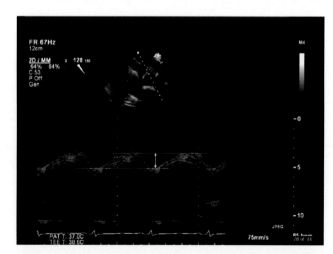

Figure 10.15. Measurement of Tricuspid Annular Systolic Excursion (TAPSE) in the transgastric inflow-outflow view using M-mode on the lateral tricuspid annulus. The thin dashed white lines delineate the movement of the leading edge of the tricuspid annulus toward the transducer. As the distance between any two vertical points is 1 cm, the TAPSE here is 16 mm.

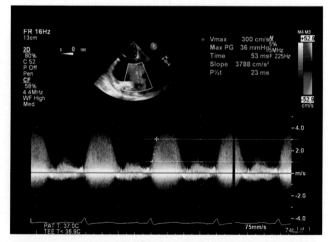

Figure 10.16. Spectral Doppler analysis of the tricuspid regurgitation jet showing calculation of dP/dT. Flow velocities of 1 and 3 m/s are marked and the time interval between them is measured (53 ms). dP/dT is calculated as 32 mm Hg/0.053 s = 600 mm Hg/s, suggesting significant RV dysfunction.

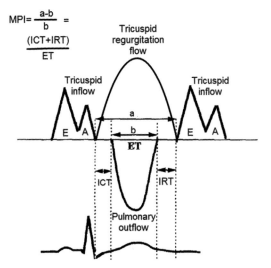

$$MPI = \frac{a-b}{b} = \frac{(ICT+IRT)}{ET}$$

Figure 10.17. Calculation of myocardial performance index (MPI) as the sum of the isovolumic contraction time (ICT) and relaxation time (IRT), divided by the right ventricular ejection time (ET). (Adapted from Tei C, Dujardin KS, Hodge DO, et al. Doppler echocardiographic index for assessment of global right ventricular function. *J Am Soc Echocardiogr* 1996;9:838–847.)

index (MPI), first introduced to evaluate LV function (36). It is defined as the sum of the two isovolumic intervals (isovolumic contraction and isovolumic relaxation), divided by the ejection time (ET) (Fig. 10.17). For the RV, the ET is measured using Doppler interrogation of PA flow while the isovolumic times are calculated by subtracting the ET from the total duration of RV systole. The systolic duration, in turn, can either be measured as the duration of a tricuspid regurgitation jet or as the interval between the end of the A wave and the start of the E wave on the tricuspid inflow spectral Doppler trace (Fig. 10.18). The MPI is a composite index

of both systolic and diastolic functions and is relatively independent of heart rate, afterload, and preload (37). Normal values for the RV range between 0.2 and 0.4. Values above 0.5 were found to be highly predictive of hemodynamic instability and mortality after cardiac valvular surgery (4).

RIGHT VENTRICULAR FUNCTION— HEMODYNAMIC ASSESSMENT

Spectral Doppler measurement of right-sided flow patterns can provide important clues to cardiac function. Cardiac output measured across the RVOT correlates well with thermodilution cardiac output values in patients without significant TV regurgitation (38). To perform this measurement, the pulsed wave sample volume is placed just below the pulmonary valve (PV) in the transgastric RV inflow-outflow view, where the RVOT diameter can also be measured (Fig. 10.19). The stroke volume is calculated as the RVOT cross-sectional area (0.7 times the diameter squared) multiplied by the RVOT velocity-time integral (VTI).

In patients with tricuspid regurgitation, continuous wave Doppler can be used to estimate RV systolic pressure, another useful index of right heart function. Measurement of the peak velocity of the tricuspid regurgitant jet allows calculation of the pressure gradient between the RV and RA, which when added to RA pressure, provides an estimate for RV systolic pressure (Fig. 10.20). In the absence of obstruction to RV outflow, RV systolic pressure provides a good estimate of PA systolic pressure. Since the vast majority of patients with pulmonary hypertension have some degree of tricuspid regurgitation even in the absence of clinical signs, this measurement has widespread application. However, when making this

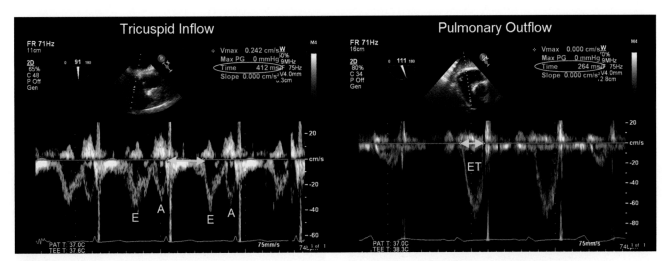

Figure 10.18. Spectral Doppler trace of the tricuspid inflow (**on the left**) with the systolic time measured between the end of the A wave to the beginning of the next E wave, and of the pulmonary outflow (**on the right**) with measurement of the ET. Here systole duration is 412 ms and ET is 264 ms. Therefore, the MPI equals (412 − 264)/264 = 0.56.

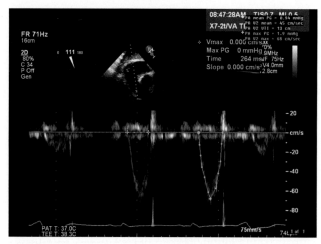

Figure 10.19. Spectral Doppler tracing of pulmonary outflow, showing the calculation of the velocity-time integral (VTI), in this case it is 13 cm. The stroke volume will be equal to the VTI multiplied by the area of the right ventricular outflow tract.

TABLE 10.2	Estimation of Right Atrial Pressure	
IVC Diameter (mm)	**IVC Collapsibility Index (%)**	**Estimated RAP (mm Hg)**
<20	>55	0–5
<20	35–55	0–10
>20	>35	10–15
>20	<35	10–20

IVC, Inferior vena cava; RAP, Right atrial pressure.
Adapted from Brennan JM, Blair JE, Goonewardena S, et al. Reappraisal of the use of inferior vena cava for estimating right atrial pressure. J Am Soc Echocardiogr 2007;20:857–861. See text for more details.

calculation, considerable care must be taken to align the ultrasound beam with the regurgitant jet to avoid underestimation of the pressure gradient.

PA diastolic pressure also can be estimated using spectral Doppler techniques. This value is calculated by measuring the end-diastolic velocity of the pulmonic regurgitation jet, which reflects the gradient between the PA and RV at end-diastole. This pressure gradient is added to RA pressure to calculate PA diastolic pressure. Unlike the estimation of PA systolic pressure from the tricuspid regurgitation jet, PA diastolic pressure measurements are less clinically useful because significant pulmonic regurgitation jets are uncommon and difficult to interrogate.

Estimation of RA pressure can be gleaned from an examination of the inferior vena cava (IVC). In spontaneously breathing patients, the IVC normally changes in size during the respiratory cycle, becoming smaller during inspiration. The combination of maximal IVC diameter during quiet breathing (normal values 17–21 mm) and the decrease in diameter in response to a forced "sniff" maneuver (collapsibility index—normal values 35%–55%) provides an estimate of RA pressure (Table 10.2) (39). IVC diameter should be measured 1 to 2 cm below the atrio-caval junction, as viewed from a transgastric approach with the probe rotated to the right (Fig. 10.21). It should be noted that while a maximal IVC diameter of less than 20 mm can accurately dichotomize RA pressure below and above 10 mm Hg, predictions of pressure within 5 mm Hg range are much less robust (39).

In mechanically ventilated patients, IVC diameter usually increases during inspiration, but this also depends upon the patient's intravascular volume status. An increase in diameter of more than 12% during the inspiratory phase of the respiratory cycle was found to accurately predict an increase in cardiac output in response to volume loading (40).

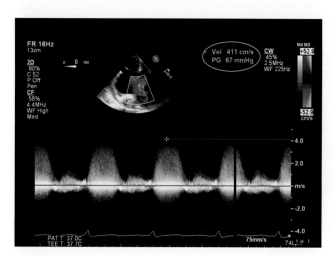

Figure 10.20. Spectral Doppler trace of the tricuspid regurgitation jet showing a right ventricle-right atrium pressure gradient of 67 mm Hg.

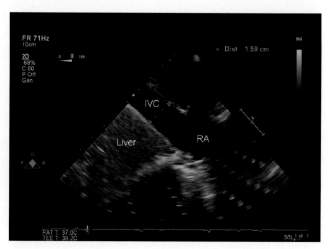

Figure 10.21. Measurement of inferior vena cara (IVC) diameter from the transgastric approach. RA, right atrium.

RIGHT VENTRICULAR DIASTOLIC FUNCTION

Measurements used to assess RV diastolic filling are similar to those used for evaluation of the left heart. Inflow velocity patterns across the TV may be used to assess E and A velocities. However, because the tricuspid annulus is larger than the mitral annulus and the duration of tricuspid inflow is longer than that of mitral inflow, the maximal velocities of RV (tricuspid) inflow are lower than the corresponding values for LV inflow (41). Normal peak E-wave velocity is 45 ± 7.5 cm/s, while peak A-wave velocity is 30 ± 8.1 cm/s (42). As with the LV, impaired relaxation of the RV results in a decreased E wave and tall A wave while restrictive RV physiology results in a tall E wave and small A wave.

Hepatic vein flow patterns provide another useful window on right heart filling pressures and global RV systolic function, analogous to the use of pulmonary vein flow patterns to assess LV function. Normal hepatic venous flow patterns have either three or four phasic components (Fig. 10.22). The decline in right atrial pressure (RAP) during systole results in an initial forward flow toward the RA and is termed the S or systolic wave. This pressure change results from atrial relaxation and apical movement of the TV during RV systole and corresponds to the x descent in atrial pressure. A fall in atrial pressure during diastole from early ventricular filling also results in forward caval flow (D wave) and corresponds to the y descent in atrial pressure. Two small retrograde waves may be seen, one of which results from the end-diastolic atrial contraction (A wave). The other small retrograde wave (V wave) is seen less often, and it appears at end-systole, prior to the y descent in RA pressure that drives the forward diastolic hepatic vein flow wave. Impaired RV systolic function is accompanied by a change in the pattern of hepatic vein flow, including blunting of the S wave and augmentation of the D wave (43). This pattern of hepatic vein flow, whether identified before or after bypass, has been shown

to predict an increased need for vasoactive drug support following surgery. In general, S-wave amplitude appears to correlate with RV systolic function (30,43,44). In addition to the influence of RV function on the hepatic venous flow velocity pattern, tricuspid regurgitation, which often accompanies systolic RV dysfunction, can obliterate the hepatic vein S wave and cause a reversed or retrograde S wave (see additional discussion in Chapter 16).

A third modality used to assess RV diastolic function is myocardial or tricuspid annular Doppler analysis. Tissue Doppler imaging of the RV free wall has shown that regional E/A velocity ratios decrease with age, although there is greater variability among younger healthy subjects than in the elderly population (6). There appears to be a good correlation between tissue Doppler parameters and RV stroke volume index when corrected for tricuspid regurgitation severity (45). However, the utility of these observations for the clinical setting is unclear.

> ### KEY POINTS
>
> ■ Evaluation of RV function is complicated by the unique anatomy of the RV.
> ■ Techniques to assess RV function include planimetry of RV size, qualitative assessment of wall motion abnormalities, calculation of TAPSE and MPI, and calculation of PA pressure.
> ■ Examination of ventricular septal motion is useful in distinguishing RV volume overload from RV pressure overload. In RV volume overload, maximal septal distortion occurs at end-diastole, while RV pressure overload produces maximal septal distortion at end-systole and early diastole, corresponding to the time of peak systolic loading of the RV.
> ■ Signs of RV infarction include akinesis or dyskinesis of the RV, RA enlargement, RV dilatation, tricuspid regurgitation, and paradoxical ventricular septal motion.

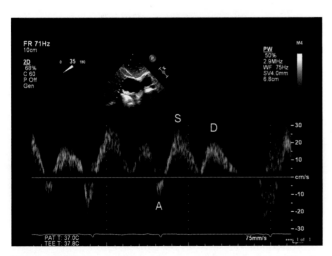

Figure 10.22. Normal hepatic venous flow pattern with the three waves: atrial (A), systolic (S), and diastolic (D).

REFERENCES

1. Voelkel NF, Quaife RA, Leinwand LA, et al. Right ventricular function and failure: report of a national heart, lung, and blood institute working group on cellular and molecular mechanisms of right heart failure. *Circulation* 2006;114:1883–1891.
2. Maslow AD, Regan MM, Panzica P, et al. Precardiopulmonary bypass right ventricular function is associated with poor outcome after coronary artery bypass grafting in patients with severe left ventricular systolic dysfunction. *Anesth Analg* 2002;95:1507–1518.
3. Coghlan JG, Davar J. How should we assess right ventricular function in 2008? *Eur Heart J Suppl* 2007;9:H22–H28.

4. Haddad F, Denault AY, Couture P, et al. Right ventricular myocardial performance index predicts perioperative mortality or circulatory failure in high-risk valvular surgery. *J Am Soc Echocardiogr* 2007;20:1065–1072.

5. Netter F. Heart. In: Yonkman F, ed. *The Ciba Collection of Medical Illustrations*. New York: Ciba Pharmaceutical Co., 1978;6:9.

6. Kukulski T, Hubbert L, Arnold M, et al. Normal regional right ventricular function and its change with age: a Doppler myocardial imaging study. *J Am Soc Echocardiogr* 2000;13:194–204.

7. Shanewise JS, Cheung AT, Aronson S, et al. ASE/SCA guidelines for performing a comprehensive intraoperative multiplane transesophageal echocardiography examination: recommendations of the American Society of Echocardiography Council for Intraoperative Echocardiography and the Society of Cardiovascular Anesthesiologists Task Force for Certification in Perioperative Transesophageal Echocardiography. *Anesth Analg* 1999;89:870–884.

8. Child JS, Krivokapich J, Abbasi AS. Increased right ventricular wall thickness on echocardiography in amyloid infiltrative cardiomyopathy. *Am J Cardiol* 1979;44:1391–1395.

9. Jiang L, Wiegers SE, Weyman AE. Right ventricle. In: Weyman AE, ed. *Principles and Practices of Echocardiography*. Philadelphia: Lea and Febiger, 1994:901–921.

10. Otto C. Echocardiographic evaluation of left and right ventricualr systolic function. In: Otto CM, ed. *Textbook of Clinical Echocardiography*. Philadelphia: W.B. Saunders Company, 2000:100–131.

11. Lang RM, Bierig M, Devereux RB, et al. Recommendations for chamber quantification: a report from the American Society of Echocardiography's Guidelines and Standards Committee and the Chamber Quantification Writing Group, developed in conjunction with the European Association of Echocardiography, a branch of the European Society of Cardiology. *J Am Soc Echocardiogr* 2005;18:1440–1463.

12. Louie EK, Rich S, Levitsky S, Brundage BH. Doppler echocardiographic demonstration of the differential effects of right ventricular pressure and volume overload on left ventricular geometry and filling. *J Am Coll Cardiol* 1992;19:84–90.

13. Jardin F, Dubourg O, Bourdarias JP. Echocardiographic pattern of acute cor pulmonale. *Chest* 1997;111:209–217.

14. Little WC, Reeves RC, Arciniegas J, et al. Mechanism of abnormal interventricular septal motion during delayed left ventricular activation. *Circulation* 1982;65:1486–1491.

15. Wilson BC, Cohn JN. Right ventricular infarction: clinical and pathophysiologic considerations. *Adv Intern Med* 1988;33:295–309.

16. Christakis GT, Fremes SE, Weisel RD, et al. Right ventricular dysfunction following cold potassium cardioplegia. *J Thorac Cardiovasc Surg* 1985;90:243–250.

17. Oh JK, Seward JB, Tajik AJ. *The Echo Manual*. 1st ed. Boston: Little, Brown and Company, 1994:82–103.

18. Sharkey SW, Shelley W, Carlyle PF, et al. M-mode and two-dimensional echocardiographic analysis of the septum in experimental right ventricular infarction: correlation with hemodynamic alterations. *Am Heart J* 1985;110:1210–1218.

19. Jugdutt BI, Sussex BA, Sivaram CA, et al. Right ventricular infarction: two-dimensional echocardiographic evaluation. *Am Heart J* 1984;107:505–518.

20. Denault AY, Chaput M, Couture P, et al. Dynamic right ventricular outflow tract obstruction in cardiac surgery. *J Thorac Cardiovasc Surg* 2006;132:43–49.

21. Bommer W, Weinert L, Neumann A, et al. Determination of right atrial and right ventricular size by two-dimensional echocardiography. *Circulation* 1979;60:91–100.

22. Graham TP Jr, Jarmakani JM, Atwood GF, et al. Right ventricular volume determinations in children. Normal values and observations with volume or pressure overload. *Circulation* 1973;47:144–153.

23. Benchimol A, Desser KB, Hastreiter AR. Right ventricular volume in congenital heart disease. *Am J Cardiol* 1975;36:67–75.

24. Ferlinz J, Gorlin R, Cohn PF, et al. Right ventricular performance in patients with coronary artery disease. *Circulation* 1975;52:608–615.

25. Panidis IP, Ren JF, Kotler MN, et al. Two-dimensional echocardiographic estimation of right ventricular ejection fraction in patients with coronary artery disease. *J Am Coll Cardiol* 1983;2:911–918.

26. Ota T, Fleishman CE, Strub M, et al. Real-time, three-dimensional echocardiography: feasibility of dynamic right ventricular volume measurement with saline contrast. *Am Heart J* 1999;137:958–966.

27. Vogel M, White PA, Redington AN. In vitro validation of right ventricular volume measurement by three dimensional echocardiography. *Br Heart J* 1995;74:460–463.

28. David J-S, Tousignant CP, Bowry R. Tricuspid annular velocity in patients undergoing cardiac operation using transesophageal echocardiography. *J Am Soc Echocardiogr* 2006;19:329–334.

29. Kaul S, Tei C, Hopkins JM, et al. Assessment of right ventricular function using two-dimensional echocardiography. *Am Heart J* 1984;107:526–531.

30. Mishra M, Swaminathan M, Malhotra R, et al. Evaluation of right ventricular function during cabg: transesophageal echocardiographic assessment of hepatic venous flow versus conventional right ventricular performance indices. *Echocardiography* 1998;15:51–58.

31. Samad BA, Alam M, Jensen-Urstad K. Prognostic impact of right ventricular involvement as assessed by tricuspid annular motion in patients with acute myocardial infarction. *Am J Cardiol* 2002;90:778–781.

32. Di Mauro M, Calafiore AM, Penco M, et al. Mitral valve repair for dilated cardiomyopathy: predictive role of right ventricular dysfunction. *Eur Heart J* 2007;28:2510–2516.

33. López-Candales A, Rajagopalan N, Saxena N, et al. Right ventricular systolic function is not the sole determinant of tricuspid annular motion. *Am J Cardiol* 2006;98:973–977.

34. Imanishi T, Nakatani S, Yamada S, et al. Validation of continuous wave Doppler-determined right ventricular peak positive and negative dP/dt: effect of right atrial pressure on measurement. *J Am Coll Cardiol* 1994;23:1638–1643.

35. Kass D, Maughan W, Guo Z, et al. Comparative influence of load versus inotropic states on indexes of ventricular contractility: experimental and theoretical analysis based on pressure-volume relationships [published erratum appears in Circulation 1988 Mar;77(3):559]. *Circulation* 1987;76:1422–1436.

36. Tei C, Ling LH, Hodge DO, et al. New index of combined systolic and diastolic myocardial performance: a simple and reproducible measure of cardiac function—a study in normals and dilated cardiomyopathy. *J Cardiol* 1995;26:357–366.

37. Tei C, Dujardin KS, Hodge DO, et al. Doppler echocardiographic index for assessment of global right ventricular function. *J Am Soc Echocardiogr* 1996;9:838–847.
38. Maslow A, Comunale ME, Haering JM, et al. Pulsed wave Doppler measurement of cardiac output from the right ventricular outflow tract. *Anesth Analg* 1996;83:466–471.
39. Brennan JM, Blair JE, Goonewardena S, et al. Reappraisal of the use of inferior vena cava for estimating right atrial pressure. *J Am Soc Echocardiogr* 2007;20:857–861.
40. Feissel M, Michard F, Faller J-P, et al. The respiratory variation in inferior vena cava diameter as a guide to fluid therapy. *Intens Care Med* 2004;30:1834–1837.
41. Feigenbaum H. *Echocardiography*. 4th ed. Philadelphia: Lea & Febiger, 1986:157–166.
42. Klein AL, Leung DY, Murray RD, et al. Effects of age and physiologic variables on right ventricular filling dynamics in normal subjects. *Am J Cardiol* 1999;84:440–448.
43. Nomura T, Lebowitz L, Koide Y, et al. Evaluation of hepatic venous flow using transesophageal echocardiography in coronary artery bypass surgery: an index of right ventricular function. *J Cardiothorac Vasc Anesth* 1995;9:9–17.
44. Carricart M, Denault AY, Couture P, et al. Incidence and significance of abnormal hepatic venous Doppler flow velocities before cardiac surgery. *J Cardiothorac Vasc Anesth* 2005;19:751–758.
45. Urheim S, Cauduro S, Frantz R, et al. Relation of tissue displacement and strain to invasively determined right ventricular stroke volume. *Am J Cardiol* 2005;96:1173–1178.

QUESTIONS

1. In patients with right ventricular (RV) volume overload, ventricular septal displacement toward the left ventricle (LV) is maximal at which point in the cardiac cycle?
   A. End-diastole
   B. End-systole
   C. Mid-diastole
   D. Mid-systole
   E. Early-diastole

2. Which of the following structures can be seen in echocardiographic images of the RV?
   A. Chiari network
   B. Crista terminalis
   C. Eustachian valve
   D. Moderator band
   E. Thebesian valve

3. Which of the following transesophageal echocardiographic scan planes allows measuring pulmonary artery (PA) systolic pressure?
   A. Midesophageal long-axis view
   B. Deep transgastric RV apical view
   C. Midesophageal four-chamber view
   D. Midesophageal RV inflow-outflow view (modified)
   E. Transgastric mid–short-axis view

4. Which of the following diagnoses is most likely in a patient whose transesophageal echocardiogram shows a 5-mm tricuspid annular plane systolic excursion (TAPSE)?
   A. Patent foramen ovale
   B. Pulmonic regurgitation
   C. RV hypertrophy
   D. RV infarction
   E. Tricuspid regurgitation

5. Which of the following echocardiographic signs would be expected in a patient with RV dilatation?
   A. Cardiac apex formed by both the RV and LV
   B. Exaggerated hepatic vein antegrade systolic inflow wave
   C. Prominent apical muscular trabeculations
   D. RV cross-sectional area equal to 50% of the LV cross-sectional area
   E. Tricuspid valve (TV) leaflet prolapse

CHAPTER 11

Assessment of Regional Ventricular Function

G. Burkhard Mackensen ■ Lori B. Heller ■ Solomon Aronson

INTRODUCTION

Assessment of global and regional ventricular function has become the cornerstone for evaluating patients with heart disease of ischemic or nonischemic origin and is an essential part of the routine perioperative transesophageal echocardiographic (TEE) examination. In the evaluation of global or regional left ventricular (LV) function, two-dimensional (2D) echocardiography is essentially a qualitative technique based on the experience of the echocardiographer to visually integrate spatial information. When using TEE to evaluate regional ventricular function, one is really attempting to make inferences about a three-dimensional (3D) structure from 2D images. Therefore, multiple images must be acquired from multiple planes, and assumptions (explicit or implicit) must be made about the shape of the ventricle and the coronary artery distribution within the ventricle.

However, recent and emerging technological advancements, such as 3D echocardiography, tissue Doppler imaging (TDI), Doppler strain imaging, and speckle tracking, have overcome certain limitations of 2D echocardiography and provide more accurate quantification of global and regional ventricular functions (1–4).

SEGMENTAL MODEL OF THE LEFT VENTRICLE

Dividing the LV into segments allows more accurate description of the location of the regional wall motion abnormalities (RWMA) detected with echocardiography and is necessary for their correlation with coronary artery anatomy.

In 1999, the Society of Cardiovascular Anesthesiologists (SCA) and American Society of Echocardiography (ASE) recommended a 16-segment model for regional LV assessment using 2D-TEE. This model divides the LV into three levels: basal, mid or papillary, and apical (Fig. 11.1). The basal and mid levels are further divided into six segments (anteroseptal, anterior, anterolateral, inferolateral, inferior, and inferoseptal), and the apical level is divided into four segments (anterior, lateral, inferior, and septal) (5). With the development of

echocardiographic contrast agents for the assessment of myocardial perfusion, the myocardial apex segment or apical cap beyond the LV cavity becomes pertinent. Therefore, in 2002, the American Heart Association Writing Group on Myocardial Segmentation and Registration for Cardiac Imaging recommended a 17-segment model with the addition of an "apical cap" segment (6) (Fig. 11.2). The 17-segment model creates a distribution of the myocardial mass of 35%, 35%, and 30% for the basal, mid-cavity, and apical thirds of the heart, respectively, which is close to the observed autopsy data (6). An advantage of using this segmental model is a common standard and terminology across different imaging modalities and in discussions about regional function of the LV.

Regional function assessment of the LV can be accomplished quickly and easily in most patients using multiplane TEE by obtaining six standard views of the LV, three from the midesophageal window and three from the transgastric window.

The first step in obtaining the midesophageal views of the LV is to position the transducer posterior to the left atrium (LA) at the mid level of the mitral valve. The imaging plane is then oriented to simultaneously pass through the center of the mitral annulus and the apex of the LV. In many patients, the esophagus is lateral to this point, and the tip of the probe must be flexed to the right to position the transducer directly posterior to the center of the mitral annulus. The LV is usually oriented with its apex somewhat more inferior to the base, and the tip of the probe must next be retroflexed to direct the imaging plane through the apex. Adequate retroflexion is best accomplished by rotating to multiplane angle 90 degrees, and then retroflexing until the apex of the LV is pointing straight down in the image display. The depth should be adjusted to include the entire LV (usually 14–18 cm). Rotating the multiplane angle to 0 degrees should keep the center of the mitral annulus and LV apex in view. The midesophageal four-chamber view is now obtained by rotating the multiplane angle forward from 0 degrees until the aortic valve is no longer in view, and the diameter of the tricuspid annulus is maximized, usually between 10 and 30 degrees. The midesophageal four-chamber view shows the inferoseptal and anterolateral walls at the basal

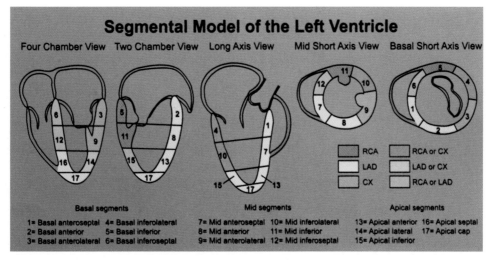

Figure 11.1. The 17-Segment Model for Regional LV Assessment and Coronary Arterial Distribution. The basal and mid levels are each divided into six segments and the apex into four. (Illustrations from ASE Guidelines Poster for Performing Multiplane Transesophageal Echocardiography, originally published by Shanewise JS, Cheung AT, Aronson S, et al. ASE/SCA guidelines for performing a comprehensive intraoperative multiplane transesophageal echocardiography examination: recommendations of the American Society of Echocardiography Council for Intraoperative Echocardiography and the Society of Cardiovascular Anesthesiologists Task Force for Certification in Perioperative Transesophageal Echocardiography. *J Am Soc Echocardiogr* 1999;12[10]:884–900.)

and mid levels, the apical septal and apical lateral walls, and the apical cap (Fig. 11.3).

The midesophageal two-chamber view can next be obtained by rotating the multiplane angle forward until the right atrium (RA) and the right ventricle (RV) disappear, usually between 90 and 110 degrees. The midesophageal two-chamber view of the LV shows the three segments in each of the anterior and inferior walls (Fig. 11.4).

Finally, the midesophageal long-axis view is developed by rotating the multiplane angle forward until the LV outflow tract, aortic valve, and the proximal ascending aorta come into view, usually between 120 and 160 degrees (Fig. 11.5). This view shows the basal and mid-anteroseptal segments, the basal and mid-inferolateral segments, as well as the apical segments. Therefore, with the imaging plane properly oriented through the center of the mitral annulus and the LV apex, one can examine the

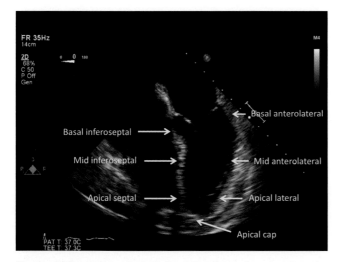

Figure 11.2. Midesophageal four-chamber view showing the basal and midinferoseptal and inferolateral segments, the apical septal and lateral segments, and the apical segment.

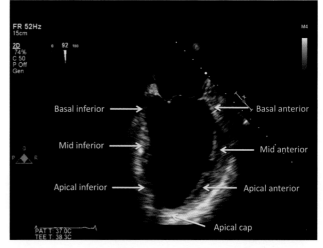

Figure 11.3. Midesophageal two-chamber view showing the basal, mid, and apical portions of the inferior and anterior walls.

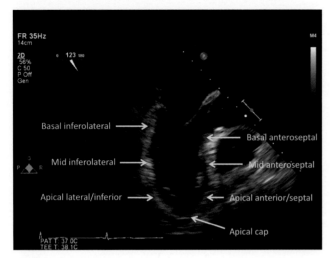

Figure 11.4. Midesophageal long-axis view of the LV showing basal and mid portions of the inferolateral and anteroseptal walls.

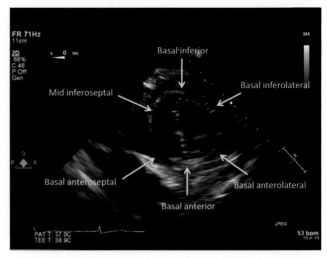

Figure 11.6. Transgastric Basal Short-Axis View. This view is obtained by withdrawing the probe from the midpapillary short-axis view until the mitral valve comes into view. It shows the basal segments of the LV walls.

entire LV without moving the probe and simply rotating the multiplane angle from 0 to 180 degrees.

The transgastric views of the LV are acquired by advancing the probe into the stomach and anteflexing the tip until the heart comes into view. At a multiplane angle of 0 degrees, a short axis of the LV should appear, and the probe is then turned to the right or left as needed to center the LV in the display. The depth should be adjusted to include the entire LV, usually 12 cm. There are three levels of transgastric views: basal, where the mitral valve is seen; mid, at the level of the papillary muscles; and apical. These transverse short-axis views have the advantage of simultaneously showing portions of the LV supplied by the right, circumflex, and the left anterior descending (LAD) coronary arteries.

The midpapillary level (Fig. 11.6), which reveals the approximate center of the LV cavity, is used to determine information regarding the cardiac function and volume status of the patient. Withdrawing the probe from the midpapillary view until the mitral apparatus appears develops the basal transgastric short-axis view (Fig. 11.7). In some patients, advancing the probe from the mid position develops the apical transgastric short-axis view, but in many the probe moves away from the heart and the image is lost.

The transgastric two-chamber view is developed from the basal transgastric short-axis view by rotating the multiplane angle forward until the apex and

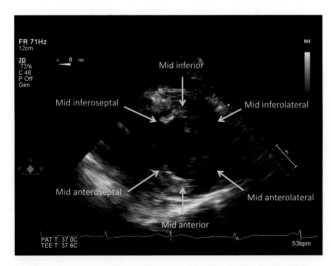

Figure 11.5. Transgastric Short-Axis View of the Mid Portion of the LV. This view is useful for its demonstration of LV preload, as well as for showing portions of the LV supplied by all three of the main coronary arteries.

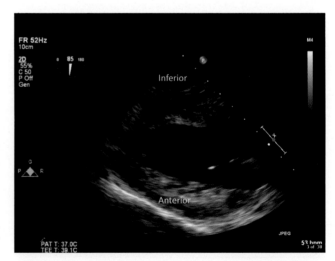

Figure 11.7. Transgastric Two-Chamber View. This view is developed by rotating the probe to 85 to 110 degrees from the basal transgastric short-axis view. This inferior wall is closest to the probe. Opposite from that is the anterior wall.

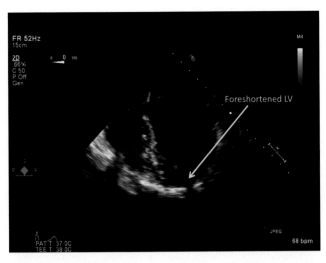

Figure 11.8. Midesophageal four-chamber view demonstrating foreshortening of the LV apex. Foreshortening occurs when the imaging plane is not correctly aligned along the axis of the chamber being examined. LV, left ventricle.

the mitral annulus come into view, usually close to 90 degrees (Fig. 11.8). The probe should be turned to the left or right as needed to open up the LV chamber, maximizing its size in the image. This view usually shows the basal and mid segments of the inferior walls but not the apex.

When assessing wall motion, it is important to recognize two artifacts of imaging that can occur with any real-time tomographic imaging technique, such as echocardiography: *foreshortening* and *pseudothickening*. Foreshortening occurs when the imaging plane is not correctly aligned along the axis of the chamber being examined, creating an image that is shorter than the true length. With TEE, this most commonly occurs at the apex of the LV (Fig. 11.9).

Pseudothickening

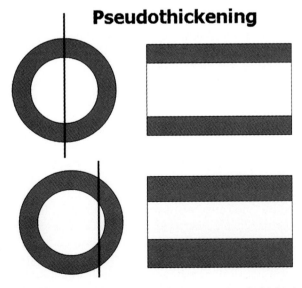

Figure 11.9. Pseudothickening of the LV. Pseudothickening occurs when the heart moves from side to side through the imaging plane, creating the illusion of a change in wall thickness.

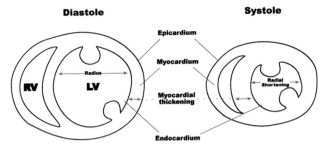

Figure 11.10. Illustration of LV radial shortening and LV thickening.

Pseudothickening occurs when the heart moves from side to side through the imaging plane, creating the illusion of a change in wall thickness (Figs. 11.9 and 11.10). In order to accurately assess wall motion and thickness, the imaging plane must be perpendicular to the region of the LV being examined.

In current clinical practice, analysis of LV segmental function is based on a qualitative visual assessment of both endocardial motion and thickening of a segment during systole. As the myocardial oxygen supply-to-demand balance worsens, graded RWMA progress from mild hypokinesia to severe hypokinesia, akinesia, and finally dyskinesia (7). The following qualitative grading scale for wall motion has been used extensively in the intraoperative TEE literature and is recommended: 1 = normal, or the endocardium moves toward the center of the LV cavity during systole greater than 30%; 2 = mildly hypokinetic, or the endocardium moves toward the center of the LV cavity less than 30%, but greater than 10% during systole; 3 = severely hypokinetic, or the endocardium moves toward the center of the LV cavity less than 10% during systole; 4 = akinetic, or the endocardium does not move or thicken; and 5 = dyskinetic, or the endocardium moves away from the center of the LV cavity during systole (Figs. 11.10 and 11.11).

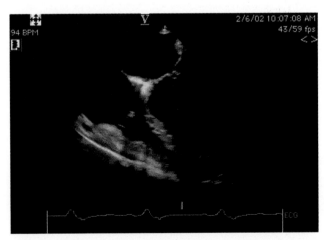

Figure 11.11. In this four-chamber midesophageal view, the lateral wall thickens and moves toward the center of the ventricle. The apical-septal wall remains still or akinetic while the basal-septal wall is dyskinetic, moving out toward the RV.

DISTRIBUTION OF CORONARY ARTERY ANATOMY

Although there is tremendous variability in the coronary artery blood supply to myocardial segments, it was believed to be appropriate to assign individual segments to specific coronary artery territories in order to facilitate the localization and reporting of coronary ischemia and to guide management. The assignment of the 17 segments to one of the three major coronary arteries is shown in Figure 11.12 (6).

A recent study investigated the correspondence between the coronary arteries distribution and the supplied myocardium according to the 17-segment model. The authors studied this relationship in a cohort of patients admitted with their first ST-segment elevation myocardial infarction who had an occluded artery at the time of primary percutaneous coronary intervention. Using cardiac magnetic resonance imaging, they were able to show that only four segments (basal anteroseptal, mid-anterior, mid-anteroseptal, or apical anterior) were completely specific for LAD artery occlusion, and none was specific for right coronary artery (RCA) or left circumflex (LCX) artery occlusion. These results emphasize the tremendous individual variability of coronary artery distribution, which is much greater than that empirically assigned to the 17-segment model segmentation. Additionally, the results of the study suggest that the apical inferior and apical inferolateral segments should be considered part of the LAD territory rather than the RCA and LCX territories as previously recommended (Fig. 11.12) (8).

CLINICAL APPLICATION OF REGIONAL WALL MOTION ANALYSIS

Regional Ventricular Function and Ischemia Detection

Although new onset of RWMA is the most common way of detecting myocardial ischemia using echocardiography, there are many other important echocardiographic features that are seen in ischemic heart disease. These include abnormal relaxation or diastolic dysfunction, mitral insufficiency with normal mitral valve anatomy, dilation of the ventricle, thin-walled myocardium, and papillary muscle dysfunction. The usefulness of echocardiography for ischemia detection should be based on all findings and not just limited to the detection of RWMA. Nevertheless, the relationship of RWMA to ischemia has been compared to changes that occur with surface electrocardiography (ECG), pulmonary capillary wedge pressure (PCWP), and the onset of chest pain. As early as 1935, Tennet and Wiggers recognized that acute myocardial ischemia results in abnormal inward motion and thickening of the affected myocardial region (9). Since then, wall motion abnormalities have been shown to occur within seconds

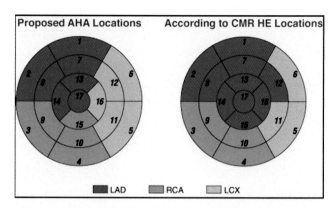

Figure 11.12. Segmentation of coronary arterial distribution within the 17-segment model as proposed by the American Heart Association (**left diagram**) and as according to the maximum specificity of cardiac magnetic resonance (**right diagram**). Results of this study suggest that the LAD artery territory in most cases supplies additional segments in the apex (segments 15 and 16) and the mid-anterolateral wall (segment 12).

of inadequate blood flow or oxygen supply (10). These abnormal contraction patterns typically occur at the same time as regional lactate production (11,12).

The precise sequence of regional functional changes that occur in the myocardium after interruption of flow has been studied in models of acute ischemia, including percutaneous transluminal coronary angioplasty (13,14). Ischemia of the heart produces a number of changes in mechanical and electrical activities. When ischemia starts, one of the first changes that occurs is abnormal relaxation of the segment involved. This is followed by a decrease in the systolic function as evidenced by a decrease in wall thickening and decrease in inward motion of the ventricular walls. As the ischemia progresses, the myocardial segment involved will progress from decreased motion (hypokinetic) to the total absence of motion (akinesis). In its most severe form, the segment involved not only fails to contract but also cannot withstand the increase in pressure in the ventricle and moves away from the segments that are contracting (dyskinetic). Systolic function is estimated qualitatively and is reflected echocardiographically by regional wall thickening and wall motion during systole. Systolic wall thickening can be calculated from the equation: $PSWT = SWT - DWT/SWT \times 100$, where $PSWT$ = percentage systolic wall thickening, SWT = end-systolic wall thickness, and DWT = end-diastolic wall thickness.

Clinical studies have indicated that abnormal changes in segmental wall motion occur earlier and are a more sensitive indicator of myocardial ischemia than the abnormal changes detected with an ECG (12,15–18) or pulmonary artery catheter (19–21). In one study (18), 30 patients undergoing percutaneous transluminal coronary angioplasty (PTCA) were simultaneously monitored with 12-lead ECG and echocardiography. All the patients had isolated obstructive lesions in their LAD coronary arteries, stable angina, normal baseline ECGs, and normal baseline myocardial function with no prior history of infarction and no angiographic evidence of collateralization. In the study, all patients developed segmental wall motion abnormalities (SWMA) approximately 10 seconds after coronary artery occlusion, and 27 of the 30 developed repolarization changes in their ECG at approximately 22 seconds.

The value of PCWP monitoring for ischemia has also been compared to changes in regional LV function assessed with TEE. In one study, PCWP, 12-lead ECG, and LV wall motion were evaluated in 98 patients before coronary artery bypass grafting (CABG) at predetermined intervals (21). Myocardial ischemia was diagnosed by TEE in 14 patients and was also detected in 10 of the 14 patients by repolarization changes on the ECG, while an increase of at least 3 mm Hg in PCWP (an indicator for ischemia) was sensitive only 33% of the time with a positive predictive value of only 16%. Overall, most studies indicate that the sensitivity of wall motion analysis for the detection of myocardial ischemia is generally superior to ECG or PCWP monitoring.

Data regarding the significance of intraoperative detection of SWMA suggest that transient abnormalities unaccompanied by hemodynamic or electrocardiographic evidence of ischemia may not represent clinically significant myocardial ischemia and are usually not associated with postoperative morbidity (22). The significance of the severity of SWMA has been studied (10,23). Hypokinetic myocardial segments appear to be associated with minimal perfusion defects compared to significant perfusion defects that accompany akinetic or dyskinetic segments. Hence, hypokinesia may be a less predictive marker for postoperative morbidity than akinesis or dyskinesis. Persistent severe SWMA, on the other hand, are clearly associated with myocardial ischemia and postoperative morbidity (16,24–26). Intraoperative wall motion abnormalities, therefore, may be spurious, reversible with or without treatment, or irreversible. The former may be associated with clinically insignificant short periods of ischemia while the latter is associated with significant ischemia or infarction.

During systole, the ventricle not only shortens and thickens but also twists around its long axis due to the contraction of the obliquely oriented epicardial and endocardial fibers. Torsion helps bring a uniform distribution of LV fiber stress and fiber shortening across the wall. Elimination of the torsion decreases epicardial shortening and increases endocardial shortening, therefore, increasing endocardial stress and strain and oxygen demand and reducing the efficiency of the LV systolic function (27). LV torsion or twist can be quantified by using some of the newer techniques in ultrasound that will be discussed later in the chapter.

LV apical rotation and torsion may be variably affected in patients who have coronary artery disease (CAD), depending on the transmural extent of myocardial ischemia. As the subepicardial fibers are the predominant source of LV torsional movement, transient ischemia predominantly confined to subendocardium may not affect LV systolic torsion to a significant extent. This has been shown in a recent study in which dobutamine-induced ischemia had no effect on global and regional systolic torsion (28). Transmural ischemia, however, results in less than normal apical rotation. In a study of patients undergoing angioplasty, Knudtson et al. demonstrated reduction in apical LV rotation due to transient ischemia caused by balloon occlusion of the LAD. The effect was confined to patients without previous myocardial infarctions because patients with previous myocardial infarctions already had compromised apical rotation with no further reduction following LAD occlusion (29). Myocardial infarction with multiregional involvement significantly alters LV systolic torsion compared to patients with infarcts confined to a single vascular territory. This may be due to the fact that patients with infarctions involving multiple vascular territories are less likely to have adequate collateral circulation and are, therefore, at greater risk for having more extensive myocardial damage (28).

During CABG, TEE has helped predict the results of surgery. Following CABG to previously dysfunctional segments, immediate improvement of regional myocardial function (which is sustained) has been demonstrated (30,31). In addition, prebypass compensatory hypercontractile segments have been reported to revert toward normal immediately following successful CABG. Persistent SWMA following CABG appear to be related to adverse clinical outcomes while lack of evidence of SWMA following CABG has been shown to be associated with a postoperative course without cardiac morbidity (19).

Although TEE appears to have many advantages over traditional intraoperative monitors of myocardial ischemia, there are potential limitations and pitfalls that can be encountered in the analysis of wall motion. The septum in particular must be given special consideration with respect to wall motion and wall thickness assessment (32–34). The septum is composed of two parts: the lower muscular portion and the basal membranous portion. The basal septum does not exhibit the same degree of contraction as the lower muscular part. At the most superior basal portion, the septum is attached to the aortic outflow track. Its movement at this level is normally paradoxical during ventricular systole. The septum is also a unique region of the LV because it is a region of the RV as well and is, therefore, influenced by forces from both ventricles. In addition, sternotomy, pericardiotomy, and cardiopulmonary bypass have been suggested to alter the translational and rotational motion of the heart within the chest that may cause changes in ventricular septal motion (33).

Another potential problem of wall motion assessment is evaluation of the uncoordinated contraction that occurs due to bundle branch block or ventricular pacing. It is paramount in these situations to evaluate not only regional endocardial wall motion but also myocardial thickening as well.

TABLE 11.1	Differential Diagnosis for RWMA
Ischemia	
Infarction	
Hibernation	
Stunning	
Bundle branch block	
Artifact	
Pacemaker	

Another limitation of SWMA analysis during surgery is that it does not differentiate stunned or hibernating myocardium from acute ischemia (35), nor does it differentiate the cause of ischemia between increased oxygen demand and decreased oxygen supply. Finally, it should be noted that areas of previous ischemia or scarring may become unmasked by changes in afterload and appear as new SWMA (36).

Regional Ventricular Function and Nonischemic Conditions

Not all SWMA are indicative of myocardial ischemia or infarction (Table 11.1). However, it is reasonable to assume that most of the time an acute change in the regional contraction pattern of the heart during surgery is likely attributable to myocardial ischemia. An important exception to this rule may apply in models of acute coronary artery occlusion. In these models, it is established that myocardial function becomes abnormal in the center of an ischemic zone, but it is also true that the myocardial regions adjacent to the ischemic zone become dysfunctional as well. Several studies have reported that the total area of dysfunctional myocardium commonly exceeds the area of ischemic or infarcted myocardium (37,38). The impairment of function in nonischemic tissue has been thought to be caused by a tethering effect. Tethering or the attachment of noncontracting tissue that mechanically impairs contraction in adjacent tissue, which is normally perfused, probably accounts for the consistent overestimation of infarct size by echocardiography when compared to postmortem studies (39).

ASSESSMENT OF MYOCARDIAL VIABILITY

Numerous clinical trials have shown that patients with multivessel CAD and LV dysfunction showed improved survival following revascularization (40,41). However, not all segments with contractile dysfunction show recovery after revascularization. Also, the high perioperative mortality and morbidity associated with ischemic heart disease

and LV dysfunction make paramount the identification of patients with jeopardized but viable myocardium who would be expected to show functional recovery.

Viable myocardium is defined as dysfunctional myocardium with reduced contractility, which improves after restoration of adequate coronary blood flow. Myocardial viability has been described in two pathologic states: myocardial stunning and myocardial hibernation. Myocardial stunning occurs when a transient ischemic insult results in contractile dysfunction that persists for a variable period of time despite adequate restoration of coronary blood flow. The postischemic contractile dysfunction may be multifactorial due to generation of oxygen free radicals, abnormalities in calcium flux, and local accumulation of neutrophils (35,42,43).

Myocardial hibernation describes a chronic contractile dysfunction due to severe CAD and chronically reduced perfusion. In the setting of chronic low flow, the myocytes are thought to reduce their metabolic requirements by adapting in such a way as to decrease contractility but to maintain cellular integrity (35). Revascularization of the hibernating myocardium results in functional recovery.

Barilla et al. (44) reported that patients with viable myocardium treated medically had less recovery of LV systolic function than those who were revascularized. Voci et al. have also shown that microvascular revascularization improves functional outcome although functional recovery does not necessarily take place immediately after CABG (45,46). Also of note has been the poor outcome (48% average event rate over 12- to 36-month follow-up periods) seen in patients with viable myocardium when these regions were not revascularized (47,48). The high rate of cardiac events was significantly lower (11%–16%) in patients with viable segments that were revascularized.

A number of noninvasive techniques have been used to identify and quantify the amount of viable myocardium. These include low-dose dobutamine stress echocardiography (DSE), myocardial contrast echocardiography, single photon emission computed tomography, positron emission tomography, cardiac magnetic resonance imaging, and computed tomography (49).

Dobutamine Stress Echocardiography

DSE induces contractility, which is a demonstration of inotropic reserve in viable myocardium, whether stunned or hibernating. This improvement in contractility forms the basis of assessing jeopardized but viable myocardium with DSE.

Dysfunctional myocardial segments can have various responses to dobutamine infusion. A myocardial segment can show initial improvement in function with low-dose dobutamine infusion (5–7.5 μg/kg/min) with worsening of function at a higher dose (>20 μg/kg/min). This represents a biphasic response and represents the presence of contractile reserve, which improves with low-dose adrenergic stimulation but is limited and results in energy depletion and ischemia at higher doses (50,51). Another possible response to dobutamine infusion is worsening of the function with the initial improvement suggesting hibernating myocardium supplied by a critically stenosed coronary artery without any contractile reserve. Normal resting wall motion and the development of hyperdynamic function with increasing doses of dobutamine are hallmarks of normally perfused myocardium. Regional segments that remain akinetic or dyskinetic despite dobutamine infusion are nonviable and likely reflect scars. Of all the possible responses to dobutamine infusion, the biphasic response has the highest predictive value for functional improvement with revascularization (50).

When used to identify patients with multivessel CAD after acute myocardial infraction, DSE has a high sensitivity (82%–85%) and specificity (86%–88%) when compared to angiography (52,53). A recent meta-analysis compared DSE with thallium scintigraphy and positron emission tomography for identification of viable myocardium in patients with chronic CAD and LV dysfunction (54). This study showed that DSE had a sensitivity of 80% and a specificity of 78% in predicting regional LV functional recovery with revascularization with studies using both low- and high-dose infusion having a similar specificity but a higher sensitivity than the studies using low-dose infusion alone.

The application of stress echocardiography intraoperatively allows for online identification of myocardial salvage and viability during coronary revascularization surgery (55,56). The ability to intraoperatively differentiate ischemia or infarction of the myocardium from stunning or hibernation of the myocardium can help define the need for revision of the surgical plan or other therapeutic options during CABG surgery, allowing more efficient utilization of resources (such as return to CPB, utilization of a mechanical assist device, or administration of vasoactive drugs).

Contrast-Enhanced Echocardiography

The use of echocardiographic contrast agents and harmonic imaging has further improved the echocardiographic assessment of LV function.

Myocardial contrast echocardiography uses high molecular weight inert gases that form microbubbles in order to assess microvascular integrity and differentiate in this way the viable from the nonviable myocardium. Contrast enhancement due to the presence of microbubbles in the myocardium suggests intact microvasculature and viability (50).

Also, opacification of the blood volume in the ventricular cavity will result in a better delineation of the endocardial border allowing for improved assessment of the ventricular function by visual estimation or techniques based on endocardial border detection (1).

EMERGING ECHOCARDIOGRAPHIC TECHNIQUES FOR ASSESSING REGIONAL VENTRICULAR FUNCTION

Tissue Doppler Imaging

The physical principles of TDI are analogous to those of conventional pulsed wave (PW) Doppler. While in conventional PW Doppler studies, the low-velocity, high-amplitude signals of wall motion are filtered out, leaving only Doppler signals from blood flow. In TDI, the opposite is true; red blood cell Doppler shifts are filtered, leaving only tissue velocity data. TDI velocities can be displayed as a spectral PW Doppler signal, as a color velocity-encoded M mode, or as a 2D color map. The high-energy signals generated by wall motion are minimally affected by tissue interfaces; thus, a high-quality 2D image is not always necessary in order to obtain adequate tissue Doppler data. The high temporal resolution of pulsed TDI allows for quantifying systolic and diastolic events during isovolumic periods. The intramyocardial velocities can easily be analyzed over the cardiac cycle, and changes with physiologic or pathologic conditions can be easily observed.

During systole, the mitral annulus descends toward the apex of the heart. The velocity of descent of the mitral annulus can be measured using TDI and correlates well with more traditional measures of LV function such as ejection fraction and the rate of rise of LV systolic pressure (dP/dt) (57,58).

Low TDI velocities correlate well with abnormal myocardial thickening (59), regional ischemia (60), and can help differentiate transmural from nontransmural infarction (1,61).

TDI has several limitations. As with all Doppler imaging, all the data are dependent on the angle of interrogation between the Doppler beam and the tissue motion. TDI is also susceptible to cardiac translational motion and myocardial tethering. In order to overcome this limitation of TDI, strain and strain rate have been developed. By isolating the region of interest, strain and strain rate allow the differentiation between passive tethering and active thickening. Strain is defined as the change in length between myocardial contraction and relaxation expressed as a percentage while strain rate measures the velocity gradient between two points giving the rate of myocardial deformation (50). Strain is dependent on the quality of the TDI data and also on the angle of interrogation. Both TDI and strain rate can be used with DSE and enhance its accuracy in determining myocardial viability (50).

Speckle Tracking

Speckle tracking–derived myocardial deformation imaging is a new echocardiographic modality, which allows quantitative analysis of segmental myocardial function on the basis of tracking of natural acoustic markers in 2D echocardiography. It is based on the tracking of unique speckle patterns created by scattering, reflection, and interference of the ultrasound beams within the myocardial tissue. Using pattern recognition, the position of these speckles can be tracked frame by frame throughout the cardiac cycle, and the distance between speckles can be measured giving information on myocardial deformation during systolic and diastolic events.

Regional myocardial strain and strain rate can also be measured by speckle tracking. Strain rate by both TDI and speckle tracking can be used to differentiate subendocardial infractions from transmural infarctions with great prognostic and clinical implications (62,63).

Three-Dimensional Echocardiography

To date, the 2D evaluation of the global and regional LV function is mainly performed by "eye-balling." This approach relies on the echocardiographer's experience and ability to integrate spatial information, and calculations of volumetric parameters are based on geometric assumptions. The introduction of a third dimension with 3D echocardiography makes geometric assumptions unnecessary and may replace imprecise estimations of global and regional LV function with more accurate quantitative assessments. The recent introduction of 3D-TEE along with semiautomated endocardial border detection systems allows for fast and accurate

measurements for global and regional LV function (64–69). However, further study is required before the superiority of 3D-TEE over 2D-TEE in assessing global and regional LV function can be confirmed.

The best mode to assess global and regional LV function by 3D-TEE is the full volume mode, which is acquired based on the midesophageal four-chamber view. Using built-in software, the 3D quantification advanced program, data for both global LV function as well as RWMA are obtained in a semiautomatic fashion. This requires a manually performed definition of the septal, lateral, anterior, inferior, and apical endocardial borders of the end-systolic and the end-diastolic frames, followed by an automatic border-tracking algorithm. The system will then calculate end-systolic as well as the end-diastolic volumes by summation of the voxels enclosed by the endocardial borders. Thereafter, global stroke volume and ejection fraction (EF) are derived. The obtained shell view is subdivided into 17 regions, which are separately analyzed by performing the "segment analysis," and 17 segmental time-volume waveforms are displayed simultaneously offering the possibility for objective wall motion comparisons and analysis of segmental myocardial contractility (Fig. 11.13).

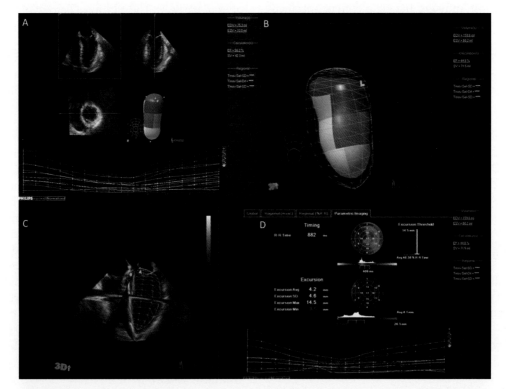

Figure 11.13. A 3D-TEE full volume of the entire heart displayed in three multiplanar reconstruction planes (MPRs; *green* = four-chamber view, *red* = two-chamber view, and *blue* = mid-papillary short axis view). Manual definition of the septal, lateral, anterior, inferior, and apical endocardial borders of the LV in end-systole and end-diastole, followed by an automatic border-tracking algorithm and segmental analysis will display the LV shell in 17 segments along with the corresponding segmental time-volume waveforms (**A**). The shell view (**B**) with an end-diastolic reference mesh and the slice plane view (**C**) are alternative options for display of the 3D LV data. Panel **D** demonstrates the new parametric imaging display that provides easy-to-use color-coded representations of regional LV segmental timing and excursion parameters displayed on the standard AHA/ASE 17-segment bull's eye display. The parametric display may be used in assisting to visualize LV regional function.

Unlike standard 2D TEE, there is no direct measurement of myocardial thickening or displacement of individual segments. However, although not yet confirmed for 3D-TEE, sensitivity and specificity of 3D-TTE in the detection and follow-up of LV RWMA have been reported to be very high (70). Alternative viewing modes provided by built-in software include the "iSlice" view that displays nine simultaneously moving short-axis views of the LV and allows verifying appropriate endocardial border detection as well as the "Slice Plane" view, which shows a moving LV surface mesh within three orthogonal axis planes (Fig. 11.13). Alternative parametric imaging provides easy-to-use color-coded representations of regional LV segmental timing and excursion parameters displayed on the standard AHA/ASE 17-segment bull's eye display (Fig. 11.13). This parametric display may be used in assisting to visualize regional ventricular function and may become clinically applicable for synchronization therapies using biventricular pacing.

TDI has not yet been integrated in commercially available 3D matrix array probes but the evaluation of possible applications of simultaneous multiple planes 3D-TTE-TDI is under investigation (71).

KEY POINTS

■ The LV is divided into 16 segments, according to guidelines established by the ASE and the SCA. The basal and mid levels of the ventricle are each divided into six segments, and the apex is divided into four with the apical cap as segment 17.

■ LV segmental function is graded on a semiquantitative scale of 1 to 5. The numbers correspond to how well the endocardium moves in toward the center of the LV cavity during systole. 1 = normal function, or that the endocardium moves in less than 30%; 2 = mildly hypokinetic, or the endocardium moves less than 30%, but greater than 10%; 3 = severely hypokinetic, or the endocardium moves less than 10%; 4 = akinetic, or the endocardium does not move in at all; and 5 = dyskinetic, or the endocardium moves away from the center of the LV cavity during systole.

■ There are two principle components to LV regional function: endocardial movement in toward the center of the chamber during systole and systolic myocardial thickening. A dilated LV cavity, ischemic mitral regurgitation, and LV thrombus offer other indirect clues for ischemia.

■ The basal septum is membranous, not muscular, and, therefore, does not exhibit the same degree of contraction as the remaining myocardium.

■ While the midpapillary short-axis view of the LV provides a relatively good indicator of overall coronary perfusion and regional wall motion, it must be recognized that not all of the segments are identified in

this view. Therefore, one may still have a considerable ischemic area despite normal endocardial motion in this single image.

■ New SWMA that persist throughout surgery imply perioperative acute myocardial infarction.

■ Low-dose DSE can aid in determining areas of limited coronary perfusion and can differentiate between viable and nonviable myocardium.

■ In addition to conventional midesophageal four-chamber, two-chamber, and long-axis views, 3D-TEE provides up to 16 parallel short axis slices that can be utilized for systematic review of SWMA. Therefore, 3D-TEE may improve the efficiency of a comprehensive intraoperative TEE examination.

■ Although the clinical value of 3D evaluation of the LV is already more established for transthoracic echocardiography, future improvements of this technology and prospective comparisons of 3D-TEE to a gold standard such as MRI will determine whether 3D-TEE can become the new intraoperative standard for accurate and reliable measurement of LV ventricular volumes, mass, regional LV function, and dyssynchrony. Other potential future 3D applications include 3D speckle tracking and use of echocardiographic contrast agents with 3D-TEE, both of which have already been introduced to transthoracic imaging.

REFERENCES

1. Marcucci C, Lauer R, Mahajan A. New echocardiographic techniques for evaluating left ventricular myocardial function. *Semin Cardiothorac Vasc Anesth* 2008;12(4):228–247.

2. Kukucka M, Nasseri B, Tscherkaschin A, et al. The feasibility of speckle tracking for intraoperative assessment of regional myocardial function by transesophageal echocardiography. *J Cardiothorac Vasc Anesth* 2009;23(4):462–467.

3. Skubas N. Intraoperative Doppler tissue imaging is a valuable addition to cardiac anesthesiologists' armamentarium: a core review. *Anesth Analg* 2009;108(1):48–66.

4. Jungwirth B, Mackensen GB. Real-time 3-dimensional echocardiography in the operating room. *Semin Cardiothorac Vasc Anesth* 2008;12(4):248–264.

5. Shanewise JS, Cheung AT, Aronson S, et al. ASE/SCA guidelines for performing a comprehensive intraoperative multiplane transesophageal echocardiography examination: recommendations of the American Society of Echocardiography Council for Intraoperative Echocardiography and the Society of Cardiovascular Anesthesiologists Task Force for Certification in Perioperative Transesophageal Echocardiography. *J Am Soc Echocardiogr* 1999;12(10):884–900.

6. Cerqueira MD, Weissman NJ, Dilsizian V, et al. Standardized myocardial segmentation and nomenclature for tomographic imaging of the heart: a statement for health care professionals from the Cardiac Imaging Committee of the Council on Clinical Cardiology of the American Heart Association. *Circulation* 2002;105(4):539–542.

7. Pandian NG, Skorton DJ, Collins SM, et al. Heterogeneity of left ventricular segmental wall thickening and excursion in

2-dimensional echocardiograms of normal human subjects. *Am J Cardiol* 1983;51(10):1667–1673.

8. Ortiz-Perez JT, Rodriguez J, Meyers SN, et al. Correspondence between the 17-segment model and coronary arterial anatomy using contrast-enhanced cardiac magnetic resonance imaging. *JACC Cardiovasc Imaging* 2008;1(3):282–293.

9. Tennant R, Wiggers CJ. The effect of coronary occlusion on myocardial infarction. *Am j Physiol* 1935;112:351–361.

10. Vatner SF. Correlation between acute reductions in myocardial blood flow and function in conscious dogs. *Circ Res* 1980;47(2):201–207.

11. Hauser AM, Gangadharan V, Ramos RG, et al. Sequence of mechanical, electrocardiographic and clinical effects of repeated coronary artery occlusion in human beings: echocardiographic observations during coronary angioplasty. *J Am Coll Cardiol* 1985;5(2 Pt 1):193–197.

12. Waters DD, Da Luz P, Wyatt HL, et al. Early changes in regional and global left ventricular function induced by graded reductions in regional coronary perfusion. *Am J Cardiol* 1977;39(4):537–543.

13. Labovitz AJ, Lewen MK, Kern M, et al. Evaluation of left ventricular systolic and diastolic dysfunction during transient myocardial ischemia produced by angioplasty. *J Am Coll Cardiol* 1987;10:748–755.

14. Massie BM, Botvinick EH, Brundage BH, et al. Relationship of regional myocardial perfusion to segmental wall motion: a physiologic basis for understanding the presence and reversibility of asynergy. *Circulation* 1978;58(6):1154–1163.

15. Battler A, Froelicher VF, Gallagher KP, et al. Dissociation between regional myocardial dysfunction and ECG changes during ischemia in the conscious dog. *Circulation* 1980;62(4):735–744.

16. Smith JS, Cahalan MK, Benefiel DJ, et al. Intraoperative detection of myocardial ischemia in high-risk patients: electrocardiography versus two-dimensional transesophageal echocardiography. *Circulation* 1985;72(5):1015–1021.

17. Tomoike H, Franklin D, Ross J Jr. Detection of myocardial ischemia by regional dysfunction during and after rapid pacing in conscious dogs. *Circulation* 1978;58(1):48–56.

18. Wohlgelernter D, Jaffe CC, Cabin HS, et al. Silent ischemia during coronary occlusion produced by balloon inflation: relation to regional myocardial dysfunction. *J Am Coll Cardiol* 1987;10(3):491–498.

19. Leung JM, O'Kelly B, Browner WS, et al. Prognostic importance of postbypass regional wall-motion abnormalities in patients undergoing coronary artery bypass graft surgery. SPI Research Group. *Anesthesiology* 1989;71(1):16–25.

20. Leung JM, O'Kelly BF, Mangano DT. Relationship of regional wall motion abnormalities to hemodynamic indices of myocardial oxygen supply and demand in patients undergoing CABG surgery. *Anesthesiology* 1990;73(5):802–814.

21. van Daele ME, Sutherland GR, Mitchell MM, et al. Do changes in pulmonary capillary wedge pressure adequately reflect myocardial ischemia during anesthesia? A correlative preoperative hemodynamic, electrocardiographic, and transesophageal echocardiographic study. *Circulation* 1990;81(3):865–871.

22. London MJ, Tubau JF, Wong MG, et al. The "natural history" of segmental wall motion abnormalities in patients undergoing noncardiac surgery. SPI Research Group. *Anesthesiology* 1990;73(4):644–655.

23. Alam M, Khaja F, Brymer J, et al. Echocardiographic evaluation of left ventricular function during coronary artery angioplasty. *Am J Cardiol* 1986;57(1):20–25.

24. Gewertz BL, Kremser PC, Zarins CK, et al. Transesophageal echocardiographic monitoring of myocardial ischemia during vascular surgery. *J Vasc Surg* 1987;5(4):607–613.

25. Roizen MF, Beaupre PN, Alpert RA, et al. Monitoring with two-dimensional transesophageal echocardiography. Comparison of myocardial function in patients undergoing supraceliac, suprarenal-infraceliac, or infrarenal aortic occlusion. *J Vasc Surg* 1984;1(2):300–305.

26. Smith JS, Roizen MF, Cahalan MK, et al. Does anesthetic technique make a difference? Augmentation of systolic blood pressure during carotid endarterectomy: effects of phenylephrine versus light anesthesia and of isoflurane versus halothane on the incidence of myocardial ischemia. *Anesthesiology* 1988;69(6):846–853.

27. Sengupta PP, Khandheria BK, Narula J. Twist and untwist mechanics of the left ventricle. *Heart Fail Clin* 2008;4(3):315–324.

28. Bansal M, Leano RL, Marwick TH. Clinical assessment of left ventricular systolic torsion: effects of myocardial infarction and ischemia. *J Am Soc Echocardiogr* 2008;21(8):887–894.

29. Knudtson ML, Galbraith PD, Hildebrand KL, et al. Dynamics of left ventricular apex rotation during angioplasty: a sensitive index of ischemic dysfunction. *Circulation* 1997;96(3):801–808.

30. Koolen JJ, Visser CA, van Wezel HB, et al. Influence of coronary artery bypass surgery on regional left ventricular wall motion: an intraoperative two-dimensional transesophageal echocardiographic study. *J Cardiothorac Anesth* 1987;1(4):276–283.

31. Topol EJ, Weiss JL, Guzman PA, et al. Immediate improvement of dysfunctional myocardial segments after coronary revascularization: detection by intraoperative transesophageal echocardiography. *J Am Coll Cardiol* 1984;4(6):1123–1134.

32. Clements FM, de Bruijn NP. Perioperative evaluation of regional wall motion by transesophageal two-dimensional echocardiography. *Anesth Analg* 1987;66(3):249–261.

33. Lehmann KG, Lee FA, McKenzie WB, et al. Onset of altered interventricular septal motion during cardiac surgery. Assessment by continuous intraoperative transesophageal echocardiography. *Circulation* 1990;82(4):1325–1334.

34. Rosenthal A, Kawasuji M, Takemura H, et al. Transesophageal echocardiographic monitoring during coronary artery bypass surgery. *Jpn Circ J* 1991;55(2):109–116.

35. Braunwald E, Kloner RA. The stunned myocardium: prolonged, postischemic ventricular dysfunction. *Circulation* 1982;66(6):1146–1149.

36. Buffington CW, Coyle RJ. Altered load dependence of postischemic myocardium. *Anesthesiology* 1991;75(3):464–474.

37. Lieberman AN, Weiss JL, Jugdutt BI, et al. Two-dimensional echocardiography and infarct size: relationship of regional wall motion and thickening to the extent of myocardial infarction in the dog. *Circulation* 1981;63(4):739–746.

38. Lima JA, Becker LC, Melin JA, et al. Impaired thickening of nonischemic myocardium during acute regional ischemia in the dog. *Circulation* 1985;71(5):1048–1059.

39. Force T, Kemper A, Perkins L, et al. Overestimation of infarct size by quantitative two-dimensional echocardiography: the role of tethering and of analytic procedures. *Circulation* 1986;73(6):1360–1368.

40. Meluzin J, Cerny J, Frelich M, et al. Prognostic value of the amount of dysfunctional but viable myocardium in revascularized patients with coronary artery disease and left ventricular dysfunction. Investigators of this Multicenter Study. *J Am Coll Cardiol* 1998;32(4):912–920.

41. Pagley PR, Beller GA, Watson DD, et al. Improved outcome after coronary bypass surgery in patients with ischemic cardiomyopathy and residual myocardial viability. *Circulation* 1997;96(3):793–800.

42. Bolli R. Myocardial 'stunning' in man. *Circulation* 1992;86(6):1671–1691.

43. Kusuoka H, Marban E. Cellular mechanisms of myocardial stunning. *Annu Rev Physiol* 1992;54:243–256.

44. Barilla F, Gheorghiade M, Alam M, et al. Low-dose dobutamine in patients with acute myocardial infarction identifies viable but not contractile myocardium and predicts the magnitude of improvement in wall motion abnormalities in response to coronary revascularization. *Am Heart J* 1991;122(6):1522–1531.

45. Voci P, Bilotta F, Caretta Q, et al. Low-dose dobutamine echocardiography predicts the early response of dysfunctioning myocardial segments to coronary artery bypass grafting. *Am Heart J* 1995;129(3):521–526.

46. Voci P, Bilotta F, Aronson S, et al. Echocardiographic analysis of dysfunctional and normal myocardial segments before and immediately after coronary artery bypass graft surgery. *Anesth Analg* 1992;75(2):213–218.

47. Di Carli MF, Davidson M, Little R, et al. Value of metabolic imaging with positron emission tomography for evaluating prognosis in patients with coronary artery disease and left ventricular dysfunction. *Am J Cardiol* 1994;73(8):527–533.

48. Lee KS, Marwick TH, Cook SA, et al. Prognosis of patients with left ventricular dysfunction, with and without viable myocardium after myocardial infarction. Relative efficacy of medical therapy and revascularization. *Circulation* 1994;90(6):2687–2694.

49. Kanderian AS, Renapurkar R, Flamm SD. Myocardial viability and revascularization. *Heart Fail Clin* 2009;5(3):333–348.

50. McLean DS, Anadiotis AV, Lerakis S. Role of echocardiography in the assessment of myocardial viability. *Am J Med Sci* 2009;337(5):349–354.

51. Nagueh SF, Vaduganathan P, Ali N, et al. Identification of hibernating myocardium: comparative accuracy of myocardial contrast echocardiography, rest-redistribution thallium-201 tomography and dobutamine echocardiography. *J Am Coll Cardiol* 1997;29(5):985–993.

52. Berthe C, Pierard LA, Hiernaux M, et al. Predicting the extent and location of coronary artery disease in acute myocardial infarction by echocardiography during dobutamine infusion. *Am J Cardiol* 1986;58(13):1167–1172.

53. Madu EC, Ahmar W, Arthur J, et al. Clinical utility of digital dobutamine stress echocardiography in the noninvasive evaluation of coronary artery disease. *Arch Intern Med* 1994;154(10):1065–1072.

54. Schinkel AF, Bax JJ, Poldermans D, et al. Hibernating myocardium: diagnosis and patient outcomes. *Curr Probl Cardiol* 2007;32(7):375–410.

55. Aronson S, Dupont F, Savage R, et al. Changes in regional myocardial function after coronary artery bypass graft surgery are predicted by intraoperative low-dose dobutamine echocardiography. *Anesthesiology* 2000;93(3):685–692.

56. Dupont FW, Lang RM, Drum ML, et al. Is there a long-term predictive value of intraoperative low-dose dobutamine echocardiography in patients who have coronary artery bypass graft surgery with cardiopulmonary bypass? *Anesth Analg* 2002;95(3):517–523, table of contents.

57. Gulati VK, Katz WE, Follansbee WP, et al. Mitral annular descent velocity by tissue Doppler echocardiography as an index of global left ventricular function. *Am J Cardiol* 1996;77(11):979–984.

58. Mishiro Y, Oki T, Yamada H, et al. Evaluation of left ventricular contraction abnormalities in patients with dilated cardiomyopathy with the use of pulsed tissue Doppler imaging. *J Am Soc Echocardiogr* 1999;12(11):913–920.

59. Gorcsan J III, Lazar JM, Schulman DS, et al. Comparison of left ventricular function by echocardiographic automated border detection and by radionuclide ejection fraction. *Am J Cardiol* 1993;72(11):810–815.

60. Derumeaux G, Ovize M, Loufoua J, et al. Doppler tissue imaging quantitates regional wall motion during myocardial ischemia and reperfusion. *Circulation* 1998;97(19):1970–1977.

61. Derumeaux G, Loufoua J, Pontier G, et al. Tissue Doppler imaging differentiates transmural from nontransmural acute myocardial infarction after reperfusion therapy. *Circulation* 2001;103(4):589–596.

62. Becker M, Hoffmann R, Kuhl HP, et al. Analysis of myocardial deformation based on ultrasonic pixel tracking to determine transmurality in chronic myocardial infarction. *Eur Heart J* 2006;27(21):2560–2566.

63. Chan J, Hanekom L, Wong C, et al. Differentiation of subendocardial and transmural infarction using two-dimensional strain rate imaging to assess short-axis and long-axis myocardial function. *J Am Coll Cardiol* 2006;48(10):2026–2033.

64. Caiani EG, Corsi C, Zamorano J, et al. Improved semiautomated quantification of left ventricular volumes and ejection fraction using 3-dimensional echocardiography with a full matrix-array transducer: comparison with magnetic resonance imaging. *J Am Soc Echocardiogr* 2005;18(8):779–788.

65. Corsi C, Lang RM, Veronesi F, et al. Volumetric quantification of global and regional left ventricular function from real-time three-dimensional echocardiographic images. *Circulation* 2005;112(8):1161–1170.

66. Sugeng L, Mor-Avi V, Weinert L, et al. Quantitative assessment of left ventricular size and function: side-by-side comparison of real-time three-dimensional echocardiography and computed tomography with magnetic resonance reference. *Circulation* 2006;114(7):654–661.

67. Arai K, Hozumi T, Matsumura Y, et al. Accuracy of measurement of left ventricular volume and ejection fraction by new real-time three-dimensional echocardiography in patients with wall motion abnormalities secondary to myocardial infarction. *Am J Cardiol* 2004;94(5):552–558.

68. Soliman OI, Krenning BJ, Geleijnse ML, et al. Quantification of left ventricular volumes and function in patients with cardiomyopathies by real-time three-dimensional echocardiography: a head-to-head comparison between two different semiautomated endocardial border detection algorithms. *J Am Soc Echocardiogr* 2007;20(9):1042–1049.

69. Chan J, Jenkins C, Khafagi F, et al. What is the optimal clinical technique for measurement of left ventricular volume after myocardial infarction? A comparative study of 3-dimensional echocardiography, single photon emission computed tomography, and cardiac magnetic resonance imaging. *J Am Soc Echocardiogr* 2006;19(2):192–201.

70. Corsi C, Coon P, Goonewardena S, et al. Quantification of regional left ventricular wall motion from real-time 3-dimensional echocardiography in patients with poor acoustic windows: effects of contrast enhancement tested against cardiac magnetic resonance. *J Am Soc Echocardiogr* 2006;19(7):886–893.

71. Marsan NA, Henneman MM, Chen J, et al. Left ventricular dyssynchrony assessed by two three-dimensional imaging modalities: phase analysis of gated myocardial perfusion SPECT and tri-plane tissue Doppler imaging. *Eur J Nucl Med Mol Imaging* 2008;35(1):166–173.

QUESTIONS

1. According to the recommended qualitative grading scale for wall motion, what numerical grade is given to dyskinesia?
   A. Grade 1
   B. Grade 2
   C. Grade 3
   D. Grade 4
   E. Grade 5

2. Which of the following statements is true regarding assessment of myocardial viability?
   A. Low-dose dobutamine will worsen function in stunned myocardium.
   B. High-dose dobutamine will worsen function in stunned myocardium.
   C. Both low- and high-dose dobutamine will improve function in stunned myocardium.
   D. Both low- and high-dose dobutamine will improve function in hibernating myocardium.
   E. High-dose dobutamine will improve function in hibernating myocardium.

3. The interventricular septum shows flattening during end-diastole on two-dimensional imaging in which of the following situations?
   A. Right ventricular volume overload
   B. Left ventricular (LV) volume overload
   C. LV pressure overload
   D. Inferoseptal ischemia
   E. Normal variant

4. Mitral annulus tissue Doppler imaging (TDI)
   A. Measures low-amplitude high-velocity signals
   B. Measures low-amplitude low-velocity signals
   C. Displays velocities higher than 15 cm/s
   D. Displays septal velocities higher than lateral velocities
   E. Can be displayed as both spectral Doppler and color map

5. What statement in regard to the transgastric midpapillary short-axis view of the LV is correct?
   A. It usually displays all segments of the LV.
   B. It is a reliable indicator of coronary perfusion and regional wall motion.
   C. It is the only transgastric view in the comprehensive TEE examination.
   D. It usually displays anteroseptal hypokinesia.
   E. It does not display all LV segments and one may still have a considerable ischemic area despite normal endocardial motion in this single image.

CHAPTER 12

Assessment of Diastolic Dysfunction in the Perioperative Setting

Alina Nicoara ■ Madhav Swaminathan

INTRODUCTION

In an increasingly ageing population, cardiovascular disease has almost acquired epidemic proportions. Indeed, heart failure is now the most common primary diagnosis of all hospitalized patients in the United States (1). Despite improvements in cardiovascular therapy, mortality and morbidity of heart failure still incur high medical costs (2) making early diagnosis paramount.

Traditionally, investigators have focused on systolic function abnormalities to explain signs and symptoms of heart failure. More recently though, with recognition of the diastolic phase as an active component of the cardiac cycle and the advent of multiple population-based epidemiologic studies, diastolic dysfunction has been recognized as an independent abnormality in heart failure and an important predictor of adverse cardiovascular events. The challenge throughout has always been diagnosing diastolic dysfunction. While systolic function is relatively easier to quantify by multiple imaging modalities, diastolic dysfunction remains best diagnosed by echocardiography.

Technically, diastolic function can be assessed by methods other than echocardiography, including invasive left-ventricular pressure-tip catheter, magnetic resonance imaging, and nuclear imaging. The measurement of the left-ventricular filling pressures in the cardiac catheterization laboratory provides an absolute number that is reproducible and can be followed in time. However, it is an invasive procedure and impractical to use in everyday clinical assessment. In the past two decades, Doppler echocardiography has emerged as a reliable and commonly used method to assess left ventricular (LV) diastolic function. The use of Doppler allows indirect measurement of LV filling patterns. With advances in computer software, Doppler is now easily used in real time with algorithms that help diagnose the severity of diastolic dysfunction and enable rapid therapeutic decisions. This method is noninvasive when used in chest wall echocardiography and adds value to a comprehensive transesophageal echocardiographic (TEE) examination in the operating room.

CLINICAL IMPORTANCE OF DIASTOLIC DYSFUNCTION

Over the past two decades, studies have shown that the epidemiologic profile of heart failure has changed. In a longitudinal population-based study, Owan et al. showed that the prevalence of preserved ejection fraction (EF) among patients with a discharge diagnosis of heart failure has increased over time from 38% to 47% to 54% in the three consecutive 5-year periods. This trend was attributed to shifts in population demographics, changes in the prevalence of risk factors for heart failure, evolution of therapeutic strategies for heart failure, and a higher likelihood of diagnosing diastolic heart failure given an improved understanding of the phenomenon (3). These findings have been supported by other epidemiologic studies, in which the diagnosis of diastolic heart failure was based on echocardiographic assessment of systolic and diastolic functions (4,5). Importantly, Owan's study showed that mortality rates associated with diastolic heart failure are still high with 65% likely to die within 5 years from the hospital discharge (3). Most studies agree that even if diastolic heart failure is associated with a marginally better survival than systolic heart failure (annual adjusted mortality of 11.2% vs. 13% in the Resource Utilization Among Congestive Heart Failure [REACH] study), the morbidity associated with these two conditions, including cardiac arrest, acute coronary syndrome, renal failure, and intensive care admission, is similar (3–11).

Diastolic dysfunction is a common, underestimated condition with a high risk of acute decompensation during the perioperative period. In a cross-sectional survey, which employed echocardiographic assessment of systolic and diastolic functions, Redfield et al. showed that diastolic dysfunction was present in almost 80% of the patients with an EF of 50% or less. The frequency of heart failure increased dramatically with increasing severity of diastolic dysfunction. However, even severe diastolic dysfunction can often be subclinical with no recognized symptoms of heart failure. In the same study, after controlling for age, gender, and EF, mild, moderate, or severe diastolic dysfunction was predictive of all-cause mortality (5).

Diastolic dysfunction in general is most commonly associated with advanced age, hypertension, ischemic heart disease, diabetes, and systolic dysfunction. According to the Acute Decompensated Heart Failure National Registry (ADHERE), patients with diastolic heart failure were older, more likely to be women, and with a higher percentage of diabetes or atrial fibrillation compared to patients with systolic heart failure (12). Diastolic dysfunction is also found in idiopathic cardiomyopathy, restrictive cardiomyopathy (amyloidosis, sarcoidosis, glycogen storage disease, hemochromatosis, fatty infiltration), hypertrophic cardiomyopathy, and pericardial disorders. While mechanisms in each of these cardiomyopathies and pericardial diseases are different, impairment of LV filling in diastole is a common theme. In the perioperative setting, diastolic dysfunction could be due to ischemia, reperfusion injury, hypothermia, myocardial edema, or pericardial effusion.

Abnormal diastolic filling patterns are frequently observed during cardiac surgery. Both LV and right ventricular diastolic dysfunction have been associated with difficulty separating from cardiopulmonary bypass and need for inotropic support, supporting the routine echocardiographic evaluation of diastolic function during the perioperative period in the patient undergoing cardiac surgery (13,14).

PHYSIOLOGY OF DIASTOLE AND PATHOPHYSIOLOGY OF DYSFUNCTION

The physiologic definition of diastole is the phase of the cardiac cycle that starts with the closure of the aortic valve and ends with the closure of the mitral valve. Hemodynamics of diastole consist of four phases: isovolumic relaxation, early filling, slow filling or diastasis, and late filling or atrial systole (Fig. 12.1). From the aortic valve closure until mitral valve opening, the LV pressure decreases without

a change in volume (isovolumic relaxation). Isovolumic relaxation ends when the LV pressure decreases below the left atrial pressure. The atrial-to-LV pressure gradient opens the mitral valve and early or rapid filling of the LV begins. As the LV fills, the pressure gradient from the left atrium (LA) to the LV apex decreases and then transiently reverses. The reversed transmitral pressure gradient decelerates and then stops the rapid flow of blood into the LV early in diastole. During the midportion of diastole (diastasis), pressures in the LA and LV equilibrate, and mitral flow nearly ceases. Late in diastole, atrial contraction increases the atrial pressure, producing a second atrial-to-LV pressure gradient that again propels blood into the LV. After atrial systole, as the LA relaxes, its pressure decreases below the LV pressure, causing the mitral valve to close. The beginning of systole produces a rapid increase in the LV pressure that seals the mitral valve and ends diastole (15).

The complexity of diastolic function arises from the multiple determinants that contribute to its physiology. Normal diastolic function allows the left ventricle to receive a large volume of blood at a rapid filling rate under low filling pressures. Numerous passive and active properties of the myocardial fibers together with physical-geometric factors contribute to the process of LV filling through three primary functions: *LV relaxation, LV compliance, and left atrial function* (16).

LV Relaxation

At the cellular level, *LV relaxation* is an active adenosine triphosphate (ATP)–dependent process with de-linking of the actin-myosin cross bridges that allows relaxation of sarcomeres. LV relaxation is accomplished by the dissociation of calcium from troponin-C and a decrease in intracellular calcium concentration by the sarcoplasmic reticulum calcium ATPase (SERCA2) pump and the sarcolemmal sodium-calcium exchanger. The rate and degree of these cellular processes dictate the rate and degree of LV relaxation. Abnormalities in the sarcolemmal channels, decreases in either the activity or level of SERCA2, changes in the phosphorylation state of the proteins that modify SERCA2, such as phospholamban, calmodulin, and calsequestrin, can cause abnormalities in both LV relaxation and LV stiffness (16–19).

LV relaxation can be quantified by three indices: isovolumic relaxation time (IVRT), peak instantaneous rate of LV pressure decline (peak –dP/dt), and the time constant of isovolumic LV pressure decline (tau). Abnormal relaxation results in prolongation of the IVRT, decrease in –dP/dt, and lengthening of the tau index (18).

The time between closure of the aortic valve and opening of the mitral valve is defined as IVRT; the volume of left ventricle during this phase is constant. This time can be obtained invasively by cardiac catheterization or by echocardiography. However, IVRT has several significant limitations. Aortic or mitral valvular insufficiencies can prolong the IVRT regardless of presence or absence of the disease. Because closure of the aortic valve largely depends

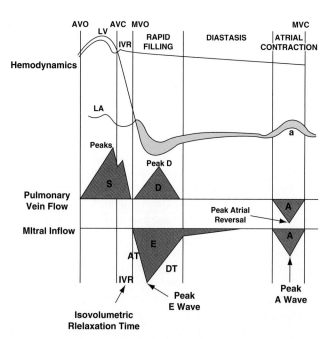

Figure 12.1. The hemodynamics of diastole consist of four phases: isovolumic relaxation, early filling, slow filling or diastasis, and atrial systole or late filling. The schematic represents the hemodynamic pressure tracings in the aorta, left ventricle (LV), and left atrium (LA); pulsed Doppler tracings of flow in pulmonary veins (PV); and pulsed Doppler tracing of mitral inflow measured at mitral valve tips by TEE approach. AVO, aortic valve opening; AVC, aortic valve closure; MVO, mitral valve opening; MVC, mitral valve closure.

on the systemic diastolic pressure, changes in afterload will affect the IVRT, and because opening of the mitral valve depends on left atrial pressure, changes in preload will affect the IVRT as well.

By using high-fidelity (micromanometer) pressure recordings taken during LV isovolumic relaxation, the peak negative rate of this pressure drop (−dP/dt) can be measured by taking the first derivative of the LV pressure tracing. With disease processes that affect diastolic function, the peak −dP/dt will be less negative. This parameter depends on systemic pressure and preload (20,21). It should also be recognized that the peak −dP/dt is taken at one point in time and does not represent the rate of pressure decline throughout the relaxation of the ventricle during diastole.

Another index of diastolic function that is based on the LV pressure decline is the time constant of relaxation (tau). LV pressure change usually is exponential between maximal −dP/dt and the time of mitral valve opening. The pressure decrease can be described by the following relationship: $P(t) = P_0 e - t/T$, where "P_0" is the LV pressure at peak dP/dt; "t" is time after onset of relaxation; and "T" is the time constant of isovolumic relaxation (22). The limitations of this index are similar to those that constrain −dP/dt: the need for invasive measurements through cardiac catheterization and the dependency on loading conditions (20,23,24).

Although LV relaxation is considered an early diastolic event, it depends on systolic events and is a part of the continuum from systole to diastole. The timing and the rate of relaxation are dependent on preload and afterload, velocity, and degree of synchrony of contraction (18). During systole, the left ventricle contracts and twists on its own axis. Myocardial fiber bundles oriented in three different directions—radial, longitudinal, and oblique—result in radial thickening, longitudinal and circumferential shortening, and LV torsion with the basal segments of the LV myocardium rotating or twisting in counterclockwise direction, while apical segments twisting clockwise (16,17,25). During isovolumic relaxation, the left ventricle untwists around its axis, creating an intraventricular pressure gradient and a suction effect responsible normally for approximately 70% of the transmitral blood flow in early diastole.

LV relaxation can be adversely influenced by cellular injury, increased cardiac mass, intraventricular conduction abnormalities and ventricular asynchrony, and impaired intracellular calcium handling due to aging or ischemia.

In addition to active relaxation, passive viscoelastic properties of the LV contribute to the process that returns the myocardium to its resting force and length (26). The passive properties of the LV include stress and strain at the level of the myocardial fiber and stiffness and compliance at the level of the ventricle.

LV Compliance

Stress is the force applied to the myocardial fiber, which in turn stretches, by a given length (strain). *LV compliance* is defined by the volume-pressure relationship during LV filling (dV/dp), and it is a function of mass and myocardial composition. Stiffness is the opposite of compliance and can be quantified by examination of the relationship between diastolic pressure and volume (dp/dV). Ventricular compliance may be influenced by intrinsic or extrinsic factors. Changes in cytoskeletal protein isoforms, density, and distribution have been shown to alter diastolic function (19,27,28). Alterations in collagen, an important constituent of the extracellular matrix, can also adversely affect LV compliance through changes in the amount, geometry, distribution, degree of cross-linking, or type of collagen. Collagen synthesis can be altered by preload or afterload, neurohumoral activation, including the renin-angiotensin-aldosterone system and sympathetic nervous system and growth factors (17,19,29,30). Extrinsic factors that influence LV compliance are pericardial constraint, interventricular dependence, and loading conditions (31).

Left Atrial Function

Although the LA acts as a reservoir of blood and as a passive conduit during early LV filling, it has an active role at end-diastole. Although younger subjects fill nearly 50% of the ventricle in the first third of diastole, elderly subjects complete only 40% of the ventricular filling even after the middle third of diastole making them much more dependent upon atrial contribution to diastolic filling (32).

Other factors that influence diastolic function are heart rate, mitral valve area, and rate of blood return through the pulmonary veins (PVs) (31).

ECHOCARDIOGRAPHIC EVALUATION OF LEFT VENTRICULAR DIASTOLIC FUNCTION

Diastolic dysfunction refers to abnormalities of diastolic distensibility, filling, or relaxation, regardless of LV ejection fraction (LVEF) or whether the patient is symptomatic. While diastolic dysfunction describes an abnormal mechanical property of the left ventricle, diastolic heart failure or heart failure with preserved EF describes a clinical syndrome (26). The Working Group for the European Society of Cardiology proposed that "A diagnosis of primary diastolic heart failure requires three obligatory conditions to be simultaneously satisfied: (a) presence of signs or symptoms of congestive heart failure (CHF); (b) presence of normal or only mildly abnormal LV systolic function; and (c) evidence of abnormal LV relaxation, filling, diastolic distensibility, or diastolic stiffness (33)." The diagnosis of abnormal LV relaxation is principally accomplished with echocardiographic imaging.

The subsequent text will describe echocardiographic methods of assessing diastolic function such as spectral Doppler flow patterns through the mitral valve and PVs, tissue Doppler imaging (TDI) and color M-mode. In addition, some newer concepts in assessment of diastolic function will be introduced.

TRANSMITRAL INFLOW VELOCITIES

Transmitral inflow velocities are acquired by employing pulsed wave (PW) Doppler in the midesophageal four-chamber (ME4C) view. The 1 to 2 mm sample volume is placed at the level of the tips of the mitral valve leaflets. Clinically useful mitral inflow parameters include flow velocities and flow durations at different times during diastole (Fig. 12.2). The early filling peak velocity (E) represents the early mitral inflow velocity and is influenced by the relative pressures between the LA and LV, which, in turn are dependent on multiple variables including LA pressure, LV compliance, and the rate of LV relaxation (34). The late filling peak velocity (A) represents the atrial contraction component of ventricular filling and is primarily influenced by LV compliance and LA contractility. The deceleration time (DT) of the E velocity is the interval from peak E to the point of intersection of the deceleration of flow with the baseline; it correlates with time of pressure equalization between the LA and LV and is a measure of the operative LV compliance (35). The duration of A wave (Adur) is important in assessing LV diastolic pressure and is measured as the interval from the beginning to the end of A wave. The duration of the mitral A wave is best acquired by moving the sampling gate into the annular plane of the mitral valve. Sometimes, in the presence of a slow heart rate, very slow mid-diastolic flow can be noticed between the E and A waves during diastasis (31,36,37). IVRT is the time interval between aortic valve closure and mitral valve opening and is recorded by continuous wave (CW) Doppler midway between left ventricular outflow tract (LVOT) and mitral valve tips in the deep transgastric long-axis view or the transgastric long-axis view (Fig. 12.3A, B).

Obtaining reproducible, high-quality flow velocity recordings require knowledge of basic Doppler principles,

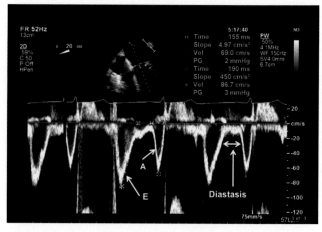

Figure 12.2. PW Doppler transmitral flow profile with sample volume placed at mitral leaflet tips. In diastole, there is a distinct early inflow (E wave) below the baseline, followed by a pause during diastasis, and a late inflow during atrial contraction (A wave).

cardiac filling mechanics, and the characteristics of the ultrasound machine used. Ultrasound beam alignment with a near-zero angle of incidence to flow minimizes errors in peak velocity (6% error at 20 degrees) and helps place the sample volume in an area of laminar flow resulting in a better-defined velocity envelope. Color flow Doppler of the blood flow though the mitral valve in diastole can be helpful in determining the initial placement of the sample volume (38). An understanding of LV filling dynamics aids proper transducer alignment and sample volume placement when performing a Doppler examination of the transmitral flow. In normal individuals, mitral inflow is directed approximately 20 degrees lateral to cardiac apex. Flow then continues down lateral wall and is directed around apex and up toward LVOT. As the left ventricle enlarges, mitral inflow is directed progressively more laterally. Improper adjustment of machine settings can markedly degrade the flow velocity

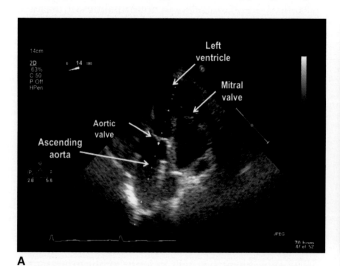

A

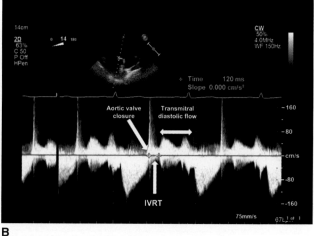

B

Figure 12.3. Deep trans-gastric echocardiographic long-axis view demonstrating the relative positions of the aortic valve and LVOT (**A**). This view is ideally suited for Doppler interrogation of aortic outflow. **B:** shows a CW Doppler flow profile through the LVOT in the same view as (**A**). The isovolumic relaxation time (IVRT) can be seen between aortic valve closure and the start of diastolic transmitral flow.

signals. It is recommended that the smallest sample volume size and lowest Doppler gain be used in order to maximize axial and lateral flow velocity resolution, as large sample volumes and excessive Doppler gain result in coarse signals, with spectral broadening of the velocity envelope that makes measurement of flow velocity and flow duration more difficult (38). The velocity scale should be adjusted according to the peak velocities of the Doppler recordings; low-frequency filters should be used to eliminate wall motion or valvular artifacts that can obscure low-velocity flow. The measurements of flow duration should be made at a monitor sweep speed of 100 mm/s while peak flow velocities can be measured at either 50 or 100 mm/s sweep speed (38).

As discussed above, mitral inflow velocities are determined by the transmitral pressure gradient and are highly dependent on age, heart rate, intrinsic properties of the myocardium, and loading conditions. There is considerable variability in normal patterns of the mitral inflow velocities induced by age. Elastic recoil and rapid LV relaxation in adolescents and young adults result in predominance of early diastolic filling (E wave) with much less filling caused by atrial contraction (E >> A). With aging, LV relaxation slows in most individuals, which results in peak E- and A-wave velocities becoming approximately equal during the seventh decade of life, with atrial filling contributing up to 35% to 40% of LV diastolic volume.

In diastolic dysfunction, three abnormal transmitral filling patterns have been described—impaired relaxation (stage I), pseudonormal (stage II), and restrictive (stage III). The restrictive pattern is further categorized as reversible restrictive (stage IIIa) and irreversible restrictive (stage IIIb).

Stage I: Impaired Relaxation Pattern

Diastolic function is very sensitive to cardiac homeostasis and often becomes abnormal prior to systemic manifestations of the disease. LV relaxation is impaired with aging, hypertension, and ischemia. In this stage, specific and reproducible changes in Doppler velocity profile are obtained at the mitral valve level. First, the impaired relaxation leads to a slower fall in intraventricular pressure at the onset of diastole, leading to a prolonged IVRT. Second, due to the continued decrease in the rate of the pressure drop between the LA and LV, a decrease in the initial hydrodynamic force that is responsible for the blood entering the LV results in a decrease in peak E velocity. Although the initial filling is decreased due to a lower transmitral pressure gradient, the overall filling will continue into late diastole, producing an increase in the DT. In order to compensate for less early filling, late filling during atrial systole will increase, producing an increase in the peak A velocity.

In summary, as the relaxation function of LV becomes less vigorous, the IVRT increases, peak E velocity decreases, E wave DT increases, peak A velocity increases, and the E/A ratio becomes less than 1 (Fig. 12.4). These changes collectively define impaired relaxation or stage I of diastolic dysfunction.

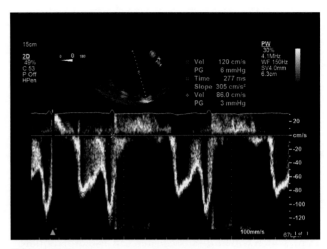

Figure 12.4. PW Doppler transmitral flow profile in a patient with impaired relaxation (see text for details).

Stage II: Pseudonormal Pattern

As diastolic function continues to deteriorate, relaxation becomes further delayed and LV compliance decreases. This leads to a requirement for higher filling pressures to maintain adequate stroke volume. The LA pressure thus gradually increases in order to adapt to this requirement. The increase in the operating LA pressure will restore the LA to LV pressure gradient, resulting in an increase in early transmitral pressure gradient. This will essentially return LV filling dynamics to resemble the baseline state (Fig. 12.5). The increased LA pressure therefore results in an increased E wave velocity and an apparently normal transmitral flow velocities pattern. This pattern of transmitral LV filling is termed "pseudonormal" and characterizes stage II of diastolic dysfunction.

Other signs may indicate higher LA pressures as an adaptive response to diastolic dysfunction. In patients with abnormal LV size, systolic dysfunction, or increased wall thickness, abnormal relaxation is expected, and a normal E/A ratio suggests elevated LA pressure, masking the

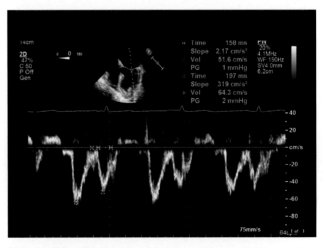

Figure 12.5. PW Doppler transmitral flow profile in a patient with a pseudonormal pattern (see text for details).

abnormal relaxation. The presence of LA enlargement in the absence of mitral valve disease also indicates elevated LV diastolic and mean LA pressure (37).

Reduction in preload or LA pressure with the Valsalva maneuver, reverse Trendelenburg position, or nitroglycerin administration will unmask the delayed relaxation pattern. In the presence of stage II diastolic dysfunction, any maneuver decreasing preload will lead to a decrease in the peak E velocity, an increase in the peak A velocity, and lengthening of the DT, resulting in an impaired relaxation (stage I) pattern. In contrast, when diastolic function is normal, the decrease in preload will result in a decrease in both peak E and A velocities. Additional echocardiographic techniques such as TDI and propagation velocity (Vp), which will be discussed later, can also differentiate a normal pattern from a pseudonormal pattern.

Stage III: Restrictive Pattern

The continuum of the disease process results in increased LV stiffness and worsening of LV compliance. Eventually, the filling pressures must overcome a very stiff LV in order to provide an adequate LV filling. At this point, patients have exercise intolerance and symptoms at rest, since an increase in heart rate also decreases the time required to fill the LV in diastole. The mitral valve inflow pattern will reflect the increased filling pressures and poor LV compliance. The increased LA pressure results in an earlier mitral valve opening, shortened IVRT, and higher initial transmitral gradient (high E velocity). The early diastolic filling into a noncompliant left ventricle results in a rapid increase in early LV diastolic pressure with rapid equalization of LV and LA pressures resulting in a shortened DT. Atrial contraction further increases LA pressure. However, A wave peak velocity is decreased and A wave duration is shortened since the increase in LV pressure is even more rapid, terminating mitral inflow prematurely resulting in a higher LV end diastolic pressure (37). When the increase in LV diastolic pressure is marked, there may even be diastolic mitral regurgitation during mid diastole or with atrial relaxation (37).

In summary, the restrictive pattern or stage III of diastolic dysfunction is characterized by mitral flow velocities that show shortened IVRT, increased E velocity, shorter E wave DT, and decreased A velocity and duration (Fig. 12.6).

Stage III (restrictive pattern) has a poor prognosis and high mortality irrespective of the status of the systolic function (39–41). There is evidence to suggest that aggressive therapeutic measures with angiotensin-converting enzyme inhibitors (ACEI) and diuresis may help reverse the restrictive pattern (stage IIIa) to pseudonormal or delayed relaxation. However, in a subset of patients, the disease process has progressed too far, and even with treatment, the mitral inflow remains restrictive. Some investigators consider this to be stage IIIb or irreversible restriction (42). The prognosis for these patients is extremely poor.

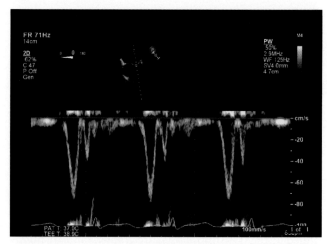

Figure 12.6. PW Doppler transmitral flow profile in a patient with restrictive pattern of diastolic dysfunction (see text for details).

PULMONARY VENOUS FLOW

Information from PV velocity curves can be used in conjunction with that from the transmitral flow velocity profile and can be obtained by PW Doppler interrogation of the flow from the PVs. The Doppler interrogation can be performed either in the left upper PV or in the right upper PV (Fig. 12.7), as they lie nearly parallel to the ultrasound beam. As with transmitral flow velocities, color flow Doppler imaging can be used to confirm the location of the PV and the presence of laminar flow; the sample volume should be placed 1 to 2 cm from the opening of the PV in the LA (31). A normal PV velocity curve (Fig. 12.8A) consists of systolic forward flow during LV systole, diastolic forward flow during early diastole, and retrograde flow during atrial contraction (43). The four variables derived from the PV flow interrogation are peak systolic flow velocity (S), peak diastolic flow velocity (D), peak atrial reversal flow velocity (AR), and AR flow duration (ARdur). The systolic forward flow sometimes has a biphasic pattern termed S1 and S2 (Fig. 12.8B).

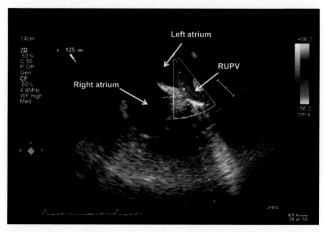

Figure 12.7. Modified midesophageal bicaval echocardiographic view showing the relative position of the right upper PV. Color flow Doppler has been used to identify flow in this vessel.

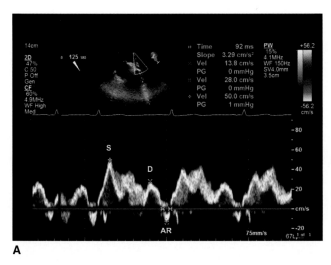
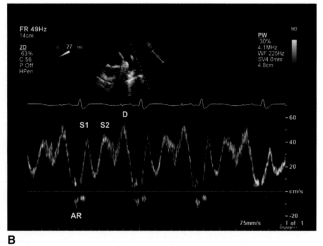

A   **B**

Figure 12.8. A: Demonstrates a PW Doppler flow profile of normal PV flow as recorded from the left upper PV. There is a forward flow in systole (S wave) followed by an early forward diastolic flow (D wave) into the LA. In late diastole, atrial contraction results in a reversed flow (AR) into the PV. **B:** Depicts two separate systolic waves (S1 and S2). See text for details.

The early systolic, or S1 wave, is associated with a fall in LA pressure probably due to the effect of atrial relaxation. The S2 wave is associated with an increase in PV forward flow due to continued descent of the LV base and decrease in LA pressure. Depression of RV function will reduce the intensity of any forward-propagating pulse, and, therefore, may reduce the S2 wave. A decrease in LA systolic function will tend to reduce the S1 wave due to delayed LA relaxation and a less marked LA pressure fall during early LV systole (44). Diastolic forward flow occurs at the time when there is an open conduit between the PV, LA, and LV and is dependent on the same factors that influence the early transmitral flow velocity (42). In late diastole, there is pulmonary venous flow reversal owing to atrial contraction, which is determined by LA contractility and the compliance of the pulmonary venous bed, LA, and LV.

The analysis of PV flow velocities complements the assessment of the transmitral flow velocity pattern but does not add incremental value in the assessment of the diastolic function, especially with the advent of TDI, which can accurately detect underlying LV relaxation abnormalities (34,43). Investigators have found that the diastolic phase of the PV flow resembles early mitral flow (E). The peak diastolic PV flow velocity and DT correlate well with those of mitral E velocity because the LA functions mainly as a passive conduit for flow during early diastole. An isolated relaxation abnormality is characterized by diminished PV diastolic forward flow and the predominant forward flow during systole (S >> D; Fig. 12.9A). Restrictive physiology is characterized by dominant diastolic forward flow velocity concomitant with an increased mitral E velocity and diminished systolic forward flow (S << D; Fig. 12.9B) (37,45).

However, the relationship between the duration of PV AR-wave and transmitral A-wave (ARdur and Adur, respectively) is of special importance in estimation of LV filling pressures. Under normal conditions, ARdur is equal

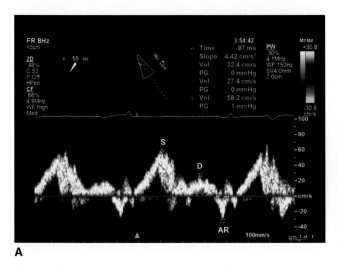
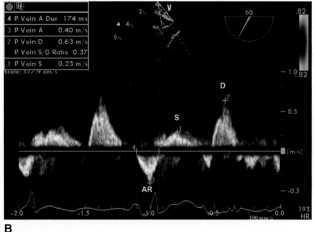

A   **B**

Figure 12.9. Two abnormal PV flow profiles are shown. **A:** Demonstrates a prominent systolic component while (**B**) shows a blunted systolic flow with predominant early diastolic forward flow.

to or less than Adur. In the presence of abnormal compliance of the LV and higher end-diastolic pressures, LV pressure rapidly equilibriates with LA pressures, terminating the transmitral A wave prematurely, resulting in a shorter Adur. However, as LA contraction continues, and transmitral flow has ceased, blood flows back into the PVs (42) resulting in an ARdur that is longer than Adur. Studies have shown that an AR velocity greater than 35 cm/s and ARdur more than 30 ms longer than Adur are indicative of an LV end-diastolic pressure greater than 15 mm Hg, regardless of the systolic function (46,47).

MITRAL ANNULUS TISSUE DOPPLER IMAGING

TDI is a relatively recently developed ultrasound imaging technique, which, instead of measuring velocities of the blood flow, focuses on the high-amplitude, low-velocity signals from the myocardium. TDI velocities can be displayed either as a PW signal or a two-dimensional (2D) color map. The movement of the mitral annulus can be easily recorded by placing the PW Doppler sample gate at the level of the lateral or septal mitral annulus in the ME4C view (Fig. 12.10A). Although the myocardial fibers have both translational and rotational components, in the ME4C view, axial motion of the left ventricle is parallel to the Doppler beam and the velocities are primarily related to LV contraction and relaxation (36). For best recordings and measurements, the filters and baseline should be adjusted for a low-velocity range with minimal gain settings at a sweep speed of 100 mm/s. The lateral mitral annulus is the location of choice since the velocities tend to be higher, are less influenced by the velocities of the blood flow, and tend to be more reproducible than the septal annulus (48). The normal mitral annulus velocity pattern obtained from TDI is similar to that of transmitral flow in patients in sinus rhythm. There is a negative systolic signal (S′) due to the descent of the annulus toward the apex and two positive signals in early (E′), and late diastole (A′) when the annulus recoils in the opposite direction (Fig. 12.10B).

In healthy subjects, the peak of E′ occurs before the peak of the transmitral flow E velocity, suggesting that E′ represents the active relaxation of the myocardium that precedes filling of the LV and is inversely related to the time constant of LV relaxation (49,50). There is ample data to suggest that TDI diastolic velocities are less preload dependent than mitral inflow velocities (50), although in normal hearts the advantage is less clear (51). The E′/A′ ratio behaves similarly to the E/A ratio obtained from the transmitral inflow velocities: it decreases with ischemia and it changes with age (52), but unlike transmitral flow it does not pseudonormalize with increased LA pressures.

An E′ value less than 8 cm/s is consistent with diastolic dysfunction (43) (Fig. 12.10C). The E/E′ ratio relates well to LV filling pressures irrespective of the LVEF (53). It has been shown that an E/E′ ratio greater than 15 was highly specific for LA pressures higher than 15 mm Hg while a ratio of less than 8 is highly specific for normal

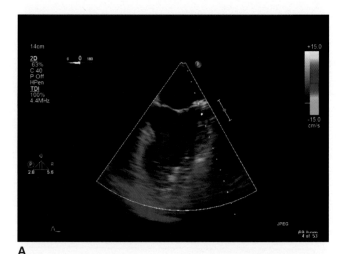

A

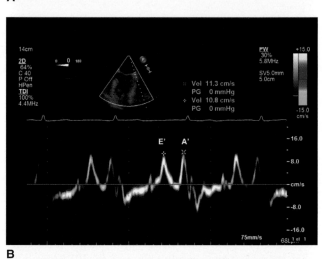

B

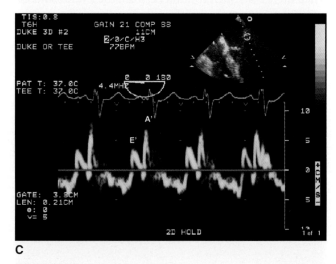

C

Figure 12.10. Tissue Doppler Imaging. **A:** A color Doppler map of tissue velocities of the left ventricle in the midesophageal four-chamber view. A normal spectral tissue velocity profile with the sample volume in the lateral mitral annulus is shown in (**B**). There is an upward motion in early diastole, marking the E′ wave, followed by a late diastolic A′ wave due to AR. **C:** A blunted E′ wave with a dominant A′ component in diastolic dysfunction.

LA pressures (43,54). The accuracy of E/E′ ratio has also been described in patients with sinus tachycardia, atrial fibrillation, hypertrophic cardiomyopathy, and after cardiac transplant in detecting early rejection (55–58). While in patients with normal EF, lateral E/E′ appears to have the highest accuracy, when regional dysfunction is present, the use of average E′ velocity is essential, and a simplified approach with the average of only septal and lateral E′ velocities provides a reasonable estimate (53,59).

Mitral annulus velocities can also be used to differentiate between constrictive pericarditis and restrictive cardiomyopathy. Both entities are characterized by elevated transmitral flow peak E wave, but while patients with constriction and normal LV relaxation have normal E′ velocities, patients with restriction have lower than normal E velocities (60,61).

However, E′ may not be a true indicator of LV relaxation and filling pressures when there are wall motion abnormalities in the basal segments of the septal and lateral LV walls, in the presence of mitral annular calcifications or after cardiac surgery in this region, such as mitral valve replacement or repair.

COLOR M-MODE DOPPLER: PROPAGATION VELOCITY

While pulsed Doppler measures blood velocity at a single specific location, color M-mode Doppler measures blood velocities at multiple locations along a scan line generating Vp, which is the velocity of the column of blood from the level of the mitral valve to the apex. Color M-mode combines the superior temporal resolution of M-mode with the spatial resolution of color Doppler to enable detection of flow velocities in multiple locations along a scan line. It should be recognized that Vp measures the Vp of early transmitral flow and is thus useful for abnormalities in early diastole.

Vp correlates well with LV relaxation, intraventricular pressure gradients, and different pathologic stages of diastolic function, as well as with the invasive measurements of diastolic function such as the time constant of LV relaxation and –dP/dt (62).

Vp should be measured in the ME4C view by applying color flow Doppler with a color sector that includes the LA, mitral valve, and LV. Attention should be paid to eliminating the foreshortening of the LV. The M-mode cursor is aligned with the mitral inflow (as identified by color Doppler) and passes from the LA through the mitral valve and toward the LV apex. The color flow Doppler scale or baseline may have to be adjusted to allow early transmitral flow to alias before it reaches the mitral leaflet tips. This way that first aliasing velocity can be tracked as it propagates through the LV cavity. The degree of adjustment depends on the existing peak transmitral flow velocities. In subjects in sinus rhythm, color M-mode Doppler generates two waves, corresponding to the mitral inflow E and A waves. In order to measure Vp, a slope should be drawn from the mitral valve at the first aliasing velocity during early filling to 4 cm distally toward the LV apex (Fig. 12.11A, B).

Although initially considered relatively insensitive to preload (63), later studies have shown that Vp is influenced by preload with either normal or depressed EF (64,65). Garcia et al. have shown that the pulmonary wedge pressure can be inferred noninvasively from the peak transmitral flow E velocity and Vp. While mitral peak E velocity is dependent on relaxation and preload, Vp is related to LV relaxation; therefore, the ratio of E to Vp, which corrects for the influence of LV relaxation on transmitral flow, should reflect the LV filling pressures. It is considered that a ratio E/Vp greater than 1.5 is associated with increased LA pressure (66). More recently, Rivas-Gotz et al. have shown a strong impact of EF on the accuracy of predicting filling pressures using the E/Vp ratio. When using this ratio in patients with a reduced

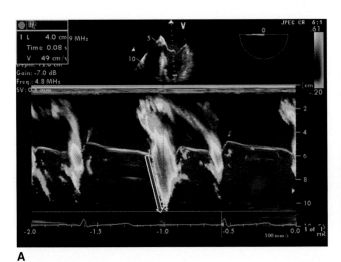
A

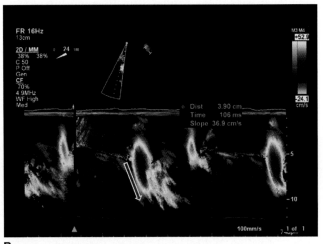
B

Figure 12.11. Myocardial Vp. A normal Vp profile is shown in (**A**), while (**B**) demonstrates a reduced Vp seen with relaxation abnormality.

TABLE 12.1	Values of Echocardiographic Parameters in Different Age Groups and in Different Stages of Diastolic Dysfunction				
	Normal (Young)	Normal (Adult)	Stage I (Delayed Relaxation)	Stage II (Pseudonormal Filling)	Stage III (Restrictive Filling)
E/A	>1	>1	<1	1–2	>2
DT (ms)	<220	<220	>220	150–200	<150
IVRT (ms)	<100	<100	>100	60–100	<60
S/D	<1	≥1	≥1	<1	<1
AR (cm/s)	<35	<35	<35	≥35	≥25
E′ (cm/s)	>10	>8	<8	<8	<8
Vp (cm/s)	>55	>45	<45	<45	<45

AR, pulmonary venous peak atrial contraction reversed velocity; DT, early filling deceleration time; E, peak early filling transmitral flow velocity; A, late filling peak transmitral flow velocity; E′, peak early diastolic myocardial velocity; IVRT, isovolumic relaxation time; S/D, systolic-to-diastolic pulmonary venous flow velocity ratio; Vp, color M-mode flow propagation velocity.
From Garcia et al. New Doppler echocardiographic application for the study of diastolic function. JACC 1998;32:865–875, with permission.

EF, a higher cutoff is needed to detect elevated filling pressures than in patients with normal EF (53). This may be related to the significant effects of stroke volume on Vp that could reduce the influence of LV relaxation. These investigators concluded that Vp was inversely related to end-systolic volume but directly to EF, stroke volume, and cardiac output. Therefore, it is possible for the Vp to fall in the normal range in patients with normal EF despite the presence of diastolic dysfunction.

Normal values of the parameters discussed above, as well as values of these parameters in various stages of diastolic dysfunction are presented in Table 12.1.

GRADING OF DIASTOLIC DYSFUNCTION

Diastolic function assessment should be an integral part of the comprehensive TEE examination. Before diastolic functional assessment, cardiac structural and functional status should be analyzed, including EF, regional wall motion abnormalities, wall thickness, LA size and contractility, valvular disease, and the pericardium.

Mitral flow PW Doppler interrogation should be the first step in the evaluation of diastolic function followed by PW Doppler analysis of pulmonary venous flow and TDI of the mitral annulus motion. Mitral flow velocities under Valsalva maneuver and color M-mode Vp of the mitral inflow can be useful adjuncts.

Using a scale of I to III, stage I identifies a patient with an abnormal relaxation pattern with normal LV filling pressures. Patients with grade I diastolic dysfunction may develop symptoms of heart failure if the contribution from atrial contraction is lost, as occurs with development of atrial fibrillation. With stage II diastolic dysfunction, there is a pseudonormalization pattern on the mitral flow velocity curves and increased filling pressures. Patients with stage III diastolic dysfunction have a restrictive filling pattern on

the mitral flow velocity curves and severe increase in filling pressures. The treatment of heart failure and decreasing preload or afterload may produce changes in the mitral flow velocity curve so that a patient with stage III diastolic dysfunction may improve to stage II or even stage I diastolic dysfunction. Some patients with severe abnormalities of ventricular compliance and end-stage heart disease maintain a severe restrictive pattern even after aggressive treatment. These are patients with the poorest prognosis; they have stage IIIb (irreversible) diastolic dysfunction (42).

It should also be recognized that diastolic dysfunction is a natural continuum, and categorization into stages is based on assumptions that help us stratify the disease process, assess risk, and tailor therapy. Not all patients will follow this categorization and its limitations should be recognized. There is a wide spectrum as a result of age, different degrees of underlying disease, changes in compliance, and loading conditions.

Khouri et al. have suggested a practical approach to evaluation diastolic function in the algorithm shown in Figure 12.12.

LIMITATIONS OF CURRENT TECHNIQUES OF ECHOCARDIOGRAPHIC ASSESSMENT OF DIASTOLIC DYSFUNCTION

Echocardiography has become a very popular tool for evaluating diastolic function. The technique is accessible, noninvasive, reproducible, and patients can be followed in time. However, several limitations preclude it from becoming the gold standard in evaluating diastolic function.

Both the transmitral and PV velocity profiles are highly dependent on the hemodynamic and physiologic states. Preload dependence has been clearly demonstrated in the velocity profiles of the mitral inflow (67,68). As diastolic function worsens, the relationship between the LV

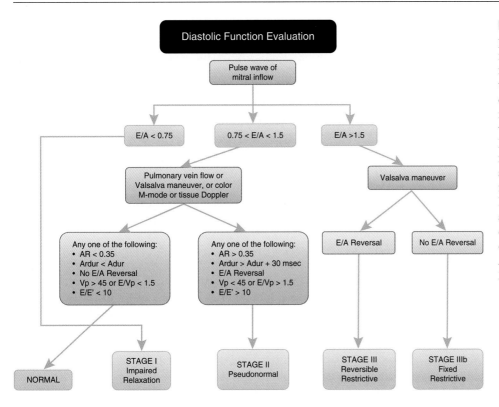

Figure 12.12. Diagram illustrates practical echocardiographic approach to evaluation of diastolic function. A, late filling peak transmitral flow velocity; Adur, duration of A wave; AR, pulmonary venous atrial reversal flow velocity; ARdur, AR duration; E, early filling peak transmitral flow velocity; E′, peak early diastolic myocardial velocity; Vp, flow propagation velocity (From Khouri SJ, Maly GT, Suh DD, et al. A practical approach to the echocardiographic evaluation of diastolic function. *J Am Soc Echocardiogr* 2004;17(3):290–297., with permission).

relaxation and mitral velocities starts to follow a parabolic function confounded by preload changes (Fig. 12.13).

Tachycardia will lead to an increase in the velocity of the transmitral flow A wave and to the fusion of the E and A waves, as atrial contraction will occur before the early filling is complete. An abnormally prolonged PR interval will result in a similar pattern. When a PR interval is abnormally short, the A wave will be terminated prematurely as a result of the beginning of the LV systole. This change may result in decreased diastolic filling and stroke volume and increased diastolic filling pressure (37).

Atrial fibrillation presents many problems, mostly related to the variability in cycle length and the absence of organized atrial contraction resulting in the absence of

the transmitral A wave and PV AR wave. Multiple studies have shown that in the setting of atrial fibrillation, mitral E wave DT can provide an accurate assessment of LV filling pressures, especially in patients with depressed systolic function (57,69). Restrictive diastolic filling has been associated with a DT < 130 ms in atrial fibrillation (70), and less beat-to-beat variability in mitral inflow parameters has been associated with increased filling pressures (57). Previously described E/Vp and E/E′ ratios can also be used to estimate LV filling pressures in atrial fibrillation.

In patients with moderate or severe aortic insufficiency, color M-mode Vp can be difficult to obtain if the regurgitant jet crosses the path of mitral inflow. Severe aortic insufficiency leads to a mitral inflow pattern characterized by an increased E wave velocity, decreased A wave velocity, and decreased E wave DT similar to a restrictive pattern and sometimes diastolic mitral regurgitation due to the rapid increase in the LV pressure.

Mitral regurgitation can influence both transmitral flow and pulmonary venous flow velocities. Increased LA pressures will result in a restrictive transmitral flow pattern and, depending on the severity of the mitral regurgitation, in blunting or even reversal of the PV flow systolic wave (31).

EMERGING TECHNIQUES FOR ASSESSING LV DIASTOLIC FUNCTION

A novel application of color TDI is the noninvasive determination of myocardial strain and strain rate (SR). Myocardial strain (S) is defined as the change in segment length (L) relative to the resting length (L_0) of muscle: $S = (L - L_0)/L_0$. SR (dS/dt) is mathematically identical to

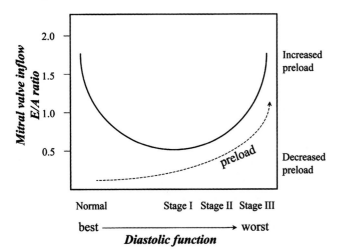

Figure 12.13. The relationship between preload and patterns of mitral valve inflow, E/A ratio. As preload increases, the E/A ratio increases to the pattern of stage III diastolic dysfunction.

the rate of change of tissue velocity over distances within the myocardium and uses tissue velocity data to calculate velocity gradients between two distinct points along the ultrasound beam. It is, therefore, theoretically less susceptible than tissue velocity to cardiac translational motion and myocardial tethering (71). SR changes with age, location (apex vs. base), and site within each segment (epicardium vs. endocardium) (72). Although most of the studies on SR have focused on systolic function, studies on diastolic function have emerged more recently. Stoylen et al. have shown that peak SR and the propagation velocities of SR are reduced during early filling in diastolic dysfunction (73). Goto et al. have also shown that peak early diastolic SR is a useful and sensitive index for regional diastolic function in hypertrophic cardiomyopathy (74).

Both strain and SR are calculated based on the measurement of tissue velocities. While tissue velocity is traditionally measured with Doppler (TDI), it is critically dependent on the angle of interrogation, as with all Doppler imaging. Advances in tissue imaging technology have enabled tracking of individual pixels or speckles within the myocardium that allows measurement of tissue velocity in two dimensions and is independent of Doppler and its limitations. Speckle tracking is a newly developed echocardiographic tool based on the tracking of unique speckle patterns created by scattering, reflection, and interference of the ultrasound beams within the myocardial tissue. These speckles, which produce tissue acoustic markers for a given myocardial region, can be tracked on a frame-by-frame basis (75) during the cardiac cycle.

Using speckle tracking, it is possible to measure several tissue motion indices, including 2D strain and SR, which can be further separated into its individual components of longitudinal, radial, and circumferential strain. In addition, rotation and displacement can also be measured in two dimensions. Wang et al. have showed recently that global SR during isovolumic relaxation (SRivr) derived by 2D speckle tracking relates well with the time constant of LV relaxation both in an animal model and in patients and is not affected by preload. Furthermore, the ratio of mitral E to SRivr can be used to predict LV filling pressures with reasonable accuracy (sensitivity 96%, specificity 82%), particularly in patients with an E/E′ ratio of 8 to 15, those with normal EF, and those with regional dysfunction (76).

The measurement of rotation with speckle tracking has enabled assessment of LV twist and untwist around its long axis. Data suggest that cardiac twist coupled with ensuing untwist plays a pivotal role in LV systolic and diastolic functions. As viewed from the apex, the LV apex rotates counterclockwise in systole, whereas the LV base rotates clockwise during the same period, which generates a twisting motion (i.e., torsional deformation) originating from the dynamic interaction between oppositely wound epicardial and endocardial myocardial fiber helices. Untwisting in the reverse direction during early diastole follows this twisting, thereby creating the temporal and spatial differences in LV relaxation required for diastolic suction (77). Apical untwisting seems to play the dominant role, whereas basal

rotation is of less importance. LV untwisting velocity has emerged as a novel index of LV diastolic function because it has a powerful relationship with intraventricular pressure gradients, which generate the force responsible for LV diastolic suction. Recent studies have linked LV torsion and LV dyssynchrony with peak untwisting velocity (78,79). In addition, delayed timing of untwisting seems to be related to LV relaxation and is a sign of early diastolic dysfunction (80). Rapid advances are being made in using these novel techniques to measure subtle changes in diastolic function. A comprehensive discussion of these techniques may be found in a review by Marcucci et al. (81).

RIGHT VENTRICULAR DIASTOLIC FUNCTION

In contrast to LV diastolic function, right ventricle (RV) diastolic function has been less investigated. By applying the same Doppler analysis, RV diastolic function can be inferred by examining RV filling patterns through transtricuspid flow and hepatic venous flow (HVF).

Transtricuspid flow velocities can be obtained with PW Doppler by placing a 2 to 3 mm sample gate between the leaflet tips either in the ME4C view or in the ME RV inflow-outflow view, whichever provides the best alignment of the blood flow with the Doppler cursor. The variables measured are similar to the transmitral flow: peak E wave velocity, E wave DT, peak A wave velocity, and E/A ratio. Because inspiration increases right ventricular filling, changes in tricuspid flow velocity are seen throughout the respiratory cycle, whereas on the left side of the heart, Doppler mitral flow variables vary only by about 5% (36).

Few studies have investigated the RV diastolic function and there is no consensus on the different patterns or stages of RV diastolic dysfunction. Some investigators have described various patterns of RV diastolic dysfunction associated with heart failure, cardiac amyloidosis and chronic obstructive pulmonary disease with pulmonary hypertension, such as abnormal relaxation patterns with increased IVRT, prolonged DT, decreased E wave velocity, increased A wave and decreased E/A ratio as well as restrictive filling patterns with shortened DT (82–84).

Assessment of the RV filling also should include the evaluation of the HVF velocities with PW Doppler (Fig. 12.14). The HVF velocities are obtained by imaging the hepatic veins at the level of the lower esophagus or stomach and by placing a 2 to 3 mm sample volume in the largest hepatic vein imaged, 1 to 2 cm distal to the confluence with the inferior vena cava. The wave pattern of normal HVF velocity consists of two forward flows and two reverse flows. Forward flow in systole (S wave) during atrial filling is influenced by right ventricular contraction in combination with atrial relaxation and descent of the tricuspid annulus toward the apex. There is a small flow reversal at the end of systole (V wave), which is influenced by RV and right atrial (RA) compliance and possibly by the recoil of the tricuspid annulus at the end of ventricular contraction. The diastolic forward flow (D wave) is a result of tricuspid valve opening

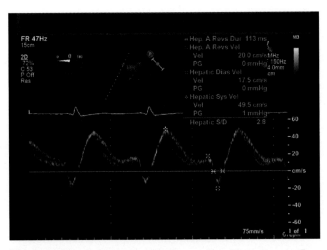

Figure 12.14. Normal PW Doppler profile of hepatic vein flow (see text for details).

and the filling of the RV. At the end of diastole following atrial contraction, there is small reversal of flow (A wave) dependent on RV and RA compliance (85). By measuring the time velocity integral (TVI) for S, V, D, and A waves, the total reverse flow integral (RF) can be calculated as a percentage of the total forward flow integral (FF): %RF/FF = (TVIa + TVIv)/(TVIs + TVId) × 100 (86).

Diastolic predominance of HVF with prominent V- and A-wave reversals is a sign of a marked decrease in right ventricular compliance and increased diastolic filling pressures (82,87). Investigators have described changes in HVF velocities after cardiac surgery with a decrease in the systolic forward flow and the S/D ratio, an increase in the reverse end-systolic flow and an increase in %RF/FF postbypass, probably due to change in compliance, decreased RV systolic function, operative procedure, poor myocardial protection (86,88,89). Most Doppler echocardiographic parameters of RV diastolic performance have been shown to be dependent on age, tricuspid regurgitation, or heart rate (90).

CLINICAL IMPLICATIONS OF DIASTOLIC DYSFUNCTION IN THE PERIOPERATIVE SETTING

The clinical management of diastolic dysfunction and diastolic heart failure is not as well characterized and evidence based as that for systolic heart failure. However, better understanding of the underlying mechanisms of disease has helped in tailoring specific therapies. For example, individuals with abnormal relaxation may become symptomatic with exercise and tachycardia as the diastolic filling period shortens. Relaxation may not be complete before the onset of atrial contraction leading to incomplete LV filling and increased filling pressures. The duration of diastole is critical for these patients, and beta-blockers or rate-slowing calcium-channel blockers often provide a favorable symptomatic response allowing more time for the ventricle to fill and for relaxation to be

completed before the atrial contraction occurs. In contrast, patients with restrictive filling pattern have a fixed stroke volume and slowing the heart rate may result in a decreased cardiac output and worsening of symptoms (34,42). In these cases, diuretics have a beneficial effect on symptoms by reducing intravascular volume and moving the LV to a more favorable position on its end-diastolic pressure-volume curve (91).

Since the renin-angiotensin-aldosterone system is involved in many of the processes associated with diastolic dysfunction (including hypertension, LV hypertrophy, myocardial fibrosis, ventricular and vascular stiffness), inhibitors of this system such as ACEI, angiotensin I receptor antagonists (ARBs) have been of particular interest as therapeutic interventions for patients with diastolic heart failure. The results in recent clinical trials have been encouraging but have not settled the issue. The CHARM-Preserved (Effects of Candesartan in Patients With Chronic Heart Failure and Preserved Left-Ventricular Ejection Fraction) trial showed a significant reduction in hospitalization for heart failure and a strong trend toward significance in the primary outcome of death or hospital admission for heart failure (11). The results of the I-PRESERVE (Irbesartan in Heart Failure with Preserved Systolic Function) trial indicate that angiotensin-receptor blockade with irbesartan is not associated with a reduction in cardiovascular mortality and morbidity in patients with heart failure and normal EF, with an increase in the incidence of observed adverse effects, including serious hyperkalemia (92). An even larger study in heart failure patients with preserved systolic function is ongoing. The Treatment Of Preserved Cardiac function heart failure with an Aldosterone anTagonist (TOPCAT) trial will examine the effects of aldosterone antagonist therapy, spironolactone versus placebo in 4,500 adult patients with heart failure and EF of at least 45% (92).

In the perioperative setting, the diagnosis of diastolic dysfunction is more commonly done with TEE and its detection can have significant implications toward clinical course and response to surgical and medical management. Diastolic dysfunction has been observed in 30% to 70% of patients planned for cardiac surgery, and in elderly patients (age > 65) planned for noncardiac surgery, the prevalence has been as high as 61% (93). Whether symptomatic or not, diastolic dysfunction carries with it an increased risk for future adverse cardiovascular events, especially in the perioperative period due to possible hemodynamic changes and the effect of anesthetic agents. Tachycardia, rhythm disturbances, myocardial ischemia, changes in loading conditions could be associated with decompensation of chronic diastolic heart failure or induction of acute diastolic dysfunction. Especially in high-risk diastolic heart failure patients, anesthesiologists should pay particular attention to avoiding acute perioperative changes in load conditions, heart rate, and myocardial oxygen balance (94).

In an echocardiographic study on a relatively heterogeneous patient population undergoing a large array of cardiac surgical procedures, Denault et al. showed that moderate to severe LV diastolic dysfunction and RV diastolic dysfunction are associated with a greater risk of difficulty in separation from cardiopulmonary bypass, greater hemodynamic abnormalities, and increased need for inotropic support (14). Recent work at Duke University Medical Center on patients undergoing on-pump coronary artery bypass surgery (CABG) has shown that, although diastolic function after CABG did not change in most of the patients (55.5%), it worsened in a small fraction (21%). Most importantly, the worsening of diastolic dysfunction was independently associated with a higher incidence of CHF and postoperative inotrope use. Since inotropic agents may adversely affect diastolic function, postoperative inotrope use may represent a powerful modifiable factor in reducing the deterioration in diastolic function after cardiopulmonary bypass (95).

Analyzing diastolic dysfunction in the perioperative setting could have significant implications on clinical decision makings and could result in improved clinical outcomes.

CONCLUSIONS

In the past three decades, our views on diastolic function have changed with better understanding of the important role it plays in the paradigm of heart failure. Echocardiography remains the most important imaging modality for diagnosing diastolic dysfunction, both in the outpatient setting and in the operating room. While traditional echocardiographic methods still provide reliable, reproducible, and accurate information, newer techniques may improve our ability to detect subtle changes in diastolic function and enhance our knowledge. A greater understanding of the mechanism of diastolic dysfunction and its importance in determining adverse outcome could lead to substantial improvement in perioperative patient care.

KEY POINTS

- Diastolic dysfunction is a common, underestimated condition with a high risk of acute decompensation during the perioperative period. Diastolic dysfunction is most commonly associated with advanced age, hypertension, ischemic heart disease, diabetes, and systolic dysfunction. In the perioperative setting, diastolic dysfunction could be due to ischemia, reperfusion injury, hypothermia, myocardial edema, or pericardial effusion.
- Diastole is often defined as the phase of the cardiac cycle that starts with the closure of the aortic valve and ends with the closure of the mitral valve. The four hemodynamics phases of diastole include isovolumic relaxation, early filling, slow filling or diastasis, and atrial systole.

- The complexity of diastolic function arises from multiple contributing factors. Numerous passive and active properties of the myocardial fibers together with physical-geometric factors contribute to the process of left ventricle (LV) filling through three primary functions: LV relaxation, LV compliance, and left atrial function.
- Echocardiographic methods of assessing diastolic function such as spectral Doppler though the mitral valve and the pulmonary veins, tissue Doppler imaging and color M-mode.
- Transmitral inflow velocities are acquired by employing pulsed wave Doppler in the mid-esophageal 4-chamber view. By measuring flow velocities and flow durations at different times during diastole, three abnormal transmitral Doppler flow velocity filling patterns have been described—impaired relaxation (stage I), pseudonormal (stage II), and restrictive (stage III).
- The analysis of the pulmonary veins flow velocities complements the assessment of the transmitral flow velocity pattern, especially in the noninvasive evaluation of the LV filling pressures.
- Tissue Doppler imaging (TDI) is a relatively recently developed ultrasound imaging technique. The parameters measured by TDI are less preload dependent, relate well to LV relaxation, and can be used to infer noninvasively LV filling pressures.
- Propagation velocity correlates well with LV relaxation, intraventricular pressure gradients, and different pathologic stages of diastolic function, as well as with the invasive measurements of diastolic function.
- Perioperative diastolic dysfunction is associated with an increased risk for postoperative adverse cardiovascular events. In high-risk patients with diastolic dysfunction, particular attention should be devoted toward avoiding acute perioperative changes in loading conditions, heart rate, and myocardial oxygen supply and demand.

REFERENCES

1. Adams KF Jr. New epidemiologic perspectives concerning mild-to-moderate heart failure. *Am J Med* 2001;110(Suppl. 7A): 6S–13S.
2. Linne AB, Liedholm H, Jendteg S, et al. Health care costs of heart failure: results from a randomised study of patient education. *Eur J Heart Fail* 2000;2(3):291–297.
3. Owan TE, Hodge DO, Herges RM, et al. Trends in prevalence and outcome of heart failure with preserved ejection fraction. *N Engl J Med* 2006;355(3):251–259.
4. Bursi F, Weston SA, Redfield MM, et al. Systolic and diastolic heart failure in the community. *JAMA* 2006;296(18):2209–2216.
5. Redfield MM, Jacobsen SJ, Burnett JC Jr, et al. Burden of systolic and diastolic ventricular dysfunction in the community: appreciating the scope of the heart failure epidemic. *JAMA* 2003;289(2):194–202.

6. Aurigemma GP, Gaasch WH. Clinical practice. Diastolic heart failure. *N Engl J Med* 2004;351(11):1097–1105.

7. Bhatia RS, Tu JV, Lee DS, et al. Outcome of heart failure with preserved ejection fraction in a population-based study. *N Engl J Med* 2006;355(3):260–269.

8. McCullough PA, Khandelwal AK, McKinnon JE, et al. Outcomes and prognostic factors of systolic as compared with diastolic heart failure in urban America. *Congest Heart Fail* 2005;11(1):6–11.

9. McMurray JJ, Ostergren J, Swedberg K, et al. Effects of candesartan in patients with chronic heart failure and reduced left-ventricular systolic function taking angiotensin-converting-enzyme inhibitors: the CHARM-Added trial. *Lancet* 2003;362(9386):767–771.

10. Smith GL, Masoudi FA, Vaccarino V, et al. Outcomes in heart failure patients with preserved ejection fraction: mortality, readmission, and functional decline. *J Am Coll Cardiol* 2003;41(9):1510–1518.

11. Yusuf S, Pfeffer MA, Swedberg K, et al. Effects of candesartan in patients with chronic heart failure and preserved left-ventricular ejection fraction: the CHARM-Preserved Trial. *Lancet* 2003;362(9386):777–781.

12. Fonarow GC. The Acute Decompensated Heart Failure National Registry (ADHERE): opportunities to improve care of patients hospitalized with acute decompensated heart failure. *Rev Cardiovasc Med* 2003;4(Suppl. 7):S21–S30.

13. Bernard F, Denault A, Babin D, et al. Diastolic dysfunction is predictive of difficult weaning from cardiopulmonary bypass. *Anesth Analg* 2001;92(2):291–298.

14. Denault AY, Couture P, Buithieu J, et al. Left and right ventricular diastolic dysfunction as predictors of difficult separation from cardiopulmonary bypass. *Can J Anaesth* 2006;53(10):1020–1029.

15. Fukuta H, Little WC. The cardiac cycle and the physiologic basis of left ventricular contraction, ejection, relaxation, and filling. *Heart Fail Clin* 2008;4(1):1–11.

16. Garcia MJ. Left ventricular filling. *Heart Fail Clin* 2008;4(1):47–56.

17. Rapp JA, Gheorghiade M. Role of neurohormonal modulators in heart failure with relatively preserved systolic function. *Cardiol Clin* 2008;26(1):23–40.

18. Zhao W, Choi JH, Hong GR, et al. Left ventricular relaxation. *Heart Fail Clin* 2008;4(1):37–46.

19. Zile MR, Brutsaert DL. New concepts in diastolic dysfunction and diastolic heart failure. Part II: causal mechanisms and treatment. *Circulation* 2002;105(12):1503–1508.

20. Chen C, Rodriguez L, Levine RA, et al. Noninvasive measurement of the time constant of left ventricular relaxation using the continuous-wave Doppler velocity profile of mitral regurgitation. *Circulation* 1992;86(1):272–278.

21. Perlini S, Meyer TE, Foex P. Effects of preload, afterload and inotropy on dynamics of ischemic segmental wall motion. *J Am Coll Cardiol* 1997;29(4):846–855.

22. Weiss JL, Frederiksen JW, Weisfeldt ML. Hemodynamic determinants of the time-course of fall in canine left ventricular pressure. *J Clin Invest* 1976;58(3):751–760.

23. Schafer S, Fiedler VB, Thamer V. Afterload dependent prolongation of left ventricular relaxation: importance of asynchrony. *Cardiovasc Res* 1992;26(6):631–637.

24. Thomas JD, Flachskampf FA, Chen C, et al. Isovolumic relaxation time varies predictably with its time constant and aortic and left atrial pressures: implications for the noninvasive evaluation of ventricular relaxation. *Am Heart J* 1992;124(5):1305–1313.

25. Rothfeld JM, LeWinter MM, Tischler MD. Left ventricular systolic torsion and early diastolic filling by echocardiography in normal humans. *Am J Cardiol* 1998;81(12):1465–1469.

26. Zile MR, Brutsaert DL. New concepts in diastolic dysfunction and diastolic heart failure. Part I: diagnosis, prognosis, and measurements of diastolic function. *Circulation* 2002;105(11):1387–1393.

27. Bell SP, Nyland L, Tischler MD, et al. Alterations in the determinants of diastolic suction during pacing tachycardia. *Circ Res* 2000;87(3):235–240.

28. Tagawa H, Wang N, Narishige T, et al. Cytoskeletal mechanics in pressure-overload cardiac hypertrophy. *Circ Res* 1997;80(2):281–289.

29. Jalil JE, Doering CW, Janicki JS, et al. Fibrillar collagen and myocardial stiffness in the intact hypertrophied rat left ventricle. *Circ Res* 1989;64(6):1041–1050.

30. Kato S, Spinale FG, Tanaka R, et al. Inhibition of collagen cross-linking: effects on fibrillar collagen and ventricular diastolic function. *Am J Physiol* 1995;269(3 Pt 2):H863–H868.

31. Groban L, Dolinski SY. Transesophageal echocardiographic evaluation of diastolic function. *Chest* 2005;128(5):3652–3663.

32. Chinnaiyan KM, Alexander D, Maddens M, et al. Curriculum in cardiology: integrated diagnosis and management of diastolic heart failure. *Am Heart J* 2007;153(2):189–200.

33. European Study Group on Diastolic Heart Failure. How to diagnose diastolic heart failure. *Eur Heart J* 1998;19(7):990–1003.

34. Lester SJ, Tajik AJ, Nishimura RA, et al. Unlocking the mysteries of diastolic function: deciphering the Rosetta Stone 10 years later. *J Am Coll Cardiol* 2008;51(7):679–689.

35. Little WC, Ohno M, Kitzman DW, et al. Determination of left ventricular chamber stiffness from the time for deceleration of early left ventricular filling. *Circulation* 1995;92(7):1933–1939.

36. Appleton CP, Firstenberg MS, Garcia MJ, et al. The echo-Doppler evaluation of left ventricular diastolic function. A current perspective. *Cardiol Clin* 2000;18(3):513–546.

37. Oh JK, Appleton CP, Hatle LK, et al. The noninvasive assessment of left ventricular diastolic function with two-dimensional and Doppler echocardiography. *J Am Soc Echocardiogr* 1997;10(3):246–270.

38. Appleton CP, Jensen JL, Hatle LK, et al. Doppler evaluation of left and right ventricular diastolic function: a technical guide for obtaining optimal flow velocity recordings. *J Am Soc Echocardiogr* 1997;10(3):271–292.

39. Moller JE, Sondergaard E, Poulsen SH, et al. Pseudonormal and restrictive filling patterns predict left ventricular dilation and cardiac death after a first myocardial infarction: a serial color M-mode Doppler echocardiographic study. *J Am Coll Cardiol* 2000;36(6):1841–1846.

40. Pinamonti B, Zecchin M, Di Lenarda A, et al. Persistence of restrictive left ventricular filling pattern in dilated cardiomyopathy: an ominous prognostic sign. *J Am Coll Cardiol* 1997;29(3):604–612.

41. Xie GY, Berk MR, Smith MD, et al. Prognostic value of Doppler transmitral flow patterns in patients with congestive heart failure. *J Am Coll Cardiol* 1994;24(1):132–139.

42. Nishimura RA, Tajik AJ. Evaluation of diastolic filling of left ventricle in health and disease: Doppler echocardiography is the clinician's Rosetta Stone. *J Am Coll Cardiol* 1997;30(1):8–18.

43. Khouri SJ, Maly GT, Suh DD, et al. A practical approach to the echocardiographic evaluation of diastolic function. *J Am Soc Echocardiogr* 2004;17(3):290–297.

44. Smiseth OA, Thompson CR, Lohavanichbutr K, et al. The pulmonary venous systolic flow pulse—its origin and relationship to left atrial pressure. *J Am Coll Cardiol* 1999;34(3):802–809.

45. Nishimura RA, Abel MD, Hatle LK, et al. Relation of pulmonary vein to mitral flow velocities by transesophageal Doppler echocardiography. Effect of different loading conditions. *Circulation* 1990;81(5):1488–1497.

46. Klein AL, Tajik AJ. Doppler assessment of pulmonary venous flow in healthy subjects and in patients with heart disease. *J Am Soc Echocardiogr* 1991;4(4):379–392.

47. Rossvoll O, Hatle LK. Pulmonary venous flow velocities recorded by transthoracic Doppler ultrasound: relation to left ventricular diastolic pressures. *J Am Coll Cardiol* 1993;21(7):1687–1696.

48. Garcia MJ, Thomas JD. Tissue Doppler to assess diastolic left ventricular function. *Echocardiography* 1999;16(5):501–508.

49. Oki T, Tabata T, Yamada H, et al. Clinical application of pulsed Doppler tissue imaging for assessing abnormal left ventricular relaxation. *Am J Cardiol* 1997;79(7):921–928.

50. Sohn DW, Chai IH, Lee DJ, et al. Assessment of mitral annulus velocity by Doppler tissue imaging in the evaluation of left ventricular diastolic function. *J Am Coll Cardiol* 1997;30(2):474–480.

51. Firstenberg MS, Vandervoort PM, Greenberg NL, et al. Noninvasive estimation of transmitral pressure drop across the normal mitral valve in humans: importance of convective and inertial forces during left ventricular filling. *J Am Coll Cardiol* 2000;36(6):1942–1949.

52. Yamada H, Oki T, Mishiro Y, et al. Effect of aging on diastolic left ventricular myocardial velocities measured by pulsed tissue Doppler imaging in healthy subjects. *J Am Soc Echocardiogr* 1999;12(7):574–581.

53. Rivas-Gotz C, Manolios M, Thohan V, et al. Impact of left ventricular ejection fraction on estimation of left ventricular filling pressures using tissue Doppler and flow propagation velocity. *Am J Cardiol* 2003;91(6):780–784.

54. Nagueh SF, Middleton KJ, Kopelen HA, et al. Doppler tissue imaging: a noninvasive technique for evaluation of left ventricular relaxation and estimation of filling pressures. *J Am Coll Cardiol* 1997;30(6):1527–1533.

55. Mankad S, Murali S, Mandarino WA, et al. Assessment of acute cardiac allograft rejection by quantitative tissue Doppler echocardiography. *Circulation* 1997;96(8S):I–342.

56. Nagueh SF, Bachinski LL, Meyer D, et al. Tissue Doppler imaging consistently detects myocardial abnormalities in patients with hypertrophic cardiomyopathy and provides a novel means for an early diagnosis before and independently of hypertrophy. *Circulation* 2001;104(2):128–130.

57. Nagueh SF, Kopelen HA, Quinones MA. Assessment of left ventricular filling pressures by Doppler in the presence of atrial fibrillation. *Circulation* 1996;94(9):2138–2145.

58. Nagueh SF, Mikati I, Kopelen HA, et al. Doppler estimation of left ventricular filling pressure in sinus tachycardia. A new application of tissue doppler imaging. *Circulation* 1998;98(16):1644–1650.

59. Wang J, Nagueh SF. Echocardiographic assessment of left ventricular filling pressures. *Heart Fail Clin* 2008;4(1):57–70.

60. Garcia MJ, Rodriguez L, Ares M, et al. Differentiation of constrictive pericarditis from restrictive cardiomyopathy: assessment of left ventricular diastolic velocities in longitudinal axis by Doppler tissue imaging. *J Am Coll Cardiol* 1996;27(1):108–114.

61. Rajagopalan N, Garcia MJ, Rodriguez L, et al. Comparison of new Doppler echocardiographic methods to differentiate constrictive pericardial heart disease and restrictive cardiomyopathy. *Am J Cardiol* 2001;87(1):86–94.

62. Takatsuji H, Mikami T, Urasawa K, et al. A new approach for evaluation of left ventricular diastolic function: spatial and temporal analysis of left ventricular filling flow propagation by color M-mode Doppler echocardiography. *J Am Coll Cardiol* 1996;27(2):365–371.

63. Garcia MJ, Smedira NG, Greenberg NL, et al. Color M-mode Doppler flow propagation velocity is a preload insensitive index of left ventricular relaxation: animal and human validation. *J Am Coll Cardiol* 2000;35(1):201–208.

64. Graham RJ, Gelman JS, Donelan L, et al. Effect of preload reduction by haemodialysis on new indices of diastolic function. *Clin Sci (Lond)* 2003;105(4):499–506.

65. Troughton RW, Prior DL, Frampton CM, et al. Usefulness of tissue Doppler and color M-mode indexes of left ventricular diastolic function in predicting outcomes in systolic left ventricular heart failure (from the ADEPT study). *Am J Cardiol* 2005;96(2):257–262.

66. Garcia MJ, Ares MA, Asher C, et al. An index of early left ventricular filling that combined with pulsed Doppler peak E velocity may estimate capillary wedge pressure. *J Am Coll Cardiol* 1997;29(2):448–454.

67. Fraites TJ Jr, Saeki A, Kass DA. Effect of altering filling pattern on diastolic pressure-volume curve. *Circulation* 1997;96(12):4408–4414.

68. Keren G, Milner M, Lindsay J Jr, et al. Load dependence of left atrial and left ventricular filling dynamics by transthoracic and transesophageal Doppler echocardiography. *Am J Card Imaging* 1996;10(2):108–116.

69. Matsukida K, Kisanuki A, Toyonaga K, et al. Comparison of transthoracic Doppler echocardiography and natriuretic peptides in predicting mean pulmonary capillary wedge pressure in patients with chronic atrial fibrillation. *J Am Soc Echocardiogr* 2001;14(11):1080–1087.

70. Hurrell DG, Oh JK, Mahoney DW, et al. Short deceleration time of mitral inflow E velocity: prognostic implication with atrial fibrillation versus sinus rhythm. *J Am Soc Echocardiogr* 1998;11(5):450–457.

71. Castro PL, Greenberg NL, Drinko J, et al. Potential pitfalls of strain rate imaging: angle dependency. *Biomed Sci Instrum* 2000;36:197–202.

72. Sun JP, Popovic ZB, Greenberg NL, et al. Noninvasive quantification of regional myocardial function using Doppler-derived velocity, displacement, strain rate, and strain in healthy volunteers: effects of aging. *J Am Soc Echocardiogr* 2004;17(2):132–138.

73. Stoylen A, Slordahl S, Skjelvan GK, et al. Strain rate imaging in normal and reduced diastolic function: comparison with pulsed Doppler tissue imaging of the mitral annulus. *J Am Soc Echocardiogr* 2001;14(4):264–274.

74. Goto K, Mikami T, Onozuka H, et al. Role of left ventricular regional diastolic abnormalities for global diastolic dysfunction in patients with hypertrophic cardiomyopathy. *J Am Soc Echocardiogr* 2006;19(7):857–864.

75. Helle-Valle T, Crosby J, Edvardsen T, et al. New noninvasive method for assessment of left ventricular rotation: speckle tracking echocardiography. *Circulation* 2005;112(20):3149–3156.

76. Wang J, Khoury DS, Thohan V, et al. Global diastolic strain rate for the assessment of left ventricular relaxation and filling pressures. *Circulation* 2007;115(11):1376–1383.

77. Sengupta PP, Khandheria BK, Korinek J, et al. Apex-to-base dispersion in regional timing of left ventricular shortening and lengthening. *J Am Coll Cardiol* 2006;47(1):163–172.

78. Notomi Y, Lysyansky P, Setser RM, et al. Measurement of ventricular torsion by two-dimensional ultrasound speckle tracking imaging. *J Am Coll Cardiol* 2005;45(12):2034–2041.

79. Saito M, Okayama H, Nishimura K, et al. Determinants of left ventricular untwisting behavior in patients with dilated cardiomyopathy: analysis by two-dimensional speckle tracking. *Heart* 2009;95:290–296.

80. Takeuchi M, Borden WB, Nakai H, et al. Reduced and delayed untwisting of the left ventricle in patients with hypertension and left ventricular hypertrophy: a study using two-dimensional speckle tracking imaging. *Eur Heart J* 2007;28(22):2756–2762.

81. Marcucci C, Lauer R, Mahajan A. New echocardiographic techniques for evaluating left ventricular myocardial function. *Semin Cardiothorac Vasc Anesth* 2008;12(4):228–247.

82. Klein AL, Hatle LK, Burstow DJ, et al. Comprehensive Doppler assessment of right ventricular diastolic function in cardiac amyloidosis. *J Am Coll Cardiol* 1990;15(1):99–108.

83. Ozer N, Tokgozoglu L, Coplu L, et al. Echocardiographic evaluation of left and right ventricular diastolic function in patients with chronic obstructive pulmonary disease. *J Am Soc Echocardiogr* 2001;14(6):557–561.

84. Yu CM, Sanderson JE, Chan S, et al. Right ventricular diastolic dysfunction in heart failure. *Circulation* 1996;93(8):1509–1514.

85. Otto C. Echocardiograpfic evaluation of ventricular diastolic filling and function. In: Otto C, ed. *Textbook of Clinical Echocardiography*. 2nd ed. Philadephia: W.B. Saunders, 2000:132–152.

86. Nomura T, Lebowitz L, Koide Y, et al. Evaluation of hepatic venous flow using transesophageal echocardiography in coronary artery bypass surgery: an index of right ventricular function. *J Cardiothorac Vasc Anesth* 1995;9(1):9–17.

87. Nagueh SF, Kopelen HA, Zoghbi WA. Relation of mean right atrial pressure to echocardiographic and Doppler parameters of right atrial and right ventricular function. *Circulation* 1996;93(6):1160–1169.

88. Mishra M, Swaminathan M, Malhotra R, et al. Evaluation of right ventricular function during CABG: transesophageal echocardiographic assessment of hepatic venous flow versus conventional right ventricular performance indices. *Echocardiography* 1998;15(1):51–58.

89. Pinto FJ, Wranne B, St. Goar FG, et al. Systemic venous flow during cardiac surgery examined by intraoperative transesophageal echocardiography. *Am J Cardiol* 1992;69(4):387–393.

90. Spencer KT, Weinert L, Lang RM. Effect of age, heart rate and tricuspid regurgitation on the Doppler echocardiographic evaluation of right ventricular diastolic function. *Cardiology* 1999;92(1):59–64.

91. Angeja BG, Grossman W. Evaluation and management of diastolic heart failure. *Circulation* 2003;107(5):659–663.

92. Massie BM, Carson PE, McMurray JJ, et al. Irbesartan in patients with heart failure and preserved ejection fraction. *N Engl J Med* 2008;359:2456–2467.

93. Phillip B, Pastor D, Bellows W, et al. The prevalence of preoperative diastolic filling abnormalities in geriatric surgical patients. *Anesth Analg* 2003;97(5):1214–1221.

94. Pirracchio R, Cholley B, De Hert S, et al. Diastolic heart failure in anaesthesia and critical care. *Br J Anaesth* 2007;98(6): 707–721.

95. Nicoara A, Phillips-Bute B, Gorrin-Rivas M, et al. Determinants of change in LV diastolic function after CABG surgery. *ASA Annual Meeting Abstracts*. San Francisco, California; 2007.

QUESTIONS

1. A 70-year-old patient with uncontrolled hypertension and moderate concentric left ventricular hypertrophy is undergoing surgical coronary artery revascularization. Spectral Doppler of transmitral flow shows E wave= 73 cm/sec, A wave=60 cm/sec, and a deceleration time=180 msec. The tissue Doppler E′ =7 cm/s, and the pulmonary vein systolic peak velocity is less than diastolic peak velocity. The propagation velocity is 28 cm/s. Which of the following most likely represents this patient's diastolic function?
   A. Normal function
   B. Impaired relaxation
   C. Pseudonormal
   D. Restrictive
   E. Cannot be determined

2. A 65-year-old patient is undergoing pericardial stripping for constrictive pericarditis. Which of the following intraoperative findings is more likely to be true?
   A. E/A ratio less than 1.5
   B. Lateral E′ lower than septal E′
   C. V_p less than 50 cm/sec
   D. E′ less than 8 cm/sec
   E. E wave DT 220msec

3. Which of the following best describes the effect of a steep reverse Trendelenburg position on the transmitral early (E) wave deceleration time (DT)?
   A. Decrease in a healthy young adult
   B. Increase in grade IIIa diastolic dysfunction
   C. Decrease in grade II diastolic dysfunction
   D. Increase in grade IIIb diastolic dysfunction

4. In a patient with left ventricular systolic dysfunction, elevation of pulmonary capillary wedge pressure is MOST likely to occur when E wave deceleration time is
   A. <420 msec
   B. >300 msec
   C. <150 msec
   D. >260 msec
   E. >365 msec

5. In a patient with an isolated relaxation abnormality and normal filling pressures, the transmitral Doppler flow pattern is most likely to show which of the following?
   A. Decreased isovolumic relaxation time
   B. Decreased E-wave velocity
   C. Increased E/A ratio
   D. Decreased E wave deceleration time
   E. Large 'L' wave

Colleen Gorman Koch

The mitral valve is aptly named because of its resemblance to a "mitre," a type of folding cap consisting of two similar parts that rise to a peak (1,2). During the Renaissance, Andreas Vesalius suggested the term mitral because of the valve's resemblance to a bishop's mitre (Fig. 13.1) (3,4). His publication of *De Humani Corporis Fabrica* in 1543 constituted a monumental achievement by presenting anatomy as a scientific discipline, ultimately advancing the knowledge of cardiology (5). The intrigue of mitral anatomy, during an age when studies were done in secret and published at risk to the anatomist, is currently captured by transesophageal echocardiography (TEE), which provides a window to real-time structure and function of the heart.

ANATOMY OF THE MITRAL VALVE

Anatomic components of the mitral valve complex include the left atrial wall, the mitral annulus, the anterior and posterior mitral valve leaflets, the chordal tendons, and the anterolateral and posteromedial papillary muscles, which attach the mitral valve to the left ventricular myocardium (6–8). The mitral annulus, which exhibits sphincteric contraction in systole, serves as a basal attachment for the mitral valve leaflets (8). The anterior mitral leaflet is somewhat triangular and subtends approximately one third of the circumference of the mitral annulus. It has a longer basal-to-margin length than the posterior mitral leaflet. Part of the annulus of the anterior mitral leaflet has a common attachment to the fibrous skeleton of the heart with the

left coronary cusp and half of the noncoronary cusp of the aortic valve. (4). The posterior mitral leaflet is shorter and subtends a greater attachment to the mitral annulus than the anterior mitral leaflet. The posterior mitral leaflet has a "true bundle of fibrous tissue," the annulus, separating the left atrium from the left ventricle (6,9,10). While morphologically different, the surface areas of the anterior and posterior mitral valve leaflets are nearly identical (4,6,8,9) and together exceed the area of the mitral annulus in a relationship of greater than two to one (4,8). The mitral valve leaflets adjoin at the sides of the valve, forming the anterolateral and posteromedial commissures (4). More than 120 chordal tendons subdivide as they project from each papillary muscle to attach to the free edge and body of both mitral valve leaflets. Subdivisions of the choral tendons can be classified as primary (first order), secondary (second order), and tertiary (third order) chordae (4).

Standard nomenclature adopted by the Society of Cardiovascular Anesthesiologists and the American Society of Echocardiography divides the anterior and posterior leaflets into three segmental regions (11). Indentations along the free margin of the posterior mitral leaflet give it a scalloped appearance, allowing identification of individual scallops P1, P2, and P3 (6). The anterior mitral leaflet is also divided into three segments located opposite the corresponding segments of the posterior mitral leaflet: A1, A2, and A3. The P1 and A1 segments are adjacent to the anterolateral commissure, while the P3 and A3 segments are adjacent to the posteromedial commissure (Fig. 13.2) (11).

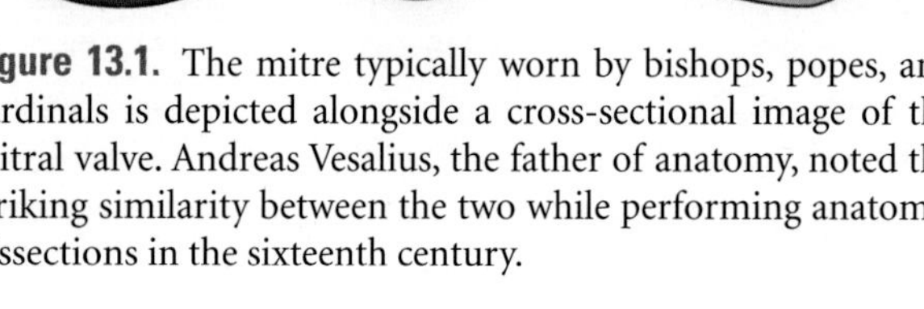

Figure 13.1. The mitre typically worn by bishops, popes, and cardinals is depicted alongside a cross-sectional image of the mitral valve. Andreas Vesalius, the father of anatomy, noted the striking similarity between the two while performing anatomic dissections in the sixteenth century.

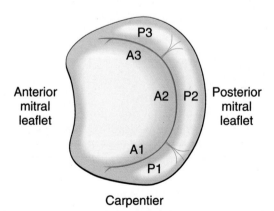

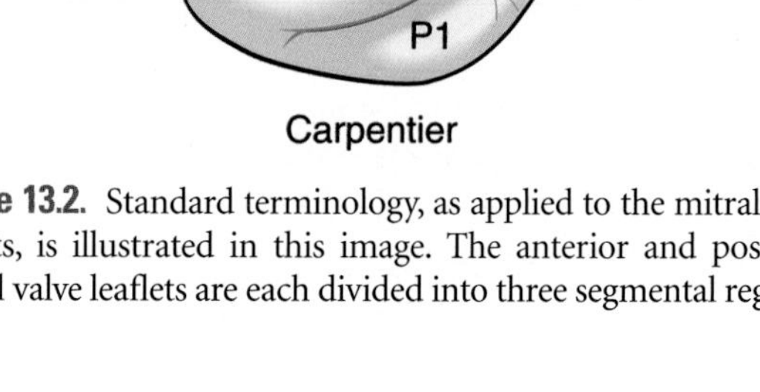

Figure 13.2. Standard terminology, as applied to the mitral valve leaflets, is illustrated in this image. The anterior and posterior mitral valve leaflets are each divided into three segmental regions.

TABLE 13.1	Etiology, Mechanism, and 2D Characteristics of Mitral Valve Dysfunction	
Etiology	**Mechanism**	**2D Echocardiographic Appearance**
Rheumatic heart disease	Retractile fibrosis of leaflet tissue and chordal tendons, resulting in failure of leaflet coaptation	Thickened leaflet tissue and chordal tendons, restricted leaflet motion, calcium deposition
Degenerative	Leaflet prolapse, malalignment of leaflet tissue	Prolapsing/flail leaflet tissue
Ischemic (infarction)	Ruptured papillary muscle	Flail leaflet
Myocardial disease	Dilatation of annulus, reduced surface area for coaptation	Normal leaflet tissue, increased annular dimensions
Congenital	Cleft leaflet, transposed valve	Cleft leaflet, tricuspid valve
Endocarditis	Destructive lesions	Perforation, flail leaflets, vegetations
Hypereosinophilic syndrome	Loss of coaptation	Reduced leaflet motion
Infiltrative disease	Thickened leaflets impair coaptation	Leaflet thickening
Marfan syndrome	Ruptured chordal tendons	Redundant tissue, prolapse, or flail of leaflet tissue
Postradiation	Leaflet thickening impairs coaptation	Thickened leaflets, restrictive leaflet motion
Carcinoid/ergot alkaloids	Fibrosis of leaflets, failure of coaptation	Leaflet thickening and restriction

Modified from Rahimtoola S, Enriquez-Sarano M, Schaff H, Frye R. Mitral valve disease. In: Fuster V, Alexander R, O'Rourke R, eds. Hurst's the Heart. 10th ed. New York: McGraw-Hill 2001, with permission.

STRUCTURAL INTEGRITY OF THE MITRAL VALVE

Mitral Regurgitation

The structural integrity of the mitral valve may be compromised by primary valve pathology or secondary disease processes affecting one or more components of the mitral valve apparatus (12). The primary etiology of mitral regurgitation in industrialized countries is from ischemic and degenerative causes (13). Table 13.1 lists a broad range of disease processes that contribute to dysfunction of the mitral valve.

Carpentier and colleagues categorized mitral valve dysfunction based on normal, excessive, or restrictive leaflet motion range (14). Mitral insufficiency with normal leaflet motion occurs in patients with congenital clefts in the leaflet tissue or those with leaflet perforation due to endocarditis. Mitral regurgitation due to excessive leaflet motion can result from chordal rupture leading to segmental leaflet prolapse. Loss of leaflet tissue from rheumatic endocarditis may lead to restricted leaflet motion and subsequent mitral insufficiency (Fig. 13.3) (15).

Severity Estimation

Echocardiographic grading of mitral regurgitation and determination of ventricular dimensions and functionare integral to clinical decision making with regard to the timing for surgical intervention. Application of severity estimation methods is dependent on the technical expertise of the imaging staff, the complexity involved with the measurement technique, associated limitations with the individual method, and time constraints.

Developed methods of estimation can be partitioned into qualitative, semiquantitative, and quantitative techniques. An integration of these techniques in conjunction with clinical features of the patient's presentation will provide an accurate assessment of regurgitant severity and need for surgical intervention.

Two-Dimensional Echocardiography

Two-dimensional (2D) echocardiography provides anatomic details to assist in delineating the underlying etiology of valve dysfunction. A complete TEE examination

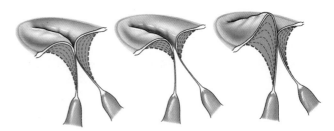

Figure 13.3. Carpentier's classification of range of mitral leaflet motion is depicted in this illustration as normal, restrictive, and excessive leaflet motion, respectively.

of the mitral valve apparatus and surrounding left ventricular myocardium aid in characterizing valve pathology. Enlargement of the left atrium and increases in the left ventricular systolic and diastolic dimensions are changes detected by 2D echocardiography. The 2D changes suggestive of severe mitral insufficiency include left atrial dimensions of ≥5.5 cm and left ventricular diastolic dimensions of 7 cm (16).

The volume overload imposed on the left ventricle is proportional to the severity of mitral regurgitation present. End-systolic chamber size is considered a sensitive marker for imminent ventricular dysfunction. In particular, it is recommended that asymptomatic and symptomatic patients with severe mitral regurgitation and left ventricular end-systolic diameter of 4.5 cm undergo corrective surgical intervention (17,18). The impact of volume overload on the left side of the heart is also dependent on the acuity of mitral regurgitation. Initial phases of severe mitral regurgitation result in a dilated left ventricle with hyperdynamic function and an end-systolic cavity volume, which is small, compared to the end-diastolic volume. Continued volume overload over time will lead to left ventricular dysfunction. Ideally, with echocardiographic guidance, corrective interventions can be implemented prior to the development of significant and irreversible ventricular dysfunction (18).

Qualitative Techniques

Continuous Wave Doppler Signal

Aligning the continuous wave Doppler (CW-Doppler) signal through the mitral regurgitant jet allows visualization of mitral regurgitant signal density and morphology. In general, the signal intensity is reflective of the severity of mitral regurgitation. Mild degrees of mitral regurgitation are detected by CW-Doppler as incomplete envelopes of low CW-Doppler signal intensity, whereas dense complete CW-Doppler signal envelopes of nearly equal intensity to mitral inflow are associated with more severe degrees of mitral regurgitation (Fig. 13.4) (16,19).

Peak E Wave Velocity

Peak E wave velocity as detected with pulsed wave Doppler of the transmitral flow velocity can be qualitatively related to mitral regurgitation severity. When the degree of mitral regurgitation increases, the added regurgitant volume across the mitral valve will increase the pressure gradient between the left atrium and the left ventricle. The increase in pressure gradient, in turn, increases the early mitral inflow velocity (20). Thomas et al. investigated the use of peak E wave velocity as an initial screening variable to identify hemodynamically significant mitral regurgitation. Peak E wave velocity was compared to a qualitative echocardiographic evaluation by an expert as well as with regurgitant fraction measurements. An

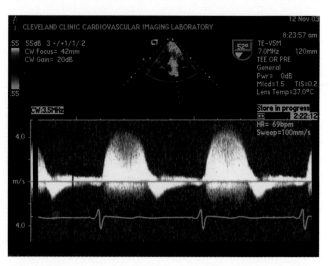

Figure 13.4. CW-Doppler displays a mitral regurgitant jet as a spectral profile represented above the baseline. This regurgitant signal is of nearly equal intensity to antegrade flow through the mitral valve. This qualitative assessment is consistent with the patient's severe degree of mitral insufficiency.

E wave velocity of greater than 1.2 m/s identified patients with severe mitral regurgitation with a sensitivity of 86%, a specificity of 86%, a positive predictive value of 75%, and a negative predictive value of 92% (20).

Semiquantitative Techniques

Spatial Area Mapping

Color flow Doppler is one of the most commonly used semiquantitative methods to estimate the severity of mitral regurgitation (21). Color flow Doppler is based on pulsed wave ultrasound techniques with different signal processing and display formats. Instead of measuring velocities at a single location as with pulsed wave Doppler, color flow Doppler has a number of gates positioned at different depths along many scan lines. Velocity is encoded into different colors based on the direction of flow to or away from the transducer (22). The extent of the velocity map displayed by color flow Doppler is reflective of the velocity of regurgitant flow rather than absolute regurgitant volume (18). In general, color Doppler can quickly differentiate mild degrees from severe grades of mitral regurgitation (Figs. 13.5 and 13.6).

Color flow Doppler estimates of mitral insufficiency correlate well with the semiquantitative angiographic grades of insufficiency (21). Castello et al. compared the correlation between color flow Doppler regurgitant jet area measurements to angiography. A maximal jet area lesser than 3 cm^2 predicted mild mitral regurgitation with a sensitivity of 96%, a specificity of 100%, and a predictive accuracy of 98%; whereas a maximal regurgitant area of greater than 6 cm^2 predicted severe regurgitation with a sensitivity of 91%, specificity of 100%, and predictive accuracy of 98% (23).

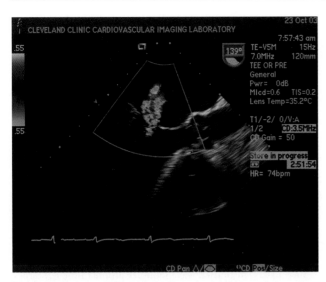

Figure 13.5. The midesophageal long-axis image of the mitral valve displays a mild grade of mitral insufficiency, as represented with color flow Doppler imaging.

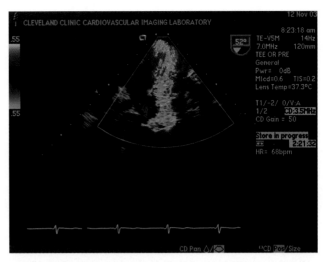

Figure 13.6. The midesophageal two-chamber view depicts severe mitral insufficiency with color flow imaging. The color flow signal extends to the posterior left atrial wall and displays an area of flow convergence on the left ventricular side of the mitral valve.

Spain et al. also reported a good correlation between maximal color flow Doppler jet area and angiographic grades of mitral insufficiency. However, they reported limited correlation between quantitative measurements of mitral regurgitant severity, such as regurgitant volume and regurgitant fraction, with maximal jet area measurements (21).

Rivera et al. compared a visual assessment method, the color flow Doppler jet area method, and regurgitant fraction measurements for grading the severity of mitral regurgitation. The visual assessment method encompassed integrating information about actual jet dimensions and jet eccentricity as well as chamber geometry to provide an educated assessment of the degree of regurgitation present. They reported that the visual grading method had a better correlation with quantitative measures of regurgitation than jet area measurements (24).

Several technical factors influence the appearance of the color flow signal within the left atrium. Among these are instrumentation settings, such as frame rate, gain settings, and transducer frequency (22). Alterations in color-scale settings impact the effect of entrainment of left atrial blood on the regurgitant jet area. Setting the color scale to the highest possible level will limit the effect of entrainment (25). Maintaining constant technical factors reduces instrumentation errors.

Alterations in intraoperative hemodynamics also influence the jet of mitral regurgitation as detected by color flow Doppler (26,27). Grewal et al. (26) reported that slightly more than half of patients with mitral insufficiency improved at least one grade with the induction of general anesthesia. Decreased intravascular volume coupled with a reduction in afterload was thought to contribute to better leaflet coaptation and reduced valvular insufficiency (26).

Compliance and size of the receiving chamber confound the relationship between the size of the regurgitant jet and

regurgitant volume (21). Patients with acute, severe mitral regurgitation may display a relatively small jet area secondary to high left atrial pressures due to limited compliance of the left atrium (18).

Eccentric regurgitant jets when imaged by color-flow mapping commonly occupy less overall area compared to jets of similar flow rates directed centrally within the left atrium (28). An eccentric jet has a different observed morphology as compared to free jets secondary to limited expansion due to impingement of the jet along the atrial wall. Consideration of jet morphology in the color flow Doppler assessment is important to avoid underestimating the degree of regurgitation (Fig. 13.7) (28).

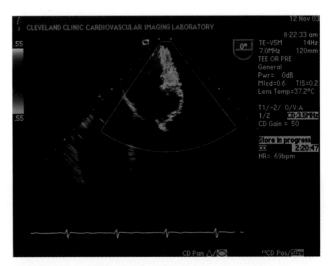

Figure 13.7. Anterior mitral leaflet prolapse results in an eccentric jet of mitral insufficiency, as displayed with color flow imaging from the midesophageal imaging plane. Note the jet of mitral insufficiency is posteriorly directed.

Pulmonary Venous Waveform Patterns

Normal pulmonary venous waveform patterns consist of a biphasic forward systolic waveform occurring during ventricular systole, a forward diastolic velocity waveform that occurs after mitral valve opening, and a retrograde atrial flow reversal waveform that occurs in response to atrial contraction (29). In general, the normal pattern of pulmonary venous flow displays the ratio of systolic waveform to diastolic waveform as greater than or equal to one. Current applications for pulmonary venous waveform patterns include differentiating constrictive pericarditis from constriction, estimation of left ventricular filling pressures, evaluation of left ventricular diastolic dysfunction, and grading the severity of mitral regurgitation (30).

Significant degrees of mitral regurgitation increase left atrial pressure and alter forward flow through the pulmonary veins. Klein et al. (31) investigated the relationship between the ratio of peak systolic to peak diastolic flow velocities in the pulmonary veins and varying degrees of mitral regurgitation as measured with TEE color-flow mapping. The ratio of peak systolic to diastolic pulmonary venous waveform velocities was categorized as having a normal pattern where the ratio of peak systolic/diastolic waveform was greater than or equal to one, a blunted pattern where the ratio of peak systolic to peak diastolic waveform was between 0 and less than 1 (Fig. 13.8), and reversed systolic waveform represented by a peak systolic velocity value of less than 0 (Fig. 13.9). The sensitivity and specificity for reversed systolic flow detecting 4-plus mitral regurgitation were 93% and 100%, respectively. Blunted systolic flow for detecting 3-plus mitral regurgitation had lower sensitivity and specificity of 61% and 97%, respectively (31).

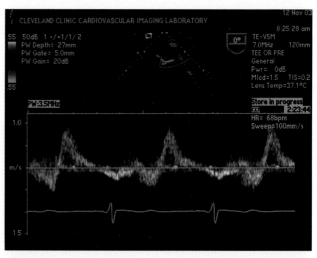

Figure 13.9. This pulsed wave Doppler profile of the left upper pulmonary vein reveals systolic flow reversal, as represented by systolic flow beneath the baseline, which is consistent with severe mitral insufficiency.

Pulmonary venous flow patterns may not be a reliable marker of valvular insufficiency for all grades of mitral regurgitation. Pu et al. evaluated the relationship between pulmonary venous flow patterns and quantitative indexes of mitral regurgitation in patients with variable degrees of left ventricular function. Quantitative Doppler measurements included regurgitant orifice area (ROA), regurgitant stroke volume, and regurgitant fraction measurements. A normal pulmonary venous waveform pattern had a sensitivity, specificity, and predictive value for detecting a small ROA of less than 0.3 cm² of 60%, 96%, and 94%, respectively. The reversed pattern was a highly specific marker for detecting a large ROA of greater than 0.3 cm² with a sensitivity, specificity, and predictive value of 69%, 98%, and 97%, respectively. The blunted pattern was seen in all grades of mitral regurgitation and had low predictive value for grading the severity of mitral regurgitation, particularly in patients with left ventricular dysfunction (32).

Hynes et al. reported similar results regarding usefulness of systolic flow reversal as an indicator of severe mitral regurgitation and a normal waveform pattern confirming the absence of significant mitral regurgitation. They reported that the blunted pulmonary venous waveform pattern was more likely associated with left ventricular abnormalities than mitral regurgitation (33).

Pulmonary venous flow patterns are influenced by a number of factors that include changes in myocardial relaxation (34), abnormal left ventricular compliance, systolic and diastolic dysfunctions, changes in loading conditions, and left atrial compliance and function (29,30,35–40). Other cardiac states that alter pulmonary vein flows include arrhythmias, such as atrial fibrillation (30,41).

Klein et al., in a separate investigation, highlighted the importance of sampling both pulmonary veins when grading mitral regurgitation by TEE. They assessed the

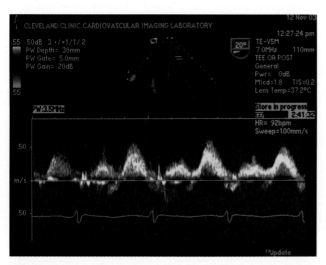

Figure 13.8. A pulsed wave Doppler sample volume placed within the left upper pulmonary vein reveals a Doppler velocity profile that displays a blunted pulmonary venous waveform pattern.

variability between left and right pulmonary venous flows in the assessment of mitral regurgitation. Discordant pulmonary venous flow as measured by PW Doppler TEE occurred between the left and right upper pulmonary veins at a rate of 37% in those patients with 4-plus mitral insufficiency (42).

Schwerzmann et al. reported that combined transmitral E wave velocity and reversed systolic pulmonary venous flow were accurate measures for the determination of moderately severe to severe mitral regurgitation as compared to regurgitant fraction. They reported that reversed systolic pulmonary venous flow with an increased E wave velocity of greater than 1 m/s had the sensitivity of 78% and a specificity of 97% for detecting severe mitral regurgitation (43).

Quantitative Techniques

Among the rationale for the use of quantitative measurements to grade mitral regurgitation are the associated limitations with semiquantitative grading methods. Others have recommended the use of quantifiable methods for patients with greater than mild degrees of mitral regurgitation (44,45).

Vena Contracta

The vena contracta is the narrowest part of the regurgitant jet as imaged with color-flow mapping as the jet emerges from the regurgitant orifice. The flow pattern in the region of the vena contracta is organized into a series of parallel flow lines. As flow gradually moves away from the vena contracta, it becomes more turbulent and disorganized secondary to entrainment of blood by the regurgitant jet within the left atrium (18).

Hall et al. compared the accuracy of the vena contracta width to regurgitant volume and ROA measurements in evaluating the severity of mitral regurgitation. They reported a good correlation between vena contracta measurements and quantitative measures of mitral regurgitation severity. In particular, a vena contracta width of 0.5 cm was always associated with a regurgitant volume greater than 60 mL and a ROA greater than 0.4 cm². A vena contracta width of ≤0.3 cm predicted a regurgitant volume of less than 60 mL and ROA of less than 0.4 cm². They reported a weak correlation between jet area and quantitative measures of mitral regurgitant severity (46).

Grayburn et al. reported that the width of the mitral regurgitant jet at its vena contracta was an accurate marker for severe mitral regurgitation. A width of greater than or equal to 6 mm identified angiographically severe mitral regurgitation with a sensitivity and specificity of 95% and 98%, respectively (47).

Limitations of vena contracta measurements include the associated difficulties with localizing the area of the vena contracta and trouble with obtaining good image quality (18). In addition, there are problems regarding axial versus lateral resolution of the ultrasound imaging system (18). This measurement technique is limited by the lateral resolution of color Doppler, which often is unable to distinguish minor variations in the width of the vena contracta (48).

Regurgitant Orifice Area

The ROA is a reliable quantitative measure of the severity of mitral regurgitation. It can be measured with 2D and pulsed Doppler echocardiography (49) or with the proximal isovelocity surface area (PISA) method (50,51). The PISA method applies the continuity principle to color Doppler mapping in the region of the mitral valve orifice where flow converges toward the mitral regurgitant orifice on the left ventricular side of the mitral valve. As blood flow converges toward the mitral regurgitant orifice, it forms a series of isovelocity shells whose surface area is hemispheric in shape (Fig. 13.10) (16,51,52–55). Color flow Doppler displays a measure of velocity at a specific distance from the regurgitant orifice (Fig. 13.11). By the law of conservation of mass, flow at each layer should be equal to orifice flow because it must all pass through the orifice (52). The maximal instantaneous flow rate can be calculated as the product of the surface area of the hemisphere and the aliasing velocity (V_a):

$$\text{Flow rate} = 2\pi r^2 \times V_a$$

where r is the distance from the regurgitant orifice to the proximal portion of the flow convergence region. Once

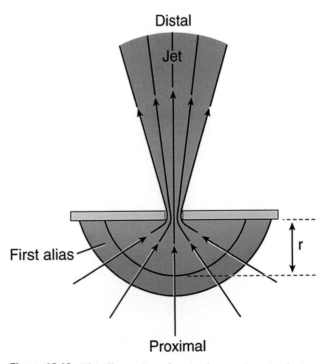

Figure 13.10. This illustration of a mitral regurgitant jet depicts the hemispheric shape of the flow convergence region, where r represents the distance from the regurgitant orifice to the first aliasing boundary.

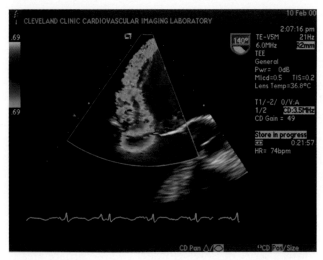

Figure 13.11. The color Doppler display from the midesophageal long-axis image of the mitral valve depicts a large proximal flow convergence region on the left ventricular side of the mitral valve.

the maximal instantaneous flow rate is calculated, the ROA can be calculated as

$$ROA = Flow\ rate / peak\ V_{MR}$$
$$ROA = 2\pi r^2 \times V_a / V_p$$

where V_{MR} is the peak regurgitant velocity of the mitral regurgitant jet. In general, an ROA 0.4 cm² is associated with severe mitral regurgitation (16).

A central assumption with the use of PISA method is that the proximal flow convergence region is hemispheric in shape. When the flow field is constrained, the flow convergence region may become eccentric and assume a non-hemispheric shape (Fig. 13.12). If the flow region is not

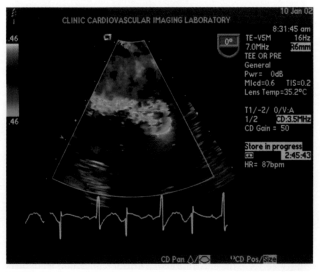

Figure 13.12. This patient with a partial flail segment of the posterior mitral leaflet displays an eccentric flow convergence region from this midesophageal view.

180 degrees and hemispheric symmetry of the flow field is assumed, there will be significant overestimation of calculated flow rates. Adjustments are needed to the equation to account for the angle subtended by the constrained flow region (56).

Improperly identifying the regurgitant orifice, when making radius measurements, will introduce errors in the flow rate and orifice area calculations (51). To circumvent the need to identify the position of the orifice, Sitges et al. introduced the concept of interaliasing distance. The flow rate at any of the multiple flow-convergence zones proximal to the orifice should be equal based on the principle of conservation of mass. With mathematical modeling, a derived radius can be calculated for use in flow convergence calculations that uses the distance between the first and second aliasing boundaries, the interaliasing distance (18,57).

To avoid problems with the variability of the regurgitant orifice throughout the cardiac cycle, use of color M-mode of the flow convergence region can provide a temporal display of the velocity throughout the cardiac cycle (48).

As real-time, three-dimensional imaging technology improves, imaging the entire geometry of the flow convergence region may reduce errors involved in the quantification of mitral regurgitation with the flow convergence method (58).

Pu et al. (59) demonstrated the accuracy of a simplified PISA method in the clinical setting. Necessary assumptions with the use of the simplified formula include assuming that the pressure difference between the left ventricle and left atrium is 100 mm Hg. Recall that when the peak mitral regurgitant jet velocity is 500 cm/s, the peak left ventricular to left atrial pressure difference is 100 mm Hg. Furthermore, if the color-aliasing velocity is set at 40 cm/s, the formula can be simplified as

$$ROA = r^2 / 2$$

where r is the radius of the proximal convergence isovelocity hemisphere.

If the peak jet velocity is greater than 500 cm/s, the ROA will be overestimated; whereas a jet velocity less than 500 cm/s will underestimate the orifice area. Associated limitations of the conventional PISA method similarly apply to the simplified formula (59).

Regurgitant Volume and Regurgitant Fraction

Regurgitant volume and regurgitant fraction are quantitative volumetric measurements that assess the amount of regurgitant volume lost from forward stroke volume. They involve measuring the difference between stroke volumes through the regurgitant mitral valve from systemic stroke volume. Measurement of flow volume through the mitral valve will be greater than volume through a competent reference valve (26). Flow across the mitral valve is calculated as the product of the mitral valve area (MVA) and time velocity integral of mitral inflow, while flow across

TABLE 13.2	Mitral Regurgitation: Severity Estimation		
Method	**Mild**	**Moderate**	**Severe**
Secondary 2D changes	Mild LAE	Moderate LAE	Severe LAE
Spatial area mapping with color Doppler	<4.0 cm²	4.0–8.0 cm²	>8.0 cm²
Pulmonary venous flow profiles	Normal pattern, S waveform ≥ D waveform	Blunted pattern, S waveform < D waveform	Systolic flow reversal, S waveform < 0
Regurgitant volume	30–40 mL	40–60 mL	>60 mL
Regurgitant fraction	10%–30%	30%–50%	>55%
Regurgitant orifice area	<0.2 cm²	0.3–0.4 cm²	>0.4 cm²
Vena contracta	≤0.3cm		0.5 cm

2D, two-dimensional; LAE, left atrial enlargement; S, systolic; D, diastolic; mL, milliliters; cm, centimeters.

the reference valve is the product of the area and time velocity integral of the reference valve (16). The absolute regurgitant volume is dependent on chamber size and hemodynamic variables, such as driving force (18,60).

The regurgitant fraction represents the percentage of stroke volume lost through the incompetent valve and is calculated by dividing the mitral valve regurgitant volume by forward mitral flow and multiplying by 100% (16). In general, a regurgitant volume of greater than 60 mL and regurgitant fraction of greater than 55% are associated with severe mitral insufficiency.

Flachskampf et al. compared color Doppler area, regurgitant jet diameter, ratio of peak systolic to peak diastolic pulmonary venous flow velocities, maximal regurgitant flow rate, and ROA to invasively determine regurgitant stroke volume. Proximal flow convergence and proximal jet diameter measurements had better discriminatory ability for distinguishing between mild and more severe forms of mitral regurgitation than pulmonary venous waveform patterns and color Doppler jet area. ROA and maximal regurgitant flow rate had the best correlation with invasively determined regurgitant stroke volume measurements; a ROA of 0.4 cm² had a 100% sensitivity, 93% specificity, 91% positive predictive value, and 100% negative predictive value for detecting angiographic grade 3 to 4 mitral regurgitation. Proximal jet diameter of 0.65 cm had a 90% sensitivity, 83% specificity, 79% positive predictive value, and a 92% negative predictive value of predicting grade 3 to 4 mitral regurgitation. Color jet area and pulmonary venous flow velocity profiles did not correlate well with invasive measurements of stroke volume in this investigation (61). Estimation methods for grading mitral regurgitation are summarized in Table 13.2.

Figure 13.13 depicts a summary of the anatomy of the regurgitant jet in relationship to a number of estimation methods. Among the techniques, specific aspects of the anatomy of the regurgitant jet are examined: the flow convergence region examines the preregurgitant orifice; the vena contracta examines the mitral regurgitant orifice; color flow disturbance in the left atrium and alterations in the pulmonary venous waveform patterns involve analysis of the postorifice aspect of the regurgitant jet.

Developments in color-coded display for three-dimensional echocardiography, electron beam–computed tomography, and the use of power-velocity integral at the vena contracta may have broader clinical applications in the future (62–64).

Mitral Stenosis

Rheumatic carditis caused by a prior episode of rheumatic fever is the leading cause of mitral stenosis in the adult patient (4,65,66). Uncommon etiologies of mitral

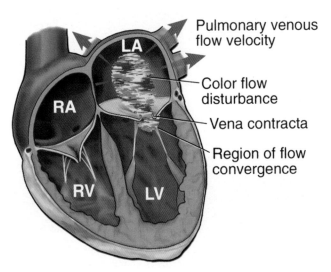

Figure 13.13. A summary of a number of estimation methods commonly used to determine the severity of mitral insufficiency is displayed in this illustration.

TABLE 13.3	Etiology, Mechanism, and 2D Appearance of Mitral Stenosis	
Etiology	**Mechanism**	**2D Appearance**
Rheumatic heart disease	Leaflet and chordal tendon fibrosis and thickening, commissural fusion	Thickened chordal tendons and leaflets, restricted leaflet motion with diastolic doming
Left atrial myxoma	Obstruction to inflow	Large mass obstructing mitral inflow
Severe mitral annular calcification	Calcium deposition	Calcium deposition from annulus to leaflet tissue
Parachute mitral valve deformity	Restricted leaflet opening, causing blood to flow through intrachordal spaces	Chordal insertion into single papillary muscle
Cor triatriatum	Restriction to mitral inflow due to partition within left atrium	Partition within the left atrium

stenosis include severe mitral annular calcification (67), obstructing lesions such as left atrial tumors (68), and congenital deformities such as a parachute mitral valve or cor triatriatum (4,65,69). Table 13.3 displays mechanisms and characteristic 2D appearances for a number of etiologies of mitral stenosis. Figures 13.14 and 13.15 demonstrate an example of subvalvular obstruction secondary to a parachute mitral valve deformity.

Although the mitral valve is the most commonly affected valve in episodes of acute rheumatic endocarditis, rheumatic heart disease may also involve the pericardium, myocardium, and other heart valves (66,69). Mitral valvulitis results in small vegetations along the mitral leaflet closure line accompanied by valve inflammation (69). Diffuse leaflet thickening results from repeated episodes of carditis interposed with episodes of healing, which results in fibrous tissue formation. In addition, a nonspecific

fibrosis and calcium deposition occur as a result of the abnormally deformed valve. There are varying degrees of fibrocalcific fusion of the commissures, contracture and scarring of the leaflet tissue, and fusion and shortening of the chordal tendons.

The rheumatic process advances to varying degrees of mitral stenosis depending upon the number and severity of episodes of rheumatic valvitis. Typically, a time interval of several years intervenes between the episode of acute carditis and the appearance of clinically symptomatic mitral stenosis (66). In advanced cases, the mitral valve may become a rigid, funnel-shaped orifice with an almost complete obliteration of the chordal spaces (4,13,65,66,69).

As the MVA becomes progressively reduced, an increase in the transvalvular pressure gradient, left atrial pressure, and area occur. The left atrial hypertension can, in turn,

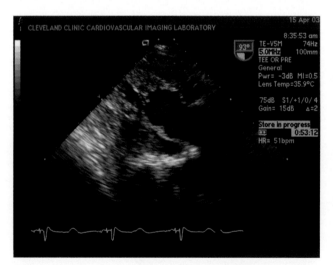

Figure 13.14. The transgastric long-axis image of the mitral valve and subvalvular apparatus is characteristic of a patient with a parachute mitral valve deformity. The chordal tendons insert into a single papillary muscle.

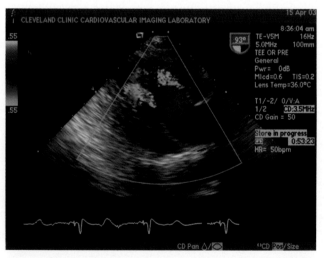

Figure 13.15. Color flow imaging displays highly turbulent inflow amid the intrachordal spaces from this transgastric long-axis imaging plane in the patient with the parachute mitral valve deformity.

result in pulmonary hypertension, right heart dysfunction, and tricuspid insufficiency (4,13,65,66,69).

Two-Dimensional Echocardiography

The 2D characteristics of rheumatic mitral stenosis follow the pathophysiologic features of rheumatic disease process. There is an enhanced echocardiographic appearance of the mitral valve leaflets due to thickening from variable degrees of tissue fibrosis and calcification. The chordal tendons also appear enhanced on the 2D examination secondary to variable degrees of thickening and contracture (4). The mitral leaflets exhibit restricted leaflet motion. Because the leaflets are anchored at the mitral annulus with fusion of the commissures, the midsection of the leaflets is the only section relatively free to move in diastole. This gives the anterior mitral leaflet an arched appearance, convex toward the left ventricular outflow tract in diastole, resulting in a characteristic diastolic doming or "hockey stick" deformity (Fig. 13.16) (70–72). In advanced degrees of leaflet deformity, the valve can become so severely rigid that there is minimal movement of the valve throughout the cardiac cycle.

Standard chamber dimensions are altered depending on the duration and degree of mitral stenosis. Typically, there is an increase in the left atrial area associated with chronic pressure overload. The presence of left atrial spontaneous echo contrast, an indicator of left atrial blood stasis, may identify patients who are at increased thromboembolic risk (Fig. 13.17) (73,74).

Right ventricular enlargement with dysfunction and tricuspid insufficiency may secondarily result from pulmonary hypertension (71). While left ventricular systolic performance in patients with severe isolated mitral stenosis is similar to that of age-matched controls, there are reductions in diastolic compliance of the left ventri-

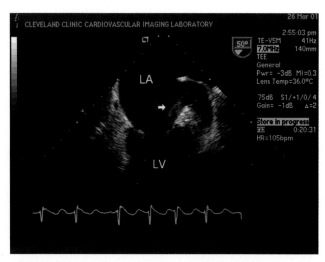

Figure 13.17. Spontaneous echo contrast or smoke is a hallmark for blood stasis within the chambers of the heart. This transesophageal echocardiographic image depicts the presence of smoke within the left atrial appendage in a patient with severe mitral stenosis. Note there is thrombus formation at the mouth of the left atrial appendage.

cle thought to be a consequence of functional restriction from tethering to a rigid mitral valve apparatus (75).

Splitability Score

Components of the splitability score, as described by Wilkins et al. (71) in 1988, are listed in Table 13.4. Wilkins et al. examined a number of clinical, hemodynamic, and echocardiographic variables to predict success following percutaneous balloon dilatation of the mitral valve. The echocardiographic variables assessed mitral leaflet mobility, leaflet thickening, subvalvular thickening, and calcification on a scale from 0 to 4. A summation of the component scores resulted in a range of possible scores of 0 to 16, where the highest score represents advanced leaflet deformity. Among the variables, the value for the echocardiographic score was the best predictor of outcome following percutaneous balloon dilatation of the mitral valve. All patients with an echocardiographic score of greater than 11 had a suboptimal result, whereas all of those patients with a score of less than 9 had an optimal result (71). While developed to determine suitability of balloon valvuloplasty, the splitability score serves as a useful intraoperative guide in assessment of the extent of valvular involvement from rheumatic endocarditis.

Severity Estimation

Pressure Gradient

The Bernoulli equation describes the relationship between velocity of blood flow and pressure gradient. Because we are unable to directly measure intravascular pressure gradients with Doppler echocardiography, the Bernoulli

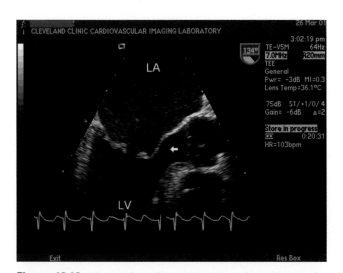

Figure 13.16. The midesophageal imaging plane depicts the classic diastolic doming or "hockey stick" deformity that characterizes leaflet restriction from the rheumatic mitral disease process.

TABLE 13.4	**Echocardiographic Scoring System**			
Grade	**Mobility**	**Subvalvular Thickening**	**Thickening**	**Calcification**
1	Highly mobile valve with only leaflet tips restricted	Minimal thickening just below the mitral leaflets	Leaflets near normal in thickness (4–5 mm)	Single area of increased echo brightness
2	Leaflet mid and base portions have normal mobility	Thickening of chordal structures extending up to one third of chordal length	Midleaflets normal, considerable thickening of margins (5–8 mm)	Scattered areas of brightness confined to leaflet margins
3	Valve continues to move forward in diastole, mainly from base	Thickening extending to the distal one third of chords	Thickening extending through the entire leaflet (5–8 mm)	Brightness extending into midportion of the leaflets
4	No or minimal forward movement of the leaflets in diastole	Extensive thickening and shortening of all chordal structures extending down to papillary muscles	Considerable thickening of all leaflet tissue (>8–10 mm)	Extensive brightness throughout much of the leaflet tissue

Reprinted from Wilkins G, et al. Percutaneous balloon dilatation of the mitral valve: an analysis of echocardiographic variables related to outcome and the mechanism of dilatation. Br Heart J 1988;60:300, with permission.

equation allows us to convert instantaneous velocity of flow across the mitral valve to an instantaneous pressure gradient (76). The Bernoulli equation is

$$P_1 - P_2 = \frac{1}{2}\rho(V_2^2 - V_1^2) + \rho 1\int_1^2 (DV/DT)DS + R(V)$$

Convective acceleration   Flow acceleration   Viscous friction

where $P_1 - P_2$ is the pressure gradient across the valve in millimeters of mercury (mm Hg), P represents the density of blood = 1.06×10^3 kg/m³, V_2 represents the instantaneous velocity of blood distal to the stenotic valve in meters per second (m/s), V_1 represents the instantaneous velocity proximal to the stenotic valve (m/s), DV is the velocity vector of the fluid element along its path, and DS is the path element. A simplification of the Bernoulli equation allows the pressure drop across a stenotic valve to be calculated from the maximal velocity, V_2, as

$$P_1 - P_2 \left(\text{mm Hg}\right) = 4V^2$$

Modification of the original formula involves eliminating terms that account for viscous losses and flow acceleration. In addition, the proximal velocity term can be ignored if the velocity proximal to the stenosis is significantly less than the velocity distal to the obstruction (26,76–78). The accuracy of the modified Bernoulli equation was demonstrated by Hatle et al. in the calculation of the gradient across a stenotic mitral valve (77). Accuracy of the equation has been demonstrated as long as the assumptions have been met: absence of long tubular stenotic lesions (26).

The mean pressure gradient is acquired by tracing the diastolic spectral profile obtained by Doppler interrogation of the inflow velocity across the mitral valve. The mean gradient is then determined by averaging instantaneous gradients across the flow period. Current ultrasound software calculates the mean gradient by integrating the area under the diastolic spectral profile curve (26).

Severe mitral regurgitation can result in high transmitral gradients, even with a mildly stenotic valve secondary to the increase in forward flow through the mitral valve in diastole (79). Technical errors involved with measuring pressure gradients with Doppler involve improper alignment of the sampling beam and the flow vector. The calculated pressure gradient will be underestimated if the angle between the flow vector and sampling beam is too large (54,77). Color-flow mapping of mitral inflow displays a turbulent jet extending at the mitral orifice into the left ventricle in diastole. Aligning the sampling beam with inflow depicted by color flow Doppler errors with improper sampling will reduce beam alignment (53). A mean gradient of greater than 10 mm Hg across the mitral valve is considered severe (16).

Valve Area Calculations

The ultimate goal with each of the methods used to calculate MVA is to provide an echocardiographic-determined valve area as close to the anatomic valve area as possible.

Planimetry

Planimetry involves the direct measurement of MVA with 2D echocardiography. The valve orifice can be visualized from a transgastric basal short-axis imaging plane, where the image is frozen in early diastole to coincide with maximal valve opening. The orifice margins are directly measured by tracing the internal margins of the mitral valve orifice to provide a valve area measurement in squared centimeters (Fig. 13.18) (80–83). Planimetry has been shown to correlate well with invasively determined valve area calculations (72,80–82).

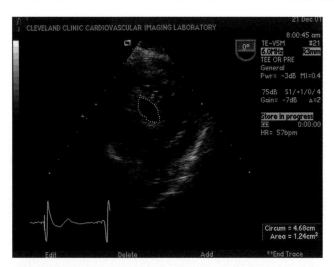

Figure 13.18. This transgastric short-axis image of the mitral valve depicts the use of planimetry as a method for MVA determination. The MVA is greater than 1.0 cm².

Limitations with this technique include technical measurement errors, instrumentation factors, and clinical situations where there is poor image quality. Image resolution is critical to obtaining accurate measurements. Calcification of the valve leaflets may result in significant acoustic shadowing that obscures the valve orifice and interferes with the accuracy of the measurement (83). Inadequate imaging plane orientation will result in errors interfering with the ability to identify the true mitral valve orifice. If the plane of the short axis is not at the tip of the mitral valve leaflets but near the body of the valve leaflet, the valve area will be overestimated (Fig. 13.19) (81–84). Scanning the mitral valve orifice superiorly to inferiorly in order to acquire the smallest orifice area will reduce improper imaging plane orientation errors (81,82,84).

The valve area may be overestimated or underestimated if the gain settings are set too low or too high. If the receiver gain settings are too low, the edges of the valve may be obscured resulting in "echo drop-out" and the valve area will be overestimated (80,84). When the gain settings are set too high, there is image saturation and the valve area is underestimated (84). Finally, valve area may be underestimated in patients who have undergone mitral valvuloplasty secondary to the inability to measure the extent of the commissural fractures with planimetry.

Pressure Half-time

The pressure gradient half-time (PHT) measures the rate of decline in the atrioventricular pressure gradient. It is defined as the time required for maximal diastolic pressure difference to decrease by one half of its initial value. In velocity terms, it is equivalent to the time required for the maximum transmitral velocity curve to decrease by a factor of the square root of 2 (16,85,86). The pressure PHT can be quantitatively related to the severity of mitral stenosis. A normal MVA of 4 cm² allows the atrioventricular flow to reduce the transmitral pressure difference to negligible values in less than 50 ms after the onset of the diastolic rise in left ventricular pressure (86). As the severity of mitral stenosis increases, there is a proportionately slower rate of pressure decline between the left atrium and left ventricle and the atrioventricular pressure gradient is maintained for a longer period of time (16,26,83,85,86). A PHT of greater than 300 m/s is associated with severe mitral stenosis (85–87).

The rate at which the left atrial and left ventricular pressures equalize is a function of the MVA. The pressure half-time method of determining MVA describes the relative diastolic pressure difference between the left atrium and the left ventricle. Increasing PHT occurs with decreasing MVA, independent of the presence of mitral regurgitation (Fig. 13.20) (86).

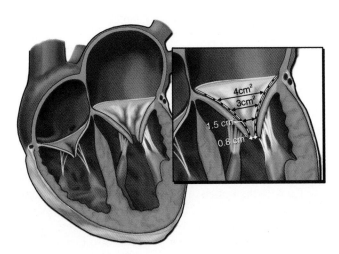

Figure 13.19. This illustration displays the funnel shape assumed by the mitral valve orifice in advanced degrees of rheumatic mitral stenosis. If measurements for planimetry are not taken from the appropriate imaging plane, the valve area will be overestimated as demonstrated in this image.

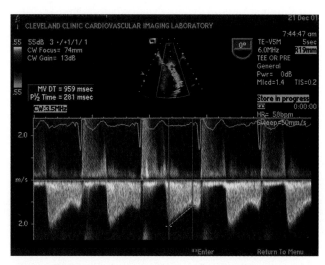

Figure 13.20. This image displays the Doppler profile of a patient with both mitral stenosis and mitral regurgitation. The Doppler spectral profile beneath the baseline depicts a pressure half-time (PHT) measurement of 281 msec, which is consistent with severe mitral stenosis.

Hatle and Angelsen (87) originally described the inverse relationship between the PHT measurement and the calculation of MVA. The mathematic relationship between PHT and MVA is described as

$$MVA\ (cm^2) = 220 / PHT\ (ms)$$

where MVA is the mitral valve area in squared centimeters and 220 is an empirically derived constant.

Potential sources of error should be considered when applying the PHT method in specific clinical settings. PHT is influenced by the peak transmitral pressure gradient and left atrial and left ventricular compliances (88). Conditions that alter left atrial or left ventricular compliance, rapid heart rates, or severe aortic insufficiency will impact the measurement accuracy. Moderate-to-severe degrees of aortic insufficiency cause a rapid rise in left ventricular diastolic pressure with a resultant shortening of the PHT and an overestimation in MVA (89–91).

The PHT may be inaccurate for predicting changes in MVA for several days following mitral valvuloplasty. The transient inaccuracies are due to the abrupt changes in left atrial pressure that occur postvalvuloplasty. Following a few days, the atrial compliance adapts to the acute decrease in atrial pressure (26). Thomas et al. demonstrated inaccuracies of the simple inverse relationship between MVA and pressure half-time in the setting of acute valvotomy. The PHT varied not only with MVA but also with chamber compliance and the peak transmitral gradient. They commented that PHT is determined by more than a simple relationship with MVA and that changes in these other hemodynamic factors contribute to the breakdown in the inverse relationship after valvotomy (92).

Other clinical conditions that limit the accuracy of the PHT method include atrial septal defects, atrial tachycardias, restrictive cardiomyopathies (16,88,91,92), and abnormal compliance, such as severe left ventricular hypertrophy, ischemia, and severe systemic hypertension (79,88,91).

Deceleration Half-time

Deceleration half-time (DHT) is another method to determine MVA by examining the decay of mitral inflow through the stenotic mitral valve. The deceleration time (DT) is defined as the time in milliseconds for the peak mitral inflow velocity to reach baseline. As with the PHT method, as the stenosis becomes more severe, the decay in the pressure gradient to baseline will be prolonged. The inverse relationship between the DHT and MVA is described as (52)

$$MVA\ (cm^2) = 759 / DT\ (ms)$$

where DT is the deceleration time in milliseconds. If the profile of the mitral DT is linear, the PHT is equal to 29% of the DT (16,83).

Continuity Equation

The continuity equation is based on the law of conservation of mass in hydrodynamics (90). Volumetric flow remains constant through the heart valves in the absence of valvular regurgitation or shunts such that flow volume at the mitral valve should equal that at a predetermined reference valve (83,90). The continuity equation is described as

$$Q\ (volumetric\ flow) = Area_1 \times velocity_1$$
$$= Area_2 \times velocity_2$$

$Area_1 \times velocity_1$ represents volumetric flow in the reference valve. The reference area ($Area_1$) is a cross-sectional area measurement that assumes the geometric model of a circle: πr^2. Mean velocities are obtained from the time velocity integrals (TVI) of the spectral profiles generated by Doppler interrogation of the reference valve ($Velocity_1$) and of the mitral valve ($Velocity_2$). The equation is rearranged to solve for the mitral stenotic area, $Area_2$:

$$Area_2 = Area_1 \times velocity_1 / velocity_2$$
$$Stenotic\ area = Flow / velocity\ across\ stenosis$$

The continuity equation provides an accurate measurement of MVA (90). It is particularly useful in clinical situations where the PHT is limited, such as in patients with moderate-to-severe degrees of aortic insufficiency (26,90). The continuity equation is theoretically independent of transvalvular pressure gradient, left ventricular compliance, and changing hemodynamic conditions, such as exercise (88–90). Limitations involve an underestimate of MVA in those patients with concomitant mitral regurgitation secondary to an augmentation of the Doppler measurement of the time velocity integral of the mitral valve (90). In addition, the continuity equation will be inaccurate in circumstances of regurgitation in the reference valve because forward volumetric flows will not be equal (90,93).

Proximal Isovelocity Surface Area Method

The flow convergence method for calculating MVA applies the use of the basic elements of the continuity equation with the addition of a correction factor to allow for constriction of the flow field by the leaflets. A truly hemispheric shell would occur if the surface of the valve was flat with the leaflets apposed at 180 degrees. The angle subtended by the mitral leaflets creates a funnel-shaped surface; an angle correction factor (α/180 degrees) adjusts the hemispheric surface area to avoid introducing errors in the calculation of the volumetric flow rate. The modified formula takes into account the funnel angle formed by the mitral leaflets, where the instantaneous flow rate

(Q) in this region can be calculated as the product of the surface area of a hemisphere ($2\pi r^2$) and the aliasing velocity at the shell (V_a):

$$Q = 2\pi r^2 \times \alpha / 180 \text{ degrees} \times V_a$$

Flow through this region should equal flow through the restricted orifice based on the continuity principle (53–55). Once the flow rate (Q) is calculated, MVA can be obtained with the use of the continuity equation:

$$MVA\ (cm^2) = Q / V_p\ (cm/s)$$

where Q = volumetric flow rate and V_p = peak transmitral inflow velocity. The flow convergence method is best applied when there are limitations associated with the continuity equation and the PHT method and in clinical circumstances in which the 2D images are technically poor, thereby limiting the use of planimetry (56). The accuracy of the flow convergence region method in assessing MVA has been validated in a number of studies (51,94). Accurate measurement of MVA can be obtained with this method in the presence of mitral insufficiency (53,95). Calculation of MVA using the flow convergence method can be time-consuming; however, its accuracy is not influenced by associated mitral or aortic regurgitation (Fig. 13.21).

Flow Area

The flow area technique for calculating MVA utilizes color Doppler to image the margins of the mitral inflow. The central laminar core of the color flow jet at the level

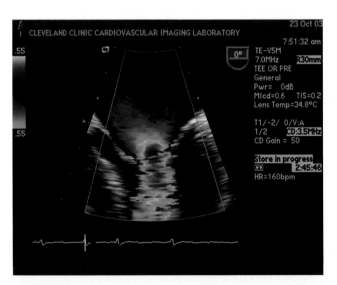

Figure 13.21. The proximal flow convergence region is detected with color flow Doppler on the left atrial side of the mitral valve in this midesophageal imaging plane. Note the area of the flow convergence region is subtended by the mitral leaflets and is not hemispheric in shape.

TABLE 13.5 Techniques for Determining MVA

Planimetry	Trace Frozen Short-Axis View in Diastole
Pressure half-time (PHT$_{msec}$)	MVA = 220/PHT
Deceleration time (DT$_{msec}$)	MVA = 759/DT
Continuity equation	MVA = (LVOT$_{area}$) × (LVOT$_{TVI}$)/(MV$_{TVI}$)
PISA	MVA = $2\pi r^2 \times \alpha$/180 degrees × V$_a$/V$_p$
Flow area	MVA = π / 4 × a × b

MVA, mitral valve area in squared centimeters; α, funnel angle; V$_a$, aliasing velocity; V$_p$, peak transmitral velocity; LVOT, left ventricular outflow tract; TVI, time velocity integral; PISA, proximal isovelocity surface area.

of the stenotic mitral orifice is imaged in two planes perpendicular to one another, producing major (a) and minor (b) diameter measurements of a presumably ellipsoid orifice. The valve area is then calculated by applying the equation for the area of an ellipse:

$$(\pi/4) \times (a \times b)$$

This technique is highly dependent on obtaining good image quality (63,84). Faletra et al. compared direct measurement of anatomic area to planimetry, PHT, PISA, and the flow area method. The flow area method was reported to be the least reliable of the four methods in this investigation (95).

Techniques for determining MVA are summarized in Table 13.5. Table 13.6 provides grades of severity for mitral stenosis with a number of estimation techniques.

TABLE 13.6 Mitral Stenosis: Severity Estimation

Mitral Stenosis Severity			
Measurement	Mild	Moderate	Severe
Mean gradient (mm Hg)	6	6–10	>10
PHT (ms)	100	200	>300
DHT (ms)	<500	500–700	>700
MVA (cm²)	1.6–2.0	1.0–1.5	<1.0

PHT, pressure half-time; DHT, deceleration half-time; MVA, mitral valve area.

■ The mitral valve complex consists of the mitral annulus, anterior and posterior mitral valve leaflets, chordal tendons, and left ventricular myocardium. Structural integrity of the mitral valve requires that all of the elements of the apparatus function appropriately.

■ The comprehensive evaluation of a patient with mitral regurgitation includes the integration of qualitative, semiquantitative, and quantitative TEE assessments along with clinical features of the patient's presentation.

■ Rheumatic heart disease continues to be the primary etiology of mitral stenosis. Characteristics include variable degrees of leaflet and subvalvular thickening, calcium deposition, and reduction in leaflet mobility.

■ The splitability score provides an overall summary score reflecting the degree of leaflet deformity in patients with rheumatic mitral stenosis. Higher scores reflect advanced leaflet deformity.

■ The PISA method may be applied to quantitatively estimate the degree of mitral regurgitation, as well as the degree of mitral stenosis. A correction factor is applied to estimate valve area for mitral stenosis as the angle subtended by the mitral leaflets creates a funnel-shaped surface.

REFERENCES

1. *The Oxford English Dictionary.* 2nd ed. Vol 9. Oxford: Clarendon Press, Oxford University Press, 1989:911.
2. *The Catholic Encyclopedia.* Vol 15. New York: The Encyclopedia Press Inc., 1913:405–406.
3. Ross DN. Historical perspective of surgery on the mitral valve. In: Duran C, Angell WW, Johnson AD, et al., eds. *Recent Progress in Mitral Valve Disease.* London: Butterworth, 1984:5–9.
4. Roberts W, Perloff J. Mitral valve disease: a clinicopathologic survey of the conditions causing the mitral valve to function abnormally. *Ann Intern Med* 1972;77:939–975.
5. Acierno L. Accurate description by dissection. In: Acierno LJ, ed. *The history of cardiology.* New York: The Parthenon Publishing Group, 1994:17–39.
6. Ranganathan N, Lam JH, Wigle ED, et al. Morphology of the human mitral valve: the valve leaflets. *Circulation* 1970;XLI:459–467.
7. Roberts WC, Perloff JK. Mitral valvular disease: a clinicopathologic survey of the conditions causing the mitral valve to function abnormally. *Ann Intern Med* 1972;77:939–974.
8. Perloff J, Roberts W. The mitral apparatus. Functional anatomy of mitral regurgitation. *Circulation* 1972;XLVI:227–239.
9. Edmunds H, Norwood W, Low D. *Atlas of Cardiothoracic Surgery. Mitral Valve Reconstruction.* Philadelphia: Lea & Febiger, 1990.
10. Ranganathan N, Lam J, Wigle E, et al. Morphology of the human mitral valve. II the leaflets. *Circulation* 1970;XLI:459–467.
11. Shanewise J, Cheung A, Aronson S, et al. ASE/SCA guidelines for performing a comprehensive intraoperative multiplane transesophageal echocardiography examination: recommendations of the American Society of Echocardiography Council for Intraoperative Echocardiography and Society of Cardiovascular Anesthesiologists Task Force for Certification in Perioperative Transesophageal Echocardiography. *J Am Soc Echocardiogr* 1999;12:884–898.
12. Gaasch W, O'Rourke R, Cohn L, et al. Mitral valve disease. In: Alexander R, Schlant R, Fuster V, eds. *Hurst's the Heart.* 9th ed. New York: McGraw-Hill, 1998:1483.
13. Rahimtoola S, Enriquez-Sarano M, Schaff H, et al. Mitral valve disease. In: Fuster V, Alexander R, O'Rourke R, eds. *Hurst's the Heart.* 10th ed. New York: McGraw-Hill, 2001:1697–1727.
14. Carpentier A, Deloche A, Dauptain J, et al. A new reconstructive operation for correction of mitral and tricuspid insufficiency. *J Thorac Cardiovasc Surg* 1971; 61:1–13.
15. Cosgrove D, Steward W. Mitral valvuloplasty. In: Cosgrove D, Steward W, eds. *Current Problems in Cardiology.* Vol 14. Chicago: Year Book Medical Publishers, Inc., 1989:353–416.
16. Oh J, Seward J, Tajik A. Valvular heart disease. In: Oh J, Steward J, Tajik A, eds. *The Echo Manual.* 2nd ed. Philadelphia: Lippincott Williams & Wilkins, 1999:103–132.
17. Bonow R, Carabello B, deLeon A, et al. ACC/AHA guidelines for the management of patients with valvular heart disease: executive summary. A report of the American College of Cardiology/American Heart Association task force on practice guidelines (committee on management of patients with valvular heart disease). *Circulation* 1998;98:1949–1984.
18. Irvine T, Li X, Sahn D, et al. Assessment of mitral regurgitation. *Br Heart J* 2002;88:11–19.
19. Utsunomiya T, Patel D, Doshi R, et al. Can signal intensity of the continuous wave Doppler regurgitant jet estimate severity of mitral regurgitation? *Am Heart J* 1992;123:166–171.
20. Thomas L, Foster E, Schiller N. Peak mitral inflow velocity predicts mitral regurgitation severity. *J Am Coll Cardiol* 1998;31:174–179.
21. Spain MG, Smith MD, Grayburn PA, et al. Quantitative assessment of mitral regurgitation by Doppler color flow imaging: angiographic and hemodynamic correlations. *JACC* 1989;13(3):585–590.
22. Edelman SK. *Understanding Ultrasound Physics: Fundamental and Exam Review.* 2nd ed. Bryan: Tops Printing, Inc., 1997:127–163.
23. Castello R, Lenzen P, Aguirre F, et al. Quantitation of mitral regurgitation by transesophageal echocardiography with Doppler color flow mapping: correlation with cardiac catheterization. *J Am Coll Cardiol* 1992;19:1516–1521.
24. Rivera J, Vandervoort P, Morris E, et al. Visual assessment of valvular regurgitation: comparison with quantitative Doppler measurements. *J Am Soc Echocardiogr* 1994;7:480–487.
25. Quinones M, Otto C, Stoddard M, et al. Recommendations for quantification of Doppler echocardiography: a report from the Doppler quantification task force of the nomenclature and standards committee of the American Society of Echocardiography. *J Am Soc Echocardiogr* 2002;15:167–180.
26. Grewal K, Malkowski M, Piracha A, et al. Effect of general anesthesia on the severity of mitral regurgitation by transesophageal echocardiography. *Am J Cardiol* 2000;85:199–203.
27. Konstadt S, Louie E, Shore-Lesserson L, et al. The effects of loading changes on intraoperative Doppler assessment of mitral regurgitation. *J Cardiothorac Vasc Anesth* 1994;8:19–23.

28. Chen C, Thomas J, Anconina J, et al. Impact of impinging wall jet on color Doppler quantification of mitral regurgitation. *Circulation* 1991;84:712–720.

29. Oh J, Seward J, Tajik A. Assessment of diastolic function. In: *The Echo Manual*. 2nd ed. Philadelphia: Lippincott Williams & Wilkins, 1999:45–57.

30. Tabitha T, Thomas J, Klein A. Pulmonary venous flow by Doppler echocardiography: revisited 12 years later. *J Am Coll Cardiol* 2003;41:1243–1250.

31. Klein A, Borski T, Stewart W, et al. Transesophageal echocardiography of pulmonary venous flow: a marker of mitral regurgitation severity. *J Am Coll Cardiol* 1991;18:518–526.

32. Pu M, Griffin B, Vandervoort P, et al. The value of assessing pulmonary flow velocity for predicting severity of mitral regurgitation: a quantitative assessment integrating left ventricular function. *J Am Soc Echocardiogr* 1999;12:736–743.

33. Hynes M, Tam J, Burwash I, et al. Predictive value of pulmonary venous flow patterns in detecting mitral regurgitation and left ventricular abnormalities. *Can J Cardiol* 1999;15:665–670.

34. Nishimura R, Abel M, Hatle L, et al. Assessment of diastolic function of the heart: background and current applications of Doppler echocardiography. *Mayo Clin Proc* 1989;64:181–204.

35. Appleton C, Gonzalez M, Basing M. Relation of left atrial pressure and pulmonary venous flow velocities: importance of baseline mitral and pulmonary venous flow patterns studied in lightly sedated dogs. *J Am Soc Echocardiogr* 1994;7:264–275.

36. Klein A, Stewart W, Bartlett J, et al. Effects of mitral regurgitation on pulmonary venous flow and left atrial pressure: an intraoperative transesophageal study. *J Am Coll Cardiol* 1992;201:345–352.

37. Hofmann T, Keck A, Antigen G, et al. Simultaneous measurement of pulmonary venous flow by intravascular catheter Doppler velocimetry and transesophageal Doppler echocardiography: relation to left atrial pressure and left atrial and left ventricular function. *J Am Coll Cardiol* 1995;26:239–249.

38. Rossvoll O, Hatle L. Pulmonary venous flow velocities recorded by transthoracic Doppler ultrasound: relation to left ventricular diastolic pressure. *J Am Coll Cardiol* 1993;21:1687–1697.

39. Pasierski T, Alton M, Person A. Transesophageal echocardiography characterization of pulmonary vein flow not due to atrial contraction or mitral regurgitation. *Am J Cardiol* 1991;68:415–418.

40. Nishimura R, Abel M, Hatle L, et al. Relation of pulmonary vein to mitral flow velocities by transesophageal Doppler echocardiography: effect of different loading conditions. *Circulation* 1990;81:1488–1497.

41. Keren G, Sonneblick E, LeJemtel T. Mitral annulus motion: relation to pulmonary venous and transmitral flow in normal subjects and in patients with dilated cardiomyopathy. *Circulation* 1988;78:621–629.

42. Klein A, Bailey A, Cohen G, et al. Importance of sampling both pulmonary veins in grading mitral regurgitation by transesophageal echocardiography. *J Am Soc Echocardiogr* 1993;6:115–123.

43. Schwerzmann M, Wustmann K, Zimmerli M, et al. Accurate determination of mitral regurgitation by assessing its influence on the combined diastolic mitral and pulmonary venous flow: just 'looking twice'. *Eur J Echocardiogr* 2001;2:277–284.

44. Pu M, Thomas J, Vandervoort P, et al. Comparison of quantitative and semiquantitative methods for assessing mitral regurgitation by TEE. *Am J Cardiol* 2001;87:66–70.

45. Enriquez-Sarano M, Tribouilloy C. Quantitation of mitral regurgitation: rationale, approach, and interpretation in clinical practice. *Br Heart J* 2002;88:1–3.

46. Hall S, Brickner E, Willett D, et al. Assessment of mitral regurgitation severity by Doppler color flow mapping of the vena contracta. *Circulation* 1997;95:636–642.

47. Grayburn P, Fehske W, Omran H, et al. Multiplane transesophageal echocardiographic assessment of mitral regurgitation by Doppler color flow mapping of the vena contracta. *Am J Cardiol* 1994;74:912–917.

48. Thomas J. Doppler echocardiographic assessment of valvular regurgitation. *Br Heart J* 2002;88:651–657.

49. Enriquez-Sarano E, Bailey K, Seward J, et al. Quantitative Doppler assessment of valvular regurgitation. *Circulation* 1993;87:841–848.

50. Bargiggia G, Tronconi L, Sahn D, et al. A new method for quantification of mitral regurgitation based on color flow Doppler imaging of flow convergence proximal to the regurgitant orifice. *Circulation* 1991;84:1481–1489.

51. Vandervoort P, Rivera J, Mele D, et al. Application of color Doppler flow mapping to calculate effective regurgitant orifice area: an in vitro study and initial clinical observations. *Circulation* 1993;88:1150–1156.

52. Weyman AE. *Left Ventricular Inflow Tract I: The Mitral Valve, Principles and Practice of Echocardiography*. 2nd ed. Malvern: Lea & Febiger, 1994:391–497.

53. Rodriguez L, Thomas JD, Monterroso V, et al. Validation of the proximal flow convergence method: calculation of orifice area in patients with mitral stenosis. *Circulation* 1993;88:1157–1165.

54. Deng Y, Matsumoto M, Wang X, et al. Estimation of mitral valve area in patients with mitral stenosis by the flow convergence region method: selection of aliasing velocity. *J Am Coll Cardiol* 1994;24:683–689.

55. Rifkin R, Harper K, Tighe D. Comparison of proximal isovelocity surface area method with pressure half-time and planimetry in evaluation of mitral stenosis. *J Am Coll Cardiol* 1995;26:458–465.

56. Pu M, Vandervoort P, Greenberg N, et al. Impact of wall constraint on velocity distribution in proximal flow convergence zone. Implications for color Doppler quantification of mitral regurgitation. *J Am Coll Cardiol* 1996;27:706–713.

57. Sitges M, Jones M, Shiota T, et al. Inter-aliasing distance of the flow convergence surface for determining mitral regurgitant volume: a validation study in a chronic animal model. *J Am Coll Cardiol* 2001;38:1195–1202.

58. Sitges M, Jones M, Shiota T, et al. Real-time three-dimensional color Doppler evaluation of the flow convergence zone for quantification of mitral regurgitation: validation experimental animal study and initial clinical experience. *J Am Soc Echocardiogr* 2003;16:38–45.

59. Pu M, Prior D, Fan X, et al. Calculation of mitral regurgitant orifice area with use of a simplified proximal convergence method: initial clinical application. *J Am Soc Echocardiogr* 2001;14:180–185.

60. Tribouilloy C, Enriquez-Sarano M, Capps M, et al. Contrasting effect of similar effective regurgitant orifice area in mitral and tricuspid regurgitation: a quantitative Doppler echocardiographic study. *J Am Soc Echocardiogr* 2002;15:958–965.

61. Flachskampf F, Frieske R, Engelhard B, et al. Comparison of transesophageal Doppler methods with angiography for evaluation of the severity of mitral regurgitation. *J Am Soc Echocardiogr* 1998;11:882–892.

62. Buck T, Mucci R, Guerrero L, et al. The power-velocity integral at the vena contracta: a new method for direct quantification of regurgitant volume flow. *Circulation* 2000;102:1053–1061.

63. Lembcke A, Wiese T, Enzweiler C, et al. Quantification of mitral valve regurgitation by left ventricular volume and flow measurements using electron beam computed tomography: comparison with magnetic resonance imaging. *J Comput Assist Tomogr* 2003;27:385–391.

64. Sugeng L, Spencer K, Mor-Avi V, et al. Dynamic three-dimensional color flow Doppler: an improved technique for the assessment of mitral regurgitation. *Echocardiography* 2003;20:265–273.

65. Olson L, Subramanian R, Ackermann D, et al. Surgical pathology of the mitral valve: a study of 712 cases spanning 21 years. *Mayo Clin Proc* 1987;62:22–34.

66. Selzer A, Cohn K. Natural history of mitral stenosis: a review. *Circulation* 1972;45:878–890.

67. Osterberger L, Goldstein S, Khaja F, et al. Functional mitral stenosis in patients with massive mitral annular calcification. *Circulation* 1981;64:472–476.

68. Nassar W, Davis R, Dillon J, et al. Atrial myxoma. *Am Heart J* 1972;83:694–704.

69. Oh J, Seward J, Tajik A. Cardiac diseases due to systemic illness, medication, or infection. In: Oh J, Steward J, Tajik A, eds. *The Echo Manual*. 2nd ed. Philadelphia: Lippincott Williams & Wilkins, 1999:169–179.

70. Otto C. *Valvular Stenosis: Diagnosis, Quantitation, and Clinical Approach, Textbook of Clinical Echocardiography*. 2nd ed. Philadelphia: WB Saunders, 2000:229–264.

71. Wilkins G, Weyman A, Abascal V, et al. Percutaneous balloon dilatation of the mitral valve: an analysis of echocardiographic variables related to outcome and the mechanism of dilatation. *Br Heart J* 1988;60:299–308.

72. Nichol PM, Gilbert BW, Kisslo JA. Two-dimensional echocardiographic assessment of mitral stenosis. *Circulation* 1977;55:120–128.

73. Daniel W, Nellessen U, Schroder E, et al. Left atrial spontaneous echo contrast in mitral valve disease: an indicator for an increased thromboembolic risk. *J Am Coll Cardiol* 1988;11:1204–1211.

74. Chen YT, Kan MN, Chen JS, et al. Contributing factors to the formation of left atrial spontaneous echo contrast in mitral valvular disease. *J Ultrasound Med* 1990;9:151–155.

75. Liu CP, Ting CT, Yang TM, et al. Reduced left ventricular compliance in human mitral stenosis: role of reversible internal constraint. *Circulation* 1992;85:1447–1456.

76. Feigenbaum H. Hemodynamic information derived from echocardiography. In: Feigenbaum H, ed. *Echocardiography*. 5th ed. Philadelphia: Lea & Febiger, 1994:181–215.

77. Hatle L, Brubakk A, Tromsdal et al. Noninvasive assessment of pressure drop in mitral stenosis by Doppler ultrasound. *Br Heart J* 1978;40:131–140.

78. Oh J, Seward J, Tajik A. Hemodynamic assessment. In: Oh J, Steward J, Tajik A, eds. *The Echo Manual*. 2nd ed. Philadelphia: Lippincott Williams & Wilkins, 1999:59–71.

79. Bruce CJ, Nishimura RA. Clinical assessment and management of mitral stenosis, valvular heart disease. In: Zoghbi WA, ed. *Cardiology Clinics*. Philadelphia: WB Saunders Co., 1998:375–403.

80. Otto C. *Valvular Stenosis: Diagnosis, Quantitation, and Clinical Approach. Textbook of Clinical Echocardiography*. 2nd ed. Philadelphia: WB Saunders, 2000:229–264.

81. Henry WL, Griffith JM, Michaelis LL, et al. Measurement of mitral orifice area in patients with mitral valve disease by real-time, two-dimensional echocardiography. *Circulation* 1975;51:827–831.

82. Wann LS, Weyman AE, Feigenbaum H, et al. Determination of mitral valve area by cross-sectional echocardiography. *Ann Intern Med* 1978;88:337–341.

83. Bruce C, Nishimura R. Newer advances in the diagnosis and treatment of mitral stenosis. In: O'Rourke R, ed. *Current Problems in Cardiology*. St. Louis: Mosby Inc., 1998:127–184.

84. Martin RP, Rakowski H, Kleiman JH, et al. Reliability and reproducibility of two-dimensional echocardiographic measurement of the stenotic mitral valve orifice area. *Am J Cardiol* 1979;43:560–568.

85. Libanoff AJ, Rodbard S. Atrioventricular pressure half-time: measure of mitral valve orifice area. *Circulation* 1968;38:144–150.

86. Hatle L, Angelsen B, Tromsdal A. Noninvasive assessment of atrioventricular pressure half-time by Doppler ultrasound. *Circulation* 1979;60:1096–1104.

87. Hatle L, Angelsen B. *Pulsed and Continuous Wave Doppler in Diagnosis and Assessment of Various Heart Lesions, Doppler Ultrasound in Cardiology: Physical Principles and Clinical Applications*. Philadelphia: Lea & Febiger, 1982:76–89.

88. Wranne B, Msee PA, Loyd D. Analysis of different methods of assessing the stenotic mitral valve area with emphasis on the pressure gradient half-time concept. *Am J Cardiol* 1990;66:614–620.

89. Braverman AC, Thomas JD, Lee R. Doppler echocardiographic estimation of mitral valve area during changing hemodynamic conditions. *Am J Cardiol* 1991;68:1485–1490.

90. Nakatani S, Masuyama T, Kodama K, et al. Value and limitations of Doppler echocardiography in the quantification of stenotic mitral valve area: comparison of the pressure half-time and the continuity equation methods. *Circulation* 1988;77:78–85.

91. Thomas JD, Weyman AE. Doppler mitral pressure half-time: a clinical tool in search of theoretical justification. *J Am Coll Cardiol* 1987;10:923–929.

92. Thomas JD, Wilkins G, Choong CYP, et al. Inaccuracy of mitral pressure half-time immediately after percutaneous mitral valvotomy: dependence on transmitral gradient and left atrial and ventricular compliance. *Circulation* 1988;78:980–993.

93. Karp K, Teien D, Eriksson P. Doppler echocardiographic assessment on the valve area in patients with atrioventricular valve stenosis by application of the continuity equation. *J Intern Med* 1989;225:261–266.

94. Degertekin M, Basaran Y, Gencbay M, et al. Validation of flow convergence region method in assessing mitral valve area in the course of transthoracic and transesophageal echocardiographic studies. *Am Heart J* 1998;135:207–214.

95. Faletra F, Pezzano A, Fusco R, et al. Measurement of mitral valve area in mitral stenosis: four echocardiographic methods compared with direct measurement of anatomic orifices. *J Am Coll Cardiol* 1996;28:1190–1197.

QUESTIONS

1. Standard nomenclature adopted by the Society of Cardiovascular Anesthesiologists and the American Society of Echocardiography applied to the anatomic description of the mitral valve is best described by which of the following?
   A. Anterior mitral leaflet is divided into two segments A1, A2, and the posterior mitral leaflet into three segments labeled P1, P2, and P3.
   B. Anterior mitral leaflet is divided into three segmental regions labeled A1, A2, and A3 and the posterior mitral leaflet into three segments labeled P1, P2, and P3.
   C. Division of the anterior and posterior mitral leaflets into two segmental regions labeled A1 and A2 and P1 and P2.
   D. Division of the leaflet segments by the distribution of the chordal tendons to the individual scallops of the leaflets.

2. Which of the following semiquantitative techniques for assessing the severity of mitral regurgitation is *most* consistent with severe mitral insufficiency?
   A. Continuous Doppler signal that is an incomplete envelope of low-signal intensity
   B. Maximal jet area as detected with color Doppler of less than 2.3 cm²
   C. Reversed systolic pulmonary venous waveform as detected with pulsed wave Doppler
   D. Peak E wave velocity of less than 0.8 m/s

3. Results from the which of the quantitative methods are most consistent with severe mitral insufficiency?
   A. Regurgitant fraction measurement of 10%
   B. Regurgitant orifice area (ROA) of 0.4 cm²
   C. Regurgitant volume of 15 mm
   D. Vena contracta width of 0.3 cm

4. Severe mitral stenosis is most likely indicated by which of the following?
   A. Mean pressure gradient of 4 mm Hg
   B. Mitral valve area (MVA) of 1.7 cm²
   C. Deceleration time (DT) of 200 ms
   D. Pressure half-time of 300 ms

5. Which of the following echocardiographic findings is most likely to lead to an overestimation of MVA?
   A. Heart rate of 120
   B. Severe aortic stenosis
   C. Severe aortic insufficiency
   D. Moderate mitral regurgitation

CHAPTER 14

Assessment of the Aortic Valve

Brenda M. MacKnight ■ Christopher A. Troianos

INTRODUCTION

Transesophageal echocardiography (TEE) is used intraoperatively to evaluate aortic valve (AV) anatomy, function, and hemodynamic perturbations secondary to disease processes. The application of Doppler echocardiography (pulsed wave, continuous wave, and color) with two-dimensional (2D) and three-dimensional (3D) imaging allows for the complete evaluation of stenotic and regurgitant lesions. Real-time 3D TEE is emerging as a new and exciting tool for evaluation of the AV intraoperatively. A recent review supports use of 3D echocardiography to assess AV morphology while identifying vegetations or post procedural changes (1). Qualitative and quantitative assessments provide information for surgical management decisions, type of intervention (repair versus replacement), correction of inadequate surgical repair, and reoperation for complications. Prebypass TEE evaluation also identifies myocardial and other valvular abnormalities associated with aortic valvular lesions and guides the surgeon in the valve size to be implanted. There are several reasons why valve sizing is important. The size of the valve is always a consideration in deciding whether a valve with only moderate stenosis should be replaced. Patients with small annular diameters may not derive a significant benefit from AV replacement. Preoperative valve sizing is also important when valves of limited availability are to be implanted, i.e., homografts (2). For patients undergoing AV replacement for aortic stenosis (AS), intraoperative TEE has been shown to alter the surgical plan in 13% of cases (Table 14.1) (3).

High-resolution images, owing to the close proximity of the valve and the esophagus, permit accurate diagnosis of the mechanism of valve dysfunction, a key aspect for determining the feasibility of repair versus replacement. The vast majority of AVs suitable for repair have regurgitant lesions rather than stenotic lesions. Valve repair for patients with aortic dissection involves resuspension of the cusps and is easily performed and highly successful in the absence of additional leaflet pathology. Valve repair techniques and pathology suitable for repair are discussed in Chapter 32. A consensus statement from the American College of Cardiology, American Heart Association, and American Society of Echocardiography gave intraoperative TEE a Class I designation ("evidence and/ or general agreement that a given procedure or treatment is useful and effective"), in patients undergoing surgical repair of valvular lesions, and a Class IIa designation ("evidence/opinion is in favor of usefulness/efficacy"), in patients undergoing valve replacement for the use of intraoperative TEE (4).

Postoperatively, TEE is used to evaluate the success of repair or function of the prosthetic valve. The degree of residual aortic regurgitation (AR) is an important aspect of valve repair evaluation. It determines the need for further surgery and possible valve replacement. AV replacement is associated with fewer regurgitant jets and smaller than the number of jets and jet area associated with mitral valve (MV) replacement, but the percentage decrease in regurgitant jet area after protamine administration is similar (5). Patients undergoing the Ross procedure for autograft replacement of their AV also require evaluation of the prosthetic pulmonic valve.

TEE evaluation of left ventricular (LV) function is important postoperatively because of the inherent low

TABLE 14.1	Impact of Intraoperative TEE During AV Replacement in 383 Patients
New Findings Before Bypass	**Surgical Impact**
Seven PFO	Two closed
Two masses (TV fibroelastoma, LVOT accessory chordae)	Two removed
Five LAA thrombi	Five removed
Ten homograft annular size measurements	Ten sized
New Findings After Bypass	**Surgical Impact**
One new wall motion abnormality	No change

PFO, patent foramen ovale; LAA, left atrial appendage; TV, tricuspid valve; LVOT, left ventricular outflow obstruction.
Source: Nowrangi S, Connolly H, et al. Impact of intraoperative transesophageal echocardiography among patients undergoing aortic valve replacement for aortic stenosis. J Am Soc Echocardiogr 2001;14:863–866.

ventricular compliance present among patients with LV hypertrophy due to long-standing AS or chronic hypertension. LV volume is more accurately determined by 2D echocardiographic assessment of LV cross-sectional area than by filling pressures measured with a pulmonary artery catheter (PAC) (6). Characteristically, patients with low LV compliance often require volume infusion despite high filling pressures in the post-bypass period, and accurate determination of optimal volume status requires TEE. Clinical information provided by TEE allows appropriate hemodynamic management of patients with AV disease undergoing AV and nonaortic valve surgery before, during, and after general anesthesia.

A comprehensive perioperative TEE examination performed in patients undergoing nonaortic valve surgery may reveal aortic valve disease in patients in whom the diagnosis was not previously apparent. It is important to identify aortic valvular disease because of the surgical and anesthetic implications associated with both AS and regurgitation. The increased population of elderly patients presenting for surgery has increased the prevalence of calcific AS. Identification of significant AS is important for anesthetic management during noncardiac surgery and for surgical management during nonaortic valve cardiac surgery. Aortic valve replacement after previous coronary artery bypass grafting is associated with higher mortality than combined aortic valve and coronary bypass surgery (7). Therefore, it is important to identify even moderate AS during coronary bypass surgery and to consider combination surgery to avoid the higher mortality associated with reoperation.

ANATOMY

A thorough understanding of the anatomy and function of the AV apparatus is important during the intraoperative echocardiographic evaluation of the AV. The AV apparatus is comprised of the left ventricular outflow tract (LVOT), valve cusps, sinuses of Valsalva, and proximal ascending aorta (Fig. 14.1). The three AV cusps are associated with three bulges or pouch-like dilations in the aortic wall called sinuses of Valsalva (Fig. 14.2). Proximal to the AV, the LVOT consists of the inferior surface of the anterior mitral leaflet, the interventricular septum, and the posterior LV free wall. The aortic root begins at the AV annulus, includes the sinuses of Valsalva, and terminates at the sinotubular junction (8). Abnormalities involving any of these structures can lead to AV dysfunction.

A normally functioning AV apparatus allows unrestricted flow of blood from the LV to the ascending aorta during systole and prevents retrograde blood flow from the aorta to the LV during diastole. The pressure change across the AV during diastole generates considerable stress within the leaflets. An intact apparatus allows distribution of this stress from the leaflets to the

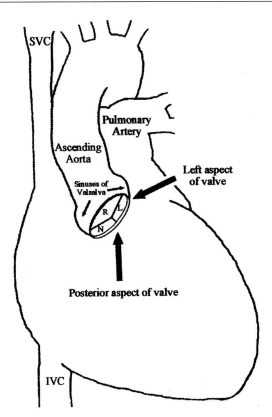

Figure 14.1. Illustration of the anatomic orientation of the AV and Sinuses of Valsalva within the heart. The AV consists of three cusps: right (R), left (L), and noncoronary (N). The right and posterior aspects of the valve are inferior to the left and anterior aspects of the valve. SVC, superior vena cava; IVC, inferior vena cava.

surrounding fibrous structure to which the leaflets are attached. The leaflets are also supported by one another along the region of coaptation on the leaflet called the lunula (Fig. 14.2). The stress is then distributed along the leaflet edges to corners of the commissures (9). Further stress reduction occurs through distribution of stress to the sinuses of Valsalva. The radius of curvature within these bulges in the aortic wall decreases between systole and diastole to accommodate the stress in accordance with LaPlace's law (9,10). The sinuses not only play an important role in leaflet closure by distributing stress, but their presence also prevents the leaflets from making contact with the aortic wall during systole. In addition, because a space is maintained between the leaflets and the aortic wall, the leaflets rapidly close at the onset of diastole (Fig. 14.3). The sinuses provide a reservoir of blood for developing vortices that move toward the ventricular arterial junction as the velocity of blood flow declines during late systole (9). These vortices within the sinuses of Valsalva prime the leaflets for closure, so that as soon as the pressure between the ventricle and aorta equalize, the leaflets rapidly close.

With atrial contraction and LV filling during late diastole, a 12% expansion of the aortic root is observed 20 to 40 ms prior to AV opening (9,11,12). Expansion

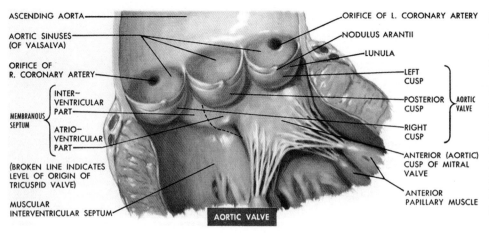

Figure 14.2. Illustration of the AV apparatus opened anteriorly to show the three cusps, LVOT, ascending aorta, and annulus. The lunula on each cusp provides overlap during coaptation and serves to distribute stress from the leaflets to the commissures. Note the close proximity of the anterior mitral valve leaflet (From Netter FH. *Heart, The Ciba Collection of Medical Illustrations*, Vol 5. New York: Ciba Pharmaceutical Company, 1978, with permission).

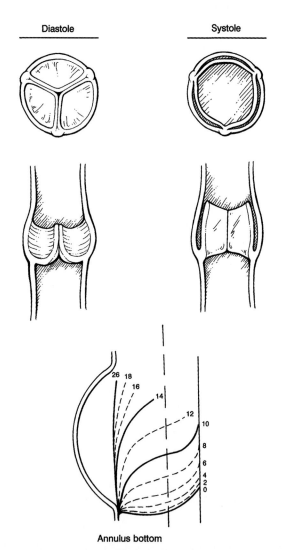

Figure 14.3. Positions of the AV leaflets at end diastole and end systole and of a single leaflet in profile during ejection as the leaflet moves from the closed position [0] to full opening [26]. Note how the fully opened leaflet tends to produce a uniform diameter above the ventricular-arterial junction to reduce turbulence that otherwise would be increased by the sinuses of Valsalva (From Mihaljevic T, Paul S, et al. Pathophysiology of aortic valve disease. In: Cohn L, Edmunds L Jr, eds. *Cardiac Surgery in the Adult*. New York: McGraw-Hill, 2003:791–810, with permission).

of the aortic root alone contributes 20% to leaflet opening (9). The effect of this aortic root expansion actually causes the leaflets to open before any positive pressure from ventricular contraction is applied (9,13). As previously mentioned, leaflet stress during diastole is distributed along the leaflet edges, to the commissures, and to the aortic root. Just before the onset of systole, with no tension within the leaflets and the aortic root expanded, the leaflets open rapidly with the onset of ventricular contraction, offering minimal resistance to LV ejection (9,14).

All components of the AV apparatus are important for the proper function and durability of the valve. Any disruption of these mechanisms within the apparatus will lead to valve dysfunction and premature deterioration. A complete understanding of these mechanisms is a requirement for both the valve-repairing surgeon and the echocardiographer. The echocardiographer must accurately interpret findings and communicate the data effectively with the surgeon. In turn, the surgeon must understand the implications of these findings and the impact of potential surgical intervention on the patient's perioperative outcome and long-term survival.

APPROACH

The AV is imaged using four cross-sectional views (15). The anatomic plane of the AV is oblique compared with the esophageal axis, which is longitudinal within the body. The right, posterior aspect of the valve is inferior to the left, anterior aspect of the valve (Fig. 14.1). The implication for TEE imaging is that the transducer must be flexed anteriorly and to the left from the transverse plane of the patient, to align the imaging plane with the plane of the AV. Alternatively, a multiplane TEE probe is rotated forward to between 30 and 60 degrees with anteflexion to develop the midesophageal AV short-axis (ME AV SAX) view (Figs. 14.4 and 14.5). A normal AV imaged with 2D and 3D TEE in the ME AV SAX view reveals three cusps of similar size and shape. The interatrial septum

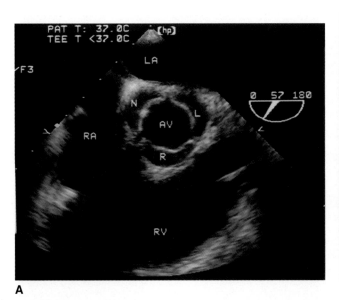

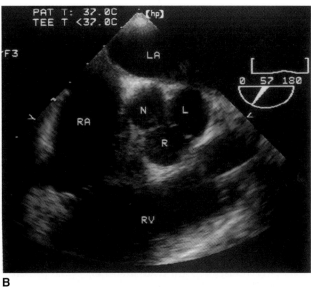

A   B

Figure 14.4. Transesophageal echocardiogram of the ME AV SAX view during systole (**A**) and diastole (**B**). A multiplane probe at 57 degrees provided this view in which all three AV cusps are similar in size and appearance, indicating a true short-axis cross section. The AV is identified by the right (R), left (L), and noncoronary (N) cusps. LA, left atrium; RA, right atrium; RV, right ventricle.

attaches to the aortic wall near the noncoronary cusp. The left coronary cusp is displayed on the right side of the screen. The right coronary cusp is the most anterior cusp and displayed below the noncoronary and left cusps on the image display. This view is important for tracing the AV orifice area using planimetry (Fig. 14.6) and for identifying the site of AR using color flow Doppler (Fig. 14.7).

Rotating the multiplane angle forward to between 110 and 150 degrees (orthogonal to the short-axis view) develops the midesophageal AV long-axis (ME AV LAX) view (Figs. 14.8 and 14.9). This view provides imaging of

the LVOT, AV, aortic root, and ascending aorta. A normal AV appears as two thin lines that open parallel to the aortic walls during systole. The far-field right coronary cusp is the most anterior cusp and is viewed along the anterior aortic wall during systole. The near-field posterior cusp is either the noncoronary cusp or the left coronary cusp depending upon probe orientation and associated structures intersected by the ultrasound beam (15). The ME AV LAX view allows the echocardiographer to differentiate between valvular from subvalvular and supravalvular pathology and provides valuable insight into the function of the AV apparatus.

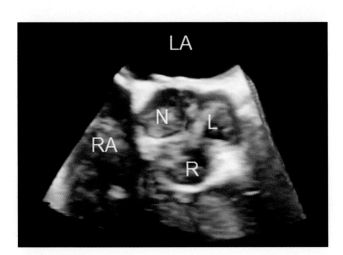

Figure 14.5. The 3D transesophageal echocardiogram of the ME AV SAX view of a normal AV during diastole. The AV is identified by the right (R), left (L), and noncoronary (N) cusps. RA, right atrium; LA, left atrium.

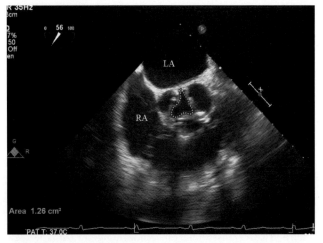

Figure 14.6. Transesophageal echocardiogram of the ME AV SAX view with the multiplane angle at 56 degrees is used for planimetry of the AV orifice in a patient with moderate AS, as indicated by the measured area of 1.26 cm². LA, left atrium; right atrium.

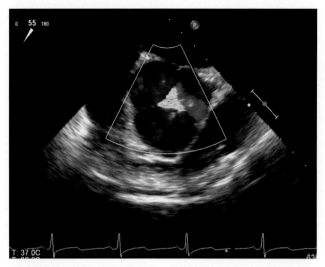

Figure 14.7. Transesophageal echocardiogram of the ME AV SAX view with the multiplane angle at 55 degrees and color flow Doppler in a patient with AR. The origin of the AR is predominantly central.

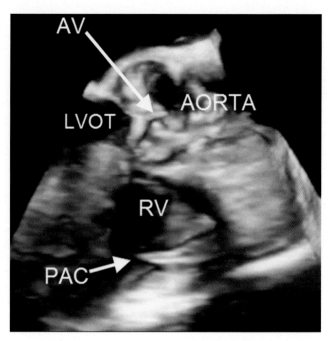

Figure 14.9. The 3D transesophageal echocardiogram of the ME AV LAX view during diastole with the AV *arrow* indicating the AV leaflet tips during diastole. LVOT, left ventricular outflow tract; RV, right ventricle; AORTA, ascending aorta; PAC, pulmonary artery catheter.

The ME AV LAX view is used to measure the AV annulus, LVOT, and aortic root dimensions (Fig. 14.10). These measurements assist with surgical management decisions and guide prosthetic valve sizing. While some use the inner-edge-to-inner-edge technique, most published echocardiographic data describe the leading edge technique and is therefore preferred. The AV annulus is measured between the leaflet hinge points, inner edge to inner edge. An American Society of Echocardiography task force on chamber quantification

recommended that all measurements be made from 2D images rather than using M-mode because the latter usually underestimates dimensions (16).

The deep transgastric long-axis (deep TG LAX) view is developed from the transgastric mid-short-axis view by

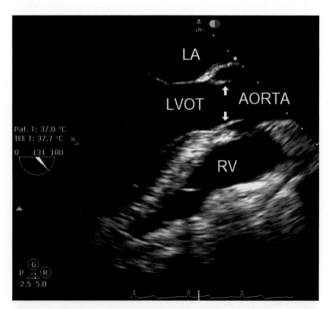

Figure 14.8. Transesophageal echocardiogram of the ME AV LAX view during systole with the multiplane angle at 131 degrees of a normal AV with leaflets (*arrows*) that open parallel to the aortic walls. The proximal ascending aorta is also imaged in this view. LA, left atrium; LVOT, left ventricular outflow tract; RV, right ventricle.

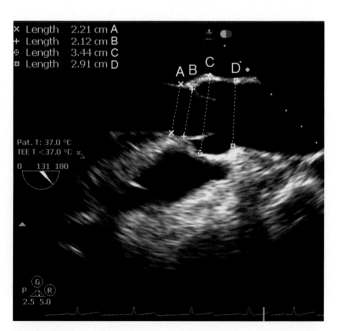

Figure 14.10. Transesophageal echocardiogram of the ME AV LAX view during systole at a multiplane angle of 131 degrees with LVOT (*A*), AV annulus (*B*), sinus of Valsalva (*C*), and sinotubular junction (*D*) measurements.

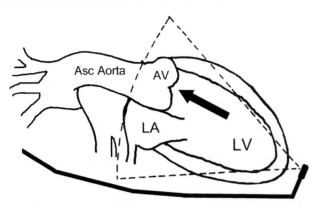

Figure 14.11. Illustration of the TEE probe position for the deep TG view of the AV that allows a parallel orientation of blood flow through the AV and LVOT (*arrow*). LA, left atrium; LV, left ventricle; Asc, ascending aorta (From Troianos CA. Aortic valve. In: Konstadt SN, Shernan S, Oka Y, eds. *Clinical Transesophageal Echocardiography: A Problem-Oriented Approach.* 2nd ed. Philadelphia, Lippincott-Williams & Wilkins, 2003, with permission).

advancing the probe and flexing the probe to the left (Fig. 14.11) until the AV is viewed in the middle or left side of the image in the far field (Fig. 14.12). The transgastric long-axis (TG LAX) view is developed from the TG mid-short-axis view by rotating the transducer forward from 0 degrees to between 90 and 120 degrees until the AV is viewed in the right far field (Fig. 14.13). Assessment of antegrade and retrograde AV velocity requires a parallel orientation of blood flow and the Doppler beam (Fig. 14.14). The ME views are not suitable for velocity measurements because blood flow is perpendicular to the Doppler beam. Conversely, the two TG views allow interrogation of flow across the AV but are

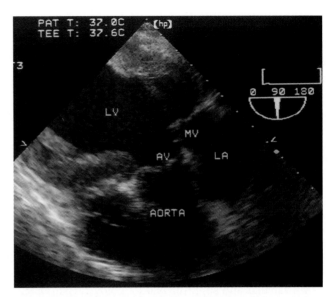

Figure 14.13. Transesophageal echocardiogram of the TG long-axis view developed at a multiplane angle of 90 degrees. AV, aortic valve; AORTA, ascending aorta; LA, left atrium; MV, mitral valve; LV, left ventricle.

not as useful for detailed 2D or 3D anatomic assessment due to the far-field location of the AV. It is important for the echocardiographer to become familiar with developing both TG views, because they are often difficult to obtain and require considerable practice and expertise. The learning curve required for measuring AV blood flow velocity with the TG approach was established by Stoddard et al., who demonstrated a 56% success rate among the first 43 patients studied as compared with an 88% success rate among the latter 43 patients studied (17).

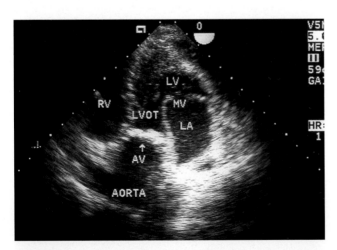

Figure 14.12. Transesophageal echocardiogram of the deep TG long-axis view developed at a multiplane angle of 0 degrees. AV, aortic valve; LA, left atrium; LV, left ventricle; LVOT, left ventricular outflow tract; AORTA, ascending aorta; MV, mitral valve, RV, right ventricle.

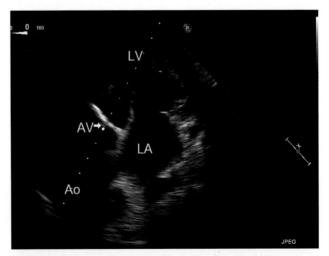

Figure 14.14. Transesophageal echocardiogram of the deep TG long-axis view of the AV, which allows parallel orientation between AV flow and the continuous wave Doppler beam. LA, left atrium; LV, left ventricle; Ao, ascending aorta.

AORTIC STENOSIS

Pathophysiology

The most common causes of AS are calcific stenosis of the elderly (Figs. 14.15 and 14.16), rheumatic valvulitis and congenital abnormalities, including bicuspid (Fig. 14.17) and rarely unicuspid (Fig. 14.18) or quadricuspid valves. An infrequent cause of AS in the United States is the commissural fusion seen with rheumatic disease, which remains a common cause of AS throughout the world. Subaortic stenosis (subaortic membrane or ridge, asymmetric septal hypertrophy) and supravalvular stenosis (narrowed aortic root) mimic AS but do not represent true valvular stenosis. Many of the echocardiographic techniques used for hemodynamic assessment of the AV, however, can also be used to evaluate the severity of subvalvular and supravalvular pathology. Asymmetric septal hypertrophy or hypertrophic obstructive cardiomyopathy is discussed in another chapter.

The mechanism of AS among elderly patients and in congenitally abnormal valves is progressive calcification of the leaflets. Distorted flow through the diseased valve leads to degenerative changes in the cusps, which predisposes the valve to progressive calcification. The rate of calcification and stenosis varies widely, although elderly men with associated coronary artery disease, and patients with a smoking history, hypercholesterolemia, and elevated serum creatinine levels, demonstrate more rapid disease progression (18–21). Many experts feel that the development of AS is an active process, which involves chronic inflammation that is fueled by atherosclerotic risk factors (22).

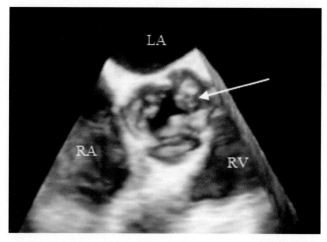

Figure 14.16. The 3D transesophageal echocardiogram of the ME AV SAX view during systole in a patient with moderate AS. Arrow, calcified AV leaflet; LA, left atrium; RA, right atrium; RV, right ventricle.

Calcific AS of the elderly typically occurs in patients older than 65 years of age while younger patients with AS typically have a congenital bicuspid aortic valve (BAV), which secondarily calcifies. BAV is the most common congenital cardiac anomaly in adults, with an incidence of 1% to 2% in the general adult population. It is associated with significant morbidity and mortality after the fourth decade of life (23).

There are three morphologic subtypes of BAV, each with prognostic implications. Type I BAV, characterized by right-left leaflet fusion, is the most common, occurring in 70% of patients with BAV (24). This subtype is associated with

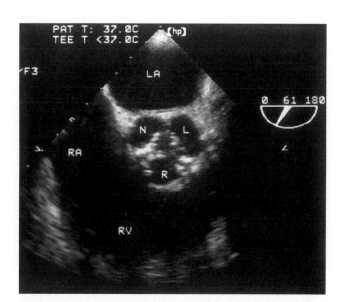

Figure 14.15. Transesophageal echocardiogram of the ME AV SAX view during systole in a patient with AS. L, left, R, right, and N, noncoronary, AV cusps; LA, left atrium; RA, right atrium; RV, right ventricle.

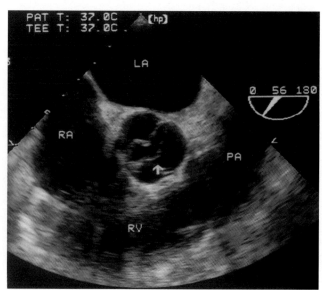

Figure 14.17. Transesophageal echocardiogram of the ME AV SAX view in a patient with a bicuspid AV. Arrow, bicuspid AV; LA, left atrium; RA, right atrium; RV, right ventricle; PA, pulmonary artery.

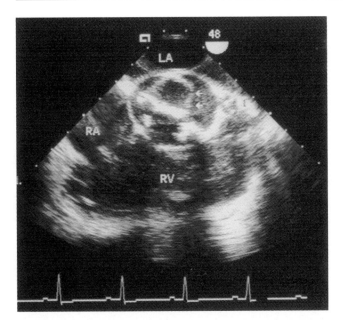

Figure 14.18. Transesophageal echocardiogram of the ME AV SAX view in a patient with a unicuspid AV as indicated by the arrows. LA, left atrium; RA, right atrium; RV, right ventricle (From Troianos CA. Perioperative echocardiography. In: Troianos CA, ed. *Anesthesia for the Cardiac Patient.* St. Louis: Mosby, 2002, with permission).

a high incidence of coarctation and cardiac anomalies, including patent ductus arteriosus, ventricular septal defects, and coronary variants (24,25). Fusion of the right and noncoronary cusps, type II BAV, is associated with more frequent valvular degeneration and greater rate of progression for both stenosis and regurgitation. Fusion of the left and noncoronary cusps, type III BAV, is quite rare (26). Although an older autopsy study demonstrated an aortic coarctation incidence of 5% among patients with a BAV (27), a more recent study in children with a BAV showed a coarctation incidence between 12% and 44%. This study also demonstrated that the incidence is higher among children with Type I BAV, as compared to Type II BAV (28). Approximately 40% of patients, diagnosed with coarctation of the aorta, will have an associated bicuspid valve (29).

A high prevalence of aortic root dilation has been demonstrated in patients with BAV, irrespective of valvular hemodynamics or age, suggesting a common developmental defect (30). BAV is also associated with increased ascending aortic diameter in patients greater than 40 years of age (31). The progression of ascending aortic dilation has been shown to continue after valve repair, leading to the suggestion that during surgery for BAV disease, consideration should be given to concomitant replacement of the ascending aorta (32).

Intraoperative echocardiography is not only critical in the evaluation of AV disease but also in the evaluation of cardiac and vascular structures that are affected by AS. Evaluation of LV function is important because patients with AS develop LV hypertrophy, decreased LV compliance, and are prone to myocardial ischemia, even in the absence of

coronary artery disease. Patients with AS commonly have LV hypertrophy, which is an adaptive mechanism in response to chronic pressure overload. Increased wall thickness reduces wall stress by distributing the pressure overload over greater myocardial mass, as indicated by La Place's Law:

$$\text{Wall stress} = \frac{\text{Pressure} \times \text{volume}}{\text{Wall thickness}}$$

The major perioperative implication is that estimates of LV filling pressure are not reliable indicators of volume loading because of the associated decreased LV compliance. The second major concern is the development of systolic anterior motion (SAM) of the MV because of the septal hypertrophy after AV replacement for AS. Although this condition is well recognized with asymmetric septal hypertrophy, SAM can also occur in patients with symmetric septal hypertrophy after AV replacement. This is usually a manifestation of the abrupt reduction in LV afterload associated with an underfilled LV in patients with septal or concentric hypertrophy. The condition usually resolves with administration of volume, phenylephrine, and discontinuation of inotropic and chronotropic medications, and the condition must be excluded in all patients after AV replacement. Echocardiographic evaluation of the MV and LVOT can predict the likelihood of SAM occurring based upon anatomic factors (33).

Patients with AS also manifest diastolic dysfunction with long-standing disease. Mitral inflow and pulmonary venous flow patterns are examined in order to determine the severity of diastolic dysfunction. Systolic function is preserved until late in the disease progression when LV dilation develops. Systolic dysfunction due to AS is usually reversible with valve replacement, but systolic dysfunction due to myocardial infarction may not improve and causes an underestimation of the severity of AS by gradient determination.

Echocardiographic Evaluation of Aortic Stenosis

Intraoperative echocardiography is used to differentiate AV disease from other conditions that lead to the development of a gradient between the LV and aorta, such as hypertrophic obstructive cardiomyopathy and supravalvular stenosis. For patients in whom the preoperative diagnosis of AV disease is well established, the intraoperative evaluation of the AV usually entails confirmation of the preoperative findings, identifying the etiology of valve dysfunction, estimating the size of the valve to be implanted, and identifying other cardiac pathology. Severe AS may simply be confirmed by a 2D echocardiographic evaluation of the valve utilizing the ME AV SAX view (Fig. 14.15). Although this view permits evaluation of leaflet motion, calcification, commissural fusion, and leaflet coaptation, multiple views, and other modalities (i.e., Doppler echocardiography) should be utilized for definitive diagnosis of AS. Application of color flow Doppler to this image can be used to identify the site of AR if present (Fig. 14.7).

This ME AV SAX view is used for measuring the AV orifice area by 2D planimetry (Fig. 14.6), which provides good correlation with other methods used for assessment of AS (34). It is important to manipulate the probe to develop the image with the smallest orifice size to ensure that the cross section is of the leaflet edges. A cross section that is oblique or inferior to the leaflet tips overestimates the orifice size (Fig. 14.19). In a true short-axis cross section, the valve should appear relatively circular and all three cusps appear equal in shape. Multiplane TEE simplifies the location of the actual orifice by imaging the AV, first in long axis to identify the smallest orifice at the leaflet tips. The orifice is centered on the image display screen and the transducer position is stabilized within the esophagus as the multiplane angle is rotated backward to the short-axis view. The smallest orifice is traced, and the 2D cross-sectional area is displayed. Planimetric measurement of the anatomic AV orifice area provides quantification of the severity of stenosis, but the leaflet edges are often difficult to identify if the valve is heavily calcified. Limitations to this technique are the inability to obtain a true short-axis view, heavy calcification, and the presence of "pinhole" AS, in which the valve orifice cannot be identified. The mere presence of these limitations suggests advanced disease and favors a decision to replace the valve. The ME AV SAX view is also useful for the identification of congenital abnormalities, including bicuspid (Fig. 14.17) and unicuspid (Fig. 14.18) valves.

Developing the ME AV LAX view by rotating the multiplane angle forward to 110–150 degrees provides imaging of AV leaflet excursion in relation to the aorta. An important sign of AS is leaflet doming during systole (Fig. 14.20).

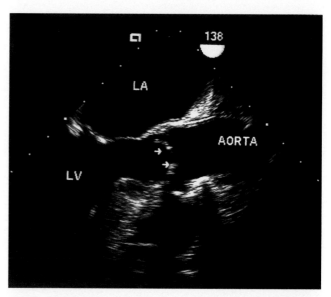

Figure 14.20. Transesophageal echocardiogram of the ME AV LAX view during systole in a patient with AS. A multiplane probe at 138 degrees provided this view of an AV with doming leaflets (*arrows*). Leaflet doming is a qualitative sign of stenosis. The proximal ascending aorta is also imaged in this view. LA, left atrium; LV, left ventricle.

The leaflets are curved toward the midline of the aorta instead of parallel to the aortic wall as demonstrated in Figure 14.8. Leaflet doming is such an important observation that this finding alone is sufficient for the qualitative diagnosis of AS. Coincident with doming is reduced leaflet separation (<15 mm), which is appreciated in both the short- and long-axis views of the AV. In the ME AV LAX view, leaflet separation less than 8 mm has a 100% predictive value of diagnosing moderate to severe AS. It is difficult to further delineate AS severity using leaflet separation because there is significant overlap between groups (35).

The 2D evaluation of the AV may confirm the diagnosis of AS in patients with severe restriction and calcification, but patients with a diagnosis of moderate AS, who are not pre-determined to undergo an AV replacement, require more sophisticated evaluation of their AV disease. Evaluation of the severity of AV disease should include more than one method and be performed by an echocardiographer with advanced training, if the findings will be used to guide surgical intervention (36). The severity of AS can be determined by planimetry using 2D echocardiography (AV area), measurement of transaortic velocity using Doppler echocardiography (gradient), and the continuity equation (AV area) with AS grading results summarized in Table 14.2 (37,38).

Measurement of antegrade and retrograde AV blood velocity requires a parallel orientation of blood flow in the LVOT and the Doppler beam to determine a gradient. As previously mentioned, the ME views used for 2D evaluation are not suitable for this measurement. Either one or both of the TG views (deep TG LAX or TG LAX) are used to measure the velocity of blood flow through the AV and LVOT because of the parallel orientation with the Doppler

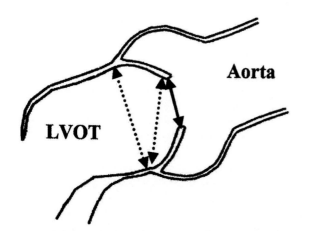

Figure 14.19. Illustration of various cross sections that may be used to perform planimetry measurements of AV orifice size. The solid line indicates the correct cross section at the tips of the aortic cusps. The two dotted lines indicate an oblique cross section and a cross section that is inferior to the leaflet tips, both would result in an overestimation of AV orifice size (From Troianos CA. Perioperative echocardiography. In: Troianos CA, ed. *Anesthesia for the Cardiac Patient.* St. Louis: Mosby, 2002, with permission).

TABLE 14.2	Grading Aortic Stenosis		
Indicator	Mild	Moderate	Severe
Peak jet velocity (m/s)	<3.0	3.0–4.0	>4.0
Mean gradient (mm Hg)	<25	25–40	>40
Valve area (cm²)	1.5	1.0–1.5	<1.0
• Planimetry			
• Continuity equation			
Valve area index (cm²/m²)			<0.6

Sources: Bonow R, Carabello B, et al. ACC/AHA 2006 guidelines for the management of patients with valvular heart disease: a report of the American College of Cardiology/American Heart Association task force on practice guidelines. J Am Coll Cardiol 2006;48:e1–e148; Oh J, Talerico C, et al. Prediction of severity of aortic stenosis by Doppler aortic valve area determination: prospective Doppler catheterization correlation in 100 patients. J Am Coll Cardiology 1988;11:1227–1234.

beam. The continuous wave Doppler cursor is aligned with the narrow, turbulent, high-velocity jet through the AV, and the spectral Doppler display is activated. Accurate localization provides a distinctive audible sound and high velocity (>3 m/s) spectral Doppler recording that exhibits a fine feathery appearance and a mid systolic peak (Fig. 14.21). Normal AVs have peak velocities of 0.9 to 1.7 m/s in adults and peak in early systole. Planimetry of the spectral envelope yields the velocity time integral (VTI) and an estimate of peak and mean AV gradients. More dominant and dense lower velocities are also evident

on the spectral Doppler display of patients with AS and represent the more laminar, lower velocities in the LVOT.

A gradient across a stenotic orifice is dynamic because of its dependence on flow. As the flow (or cardiac output) through the valve decreases, the gradient also decreases. Conversely, as flow or the force of contraction increases, the gradient also increases. Pressure gradients preoperatively obtained with transthoracic echocardiography utilize the same principles as intraoperative TEE. However, the intraoperative loading conditions, heart rate, and force of contraction may differ markedly from preoperative conditions, yielding disparate gradient data. Doppler-derived gradients also differ from gradients obtained in the cardiac catheterization lab because of the differing techniques employed for gradient determination. A Cath-lab gradient is usually a peak-to-peak gradient, which represents the difference between the peak LV pressure and the peak aortic pressure. A Doppler gradient, however, is a "peak instantaneous" gradient, which is greater than the peak-to-peak gradient (Fig. 14.22). It is also important to correctly identify the origin of the gradient between the LV and aorta as either valvular, subvalvular, or supravalvular based upon 2D imaging. The shape of the spectral Doppler display differs depending on the etiology of the outflow obstruction. AS produces a rounded pattern with a midsystolic peak (Fig. 14.21), while LVOT obstruction produces a dagger-shaped pattern (Fig. 14.23). Limitations

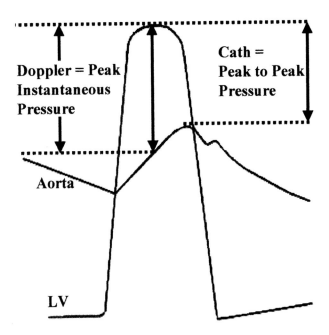

Figure 14.22. Illustration of the pressure tracings obtained during cardiac catheterization in a patient with AS. The pressure gradient obtained with Doppler echocardiography is reflective of the peak instantaneous gradient. The cardiac catheterization gradient is the difference between the peak LV and peak aortic pressures. (From Troianos CA. Perioperative echocardiography. In: Troianos CA, ed. *Anesthesia for the Cardiac Patient.* St. Louis: Mosby, 2002, with permission).

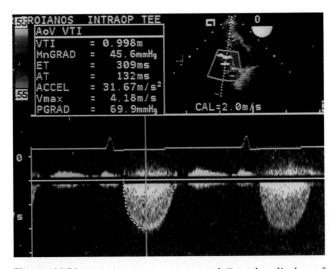

Figure 14.21. Continuous wave spectral Doppler display of velocities through a stenotic AV. The fine, feathery appearance of the high (4.18 m/s) velocities with a mid-systolic peak indicates flow through a stenotic AV. The denser lower velocities near the baseline indicate flow through the LVOT.

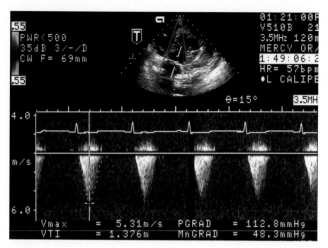

Figure 14.23. Continuous wave spectral Doppler display of LVOT and AV flow velocities in a patient with LVOT obstruction. The characteristic "shark tooth" appearance indicates increased jet acceleration as velocity increases.

to assessing the severity of stenosis by transvalvular velocity measurement are listed in Table 14.3.

Doppler echocardiography is used to quantify the severity of AS by measuring transvalvular blood velocity. The peak pressure gradient is estimated from the peak velocity measurement using the simplified Bernoulli equation:

$$\text{Aortic valve peak gradient} = 4 \times (\text{aortic valve velocity})^2$$

$$\text{Aortic valve mean gradient} = 2.4 \times (\text{aortic valve velocity})^2$$

The simplified Bernoulli equation is based on the assumption that velocity proximal to the narrowed orifice is insignificant (<1.0 m/s). The more proximal velocity in

the LVOT cannot be ignored in clinical conditions of increased transaortic blood flow during systole, such as combined AS and regurgitation, where the proximal velocity may exceed 1.0 m/s because the peak gradient will be overestimated. For example, a patient with an AV peak velocity of 4.5 m/s and an LVOT peak velocity of 1.5 m/s has a calculated gradient of $4 \times ([4.5]^2 - [1.5]^2) = 72$ mm Hg using the modified Bernoulli equation while the calculated AV peak gradient using the simplified Bernoulli equation is $4 \times (4.5)^2 = 81$ mm Hg. The presence of mitral stenosis causes an underestimation of the AS gradient because of decreased transaortic blood flow.

AV area is considered a more constant and less dynamic assessment of AS. The continuity equation calculation of valve area is based on the assumption that blood flowing through sequential areas of a continuous, intact vascular system must be equal. Blood flowing through the LVOT is thus equated with blood flow through the AV.

$$\text{Aortic valve}_{\text{blood flow}} = \text{LVOT}_{\text{blood flow}}$$

Substitution of blood flow with the product of velocity (VTI) and cross-sectional area yields

$$\text{Aortic valve area} \times \text{aortic valve}_{\text{VTI}} = \text{LVOT area} \times \text{LVOT}_{\text{VTI}}$$

AV area is then calculated as

$$\text{Aortic valve area} = \frac{\text{LVOT}_{\text{area}} \times \text{LVOT}_{\text{VTI}}}{\text{Aortic valve}_{\text{VTI}}}$$

LVOT_{VTI} is measured by placing the pulsed wave Doppler sample volume in the LVOT just inferior to the AV and tracing the spectral Doppler envelope. $\text{LVOT}_{\text{area}}$ is determined using the ME AV LAX view and measuring the LVOT diameter (d) near the AV annulus, approximating the same anatomic location as the pulsed wave Doppler recording of LVOT velocity. $\text{LVOT}_{\text{area}}$ is calculated by assuming the LVOT is circular and using the formula

$$\text{Area} = \pi \times (d/2)^2$$

Calculation of $\text{LVOT}_{\text{area}}$ provides the greatest source of error in the continuity equation for valve area calculation. Erroneously foreshortened measurements of LVOT diameter are squared to significantly underestimate the true $\text{LVOT}_{\text{area}}$ and subsequently underestimate actual AV area.

Another source of error using the continuity equation for determination of AV area is the patient with an irregular cardiac rhythm, such as atrial fibrillation. The equation is based on the conservation of mass, with the assumption that flow through the LVOT is equal to flow through the AV. Different cardiac beats in a patient with an irregular rhythm have different stroke volumes. It is imperative to measure VTI for both the AV and LVOT using the same cardiac beat. The AV VTI is traced around the trailing

TABLE 14.3	Limitations to Assessing the Severity of Aortic Stenosis by Transvalvular Velocity Measurement	
Etiology of Limitation	**Consequence**
Decreased transvalvular flow	Decreased pressure gradient
• Severe LV dysfunction	
• Severe mitral regurgitation	
• Left to right intracardiac shunt	
• Low cardiac output	
Increased transvalvular flow	Increased pressure gradient
• Hyperdynamic LV function	
• Sepsis	
• Hyperthyroidism	

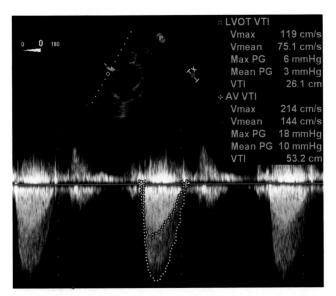

Figure 14.24. Planimetry of both the AV and LVOT velocities is performed on the same cardiac beat using continuous wave spectral Doppler. This is known as the double envelope technique.

edge of the higher velocity envelope of the continuous wave spectral Doppler display as previously described. However, instead of using pulsed wave Doppler to measure LVOT velocity, the $LVOT_{VTI}$ is traced from the same continuous wave spectral Doppler display as the AV VTI, tracing the denser lower velocities within the same cardiac beat (Fig. 14.24). This "double envelope" technique (39) circumvents the problem of different stroke volumes for different beats but can also be used for patients with a regular rhythm. Pulsed wave Doppler for $LVOT_{VTI}$ measurements in patients with a regular rhythm is preferred when the continuous wave Doppler beam used to measure AV VTI does not precisely intercept the AV and LVOT flow in the same imaging plane or beam intercept angle. An alternative to measuring AV and $LVOT_{VTI}$ from the same cardiac beat in patients with an irregular rhythm is to measure aortic $valve_{VTI}$ and $LVOT_{VTI}$ of several (seven or more) cardiac beats and take the average VTI for each in calculation of AV area.

Calculated AV area is affected by stroke volume even among patients with a regular sinus rhythm. Increased stroke volume with a dobutamine infusion yields a slightly larger area that is related to the continuity equation area calculation rather than an actual change in valve area (40,41). Recent evidence indicates that more pliable valves, such as moderately stenotic or nonrheumatic valves, may enlarge the orifice size with increased contractility (42).

Many patients with AS also have AR. The diastolic regurgitation of blood into the LV increases transaortic blood flow during systole, yielding a higher gradient for a given AV orifice. The presence of AR, however, does not affect continuity equation area calculations because the measurements of systolic flow in the LVOT and the AV both account for the increased systolic flow. Limitations to determination of AV area by the continuity equation are summarized in Table 14.4.

The continuity equation is a reliable method to determine AV area unless poor image quality introduces error into the calculation, especially with measurement of the LVOT diameter. A modified continuity equation that uses Simpson's biplane method of disks to determine stroke volume attempts to reduce this error:

$$\text{Aortic valve area} = \frac{\text{LVDv} - \text{LVSv}}{\text{Aortic valve}_{VTI}}$$

Simpson's biplane method of disks from ME images is used to determine the left ventricular diastolic volume (LVDv) and left ventricular systolic volume (LVSv). The difference determines the stroke volume or flow while transvalvular aortic flow or aortic $valve_{VTI}$ using continuous wave Doppler from deep TG LAX or TG LAX determines the aortic valve velocity–time integral.

This modified method has an 80% correlation with the standard continuity equation and is most useful when measurements of the LVOT diameter and flow are difficult to obtain. Another important aspect of the modified continuity equation is accurate aortic valve

TABLE 14.4	Limitations to Determination of AV Area by the Continuity Equation	
Limitation	**Etiology**	**Consequence**
Inadequate TG view	Patient anatomy	Inability to position Doppler beam parallel to blood flow for velocity measurements
Inability to identify high velocity jet	Pinhole AS	Inability to measure transvalvular flow
Inability to measure an accurate LVOT diameter	Anatomic relation between LVOT and esophagus	Error in valve area calculations

area measurement in the presence of accelerated LVOT flow (>1.5 m/s), which may occur with combined AR and stenosis. Although the numbers were small, the modified continuity equation correlated better with cardiac catheterization data in the presence of increased LVOT flow (43). This is an important option for determining aortic valve area, although the standard continuity equation has more data to support its use and should be used preferentially when feasible.

The velocity ratio, expressed as the ratio of the LVOT velocity and aortic valve velocity, is also a useful measure of stenosis that is independent of body size. This dimensionless index is derived from the continuity equation and represents the ratio of the AV area to the LVOT area.

$$\text{Aortic valve}_{area} \times \text{aortic valve}_{VTI} = \text{LVOT}_{area} \times \text{LVOT}_{VTI}$$

$$\frac{\text{Aortic valve}_{area}}{\text{LVOT}_{area}} = \frac{\text{LVOT}_{VTI}}{\text{Aortic valve}_{VTI}}$$

If the AV area is equivalent to the LVOT area (normal AV), then the blood flow velocities through the LVOT and AV should also be equivalent, which yields a ratio of 1.0. An LVOT/AV velocity ratio of 0.5 indicates that the AV area is half that of the LVOT area. A velocity ratio less than 0.25 indicates that the AV area is less than one fourth that of the LVOT, and reliably indicates the presence of severe AS (38). The importance of using a dimensionless index is illustrated among patients with varying body surface areas. For example, a small patient with a body surface area of 1.3 m² and an AV area of 0.9 cm² may not have critical AS, whereas a large patient with a body surface area of 2.5 m² with the same 0.9 cm² valve area will most likely have critical AS. The dimensionless index of the larger patient with an LVOT$_{area}$ of 3.7 cm² would have a Aortic valve$_{area}$/LVOT$_{area}$ ratio (and hence a LVOT$_{VTI}$/Aortic valve$_{VTI}$ ratio) of 0.24, indicating severe AS. The smaller patient with an LVOT$_{area}$ of 2.5 cm² would have a ratio of 0.4, which is not indicative of severe stenosis. So, although both patients have an AV area of 0.9 cm², the larger patient has severe stenosis based upon the velocity ratio of less than 0.25. This technique of solely utilizing VTI measurements circumvents the need to determine LVOT$_{area}$, which is necessary for assessment of AS using the continuity equation and is the measurement most prone to error.

A small transthoracic study reported use of continuous wave Doppler pattern in the descending thoracic aorta to identify patients with significant AS (Fig. 14.25). Two general patterns are elucidated, biphasic or uniphasic, with velocity interrogation distal to the left subclavian artery and parallel to blood flow. All patients with a biphasic S1/S2 ratio less than 0.5 have severe AS while no patients with an AV area less than 1.5 cm² have a uniphasic signal (44).

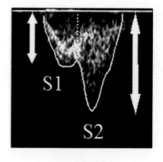 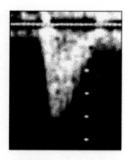

Biphasic **Uniphasic**

Figure 14.25. Transthoracic continuous wave Doppler of flow in the descending thoracic aorta just distal to the subclavian artery. Biphasic image with two separate systolic velocities, S1 and S2, indicative of moderate to severe AS. Uniphasic image with a single systolic velocity indicative of an AV are greater than 1.5 cm² (From Hansen W, Behrenbeck T, Spittell PC, et al. Biphasic Doppler pattern of the descending thoracic aorta: a new echocardiographic finding in patients with AV stenosis. *J Am Soc Echocardiogr* 2005;18:860–864, with permission).

A recent study indicated that mitral annular tissue Doppler echocardiographic (TDE) indices may better reflect the physiologic consequences of afterload burden of AS on the LV than body surface area–indexed AV area (45). This technique involves measurement of peak systolic and early and late diastolic TDE velocities at the septal and lateral mitral annulus in the four-chamber view and with derivation of the respective mitral E/E' ratios. These TDE indices correlate better with plasma N-terminal pro-B-type natriuretic peptide (NT-proBNP) levels than body surface area–indexed AV area (AVAI). TDE indices predict adverse cardiovascular outcomes better than NT-proBNP levels and AVAI (45).

The recent introduction of 3D echocardiography into clinical practice allows a more detailed evaluation of the LVOT and AV area, compared with 2D echocardiography. Direct measurement of the AV orifice and LVOT using offline selection of specific planes allows the echocardiographer to precisely measure the desired orifice. The 3D determination of AV orifice area has less deviation from invasive or planimetry measured areas than conventionally calculated areas using the continuity equation (46). Real-time intraoperative 3D echocardiography is also useful for identifying AV abnormalities that are missed with 2D echocardiography such as a quadricuspid AV (47).

AORTIC REGURGITATION

Pathophysiology

AR is caused by either intrinsic disease of the aortic cusps or secondarily from diseases affecting the ascending aorta. Intrinsic valvular problems include rheumatic, calcific, myxomatous disease, endocarditis, traumatic injury, and congenital abnormalities. Conditions affecting the ascending aorta that lead to AR include annular dilation and aortic dissection (secondary to blunt trauma or hypertension), mycotic aneurysm, cystic medial necrosis, connective tissue disorders (Marfan's syndrome), and chronic hypertension. The most common cause of pure AR is no longer post-inflammatory with the decreasing prevalence of rheumatic heart disease among cardiac surgical patients. Aortic root dilation (Fig. 14.26) is now the most common etiologic factor due to the increased prevalence of degenerative disease, followed by post-inflammatory and bicuspid valve disease (48).

Chronic LV volume overload causes progressive LV dilation over many years, while systolic function is preserved. Ejection fraction is initially normal while end-diastolic dimensions are increased. In contrast to AS, the ventricle remains relatively compliant until systolic dysfunction ensues late in the course of disease progression. Another contrasting feature is that systolic dysfunction is not reversible. Acute AR is not associated with LV dilation because the adaptive LV dilation has not yet occurred (49). This lack of adaptation is associated with decreased LV compliance and a rapid onset of symptoms. Other echocardiographic findings of chronic AR include premature MV closure and fluttering of the MV leaflets, most effectively demonstrated using M-mode echocardiography. Depending on the etiology of the AR, aortic root abnormalities may also be present, including aortic dissection or aneurysm.

AR causes an overestimation of MV area by the pressure half-time (PHT) method of determining mitral orifice size. The PHT method exploits the relation between mitral inflow deceleration and MV area. Deceleration is based on the equalization of pressure in the left atrium (LA) and the LV and is prolonged as mitral orifice size decreases. In the absence of AR, LV volume (and subsequently left pressure) increases via mitral inflow alone. In the presence of AR, LV volume increases by both mitral inflow and AR, giving the impression that mitral inflow is better than it actually is, underestimating the severity of mitral stenosis.

Echocardiographic Evaluation of Aortic Regurgitation

The AV, ascending aorta, and LVOT are inspected using the ME AV LAX view. Normal leaflets are often not visible during diastole, because they are parallel to the Doppler beam when closed. Stenotic leaflets, which dome during systole, often do not completely coapt during diastole leading to AR. The diagnosis of leaflet prolapse is made when aortic leaflet tissue is imaged in the LVOT below the annular plane during diastole (Fig. 14.27). An aortic dissection in the aortic root causes disruption of leaflets from the aortic annulus and may also cause leaflet prolapse. The 2D echocardiography is used to determine the etiology of the AR by identifying structural abnormalities of the leaflets or aortic root.

Although 2D echocardiography is not useful for quantifying the severity of AR, there are several associated echocardiographic features. The LV is dilated and more spherical in shape with chronic AR but not necessarily with acute AR. The MV exhibits premature closure and fluttering of the anterior mitral leaflet during diastole. An eccentric AR jet directed toward the anterior MV leaflet may cause doming of the anterior leaflet with convexity toward the left atrial side of the MV (Fig. 14.28).

Doppler echocardiography is used to quantify the severity of AR by several techniques that involve color, pulsed wave, and continuous wave Doppler. These techniques are sensitive and reliable, but all have limitations. Color Doppler applied

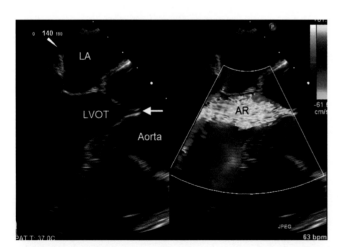

Figure 14.26. **Left:** Transesophageal echocardiogram of the ME AV LAX view in a patient with aortic root dilation leading to incomplete closure of the AV (*arrow*). LA, left atrium; LVOT, left ventricular outflow tract; Aorta, ascending aorta. **Right:** Color comparison of same image with color flow Doppler showing the incomplete valve closure leading to severe AR.

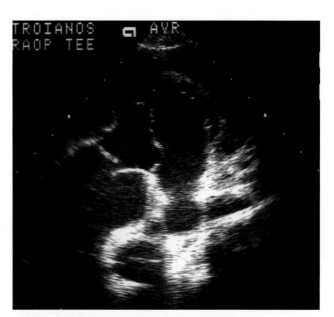

Figure 14.27. Transesophageal echocardiogram of an AV with single leaflet prolapse using the deep TG view.

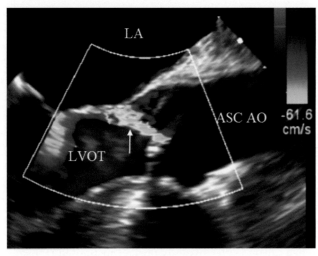

Figure 14.28. Transesophageal echocardiogram with color flow Doppler in a patient with eccentric AR. The AR is identified by the color flow disturbance (*arrow*) that originates from the AV and directed toward the anterior MV leaflet. LA, left atrium; LVOT, left ventricular outflow tract; ASC AO, ascending aorta.

to ME AV SAX is useful for localizing the site of regurgitation (Fig. 14.7). Despite the orthogonal relationship between the AV flow and Doppler beam in this short-axis view, the regurgitant orifice is identifiable because the AR jet is usually not completely orthogonal to the Doppler beam, particularly if the jet is eccentric. Utilizing the ME AV SAX, the cross-sectional area of the regurgitant jet can be measured by planimetry within 1 cm of the valve. The cross-sectional area of the jet and its ratio to the LVOT area can be used to quantify the severity of AR (50). This method defines severe AR as a ratio ≥0.6 illustrated in Table 14.5 (49).

The ME AV LAX view is the most useful for quantifying the severity of AR. Color Doppler reveals a flow disturbance in the LVOT originating from the AV and directed into the LV (Fig. 14.26). A central jet is usually caused by aortic root dilatation whereas an eccentric jet usually implies a leaflet problem. The width of the jet at the orifice compared to the width of the LVOT correlates with angiographic determinants of AR (Fig. 14.29) (50). A jet width/LVOT width ratio of less than 0.25 is mild AR, and a ratio ≥0.65 is indicative of severe AR (49). The length of the AR jet into the receiving chamber does not correlate with the AR severity (50).

Limitations to the use of color flow Doppler echocardiography to estimate severity of AR are listed in Table 14.6. One such limitation to this technique is that the regurgitant jet orifice and the true LVOT diameter (not foreshortened) may not be in the same imaging plane (51). This limitation is most apparent if "color M-mode" is used to determine the jet/LVOT ratio. Color M-mode refers to the application of M-mode imaging to a color flow Doppler image. M-mode evaluation of the LVOT in the patient with AR is more useful for determination of the duration of AR into the diastolic phase rather than the jet/LVOT ratio. Another limitation to the jet/LVOT ratio method of assessing AR is that the shape of the regurgitant orifice may not be circular or symmetric. An irregularly shaped regurgitant orifice may cause the jet to appear wider in one imaging plane than another (52), hence the importance of examining multiple imaging planes. The AR jet may also be eccentric or converge with the MV inflow, rendering the jet particularly difficult to evaluate in patients with mitral stenosis (53). An eccentric AR jet directed toward the anterior MV leaflet tends to underestimate severity with the jet width/LVOT width ratio method (54). If color Doppler cannot

TABLE 14.5	Grading Aortic Regurgitation			
Indicator	**Mild**	**Moderate**		**Severe**
Angiographic grade	1+	2+	3+	4+
Color Doppler jet width/LVOT width	<0.25	0.25–0.46	0.47–0.64	≥0.65
Doppler vena contracta width (cm)	<0.3	0.3–0.6		>0.6
Deceleration slope (m/s²)				>3
PHT (ms)	>500	500–200		<200
Regurgitant volume (mL/beat)	<30	30–59		≥60
Regurgitant fraction (%)	<30	30–49		≥50
Regurgitant orifice area (cm²)	<0.10	0.10–0.29		≥0.30

Sources: Bonow R, Carabello B, et al. ACC/AHA 2006 guidelines for the management of patients with valvular heart disease: a report of the American college of cardiology/American heart association task force on practice guidelines. J Am Coll Cardiol 2006;48:e1–e148; Zoghbi W, Enriquez-Sarano M, et al. Recommendations for evaluation of the severity of native valvular regurgitation with two-dimensional and Doppler echocardiography. J Am Soc Echocardiogr 2003;16:777–802.

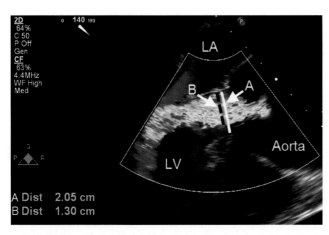

Figure 14.29. Transesophageal echocardiogram of the ME AV LAX view with color flow Doppler in a patient with AR. **A:** LVOT width measures 2.05 cm; **B:** AR jet width measures 1.30 cm. Ratio of Jet width 1.30 cm/LVOT width 2.05 cm = 0.63. LA, left atrium; LV, left ventricle; Aorta, ascending aorta.

be applied to the LVOT from the ME AV LAX view because of annular calcification or shadowing of the LVOT from a prosthetic mitral or AV, a deep TG LAX or TG LAX view is used. The AR jet in this view appears red or mosaic in color with the jet directed away from the AV toward the LV cavity (Fig. 14.30). Multiple imaging planes should be utilized to appreciate the 3D character of the jet.

While in the ME AV LAX the vena contracta can also be measured. The vena contracta is slightly different than the jet width in that it is the smallest diameter of regurgitant color flow at the level of the AV and is usually smaller than the jet width in the LVOT (Fig. 14.31). Some consider the vena contracta measurement to be a stronger measurement than the jet width/LVOT ratio (55). Despite the simplicity of the vena contracta measurement in estimating

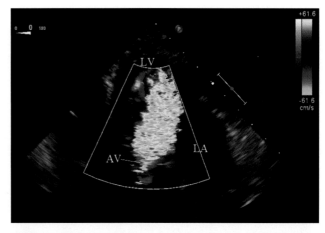

Figure 14.30. Transesophageal echocardiogram of the deep TG view with color flow Doppler in a patient with AR. AV, aortic valve; LA, left atrium; LV, left ventricle.

the severity of AR, there are few limitations, such as the presence of multiple or abnormally shaped regurgitant jets and the inability to accurately determine the annular plane of the AV due to pathology.

Although the jet width/LVOT width and vena contracta methods are easy to use and provide useful information for making clinical decisions, there are other methods to evaluate patients with AR. Continuous wave Doppler is used to determine the severity of AR by measuring the deceleration slope of the regurgitant jet and by calculating PHT. PHT is the time required for the peak regurgitant pressure to decrease to half of its maximum value and is measured in milliseconds. A deep TG LAX or TG LAX view aligns the regurgitant jet with the Doppler beam. Color Doppler is used to identify the location and direction of the AR jet while the continuous wave Doppler cursor is placed within the jet to obtain the continuous wave spectral velocity profile (Fig. 14.32). The velocity of the regurgitant jet declines more rapidly

TABLE 14.6	Limitations to Estimating the Severity of Aortic Regurgitation with Color Flow Doppler		
Limitations	**Etiology**	**Consequence**
Shadowing of LVOT	Prosthetic aortic or MV Mitral annular calcification	Inability to image LVOT or AR jet
AR jet is wider in one plane versus another	Regurgitant orifice asymmetric in its 3D shape	Inaccurate estimate of AR jet width and vena contracta
Eccentric jet causing swirling of flow disturbance	Leaflet prolapse	AR jet appears wider than orifice size

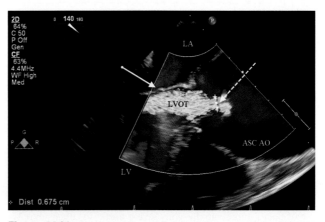

Figure 14.31. Transesophageal echocardiogram of the ME AV LAX view with color flow Doppler in a patient with AR. The vena contracta at the AV (*dashed arrow*) measuring 0.675 cm indicates severe AR. LA, left atrium; LV, left ventricle; LVOT, left ventricular outflow tract; ASC AO, dilated ascending aorta; solid arrow, anterior leaflet of the MV.

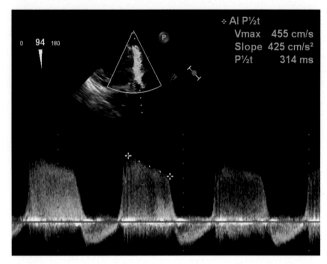

Figure 14.32. Continuous wave spectral Doppler velocities within the LVOT of a patient with AR. The slope of the velocity deceleration (AR slope = 4.25 m/s²) and the pressure half time (314 ms) indicates the severity of the AR.

TABLE 14.7	Limitations to Estimating the Severity of Aortic Regurgitation Using the Deceleration Slope
Limitations	**Consequence**
Increased systemic vascular resistance	Steeper slope overestimating AR
Decreased LV compliance	Steeper slope overestimating AR
Eccentric AR jet	Cannot align Doppler beam with AR jet

in patients with severe AR because the larger regurgitant orifice allows a more rapid equilibration of the aortic and LV pressures. In other words, if the pressure difference between the aorta and LV approaches zero rapidly, the regurgitant jet velocity also approaches zero rapidly, creating a steeper slope (Fig. 14.33). A regurgitant velocity slope greater than 3 m/s² is indicative of advanced (3 or 4+) AR (56).

Factors other than regurgitant orifice size may influence the deceleration slope (Table 14.7). Systemic vascular

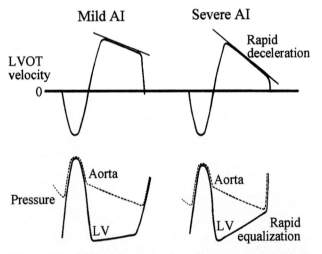

Figure 14.33. Illustration of the association between the LVOT deceleration slope and the pressure difference between the aorta and LV during diastole. The deceleration slope is steeper and approaches zero velocity more rapidly with severe aortic insufficiency (AI) as the pressures in the aorta and LV equalize more rapidly (From Troianos CA. Perioperative echocardiography. In: Troianos CA, ed. *Anesthesia for the Cardiac Patient*. St. Louis, Mosby, 2002, with permission and adapted from Feigenbaum H. *Echocardiography*. 5th ed. Philadelphia: Lea & Febiger, 1994:286, with permission).

resistance and LV compliance affect the rate of deceleration, irrespective of the regurgitant orifice size (57). Decreased systemic vascular resistance (sepsis) and reduced LV compliance (ischemia, cardiomyopathy, acute AR) cause a steeper deceleration slope because aortic and LV pressures equalize more rapidly in these conditions. Another limitation to this technique is that measurement of regurgitant jet velocity is difficult and unreliable in patients with eccentric jets, because it is difficult to align the Doppler beam with the regurgitant jet.

Pulsed wave Doppler is used to detect retrograde flow in the aorta during diastole. Holodiastolic flow reversal in the abdominal aorta is both sensitive and specific for severe AR. Detection of holodiastolic retrograde flow in the proximal descending thoracic aorta and aortic arch is a sensitive indicator of AR but is not specific for severe AR. The short-axis TEE view of the descending thoracic aorta is used for placement of the pulsed wave sample volume distal in the aorta, near the diaphragm. Despite the orthogonal relationship between the aortic flow and Doppler beam in this short-axis view, the flow in the aorta is identifiable because the blood in the aorta tends to swirl as it travels down the aorta. The spectral Doppler display is examined for the duration of diastolic flow. Retrograde flow throughout diastole (holodiastolic) in the distal descending (58) or abdominal aorta (59) indicates severe AR (Fig. 14.34).

Regurgitant volume and regurgitant fraction can also be used to evaluate the severity of AR. Regurgitant volume is the difference between the systolic flow across the AV and "net forward" cardiac output. In the absence of intracardiac shunts and mitral regurgitation, flow through the pulmonary artery (PA) or MV is equivalent to (net) cardiac output. PA blood flow is reliably measured with TEE by measuring the PA diameter (d), calculating its area [$\pi (d/2)^2$], and multiplying the area by the PA VTI and heart rate (60). AV systolic flow is the product of AV area and VTI. The aortic regurgitant volume is the difference between AV systolic flow and pulmonary blood flow (cardiac output). Regurgitant fraction is expressed as the

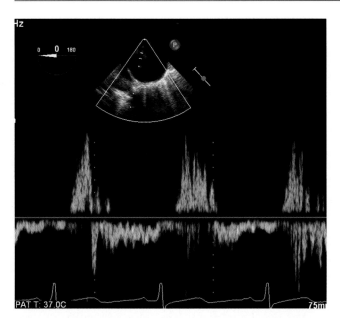

Figure 14.34. Pulse wave Doppler spectral velocity of blood flow in the descending thoracic aorta. The retrograde flow throughout diastole is termed holodiastolic and is associated with severe AR.

proportion of AV systolic flow that is regurgitant volume and indicates the severity of AR listed in Table 14.5 (61).

$$\text{Regurgitant volume} = \text{Aortic valve systolic flow} - \text{cardiac output}$$

$$\text{Regurgitant fraction} = \frac{\text{Regurgitant volume}}{\text{Aortic valve systolic flow}}$$

The continuity equation could be theoretically used to determine regurgitant orifice size. Diastolic velocities just above (aortic root-VTI) and through the AV (AV-VTI) measured with Doppler echocardiography and the cross-sectional area of the aortic root measured with 2D echocardiography are used in this calculation (62,63). This theoretical technique has not been widely accepted or validated.

$$\text{Aortic valve regurgitant orifice} = \frac{\text{Aortic root}_{\text{area}} \times \text{aortic root diastolic}_{\text{VTI}}}{\text{Aortic valve regurgitant jet}_{\text{VTI}}}$$

As the utility of 3D echocardiography of the AV is becoming more apparent for evaluation of structural anatomy among patients with AS, its use is also becoming more apparent among patients with AR. Online or offline software systems, that allow planimetry measurements of area, may also provide accurate measurements of vena contracta and vena contracta area. The 3D echocardiography can be used to identify and measure multiple jets, which can then be summated to accurately determine a true 3D vena contracta (64).

KEY POINTS

■ The close anatomic proximity between the AV and the esophagus permits accurate diagnosis of the mechanism of AV dysfunction, valve sizing for valve replacement, and identification of associated lesions.

■ Complete evaluation of the AV utilizes 2D and 3D imaging and pulsed wave, continuous wave, and color Doppler for quantitative evaluation of stenotic and regurgitant lesions.

■ Velocity measurement of AV flow provides an estimate of valve gradient using the modified Bernoulli equation. Transvalvular velocities increase as orifice size decreases and as the force of ventricular contraction and transaortic blood flow increases. The severity of AS is underestimated in patients with severe LV dysfunction. These patients require area determination to assess the severity of AS.

■ There is often a discrepancy between Doppler and cardiac catheterization derived gradient measurements due to differences in technique and measurements. Doppler-derived measurements usually exceed catheterization measurements.

■ AV area is determined by planimetry and by the continuity equation.

■ AR is caused by conditions affecting the aortic cusps or secondarily from diseases affecting the ascending aorta.

■ The 2D echocardiography is useful for identifying the etiology of AR and associated lesions but not for assessing the severity of regurgitation.

■ Color, pulsed wave, and continuous wave Doppler are used to quantify the severity of regurgitation, but each technique has its own limitations.

REFERENCES

1. Hung J, Lang R, et al. 3D Echocardiography: a review of the current status and future directions. *J Am Soc Echocardiogr* 2007;20:213–233.

2. Oh C, Click R, et al. Role of intraoperative transesophageal echocardiography in determining aortic annulus diameter in homograft insertion. *J Am Soc Echocardiogr* 1998;11:638–642.

3. Nowrangi S, Connolly H, et al. Impact of intraoperative transesophageal echocardiography among patients undergoing aortic valve replacement for aortic stenosis. *J Am Soc Echocardiogr* 2001;14:863–866.

4. Cheitlin M, Armstrong W, et al. ACC/AHA/ASE 2003 Guideline update for the clinical application of echocardiography. Summary article: a report of the American college of cardiology/American hart association task force on practice guidelines (ACC/AHA/ASE committee to update the 1997 guidelines for the application of echocardiography). *J Am Coll Cardiol* 2003;42:954–970.

5. Morehead J, Firstenberg S, et al. Intraoperative echocardiographic detection of regurgitant jets after valve replacement. *Ann Thorac Surg* 2000;69:135–139.

6. Swenson J, Bull D, Stringham J. Subjective assessment of left ventricular preload using transesophageal echocardiography: corresponding pulmonary artery occlusion pressures. *J Cardiothorac Vasc Anesth* 2001;15:580–583.

7. Odell J, Mullany C, et al. Aortic valve replacement after previous coronary artery bypass grafting. *Ann Thorac Surg* 1996;62:1424–1430.

8. Pantin E, Cheung A. Thoracic aorta. In: Kaplan J, Reich D, Lake C, Konstadt S, eds. *Kaplan's Cardiac Anesthesia.* 5th ed. Philadelphia: Saunders Elsevier, 2006:723–764.

9. Mihaljevic T, Paul S, Cohn LH, Wechsler A. Pathophysiology of aortic valve disease. In: Cohn L, Edmunds L Jr, eds. *Cardiac Surgery in the Adult.* New York: McGraw-Hill, 2003:791–810.

10. Thubrikar M, Nolan SP, et al. Stress sharing between the sinus and leaflets of canine aortic valve. *Ann Thorac Surg* 1986;42:434–440.

11. Deck J, Thubrikar M, et al. Structure, stress, and tissue repair in aortic valve leaflets. *Cardiovasc Res* 1988;22:7–16.

12. Thubrikar M, Harry R, Nolan S. Normal aortic valve function in dogs. *Am J Cardiol* 1977;40:563–568.

13. Gnyaneshwar R, Kumar R, Komarakshi R. Dynamic analysis of the aortic valve using a finite element model. *Ann Thorac Surg* 2002;73:1122–1129.

14. Mercer J. The movements of the dog's aortic valve studied by high speed cineangiography. *Br J Radiol* 1973;46:344–349.

15. Shanewise J, Cheung A, et al. ASE/SCA guidelines for performing a comprehensive intraoperative multiplane transesophageal echocardiography examination: recommendations of the American Society of Echocardiography Council for Intraoperative Echocardiography and the Society of Cardiovascular Anesthesiologists Task Force for Certification in Perioperative Transesophageal Echocardiography. *Anesth Analg* 1999;89:870–884.

16. Lang R, Bierig M, et al. Recommendations for chamber quantification: a report from the American Society of Echocardiography's guidelines and standards committee and the chamber quantification writing group, developed in conjunction with the European Association of Echocardiography, a branch of the European Society of Cardiology. *J Am Soc Echocardiogr* 2005;18:1440–1463.

17. Stoddard M, Hammons R, Longaker R. Doppler transesophageal echocardiographic determination of aortic valve area in adults with aortic stenosis. *Am Heart J* 1996;132:337–342.

18. Peter M, Hoffman A, et al. Progression of aortic stenosis. *Chest* 1993;103:1715–1719.

19. Bahler R, Desser D, et al. Factors leading to progression of valvular aortic stenosis. *Am J Cardiol* 1999;84:1044–1048.

20. Palta S, Pai A, et al. New insights into the progressions of aortic stenosis: implications for secondary prevention. *Circulation* 2000;101:2497–2502.

21. Kume T, Kawamoto T, et al. Rate of progression of valvular aortic stenosis in patients undergoing dialysis. *J Am Soc Echocardiogr* 2006;19:914–918.

22. Mohler E III. Are atherosclerotic processes involved in aortic-valve calcification? *Lancet* 2000;356:524–525.

23. Hoffman J, Kaplan S. The incidence of congenital heart disease. *J Am Coll Cardiol* 2002;39:1890–1900.

24. Fernandes S, Sanders S, et al. Morphology of bicuspid aortic valve in children and adolescents. *J Am Coll Cardiol* 2004;44:1648–1651.

25. Ciotti G, Vlahos A, Silverman N. Morphology and function of the bicuspid aortic valve with and without coarctation of the aorta in the young. *Am J Cardiol* 2006;98:1096–1102.

26. Schaefer B, Lewin M, et al. An integrated phenotypic classification of leaflet morphology and aortic root shape. *Heart* 2008;94:1634–1638.

27. Roberts W. The congenitally bicuspid aortic valve. A study of 85 autopsy cases. *Am J Cardiol* 1970;26:72–83.

28. Fernandes S, Khairy P, et al. Bicuspid aortic valve morphology and interventions in the young. *J Am Coll Cardiol* 2007;49:2211–2214.

29. Laks H, Marelli D, Drinkwater D Jr. Surgery for adults with congenital heart disease. In: Edmunds LH Jr, ed. *Cardiac Surgery in the Adult.* New York: McGraw-Hill, 1997:1368.

30. Hahn R, Roman M, et al. Association of aortic dilation with regurgitant, stenotic and functionally normal bicuspid aortic valves. *J Am Coll Cardiol* 1992;19:283–288.

31. Cecconi M, Manfrin M, et al. Aortic dimensions in patients with bicuspid aortic valve without significant valve dysfunction. *Am J Cardiol* 2005;95:292–294.

32. Borger M, Preston M, et al. Should the ascending aorta be replaced more frequently in patients with bicuspid aortic valve disease? *J Thorac Cardiovasc Surg* 2004;128:677–683.

33. Maslow A, Regan M, et al. Echocardiographic predictors of left ventricular outflow tract obstruction and systolic anterior motion of the mitral valve after mitral valve reconstruction for myxomatous valve disease. *J Am Coll Cardiol* 1999;34:2096–2104.

34. Hoffmann R, Flachskampf F, Hanrath P. Planimetry of orifice area in aortic stenosis using multiplane transesophageal echocardiography. *J Am Coll Cardiol* 1993;22:529–534.

35. Godley R, Green D, et al. Reliability of two-dimensional echocardiography an assessing the severity of valvular aortic stenosis. *Chest* 1981;79:657–662.

36. Cahalan M, Abel M, Goldman M, et al. American Society of Echocardiography; Society of Cardiovascular Anesthesiologists. American Society of Echocardiography and Society of Cardiovascular Anesthesiologists task force guidelines for training in perioperative echocardiography. *Anesth Analg* 2002;94:1384–1388.

37. Bonow R, Carabello B, et al. ACC/AHA 2006 guidelines for the management of patients with valvular heart disease: a report of the American college of cardiology/American heart association task force on practice guidelines. *J Am Coll Cardiol* 2006;48:e1–e148.

38. Oh J, Talerico C, et al. Prediction of severity of aortic stenosis by Doppler aortic valve area determination: prospective Doppler catheterization correlation in 100 patients. *J Am Coll Cardiol* 1988;11:1227–1234.

39. Maslow A, Mashikian J, et al. Transesophageal echocardiographic evaluation of native aortic valve area: utility of the double-envelope technique. *J Cardiothorac Vasc Anesth* 2001;15:293–299.

40. Rask L, Karp K, Eriksson N. Flow dependence of the aortic valve area in patients with aortic stenosis: assessment by application of the continuity equation. *J Am Soc Echocardiogr* 1996;9:295–299.

41. Lin S, Roger V, et al. Dobutamine stress Doppler hemodynamics in patients with aortic stenosis: feasibility, safety, and surgical correlations. *Am Heart J* 1998;136:1010–1016.

42. Shively B, Charlton G, et al. Flow dependence of valve area in aortic stenosis: Relation to valve morphology. *J Am Coll Cardiol* 1998;31:654–660.

43. Dumont Y, Arsenault M. An alternative to standard continuity equation for the calculation of aortic valve area by echocardiography. *J Am Soc Echocardiogr* 2003;16:1309–1315.

44. Hansen W, Behrenbeck T, et al. Biphasic Doppler pattern of the descending thoracic aorta: a new echocardiographic finding

in patients with aortic valve stenosis. *J Am Soc Echocardiogr* 2005;18:860–864.

45. Poh K, Chan M, et al. Prognostication of valvular aortic stenosis using tissue Doppler echocardiography: underappreciated importance of late diastolic mitral annular velocity. *J Am Soc Echocardiogr* 2008;21:475–481.

46. Khaw A, von Bardeleben R, et al. Direct measurement of left ventricular outflow tract by transthoracic real-time 3D-echocardiography increases accuracy in assessment of aortic valve stenosis. *Int J Cardiol* 2008, doi:10.1016/j.ijcard.2008.04.070.

47. Armen T, Vandse R, et al. Three-dimensional echocardiographic evaluation of an incidental quadricuspid aortic valve. *Eur J Echocardiogr* 2008;9:318–320.

48. Cosgrove D, Rosenkranz E, et al. Valvuloplasty for aortic insufficiency. *J Thorac Cardiovasc Surg* 1991;102:571–577.

49. Zoghbi W, Enriquez-Sarano M, et al. Recommendations for evaluation of the severity of native valvular regurgitation with two-dimensional and Doppler echocardiography. *J Am Soc Echocardiogr* 2003;16:777–802.

50. Perry G, Helmcke F, et al. Evaluation of aortic insufficiency by Doppler color flow mapping. *J Am Coll Cardiol* 1987;9:952–959.

51. Reynolds T, Abate J, et al. The JH/LVOH method in the quantification of aortic regurgitation: how the cardiac sonographer may avoid an important potential pitfall. *J Am Soc Echocardiogr* 1991;4:105–108.

52. Taylor A, Eichhorn E, et al. Aortic valve morphology: an important in vitro determinant of proximal regurgitant jet width by Doppler color flow mapping. *J Am Coll Cardiol* 1990;16:405–412.

53. Masuyama T, Kitabatake A, Kodama K, et al. Semiquantitative evaluation of aortic regurgitation by Doppler echocardiography: effects of associated mitral stenosis. *Am Heart J* 1989;117:133–139.

54. Cape E, Yoganathan A, et al. Adjacent solid boundaries alter the size of regurgitant jets on Doppler color flow maps. *J Am Coll Cardiol* 1991;17:1094–1102.

55. Tribouilloy C, Enriquez-Sarano M, et al. Assessment of severity of aortic regurgitation using the width of the vena contracta: a clinical color Doppler imaging study. *Circulation* 2000;102:558–564.

56. Grayburn P, Handshoe R, et al. Quantitative assessment of the hemodynamic consequences of aortic regurgitation by means of continuous wave Doppler recordings. *J Am Coll Cardiol* 1987;10:135–141.

57. Griffin B, Flachskampf F, et al. The effects of regurgitant orifice size, chamber compliance, and systemic vascular resistance on aortic regurgitant velocity slope and pressure half-time. *Am Heart J* 1991;122:1049–1056.

58. Sutton D, Kluger R, et al. Flow reversal in the descending aorta: a guide to intraoperative assessment of aortic regurgitation with transesophageal echocardiography. *J Thorac Cardiovasc Surg* 1994;108:576–582.

59. Takenaka K, Sakamoto T, et al. Pulsed Doppler echocardiographic detection of regurgitant blood flow in the ascending, descending, and abdominal aorta of patients with aortic regurgitation. *J Cardiol* 1987;17:301–309.

60. Savino J, Troianos C, et al. Measurement of pulmonary blood flow with transesophageal two-dimensional and Doppler echocardiography. *Anesthesiology* 1991;75:445–451.

61. Kitabatake A, Ito H, et al. A new approach to noninvasive evaluation of aortic regurgitant fraction by two-dimensional Doppler echocardiography. *Circulation* 1985;72:523–529.

62. Reimold S, Ganz P, et al. Effective aortic regurgitant orifice area: description of a method based on the conservation of mass. *J Am Coll Cardiol* 1991;18:761–768.

63. Yeung A, Plappert T, St. John Sutton M. Calculation of aortic regurgitation orifice area by Doppler echocardiography: an application of the continuity equation. *Br Heart J* 1992;68:236–240.

64. Mallavarapu R, Nanda N. Three-dimensional transthoracic echocardiographic assessment of aortic stenosis and aortic regurgitation. *Cardiol Clin* 2007;25:327–334.

QUESTIONS

1. An 80-year-old patient with a 15% left ventricular (LV) ejection fraction presents for coronary artery bypass grafting and possible aortic valve replacement. Preoperative cardiac catheterization revealed a LV to aorta gradient of 20 mm Hg. What is the best way to determine the severity of aortic stenosis (AS) in this patient?
   A. Determine aortic valve (AV) area using the continuity equation.
   B. Determine mean AV gradient using the modified Bernoulli equation.
   C. Measure maximal AV cusp separation via the AV long-axis view.
   D. Measure peak transaortic valve velocity using continuous wave Doppler via the deep trans-gastric (TG) view.

2. A patient with AS was found to have a 30 mm Hg AV gradient via cardiac catheterization but a 50 mm Hg gradient using continuous wave Doppler echocardiography via the deep TG view. What is the most likely explanation for this discrepancy?

   A. Doppler beam-AV flow angle greater than 20 degrees
   B. Peak-to-peak cardiac catheter pressure gradient determination versus peak instantaneous pressure gradient determination via echo
   C. "Pin-hole" AS
   D. Severe aortic regurgitation (AR) associated with AS

3. The etiology of AR is best determined with
   A. color flow Doppler echocardiography
   B. continuous wave Doppler echocardiography
   C. pulsed wave Doppler echocardiography
   D. two-dimensional (2D) echocardiography

4. Which of the following would cause an AV regurgitant velocity deceleration slope of 5 m/s?
   A. Increased LV compliance
   B. Mild aortic insufficiency (AI)
   C. Phenylephrine administration to a patient with a competent AV
   D. Severe AR

CHAPTER 15

Assessment of the Tricuspid and Pulmonic Valves

Atilio Barbeito ■ Rebecca A. Schroeder ■ Shahar Bar-Yosef ■ Jonathan B. Mark

INTRODUCTION

The primary function of the tricuspid and pulmonic valves is to regulate blood flow from the periphery to the pulmonary vascular bed and to maximize the efficiency of the right ventricle (RV). Although these valves lie more anteriorly in the chest, transesophageal echocardiographic (TEE) evaluation can still be accomplished easily and often adds useful clinical information. A systematic examination of the right heart chambers, including the tricuspid and pulmonic valves, should be part of any routine TEE study.

STRUCTURE AND FUNCTION OF THE TRICUSPID AND PULMONIC VALVES

Structure and Function of the Tricuspid Valve

The tricuspid valve (TV) has several important characteristics that differentiate it from the other cardiac valves. The area of the TV, 7 to 9 cm^2, is significantly greater than

that of any other valve (1). It consists of a large anterior leaflet and smaller septal (or medial) and posterior leaflets, each attached to papillary muscles by way of chordae tendineae and affixed to the annulus and a portion of the RV free wall (Fig. 15.1). These three thin membranous leaflets, separated more by indentations in a continuous sheet of tissue rather than true commissures, are much less distinct than the leaflets of the mitral valve (MV).

The tricuspid annulus lies in a slightly more apical position than the mitral annulus, with its inferior margin near the entrances of the inferior vena cava (IVC) and coronary sinus (CS) into the right atrium (RA). It has a complex, nonplanar three-dimensional (3D) shape, different from the saddle-shaped mitral annulus, its highest point being the anteroseptal commissure (near the right ventricular outflow tract [RVOT] and the aortic valve [AV]) and the lowest segment being the posteroseptal one (2). The base of the septal leaflet rests on the medial portion of the tricuspid annulus, which is reinforced by the right fibrous trigone while the remainder of the valve is attached to the thinner anterior and posterior portions of the annulus.

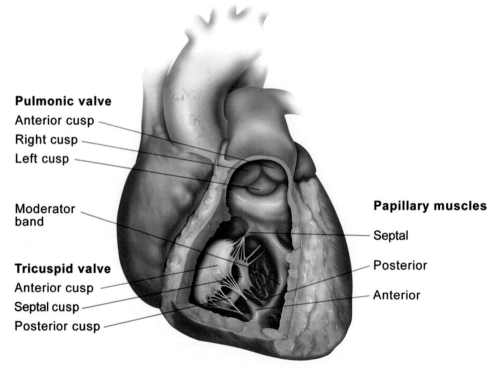

Figure 15.1. Anatomic drawing of RV with valves labeled, anterior view (Modified and reprinted from Konstadt SN, Shernan S, Oka Y, eds. *Clinical Transesophageal Echocardiography: A Problem Oriented Approach*. 2nd ed. Philadelphia: Lippincott Williams & Wilkins, with permission).

Pulmonic valve
Anterior cusp
Right cusp
Left cusp

Moderator band

Tricuspid valve
Anterior cusp
Septal cusp
Posterior cusp

Papillary muscles
Septal
Posterior
Anterior

Contraction of longitudinal muscle fibers of the RV causes motion of the tricuspid annulus toward the RV apex. Because the septal attachment of the tricuspid annulus is relatively fixed, the majority of tricuspid annular motion occurs in its lateral aspect. This gives the motion of the tricuspid annulus a hinge-like appearance, moving more laterally than medially. This motion contrasts with that of the mitral annulus, which has a more symmetrical or piston-like appearance during systole. *Tricuspid annular plane systolic excursion (TAPSE)* describes this long-axis systolic excursion of the lateral aspect of the tricuspid annulus and has been validated as a useful additional measure of global RV systolic function (see Chapter 10 on RV function).

The TV annulus also exhibits a horizontal, sphincter-like motion during RV contraction. In healthy subjects, the TV annular area is maximal during atrial contraction in late diastole, then decreases during early and midsystole, and increases again during late systole and early diastole (3). With more of its circumference in contact with the right ventricular myocardium, the tricuspid annulus exhibits an increased systolic area reduction when compared with the MV annulus (mean 33% reduction vs. 26% reduction) (3). The difference between the systolic and diastolic annular diameters expressed as a fraction of the maximal (diastolic) diameter is known as *tricuspid annulus fractional shortening (TAFS)* and provides additional information regarding RV systolic function (4,5).

The subvalvular apparatus of the TV, while similar to that of the MV, is more complex and variable in structure. The anterior papillary muscle is the largest muscle supporting the TV leaflets. It arises from the *moderator band*, a linear band of cardiac muscle that runs perpendicular to the papillary muscle, attaches to the ventricular septum near the apex of the RV, and may be mistaken for an intracardiac mass (Fig. 15.2). The posterior papillary muscle is frequently small and at times even absent. A diminutive

septal papillary muscle is also present (Fig. 15.1). An alternative nomenclature describes two papillary muscles: a right anterior muscle and a posterior muscle that may have multiple heads.

Structure and Function of the Pulmonic Valve

The pulmonic valve (PV) is most similar in structure and function to the AV. Due to its position on the lower pressure right side of the heart, the pulmonic leaflets are somewhat thinner than those of the AV. The three PV leaflets are termed anterior, left, and right. The latter two are situated posterior to the anterior leaflet and may be more correctly termed the right posterior and left posterior (Fig. 15.1).

The valvular apparatus of the PV consists of the three leaflets or cusps, their associated sinuses of Valsalva, and a sinotubular junction, similar to that of the AV. This structural similarity is a consequence of their common embryologic origin. Both semilunar valves develop from ridges of subendocardial tissue that form at the orifices of the aorta and the pulmonary trunk after partition of the bulbus cordis and the truncus arteriosus has occurred (6). The annulus of the PV is much more ill defined and distensible than that of the AV because the pulmonary root attaches directly to RV muscle rather than to a fibrous annular ring. The geometric relationships between the valve annulus and sinotubular junction are similar on the right and left sides of the heart, resulting in a pulmonic sinotubular junction that is 10% to 15% smaller than the PV annulus diameter (7). The PV area is similar to that of the AV, approximately 2 cm^2/m^2 body surface area. The anterior and right posterior PV leaflets and their associated sinuses of Valsalva are slightly larger than the left posterior (8). Other features common to both the PV and the AV are the *nodulus Arantii* (small fibrous nodules in the free margin of the cusp) and the *lunula* (thin half-moon–shaped areas along the free edge of each cusp that can have perforations not considered clinically important) (9).

TRANSESOPHAGEAL ECHOCARDIOGRAPHIC EVALUATION OF THE TRICUSPID AND PULMONIC VALVES

Two-Dimensional and Color Flow Doppler Examination

A complete evaluation of the right-sided valves includes standard two-dimensional (2D) views, color flow Doppler (CFD), and spectral Doppler examination of the right-sided chambers, TV, PV, vena cavae, hepatic veins, and proximal main pulmonary artery (PA). TEE may prove less effective in visualizing the TV and PV compared to the MV and AV due to the anterior location of the right-sided valves. Examination of the TV may be especially difficult in the presence of a calcified or prosthetic aortic or mitral annulus or a thickened interatrial

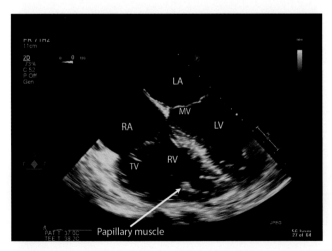

Figure 15.2. TEE image of a modified ME 4-C view showing a prominent papillary muscle in the RV near the apex. RA, right atrium; LA, left atrium; RV, right ventricle; LV, left ventricle; TV, tricuspid valve; MV, mitral valve.

TABLE 15.1	Suggested Views for Imaging Tricuspid and Pulmonic Valves	
View	**Transducer Position (degrees)**	**Right-Sided Structures Imaged**
ME 4-C	0–10	RA, RV, TV, IAS, IVS
Midesophageal RV inflow-outflow	60–90	TV, RV, RVOT, PV
Modified midesophageal bicaval	90–120	RA, IAS, SVC, IVC, CS, TV
Modified midesophageal ascending aortic short axis	0–10	PV, main PA, right PA
UE aortic arch short axis	60–100	PA, PV, aortic arch
TG TV short axis	0–20	TV (anterior, posterior, and septal leaflets)
TG RV inflow	100–120	RV, RA, TV, chordae, papillary muscles
TG RV outflow	120–145	RA, TV, RV, RVOT, PV
TG hepatic	0–120 (variable)	Hepatic veins
Deep TG RV inflow	0	RA, IAS, TV, RV, IVS

PA, pulmonary artery; PV, pulmonic valve; RA, right atrium; RV, right ventricle; TV, tricuspid valve; IAS, interatrial septum; IVS, interventricular septum; RVOT, right ventricular outflow tract; SVC, superior vena cava; IVC, inferior vena cava; CS, coronary sinus.

septum. Furthermore, visualization of all three leaflets of the PV is difficult with either transthoracic echocardiography (TTE) or TEE. The Society of Cardiovascular Anesthesiologists, in collaborative effort with the American Society of Echocardiography (SCA/ASE), has published TEE practice guidelines detailing standard imaging planes useful for evaluating the TV and the PV (10). The relevant views for examination of these right heart structures are listed in Table 15.1.

The midesophageal four-chamber (ME 4-C) view is the starting point for assessing the TV. In this view, the atria and ventricles, the atrioventricular valves, and the atrial and ventricular septa are well seen. The TV septal leaflet is displayed to the right of the screen, with either the anterior or posterior leaflets to the left, depending on the degree of TEE probe retroflexion (Fig. 15.3A,B). It may be necessary to advance the probe slightly to optimize this view if the TV is obscured by a calcified or prosthetic AV.

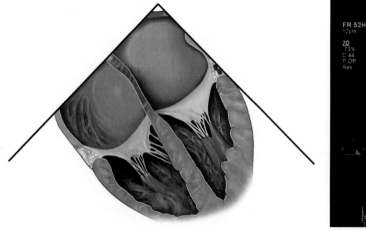

A

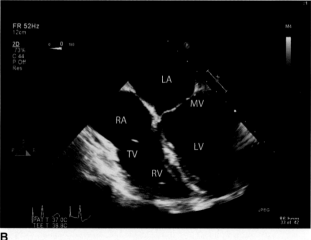

B

Figure 15.3. **A:** Anatomic drawing of the ME 4-C view (Modified and reprinted from Konstadt SN, Shernan S, Oka Y, eds. *Clinical Transesophageal Echocardiography: A Problem Oriented Approach.* 2nd ed. Philadelphia: Lippincott Williams & Wilkins, with permission). **B:** TEE image of a ME 4-C view. RA, right atrium; LA, left atrium; RV, right ventricle; LV, left ventricle; TV, tricuspid valve; MV, mitral valve.

Anatomic abnormalities of the TV are easily seen, as well as the relative sizes of the RA and ventricle that may result from TV pathology. Other relevant information that may be obtained from this view includes the tricuspid annular diameter in systole and diastole and qualitative and quantitative assessments of the tricuspid annular motion.

CFD examination of the TV allows assessment of tricuspid regurgitation (TR). The valve should be interrogated throughout its superior-to-inferior aspect and across its transverse dimension (0, 30, and 60 degrees) to completely map the TR jet and determine the severity of regurgitation. Spectral Doppler examination of the valve may be attempted in this imaging plane, but the angle of interception between the direction of flow and the ultrasound beam may preclude an accurate result. The PV is not visualized in the ME 4-C view.

At the same midesophageal level, advancement of the transducer multiplane angle (60–90 degrees) will display the midesophageal RV inflow-outflow view. In this view, the TV will appear to the left side of the screen display,

with the posterior leaflet to the left and the anterior leaflet to the right. In the right far field, the PV is visible, separating the proximal PA and RVOT (Fig. 15.4A–C). Rotation of the probe to the left (counterclockwise) may improve the image of the proximal main PA, allowing evaluation of its first few centimeters for abnormalities. Of note, although the PV leaflets may not be clearly imaged in this view, CFD may still be used to detect pulmonic regurgitation (PR) (Fig. 15.4D).

A third imaging plane for examining RV inflow can be acquired beginning with the midesophageal bicaval view (90–110 degrees), then advancing the multiplane angle further to 120–140 degrees and applying slight counterclockwise probe rotation (Fig. 15.5A,B). The Eustachian valve and CS are often well seen on the left side of the display. In this modified bicaval view, sometimes referred to as an RV inflow/CS view, the basal RV and portions of the TV appear in the left far field and allow evaluation of TV inflow and regurgitation. The direction of blood flow and the ultrasound beam vector are closely aligned

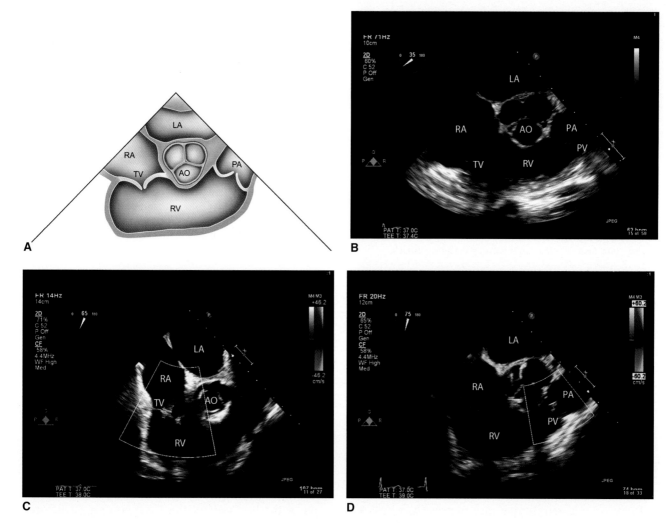

Figure 15.4. A: Anatomic drawing of the midesophageal right ventricular inflow-outflow view. **B:** TEE image of a right ventricular inflow-outflow view. **C:** CFD interrogation of the TV showing mild TR. **D:** CFD interrogation of the PV showing trivial TR. RA, right atrium; LA, left atrium; RV, right ventricle; AO, aortic valve; TV, tricuspid valve; PV, pulmonary valve; PA, pulmonary artery.

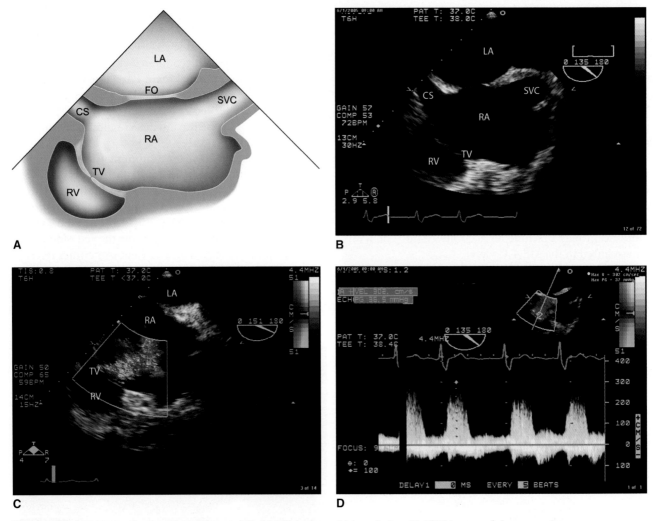

Figure 15.5. **A:** Anatomic drawing of the modified midesophageal bicaval view. **B:** TEE image of the same view. **C:** CFD interrogation of the TV showing moderate TR in the same view. **D:** Spectral Doppler interrogation of the TV. Note peak TR jet velocity of 302 cm/s, which corresponds to a peak systolic transvalvular pressure gradient of 36.5 mm Hg. RA, right atrium; LA, left atrium; FO, fossa ovalis; CS, coronary sinus; SVC, superior vena cava; IVC, inferior vena cava; TV, tricuspid valve; RV, right ventricle.

in this view, thereby allowing accurate spectral Doppler assessment of transvalvular flow (Fig. 15.5C). Continuous wave (CW) Doppler analysis of TR peak jet velocity allows estimation of RV and PA systolic (PAs) pressures (Fig. 15.5D). This view is also useful for TEE-guided percutaneous placement of CS catheters.

Also useful for PV imaging is the upper esophageal (UE) aortic arch short-axis view. In this window, the PA and the PV appear on the left side of the screen, with PV flow well aligned with the ultrasound beam vector (Fig. 15.6A). Hence, it is one of the best views for assessing the severity of pulmonic stenosis (PS) and PR (Fig. 15.6B,C). Turning the probe slightly to the left (counterclockwise) and retroflexing may improve the view of the PV. This view provides the best longitudinal assessment of the main PA.

Transgastric (TG) views of the right-sided heart valves are useful, although slightly more difficult to obtain.

A short axis of the RV is obtained by visualizing the short axis of the LV and rotating the probe to the right (clockwise). By anteflexing the probe and withdrawing slightly, the three leaflets of the TV come into view in a manner somewhat analogous to that of the short axis of the leaflets of the MV (Fig. 15.7). The anterior leaflet appears in the left far field, the posterior leaflet in the left near field, and the septal leaflet to the right of these.

The TG RV inflow view is also developed from the TG midpapillary, short-axis view of the left ventricle (LV) by turning the probe slightly rightward (clockwise), centering the RV on the display, and advancing the multiplane angle to 90–110 degrees (Fig. 15.8A,B). This scan plane provides the best view of the TV supporting structures, including the chordae tendineae and papillary muscles. The RV appears on the left and the RA on the right of the display screen. Improved views of the PV and the RVOT may be obtained by advancing the multiplane angle further

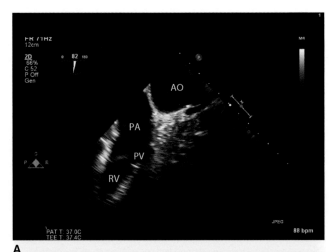

A

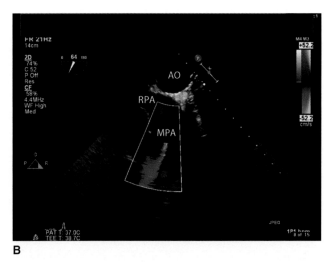

B

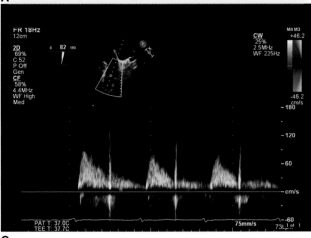

C

Figure 15.6. **A:** TEE image of an UE aortic arch short-axis view. **B:** CFD interrogation of the PV valve in diastole in the same view demonstrating mild PR. **C:** Spectral Doppler interrogation of the PV. RV, right ventricle; PV, pulmonary valve; PA, pulmonary artery; MPA, main pulmonary artery; RPA, right pulmonary artery; AO, aorta.

and anteflexing the probe, in what is sometimes referred to as the TG RV *outflow* view. This brings PV and the RVOT into view somewhere between 100 and 145 degrees (Fig. 15.8C,D) (10–12). At times, the AV may appear just to the right of the PV, demonstrating the intimate relationship

between the two semilunar valves. Measurements of the tricuspid annulus in this view correlate best with intraoperative surgical measurements (12). From this scan plane, the TEE probe can be rotated further rightward (clockwise) to image the hepatic veins, most easily identified with CFD. Pulsed wave (PW) Doppler can then be used to evaluate hepatic venous flow velocities (Fig. 15.9A,B). Adjustment of the multiplane angle (0–120 degrees) is often required to provide optimal hepatic vein alignment for spectral Doppler measurements.

Finally, further advancing the TEE probe to the deep TG position at 0 degrees, rightward (clockwise) probe rotation, and anteflexion will reveal another view of the RV and the TV. CFD and spectral Doppler evaluation of TR jets is also possible in this view (Fig. 15.10A,B).

An additional view for assessment of right-sided heart valve pathology, while not directly focused on TV or PV imaging, is a view of the short axis of the aorta, the main and right pulmonary arteries, and superior vena cava (SVC) at the base of the heart. This view is developed from the AV short-axis view by slow withdrawal of the TEE probe until these structures come into view. In this modification of the midesophageal ascending aortic short axis view, the distal portion of the main PA is seen to the right of the screen and the proximal right PA is seen in long

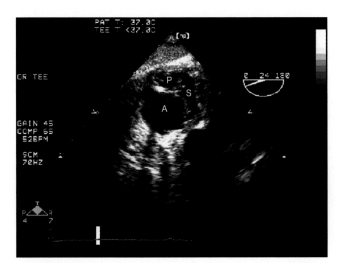

Figure 15.7. TEE image of a TG TV short-axis view. Note the location of the large anterior leaflet (A) and smaller posterior (P) and septal (S) leaflets with respect to the TEE transducer.

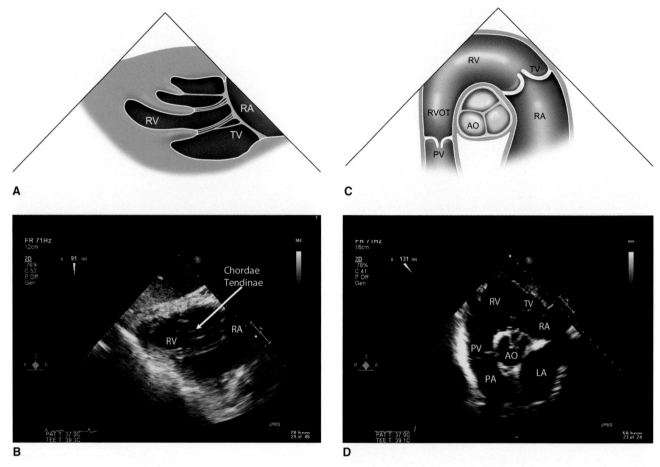

Figure 15.8. **A:** Anatomic drawing of the TG right ventricular inflow view with subvalvular apparatus of the TV prominent. **B:** TEE image of a midesophageal RV inflow view focusing on the TV subvalvular apparatus. **C:** Anatomic drawing of the TG right ventricular outflow view. **D:** TEE view of a TG RV outflow view with focus on the RVOT and PV. Note the intimate relationship between the two semilunar valves. RA, right atrium; LA, left atrium; RV, right ventricle; AO, aortic valve; TV, tricuspid valve; RVOT, right ventricular outflow tract; PV, pulmonary valve; PA, pulmonary artery.

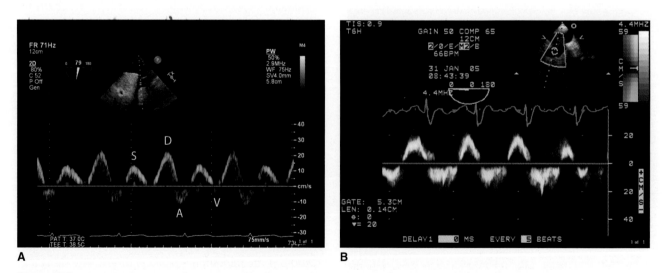

Figure 15.9. **A:** Normal PW Doppler pattern of hepatic vein flow velocity. **B:** Hepatic venous flow in demonstrating TR. Note S wave reversal.

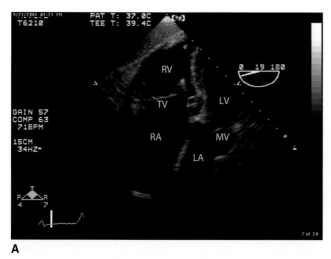 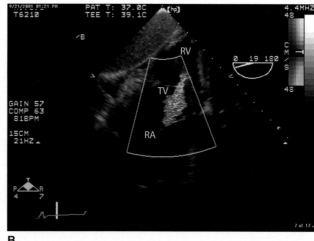

A   B

Figure 15.10. A: TEE image of the deep TG right ventricular inflow view. **B:** CFD demonstrating TV regurgitation. RA, right atrium; LA, left atrium; RV, right ventricle; LV, left ventricle; TV, tricuspid valve; MV, mitral valve.

axis at the top of the screen. When properly positioned, a PA catheter can be seen in both the SVC and the right main PA in this view. The left PA is usually obscured by the bronchial structures (Fig. 15.11).

Any of the echocardiographic imaging artifacts may confound evaluation of the TV and the PV. Especially pertinent to imaging of the right-sided structures, however, are pacing wires and intracardiac catheters that may cause acoustic shadowing or be misinterpreted as intracardiac masses, clots, or vegetations (Fig. 15.12) (13).

Spectral Doppler Examination

Evaluation of flow through the TV and PV is performed using spectral Doppler techniques. Analysis of tricuspid flow is optimally performed using the modified bicaval view, the ME RV inflow-outflow view, or the ME 4-C view, depending on which view provides the best alignment of flow with the ultrasound beam. The sample volume should be placed between the TV leaflet tips during diastole to assess diastolic filling patterns. Analogous to transmitral flow, characteristic early (E) wave and atrial (A) wave Doppler peaks correspond, respectively, to early ventricular filling and late diastolic filling from atrial contraction. From these recordings, E velocity, A velocity, E/A velocity ratio, and E-wave deceleration time may be measured or calculated. Typical pathologic patterns of diastolic dysfunction include impaired relaxation (E < A) and restriction (E >> A) of RV filling. It is important to note that tricuspid inflow patterns have lower absolute velocities than the corresponding mitral inflow velocities owing to the larger cross-sectional area of the TV.

Useful information concerning TV and RV function may often be obtained by the analysis of hepatic venous

Figure 15.11. TEE image of the UE aortic short-axis view. The PV, main PA (MPA), and PA bifurcation are clearly seen. The right PA (RPA) is seen traversing posterior to the ascending aorta (AO).

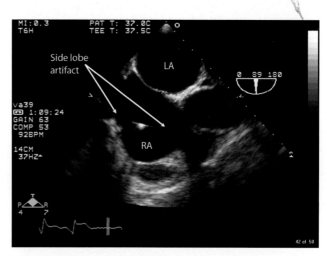

Figure 15.12. Midesophageal bicaval view showing a PA catheter in the RA. RA, right atrium; LA, left atrium.

flow patterns. Normal venous flow in the hepatic veins is similar to pulmonary venous flow, with antegrade systolic (S) and diastolic (D) waves, and a retrograde atrial (A) wave resulting from atrial contraction (Fig. 15.9A). At times, an additional small retrograde wave appears at end systole and is termed a *V-wave*. This additional retrograde wave likely results from tricuspid annular recoil motion toward the base of the heart at end systole. When right atrial pressure is increased, the S-wave and the S/D ratio decrease while the A-wave increases. Severe TR eliminates the normal antegrade S-wave and produces a reversed flow signal during systole (Fig. 15.9B). In patients with atrial fibrillation, no A-wave is seen in the hepatic venous or TV inflow patterns.

Spectral Doppler assessment of the TV may provide a great deal of pertinent hemodynamic information. As mentioned earlier, PAs pressure may be estimated by measuring the peak velocity of the TR jet, using the simplified Bernoulli equation to estimate the transvalvular gradient, and adding an estimate of RA pressure to derive RV (or PA) systolic pressure (Fig. 15.5D; Table 15.2). In spontaneously breathing patients, RA pressure can be estimated by measuring the size and respiratory variation in IVC dimensions (see Chapter 10 on RV function, Table 2).

For accurate results, quantitative spectral Doppler measurements must be made carefully, assuring that the ultrasound beam is parallel to the flow vector. Misinterpretation may result when the TR Doppler signal is contaminated by a high velocity jet of mitral regurgitation or aortic stenosis and not differentiated from these other high velocity signals. The TR jet may be distinguished by identifying the accompanying low-velocity antegrade diastolic flow signal that results from flow through the TV. Contrast enhancement of the TR jet with agitated saline injection may also help make the signal envelope more visible.

Spectral Doppler assessment of PV flow usually follows CFD assessment of PR and PS and is best accomplished in the UE aortic arch short-axis view or the TG view of the RVOT and the PV (Figs. 15.6C and 15.8D). CFD is helpful to define the direction of flow and assist in alignment of the Doppler beam for PW and CW techniques. Because flow through the PV is roughly perpendicular to that through the AV, the two are rarely confused. Normal blood flow through the PV is directed in an anterior-to-posterior direction and slightly right-to-left direction with respect to the patient. PS is considered mild when the peak gradient across the PV is less than 30 mm Hg, moderate when the gradient is 30 to 50mm Hg, and severe when the gradient is greater than 50 mm Hg (14). It is important to remember that Doppler techniques measure peak instantaneous gradients, while catheter-based techniques measure peak-to-peak gradients and that variables such as different hemodynamic states, viscous forces, and flow acceleration effects affect these measurements differently. Correlation studies on patients with different degrees of severity of pulmonary stenosis have shown that *mean* Doppler and catheter-based gradients correlate better than *peak* gradients (15).

Doppler patterns of regurgitant flow may also be used to estimate PA pressures. In the absence of PS, PAs pressure equals RV systolic pressure. The RV systolic pressure can be obtained from measuring the pressure gradient between the RV and RA from the TR jet peak velocity using the simplified Bernoulli equation, and then adding the RA pressure. The diastolic PA (PAd) pressure can be calculated from the end-diastolic PR jet velocity as follows: at end diastole, the RV pressure equals RA pressure. Since the gradient between the PA and the RV at end diastole may be calculated using the end-diastolic PR jet velocity, the PAd can then be deduced (Table 15.2). Several different formulas are available for the calculation of mean PA (PAm) pressure. In addition to the standard calculation of mean pressure as 2/3 of the diastolic pressure plus 1/3 of the systolic pressure, PAm pressure can also be derived from measurement of RV acceleration time, which becomes proportionally shorter as pulmonary pressures increase (16). Of the other formulas available, the one derived by Chemla et al. and confirmed by others appears to be the most accurate and simple to use (Table 15.2) (17). PW Doppler can be used to assess RV stroke volume, and to calculate regurgitant and shunt fractions (Table 15.2) (11,18).

Three-Dimensional Examination

The 3D examination of the TV may add clinically relevant information to the standard 2D assessment. Since traditional 2D imaging cannot provide a real-time view of the entire valve, an anterior to posterior sweep of the TEE transducer is required for the echocardiographer to mentally envision valve anatomy. A 3D *en face* view

TABLE 15.2	Formulas Useful for Assessing the TV, PV, and PA Blood Flow

PAs (RVSP) = $4V^2$ + CVP

   V = peak systolic velocity of the tricuspid regurgitant jet

PAd = $4V^2$ + RVDP or CVP

   V = end-diastolic velocity of the pulmonary regurgitant jet

PAm = $0.61 \times$ PAs + 2 mm Hg (17)

RV SV = PV area $\times$ VTI_{PV}

RV SV = $0.785 \times$ (PV diameter)^2 $\times$ VTI_{PV}

RV, right ventricle; RA, right atrium; PA, pulmonary artery; V, velocity; RVSP, right ventricle systolic pressure; PAs, pulmonary artery systolic pressure; CVP, central venous pressure; PAd, pulmonary artery diastolic pressure; RVDP, right ventricle diastolic pressure; SV, stroke volume; PAm, pulmonary artery mean pressure; VTI, velocity time integral; PV, pulmonic valve.

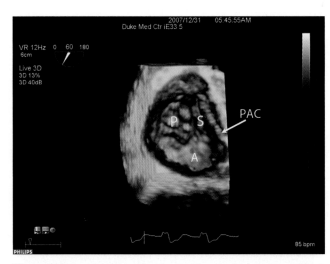

Figure 15.13. The 3D *en face* view of the TV from the atrial perspective. A, anterior leaflet; S, septal leaflet; P, posterior leaflet; PAC, pulmonary anrtery catheter.

of the TV eliminates the need for probe manipulation and mental reconstruction of valve anatomy and provides a simultaneous view of the anatomical relationship between the three valve leaflets, their points of coaptation, and movements during the cardiac cycle (Fig. 15.13) (19). The 3D imaging may reduce interobserver variability and may allow the diagnosis of unusual TV variants, such as a bileaflet TV (20). Other reports highlight the incremental value of real-time 3D transthoracic and TEE over the 2D technique in carcinoid disease, Ebstein's anomaly, chordal rupture, rheumatic tricuspid disease, prolapsing Chiari network, and other uncommon valvular pathology (19,21,22,22a). Although also technically challenging, 3D examination of the PV has been reported to provide additional information in some cases (23).

The morphology of the TV and PV leaflets and annulae is generally best assessed using the real-time 3D zoom mode. The 3D full volume mode images may provide additional information regarding the RV walls and papillary muscles, and the 3D color full volume mode may be useful to assess TR jets.

In spite of these reported benefits, 3D examination of the right-sided valves remains difficult with current ultrasound technology, likely due to the anterior location and thin leaflets of these valves. In one recent report, optimal visualization of the tricuspid leaflets from both the atrial and ventricular perspectives was only possible in 11% of cases (24).

Tricuspid Regurgitation

TR is by far the most common right heart valvular abnormality. Assessment should include quantification of TR severity and description of its underlying mechanism. Mild TR is extremely common in the normal population. It has an overall incidence of 65% but may be seen in up to 93% of patients over 70 years of age (25). This

"physiologic" TR, however, should have a high-velocity, turbulent, small CFD jet.

The most common causes of clinically significant TR are annular dilation and altered RV anatomy that result from pulmonary hypertension (PHTN), constrictive pericarditis, PS, or RV ischemia or infarction. Moderate or severe TR may also develop in patients with rheumatic disease, endocarditis, carcinoid heart disease, tumors, endomyocardial fibrosis, or mechanical valve damage resulting from trauma or iatrogenic injury from cardiac catheters (26–28).

Assessing severity of TR and deciding whether it is physiologic or pathologic may be difficult. Normal TR jet velocity is 2.0 to 2.5 m/s (29). Higher velocities indicate PHTN or PS, both of which increase RV systolic pressure and TR jet velocity. Note that TR jet velocity is directly related to RV systolic pressure; it is not related to the severity of TR. Consequently, lower TR jet velocities often accompany more severe degrees of regurgitation, and a large TR CFD jet area with a laminar regurgitant flow pattern indicates unrestricted, severe TR.

There are several alternative, complementary methods used to evaluate TR. Right ventricular volume overload suggests severe TR unless another etiology is identified. Echocardiographic signs include RV and RA enlargement, flattening of the ventricular septum, dilatation of the tricuspid annulus, SVC, IVC, or hepatic veins, and leftward displacement of the atrial septum. The proximal isovelocity surface area (PISA) method of determining the size of the regurgitant orifice may be useful in quantifying the degree of TR, although this is rarely done (30). In addition, PWD analysis of the hepatic veins may show reversed flow during systole (Fig. 15.9B). As always, clinical correlation is extremely important because chronic valvular disease can increase RA compliance and obviate many of these findings.

Several CFD grading systems for TR have been reported in the literature (Table 15.3). The first focuses on the longitudinal extension of the jet into the RA and the other two focus on estimation of the CFD regurgitant jet area. All three systems classify TR into three or four grades: trace or trivial, mild, moderate, and severe regurgitation (31–33). Although these grades of TR correlate well with

TABLE 15.3	TR Classification Schemes		
	RA Area (%)	TR Jet Area (cm²)	Length of TR Jet (cm)
Trace		<2	<1.5
Mild	≤20	2–4	1.5–3.0
Moderate	21–33	4–10	3.0–4.5
Severe	≥33	>10	>4.5

TR, tricuspid regurgitation; RA, right atrium.

angiographic measurements, it is important to remember that all of these methods are semiquantitative and subject to technical and physiologic factors that affect jet length and area.

Pulmonic Regurgitation

As with other regurgitant lesions, trace amounts of PR are normally seen in healthy persons, with a higher prevalence in the elderly. Clinically relevant PR in the adult is usually the result of PHTN, carcinoid disease, endocarditis, or surgery involving the RVOT or PV itself, as in repair of Tetralogy of Fallot.

CFD analysis is used to map the extent of the PR jet into the RVOT. Trace and mild degrees of PR, of minimal clinical significance, are diagnosed when the PR jet is less than one centimeter in length and only appears in late diastole (Figs. 15.4D and 15.6B). Most PR jets are central, although a prolapsed or restricted pulmonic leaflet may produce an eccentric jet. Regurgitant jets that are pandiastolic and of greater dimension are generally considered pathologic. However, PR is considered clinically significant only when the jet extends more than two centimeters into the RVOT or reaches within one centimeter of the TV (34,35). When assessed using PWD or CWD, severe PR can be recognized because it results in rapid equalization of the RV and PA end diastolic pressures. As a result, the PR Doppler signal, which is normally sustained throughout diastole, is greatly shortened, returning to the baseline (zero flow) well before the onset of the next systole.

As in the case of TR jets, PR jet velocity is not related to the severity of valvular regurgitation. In addition, owing to the small pressure gradient between the PA and the RV, even small PR jets may not appear turbulent, and jet velocity may vary greatly with respiration. Hence, accurate and meaningful measurements of PR jet velocity must include averaging over several cardiac cycles. In the setting of tachycardia, color M-mode of the RVOT may be a useful method to measure the width of the PR jet in relation to the diameter of the RVOT (36).

Tricuspid Stenosis

Tricuspid stenosis (TS) is most commonly of rheumatic etiology, and in these cases, the MV is invariably involved. Other causes of TS include congenital anomalies, endocarditis, methysergide toxicity, carcinoid heart disease, and endomyocardial fibrosis. On 2D examination, characteristic findings of rheumatic TS include doming of the leaflets during diastole, thickening of the leaflet tips, restricted leaflet motion, and commissural fusion (Fig. 15.14). Doppler evaluation of TV inflow will show increased peak velocities (E waves > 1.5 m/s) (37,38). Of note, when TS results from carcinoid syndrome, the leaflets appear more fixed and retracted and do not display the typical doming seen in rheumatic TS.

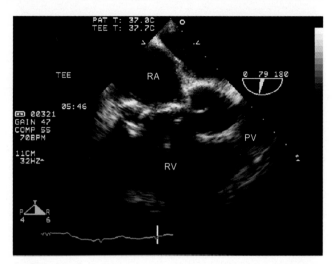

Figure 15.14. Midesophageal RV inflow outflow view demonstrating severe TS. RA, right atrium; RV, right ventricle; PV, pulmonary valve.

Pulmonic Stenosis

Similarly to TS, PS is characterized by leaflet doming due to commissural fusion, leaflet thickening, and restricted systolic motion. Other relevant echocardiographic findings that may confirm the clinical significance of stenosis include poststenotic dilatation of the main PA and its primary branches. Interestingly, the left PA will often be more dilated than the right (34,38). Hypertrophy of the RV, flattening of the ventricular septum producing a characteristic D-shaped LV, RA enlargement, and moderate-to-severe TR all suggest RV pressure overload. In this setting, a search for coexisting congenital anomalies is important.

The peak pressure gradient across the PV indicates PS severity and is often classified as mild (gradient < 30 mm Hg), moderate (gradient = 30–50 mm Hg), or severe (gradient > 50 mm Hg) (14). PS should be easily detectable with CFD mapping of the PV and proximal PA, which should reveal a highly turbulent PA jet with marked aliasing of the color flow signal.

M-mode echocardiography may be useful in differentiating valvular PR and PS from severe PHTN as a cause of right-sided valvular dysfunction or RV failure, by helping identify structural leaflet pathology in patients with PS. Early systolic closure of the PV and an absent A wave occur with severe PHTN but not with valvular PS.

CONGENITAL DISEASES OF THE TRICUSPID AND PULMONIC VALVES

Ebstein's Anomaly

Ebstein's anomaly of the TV is a rare congenital disorder that occurs in approximately 1 per 210,000 live births (39). Echocardiography is the diagnostic test of choice for this heterogeneous condition, in which there is inadequate delamination of the TV leaflets from the endocardium of the RV. This results in features that are characteristic of this anomaly, which include apical displacement of the leaflets, particularly the septal leaflet, with associated TR and right ventricular dysfunction (Fig. 15.15). The cardinal echocardiographic feature is apical displacement of the insertion point of the septal leaflet of the TV relative to the insertion of the anterior leaflet of the MV by at least 8 mm/m^2 body surface area (40). Other features include dilation of the "atrialized" portion of the RV, redundancy, fenestrations and tethering of the anterior TV leaflet, and dilation of the true tricuspid annulus (9,30,41). An atrial septal defect or patent foramen ovale is commonly seen in these patients, most likely due to increased right atrial pressures (42). Other associated findings in patients with Ebstein's anomaly include MV prolapse, bicuspid AV, coarctation of the aorta, ventricular septal defects, pulmonary stenosis, and hypoplastic PA. Clinical presentation is highly variable and dependent on the degree of apical displacement of the TV and distortion of RV anatomy and function. The cardinal symptoms of the disease include cyanosis, right ventricular failure, and arrhythmias (43). Generally, greater degrees of valvular displacement and smaller portions of residual normal RV cavity result in more severe symptoms and a worse prognosis.

Tricuspid dysplasia may sometimes be seen in Ebstein's anomaly and is defined as irregularity, thickening, and nodularity of the TV leaflets. The valve may be described as tethered when three or more accessory attachments of the leaflet to the RV wall exist and restrict leaflet motion. Other features include RV dysplasia (thinning, dilation, and hypokinesis or dyskinesis) and marked enlargement of the RA (43).

The characteristics of the anterior leaflet of the TV and the size of the RV relative to the remaining three chambers are especially important to note during the

echocardiographic assessment of Ebstein's anomaly. A tethered anterior leaflet with restricted motion and a small functional RV (ratio of functional to total RV cavity dimension <35% in the ME 4-C view) are indications for valve replacement. Plastic repair may be considered if the anterior TV leaflet is elongated, has no fenestrations, and shows large excursion (44).

Limitations of 2D echocardiography include inability to adequately characterize the posterior TV leaflet and identify fenestrations or perforations in the anterior TV leaflet (44). By allowing an *en face* view of the entire valve, real-time 3D TEE overcomes some of these difficulties and may provide a more precise description of the anomalies present in this condition (45,21).

Tricuspid Atresia

In tricuspid atresia, there is no normal flow through the tricuspid annulus, and the only egress from the RA is via the foramen ovale or an atrial septal defect. Pulmonary blood flow is supplied through a patent ductus arteriosus or a ventricular septal defect and is highly dependent on the size of these connections. Most patients present in the first months of life with cyanosis, but if the sizes of these left-to-right shunts are optimal, this condition may remain clinically stable for many years and present first in young adulthood. In such cases, congestive heart failure from long-standing left ventricular volume overload brings these patients to clinical attention (6).

Congenital Anomalies of the Pulmonic Valve

Congenital PS usually presents in newborns although it may remain undiagnosed into adulthood. The obstruction may be above, below, or at the level of the PV. Valvular PS is the most common form and accounts for 10% to 12% of all congenital heart disease in the United States (8). In the neonate, complete RVOT obstruction from critical PS or pulmonary atresia cannot occur as an isolated lesion (46). These patients require a shunt or other corrective procedure to palliate or repair the condition.

ACQUIRED DISEASES OF THE TRICUSPID AND PULMONIC VALVES

Functional Tricuspid Regurgitation

The most common cause of clinically significant TR is annular dilation and altered RV anatomy that results from PHTN, (primary or secondary to left-sided valvular disease or ventricular failure), chronic RV ischemia, cardiomyopathy, or volume overload (26–28). Often termed "functional" TR because there is no intrinsic pathology of the TV leaflets, this form of TR results from dilatation of the TV annulus, dysfunction of the supporting apparatus, and malcoaptation of the valve leaflets. Multiple regurgitant jets are commonly seen. Classically,

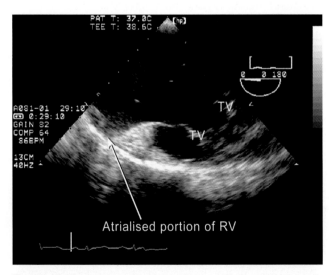

Figure 15.15. TEE image of a patient with Ebstein's anomaly showing apical displacement of the TV leaflet and the thin, "atrialized" portion of the affected right ventricular wall. TV, tricuspid valve.

the annulus dilates asymmetrically in the septal to lateral and anteroseptal to posterolateral directions, resulting in a more circular shape (2,46a). With severe annular dilation, the TV is more dependent on annular shortening for adequate leaflet coaptation to prevent regurgitation. As RV dysfunction progresses, the sphincter-like function of the TV is lost and TAFS is reduced.

Transthoracic echocardiographic studies have proposed a maximal (diastolic) annular diameter of greater than 21 mm/m² and a TAFS of less than 25% (as measured using apical four-chamber and parasternal short-axis imaging planes) to be indications for repair irrespective of TR severity (4,47), but these measurements have not been tested using TEE. The tricuspid annulus should be evaluated in multiple views and measurements obtained in the TG RV inflow view, since these correlate best with intraoperative tricuspid annular measurements on the arrested heart (12). Obtaining three separate measurements at end-expiration and averaging them provides the most accurate results.

Endocarditis

Echocardiography is the diagnostic test of choice for detecting vegetations and perivalvular abscesses. Furthermore, TEE is often preferable to TTE due to the low negative predictive value of the latter (48,49). Vegetations vary in appearance from flat, small sessile lesions involving a single leaflet to large bulky, friable, echodense, or oscillating masses that may obstruct flow through the valve. These larger vegetations are more common in tricuspid endocarditis (Fig. 15.16). The most common organisms are *Staphylococcus aureus* and *Streptococcus viridans*. Tricuspid endocarditis is less common than mitral or aortic endocarditis, except among intravenous drug abusers (48,50,51). When using TEE to evaluate endocarditis, it is important to evaluate the chordae tendineae and other supporting structures because these may be involved in the infectious/inflammatory process (48,50,51).

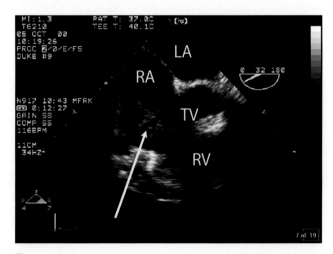

Figure 15.16. Modified ME 4-C TEE view demonstrating a TV vegetation in a patient with endocarditis. RA, right atrium; LA, left atrium; RV, right ventricle; TV, tricuspid valve.

Even rarer than tricuspid disease is isolated endocarditis of the PV. In addition, the PV is the least commonly involved valve in cases of multivalvular endocarditis and usually occurs in patients with other predisposing factors, such as a structurally abnormal PV, immunosuppression, or intravenous drug abuse (52,53). Indwelling intravascular catheters or wires are another risk factor for right-sided endocarditis (54,55). Complications of tricuspid and pulmonic endocarditis include septic pulmonary emboli or infarcts and RV failure.

Carcinoid Heart Disease

Carcinoid tumors are rare malignancies that originate from enterochromaffin cells located most frequently in the gastrointestinal tract. Carcinoid heart disease occurs almost exclusively in patients with primary carcinoid tumors that do not drain into the portal circulation, such as ovarian tumors, or in patients with hepatic metastases of their primary gastrointestinal carcinoid tumors. Vasoactive amines, such as serotonin and bradykinin, are chronically secreted and lead to fibrosis, chronic inflammation, and neovascularization of the surface of the right heart valves predominantly. Characteristic carcinoid plaque deposition occurs on the "downstream" endocardial surfaces of the valves (ventricular surface of the TV and the pulmonary arterial surface of the PV) initially, eventually encasing the entire free edge of the valve and extending to the chords and papillary muscles (56). Right-sided cardiac valve involvement occurs in 50% of patients with carcinoid tumors and can be rapidly progressive (57). Of note, TEE has been used to monitor somatostatin analog therapy in patients with carcinoid heart disease (58). Cardiac surgical intervention is indicated for severe valvular disease because carcinoid is a slow-growing tumor and carcinoid-related death more commonly results from cardiac failure than primary tumor growth.

Echocardiographically, carcinoid heart disease produces short, thickened, retracted TV leaflets that eventually become immobile and often remain fixed in the open position, resulting in severe TR (Fig. 15.17). As mentioned above, the typical doming seen in rheumatic TS is not seen in carcinoid heart disease. Interestingly, the PV changes in carcinoid heart disease more often result in valvular stenosis with or without PR.

Rheumatic Heart Disease

The right heart valves can be affected by rheumatic heart disease in several ways. Rheumatic mitral stenosis and/or regurgitation may produce PHTN, resulting in RV enlargement, tricuspid annular dilatation, and functional TR. Acute rheumatic carditis is characterized by myocardial and valve leaflet edema and leukocyte infiltration with eventual erosion of the leaflet tips. Ultimately, bead-like vegetations develop along the line of valve coaptation. Capillaries invade the vegetations during the healing phase, and fibrous nodules develop, frequently involving scarring

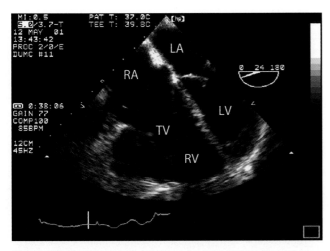

Figure 15.17. TEE image demonstrating TV leaflet thickening and retraction in a patient with carcinoid heart disease. RA, right atrium; LA, left atrium; RV, right ventricle; LV, left ventricle; TV, tricuspid valve.

and fusion of the chordae tendineae. The free edges of the cusps become shortened at the site of healed vegetations, and chordal contracture and commissural fusion develop. TR rather than TS usually results (30). There have been a few case reports of PV involvement in rheumatic heart disease, including one involving all four cardiac valves, but in general, rheumatic PV disease is rare (59).

Echocardiographic features of rheumatic valvular disease include leaflet doming, thickening, and restriction. A reduction of the TV orifice diameter is sometimes present. CW Doppler allows estimation of the transvalvular pressure gradient. Commissural fusion, calcification, and thickening of the subvalvular apparatus are best seen in the TG short and long-axis views of the RV.

Other Pathologic Conditions

TV prolapse is uncommon and rarely found as an isolated condition. Prolapse of both atrioventricular valves usually coexists and is most commonly seen in patients with floppy valve syndromes, such as Ehlers-Danlos syndrome, Marfan's syndrome, Ebstein's anomaly, or septum secundum atrial septal defect. The anterior and septal TV leaflets are most commonly involved, and the resulting regurgitant jet is often eccentric. Diagnosis of TV prolapse is made by identifying displacement of valve leaflet tissue beyond the annular plane into the RA (30).

Heart disease associated with systemic lupus erythematosus is characterized by myocarditis, pericarditis, and endocarditis that may involve the TV. Valvular leaflets may become thickened and stenotic after multiple episodes of lupus endocarditis. Lesions are small, berry-shaped excrescences that appear on both the atrial and ventricular sides of the leaflets as well as on the chordae tendineae, papillary muscles, and the mural endocardium. Characteristic vegetations located on both sides of the TV differentiate lupus endocarditis from rheumatic disease in which the valvular lesions appear preferentially on the atrial side of the TV (60).

Papillary fibroelastomas are rare benign cardiac tumors that usually involve the AV, although they may occasionally appear on the mitral, pulmonic, or TVs. These lesions appear as small, mobile, echodense masses attached to the valve leaflets and may be difficult to differentiate from clot or endocarditis. In general, however, these tumors do not cause TR or PR (61,62).

Twenty percent of all cardiac myxomas occur in the right heart chambers, with three quarters of these originating from the RA. These can affect the TV by prolapsing into the valvular annulus and causing dynamic RV inflow obstruction (37). Renal cell carcinomas may encroach upon the RA and TV and cause obstructive symptoms. Traumatic disruption of the TV causing acute TR, while uncommon, may result from deceleration injuries and produce endothelial tears, hemorrhage into valvular cusps, or rupture of the papillary muscles (63). Either the TV or the PV may be injured iatrogenically during catheterization procedures, although routine PA catheter placement has not been shown to cause significant right-sided valvular dysfunction (64).

In the adult, RVOT obstruction that results from valvular PS may be caused by commissural fusion, leaflet dysplasia, congenital bicuspid valve, rubella embryopathy, rheumatic heart disease, and senile calcification. TEE is particularly useful for monitoring patients, with these conditions, undergoing balloon valvuloplasty (65). Laminar antegrade flow on CFD and a reduced transvalvular peak gradient assessed by CWD provide echocardiographic evidence of a successful procedure. Other uncommon causes of RVOT obstruction include a right sinus of Valsalva aneurysm that encroaches on the RVOT, postoperative mediastinal hematomas, primary sarcomas, pericardial cysts, and iatrogenic obstruction following repair of complex cardiac abnormalities (66,67).

Perhaps the most common cause of RVOT obstruction in adults is dynamic obstruction seen in cardiac surgical patients, many of whom are hypovolemic and receiving inotropic drug infusions (see Ref. 20 in Chapter 10).

The Ross Procedure

In certain cases, the PV may be used to replace another valve, most often the AV, in a procedure known as the PV autograft or Ross procedure. The PV has been used to replace the MV as well, although this is much less common (68,69). Prior to the surgical procedure, TEE is used to exclude any congenital or acquired abnormality of the PV that would preclude successful autotransplantation. The diameter of the PV annulus should be 10% to 15% larger than the diameter of its adjacent sinotubular junction, as measured by TEE. Similar measurements are made of the AV. The sizes of the donor and the recipient site should be within 2 mm of each other to avoid distortion of either the transplanted valve annulus or the recipient site sinotubular junction. Size mismatch may result in autograft valvular incompetence. In a series of 81 patients undergoing this procedure, David et al. reported the range of AV annulus diameters to be

19 to 35 mm and the PV annulus diameters to be 19 to 27 mm (7). In cases with size discrepancies, the aortic annulus diameter can be reduced by plication of the annulus and annuloplasty to achieve geometric parity (70). After the harvested PV has been placed in the aortic position, a PV cadaveric homograft is implanted. TEE measurements are also used for appropriate sizing of this graft. Postoperatively, suture lines of the PV homograft are visible with TEE, but there are few other visible echocardiographic changes. However, PR or even PS may develop postoperatively, necessitating balloon valvuloplasty, PA stenting, or even PV replacement with a bioprosthetic or mechanical valve (71).

A variation of the Ross procedure, known as the "semilunar valve switch," is an operation in which the native AV is repaired and reimplanted into the pulmonic position rather than using a cadaveric homograft for the PV. However, in one report, neopulmonic valvular stenosis was present in 54% of patients undergoing this procedure (72).

KEY POINTS

- The TV apparatus is distinguished by its poorly defined annulus, its large anterior and small septal and posterior leaflets, and its corresponding large anterior, small septal, and posterior papillary muscles.
- Compared to the structure of the AV, the PV has an ill-defined apparatus and slightly smaller size.
- The best views in which to evaluate the TV are the ME 4-C view, the RV inflow-outflow view, the midesophageal modified bicaval view, and the TG RV inflow view.
- Most useful views for evaluation of the PV are the midesophageal RV inflow-outflow view, the TG RV outflow view, and the UE aortic arch short-axis view.
- The ascending main PA can be well visualized in multiple views, allowing anatomic assessment of this structure. The right main PA can also be visualized and assessed for pathology, as well as positioning of a PA catheter.
- Differentiation of physiologic TR from pathologic TR involves examination of systolic and diastolic tricuspid annular diameters, right ventricular function, hepatic venous flow patterns, peak TR jet velocity, relative right ventricular and atrial sizes, and pattern on CFD analysis.
- Clinically significant TR is most commonly secondary to left-sided pathology or PHTN.
- Estimations of PAs pressure are best made from the midesophageal modified bicaval view. By this approach, the direction of TR flow is best aligned with the direction of the ultrasound beam.
- In the Ross procedure, the PV is transplanted in the AV position and replaced with a homograft.

REFERENCES

1. Hauck AJ, Freeman DP, Ackermann DM, et al. Surgical pathology of the tricuspid valve: a study of 363 cases spanning 25 years. *Mayo Clin Proc* 1988;63:851–863.
2. Fukuda S, Saracino G, Matsumura Y, et al. Three-dimensional geometry of the tricuspid annulus in healthy subjects and in patients with functional tricuspid regurgitation: a real-time, 3-dimensional echocardiographic study. *Circulation* 2006;114:I492–I498.
3. Tei C, Pilgrim JP, Shah PM, et al. The tricuspid valve annulus: study of size and motion in normal subjects and in patients with tricuspid regurgitation. *Circulation* 1982;66:665–671.
4. Colombo T, Russo C, Ciliberto GR, et al. Tricuspid regurgitation secondary to mitral valve disease: tricuspid annulus function as guide to tricuspid valve repair. *Cardiovasc Surg* 2001;9:369–377.
5. Anwar AM, Soliman OI, Nemes A, et al. Value of assessment of tricuspid annulus: real-time three-dimensional echocardiography and magnetic resonance imaging. *Int J Cardiovasc Imaging* 2007;23:701–705.
6. Gersony W, Pruitt A, Riemenschneider T. The cardiovascular system. In: Behrman R, Kliegman R, Nelson W, et al., eds. *Nelson Textbook of Pediatrics*. 13th ed. Philadelphia: W.B. Saunders, 1987:943–1032.
7. David TE, Omran A, Webb G, et al. Geometric mismatch of the aortic and pulmonary roots causes aortic insufficiency after the Ross procedure. *J Thorac Cardiovasc Surg* 1996;112:1231–1237; discussion 1237–1239.
8. Brickner ME, Hillis LD, Lange RA. Congenital heart disease in adults. First of two parts. *N Engl J Med* 2000;342:256–263.
9. Netter F. Atria and ventricles. In: Yonkman F, ed. *The Heart*. New York: CIBA-GEIGY Corporation, 1981:8.
10. Shanewise JS, Cheung AT, Aronson S, et al. ASE/SCA guidelines for performing a comprehensive intraoperative multiplane transesophageal echocardiography examination: recommendations of the American Society of Echocardiography Council for Intraoperative Echocardiography and the Society of Cardiovascular Anesthesiologists Task Force for Certification in Perioperative Transesophageal Echocardiography. *Anesth Analg* 1999;89:870–884.
11. Maslow A, Comunale ME, Haering JM, et al. Pulsed wave Doppler measurement of cardiac output from the right ventricular outflow tract. *Anesth Analg* 1996;83:466–471.
12. Maslow AD, Schwartz C, Singh AK. Assessment of the tricuspid valve: a comparison of four transesophageal echocardiographic windows. *J Cardiothorac Vasc Anesth* 2004;18:719–724.
13. Song MH, Usui M, Usui A, et al. Giant vegetation mimicking cardiac tumor in tricuspid valve endocarditis after catheter ablation. *Jpn J Thorac Cardiovasc Surg* 2001;49:255–257.
14. Warnes CA, Williams RG, Bashore TM, et al. ACC/AHA 2008 guidelines for the management of adults with congenital heart disease: a report of the American College of Cardiology/American Heart Association Task Force on Practice Guidelines (Writing Committee to Develop Guidelines on the Management of Adults With Congenital Heart Disease). Developed in Collaboration With the American Society of Echocardiography, Heart Rhythm Society, International Society for Adult Congenital Heart Disease, Society for Cardiovascular Angiography and Interventions, and Society of Thoracic Surgeons. *J Am Coll Cardiol* 2008;52:e1–e121.

15. Silvilairat S, Cabalka AK, Cetta F, et al. Echocardiographic assessment of isolated pulmonary valve stenosis: which outpatient Doppler gradient has the most clinical validity? *J Am Soc Echocardiogr* 2005;18:1137–1142.

16. Kitabatake A, Inoue M, Asao M, et al. Noninvasive evaluation of pulmonary hypertension by a pulsed Doppler technique. *Circulation* 1983;68:302–309.

17. Chemla D, Castelain V, Provencher S, et al. Evaluation of various empirical formulas for estimating mean pulmonary artery pressure by using systolic pulmonary artery pressure in adults. *Chest* 2008;135:760–768.

18. Goodman DJ, Harrison DC, Popp RL. Echocardiographic features of primary pulmonary hypertension. *Am J Cardiol* 1974;33:438–443.

19. Ahlgrim AA, Nanda NC, Berther E, et al. Three-dimensional echocardiography: an alternative imaging choice for evaluation of tricuspid valve disorders. *Cardiol Clin* 2007;25:305–309.

20. Anwar AM, Attia WM, Nosir YF, et al. Unusual bileaflet tricuspid valve by real time three-dimensional echocardiography. *Echocardiography* 2008;25:534–536.

21. Ahmed S, Nanda NC, Nekkanti R, et al. Transesophageal three-dimensional echocardiographic demonstration of Ebstein's anomaly. *Echocardiography* 2003;20:305–307.

22. Betrian Blasco P, Sarrat Torres R, Pijuan Domenech MA, et al. Three-dimensional imaging of redundant Chiari's network prolapsing into right ventricle. *J Am Soc Echocardiogr* 2008;21:188. e1—188.e2.

22a. Pothineni RK, Duncan K, Yelamanchili P, et al. Live/real time three-dimensional transthoracic echocardiographic assessment of tricuspid valve pathology: incremental value over the two-dimensional technique. *Echocardiography* 2007;24(5): 541–552.

23. Lee KJ, Connolly HM, Pellikka PA. Carcinoid pulmonary valvulopathy evaluated by real-time 3-dimensional transthoracic echocardiography. *J Am Soc Echocardiogr* 2008;21:407.e1–407.e2.

24. Sugeng L, Shernan SK, Salgo IS, et al. Live 3-dimensional transesophageal echocardiography initial experience using the fully-sampled matrix array probe. *J Am Coll Cardiol* 2008;52:446–449.

25. Klein AL, Burstow DJ, Tajik AJ, et al. Age-related prevalence of valvular regurgitation in normal subjects: a comprehensive color flow examination of 118 volunteers. *J Am Soc Echocardiogr* 1990;3:54–63.

26. Braunwald E. Valvular heart disease. In: Braunwald E, Zipes D, Licina M, eds. *A Textbook of Cardiovascular Medicine*. 6th ed. Philadelphia: W.B. Saunders Company, 2001:1643–1722.

27. Cohen SR, Sell JE, McIntosh CL, et al. Tricuspid regurgitation in patients with acquired, chronic, pure mitral regurgitation. I. Prevalence, diagnosis, and comparison of preoperative clinical and hemodynamic features in patients with and without tricuspid regurgitation. *J Thorac Cardiovasc Surg* 1987;94:481–487.

28. Morrison DA, Ovitt T, Hammermeister KE. Functional tricuspid regurgitation and right ventricular dysfunction in pulmonary hypertension. *Am J Cardiol* 1988;62:108–112.

29. Oh J, Seward J, Tajik A, eds. *The Echo Manual*. 1st ed. Boston: Little, Brown and Company, 1994:177–178.

30. Zaroff JG, Picard MH. Transesophageal echocardiographic (TEE) evaluation of the mitral and tricuspid valves. *Cardiol Clin* 2000;18:731–750.

31. Miyatake K, Okamoto M, Kinoshita N, et al. Evaluation of tricuspid regurgitation by pulsed Doppler and two-dimensional echocardiography. *Circulation* 1982;66:777–784.

32. Rivera JM, Vandervoort PM, Morris E, et al. Visual assessment of valvular regurgitation: comparison with quantitative Doppler measurements. *J Am Soc Echocardiogr* 1994;7:480–487.

33. Nagueh SF. Assessment of valvular regurgitation with Doppler echocardiography. *Cardiol Clin* 1998;16:405–419.

34. Kerut E, McIlwain E, Plotkin G. *Handbook of Echo-Doppler Interpretation*. Armonk, NY: Futura Publishing Company, 1996:117.

35. Reynolds T. Values and formulas. In: Reynolds T, ed. *The Echocardiographer's Pocket Reference*. 2nd edn. Phoenix, Arizona: Heart Institute, 2000:410.

36. Frasco PE, deBruijn NP. Valvular heart disease. In: Estefanous EF, Barash JG, Reves JG, eds. *Cardiac Anesthesia: Principles and Clinical Practice*. Philadelphia: Lippinott Williams & Wilkins, 2001:557–584.

37. Otto C. Echocardiographic evaluation of ventricular diastolic filling and function. In: Otto C, ed. *Textbook of Clinical Echocardiography*. 2nd edn. Philadelphia: W.B. Saunders Company, 2000:329–359.

38. Rumbak MJ, Scott M, Walsh FW. Left hilar mass in a 62-year-old man: severe pulmonary valvular stenosis with a poststenotic aneurysm. *South Med J* 1996;89:824–825.

39. Boston US, Dearani JA, O'Leary PW, et al. Tricuspid valve repair for Ebstein's anomaly in young children: a 30-year experience. *Ann Thorac Surg* 2006;81:690–695; discussion 695–696.

40. Oechslin E, Buchholz S, Jenni R. Ebstein's anomaly in adults: Doppler-echocardiographic evaluation. *Thorac Cardiovasc Surg* 2000;48:209–213.

41. Attenhofer Jost CH, Connolly HM, Dearani JA, et al. Ebstein's anomaly. *Circulation* 2007;115:277–285.

42. Watson H. Natural history of Ebstein's anomaly of tricuspid valve in childhood and adolescence. An international co-operative study of 505 cases. *Br Heart J* 1974;36:417–427.

43. Attenhofer Jost CH, Connolly HM, Edwards WD, et al. Ebstein's anomaly—review of a multifaceted congenital cardiac condition. *Swiss Med Wkly* 2005;135:269–281.

44. Shiina A, Seward JB, Tajik AJ, et al. Two-dimensional echocardiographic—surgical correlation in Ebstein's anomaly: preoperative determination of patients requiring tricuspid valve plication versus replacement. *Circulation* 1983;68:534–544.

45. Parranon S, Abadir S, Acar P. New insight into the tricuspid valve in Ebstein anomaly using three-dimensional echocardiography. *Heart* 2006;92:1627.

46. Vargas-Barron J, Espinola-Zavaleta N, Rijlaarsdam M, et al. Tetralogy of Fallot with absent pulmonary valve and total anomalous pulmonary venous connection. *J Am Soc Echocardiogr* 1999;12:160–163.

46a. Dreyfus GD, Corbi PJ, Chan KM, Bahrami T. Secondary tricuspid regurgitation or dilatation: which should be the criteria for surgical repair? *Ann Thorac Surg* 2005;79(1):127–132.

47. Chopra HK, Nanda NC, Fan P, et al. Can two-dimensional echocardiography and Doppler color flow mapping identify the need for tricuspid valve repair? *J Am Coll Cardiol* 1989;14:1266–1274.

48. Ryan EW, Bolger AF. Transesophageal echocardiography (TEE) in the evaluation of infective endocarditis. *Cardiol Clin* 2000;18:773–787.

49. Birmingham GD, Rahko PS, Ballantyne F III. Improved detection of infective endocarditis with transesophageal echocardiography. *Am Heart J* 1992;123:774–781.

50. San Roman JA, Vilacosta I, Zamorano JL, et al. Transesophageal echocardiography in right-sided endocarditis. *J Am Coll Cardiol* 1993;21:1226–1230.

51. Clifford CP, Eykyn SJ, Oakley CM. Staphylococcal tricuspid valve endocarditis in patients with structurally normal hearts and no evidence of narcotic abuse. *QJM* 1994;87:755–757.

52. Schaefer A, Meyer GP, Waldow A, et al. Images in cardiovascular medicine: Pulmonary valve endocarditis. *Circulation* 2001;103:E53–E54.

53. Akram M, Khan IA. Isolated pulmonic valve endocarditis caused by group B streprococcus (*Streptococcus agalactiae*)—a case report and literature review. *Angiology* 2001;52:211–215.

54. Kamaraju S, Nelson K, Williams DN, et al. *Staphylococcus lugdunensis* pulmonary valve endocarditis in a patient on chronic hemodialysis. *Am J Nephrol* 1999;19:605–608.

55. Hearn CJ, Smedira NG. Pulmonic valve endocarditis after orthotopic liver transplantation. *Liver Transpl Surg* 1999;5:456–457.

56. Simula DV, Edwards WD, Tazelaar HD, et al. Surgical pathology of carcinoid heart disease: a study of 139 valves from 75 patients spanning 20 years. *Mayo Clin Proc* 2002;77:139–147.

57. Moyssakis IE, Rallidis LS, Guida GF, et al. Incidence and evolution of carcinoid syndrome in the heart. *J Heart Valve Dis* 1997;6:625–630.

58. Denney WD, Kemp WE Jr, Anthony LB, et al. Echocardiographic and biochemical evaluation of the development and progression of carcinoid heart disease. *J Am Coll Cardiol* 1998;32:1017–1022.

59. Kumar N, Rasheed K, Gallo R, et al. Rheumatic involvement of all four heart valves—preoperative echocardiographic diagnosis and successful surgical management. *Eur J Cardiothorac Surg* 1995;9:713–714.

60. Roldan CA, Shively BK, Crawford MH. An echocardiographic study of valvular heart disease associated with systemic lupus erythematosus. *N Engl J Med* 1996;335:1424–1430.

61. Saad RS, Galvis CO, Bshara W, et al. Pulmonary valve papillary fibroelastoma. A case report and review of the literature. *Arch Pathol Lab Med* 2001;125:933–934.

62. Wolfe JT III, Finck SJ, Safford RE, et al. Tricuspid valve papillary fibroelastoma: echocardiographic characterization. *Ann Thorac Surg* 1991;51:116–118.

63. Leszek P, Zielinski T, Rozanski J, Klisiewicz A, et al. Traumatic tricuspid valve insufficiency: case report. *J Heart Valve Dis* 2001;10:545–547.

64. Sherman SV, Wall MH, Kennedy DJ, et al. Do pulmonary artery catheters cause or increase tricuspid or pulmonic valvular regurgitation? *Anesth Analg* 2001;92:1117–1122.

65. Tumbarello R, Bini RM, Sanna A. Omniplane transesophageal echocardiography: an improvement in the monitoring of percutaneous pulmonary valvuloplasty. *G Ital Cardiol* 1997;27:168–172.

66. Shively BK. Transesophageal echocardiographic (TEE) evaluation of the aortic valve, left ventricular outflow tract, and pulmonic valve. *Cardiol Clin* 2000;18:711–729.

67. Liau CS, Chu IT, Ho FM. Unruptured congenital aneurysm of the sinus of Valsalva presenting with pulmonary stenosis. *Catheter Cardiovasc Interv* 1999;46:210–213.

68. Kouchoukos NT, Davila-Roman VG, Spray TL, et al. Replacement of the aortic root with a pulmonary autograft in children and young adults with aortic-valve disease. *N Engl J Med* 1994;330:1–6.

69. Kabbani SS, Ross DN, Jamil H, et al. Mitral valve replacement with a pulmonary autograft: initial experience. *J Heart Valve Dis* 1999;8:359–366; discussion 366–357.

70. Azari DM, DiNardo JA. The role of transesophageal echocardiography during the Ross procedure. *J Cardiothorac Vasc Anesth* 1995;9:558–561.

71. Hokken RB, Bogers AJ, Taams MA, et al. Does the pulmonary autograft in the aortic position in adults increase in diameter? An echocardiographic study. *J Thorac Cardiovasc Surg* 1997;113:667–674f.

72. Roughneen PT, DeLeon SY, Eidem BW, et al. Semilunar valve switch procedure: autotransplantation of the native aortic valve to the pulmonary position in the Ross procedure. *Ann Thorac Surg* 1999;67:745–750.

QUESTIONS

Pick the false statement in each of the numbered items below.

1. The pulmonic valve (PV)
   A. is well seen in the deep trans-gastric (TG) RV outflow view
   B. is embryologically derived from the same structure as the aortic valve (AV)
   C. is replaced with a mechanical valve as part of the Ross procedure
   D. may have *nodulus arantii*

2. Tricuspid regurgitation (TR)
   A. is always pathologic
   B. may be used to assess intracardiac pressures
   C. is graded by color flow jet extension into the right atrium (RA)
   D. is graded by reversal of hepatic venous flow
   E. its severity is unrelated to the velocity of the regurgitant jet

3. Carcinoid heart disease
   A. is characterized by right-sided cardiac valvular lesions
   B. may be monitored by TEE for regression of disease with medical therapy
   C. is an uncommon cause of death in patients with carcinoid syndrome
   D. results in fixed immobile valves characterized by regurgitation and stenosis
   E. tends to occur on the ventricular surface of the TV and the arterial surface of the PV

4. Stenotic right-sided cardiac valves
   A. are characterized by leaflet doming for all disease processes
   B. may be assessed by the velocity of the regurgitant jet
   C. are commonly associated with rheumatic heart disease
   D. are suggested by right atrial enlargement
   E. may involve commissural leaflet fusion

CHAPTER 16

Assessment of Prosthetic Valves

Michelle Capdeville ■ Michael G. Licina

The first clinical artificial heart valve was introduced more than 45 years ago. Mechanical and biological prostheses developed in parallel. In 1953, Huffnagel treated aortic regurgitation by placing a caged ball valve in the descending thoracic aorta (1). In 1956, Murray implanted a cadaveric aortic valve in a similar fashion (2). With the subsequent development of cardiopulmonary bypass techniques, intracardiac valve replacement became possible, with Starr and Edwards performing the first successful valve replacement using a caged ball prosthesis in 1960 (3).

TYPES OF PROSTHETIC VALVES

Currently available prosthetic heart valves can be divided into two broad categories: mechanical and bioprosthetic. Multiple sizes are available for each valve type (Table 16.1). With prolonged implantation of a prosthetic valve, regardless of type, one can expect to see some degree of malfunction or failure, making this a form of palliative treatment (4,5). The overall complication rate with appropriate management is approximately 3% per year (6).

Mechanical Valves

The term "profile" is frequently used when describing prosthetic valves and refers to the height from the base of the prosthesis to the top of the struts.

High-Profile Valves

Ball-cage valves

Ball-cage valves were the earliest mechanical valves used. The Starr-Edwards valve is the only ball-cage valve that is still occasionally seen in patients who had remote implantation in the United States. Other modifications of this valve have included the Smeloff-Sutter valve and the Magovern-Cromie sutureless valve.

Starr-Edwards valve

The Starr-Edwards prosthesis is the most well-known caged ball valve, having the longest history and most extensive follow-up. It was designed in 1960 and consists of a metal cage and a round silastic ball (poppet or occluder) with a circular sewing ring. Over the years, this valve has undergone constant modification to eliminate problems, such as thrombogenicity, noise, and hemolysis (Fig. 16.1) (7).

When blood flows across the valve, the ball moves to the apex of the cage; the ball moves to the base of the cage to close the valve and prevent regurgitation. The motion of the ball, with its continually changing points of contact, is thought to reduce the risk of thrombus formation. These valves have a high profile with the potential for left ventricular outflow tract (LVOT) obstruction in the mitral position. They also have a relatively small orifice and can cause some degree of hemolysis, though the latter is relatively insignificant in the absence of a perivalvular

TABLE **16.1** Prosthetic Valve Types	
Advantages	**Disadvantages**
Mechanical valves	
Durability	Higher incidence of thromboembolism
Low profile (bileaflet and tilting disc models)	Anticoagulant-related hemorrhage Hemolysis
Low incidence of structural failures	Higher incidence of perivalvular leak
Bioprosthetic valves	
Reduced incidence of thromboembolism	Tissue degeneration (worse in younger patients)
Lower incidence of perivalvular leak	More flow obstruction with smaller sizes (especially stented valves)
Fewer bleeding complications	Poor long-term durability

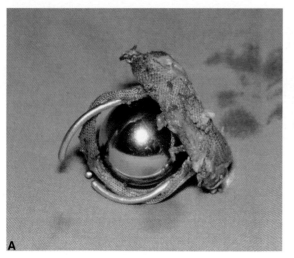
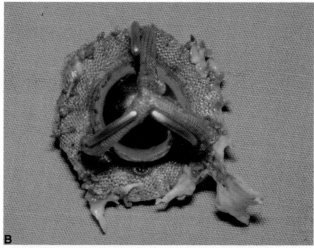
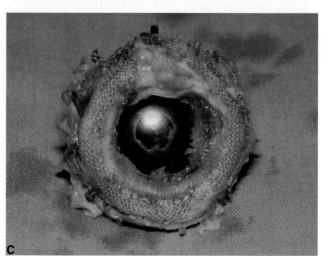

Figure 16.1. A–C: Various views of an excised Starr-Edwards valve with surgically bent strut.

leak. Axisymmetrical and turbulent flow occurs because of the central obstruction by the ball and flow around its edges (flow downstream remains evenly distributed and converges). Stagnation can occur behind the ball, predisposing to thromboembolism. These valves have a very small regurgitant volume.

The Starr-Edwards valve has three orifices: a primary orifice at the annulus; a secondary orifice at the angle made by the ball in the open position and the annular opening; and a tertiary orifice between the ball perimeter and the ventricular or aortic walls. Therefore, a large primary orifice can result in a small tertiary orifice because of the larger size ball. This occurs because the ball must be larger than the valve opening in order for it to occlude the orifice completely. Consequently, in the mitral position, a relatively large ball lying in the middle of the ventricle partially obstructs blood flow. Compared to other mechanical valves, the inlet orifice diameter compared to the overall valve diameter is less favorable. Effective orifice size may not reflect the actual (larger) measured orifice because the former is affected by the shape of the valve orifice (Fig. 16.2).

Caged disc valves

Caged disc valves include the Cooley-Cutter, the Beall, the Cross-Jones, the Harken, the Starr-Edwards (6500 series), the Kay-Suzuki, and the Kay-Shiley. Although these valves

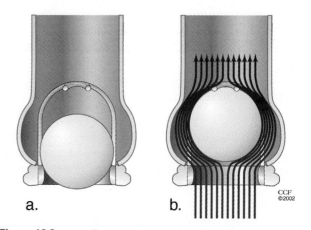

Figure 16.2. A: Ball-cage valve in a closed position. **B:** Complex flow around a ball-cage valve. This illustrates how the EOA is affected by a high-profile valve.

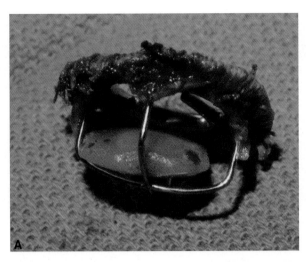
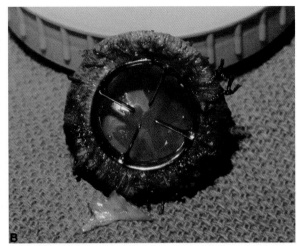

Figure 16.3. **A, B:** Various views of a surgically excised Kay-Suzuki valve (disc-cage).

have all been discontinued, some are still functional more than 20 years after implantation (Fig. 16.3).

Low-Profile Valves

The introduction of low-profile valves reduced the "mass to orifice ratio," thereby improving hemodynamics. Most low-profile mechanical valves are made of pyrolitic carbon to reduce thrombogenicity and improve durability.

Tilting disc valves

Tilting disc valves were introduced in 1967 with the goal of achieving a low profile and reducing bulk within the left ventricular (LV) cavity. They have an intermediate range of valve obstruction. The circular disc of the valve is attached to the sewing ring by way of an eccentric strut/hinge mechanism. Back pressure on the larger portion of the disc causes the valve to close. The opening angle of the disc is important because the gradient will increase when the angle is less than 60 degrees from the sewing ring. The opening angle is typically 60 to 70 degrees. To ensure proper valve closure, this angle must be less than 90 degrees. If the opening angle is too great, the regurgitant volume will increase. A certain amount of valvular insufficiency is felt to be beneficial as it reduces the problem of periprosthetic flow stagnation, which could lead to thrombosis. In the open position, there is an area of stagnation behind the valve because the opening angle is less than 90 degrees. Flow across tilting disc valves is complex. These valves have a major orifice (70% of flow) and a minor orifice. The orientation of the orifice is important because it affects flow dynamics. As blood flow opens the disc, it is directed laterally through each orifice (Figs. 16.4 and 16.5) (8–11).

Bjork-Shiley valve

The Bjork-Shiley convexoconcave valve was originally manufactured in 1969. It was removed from the United States market because of problems with strut fractures

due to weld fractures and disc embolization. It consists of a free-floating disc, which is suspended in a stellite cage with a major inflow and a minor outflow C-shaped strut.

The Bjork-Shiley Monostrut valve was subsequently developed and eliminated the two-armed welded outflow strut entirely; instead, it has a single thick arm, which is part of the single piece housing. It is currently used in some ventricular assist devices.

Medtronic Hall valve

The Medtronic Hall valve, previously known as the Hall-Kaster valve, was developed in 1975. It became the most commonly implanted single-disc valve in the United States. It consists of a disc, housing, struts, and ring. The disc moves up and down on the S-shaped guide strut (Fig. 16.4).

OmniScience valve

The OmniScience valve is a descendant of the Lillehei-Kaster disc valve. It was manufactured in 1978. It has a curved pivoting disc, a one-piece cage, and a sewing ring.

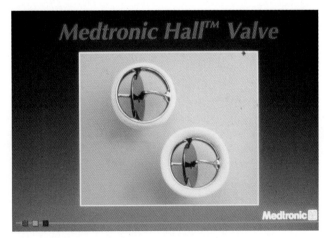

Figure 16.4. An example of Medtronic's single-disc valve.

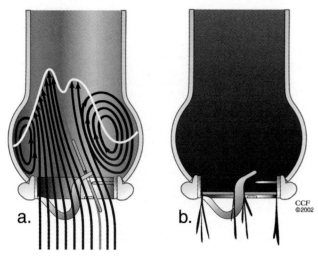

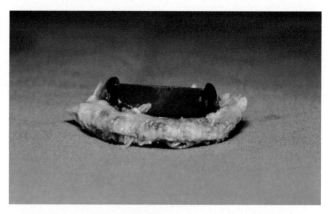

Figure 16.7. Surgically excised St. Jude valve revealing its low-profile nature.

Figure 16.5. A: Complex flow pattern around a single-disc valve with a major and a minor orifice flow pattern represented. **B:** Closed single-disc valve shows the characteristic regurgitant (washing) jets.

Wada-Cutter valve

The Wada-Cutter valve is a single-disc valve with two metal struts at the sides of the valve housing to hold the disc in place. It was manufactured in 1967 and subsequently discontinued in 1972.

Bileaflet valves

Bileaflet valves have the advantage of being less obstructive (flow is across three orifices) and have the lowest pressure gradients, especially with the smaller sizes. They also have the greatest regurgitant fraction (10%), due in part to asynchronous closure of the leaflets and a long closing arc. Advantages of the bileaflet prostheses over the tilting disc valves include a reduced area of stagnation and a larger unobstructed and symmetrical flow area.

Bileaflet valves make up approximately 90% of the mechanical valve market share in the United States. The

St. Jude valve is the prototype "gold standard" against which all mechanical prostheses are compared (Figs. 16.6–16.8).

St. Jude valve

The St. Jude valve was manufactured in 1977. It has two semicircular leaflets attached to a sewing ring by a midline hinge mechanism. The leaflets pivot open (no rotation) during valve opening. When the valve opens, there are two large lateral semicircular openings and a smaller central rectangular opening. The leaflets open to 85 degrees from horizontal and the angle of closure is at 30 to 35 degrees to the orifice plane (varies with valve size). Because of the large opening angle, the effective valve orifice closely approximates the area of the sewing ring. This wide angle of excursion, however, allows for significant backflow across the valve (~10% regurgitant volume) (12).

Carbomedics valve

The Carbomedics valve was introduced in 1986. It is structurally different from the St. Jude valve but has the same echocardiographic characteristics. Pressure gradients across this prosthesis are similar to the St. Jude valve.

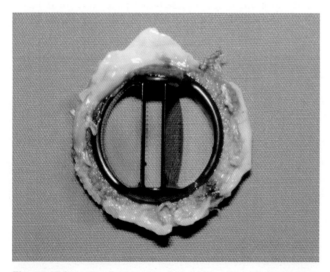

Figure 16.6. A surgically excised St. Jude valve with the leaflets in the open position.

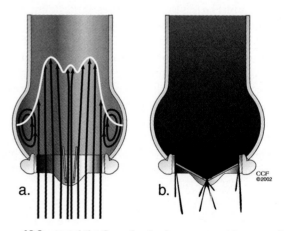

Figure 16.8. A: A bileaflet valve in the open position revealing the near laminar flow pattern. **B:** A bileaflet valve in the closed position showing the characteristic regurgitant (washing) jets.

On-X valve

The On-X valve was manufactured in 1996. It is a second generation bileaflet prosthesis that is made with pure, unalloyed pyrolitic carbon material, which is an improvement over the silicon alloying previously used in pyrolitic carbon valves. This material has better strength and deformability (13). The On-X valve is characterized by straight leaflets that open at 90 degrees, a flared inlet, a length-to-diameter ratio of 0.6, decreased closing contact velocity, and stasis-free hinges. It opens more quickly than the St. Jude mechanical valve and has a wider opening area when fully open. It has strong flow through all orifices, unlike the St. Jude valve, where most flow is across the lateral orifices (14,15). The On-X valve has a cylindrical housing that shelters most of the leaflet motion and is believed to improve the transvalvular flow pattern. In the case of mitral valve replacement (MVR), a small annulus or significant fibrosis/calcification of the subvalvular apparatus can interfere with mechanical prosthetic leaflet motion. Excision of the subvalvular apparatus is generally necessary if there is severe leaflet disease and subvalvular calcification or scarring. Unfortunately, this latter approach has a negative effect on LV function (16,17). Whenever possible, it is desirable to preserve the chordal apparatus in order to maintain LV geometry and function. Preservation of the subvalvular apparatus is thought to result in smaller LV size and decreased end-systolic stress, as well as maintain a more ellipsoid shape versus spherical LV shape (18). The cylindrical housing of the On-X valve can prevent the need to resect the native valve leaflets. When the mitral annulus is small and/or calcified, and preservation of the posterior mitral valve leaflet is preferred, MVR can be facilitated by positioning the prosthesis outside the native annulus. The On-X conform-X prosthesis was developed for atrialized MVR and was modified to include a newly developed asymmetrical sewing ring that allows easier anchoring and increased flexibility to adapt to all native annulus diameters greater than 25 mm (19). For valves in the aortic position (25 mm or smaller), the sewing ring is implanted in a supra-annular location. Patients receiving the On-X valve have exhibited less hemolysis, low adverse event rates, and favorable hemodynamics (20). Leaflet guards and the length of the orifice may help prevent the development of pannus ingrowth.

Other bileaflet valves

Other manufactured bileaflet mechanical prostheses include the Edwards Duromedics valve (withdrawn due to disc fractures), the Medtronic Parallel valve (withdrawn due to a high incidence of thromboembolism), and the Edwards MIRA valve, which has circumferentially curved leaflets.

Bioprosthetic Valves

The first use of intracardiac tissue valves occurred in 1962 when Heimbecker et al. (21) implanted a stentless cadaveric aortic valve in the mitral position, and Ross implanted the same in the aortic position (22,23). The low availability of these cadaveric valves led to the subsequent use of heterografts in 1965 by Binet et al. (24). Limited durability was improved by the use of glutaraldehyde preservation as described by Carpentier et al. in 1969 (25); ease of implantation was facilitated by mounting these valves on a stent as described by Reis et al. in 1971 (26).

Tissue valves are distinguished by their tissue composition. They are typically made of animal (heterograft, xenograft) or human (homograft) tissue, and the tissue can be of valvular or nonvalvular origin. Today's bioprosthetic valves are made of biologic material and include homograft valves, porcine aortic valves, and bovine pericardial tissue valves. These valves are well suited for patients at risk for hemorrhage, women who plan to bear children, and those who will not reliably follow a strict anticoagulation regimen. Unfortunately, the bioprostheses have a limited durability. This is generally due to progressive collagen disruption and calcification, leading to stenosis and eventual leaflet disruption. Valve longevity appears to be inversely related to patient age (27,28). It is believed that the lower rate of valve failure in older patients is due in part to decreased activity levels. In patients with end-stage renal disease, accelerated valve calcification tends to occur with increased frequency with the use of biological prostheses. The newer second generation porcine valves and pericardial valves appear to have greater durability than the earlier first generation porcine valves (29), and newer stentless valves may prove to be even more advantageous in this respect (30).

Mitral bioprostheses have a higher failure rate than aortic bioprostheses. This is believed to be related to mechanical closure stress, bending of the struts by LV contraction, and atrial fibrillation. A greater back pressure between the LV and LA in systole compared to the LA and LV in diastole has also been implicated. There is a 30% to 35% failure rate of porcine heterograft prostheses within 10 to 15 years of implantation (mitral 44%; aortic 26%) (27). Current third generation bioprostheses (see below) appear to be more resistant to structural failure compared to earlier generation valves (31).

Smaller sized valves have a greater obstruction to flow. Flow characteristics are improved in the larger sized valves when compared to mechanical prostheses, and there is less shear stress to blood elements. Valve orientation during insertion is unimportant because the orifice is central. Care must be taken, however, to ensure that the struts do not impinge on the LVOT for mitral prostheses.

Mitral Homograft Valves

Homografts are cryopreserved human cadaveric valves, either stented or unstented. They are harvested shortly after death (when the endothelium is still viable). Stented mitral homografts have not proven very successful, with a high incidence of failure within 5 years due to leaflet thickening, calcification, and the development of valvular insufficiency.

Mitral homografts are more difficult to implant, and the patient's valve size must be known beforehand. Early attempts at homograft MVR yielded a high failure rate because of technical problems, including inadequate sizing of the graft and early dehiscence of the papillary muscle anastomosis. The technique appears to be limited by technical difficulty and lack of standardization of the operation, early valve dysfunction secondary to mismatch, and risk of late deterioration resulting in valvular stenosis. Good results have been reported in Europe, though mitral homograft durability is decreased in younger patients (32–37).

Aortic Homograft Valves

Aortic homografts are cryopreserved human cadaveric aortic valves (38). Typically, a mini root replacement is done with reimplantation of the coronary ostia. This is an attractive alternative for younger patients and patients with endocarditis. Another advantage of these valves is a notable resistance to infection. In patients with active prosthetic valve endocarditis (PVE), a homograft is considered the most reasonable re-replacement valve. Earlier methods of chemical preservation led to early valve failure (39). Antibiotic sterilization and cryopreservation have resulted in significant improvements in long-term valve performance (40). Size limits the availability of this type of valve because the patient's annulus must match that of the homograft. There is a 10% to 20% failure rate within 10 to 15 years of implantation (38).

The Ross procedure is a double valve procedure in which the patient's pulmonic valve is placed in the aortic position as an autograft, and the pulmonic valve is then replaced with an aortic homograft (41). The right and left coronary ostia must be reimplanted. (Some surgeons use an inclusion technique where the pulmonic valve is inserted into the aortic root without removing the coronary ostia.) A major concern with this procedure is the risk of injury to the first septal perforator (near the base of the pulmonic valve), which can lead to high septal infarction and death. The procedure is well suited to younger, growing patients because the autograft can continue to grow with the cardiovascular tree (Fig. 16.9) (38).

Stented Porcine Valves

The stented porcine bioprostheses in current use are the Carpentier-Edwards and Hancock valves. These valves consist of a stented preserved porcine aortic valve attached to a sewing ring. Prior to mounting, the valve leaflets are treated with glutaraldehyde, which reduces their antigenicity. These leaflets are stiffer than those on a homograft because the tissue is nonviable. As a result of this stiffness, incomplete valve opening occurs at low flow rates.

The greatest disadvantage of these valves is their lack of long-term durability. Patient age greatly affects the rate of degeneration, with the highest failure rates occurring in patients under 20 years of age. This is thought to be due to a more active immune reaction to the foreign tissue. Valve failure is generally due to stenosis (cusp calcification), leaflet thickening, leaflet fracturing, or insufficiency (torn leaflets).

Porcine valve degeneration usually occurs gradually but can also have an acute onset. The valve surface tends to undergo endothelial denudation with basement membrane exposure, leading to the deposition of fibrin, platelet aggregates, activated leukocytes, and small focal calcium deposits. The fixation process also makes the collagen more brittle. Approximately 10% of these valves have some degree of central regurgitation. With mitral annular calcification, the sewing ring may be distorted, leading to regurgitation (Fig. 16.10) (42–50).

Hancock porcine valve

The Hancock valve, a treated stented porcine aortic valve, was the first commercially successful bioprosthetic valve. It was manufactured in 1970 and is still widely used.

Carpentier-Edwards porcine valve

The Carpentier-Edwards treated aortic porcine valve has been on the market since 1976 and is the most frequently implanted biological valve. The frame is flexible and the sewing ring is saddle shaped.

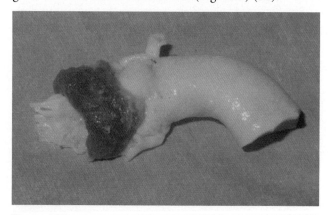

Figure 16.9. Aortic valve homograft. Please note a portion of the LVOT muscle with the anterior mitral valve leaflet attached along with a section of the ascending aorta.

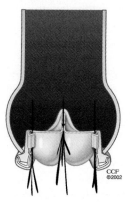

Figure 16.10. A cross-sectional view of a stented bioprosthetic valve showing the characteristic regurgitant (washing) jets.

Bovine Pericardial Valves

Pericardial valves make up approximately 40% of the U.S. tissue valve market and 16% of all valves implanted in the United States. Their first clinical use was in 1971. Bovine pericardial valves are similar to porcine valves; however, the three leaflets are made from bovine pericardium. The advantages over porcine valves include unlimited size and easy modification of valve design.

The most common causes of pericardial valve failure were abrasion of the leaflets by the support frame and leaflet calcification leading to valvular incompetence. Cusp tears tended to occur along the free edges of the cusp and at the leaflet crease. The cloth covering of the stents was believed to cause abrasion of the pericardial commissures and cusps. Cusp perforations were also caused by long suture ends. Calcification of pericardial valves tended to occur in the line of flexion parallel to the annulus (porcine valves tend to become calcified at the commissures) (Fig. 16.11) (51,52).

Ionescu-Shiley Valve

The Ionescu-Shiley valve is the prototype and was first manufactured in 1976. Premature failure typically occurred after 6 to 8 years. Some of the failures were due to tears occurring along the suture line of the valve leaflets to the stent posts. This valve is no longer commercially available.

Carpentier-Edwards Perimount Valve

The Carpentier-Edwards (CE) Perimount pericardial bioprosthesis was introduced clinically in 1981 and approved for commercial use in the United States in 1991. Its design is similar to the CE porcine valve, with thicker leaflets. It is made for use in both the aortic position and the mitral position. The valve shows a similar durability profile to the porcine valve. In 2002, the Carpentier-Edwards Perimount Magna valve was introduced, as a modification of the standard Perimount valve. Modifications of the newer valve include a reduced sewing ring width,

resulting in a reduction in external diameter of 2 mm. This, in turn, might allow the implantation of a prosthesis one size larger compared to the standard Perimount valve. The sewing cuff is also more flexible and scalloped to facilitate proper seating and minimize the possibility of a dehiscence. The sewing cuff is displaced upstream, placing the sewing cuff and leaflets in a complete supra-annular position. This maximizes clearance of the aortic valve orifice (53).

Third Generation "Lower Profile" Stented Bioprostheses

St. Jude medical Biocor

The Biocor stented porcine bioprosthesis is a third generation valve that has reduced stiffness and improved flexibility of the valve cusps, in the hope of improving valve lifespan relative to previous biological valves. Low stent posts (9–11 mm) provide an overall lower profile, thereby reducing the risk of LVOT obstruction in the mitral position, and aortic wall protrusion in the aortic position. A low stent base allows for optimal coronary ostial clearance. The scalloped inflow edge optimizes valve seating. It is preserved in glutaraldehyde. There are age-dependent risks of structural valve degeneration that can be seen as early as 7 years postimplantation in patients under 65 years of age for aortic prostheses, however, there is a low incidence of valve-related complications and overall excellent durability (70.3% ± 10.9% freedom from structural failure at 20 years) (54). In the mitral position, freedom from structural valve deterioration was low at 15 years postimplant (51.8% ± 13.8%, <50 years; 88.7% ± 5.1%, 51–60 years; 84.0% ± 9.8%, 61–80 years) (55).

Medtronic Mosaic heart valve

The Medtronic Mosaic bioprosthesis is a third-generation stented porcine valve that has been available since 1994. It is treated with alpha-amino oleic acid (AOA), which covalently binds to glutaraldehyde pretreated bioprostheses and diminishes calcium diffusion into tissue. During the fixation process, a net zero pressure differential across the leaflets helps to preserve leaflet morphology and function. The flexible polymer stent is low profile and is suitable for patients with a small aortic root diameter (56). The rate of structural valve deterioration after 6 years is reported as zero in the aortic position for patients less than 60 years old and zero in the mitral position for patients less than 60 years old (57).

Stentless porcine valves

Several stentless aortic valve prostheses have entered the market since the introduction of the Medtronic Freestyle stentless aortic xenograft and the St. Jude Medical Toronto stentless porcine valve (SPV).

Because mechanical and stented aortic prostheses are relatively stenotic, the stentless valves were developed in an effort to provide a larger effective orifice area (EOA)

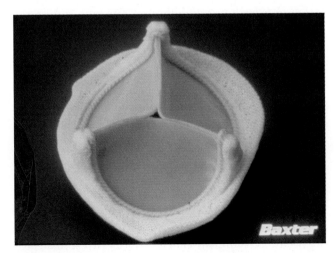

Figure 16.11. The Baxter pericardial valve.

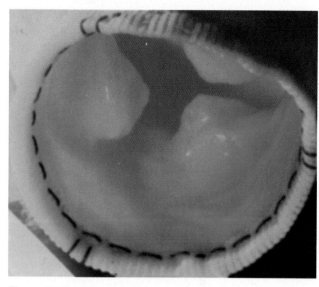

Figure 16.12. The Medtronic Freestyle stentless aortic valve.

and a superior hemodynamic profile. Benefits of these stentless valves include regression of LV hypertrophy, a factor that has been linked to survival (58–61). It has been shown that LV mass regression occurs at the greatest rate during the first postoperative year, and that the strongest predictor of this is baseline ventricular mass (62). The Medtronic Freestyle and Toronto SPV valves are derived from the porcine aortic root and lack any sewing ring or supporting struts. They have a single layer of polyester covering around the outer base of the valve (Fig. 16.12). The Medtronic Freestyle valve is fixed in glutaraldehyde at zero pressure, and the cusps are treated with AOA (63). The Prima valve is another stentless valve undergoing clinical trials, but it is not yet commercially available.

The Sorin Freedom Solo stentless pericardial valve, released in June 2004, was designed to adapt to dilatation of the sinotubular (ST) junction since valve continence is highly dependent on implantation technique, annular symmetry, and ST junction dimensions. It is made of bovine pericardium, has a large coaptation surface, and was designed for supra-annular implantation with a single running suture (64). In vitro, this valve has been shown to prevent residual valvular regurgitation for a greater range of ST junction mismatch versus SPVs (65). In vivo, this valve has shown good hemodynamic performance, with early LV mass regression (66).

ECHOCARDIOGRAPHIC EVALUATION OF PROSTHETIC HEART VALVES

Because of the large number of prostheses, a wide range of sizes, and a wide variety of pathologic findings, the echocardiographer must have a good understanding of the appearance and function of the commonly implanted prosthetic heart valves.

A complete examination should include evaluation of

1. Function of the prosthesis
2. Chamber size
3. Presence of intracardiac densities (e.g., thrombus, vegetations, pannus formation)
4. Ventricular function
5. Valvular lesions
6. Hemodynamic measurements (gradients, EOA)
7. Regurgitant jets (normal vs. pathologic)

The two-dimensional (2D) and color flow Doppler examination of prosthetic valves can be challenging because of

1. Dense reverberations
2. Dense sewing ring
3. Sound beam attenuation by prosthesis (flow masking) (67–69)

NORMAL IMAGING

Prosthetic heart valves have characteristic echo appearances. They produce a certain degree of acoustic shadowing and characteristic reverberations. Acoustic shadowing occurs because of the highly reflective material in prosthetic valves and usually occurs on the opposite side of the prosthesis. Reverberations need to be distinguished from vegetations or thrombus.

The elongated appearance of parts of the prosthesis on the echo examination is due to the differential speed of sound through the dense prosthesis versus through the tissue. The valve's occluding mechanism determines the pattern of flow and shadowing/artifact. The sewing ring should be examined closely for stability (i.e., no rocking motion), and disc/leaflet/poppet motion should be thoroughly evaluated. All valves should be scanned from multiple views and planes.

Baseline function should be determined after valve replacement prior to hospital discharge. (Immediate postcardiopulmonary bypass results may be different from findings prior to hospital discharge.) This allows monitoring of valve function over time. The type and size of valve should be documented, as well as previously measured gradients and duration of implantation (70,71).

HEMODYNAMIC MEASUREMENTS

Normal Doppler hemodynamic measurements for the prosthetic mitral valve include

1. Early peak velocity (E wave) of mitral inflow
2. Mean gradient
3. End-diastolic gradient
4. Pressure half-time
5. Estimated valve orifice area
6. Tricuspid regurgitation (TR) velocity (to estimate pulmonary artery [PA] pressure)

Normal Doppler hemodynamic measurements for the prosthetic aortic valve include

1. Peak and mean gradients
2. Dimensionless ratio

Valve Gradients by CW Doppler

Each valve type and size has its own hemodynamic characteristics. Even though peak and mean transvalvular gradients are only grossly correlated to the size of the prosthesis, such measurements are important in practice. They can reflect increased stroke work and can be abnormally elevated because of pathologic stenosis/obstruction, a high cardiac output state, increased stroke volume (e.g., regurgitation), or a mismatch between prosthesis size and body size. With the exception of the Starr-Edwards valve, the diameter of the valve is generally the size of the sewing ring. The point to remember is that transvalvular gradients obtained by Doppler are very flow dependent. With increasing prosthetic valve size there is a notable decrease in peak velocity and mean gradient for all valve types (72,73).

There is generally a good correlation between simultaneous Doppler mean and catheter gradients using the simplified Bernoulli equation (74). In a simultaneous Doppler/catheter study, left atrial pressure (LAP) by transseptal puncture correlated well with the mean Doppler gradient; however, pulmonary capillary wedge pressure (PCWP) significantly overestimated the mean gradient in several cases.

Normal prosthetic gradients depend on the size and type of prosthesis, valve location, and ventricular function. For all measurements, an average of several beats should be taken (especially when there is an irregular cardiac rhythm). Furthermore, measurement of exercise hemodynamics can uncover mild dysfunction and may augment the differences noted between different prostheses (75,76).

Pressure Recovery

The phenomenon of "pressure recovery" must be considered because it can become a source of error during prosthetic valve gradient measurements (77). Pressure recovery is a term used in physics to describe the phenomenon of conservation of energy when fluid flows through a narrow orifice and accounts for the differences between Doppler- and catheter-derived gradients. The law of conservation of energy states that the total amount of energy in an isolated system remains constant, although it may change its form. In 1638, Galileo published several concepts, including the celebrated "interrupted pendulum," which can be described as the conversion of potential energy into kinetic energy, and back again. This idea forms the basis for pressure recovery. Simply stated, the total energy of a system is equal to the sum of the kinetic and potential energies.

When echocardiography is used to evaluate a prosthetic valve, the modified Bernoulli equation is used to calculate the pressure gradient across the valve.

Modified Bernoulli Equation

$$\text{Pressure gradient} = 4V^2$$

$$\underset{\text{Convective acceleration}}{\text{Pressure gradient}(P_1 - P_2) = \rho(V_2^2 - V_1^2)} \underset{\text{Flow acceleration}}{} + \underset{\text{Viscous friction}}{\rho(DV/DT)(DS) + RV}$$

In most clinical studies, flow acceleration and viscous friction can be ignored, as they represent small values. Therefore, the equation becomes simplified to

$$P_1 - P_2 = 1/2\rho(V_2^2 - V_1^2)$$

$V_1 << V_2$, therefore, V_1 can be ignored; ρ = mass density of blood (1.06×10^3 kg/m³)

$$\Delta P = 4(V_2)^2$$

ΔP is the instantaneous or maximal pressure gradient. Many assumptions are made when using this equation, and V_2 is the maximum velocity that can be recorded with continuous wave (CW) Doppler. In the catheterization laboratory, valve gradients are measured by catheters that are placed proximal and distal to the valve. Most outcome studies have been based on this method. The concept of pressure recovery accounts for differences that can be seen between catheter-derived and Doppler-derived gradients.

Figure 16.13A illustrates the LVOT (1), valve (2), and aorta (3). If a catheter is withdrawn from point 1 to point 3, and the pressures are measured, then by the law of energy conservation, the LVOT will show a high pressure (increased potential energy) and a low velocity (smaller amount of kinetic energy); the valve will show a high velocity (increased kinetic energy) and very low pressure (little to no potential energy); and the aorta will show a return of kinetic energy to potential energy. The area at point 2 (i.e., the valve) is the vena contracta (minimum jet cross section). The point of highest velocity and lowest pressure occurs at the narrowest point in a prosthetic valve or at the vena contracta downstream. Velocity decreases and pressure increases ("pressure recovery") as one moves further from the prosthesis because of re-expansion of flow downstream. The pressure gradient will therefore depend on where the pressure is sampled. "Pressure recovery" is more significant in prosthetic than native valves (especially aortic prostheses). For an aortic prosthesis, pressure measured at the LVOT decreases at the aortic valve level and "recovers" at the proximal ascending aorta. Using spectral Doppler, one can obtain the maximum pressure gradient between the LVOT and the prosthetic valve orifice (vena contracta) while catheter measurements provide the gradient between the LVOT and the proximal ascending aorta, where the pressure beyond the vena contracta is recovered.

Location	Proximal to Valve (*1*)	Valve (*2*)	Aorta (*3*)
Amount of kinetic energy (velocity)	+	++++	++
Amount of potential energy (pressure)	++++	+	+++

Figure 16.13B illustrates the pressure gradients. Point *1* has the highest pressure and point *2* the lowest pressure. P_{1-2} is the peak, or maximal pressure gradient, which represents the gradient obtained with Doppler and the Bernoulli equation. P_{1-3} is the gradient that would be obtained in the catheterization laboratory using the catheter-based technique. P_{3-2} represents the recovered pressure. This

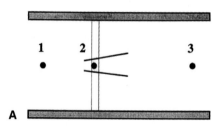

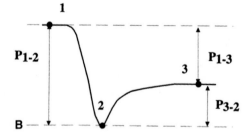

P_{1-2}: Peak catheter gradient
P_{3-2}: Pressure recovery
P_{1-3}: Net catheter gradient

Figure 16.13. A: Diagram illustrating the LVOT (*1*), aortic valve (*2*), and aorta (*3*). The area around point *2* represents the vena contracta. **B:** Pressure gradients are shown, including P_{1-2} (peak catheter gradient), P_{3-2} (pressure recovery), and P_{1-3} (net catheter gradient). The maximum pressure change occurs at the valve level.

pressure recovery is dependent on the location of the catheter within the aorta (point *3*). If the catheter is closer to the valve (point *2*), results can vary. Figure 16.13B shows that the maximum pressure change occurs at the level of the valve and that as one moves away from the valve, there is a change in slope to a relative plateau.

In general, all narrowed areas show some degree of pressure recovery. In 1989, Doppler versus dual catheter measurements were studied at the Mayo Clinic in patients with prosthetic valves. A good correlation was found between the measurements. Valve types studied included ball and cage, disc, tilting disc, bioprosthetic valves, and lesser numbers of bileaflet valves (74).

In 1990, Baumgartner et al. (78) used an in vitro model to study the observed discrepancy between Doppler- and catheter-based pressure gradients in five sizes (19–27 mm) of St. Jude mechanical and Hancock porcine bioprosthetic valves. In the case of St. Jude valves, central jet flow (between the open leaflets) and side flow (between the leaflets and side wall) were studied (Figs. 16.6 and 16.8). Higher velocity of blood flow was seen across the smaller central rectangular orifice compared to the larger semicircular side orifices. The authors measured catheter gradients at multiple sites distal to the valves, while measuring simultaneous Doppler gradients. For St. Jude valves, significant differences were noted between the two methods when the catheter was located 30 mm from the valve, within the aorta. In this situation, Doppler measurements were at least 10 mm Hg greater than peak and mean catheter measurements in 81% and 71% of cases, respectively. The greatest discrepancy occurred with smaller valve sizes. The gradients also decreased 22% when the catheter was moved from a central position to the side orifice.

St. Jude Valves: Peak and Mean Gradients Measured by Doppler and Catheter (at 30 mm from Valve Level)

Size (mm)	Peak Doppler (mm Hg)	Peak Catheter (mm Hg)	Mean Doppler (mm Hg)	Mean Catheter (mm Hg)
19	42.7 ± 13.6	26.4 ± 10.0	24.7 ± 8.5	14.6 ± 5.2
21	26.6 ± 11.0	14.4 ± 8.3	14.4 ± 6.2	7.2 ± 2.2
23	17.8 ± 8.1	4.9 ± 4.0	9.7 ± 4.6	3.4 ± 2.6
25	7.8 ± 3.2	3.8 ± 1.6	4.3 ± 1.6	2.9 ± 1.2
27	4.8 ± 2.0	0.7 ± 0.7	3.1 ± 1.1	0.7 ± 0.7
Values are mean ± SD.				

For Hancock valves, although Doppler gradients were higher, the degree of discrepancy was less. Peak and mean catheter gradients of 10 mm Hg or more occurred in 18% and 13%, respectively.

Hancock Valves: Peak and Mean Gradients Measured by Doppler and Catheter (at 30 mm from Valve Level)

Size (mm)	Peak Doppler (mm Hg)	Peak Catheter (mm Hg)	Mean Doppler (mm Hg)	Mean Catheter (mm Hg)
19	38.7 ± 12.4	35.0 ± 13.3	23.5 ± 6.9	21.0 ± 7.4
21	23.7 ± 8.2	18.7 ± 7.0	14.9 ± 5.7	12.0 ± 4.1
23	16.5 ± 5.0	13.5 ± 6.6	10.4 ± 3.5	9.3 ± 3.2
25	12.4 ± 4.1	10.8 ± 3.4	7.2 ± 2.7	7.5 ± 2.3
27	17.7 ± 4.7	14.9 ± 6.0	10.5 ± 2.7	9.7 ± 3.1

Values are mean ± SD.

Therefore, clinically relevant pressure recovery occurs in low-profile bileaflet valves, especially with smaller sizes. In order to minimize the pressure recovery effect, CW Doppler measurements should be made at the side orifices, which can be clinically challenging with transesophageal echocardiography (TEE).

In 1991, Baumgartner et al. (79) examined Doppler-derived velocities and gradients and compared them to catheter-derived gradients in five valve sizes of bileaflet, single tilting disc, ball and cage, and bioprosthetic valves, using a pulsatile in vitro model. Doppler peak and mean gradients correlated well with catheter peak and mean gradients in all four valve types. The relationship between techniques was good for the single disc and bioprosthetic valves. For the bileaflet and caged ball valves, the Doppler gradients significantly and consistently exceeded the catheter gradients, with a difference of up to 44 mm Hg. These Doppler-derived gradients were also very dependent on high flow rates (e.g., higher flow rates increased the Doppler gradient). Therefore, under conditions where high flow rates exist, such as immediately post–valve replacement, the Doppler gradients may mimic prosthetic valvular stenosis. Furthermore, pressure recovery plays an important role in bileaflet and caged ball valve gradient measurements. Valve design and size will influence the extent of pressure recovery. As a result, Doppler-derived gradients can be misleading (80). As such, peak velocities should be measured using CW Doppler across a lateral orifice for bileaflet valves. If velocity is measured across a central orifice, it may lead to an overestimation of the degree of stenosis.

In 1992, Baumgartner et al. (80) compared Doppler-estimated prosthetic valve area to Gorlin catheter EOA and its dependence on flow. Again, five valve sizes were studied. Doppler valve areas were calculated using three different methods: standard continuity equation; standard continuity equation with simplified modifications (peak flow/peak velocity); and Gorlin equation using Doppler pressure gradients. The results were compared with the Gorlin EOA derived from direct flow and catheter pressure measurements. The authors found excellent correlation between all three methods. They concluded that Doppler echocardiography allows the use of either the continuity equation or the Gorlin formula for in vitro calculations of the single disc or bioprosthetic valves but that it underestimates valve areas in bileaflet valves.

In an in vitro and in vivo study of bileaflet valves, Vandervoort et al. (81) demonstrated that pressure recovery does occur. The authors noted that 36% of the pressure drop was recovered between the valve leaflets. Side orifice velocities were 85% of centerline velocities, and pressure recovery was more pronounced in the aortic than the mitral position. The authors concluded that in order to compare Doppler measurements to catheter measurements, Doppler measurements needed to be based on side orifice measurements. Otherwise, a pressure loss coefficient (experimentally derived, K = 0.64) must be used when central orifice velocities are recorded (Pressure gradient = $4V^2 \times 0.64$).

In 2000, Bech-Hanssen et al. (82) compared bileaflet (St. Jude), monoleaflet (Omnicarbon), and stented porcine (Biocor) valves. They performed Doppler and catheter measurements on the central and side orifices of the St. Jude valve, the major and minor orifices of the Omnicarbon valve, and the single orifice of the Biocor valve. Pressure recovery data showed the following: 53% for the central and 29% for the side orifices of the St. Jude valve; 20% for the major and 23% for the minor orifices of the Omnicarbon valve; and 18% for the Biocor valve. The Omnicarbon valve had similar Doppler gradients to the St. Jude valve but less pronounced pressure recovery and higher net pressure gradients. With increasing size, the St. Jude valve showed more pressure recovery in terms of percentage of peak gradient. Therefore, if there is a significant pressure recovery gradient, comparison outcomes are likely to be better. It is difficult to compare these gradients between different valve types.

In 2003, Bech-Hanssen et al. (83) compared different sizes of St. Jude and Biocor valves using an in vitro model. They studied pressure recovery in the valves and aorta and demonstrated that pressure recovery in the valve was dependent on valve size, showing less recovered pressure with smaller valve sizes (19,21). This occurred because of more turbulent flow and energy loss. Furthermore, pressure recovery in the St. Jude valve was due primarily to the valve itself, with a small contribution from the aorta. For the Biocor valve, pressure recovery was significant and only due to the aorta. A narrow aorta was shown to promote pressure recovery because the flow is less turbulent and the energy loss is less pronounced.

In 2006, Dohmen et al. (84) studied pressure recovery in the Omnicarbon valve and showed that it ranged from 42% to 74%. These values are higher than in the above study and may indicate a more favorable performance of these valves than previously reported.

In summary, pressure recovery is dependent on the valve type, size position, and aorta size.

Effective Orifice Area

EOA is superior to transvalvular gradients as a measure of prosthetic valve function and performance. All valve prostheses are mildly stenotic, and the EOA is always less than the anatomic area. The prosthesis EOA gives a more flow-independent measure of resistance, as with stenotic native valves. Gradients, on the other hand, are more dependent on flow, diastolic filling time, heart rate, valve size, and valve type. Unfortunately, measurement of EOA for mitral prostheses has been imprecise (85–96). For native mitral valves, it is generally measured using the pressure half-time method as described by Hatle (86):

$$EOA = 220/T_{1/2}$$

The pressure half-time method, however, has not been validated for prosthetic valves (mechanical or bioprosthetic), and it has been shown in some studies to overestimate the true EOA of mitral bioprostheses (87,97,98). Pressure half-time probably cannot detect early prosthetic obstruction; however, it can differentiate a high peak velocity secondary to stenosis from that due to a high stroke volume. Increased flow velocity across a prosthetic valve does not always indicate obstruction. For example, a high output state or severe prosthetic regurgitation can cause an increase in velocity. With a mitral prosthesis, the pressure half-time is useful in distinguishing whether an increased gradient (i.e., velocity) is secondary to increased flow or obstruction. Obstruction of an aortic prosthesis will lead to an increased velocity unless the cardiac output is decreased.

Data provided by the manufacturer about pressure and flow suggest that the EOA increases with increasing pressure and flow, and that there is not a unique area for each prosthesis. The explanation for this finding is that bioprosthetic leaflet inertia occurs at low flow. Dumesnil et al. (87) suggests that the overestimation of EOA by pressure half-time seen in most patients with bioprostheses is due to opening inertia of the prosthesis early in diastole, leading to a higher initial gradient and steeper deceleration slope when the valve opens. Bileaflet mechanical prostheses, on the other hand, open fully at low flows, with minimal variation in orifice area between valves. Therefore, EOA and measured manufacturer's area should be similar.

For patients with no aortic or mitral regurgitation (MR), and an aortic or mitral prosthesis, the continuity equation can be used:

$$EOA = \frac{(\text{LVOT area}) \times (\text{LVOT TVI})}{(\text{Prosthesis TVI})}$$

The continuity equation is the preferred method with prostheses, provided there is no significant aortic insufficiency (AI) or MR. Areas calculated with the continuity equation correlate well with areas derived from an in vitro hydraulic model while those calculated using the pressure half-time method do not (95,98). Note that time velocity integral (TVI) must be used in the equation (not velocity) for mitral prostheses, and LVOT area is calculated from the external diameter of the sewing ring for aortic prosthesis calculations. The LVOT diameter is generally within 1 to 2 mm of the external sewing ring diameter (99,100). The simplified continuity equation has been validated for aortic prostheses using velocity in the formula (99,101,102); however, the software on newer instruments allows for TVI to be easily measured.

An alternate continuity equation method (103) has also been described and can be used in the presence of aortic or MR for mitral or tricuspid prosthesis EOA. The external sewing ring diameter is used to approximate left atrial (LA) diameter near the sewing ring; pulse wave (PW) Doppler is used to measure LA TVI with the sample volume just above the sewing ring; CW Doppler is used to measure MVR TVI:

$$EOA = \frac{(\text{Sewing ring D})^2 \times (0.785) \times \text{LA TVI}}{\text{MVR TVI}}$$

This latter method compares favorably with the standard continuity equation method but neither compares well with the pressure half-time method.

The proximal isovelocity surface area (PISA) method (104) has also been used to calculate forward flow and estimate the EOA of St. Jude mitral prostheses:

$$Q = \frac{2\pi r^2 v_a \cdot v}{v - v_a}$$

and

$$EOA = \frac{Q}{v}$$

where Q is instantaneous flow rate; r is radius from orifice (measured to the level of the prosthetic annulus); v_a is aliasing velocity; v is peak transorifice velocity (across lateral orifice of St. Jude prosthesis, measured with CW). $v/(v - v_a)$ is a correction factor for flow underestimation (isotach flattening near orifice secondary to finite size and low transorifice velocity of the prosthesis). The valve orifice is assumed to be at the level of the prosthetic annulus. It is suggested that this method might improve the noninvasive assessment of prosthetic mitral valve obstruction.

The modified continuity equation has proven to be an unreliable substitute for the standard method in the assessment of normally functioning On-X valves (105).

The dimensionless ratio, also known as the Doppler velocity index (DVI), velocity ratio (VR), or dimensionless obstructive index (DOI), is the ratio of the velocity or velocity time integral of the LVOT to the aortic prosthesis (99,106).

$$DOI = \frac{v_{LVOT}}{v_{max}}$$

or

$$DOI = \frac{TVI_{LVOT}}{TVI_{prosthesis}}$$

It is useful to help differentiate increased velocity across an aortic prosthesis, which is secondary to obstruction (DOI ≤ 0.25), from increased velocity due to AI (DOI ≥ 0.3). This ratio remains unchanged unless either the LVOT dimension changes (a less likely occurrence) or the dimension of the prosthetic aortic valve orifice changes.

A double-envelope technique has been described for the evaluation of prosthetic aortic valves. With this method, LVOT velocity and aortic valve velocity are simultaneously obtained from transgastric views using CW Doppler. It was suggested that obtaining subvalvular and valvular peak velocities from the same Doppler trace might reduce the beat-to-beat variability that can occur with nonsimultaneous measurements and might simplify use of the continuity equation (107).

Three-dimensional (3D) TEE is a newer ultrasonic modality that has been used for quantitative assessment of mechanical prosthetic valve area. Orifice area assessment by 3D TEE offers the advantage of being independent of flow, heart rate, MR, AI, systolic, and diastolic LV function. Further study is warranted with this newer technology (108).

Normal Prosthetic Mean Gradients from the Mayo Clinic Prosthesis Project

Mitral Prosthesis	N	Peak Velocity (m/s)	Mean Gradient (mm Hg)	EOA (cm²) (Pressure Half-Time)	% Valves with Trivial or Mild MR
Ball-Cage	161	1.8 ± 0.3	4.9 ± 1.8	2.4 ± 0.7	7.5
Bjork-Shiley	79	1.7 ± 0.3	4.1 ± 1.6	2.6 ± 0.6	20.3
Heterograft	150	1.6 ± 0.3	4.1 ± 1.5	2.3 ± 0.7	24.7
St. Jude	66	1.6 ± 0.4	4.0 ± 1.8	3.0 ± 0.8	24.2
Total	456	1.7 ± 0.3	4.4 ± 1.7	2.5 ± 0.7	17.8

For all mitral prostheses, as size increases the gradient decreases.

Aortic Prosthesis	N	Peak Velocity (m/s)	Mean Gradient (mm Hg)	Dimensionless Obstructive Index
Heterograft	215	2.4 ± 0.5	13.3 ± 6.1	0.42 ± 0.12
Ball-Cage	158	3.2 ± 0.6	22.8 ± 8.6	0.32 ± 0.09
Bjork-Shiley	142	2.5 ± 0.6	13.7 ± 7.0	0.40 ± 0.10
St. Jude	74	2.6 ± 0.6	15.1 ± 7.3	0.39 ± 0.10
Homograft	33	1.9 ± 0.4	7.8 ± 2.7	0.56 ± 0.12
Medtronic Hall	24	2.6 ± 0.4	15.1 ± 5.2	0.39 ± 0.08
Total	646	2.6 ± 0.7	15.7 ± 8.2	0.39 ± 0.12

With the exception of the ball-cage prostheses, prosthetic aortic gradients decreased with increasing valve size.

Tricuspid Prosthesis	N	Peak Velocity (m/s)	Mean Gradient (mm Hg)	Pressure Half-Time (ms)	% Valves with Trivial or Mild TR
Heterograft	43	1.3 ± 0.2	3.2 ± 1.1	145 ± 37	20.9
Ball-Cage	35	1.3 ± 0.2	3.2 ± 0.8	140 ± 48	8.6
St. Jude	7	1.2 ± 0.3	2.7 ± 1.1	108 ± 32	28.6
Bjork-Shiley	1	1.3	2.2	144	0
Total	86	1.3 ± 0.2	3.1 ± 1.0	140 ± 42 (N = 69)	16.3

For tricuspid prostheses, respiratory variation accounted for average differences between maximum and minimum values for peak velocity (0.5 ± 0.2 m/s), mean gradient (0.3 ± 0.2 mm Hg), and pressure half-time (81.6 ± 36.9 ms) (109–111).

In a review of 129 studies, published information about Doppler findings in normally functioning aortic prostheses was reviewed. Information available to the end of 2005 was summarized, and it showed that caged-ball valves were the most obstructive, followed by stented porcine and single tilting disc valves. Bovine pericardial valves were somewhat less obstructive, as were intra-annular bileaflet mechanical valves. Stentless valves and reduced-cuff mechanical bileaflet valves were still less obstructive while homografts were the least obstructive (112).

Prosthetic Valve Regurgitation

Degree of prosthetic aortic regurgitation is difficult to assess by color flow Doppler. For aortic prostheses, a low-pressure half-time (≤250 ms), a restrictive mitral inflow pattern, an increased LVOT velocity (>1.5 m/s), and diastolic flow reversal in the aorta are suggestive of severe aortic regurgitation. For a mitral prosthesis, a normal pressure half-time (≥150 ms), reversal of flow in the pulmonary veins, and an increased peak inflow velocity (≥2.5 m/s) are suggestive of severe MR.

ECHOCARDIOGRAPHIC CHARACTERISTICS OF SPECIFIC VALVE TYPES

Unless otherwise specified, the descriptions below will focus on prosthetic valves in the mitral position.

Starr-Edwards Valve

During diastole, blood entering the LA goes around the ball. The ring, tip of the cage, and the leading and trailing edges of the ball give off strong echoes. In systole, the trailing edge of the ball has an artifactual elongated appearance with a large portion extending outside the cage (into the LA). The ring can be seen, as can the tip of the cage, the leading edge of the ball within the cage, and the trailing edge of the ball. In diastole, reverberations from the prosthesis are seen in the LA.

The "closing volume" of the prosthesis is the volume displaced by the ball in early systole as the ball moves toward the sewing ring. This is seen as a small central early systolic regurgitant volume in the LA. This needs to be distinguished from pathologic regurgitation, which is holosystolic. CW gradients should be measured around the periphery of the ball where flow velocities are the highest.

Echocardiography has been used to detect cloth cover tears in the fully covered Starr-Edwards valve (Fig. 16.14). Such tears appeared as elongated echogenic masses attached to the cage and floating downstream, with normal transvalvular gradients (113). There is little information available about the normal hemodynamic profile derived from Doppler measurements, most notably for prostheses in the mitral position. Typically, Doppler measurements have been limited to the EOA derived from

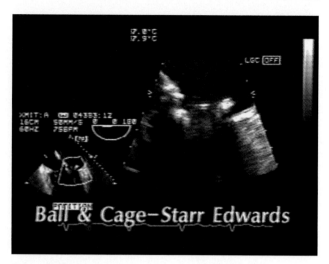

Figure 16.14. Starr-Edwards valve in the mitral position.

the pressure half-time, peak and mean gradients, and the maximum E wave for diastolic mitral inflow (114). A study from the Mayo Clinic sought to define the normal hemodynamic profile of the Starr-Edwards valve in the mitral position using all standard Doppler-derived measurements, as well as the correlation between in vivo Doppler-derived EOA and the in vitro geometric orifice provided by the manufacturer (115). The authors found that EOA measurements were higher using the pressure half-time method versus the continuity equation, a finding that has also been described in St. Jude mitral prostheses (116). Dumesnil et al. (87) have previously shown that the pressure half-time method tends to overestimate the in vitro–derived EOA, and that a better correlation can be obtained using the continuity equation method. In the Mayo Clinic study, the authors recommended TEE study to rule out thrombus or pannus formation, and to assess occluder motion if the pressure half-time exceeded 130 ms. They also suggested that if the E velocity was greater than 2 m/s, or if the ratio of the velocity-time integral (VTI) of the mitral prosthesis to the VTI of the LVOT was greater than or equal to 2.2 in the presence of a pressure half-time less than 130 ms, then TEE is recommended to rule out significant valvular or paravalvular regurgitation.

Disc Valves

Bjork-Shiley Valve

During systole, when the disc closes, a characteristic rectangular reverberation is seen in the LA. In diastole, there is flow across the major and minor orifices of the valve, with convergence of the two jets into one as they pass the tip of the disc.

In this valve, only peripheral regurgitant jets are seen (only one disc without a central hole). The jets are narrow (<10 mm) and short (<30 mm). Knowledge of the specific type of Bjork-Shiley valve is important as "normal" jet sizes differ (Fig. 16.15; see also Fig. 16.5B) (117–120).

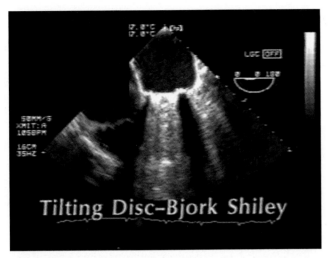

Figure 16.15. Tilting-disc valve in the mitral position showing reverberation and acoustic shadowing artifacts.

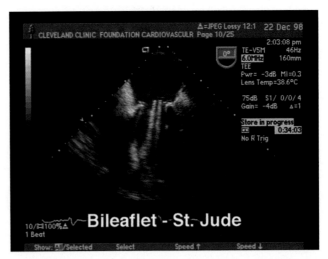

Figure 16.16. Open bileaflet valve in the mitral position. Notice the acoustic shadowing and reverberation artifacts in the LV cavity.

Medtronic-Hall Valve

The ring, which is located just inside the mitral annulus, causes acoustic shadowing (increased echogenicity adjacent to the annulus). The strut is seen as a strong echo dot with side lobes just above the annulus level between the dot and the ring. The disc is seen as a strong echo line in the LA. Disc reverberations are more prominent in systole.

There are usually two peripheral jets and one central regurgitant jet. The central jet originates at the small gap formed between the strut and central hole of the disc. Peripheral jets occur at the gap between the ring and disc. These "normal" regurgitant jets are usually small and narrow. These washing jets eliminate stagnation on the underside of the valve.

Bileaflet Valves

St. Jude Valve

Regurgitant jets in the St. Jude valve occur at the hinge points. There is one central jet and two peripheral jets. The central jet is due to the gap between the disc leaflets. Color flow Doppler mapping of the St. Jude valve shows regurgitant flow at the periphery (between the disc and sewing ring) and centrally (between the leaflets). These jets are 3D and therefore can appear convergent or divergent, depending on the imaging plane. The CW Doppler beam should be directed through the lateral orifices of the valve. The phenomenon of "pressure recovery" (see above) occurs across St. Jude prostheses and can lead to an overestimation of the true valve gradient when the central orifice is used. This occurs because some of the gradient recorded by Doppler is "recovered" as flow emerges from the valve. Pressure recovery is limited to the central orifice of the valve (84). The gradient measured across the central orifice can be 40% to 50% higher than that measured across the lateral orifices, which are the preferred measurement sites (Figs. 16.9, 16.16, and 16.17) (81,121).

CarboMedics Valve

Color flow Doppler of the CarboMedics valve normally shows four washing jets, one on either side of each pivot point. One jet is often more prominent than the others. Regurgitant jets are more significant compared to the St. Jude valve (122–124). Normal valve function is characterized by opening and closing clicks and separation of E and A waves of mitral inflow (125).

Stented Bioprosthetic Valves

Valve stents are usually oriented toward the septum in a mitral prosthesis. It is important to look for extraneous echoes, leaflet excursion, leaflet thickening, leaflet prolapse/flail, and stability of the sewing ring. It is also important to make sure the stents do not create an obstruction by impinging upon the LVOT. Perimount

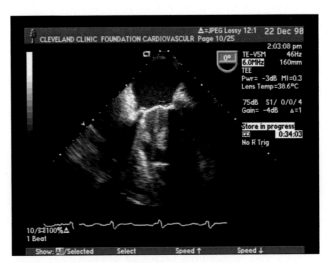

Figure 16.17. Closed bileaflet valve in the mitral position. Notice the acoustic shadowing and reverberation artifacts.

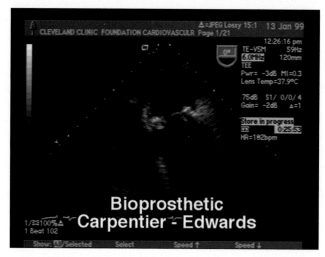

Figure 16.18. Bioprosthetic Carpentier-Edwards valve in the mitral position. A thin leaflet can be seen along the lateral wall and a strut in the LV cavity.

bovine pericardial valves have prominent washing jets (central where the three leaflets coapt and between the leaflets where they attach to the sewing ring), which may be considered excessive if you are not familiar with the normal color flow of this valve (Figs. 16.11, 16.18, and 16.19) (126,127).

Stentless Bioprosthetic Valves

Depending on the method of valve implantation, the echocardiographic appearance of stentless aortic bioprostheses will vary. If the valve has been implanted using a subcoronary or root inclusion technique (where the bioprosthesis is within the native aortic root), a space can be detected between the native aortic wall and the porcine aortic wall. This is a normal finding, provided there is no detectable color flow within this space. The presence of color flow within this space is suggestive of a dehiscence of the proximal or the distal suture line. This space

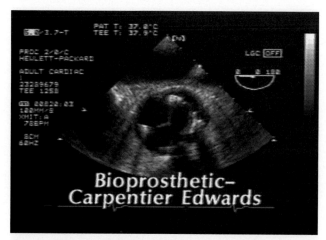

Figure 16.19. Bioprosthetic Carpentier-Edwards valve in the aortic position. You can see the three cusps, which are closed, and the three struts with the annular ring around the valve.

generally disappears within 6 months when the porcine wall becomes fully adherent to the native aortic wall. With a valve dehiscence, hematoma forms between the porcine aortic wall and the native aortic wall, leading to disruption of the normal 3D structure of the valve and structural valve deterioration (128). Valve competence is dependent on proper matching between the aortic annulus and the sinotubular junction. Any mismatch between these variables is a contraindication for the subcoronary implantation technique. If the ST junction is dilated, the prosthetic valve commissures become pulled apart, and the coaptation surface becomes reduced, resulting in leaflet tethering and central regurgitation. Conversely, if the ST junction dimension is reduced, leaflet prolapse occurs, and the coaptation height becomes reduced.

If the valve has been implanted using the root replacement technique, the coronary ostia are reimplanted. In this case, the echocardiographic appearance is very similar to that of an aortic valve homograft (58,129). The implantation technique is dependent on the anatomy of the aortic root. Distortion of the prosthesis during subcoronary implantation can affect valve competency and can lead to accelerated cusp fibrosis and calcification, with early prosthesis failure (130).

Aortic Valve Homografts

The unstented homografts placed in the aortic position are nearly identical in appearance and flow characteristics to the native aortic valve. In a normally functioning aortic valve homograft, the only distinguishing echocardiographic feature is an increase in echo density around the suture line.

PROSTHETIC VALVE DYSFUNCTION AND COMPLICATIONS

Prosthetic Valve Stenosis

Compared to native valves, prosthetic valves are relatively obstructive, with the degree of obstruction being a function of valve type and size. Because there is such a wide range of normal velocities across prosthetic valves, the diagnosis of prosthetic valve stenosis can prove challenging.

Degree of stenosis is generally assessed by measuring peak velocity, mean velocity, velocity time integral, valve area (pressure half-time), and effective valve orifice area (continuity equation and Gorlin formula) for mitral prostheses. For aortic prostheses, peak and mean velocities, velocity time integral, and dimensionless ratio are measured. Even though Doppler gradients can be indicative of prosthetic valve obstruction, one must keep in mind that transvalvular gradients obtained by Doppler are very flow dependent. Prosthetic orifice area gives a more flow-independent measure of resistance, as with stenotic native valves.

In order to determine if a prosthetic valve is stenotic, it is best to compare Doppler-derived estimates of gradients or valve areas to the expected value for a valve of particular size and type. When a prosthetic valve has been implanted, a baseline echocardiographic study should be obtained prior to hospital discharge. Gradient values can be used for future follow-up comparison. Measurements and calculations should be made in the same manner, specifying the method and mathematical formula employed. Trends and deviation from baseline values may be more revealing than absolute numbers. And of course, 2D echo information can provide information on the etiology of prosthetic valvular stenosis (131,132).

The simplified form of Bernoulli's equation ($P = 4V_2^2$) is frequently used to measure the pressure gradient across aortic valve prostheses. This can be a source for error in some situations, leading to an overestimation of the gradient (133). In 1982, Bird et al. described the association of significant subvalvular gradients without subvalvular obstruction in patients with aortic stenosis. This finding illustrated that omitting the V_1 component of the modified Bernoulli equation could lead to a significant overestimation of the pressure gradient (134). Thrombosis and pannus formation are the most common causes of prosthetic valve stenosis in mechanical valves (135,136). Thrombosis is the most common cause of prosthetic valve obstruction. Mitral valve thrombosis occurs with twice the frequency of aortic valve thrombosis (137). Pannus formation is fibroconnective tissue ingrowth from the sewing ring and typically occurs after many years of valve implantation. It tends to occur more commonly with aortic prostheses. It can interfere with valve closure and opening by impinging on the hinge mechanism of a mechanical valve. This can lead to flow obstruction (restricted opening) or regurgitation (restricted closure). Its formation is unaffected by routine anticoagulation. Obstruction with normal disc motion has also been demonstrated in a patient with a Bjork-Shiley aortic prosthesis who developed annular pannus ingrowth (138). Doppler findings consistent with a bileaflet valve occlusion include fusion of E and A waves (with decreased pressure half-time and increased deceleration time) and lack of opening and closing valve clicks, which are seen as bright vertical lines at the opening and closing points on the Doppler trace and increased E wave velocity. Stenosis can also be due to an undersized prosthesis or other structural problems, such as the leaflet being stuck in the closed position. Differentiation of thrombus from pannus can prove difficult. Thrombus has more of a tendency to be mobile, associated with stasis, and is generally less echodense than pannus. Pannus is generally strongly echogenic and tends to be fixed and immobile. Proximal flow convergence and color flow aliasing can be suggestive of pannus ingrowth (139). Acute disc or leaflet immobilization has been described in mechanical prostheses (140–145). Restricted occluder motion can be complete, partial, or intermittent. The occluder may be fixed in the open or closed position. If sutures are not cut short enough, or become unraveled, they can get caught in the valve housing and cause sticking. Mitral chordal remnants and even the LV wall can interfere with proper

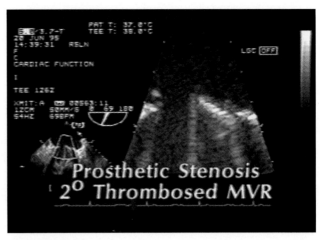

Figure 16.20. A St. Jude mitral valve with one leaflet in the open position and the other leaflet in the closed position secondary to thrombosis.

disc/leaflet motion. LVOT obstruction can occur with retention of the anterior mitral leaflet during MVR. With ball-cage valves, one can see ball variance, where the ball swells and becomes partially stuck in the cage.

Identification of thrombus on a prosthetic valve can be difficult, especially if it is nonobstructive. TEE can be used to monitor thrombolysis of thrombosed prosthetic valves (146–149). TEE can help assess thrombus size, location, and aid in treatment decisions, such as thrombolysis, anticoagulation, and surgery.

Opening angle can sometimes be measured. The echocardiographer should have an understanding of normal occluder motion for each type of prosthesis (Figs. 16.20–16.22).

Prosthetic Valve Regurgitation

Because of the location of the TEE transducer behind the LA, prosthetic MR can be well visualized with color flow Doppler (118,150–156). TEE is far superior to

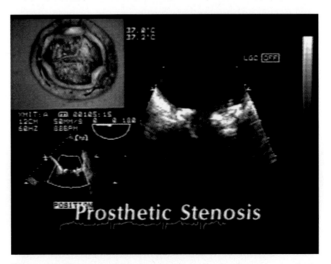

Figure 16.21. The stenosis of a mitral CE valve. It shows calcification and thickening of the leaflets.

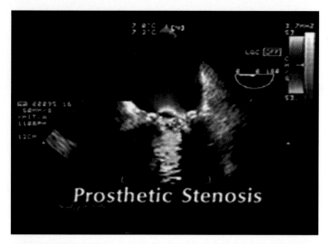

Figure 16.22. Prosthetic stenosis of a bioprosthetic valve. Note the large PISA on the LA side of the valve indicating severe prosthetic stenosis

transthoracic echocardiography (TTE) (157) in the evaluation of prosthetic MR (28% vs. 95% mitral, 29% vs. 44% aortic). Prosthetic aortic regurgitation originating from the posterior side of the prosthesis can be well appreciated by TEE while anteriorly located AI may be difficult to visualize, especially if there is shadowing from a mitral prosthetic valve or ring, or dense mitral annular calcification.

An understanding of normal prosthetic regurgitation is necessary. "Normal" regurgitant jets are short, narrow, flame-like, laminar, and of low velocity. This type of regurgitation can be subdivided into two categories based on timing of flow. "Closure backflow" occurs during valve closure as the prosthetic disc or ball displaces blood into the LA for a mitral prosthesis. "Leakage backflow" can be transvalvular or paravalvular and occurs after valve closure (158). With the exception of the Starr-Edwards caged ball prosthesis, which demonstrates only closure backflow jets, all mechanical prostheses show some degree of closure and leakage backflow due to their design. Leakage backflow occurs at hinge points, around struts, or between the ring and central occluder (159). Most often, these regurgitant jets are of no hemodynamic significance. Pathologic jets tend to show increased color variance and are longer and broader than normal physiologic jets.

Regurgitation can be quantified by examining volume of color jet in LA, density of CW signal, PISA on ventricular side of regurgitant orifice, and systolic reversal of flow in pulmonary vein(s). Flow convergence should be looked for on the ventricular side of the regurgitant prosthesis (104). This proximal flow acceleration is indicative of significant valvular regurgitation.

Regurgitation can be perivalvular, transvalvular, or a combination of both. Both etiologies can lead to shearing of red blood cells and intravascular hemolysis (see below). It is more commonly seen with mechanical than biological prostheses, and is believed to be due in part to the inflexibility of the mechanical valve annulus. Endocarditis is also

an important cause of periprosthetic leaks and should be ruled out.

With valvular regurgitation secondary to prosthetic valve dehiscence, there is a rocking motion of the prosthesis at its site of attachment. A perivalvular leak originates at the junction of the annulus and prosthetic sewing ring. Systolic and diastolic flows should be sought across a suspected periprosthetic defect.

Preservation of the mitral subvalvular apparatus during MVR is commonly performed and has been associated with improved long-term survival and better preservation of LV function (160). MR secondary to obstruction of a St. Jude mitral prosthesis by entrapment of preserved subvalvular mitral tissue several years after implant has been described (161).

Surgical technique has also been implicated, especially with the use of running, small-sized sutures (leads to suture fracture). Oversizing and undersizing of the valve can lead to valve dehiscence, as can severe annular calcification, which makes suture placement and proper valve seating difficult. In some instances, the surgeon will bend the prosthetic ring to make it fit.

Disc escape or embolization, most commonly associated with the Bjork-Shiley valve, has been described for several mechanical prostheses and is generally a fatal complication (Figs. 16.23–16.25) (162,163).

With bioprostheses, transvalvular regurgitation is usually due to cusp degeneration. With mechanical valve, transvalvular regurgitation may be caused by a thrombus, which prevents proper mechanical disc motion or proper seating of the valve poppet; it may also be caused by variance in the shape of the mechanical ball or disc.

Immediately after prosthetic valve insertion, perivalvular leaks are frequently seen. Most leaks usually disappear in approximately 2 weeks when the sewing ring has become endothelialized. Some jets decrease in size after insertion with the reversal of heparin with protamine

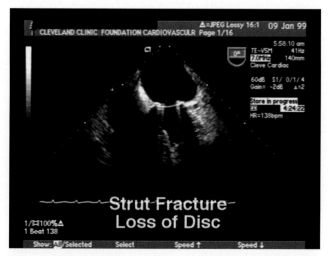

Figure 16.23. This image shows a single-disc mitral valve in which the disc is absent and the picture shows the annular ring with an echo lucency where the disc should be.

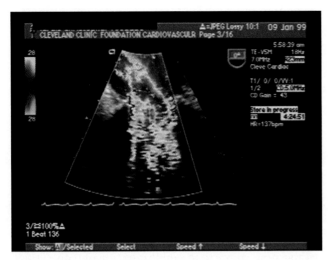

Figure 16.24. This image shows the regurgitation secondary to loss of the single-disc valve.

following cardiopulmonary bypass. Mild paravalvular AI has been described immediately following the implantation of stentless aortic valves. One study found that small AI paraprosthetic jets measuring 0.3 cm or less in width at the vena contracta resolved in a predictable manner following protamine administration (164). Most perivalvular leaks that are noted early on are generally trivial to mild, and generally do not progress (165,166). Late onset, severe periprosthetic regurgitation should raise concern over possible structural failure of the prosthesis, or infection. In a study of 134 patients with nonstenotic mitral prostheses (pressure half-time < 130 ms), a peak velocity across the prosthesis greater than 1.9 m/s or a ratio of the peak diastolic transmitral flow to LVOT velocity greater than 2.2 was highly suggestive of prosthetic MR. Likewise, if the peak transmitral flow was lesser than 1.9, and the ratio was lesser than 2.2, then there was a 98% likelihood that the prosthesis was normal (i.e., no stenosis or regurgitation) (167).

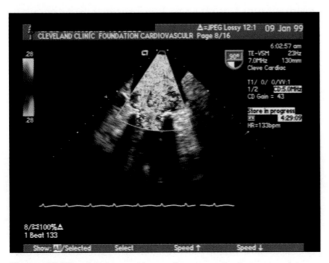

Figure 16.25. This image shows the regurgitation secondary to loss of the single-disc valve.

Patient Prosthesis Mismatch

The term "patient prosthesis mismatch" (PPM) was originally coined by Rahimtoola in 1978, when he described the condition in which the orifice area of implanted aortic prostheses was smaller than that of the native valve (168). This is generally due to the reduction in available orifice area created by the presence of struts, sewing ring, and leaflet housing. PPM occurs when the valve prosthesis is too small relative to the patient's size. It is typically seen as high transvalvular pressure gradients in normally functioning aortic valves and can lead to incomplete LV mass regression (169).

Reportedly, the most reliable method to determine PPM is to use the projected EOA derived from the published normal values of in vivo EOA measurements. The indexed effective orifice area (EOAi) is used to assess degree of patient PPM and is obtained by dividing the EOA by the body surface area. This parameter has been validated for the identification of PPM (170,171). Moderate PPM is defined as EOAi $\leq$ 0.85 cm^2/m^2 body surface area, and severe PPM is defined as EOAi < 0.65 cm^2/m^2. Values greater than 0.85 cm^2/m^2 are generally considered as clinically insignificant, or no PPM. High transvalvular gradients across a normally functioning prosthesis become cause for concern. The correlation between indexed EOA and mean transprosthetic pressure gradients is greater for aortic prostheses (r > 0.75) compared to mitral prostheses (r < 0.50) (87).

PPM is a relatively common occurrence following aortic valve replacement, with a reported incidence of 20% to 70% (172–174). The significance of moderate PPM on patient outcomes remains controversial. Several studies have suggested that moderate PPM leads to increased morbidity and mortality (175,176), as well as reduced exercise tolerance (177) while others show no effect on long-term outcomes (173,178). One study examined the effect of PPM on physical capacity in patients who underwent aortic valve replacement with a bioprosthesis (179). The incidence of PPM was 34.3%, and the authors found that PPM had a significant impact on physical capacity as determined by exercise testing. Another large study showed that most patients reported improvement in functional quality of life at an average of 8.3 months following aortic valve replacement, and that other factors (e.g., age, gender, transfusion) may be responsible for the poor functional recovery described in the postoperative period (180). LV ejection fraction has been shown to be an important predictor of risk following aortic valve replacement (181,182). In a study of 1,266 consecutive patients undergoing aortic valve replacement, 38% of patients were noted to have moderate or severe PPM, with an overall associated 30-day mortality of 4.6%. In this study, a LV ejection fraction less than 40% was an independent predictor of risk (183).

A number of frequently cited studies were published prior to the introduction of newer supra-annular prostheses, which were developed to optimize hemodynamic performance of aortic prostheses. More recent valve design includes lower profile, thinner sewing rings, and superior hemodynamic performance (184,185), and it is believed that these improvements will reduce the incidence of PPM. Supra-annular seating of aortic valve prostheses maximizes flow by optimizing alignment of the valve orifice to the native annulus (186), and was shown in one study to significantly reduce the incidence of PPM from 50% to 34% (187).

Freestyle stentless bioprostheses are well recognized for superior hemodynamic performance and more effective regression of LV hypertrophy compared to stented bioprostheses. In a study of 419 patients who underwent Freestyle stentless valve subcoronary implant, PPM was found in 91% and 80% of patients receiving 19 and 21-mm prostheses, and severe mismatch was present in 58% and 17%, respectively (188). For Freestyle valves, it has also been shown that higher postoperative transvalvular gradients can lead to impaired physical mobility. One study identified indexed geometric orifice area, subcoronary implantation technique (vs. full root), and individual surgeons as predictors of elevated gradients (189).

The use of a fixed value for the in vivo measured EOA was previously suggested by Pibarot and Dumesnil (190). The EOA of mitral prostheses is frequently small relative to body size, leading to a mismatch with transvalvular flow (191). The result of this is normally functioning prostheses with transvalvular gradients found in patients with mild-to-moderate native mitral stenosis (76,192). This can in turn lead to postoperative pulmonary hypertension (193,194). Some studies have suggested that severe PPM, based on EOAi, leads to worse survival when compared to moderate or nonsignificant PPM (195,196). Criticism of these studies has included failure to separate results between patients being treated for MR versus stenosis and the relation of cardiopulmonary bypass and cross-clamp times between groups. The impact of PPM on PA pressure following MVR was studied in 56 patients with normally functioning prostheses (193). Fifty-four percent of patients had pulmonary hypertension, defined as systolic PA pressure greater than 40 mm Hg, and 71% of patients had PPM, defined as EOAi $\leq$ 1.2 cm^2/m^2. Systolic PA pressure correlated strongly with EOAi (r = 0.64), and by multivariate analysis, EOAi was the strongest predictor of systolic PA pressure.

It has been suggested that patients with lower stroke volumes might benefit more from a porcine bioprosthesis because of the greater tissue pliability while patients with a higher stroke volume might derive more benefit from pericardial valves (197). PPM may be related to valve type, with bioprosthetic valves having a stronger association (198). In a study of 1,400 patients, PPM was noted in 51% of patients receiving bioprostheses versus 11% of mechanical valve recipients (PPM was defined as EOAi < 0.75 cm^2/m^2). For patients less than 60 years of age

having PPM, 10-year survival was less (68% vs. 75% for bioprosthetic valves; 62% vs. 79% for mechanical valves) compared to older patients.

Prosthetic Valve Endocarditis

PVE is a devastating complication of valve replacement. Early detection and treatment rely on accurate diagnosis. With early infection, bacterial pathogens gain direct access to perivalvular tissue along suture lines and the prosthesis-annulus interface. These areas are targets for infectious invasion because they are not endothelialized early on after valve implantation. Endothelialization occurs over a period of several months. With late infection, the sites for microorganism invasion are altered, and the pathogenesis comes to resemble infection of native valves. Platelet-fibrin thrombi may serve as a nidus for infection. Late infections (>12 months) are generally less invasive than early infections, and perivalvular abscess formation and valve dehiscence are less common in comparison (199–201). The risk of PVE is highest in the first three postoperative months and falls gradually after 6 months. The rate of infection is similar for mitral and aortic prostheses. In the first postoperative year, mechanical and bioprostheses have similar infection rates; however, after 18 months, bioprostheses show a greater risk of late infection (202). TEE is considered the best approach for defining anatomic valve abnormalities, dysfunction, periprosthetic leak, fistulous communications, and abscess formation. When a prosthetic valve dehiscence occurs, hypermobility of the prosthesis secondary to suture disruption can be a surgical emergency. Perivalvular invasion is seen as any of the following: perivalvular abscess, valve dehiscence, fistula formation, and aortic aneurysm or pseudoaneurysm (203). More invasive infection tends to occur when the infection occurs within 12 months of the original valve implant, or if the prosthesis is in the aortic position (204). The sensitivity of TEE in the detection of PVE is 85% to 90% (five times more sensitive than TTE). With TTE, reverberations from the prosthesis make it very difficult to see vegetations. TEE is indicated in all patients suspected of having PVE.

Vegetations are seen as echodense, mobile, "shaggy" appearing structures representing infected material containing bacteria, fibrin, platelets, and white and red blood cells. The rate of PVE is similar between mechanical and biological prostheses. Ring abscesses and septal muscle abscesses are more common in prosthetic valvular than native valvular endocarditis. All parts of the prosthesis must be inspected for vegetations and disruption. The initial infective growth tends to occur on the sewing ring of mechanical valves. Bioprosthetic valves tend to have vegetations on diseased or disrupted leaflets.

Differentiation of thrombus from vegetation (diagnosis based on clinical picture) can be quite difficult, particularly with mechanical valves and small lesions. The entire perivalvular region must be scanned to rule out multicentric abscesses. A torn or disrupted sewing ring cloth can be mistaken for vegetations.

A perivalvular abscess has the appearance of an echolucent or echodense region within the annulus or perivalvular tissue. Early on, a perivalvular abscess may appear homogeneous. Later, necrosis can lead to an echolucent and heterogeneous appearance. Some abscesses may be multicentric; some may form fistulae with other cardiac chambers or vascular spaces (best seen with color flow Doppler). Systolic motion of an abscess cavity is suggestive of communication with a cardiac chamber or great vessel. Color flow Doppler imaging facilitates the diagnosis of such communications (Figs. 16.26–16.29) (205–210). With aortic valve PVE, the infection can extend through the annulus and into the membranous portion of the interventricular septum, leading to conduction block. New-onset first degree AV block in a patient with aortic PVE is highly suspect for a periaortic abscess. Pericarditis can also result from the infection (211).

Structural Abnormalities

Fibrin strands are often seen on otherwise structurally and functionally normal mechanical or biologic prostheses. They are more commonly seen on the atrial side of St. Jude mechanical valves and are not clearly associated with endocarditis, thrombosis, or embolization (212,213). They have been identified adherent to the mechanical disk or associated with the prosthetic annulus (214). These strands are echodense, generally less than 1 mm wide, mobile, linear, and of variable length. Their etiology, incidence, and significance remain unclear, and many still consider them a potential source of embolization. In one report, a strand from a degenerated mitral bioprosthetic valve was analyzed and found to consist of a sparsely cellular component with extracellular amorphous of fibrillary areas (predominantly collagen) (215). Valvular strands have also been detected during thrombolytic therapy, suggesting a fibrotic or thrombotic origin.

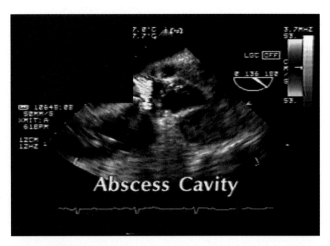

Figure 16.27. This image shows aortic regurgitation secondary to this abscess of the aortic homograft.

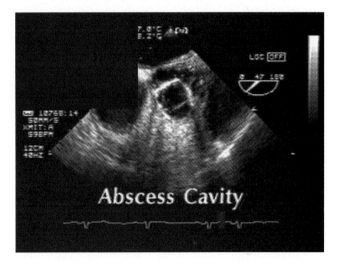

Figure 16.28. This image shows a cross section of the infected abscessed aortic homograft. Superiorly you may see part of the ring abscessed cavity.

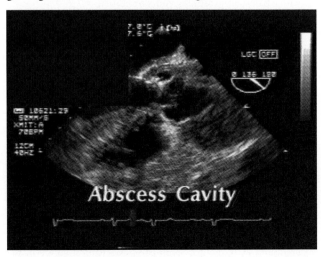

Figure 16.26. This image shows an abscess cavity with a ring abscess around an aortic homograft.

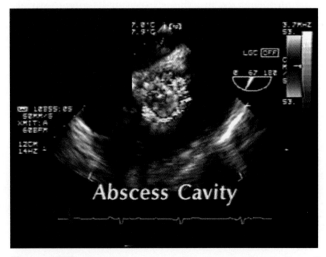

Figure 16.29. This image shows the cross-sectional view of the infected abscess cavity and aortic homograft and the color shows the ring abscess around this valve.

ASSOCIATED COMPLICATIONS

Thromboembolism

Thromboembolism continues to be one of the major drawbacks of mechanical prostheses. It includes systemic emboli, nonhemorrhagic strokes, and transient ischemic attacks. It is believed to be due to a combination of flow stasis at hinge points and the sewing ring and a lack of endothelialization (216).

A number of factors contribute to this complication including adequacy of anticoagulation, atrial fibrillation, low cardiac output, multiple valve replacement, endocarditis, and previous history of thromboembolism.

Hemorrhage

Hemorrhage is generally related to anticoagulation.

Hemolysis

Hemolysis from prosthetic regurgitation is related to high shear stress, which is in turn related to the configuration of the resulting flow disturbance. Regurgitant flow patterns seen in patients with hemolysis secondary to a mitral prosthesis have been shown to be associated with rapid acceleration/deceleration, high peak shear rates, or both. (In vitro shear stresses >3,000 dynes/cm² can cause red blood cell destruction.) The site of origin of the flow disturbance (central vs. paravalvular) and type of prosthesis are less important than the nature of the flow disturbance produced by the regurgitant lesion and the resulting increased shear stress.

The development of hemolytic anemia with valve prostheses has been attributed to high shear stresses, pressure fluctuations, turbulent flow, the interaction of red blood cells with foreign surfaces, and abnormalities of the red cell membrane. Perivalvular regurgitant jets can denude an endothelialized prosthesis, exposing its foreign surface and increasing the risk of hemolysis. With the early ball-cage valves, the incidence of hemolysis was as high as 6% to 15%. Improved design reduced this frequency. Hemolysis is more significant with malfunctioning prostheses than normal prostheses.

Evidence suggests that acceleration and deceleration may be important causes of hemolysis, the absence of a perivalvular leak does not preclude the development of clinical hemolysis, and hemolysis is not related to the severity of MR. Collision with rapid deceleration was the most common pattern associated with hemolysis. Regurgitation through small single or multiple orifices and flow fragmentation or collision were associated with more hemolysis than flow through larger single orifices. This was thought to be due to the greater flow acceleration across smaller orifices. Collision with rapid deceleration was found to be the most common mechanism associated with hemolysis (217).

KEY POINTS

■ The echocardiographic evaluation of prosthetic heart valves is complex and requires a thorough knowledge of the different types of valves available, how they function, and their echocardiographic appearance during normal function and dysfunction.
■ The echocardiographic examination of all prosthetic valves can be limited by acoustic shadowing and reverberations by the echodense areas of the valve.
■ TEE and TTE are complementary in the evaluation of all prosthetic heart valves.
■ Causes of prosthetic valve dysfunction include the following: degeneration, thrombosis, dehiscence, obstruction, and infection.
■ The Doppler examination of prosthetic valves can be used to assess gradients, keeping in mind that each type of valve has its own degree of obstruction and that gradients are highly dependent on valve type, size, location, flow, and cardiac function.
■ EOA is a superior measure of prosthetic valve performance compared to transvalvular gradients because it is a flow-independent measurement.
■ All prosthetic valves (with perhaps the exception of SPVs and aortic homografts) are relatively stenotic compared to native valves and have distinct "normal" regurgitant flow patterns.

REFERENCES

1. Huffnagel CA, Harvey WP. The surgical correction of aortic insufficiency. Preliminary report. *Bull Georgetown Univ Med Cent* 1953;6:60–61.
2. Murray G. Homologous aortic-valve-segment transplants as surgical treatment for aortic and mitral insufficiency. *Angiology* 1956;7:466–471.
3. Starr A, Edwards ML. Mitral replacement: clinical experience with a ball valve prosthesis. *Ann Surg* 1961;154:726–740.
4. Grunkemeier GL, Starr A, Rahimtoola SH. Prosthetic heart valve performance: Long-term follow-up. *Curr Probl Cardiol* 1992;17:335–406.
5. Whittlesey D, Geha AS. Selection and complications of cardiac valvular prostheses. In: Baue AE, Geha AS, Hammond GL, et al., eds. *Glenn's Thoracic and Cardiovascular Surgery*. Norwalk: Appleton and Lange CN, 1991:1719–1728.
6. Vongpatanasin W, Hillis LD, Lange RA. Prosthetic heart valves. *N Engl J Med* 1996;335:407–416.
7. Pluth JR. The Starr-Edwards mitral valve. In: Ionescu MI, Cohn LH, eds. *Mitral Valve Disease: Diagnosis and Treatment*. London: Butterworth and Co. (Publishers) Ltd., 1985:217–220.
8. Lepley D Jr, Flemma RJ, Mullen DC. The Bjork-Shiley tilting disc valve in the mitral position. In: Ionescu MI, Cohn LH, eds. *Mitral Valve Disease: Diagnosis and Treatment*. London: Butterworth and Co. (Publishers) Ltd., 1985:221–232.
9. Lindblom D, Bjork VO, Semb BKH. Mechanical failure of the Bjork-Shiley valve. Incidence, clinical presentation, and management. *J Thorac Cardiovasc Surg* 1986;92:894–907.

10. Sugita T, Yasuda R, Watarida S, et al. Minor strut fracture of the Bjork-Shiley mitral valve. *Nippon Kyobu Geka Zasshi* 1990;38:1049–1052.

11. Bjork VO, Lindblom D, Henze A. The monostrut strength. *Scand J Thorac Cardiovasc Surg* 1985;19:13–19.

12. Matloff JM, Chaux A, Czer LSC, et al. A four year experience with the St. Jude mitral valve prosthesis. In: Ionescu MI, Cohn LH, eds. *Mitral Valve Disease: Diagnosis and Treatment*. London: Butterworth and Co. (Publishers) Ltd., 1985: 233–234.

13. Ely JL, Emken MR, Accuntius JA, et al. Pure pyrolitic carbon: preparation and properties of a new material, On-X carbon for mechanical heart valve prostheses. *J Heart Valve Dis* 1998;7:626–632.

14. Tossios P, Reber D, Oustria M, et al. Single-center experience with the On-X prosthetic heart valve between 1996 and 2005. *J Heart Valve Dis* 2007;16:551–557.

15. Ozyurda U, Akar AR, Uymaz O, et al. Early clinical experience with the On-X prosthetic heart valve. *Interact Cardiovasc Thorac Surg* 2005;4:588–594.

16. Lee EM, Shapiro LM, Wells FC. Superiority of mitral valve repair in surgery for degenerative mitral regurgitation. *Eur Heart J* 1997;18:655–663.

17. Rozich JD, Carabello BA, Usher BW, et al. Mitral valve replacement with and without chordal preservation in patients with chronic mitral regurgitation. Mechanisms for differences in postoperative ejection performance. *Circulation* 1992;86:1718–1726.

18. Goldfine H, Aurigemma GP, Zile MR, et al. Left ventricular length-force shortening relations before and after surgical correction of chronic mitral regurgitation. *J Am Coll Cardiol* 1998;31:180–185.

19. Wippermann J, Albes JM, Madershahian N, et al. Three years' experience with the On-X conform-X bileaflet prosthesis for 'atrialized' mitral valve replacement: a preliminary report. *J Heart Valve Dis* 2005;14:637–643.

20. Palatianos GM, Laczkovics AM, Simon P, et al. Multicentered European study on safety and effectiveness of the On-X prosthetic heart valve: intermediate follow-up. *Ann Thorac Surg* 2007;83:40–46.

21. Heimbecker RO, Baird RJ, Lajox TZ, et al. Homograft replacement of the human mitral valve: a preliminary report. *Can Med Assoc J* 1962;86:805–809.

22. Ross DN. Homograft replacement of the aortic valve. *Lancet* 1962;2:487.

23. Duran CMG, Gunning AJ. A method for placing a total homologous aortic valve in the subcoronary position. *Lancet* 1962;2:488–489.

24. Binet JP, Duran CMG, Carpentier A, et al. Heterologous aortic valve transplantation. *Lancet* 1965;2:1275.

25. Carpentier A, Lemaigre G, Robert L, et al. Biological factors affecting long term results of valvular heterografts. *J Thorac Cardiovasc Surg* 1969;58:467–483.

26. Reis RL, Hancock WD, Yarbrough JW, et al. The flexible stent: a new concept in the fabrication of tissue heart valve prostheses. *J Thorac Cardiovasc Surg* 1971;62:683–689.

27. Hammermeister K, Sethi GK, Henderson WG, et al. Outcomes 15 years after valve replacement with a mechanical versus bioprosthetic valve: final report of the Veterans Affairs randomized trial. *J Am Coll Cardiol* 2000;36:1152–1158.

28. Rahimtoola SH. Choice of prosthetic heart valve for adult patients. *J Am Coll Cardiol* 2003;41:893–904.

29. Poirier NC, Pelletier LC, Pellerin M, et al. 15 year experience with Carpentier-Edwards pericardial bioprosthesis. *Ann Thorac Surg* 1998;66(6 Suppl.):S57–S61.

30. Bach DS, Metras J, Doty JR, et al. Freedom from structural valve deterioration among patients aged < or = 60 years undergoing Freestyle stentless aortic valve replacement. *J Heart Valve Dis* 2007;16:649–655.

31. Bonow RO, Carabello BA, Chatterjee K, et al. ACC/AHA 2006 guidelines for management of patients with valvular heart disease: a report of the American College of Cardiology/American Heart Association Task Force on Practice Guidelines (writing Committee to Revise the 1998 guidelines for the management of patients with valvular heart disease) developed in collaboration with the Society of Cardiovascular Anesthesiologists endorsed by the Society for Cardiovascular Angiography and Interventions and the Society of Thoracic Surgeons. *J Am Coll Cardiol* 2006;48:e1-148.

32. Reardon MJ, Oury JH. Evolving experience with cryopreserved mitral valve allografts. *Curr Opin Cardiol* 1998;13:85–90.

33. Kumar AS, Kumar DA, Chander H, et al. Experience with homograft mitral valve replacement. *J Heart Valve Dis* 1998;7:225–228.

34. Acar C. Mitral valve homograft. *Adv Card Surg* 1997;9:1–13.

35. Vrandecic M, Gontijo B, et al. Homograft replacement of the mitral valve. *J Thorac Cardiovasc Surg* 1996;112:678–679.

36. Acar C, Ali M. Homologous transplantation of the mitral valve. A review. *J Cardiovasc Surg (Torino)* 2004;45:455–464.

37. Ali M, Iung B, Lansac E, et al. Homograft replacement of the mitral valve: eight-year results. *J Thorac Cardiovasc Surg* 2004;128:529–534.

38. Yacoub M, Rasmi NRH, Sundt TM, et al. Fourteen year experience with homovital homografts for aortic valve replacement. *J Thorac Cardiovasc Surg* 1995;110:186–194.

39. Cohen DJ, Myerowitz PD, Young WP, et al. The fate of aortic valve homografts 12 to 17 years after implantation. *Chest* 1988;93:482–484.

40. Kirklin JK, Smith D, Novick W, et al. Long-term function of cryopreserved aortic homografts: a ten year study. *J Thorac Cardiovasc Surg* 1993;106:154–166.

41. Oury JH. Clinical aspects of the Ross procedure: indications and contraindications. *Semin Thorac Surg* 1996;65:496–502.

42. DiSesa VJ, Collins JJ Jr, Cohn LH. Mitral valve replacement with the porcine bioprosthesis. In: Ionescu MI, Cohn L, eds. *Mitral Valve Disease: Diagnosis and Treatment*. London: Butterworth and Co. (Publishers) Ltd., 1985:243–252.

43. Jones M, Rodriguez ER, Eidbo EE, et al. Cuspal perforations caused by long suture ends in implanted bioprosthetic valves. *J Thorac Cardiovasc Surg* 1985;90:557–563.

44. Orszulak TA, Schaff HV, Danielson GK, et al. Results of reoperation for periprosthetic leakage. *Ann Thorac Surg* 1983;35:584–589.

45. Thiene G, Bortolotti U, Valente M, et al. Mode of failure of the Hancock pericardial valve xenograft. *Am J Cardiol* 1989;63:129–133.

46. Riddle JM, Magilligan DJ, Stein PD. Surface morphology of degenerated porcine bioprosthetic valves four to seven years following implantation. *J Thorac Cardiovasc Surg* 1981;81:279–287.

47. Ishihara T, Ferrans VJ, Boyce SW, et al. Structure and classification of cuspal tears and perforations in porcine bioprosthetic cardiac valves implanted in patients. *Am J Cardiol* 1981;48:665–678.

48. Thubrikar MJ, Deck JD, Aouad J, et al. Role of mechanical stress in calcification of aortic biprosthetic valves. *J Thorac Cardiovasc Surg* 1983;86:115–125.

49. Magilligan DJ, Lewis JW Jr, Tilley B, et al. The porcine bioprosthetic valve: twelve years later. *J Thorac Cardiovasc Surg* 1985;89:499–507.

50. Curcio CA, Commerford PJ, Rose AG, et al. Calcification of glutaraldehyde-preserved porcine xenografts in young patients. *J Thorac Cardiovasc Surg* 1981;81:621–625.

51. Kopf GS, Geha AS, Hellerbrand WE. Fate of left-sided cardiac bioprosthesis valves in children. *Arch Surg* 1986;121:488–490.

52. Ionescu MI, Silverton NP, Tandon AP. The pericardial xenograft in the mitral position. In: Ionescu MI, Cohn LH, eds. *Mitral Valve Disease: Diagnosis and Treatment.* London: Butterworth and Co. (Publishers) Ltd., 1985:243–252.

53. Dalmau MJ, Gonzalez-Santos JM, Lopez-Rodriguez J, et al. The Carpentier-Edwards Perimount Magna aortic xenograft: a new design with an improved hemodynamic performance. *Interact Cardiovasc Thoracic Surg* 2006;5:263–267.

54. Eichinger WB, Hettich IM, Ruzicka DJ, et al. Twenty-year experience with the St. Jude medical Biocor bioprosthesis in the aortic position. *Ann Thorac Surg* 2008;86:1204–1210.

55. Pomerantzeff PM, Brandao CM, Albuquerque JM, et al. Long-term followup of the Biocor porcine bioprosthesis in the mitral position. *J Heart Valve Dis* 2006;15:763–766.

56. Riess FC, Bader R, Cramer E, et al. Hemodynamic performance of the Medtronic Mosaic porcine bioprosthesis up to ten years. *Ann Thorac Surg* 2007;83:1310–1318.

57. Jamieson WR, Fradet GJ, MacNab JS, et al. Medtronic mosaic porcine bioprosthesis: Investigational center experience to six years. *J Heart Valve Dis* 2005;14:54–63.

58. Bach DS. Echocardiographic assessment of stentless aortic biprosthetic valves. *J Am Soc Echocardiogr* 2000;13:941–948.

59. Del Rizzo DF, Abdoh A. Clinical and hemodynamic comparison of the Medtronic Freestyle and Toronto SPV stentless valves. *J Card Surg* 1998;13:398–407.

60. Jin XY, Westaby S, Gibson DG, et al. Left ventricular remodeling and improvement in Freestyle stentless valve haemodynamics. *Eur J Cardiothorac Surg* 1997;12:63–69.

61. Pibarot P, Dumesnil JG, Leblanc MH, et al. Changes in left ventricular mass and function after aortic valve replacement: a comparison between stentless and stented biprosthetic valves. *J Am Soc Echocardiogr* 1999;12:981–987.

62. Lim E, Theodorou P, Sousa I, et al. Longitudinal study of the profile and predictors of left ventricular mass regression after stentless aortic valve replacement. *Ann Thorac Surg* 2008;85:2026–2029.

63. Chen W, Schoen FJ, Levy RJ. Mechanism of efficacy of 2-amino oleic acid for inhibition of calcification of glutaraldehyde-pretreated porcine biprosthetic heart valves. *Circulation* 1994;90:323–329.

64. Beholz S, Dushe S, Konertz W. Continuous suture technique for freedom stentless valve: reduced crossclamp time. *Asian Cardiovasc Thorac Ann* 2006:14:128–133.

65. Weltert L, DePaulis R, Maselli D, et al. Sorin Solo stentless valve: extended adaptability for sinotubular junction mismatch. *Interact Cardiovasc Thorac Surg* 2008;7:548–551.

66. Da Col U, Di Bella I, Bardelli G, et al. Short-term hemodynamic performance of the Sorin Freedom SOLO stentless valve. *J Heart Valve Dis* 2007;16:546–550.

67. Feigenbaum H. Acquired valvular heart disease: prosthetic valves. In: Feigenbaum H, ed. *Echocardiography.* 5th ed. Baltimore: Williams & Wilkins, 1993:297–314.

68. Oka Y, Kato M, Strom J. Mitral valve. In: Oka Y, Goldiner PL, eds. *Transesophageal Echocardiography.* Philadelphia: Lippincott Williams & Wilkins, 1992:99–151.

69. Clements FM, de Bruijn NP. Interventional echocardiography and the mitral valve. In: Clements FM, de Bruijn NP, eds. *Transesophageal Echocardiography.* Boston: Little, Brown and Co., 1991:111–131.

70. Renee BA, Brink VD, Visser CA. Comparison of transthoracic and transesophageal color Doppler flow imaging in patients with mechanical prostheses in the mitral valve position. *Am J Cardiol* 1989;63:1471–1474.

71. Khandheria BK, Seward JB, Oh JK, et al. Value and limitations of transesophageal echocardiography in assessment of mitral valve prostheses. *Circulation* 1991;83:1956–1968.

72. Levine RA, Jimoh A, Cape EG, et al. Pressure recovery distal to a stenosis: Potential cause of gradient "overestimation" by Doppler echocardiography. *J Am Coll Cardiol* 1989;13:706–715.

73. Reisner SA, Meltzer RS. Normal values of prosthetic valve Doppler echocardiographic parameters: a review. *J Am Soc Echocardiogr* 1988;1:201–210.

74. Burstow DJ, Nishimura RA, Bailey KR, et al. Continuous wave Doppler echocardiographic measurement of prosthetic valve gradients: a simultaneous Doppler-catheter correlative study. *Circulation* 1989;80:504–514.

75. Tatineni S, Barner HB, Pearson AC, et al. Rest and exercise evaluation of St. Jude Medical and Medtronic Hall prostheses: influence of primary lesion, valvular type, valvular size, and left ventricular function. *Circulation* 1989;80(3 Pt I):I-16–I-23.

76. Leavitt JI, Coats MH, Falk RH. Effects of exercise on transmitral gradient and pulmonary artery pressure in patients with mitral stenosis or a prosthetic mitral valve: a Doppler echocardiographic study. *J Am Coll Cardiol* 1991;17:1520–1526.

77. Garcia D, Dumesnil JG, Giles Durand LG, et al. Discrepancies between catheter and Doppler estimates of valve effective orifice area can be predicted from the pressure recovery phenomenon: practical implications with regard to quantification of aortic stenosis severity. *J Am Coll Cardiol* 2003;41:435–442.

78. Baumgartner H, Khan, S, Derobertis M, et al. Discrepancies between Doppler and catheter gradients in aortic prosthetic valves in vitro. *Circulation* 1990;82:1467–1475.

79. Baumgartner H, Khan S, DeRobertis M, et al. Effect of prosthetic aortic valve design on the Doppler-catheter gradient correlation: an in vitro study of normal St. Jude, Medtronic-Hall, Starr-Edwards and Hancock valves. *J Am Coll Cardiol* 1992;19:324–332.

80. Baumgartner H, Khan SS, DeRobertis M, et al. Doppler assessment of prosthetic valve orifice area. An in vitro study. *Circularion* 1992;85:2275–2283.

81. Vandervoort PM, Greenberg NL, Pu M, et al. Pressure recovery in bileaflet heart valve prostheses. Localized high velocities and gradients in central and side orifices with implications for Doppler-catheter gradient relation in aortic and mitral position. *Circulation* 1995;92:3464–3472.

82. Bech-Hanssen O, Caidahl K, Wallentin I, et al. Aortic prosthetic valve design and size: relation to Doppler echocardiographic

findings and pressure recovery—An in vitro study. *J Am Soc Echocardiogr* 2000;13:39–50.

83. Bech-Hanssen O, Gjertsson P, Houltz E, et al. Net pressure gradients in aortic prosthetic valves can be estimated by Doppler. *J Am Soc Echocardiogr* 2003;16:858–866.

84. Dohmen G, Schmitz C, Langebartels G, et al. Impact of pressure recovery in the evaluation of the Omnicarbon tilting disc valve. *Thorac Cardiovasc Surg* 2006;54:173–177.

85. Cooper DM, Stewart WJ, Schiavone WA, et al. Evaluation of normal prosthetic valve function by Doppler echocardiography. *Am Heart J* 1987;114:576–582.

86. Hatle L, Angelsen B, Tromsdal A. Noninvasive assessment of atrioventricular pressure half-time by Doppler ultrasound. *Circulation* 1979;60:1096–1104.

87. Dumesnil JG, Honos GN, Lemieux M, et al. Validation and applications of mitral prosthetic valvular areas calculated by Doppler echocardiography. *Am J Cardiol* 1990;65: 1443–1448.

88. Henneke KH, Pongratz G, Bachmann K. Limitations of Doppler echocardiography in the assessment of prosthetic valve hemodynamics. *J Heart Valve Dis* 1995;4:18–25.

89. Nakatani S, Masuyama T, Kodama K, et al. Value and limitations of Doppler echocardiography in the quantification of stenotic mitral valve area: comparison of the pressure half-time and the continuity equation methods. *Circulation* 1988;77:78–85.

90. Bitar JN, Lechin ME, Salazar G, et al. Doppler echocardiographic assessment with the continuity equation of St. Jude Medical mechanical prostheses in the mitral valve position. *Am J Cardiol* 1995;76:287–293.

91. Cha R, Yang SS, Salvucci T, et al. Doppler echocardiography in normal functioning valve prostheses. *N J Med* 1994;91:597–602.

92. Chambers JB, Jackson G, Jewitt DE. Limitations of Doppler ultrasound in the assessment of the function of prosthetic mitral valves. *Br Heart J* 1990;63:189–194.

93. Loyd D, Ask P, Wranne B. Pressure half-time does not always predict mitral valve area correctly. *J Am Soc Echocardiogr* 1988;1:313–321.

94. Leung DY, Wong J, Rodriguez L, et al. Application of color Doppler flow mapping to calculate orifice area of St. Jude mitral valve. *Circulation* 1998;98:1205–1211.

95. Mohan JC, Agrawal R, Arora R, et al. Improved Doppler assessment of the Bjork-Shiley mitral prosthesis using the continuity equation. *Int J Cardiol* 1994;43:321–326.

96. Williams GA, Labovitz AJ. Doppler hemodynamic evaluation of prosthetic (Starr-Edwards and Bjork-Shiley) and bioprosthetic (Hancock and Carpentier-Edwards) cardiac valves. *Am J Cardiol* 1985;56:325–332.

97. Chambers JB, Cochrane T, Black MM, et al. The effect of flow on Doppler estimates of bioprosthetic mitral valve function in vitro. *Cardiovasc Res* 1989;1007–1014.

98. Chambers JB. Mitral pressure half-time: is it a valid measure of EOA in artificial heart valves? *J Heart Valve Dis* 1993;2:571–577.

99. Chambers J, Deveral P, Jackson G, et al. The Hatle orifice area formula tested in normal bileaflet mechanical mitral prostheses. *Int J Cardiol* 1992;35:397–404.

100. Rothbart RM, Castriz JL, Harding LV, et al. Determination of aortic valve area by two-dimensional and Doppler echocardiography in patients with normal and stenotic bioprosthetic valves. *J Am Coll Cardiol* 1990;15:817–824.

101. Chafizadeh ER, Zoghbi WA. Doppler echocardiographic assessment of the St. Jude Medical prosthetic valve in the aortic position using the continuity equation. *Circulation* 1991;83:213–223.

102. Dumesnil JG, Honos GN, Lemieux M, et al. Validation and applications of indexed aortic prosthetic valve areas calculated by Doppler echocardiography. *J Am Coll Cardiol* 1990;16:637–643.

103. Miller FA Jr, Khanderia BK, Freeman WK, et al. Mitral prosthesis effective orifice area by a new method using continuity of flow between left atrium and prosthesis. *J Am Coll Cardiol* 1992;193:214A.

104. Cohen GI, Davison MB, Klein AL, et al. A comparison of flow convergence with other transthoracic echocardiographic indexes of prosthetic mitral regurgitation. *J Am Soc Echocardiogr* 1992;5:620–627.

105. Chambers J, Ely J. A comparison of the classical and modified forms of the continuity equation in the On-X prosthetic heart valve in the aortic position. *J Heart Valve Dis* 2000;9:299–301.

106. Saad RM, Barbetseas J, Ohnos L, et al. Application of the continuity equation and valve resistance to the evaluation of St. Jude Medical prosthetic aortic valve dysfunction. *Am J Cardiol* 1997;80:1239–1242.

107. Maslow AD, Haering JM, Heindel S, et al. An evaluation of prosthetic aortic valves using transesophageal echocardiography: the double-envelope technique. *Anesth Analg* 2000;91:509–516.

108. Mannaerts H, Li Y, Kamp O, et al. Quantitative assessment of mechanical prosthetic valve area by 3-dimensional transesophageal echocardiography. *J Am Soc Echocardiogr* 2001;14:723–731.

109. Lengyel M, Miller FA Jr, Taylor CL, et al. Doppler hemodynamic profiles of 456 clinically and echo-normal mitral valve prostheses. *Circulation* 1990;82(Suppl. 3):III-43(abst).

110. Miller FA, Callahan JA, Taylor CL, et al. Normal aortic valve prosthesis hemodynamics: 609 prospective Doppler examinations. *Circulation* 1989;80(Suppl. 2): II-169(abst).

111. Connolly H, Miller FA Jr, Taylor CL, et al. Doppler hemodynamic profiles of 82 clinically and echocardiographically normal tricuspid valve prostheses. *Circulation* 1993;88:2722–2727.

112. Rajani R, Mukherjee D, Chambers JB. Doppler echocardiography in normally functioning replacement aortic valves: a review of 129 studies. *J Heart Valve Dis* 2007;16: 519–535.

113. Shapira Y, Feinberg MS, Hirsch R, et al. Echocardiography can detect cloth tears in fully covered Starr-Edwards valves: a long-term clinical and echocardiographic study. *Am Heart J* 1997;134:665–671.

114. Nihoyannopoulos P, Kambouroglou D, Athanassopoulos G, et al. Doppler hemodynamic profiles of clinically and echocardiographically normal mitral and aortic valve prostheses. *Eur Heart J* 1992;13:348–355.

115. Malouf JF, Ballo M, Hodge DO, et al. Doppler echocardiography of normal Starr-Edwards mitral prostheses: a comprehensive function assessment including continuity equation and time-velocity integral ratio. *J Am Soc Echocardiogr* 2005;18:1399–1403.

116. Malouf JF, Ballo M, Connolly HM, et al. Doppler echocardiography of 119 normal functioning St. Jude medical mitral valve prostheses: a comprehensive assessment including

time-velocity integral ratio and prosthesis performance index. *J Am Soc Echocardiogr* 2005;18:252–256.

117. Temesvari A, Mohl W, Kupilik N. Characterization of normal leakage flow of monostrut tilting disc prosthetic mitral valves by multiplane transesophageal echocardiography. *J Am Soc Echocardiogr* 1997;10:155–158.

118. Lindower PD, Dellsperger KC, Johnson B, et al. Variability of regurgitation in Bjork-Shiley mitral valves and relationship to disc occluder design: an in vitro two-dimensional color-Doppler flow mapping study. *J Heart Valve Dis* 1996;5(Suppl. 2):S178–S183.

119. Holen J, Simonsen S, Froysaker T. An ultrasound Doppler technique for the noninvasive determination of the pressure gradient in the Bjork-Shiley mitral valve. *Circulation* 1979;9:436–442.

120. Dittrich H, Nicod P, Hoit B, et al. Evaluation of Bjork-Shiley prosthetic valves by real-time two dimensional Doppler echocardiographic flow mapping. *Am Heart J* 1988;115:133–138.

121. Panidis IP, Ren JF, Kotler MN, et al. Clinical and echocardiographic evaluation of the St. Jude cardiac valve prostheses: follow-up of 126 patients. *J Am Coll Cardiol* 1984;4:454–462.

122. Chambers J, Cross J, Deverall P, et al. Echocardiographic description of the CarboMedics bileaflet prosthetic heart valve. *J Am Coll Cardiol* 1993;21:398–405.

123. Soo CS, Ca M, Tay M, et al. Doppler echocardiographic assessment of CarboMedics prosthetic valves in the mitral position. *J Am Soc Echocardiogr* 1994;7:159–164.

124. Chakraborty B, Quek S, Pin DZ, et al. Evaluation of normal hemodynamic profile of CarboMedics prosthetic valves by Doppler echocardiography. *Angiology* 1997;48:1055–1061.

125. Bjornerheim R, Ihlen H, Simonson S, et al. Hemodynamic characterization of the CarboMedics mitral valve prosthesis. *J Heart Valve Dis* 1997;6:115–122.

126. Fawzy ME, Halim M, Ziady G, et al. Hemodynamic evaluation of porcine bioprostheses in the mitral position by Doppler echocardiography. *Am J Cardiol* 1987;59:643–646.

127. Firstenberg MS, Morehead AJ, Thomas JD, et al. Short-term hemodynamic performance of the mitral Carpentier-Edwards Perimount Pericardial Valve. *Ann Thorac Surg* 2001;71:S285–S288.

128. Takami Y, Masumoto H, Fyfe-Kirschner B. Late disruption of a Freestyle stentless bioprosthesis used for repair of sinus of Valsalva aneurysm of non-coronary cusp. *Ann Thorac Surg* 2007;83:2210–2212.

129. Baur LHB, Jin XY, Houdas Y, et al. Echocardiographic parameters of the Freestyle bioprosthesis in aortic position: the European experience. *J Am Soc Echocardiogr* 1999;12:729–735.

130. van Nooten G, Ozaki S, Herijgers P, et al. Distortion of the stentless porcine valve induces accelerated leaflet fibrosis and calcification in juvenile sheep. *J Heart Valve Dis* 1999;8:34–41.

131. Lytle BW, Cosgrove DM, Taylor PC, et al. Reoperations for valve surgery: Perioperative mortality and determinants of risk for 1,000 patients, 1958–1984. *Ann Thorac Surg* 1986;432:632–643.

132. Roberts WC, Sullivan MF. Clinical and necropsy observations early after simultaneous replacement of the mitral and aortic valves. *Am J Cardiol* 1986;58:1067–1084.

133. Schroeder RA, Mark JB. Is the valve ok or not? Immediate evaluation of a replaced aortic valve. *Anesth Analg* 2005;101:1288–1291.

134. Bird JJ, Murgo JP, Pasipoularides A. Fluid dynamics of aortic stenosis: Subvalvular gradients without subvalvular obstruction. *Circulation* 1982;66:835–840.

135. Cannegieter SC, Rosendaal FR, Briet E. Thromboembolic and bleeding complications in patients with mechanical heart valve prostheses. *Circulation* 1994;89:635–641.

136. Barbetseas J, Pistavos C, Lalos S, et al. Partial thrombosis of a bileaflet mitral prosthetic valve: diagnosis by transesophageal echocardiography. *J Am Soc Echocardiogr* 1993;6:91–93.

137. Dinarevic S, Redington A, Rigby M, et al. Left ventricular pannus causing inflow obstruction late after mitral valve replacement for endocardial fibroelastosis. *Pediatr Cardiol* 1996;17:257–259.

138. Nakatani S, Andoh M, Okita Y, et al. Prosthetic valve obstruction with normal disc motion: usefulness of transesophageal echocardiography to define cause. *J Am Soc Echocardiogr* 1999;12:537–539.

139. Barbetseas J. Differentiating thrombus from pannus formation in obstructed mechanical prosthetic valves. An evaluation of clinical, transthoracic, and TEE parameters. *J Am Coll Cardiol* 1998;32:1410–1417.

140. Van Son JA, Steinseifer U, Reul H, et al. Jamming of prosthetic heart valves by suture trapping: experimental findings. *J Thorac Cardiovasc Surg* 1989;37:288–293.

141. Waggoner AD, Perez JE, Barzilai B, et al. Left ventricular outflow obstruction resulting from insertion of mitral prostheses leaving the native leaflets intact: adverse clinical outcome in seven patients. *Am Heart J* 1991;122:483–488.

142. Shahid M, Sutherland G, Hatle L. Diagnosis of intermittent obstruction of mechanical mitral valve prostheses by Doppler echocardiography. *Am J Cardiol* 1995;76:1305–1309.

143. Jaggers J, Chetham PM, Kinnard TL, et al. Intraoperative prosthetic valve dysfunction: detection by transesophageal echocardiography. *Ann Thorac Surg* 1995;59:755–757.

144. Vesely L, Boughner D, Song T. Tissue buckling as a mechanism of bioprosthetic valve failure. *Ann Thorac Surg* 1988;46:302–308.

145. Pai GP, Ellison RG, Rubin JW, et al. Disc immobilization of Bjork-Shiley and Medtronic Hall valves during and immediately after valve replacement. *Ann Thorac Surg* 1987;44:73–76.

146. Young E, Shapiro SM, French WJ, et al. Use of transesophageal echocardiography during thrombolysis with tissue plasminogen activator of a thrombosed prosthetic mitral valve. *J Am Soc Echocardiogr* 1992;5:153–158.

147. Lee TM, Chu SH, Wang LC, et al. Thrombolysis for obstructed CarboMedics mitral valve prosthesis. *Ann Thorac Surg* 1995;59:509–511.

148. Oliver JM, Gallego P, Gonzalez A, et al. Bioprosthetic mitral valve thrombosis: clinical profile, transesophageal echocardiographic features, and follow-up after anticoagulant therapy. *J Am Soc Echocardiogr* 1996;9:691–699.

149. Gueret P, Vignon P, Fournier, et al. Transesophageal echocardiography for the diagnosis and management of nonobstructive thrombosis of mechanical mitral valve prosthesis. *Circulation* 1995;9:103–110.

150. Meloni L, Aru G, Abbruzzese PA, et al. Regurgitant flow of mitral valve prostheses: an intraoperative transesophageal

echocardiographic study. *J Am Soc Echocardiogr* 1994;7: 36–46.

151. Chen YT, Kan MN, Chen JS, et al. Detection of prosthetic mitral valve leak: a comparative study using transesophageal echocardiography, transthoracic echocardiography, and auscultation. *J Clin Ultrasound* 1990;18:557–561.

152. Yoshida K, Yoshikawa J, Akasaka T, et al. Value of acceleration flow signals proximal to the leaking orifice in assessing the severity of prosthetic mitral valve regurgitation. *J Am Coll Cardiol* 1992;19:333–338.

153. Foster GP, Isselbacher EM, Rose GA, et al. Accurate localization of mitral regurgitant defects using multiplane transesophageal echocardiography. *Ann Thorac Surg* 1998;65: 1025–1031.

154. Hixson CS, Smith MD, Mattson MD, et al. Comparison of transesophageal color flow Doppler imaging of normal mitral regurgitant jets in St. Jude Medical and Medtronic Hall cardiac prostheses. *J Am Soc Echocardiogr* 1992;5: 57–62.

155. Dhasmana JP, Blackstone EH, Kirklin JW, et al. Factors associated with periprosthetic leakage following primary mitral valve replacement with special consideration of the suture technique. *Ann Thorac Surg* 1983;35:170–178.

156. Bedderman C, Borst HG. Comparison of two suture techniques and materials: relationship to perivalvular leaks after cardiac valve replacement. *Cardiovasc Dis (Bull Tex Heart Inst)* 1978;5:354–359.

157. Mohr-Kahaly S, Kupferwasser I, Erbel R, et al. Regurgitant flow in apparently normal valve prostheses: improved detection and semiquantitative analysis by transesophageal two-dimensional color-coded Doppler echocardiography. *J Am Soc Echocardiogr* 1990;3:187–195.

158. Dellsperger KC, Wieting DW, Baehr DA, et al. Regurgitation of prosthetic heart valves: dependence on heart rate and cardiac output. *Am J Cardiol* 1983;51:321–328.

159. Flachskampf FA, Guerrero JL, O'Shea JP, et al. Patterns of normal transvalvular regurgitation in mechanical valve prostheses. *J Am Coll Cardiol* 1991;18:1493–1498.

160. Popovic Z, Barac I, Jovic M, et al. Ventricular performance following valve replacement for chronic mitral regurgitation: importance of chordal preservation. *J Cardiovasc Surg* 1999;40:183–190.

161. Agostini F, Click RL, Mulvagh SL, et al. Entrapment of subvalvular mitral tissue causing intermittent failure of a St. Jude mitral prosthesis. *J Am Soc Echocardiogr* 2000;13:1121–1123.

162. van der Graaf Y, de Waard F, van Herwerden LA, et al. Risk of strut fracture of Bjork-Shiley valves. *Lancet* 1992;339: 257–261.

163. Novaro GM, Robbins MA, Firstenberg MS, et al. Disc embolization of a Bjork-Shiley convexo-concave mitral valve: a cause of sudden cardiovascular collapse and mesenteric ischemia. *J Am Soc Echocardiogr* 2000;13:417–420.

164. Lau WC, Carroll JR, Deeb M, et al. Intraoperative transesophageal echocardiographic assessment of the effect of protamine on paraprosthetic aortic insufficiency immediately after stentless tissue aortic valve replacement. *J Am Soc Echocardiogr* 2002;15:1175–1180.

165. O'Rourke DJ, Palac RT, Malenka DJ, et al. Outcome of mild periprosthetic regurgitation detected by intraoperative transesophageal echocardiography. *J Am Coll Cardiol* 2001;38:163–166.

166. Rallidis LS, Moyssakis IE, Ikonomidis I, et al. Natural history of early aortic paraprosthetic regurgitation: a five-year follow-up. *Am Heart J* 1999;138:351–357.

167. Fernandes V, Olmos L, Nagueh SF, et al. Peak early diastolic velocity rather than pressure half-time is the best index of mechanical prosthetic mitral valve function. *Am J Cardiol* 2002;15:704–710.

168. Rahimtoola SH. The problem of valve prosthesis-patient mismatch. *Circulation* 1978;58:20–24.

169. Pibarot P, Dumesnil JG, Lemieux M, et al. Impact of prosthesis-patient mismatch on hemodynamic and symptomatic status, morbidity and mortality after aortic valve replacement with a bioprosthetic heart valve. *J Heart Valve Dis* 1998;7:211–218.

170. Pibarot P, Dumesnil JG. Prosthesis-patient mismatch. Definition, clinical impact, and prevention. *Heart* 2006;92: 1022–1029.

171. Dumesnil JG, Pibarot P. Prosthesis-ptient mismatch and clinical outcomes: the evidence continues to accumulate. *J Thorac Cardiovasc Surg* 2006;131:952–955.

172. Flameng W, Meuris B, Herijgers P, et al. Prosthesis-patient mismatch is not clinically relevant in aortic valve replacement using the Carpentier-Edwards Perimount valve. *Ann Thorac Surg* 2006;82:530–536.

173. Fuster RG, Montero JA, Albarran IR. Patient-prosthesis mismatch in aortic valve replacement: really tolerable? *Eur J Cardiothorac Surg* 2005;27:441–449.

174. Mohty-Echahidi D, Malouf JF, Girard SE, et al. Impact of prosthesis-patient mismatch on long-term survival in patients with small St. Jude Medical mechanical prostheses in the aortic position. *Circulation* 2006;113:420–426.

175. Pibarot P, Dumesnil JG, Cartier PC, et al. Patient-prosthesis mismatch can be predicted at the time of operation. *Ann Thorac Surg* 2001;71:S265–S268.

176. Bonow RO, Carabello B, de Leon AC Jr, et al. Guidelines for the menegement of patients with valvular heart disease: executive summary: a report of the American College of Cardiology/American Heart Association Task Force on Practice Guidelines (Committee on management of patients with valvular heart disease). *Circulation* 1998;98:1949–1984.

177. Rahimtoola SH. Is severe valve prosthesis-patient mismatch (VP-PM) associated with a higher mortality? *Eur J Cardiothorac Surg* 2006;31:1.

178. Mascherbauer J, Rosenhek R, Fuchs C, et al. Moderate patient-prosthesis mismatch after valve replacement for severe aortic stenosis has no impact on short- and long-term mortality. *Heart Online* 2008; http://heart.bmj.com/cgi/content/full/ hrt.2008.142596v1.

179. Bleiziffer S, Eichinger WB, Hettich I, et al. Impact of patient-prosthesis mismatch on exercise capacity in patients after bioprosthetic aortic valve replacement. *Heart* 2008;94:637–641.

180. Koch CG, Khandwala F, Estafanous FG, et al. Impact of prosthesis-patient size on functional recovery after aortic valve replacement. *Circulation* 2005;n:3221–3229.

181. Taggart DP. Prosthesis patient mismatch in aortic valve replacement: possible but pertinent? *Eur Heart J* 2006;27: 644–646.

182. Ruel M, Al-Faleh H, Kulik A, et al. Prosthesis-patient mismatch after aortic valve replacement predominantly affects patients with preexisting left ventricular dysfunction: effect on survival, freedom from heart failure, and left ventricular

mass regression. *J Thorac Cardiovasc Surg* 2006;131: 1036–1044.

183. Blais C, Dumesnil JG, Baillot R, et al. Impact of valve prosthesis-patient mismatch on short-term mortality after aortic valve replacement. *Circulation* 2003;108:e9014–e9015.

184. Bottio T, Caprili L, Casarotto D, et al. Small aortic annulus: the hydrodynamic performances of 5 commercially available bileaflet mechanical valves. *J Thorac Cardiovasc Surg* 2004;128:457–462.

185. Fuster RG, Estevez V, Rodriguez I, et al. Prosthesis patient mismatch with latest generation supra-annular prostheses. The beginning of the end? *Interact CardioVasc Thorac Surg* 2007;6:464–469.

186. Botzenhardt F, Eichinger WB, Bleiziffer S, et al. Hemodynamic comparison of bioprostheses for complete supra-annular position in patients with small aortic annulus. *J Am Coll Cardiol* 2005;45:2054–2060.

187. Badano LP, Pavoni D, Musumeci S, et al. Stented bioprosthetic valve hemodynamics: is the supra-annular implant better than the intra-annular? *J Heart Valve Dis* 2006;15: 238–246.

188. Lopez S, Mathieu P, Pibarot P, et al. Does the use of stentless aortic valves in a subcoronary position prevent patient-prosthesis mismatch for small aortic annulus? *J Card Surg* 2008;23:331–335.

189. Albert A, Florath I, Rosendahl U, et al. Effect of surgeon on transprosthetic gradients after aortic valve replacement with Freestyle stentless bioprosthesis and its consequences: a follow-up study in 587 patients. *J Cardiothorac Surg* 2007;2:40.

190. Pibarot P, Dumesnil JG. Hemodynamic and clinical impact of prosthesis-patient mismatch in the aortic valve position and its prevention. *J Am Coll Cardiol* 2000;36:1131–1141.

191. Dumesnil JG, Yoganathan AP. Valve prosthesis hemodynamics and the problem of high transprosthetic pressure gradients. *Eur J Cardiothorac Surg* 1992;6:S34–S38.

192. Reisner SA, Lichtenberg GS, Shapiro JR, et al. Exercise Doppler echocardiography in patients with mitral prosthetic valves. *Am Heart J* 1989;118:755–759.

193. Li M, Dumesnil JG, Mathieu P, et al. Impact of valve prosthesis-patient mismatch on pulmonary arterial pressure after mitral valve replacement. *J Am Coll Cardiol* 2005;45:1034–1040.

194. Crawford FA Jr. Residual pulmonary artery hypertension after mitral valve replacement: size matters! *J Am Coll Cardiol* 2005;45:1041–1042.

195. Magne J, Mathieu P, Dumesnil JG, et al. Impact of prosthesis-patient mismatch on survival after mitral valve replacement. *Circulation* 2007;115:1417–1425.

196. Bolman RM III. Survival after mitral valve replacement: does the valve type and/or size make a difference? *Circulation* 2007;115:1336–1338.

197. Kuehnel RU, Puchner R, Pohl A, et al. Characteristic resistance curves of aortic valve substitutes facilitate individualized decision for a particular type. *Eur J Cardiothorac Surg* 2005;27:450–455.

198. Moon MR, Pasque MK, Munfakh NA, et al. Prosthesis-patient mismatch after aortic valve replacement: impact of age and body size on late survival. *Ann Thorac Surg* 2006;81:481–488.

199. Horstkotte D, Piper C, Niehues R, et al. Late prosthetic valve endocarditis. *Eur Heart J* 1995;16(Suppl. B):39–47.

200. Agnihotri AK, McGiffin DC, Galbraith AJ, et al. The prevalence of infective endocarditis after aortic valve replacement. *J Thorac Cardiovasc Surg* 1995;110:1708–1720.

201. Blumberg EA, Karalis DA, Chandrasekaran K, et al. Endocarditis-associated paravalvular abscesses. Do clinical parameters predict the presence of abscess? *Chest* 1995;107: 898–903.

202. Grover FL, Cohen DJ, Oprian C, et al. Determinants of occurrence and survival from prosthetic valve endocarditis. Experience of the Veterans Affairs Cooperative Study on Valvular Heart Disease. *J Thorac Cardiovasc Surg* 1994;108:207–214.

203. Karchmer AW, Dismukes WE, Buckley MJ, et al. Late prosthetic valve endocarditis: clinical features influencing therapy. *Am J Med* 1978;64:199–206.

204. Calderwood SB, Swinski LA, Karchmer AW, et al. Prosthetic valve endocarditis: analysis of factors affecting outcome of therapy. *J Thorac Cardiovasc Surg* 1986;92:776–783.

205. Parker FB Jr, Greiner-Hayes C, Tomar RH, et al. Bacteremia following prosthetic valve replacement. *Ann Surg* 1983;197:147–151.

206. Rutledge R, Kim J, Applebaum RE. Actuarial analysis of the risk of prosthetic valve endocarditis in 1,598 patients with mechanical and bioprosthetic valves. *Arch Surg* 1985;120: 469–472.

207. Lytle BW. Surgical treatment of prosthetic valve endocarditis. *Semin Thorac Cardiovasc Surg* 1995;7:13–19.

208. Mugge A, Daniel WG, Frank G, et al. Echocardiography in infective endocarditis: reassessment of prognostic implications of vegetation size determined by transthoracic and transesophageal approach. *J Am Coll Cardiol* 1989;14: 631–638.

209. Shively BK, Gurule FT, Rolden CA, et al. Diagnostic value of transesophageal compared with transthoracic echocardiography in infective endocarditis. *J Am Coll Cardiol* 1991;18: 391–397.

210. Stoddard MF, Dawkins PR, Longaker RA. Mobile strands are frequently attached to the St. Jude Medical mitral valve prosthesis as assessed by two-dimensional transesophageal echocardiography. *Am Heart J* 1992;124:671–674.

211. Anderson DJ, Bulkley BH, Hutchins GM. A clinicopathologic study of prosthetic valve endocarditis. *Am Heart J* 1977;94:325–332.

212. Narins CR, Eichelberger JP. The development of valvular strands during thrombolytic therapy detected by transesophageal echocardiography. *J Am Soc Echocardiogr* 1996;9: 888–890.

213. Isada LR, Torelli JN, Stewart WJ, et al. Detection of fibrous strands on prosthetic mitral valves by transesophageal echocardiography: another potential embolic source. *J Am Soc Echocardiogr* 1994;7:641–645.

214. Rozich JD, Edwards WD, Hanna RD, et al. Mechanical prosthetic valve-associated strands: pathologic correlates to transesophageal echocardiography. *J Am Soc Echocardiogr* 2003;16:97–100.

215. Ionescu AA, Newman GR, Butchart EG, et al. Morphologic analysis of a strand recovered from a prosthetic mitral valve: no evidence of fibrin. *J Am Soc Echocardiogr* 1999;641–651.

216. Cohn LH. Thromboembolism after mitral valve replacement. Recent progress. In: Duran CMG, Angell W, Johnson A, et al., eds. *Mitral Valve Disease*. London: Butterworth, 1984:330–339.

217. Garcia MJ, Vandervoort P, Stewart WJ, et al. Mechanisms of hemolysis with mitral prosthetic regurgitation: study using transesophageal echocardiography and fluid dynamic simulation. *J Am Coll Cardiol* 1996;27:399–406.

1. Low-profile mechanical valves
   A. have an increased mass-to-orifice ratio
   B. are bileaflet valves, such as the St. Jude and Carbomedics valves, which are less obstructive than tilting-disc valves
   C. are not MRI compatible
   D. are less durable than porcine bioprostheses
2. Stentless porcine valves (SPV), such as the Medtronic Freestyle and St. Jude SPV valves, are characterized by
   A. a smaller effective orifice area (EOA) than stented porcine bioprostheses
   B. a sewing ring with supporting struts
   C. earlier regression of left ventricular (LV) hypertrophy
   D. uniform echocardiographic appearance regardless of implantation technique
3. A prosthetic perivalvular leak
   A. originates within the sewing ring
   B. demonstrates diastolic but not systolic color flow across the defect
   C. is always caused by endocarditis
   D. is seen as a rocking motion of the prosthesis at its site of attachment
4. Transvalvular gradients obtained by Doppler are
   A. flow dependent
   B. flow independent
   C. unrelated to ventricular function
   D. unaffected by valvular regurgitation
5. The sensitivity of TEE in the detection of prosthetic valve endocarditis (PVE) is
   A. 25% to 40%
   B. 40% to 50%
   C. 60% to 75%
   D. 85% to 90%

CHAPTER 17 Assessment of Cardiac Masses

Dilip R. Thakar ■ Andrew D. Shaw ■ Juan C. Plana

Echocardiography remains the principal modality for the identification of intracardiac masses Transesophageal echocardiography (TEE) provides an unparalleled and generally unobstructed window into the heart, and, given the higher frequency and closer proximity of TEE (compared to transthoracic) probes, TEE offers superior evaluation of most normal and abnormal intracardiac structures. In general, compared to transthoracic echocardiography (TTE), TEE allows improved definition of mass size, shape, and mobility (1–9). In addition, clarification of mass location, attachment, extent, and myocardial involvement are easily accomplished with TEE (5,7,10–12). The benefit of TEE is particularly striking for the evaluation of masses in the left atrial appendage (LAA), right atrium (RA), and aorta. TEE also offers imaging advantages in those patients with technically limited TTE images (1,7,9). TEE can be performed at the patient's bedside and still provide immediate and dynamic evaluation of intracardiac mass and associated abnormalities of the valves. Magnetic resonance imaging (MRI) and computerized tomography (CT) scans provide better tissue characterization, especially when ultrasound artifacts are present (Fig. 17.1). Occasionally echo contrast enhancement is helpful to delineate the vascularity and answer the question of intracardiac mass versus extracardiac extension. Three-dimensional (3D) reconstruction from the TEE images allows dynamic presentation of views simulating intraoperative visualization of cardiac masses (Fig. 17.2) (13,14).

Cardiac surgery for intracardiac masses is recognized as a category two indication for perioperative TEE (15). Although patients may have had preoperative TTE and even TEE examinations, a complete intraoperative evaluation is paramount for complete characterization of the mass prior to surgical exploration (15–17). Likewise, rapid and accurate interpretation after the discovery of an unsuspected cardiac mass in the operating room is essential (18–20). Once a cardiac mass is confirmed, intraoperative TEE (IO-TEE) is useful for guiding the surgical approach for removal (10,21–23). In addition, placement of vascular or intracardiac cannula in the presence of cardiac masses, whether in the inferior vena cava (IVC), superior vena cava (SVC), or aorta, may be guided using TEE (17,24). Often, assessment of the hemodynamic effects of a cardiac mass with IO-TEE can prove invaluable. Lastly, IO-TEE allows immediate and real-time assessment of the surgical intervention and repair. IO-TEE permits evaluation for residual mass as well as unintentional surgical sequelae of mass removal such as ventricular septal defect, atrial septal defect (ASD), as well as valvular and myocardial function at the end of surgery (15).

The value of IO-TEE during surgery for cardiac masses was highlighted in a recent series by Dujardin et al. in 2000 (17). In this study, IO-TEE provided new prebypass

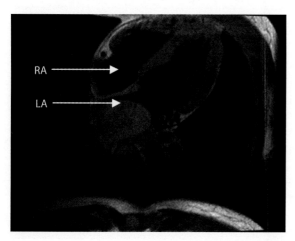

Figure 17.1. Larger mass pushing the LA wall is paraganglioma. The images generated by cardiac MRI are remarkably complete, detailed, and precise.

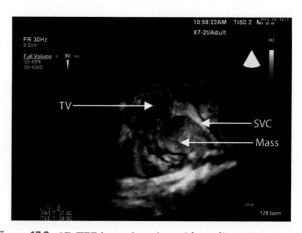

Figure 17.2. 3D TEE in conjunction with cardiac MRI can provide additional information for surgical management of cardiac masses. 3D image shows mass SVC and tricuspid valve (TV).

information in 6 of 75 (8%) patients presenting for mass removal, altering the surgical plan for all 6. Two patients had patent foramen ovale, which was closed. One patient had a second myxoma, one patient required mitral valve repair, in one patient no mass was found and surgery was cancelled, and TEE confirmed cannulation of IVC in one patient. In 10 patients, new post bypass information was found, which required return to bypass for valve repair in 3 patients, altered nonsurgical management in 3 patients, and did not change the plan in 4 patients. Thus, in 12 out of 75 (16%) patients, IO-TEE affected surgical management.

APPROACH/STRUCTURES

For TEE, the echocardiographer must possess a complete and thorough understanding of the examination technique, normal structures, anatomic variants, and both tissue and ultrasound artifacts encountered during a TEE examination since normal structures or variants can be mistaken for a pathologic finding. Detailed knowledge of these normal findings prevents unwarranted concern or delay in the operative setting to pursue further evaluation or solicit opinions regarding a structure, which is, in fact, a normal variant. Correct interpretation of normal intracardiac findings can prevent surgical evaluation or inappropriate medical therapy for these structures. Some patients referred for surgical removal of intracardiac masses have been spared operation by a thorough and knowledgeable intraoperative TEE examination. In fact, some of the structures, like in Table 17.1, have been confused with pathology at one time or another (3,8). In this chapter, the first half describes normal anatomic and embryonic variants that can easily be confused with primary mass lesion. The second half of the chapter describes specific features of the pathologic cardiac masses.

IVC/SVC/RIGHT ATRIUM

The RA and vena cava can be imaged in a midesophageal bicaval view, which displays a long axis view of the vena cava as it enters the RA cavity. In this view, the eustachian valve, crista terminalis, Chiari network, thebesian valve, and cor triatriaum dexter can be seen. These are remnants of the various portions of the embryonic right venous valve of the right horn of sinus venosus. In the development of RA, there are two portions; the auricular portion or rough RA and the sinus venosus or smooth RA. The sinus venosus is initially made up of right and left horns. The right valve of the sinus venosus separates the rough and smooth portions, in essence creating two RA chambers. With fetal development, the left horn becomes the coronary sinus and the right becomes the SVC, IVC, and remainder of the smooth RA. The right valve regresses and persists as the crista terminalis, the thebesian valve, and the

TABLE 17.1	Normal Structures that Mimic Cardiac Tumors
Eustachian valve	
Chiari network	
Lipomatous hypertrophy of interatrial septum	
RA trabeculation	
Pacemaker wire, central line, swan-genz catheter	
Thebacian valve	
Epicardial fat	
Fat deposit in tricuspid annulas	
Nodules of Arantius	
Lambl's excrescences	
Base of aortic valve en face	
Coumadin ridge	
Suture line after cardiac transplant	
Moderator band	
Mitral annular calcification	
Papillary muscle hypertrophy	
Dilated coronary and transverse sinus	
Artifact	
Hiatal hernia	

eustachian valve. The chiari network is a membrane that pathologically persists and joins these three structures. It is often fenestrated or strand-like, and rarely causes problems although it may obstruct flow or become infected. The eustachian valve can be found at the juncture of the IVC and RA. This structure projects into the RA cavity and can be mistaken for an intracardiac mass. There is wide variation in eustachian valves among patients, and, although typically thin and mobile, eustachian valves may be thick and rigid. It is the typical location of the eustachian valve that allows it to be discerned from a pathologic structure. A giant eustachian valve should be differentiated from a Cor triatriaum dexter.

One might also see a Chiari network in the RA. This structure consists of a meshwork of fibers originating at the margin of the eustachian and thebesian valves and attaching at the area of the crista terminalis. Echocardiographically, a Chiari network appears as an echogenic, long filamentous, highly mobile structure having whip-like motion within the RA (Fig. 17.3) (25–27). The anatomic variation in Chiari networks is quite wide with many patients having no visible Chiari network and others having prominent ones. Distinction of this structure from an intracardiac mass is made by its typical echocardiographic appearance and by noting that this structure is tethered at its margins although the body is mobile. Chiari remnants are seldom clinically important but have

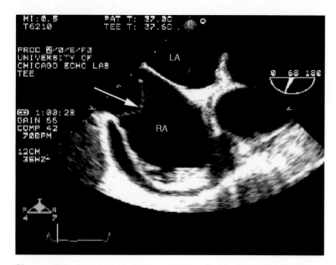

Figure 17.3. This linear RA is a Chiari network, which is a normal variant. LA, left atrium.

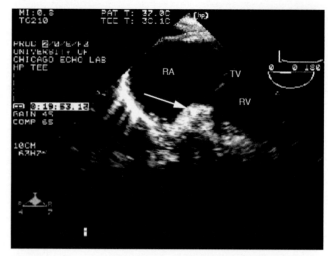

Figure 17.4. A view of the right atrium (RA), tricuspid value (TV), and right ventricle (RV), showing a prominent tricuspid annulus (*arrow*), which can be confused with an intracardiac mass.

been reported as sources of entrapment for emboli and right heart catheters (28,29).

Within the body of the RA itself, several structures are noteworthy for potential confusion with pathologic masses. The RA wall is trabeculated with pectinate muscles that must be recognized as normal variants. Pectinate muscles are distinguished by their perpendicular alignment from the RA wall and their regular spacing from one another. When the SVC is viewed in long axis, there is a prominent ridge at the juncture of the SVC and the RA, the crista terminalis. There is somewhat wide anatomic variation in this ridge, and it may appear quite prominent in some patients. Its location adjacent to the right atrial appendage (RAA) can sometimes be confused with a RAA thrombus. Crista terminalis is an important anatomical structure, shown to be the site of RA tachyarrhythmias, and frequently referred to as "crystal tachycardia".

In the process of a loculated pericardial effusion behind the RA, the RA wall may appear to be an intracardiac linear density. This abnormality can be readily discerned with the intravenous injection of agitated saline, which easily delineates the RA cavity. The tricuspid annulus may accumulate fat and become prominent. Particularly when imaged off-axis, this may appear to represent an intracardiac mass between the RA and RV. Imaging in multiple planes might help delineate the smooth continuity of this fatty accumulation with the rest of the cardiac structures, preventing an incorrect diagnosis of intracardiac tumor (Fig. 17.4).

Two normal anatomic variants (lipomatous hypertrophy, interartrial septal aneurysm) of the interatrial septum can also be confused with intracardiac masses. Pathologically, lipomatous hypertrophy represents a benign proliferation in which mature adipocytes infiltrate the interatrial septum. This fatty involvement is more prominent at the cephalad and caudal ends sparing the fossa ovalis, giving the interatrial septum a dumb-

bell–shaped appearance (Fig. 17.5). Fatty infiltration of the interatrial septum is denoted not only by its typical pattern of involvement but also by the hyperrefractile nature of the fatty deposits that may cast a prominent acoustic shadow. Although this disorder represents a spectrum of interatrial septal thickening, diagnostic thickness criteria of 1.5 to 2.0 cm have been proposed (30–33). At the other end of the spectrum, lipomatous hypertrophy can reach massive proportions and infiltrations several centimeters in diameter have been reported (34,35).

An interatrial septal aneurysm, which has a prevalence of between 2% and 10%, is another anatomic variant that can mimic an intracardiac mass (36–38). The definitions of redundant septum and aneurysmal septum are somewhat arbitrary. Published criteria define an interatrial septal aneurysm as a redundancy of at least 1.5 cm of the septum, with a displacement past the

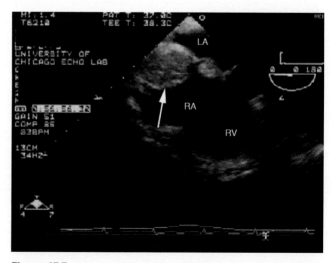

Figure 17.5. Interatrial septum with lipomatous hypertrophy (*arrow*). Note the sparing of the fossa ovalis.

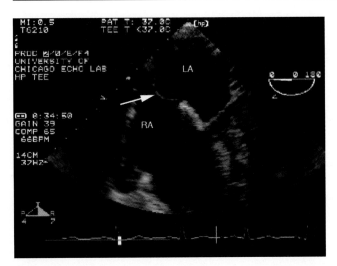

Figure 17.6. Midesophageal four-chamber view, demonstrating an interatrial septal aneurysm (*arrow*).

midline of at least 1 cm (36,39). In some patients, the redundancy of the interatrial septum is prominent with excursions of several centimeters into the left atrium (LA) or RA depending on interatrial pressures (Fig. 17.6). When imaging off-axis, the aneurysmal portion of the septum may protrude into and out of plane giving the appearance of a mobile interatrial mass. This may present during intraoperative TEE as an unexpected mass, despite a preoperative transthoracic echocardiogram, because of TEE's superior rate of detection for this lesion (37,39). In some patients, an interatrial septal aneurysm might be associated with a patent foramen ovale, ASD, and systemic embolization.

RIGHT VENTRICLE/PULMONARY ARTERY

There are several normal structures within the right ventricle (RV) and RV outflow track that can be confused with pathologic intracardiac masses. Within the RV chamber itself, the primary structures to beware of are the ventricular trabeculations. The RV is a heavily trabeculated chamber and in the setting of RV pressure overload, these trabeculations may become quite prominent. Even in the normal RV, there is a prominent muscular band, the moderator band, which is a normal finding. Catheters and pacemaker leads within the RV must be discerned from intracardiac masses. Although this would seem straightforward, because catheters are curvilinear structures being interrogated with a flat imaging plane, only small portions of the catheter may be visualized at any one time. This may give the appearance of small mobile intracardiac echodensities. In addition, because catheters are echodense, they are prone to forming reverberation and side lobe artifacts, which must not be mistaken for pathologic structures.

The presence of the ultrasound clutter in the pulmonary artery should not be mistaken for an intraluminal mass. The main pulmonary artery (MPA) is typically imaged in the midesophageal RV inflow-outflow view. This puts the PA in the far field where, because of ultrasound beam spreading, there is often prominent clutter. With adjustment of the ultrasound imaging controls, such as gain and focus, as well as manipulating the probe itself, this clutter artifact can usually be "cleaned up." Clutter artifact is also prominent in near field. When the right pulmonary artery (RPA) is being imaged from the midesophageal ascending aortic short-axis view, it often projects prominent clutter. Again, adjusting focus and gain can minimize this artifact and avoid the false interpretation of an RPA thrombus.

PULMONARY VEINS/LEFT ATRIUM/LEFT ATRIAL APPENDAGE

A normal structure that can be confused with an intracardiac mass in the LA is the fold of tissue between the left upper pulmonary vein and the LA itself. This ridge has anatomic variation and may be prominent. In addition, though this ridge is typically linear, the end of the ridge may appear somewhat bulbus giving it a "Q-tip" appearance, also called a "coumadin" ridge. This structure has also been confused with an LA or LAA thrombus. Another structure that can lead to the erroneous diagnosis of an LAA mass is the transverse sinus. When there is fluid in this pericardial reflection, it may appear to be continuous with the LAA cavity. The LAA wall may then appear to be a linear mass. In addition, this structure often has echodense fibrinous material in it that can be confused with an LAA thrombus.

The LAA is a structure that commonly has echocardiographic features suggesting an intracardiac mass. The LAA has pectinate muscles that may simulate LAA thrombus. Pectinate muscles typically have a tissue characterization more similar to muscle than thrombus. In addition, the pectinate muscles typically emanate perpendicularly from the LAA wall and appear multiple in a somewhat regularly spaced pattern. A multiplane approach to the evaluation of LAA is essential. The LAA often has multiple lobes (40), and the tissue separating these infoldings may be confused with thrombus.

Another phenomenon, although not truly a normal anatomic finding, is LA spontaneous echo contrast or "smoke," which sometimes is confused as an intra-atrial mass. Spontaneous echo contrast in the LA chamber is noted by its echodense swirling pattern. Presence of SEC in the LAA, particularly in situations of low appendage flow such as mitral stenosis, atrial fibrillation and severe heart failure is a common echo finding. Dense spontaneous echo contrast can be very difficult to discern from intra-appendage thrombus (Fig. 17.7). Multiplane analysis to confirm the presence of a thrombus can be helpful to prevent misinterpretations.

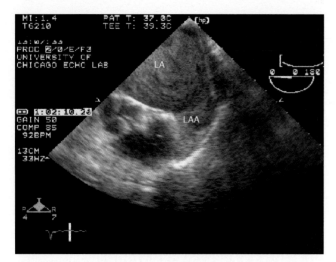

Figure 17.7. Spontaneous echo contrast in a patient with severe mitral stenosis. Though the LAA appears to have a thrombus, this actually represents dense spontaneous echo contrast.

LEFT VENTRICLE

Several normal structures within the left ventricular (LV) cavity, when imaged along tangential planes, can lead to the false diagnosis of an intracardiac mass. The LV papillary muscles are usually easily discerned from pathologic masses by their location and attachments to the submitral apparatus, as well as having a tissue characterization that is similar to that of the myocardium. When imaging from a midesophageal four-chamber view, the base of the interventricular septum may appear prominent, suggesting an intramyocardial mass. However, far more common is the presence of sigmoid septum. This is a normal variant of aging, in which remodeling of the LV cavity projects the basilar interventricular septum into the LV outflow tract.

The LV cavity can also have thick, fibrous, band-like, highly refractile structures, which cross the chamber, particularly near the LV apex. These false tendons pass between papillary muscle, septum, and free wall of the LV. They are common normal anatomic variants. Lastly, the LV apex is often foreshortened and difficult to completely image from a midesophageal four-chamber view. This foreshortening can give the appearance that the apex contains thrombus material, thus leading to the erroneous conclusion of an LV apical thrombus. When evaluating the LV apex using TEE, care must be taken to retroflex the probe to fully visualize the LV cavity. Additional imaging from the transgastric long-axis and inverted four-chamber views may be helpful.

AORTA/VALVES

False positive masses in the thoracic aorta result primarily from linear beam width, side lobe, and reverberation ultrasound artifacts. The aorta is in the near field when imaging from the esophagus and near-field clutter is common, so it must be distinguished from intra-aortic thrombus or atheroma. The mechanism of these artifacts has been elucidated, and distinction from true pathology is often possible (41). Certain valvular structures can be confused with mass lesions as well, including the nodules of Arantius and thread-like Lambl's excrescence, which are commonly found on the aortic valve in patients older then 60 years. A large vegetation on the valve can be confused with mass. Vegetations are usually echodense, highly mobile, and attached to the atrial side of the mitral valve and the ventricular side of the aortic valve. Associated findings may include destruction of valve leaflet or abscess.

PATHOLOGY

Most pathologic cardiac masses represent thrombus, infection, or tumor. A TEE examination cannot definitively diagnose an intracardiac mass as this requires histologic confirmation. However, a reasonably accurate diagnosis can usually be made by incorporating the echocardiographic location and appearance of the mass with available clinical data. In addition, there may be associated echocardiographic findings that substantially alter the differential diagnostic choices for an intracardiac mass.

Cardiac involvement by malignancy may be primary (origin within the heart) or secondary/metastatic (Fig. 17.8). Metastatic neoplasms are far more common than are primary tumors by a 20–30:1 ratio (42–44). Although most secondary involvement of the heart by malignancy is pericardial (~75%), this chapter focuses on the myocardial and intracardiac involvement because these structures will present as cardiac masses.

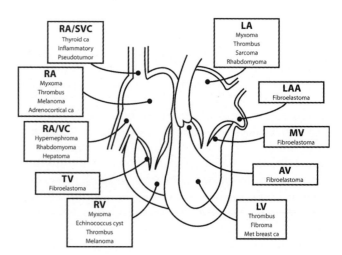

Figure 17.8. Diagram illustrating the distribution and pathologic characteristics of the masses according to intracardiac location site. (*J Am Soc Echocardiography* 2000;13:1080–1083.)

For metastatic involvement of the heart, the most common tumors are lung, breast, melanoma, and lymphoma followed by esophageal and uterine (42–44). Cardiac involvement may occur from direct invasion or hematogenous metastatic spread from distant disease. Certain tumors, such as melanoma, have a predilection for metastasizing to the heart. IO-TEE evaluation of metastatic disease of the heart is not simply an imaging exercise. Patients with metastatic tumors of the heart who have made it to the operating room may be there for attempt at surgical cure. In this case, careful TEE evaluation of tumor extent and myocardial infiltration is crucial. If intraoperative and preoperative tumor staging differ, the surgical approach may be aborted or altered (45). In addition, patients may be undergoing palliative surgery to relieve the hemodynamic effects of tumor involvement (e.g., intracardiac obstruction). Intraoperative evaluation of hemodynamic improvement after tumor resection is vital to operative success. For example, 5-year survival after successful removal of intracardiac extension of renal cell cancer is about 80%.

Primary cardiac tumors are less commonly found with an incidence of 0.1% to 0.3% in autopsy series (42,44,46). Most tumors (75%–80%) are benign; more than one half of these are myxomas in adults. The most common benign cardiac tumors in young patients include rhabdomyoma, fibroma, papilloma, hemangioma, and familial myxoma. Primary malignant cardiac tumors are almost exclusively sarcoma (>95%) (47–49), and of the sarcomas, angiosarcoma and rhabdomyosarcoma are the most common (50). Tumors which are suitable for primary resection can be evaluated with IO-TEE to guide surgical resection.

Cardiac involvement by tumors may be asymptomatic or cause significant morbidity, such as pericardial tamponade, arrhythmias, or congestive heart failure. The lack of malignant potential does not always indicate a "benign" clinical course because nonmalignant intracavitary tumors may produce obstruction to blood flow or partially dislodge, thus causing embolization.

IVC/SVC/RIGHT ATRIUM

The most common intracardiac mass in the vena cava and RA is a thrombus. RA thrombi occur in several settings. Thrombi from the deep venous system may embolize and become entrapped in the RA (51). This clinical scenario probably happens far more frequently than detected, as most thromboemboli rapidly pass through the RA. Thromboemboli originally from peripheral veins appear as mobile serpiginous irregular masses in the RA that do not have a point of attachment to the RA wall. These thrombi may become entrapped in the foramen ovale, which is a potential mechanism for paradoxical embolization (1,52).

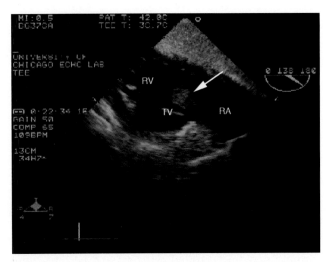

Figure 17.9. Transgastric long-axis view of the TV, showing a large RA thrombus (*arrow*) prolapsing through the TV.

Another cause of RA thrombus is in situ formation, which occurs in conditions with low atrial blood flow, such as atrial fibrillation or RA dilatation in cardiomyopathic states. In situ thrombi typically are homogenous echodensities adherent to the RA wall with a broad base of attachment. Although RA thrombi have been reported along the interatrial septum, this presentation is unusual. RA thrombi commonly have mobile irregularities extending from their surface. These projections may be large enough to prolapse into the RV cavity during diastole (Fig. 17.9).

RA thrombi associated with atrial fibrillation typically form on the RA free wall or within the RAA (Fig. 17.10). In patients with atrial fibrillation, approximately 15% of cardiac thrombi are located within the RAA. RAA thrombi are best visualized in a midesophageal bicaval view. Careful movement of the probe into and out of the esophagus is required to interrogate the entire body of the RAA.

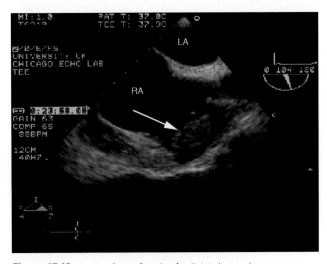

Figure 17.10. Large thrombus in the RAA (*arrow*).

A special case of in situ RA thrombus formation is that associated with intracardiac catheters. SVC catheters, particularly hemodialysis catheters that are stiff and have higher flows, may lead to endocardial damage that serves as a nidus for mural thrombus formation. Given the orientation of the vena cava and RA, SVC catheter-associated thrombi most commonly form near the IVC-RA, often on or near the eustachian valve (Fig. 17.11). RA thrombi in this location and others, associated with patients who have chronic renal failure, are typically less homogenous and partially calcified.

Lastly, RA thrombi may form around a foreign body, such as catheter or electrode (Fig. 17.12). Small mobile echodensities are commonly associated with functioning catheters in asymptomatic patients. More substantial thrombi may form around catheters and become quite large. A catheter-associated thrombus may involve and extend into the SVC, leading to partial obstruction. Differentiation of an atrial thrombus from other RA masses is done by noting the typical location of thrombi and the presence of associated thrombogenic conditions. Additionally, thrombi may appear laminated and partially calcified.

RA masses may also represent primary cardiac tumors. Of these, the most common is a myxoma. When myxoma appears at an atypical site, multiple or recurrent, there is a high probability of familial myxoma syndrome (Carneys' complex). The familial form may be characterized by associated findings such as breast adenoma, pituitary adenoma, skin pigmentation, skin myxoma, and neurofibroma. Myxoma typically have well-defined borders and possess somewhat globular (grape-like) shape with heterogeneous tissue characterization (Fig. 17.13). RA myxomas represent 20% to 25% of all cardiac myxomas (42,53,54). Like LA tumors, RA myxomas usually are mobile,

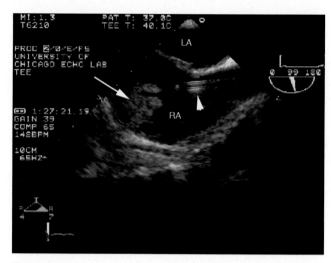

Figure 17.12. Bicaval view of the RA with a catheter (*arrowhead*) in the SVC protruding into the RA cavity. There is a large thrombus (*arrow*) in the RA formed around the catheter.

pedunculated, and echodense masses. If large enough, they may obstruct the tricuspid orifice in diastole, producing a tumor "plop," which can be clinically misdiagnosed as mitral stenosis (Fig. 17.14). RA myxomas can be imaged from the midesophageal four-chamber and bicaval views as well as the transgastric RV inflow view. Complete TEE assessment of RA myxomas includes evaluation of tumor attachment, size, and mobility as well as tricuspid valve function (55).

Other primary benign tumors of the heart infrequently involve the RA. Of the primary malignant cardiac tumors, angiosarcoma is the most common (Fig. 17.15) (56). This tumor originates in the RA in 80% of cases and presents as a large mural mass that frequently extends into the pericardium and vena cava. Usual echo findings are thickening of atrial wall. Pericardial

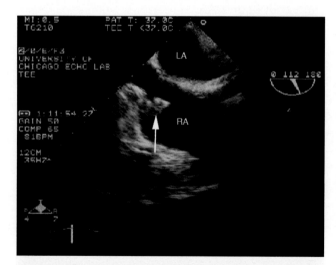

Figure 17.11. Bicaval view of the RA, demonstrating a mural thrombus (*arrow*) at the junction of the IVC. The location of this thrombus is typical for patients with dialysis catheters in the SVC, which causes endothelial injury of the RA wall.

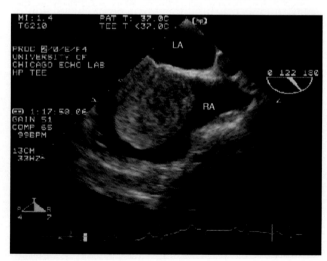

Figure 17.13. Large RA myxoma. The characteristic shape and attachment of this mass to the interatrial septum in the area of the fossa ovalis make a myxoma very high on the differential.

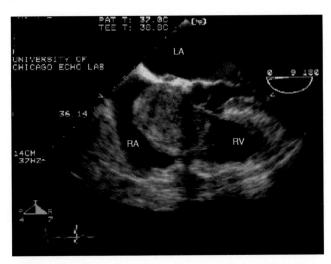

Figure 17.14. Large RA myxoma prolapsing into the TV. Transesophageal evaluation of the hemodynamic effects of this mass would be essential.

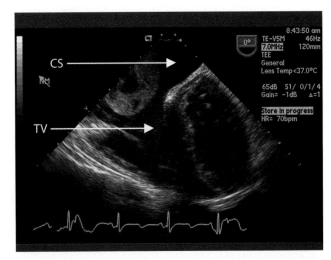

Figure 17.16. Midesophageal four-chamber view demonstrating a renal cell carcinoma extending up to RA. CS, coronary sinus.

effusion or tamponade is due to hemopericardium (47–49,56,57).

RA masses may also represent secondary involvement of the RA by malignancy. This may happen through intravascular extension or extracardiac invasion of the RA. Tumor extension along the IVC into the RA is a common form of secondary cardiac involvement in certain malignancies, such as renal cell carcinoma, Wilms' tumor, hepatoma, and uterine leiomyomatosis (10,58–63). These tumors appear as elongated mobile masses protruding into the RA cavity from the IVC. These tumors may become quite large, occupying most of the RA cavity causing tricuspid valve obstruction (64). Mobile tumor components may prolapse across the tricuspid valve into the RV cavity.

IO-TEE may be useful during resection of these IVC and RA tumors (Fig. 17.16). Using the midesophageal bicaval view, the distal IVC and RA chamber can be well visualized. By advancing the probe in this view, more proximal aspects of the IVC and hepatic vein (HV) may be visualized (Fig. 17.17). The intraoperative examination should define the cephalic extent of the tumor, extent of caval occlusion, its relation with the HV, and the mobility of the tumor, all of which help plan a surgical strategy (Fig. 17.18) (61–63,65). During resection, IO-TEE allows monitoring for embolization as well as positioning of cannula (10,45,50,66–70). Once resection is complete, IO-TEE is essential to look for residual tumor and IVC patency.

Direct invasion of the RA and great venous vessels is also possible. Usually this occurs from breast, lung, and esophageal cancers. Invasion of the RA or vena cava from extracardiac tumors is noted echocardiographically by careful inspection of the wall. Finding continuity between an intra-atrial and an extracardiac mass, which are similar in tissue characterization, is highly suggestive of tumor invasion.

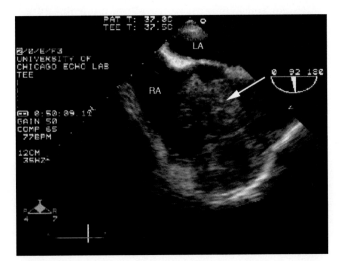

Figure 17.15. Although the location of this mass (*arrow*) in the RAA protruding into the RA cavity would suggest thrombus, this in fact, was pathologically shown to be an angiosarcoma.

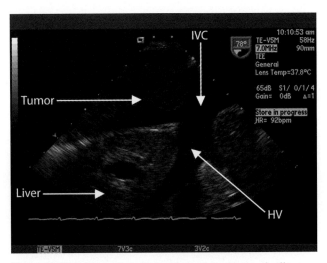

Figure 17.17. Midesophageal view demonstrating renal cell tumor extension in the IVC. HV is an important surgical landmark.

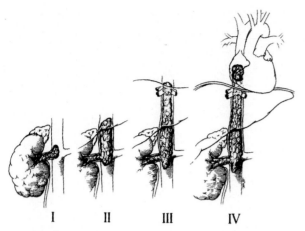

Figure 17.18. Classification system depicting the level of IVC involvement by tumor thrombus. (*Ann Thoracic Surg* 1997;63: 1592–1600.)

RIGHT VENTRICLE/PULMONARY ARTERY

The RV and PA are relatively uncommon sites for intracardiac masses, although in situ RV thrombi may occur in pulmonary hypertension, RV infarction, and RV contusion. This should be differentiated from carcinoid heart disease, which in a typical case is characterized by plaque-like fibrous thickening of endocardium that causes retraction and fixation of the tricuspid and pulmonary valve leaflets. Tricuspid regurgitation and pulmonic stenosis are the usual echocardiographic findings. Identification of RV thrombus can be challenging in the heavily trabeculated RV. Thrombi are most likely to form in situations of low flow states or in the presence of RV regional wall motion abnormalities. RV thrombi are most likely to be located in the apex and have ultrasound characteristics distinctly different from the myocardium (Fig. 17.19). The RV apex should be viewed from both the midesophageal four-chamber and transgastric RV inflow views to confirm the presence of a RV thrombus.

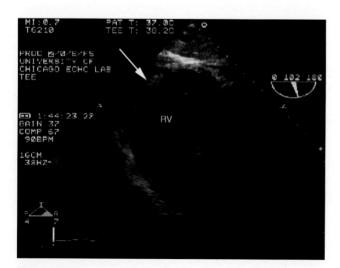

Figure 17.19. Transgastric long axis of the TV showing a large apical RV thrombus (*arrow*).

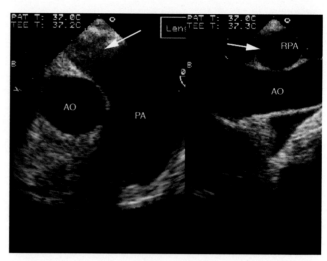

Figure 17.20. The first panel shows the short axis of the ascending thoracic aorta (AO) with pulmonary artery (PA) bifurcation. The RPA has an intraluminal mass consistent with thrombus (*arrow*). The second panel shows the ascending aorta in long axis with a cross section of the RPA demonstrating thrombus.

Thrombi in the PA are exclusively the result of emboli from the deep venous system and can be visualized using TEE (71–74). Evaluation of the PA and pulmonary branches is critical in hemodynamically unstable patients, as the specificity of a PA thrombus detected with TEE is very high (Fig. 17.20) (72,75–77). In addition, IO-TEE to detect residual emboli during pulmonary embolectomy is beneficial. IO-TEE may document residual thrombus in up to 30% of embolectomy procedures (15). The MPA can be visualized using the midesophageal RV inflow-outflow and ascending aortic short-axis views. The proximal left pulmonary artery (LPA) and initial 4 to 6 cm of the RPA can be visualized from the midesophageal ascending aortic short- and long-axis views.

Benign and malignant primary tumors of the RV are uncommon, but nearly all types, including myxoma, rhabdomyoma, fibroma, and rhabdomyosarcoma, have been noted (47–49,78). Like other cardiac chambers, direct invasion of the RV from extracardiac tumor can result in myocardial replacement and intracardiac extension of tumor (Fig. 17.21).

Although involvement of the PA by lung carcinoma is infrequent, this typically involves external compression rather than presenting as an intracardiac mass (79). Inspection of the PA for hemodynamically significant compression using IO-TEE in lung cancer patients is pertinent. Tumor may also involve the PA via embolization. Intracardiac RA tumors may partially dislodge spontaneously or during surgical manipulation (70). These tumor emboli may become entrapped in the proximal pulmonary arterial tree and be visualized using TEE as heterogeneous, irregular intraluminal masses (69,80).

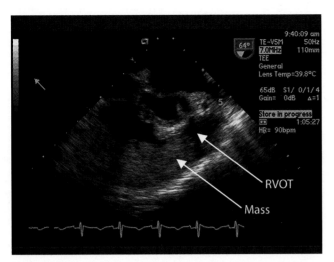

Figure 17.21. Involvement of RV by metastatic lymphoma mass is occupying almost 70% of RV outflow tract (RVOT).

PULMONARY VEINS/LEFT ATRIUM/LEFT ATRIAL APPENDAGE

The majority of intracardiac masses in the LA are cardiac thrombi, and although LA thrombi can be located in any portion of this chamber (Figs. 17.22 and 17.23), the vast majority are located in the LAA. Complete visualization of the LAA requires careful multiplane interrogation as the LAA often demonstrates complex multilobed structures (81). LA thrombi have a tissue characterization that differs from the surrounding cardiac structures. LA clots often appear laminated and have irregular or lobulated borders. Although the base of attachment to the LA wall is broad, LA thrombi may be mobile or have mobile projections. Rarely, thrombi may detach from the LA wall after they become so large that they cannot escape the LA cavity and become free floating (82).

In addition to echocardiographic appearance and location, the clinical setting influences differentiation of thrombus from other LA masses. In patients with risk factors for atrial stasis, such as atrial fibrillation, mitral

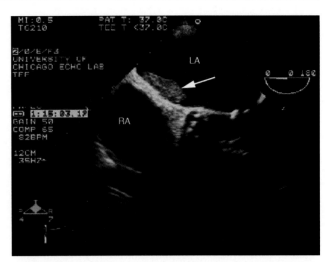

Figure 17.23. Atypical LA thrombus (*arrow*) located on the interatrial septum. Because of the location of this mass, it would be difficult to distinguish from a myxoma with certainty.

stenosis, or LV dysfunction, thrombus should be high on the differential list of a LA mass. This is especially true when there is TEE evidence of atrial stasis, such as spontaneous echo contrast. Using IO-TEE in patients with atrial fibrillation, one may expect to find a thrombus in 5% to 15% of cases (83,84). Although initially thought to be uncommon in atrial flutter, LA thrombi are also present in that disorder (85). TEE is both highly sensitive and specific for thrombus detection in the LA and LAA (86–88).

The most common primary cardiac tumor in adult is an atrial myxoma, which occurs 75% to 80% of the time in the LA (42,53,54,89). LA myxomas characteristically appear as rounded or oval structures. Although they may appear fairly smooth, close inspection often reveals multiple villous grape-like projections (Fig. 17.24). Most LA myxomas (~90%) arise from the interatrial septum, though they may arise from nearly any location in the atrium, including the appendage (Fig. 17.25) (90). Myxomas are typically attached to the atrial septum via a stalk that arises from or near the fossa ovalis. However, the presence of a stalk is not essential for the diagnosis, because up to 10%

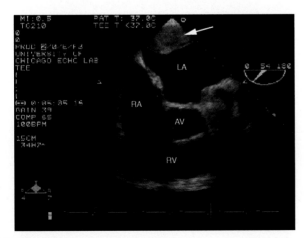

Figure 17.22. Short-axis view of the aortic valve (AV). A large mural thrombus (*arrow*) can be noted in the LA chamber.

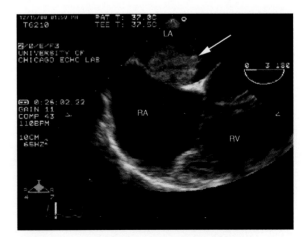

Figure 17.24. LA myxoma (*arrow*) attached to the interatrial septum. Note the projections from the main body of the myxoma.

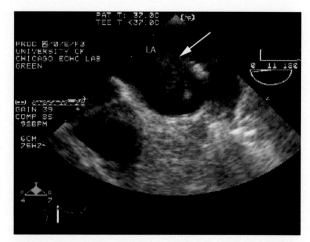

Figure 17.25. Atypical LA myxoma attached near the mouth of the LAA (*arrow*).

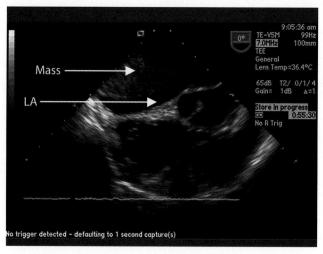

Figure 17.27. Extracardiac paraganglioma invading the LA wall.

of myxomas may be sessile (91). Pedunculated myxomas with long stalks may be quite mobile and move toward the mitral valve during diastole and back into the LA chamber in systole. A very large myxoma can, in fact, occupy most of the LA volume and interfere with LV inflow.

Atrial myxomas are typically distinguished from other LA masses by their characteristic shape and appearance, as well as their site of origin. However, final diagnosis requires histologic confirmation. Intraoperatively, the TEE operator must confirm the presence of a myxoma and identify the extent of involvement of the interatrial septum. Careful inspection of the remaining atrium and contralateral atrium is essential as these tumors may occasionally be multiple or biatrial. IO-TEE is also used to identify mitral valve dysfunction (both obstruction and regurgitation) resulting from the myxoma. Evaluation of the integrity of the mitral valve and interatrial septum after resection prior to leaving the operating room is also important. Recently, 3D TEE has allowed superior visualization of the size and attachment, as well as mitral involvement of LA myxomas (13,14).

Other primary cardiac tumors such as sarcoma are unusual within the LA, but they have been reported on

occasion (92). Secondary involvement of the LA by cardiac tumors occurs in two manners. The first is by invasion of the LA from extracardiac extension of a tumor, most commonly from breast, lung, or esophageal cancer (Fig. 17.26). Lung carcinomas may also invade the LA hematogenously through one of the pulmonary veins (93,94). A homogeneous mass filling a pulmonary vein and entering the LA should be considered highly suspicious for bronchogenic carcinoma. Malignant tumors of the LA have proven to be problematic due to their posterior location and difficulty of surgical exposure. The technique of autotransplantation is the surgical procedure of choice, and preoperative TEE and MRI are extremely valuable diagnostic tools for planning the surgical technique (Figs. 17.27 and 17.28).

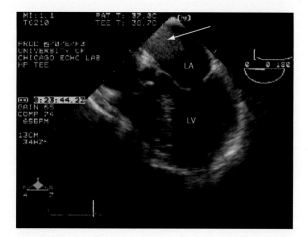

Figure 17.26. Infiltration into the LA of a lung carcinoma (*arrow*).

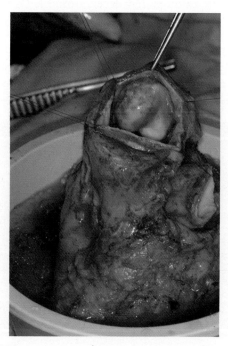

Figure 17.28. Autotransplant is the surgical procedure of choice in some of the cardiac tumors.

LEFT VENTRICLE

Many different types of masses can be found within the LV cavity; however, the most common are thrombi. Thrombi occur primarily in one of two situations, either in global LV systolic dysfunction or regional akinesis/dyskinesis of the ventricular apex. Less commonly, thrombi may also be seen in inferobasilar aneurysms. Apical LV thrombi appear as masses with increased echogenicity and clearly delineated borders adjacent to but distinct from the endocardium (Fig. 17.29). The acoustic quality of thrombi is distinctly different from the surrounding myocardium. Thrombi should be visualized in both systole and diastole, as well as in more than one view, to ensure differentiation from artifact and tangential cuts through the LV apex. Although large pedunculated thrombi are easy to visualize, small thrombi and mural thrombi may be difficult to differentiate from wall thickening due to apical hypertrophy, endomyocardial fibrosis, and hypereosinophilic syndrome. The wall motion may appear normal by TEE, especially when infarction is subendocardial.

Complete visualization of the LV apex from the midesophageal two- and four-chamber views requires significant retroflexion such that maintaining contact may be difficult. Despite this, several studies have shown the superiority of TEE over TTE for visualization of apical thrombus (7,95), although others have not (1). Intraoperative assessment of the LV for thrombus may be particularly helpful in patients with TTE examinations that are equivocal for apical thrombus. In this group, TEE confirms the presence of a clot in more than 50% of cases (95). Use of the transgastric two-chamber and the deep transgastric long-axis views may be useful to visualize the LV apex. Intraoperative identification of an apical clot may allow alteration of the surgical procedure to minimize LV manipulation or even remove the clot. Because apical thrombi may be dislodged or fragmented during bypass surgery, careful inspection of the LV apex in susceptible

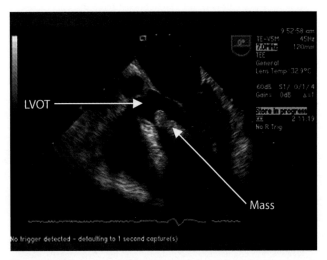

Figure 17.30. Metastatic melanoma of the LV. Tumor mass is seen occupying majority of LV outflow tract (LVOT) in five-chamber view.

patients prior to removal of the cross-clamp may prevent intraoperative embolization (19).

There are several primary tumors that involve the LV. Unlike atrial tumors, primary tumors of the LV tend to be intramural. Rhabdomyomas are the most common primary cardiac tumors in pediatric patients and are often multiple (42,47–49). These are primarily ventricular tumors with nearly equal frequency in the right and LVs. Rhabdomyomas typically are more echodense than the myocardium and may be intramural or intracavitary. Fibroma are the second most common tumors in the LV and most frequently are intramural, involving the interventricular septum or anterior free wall. These tumors range in size from 3 to 10 cm, and central calcification is common, usually involving the conduction system (96,97). LV myxomas are uncommon (98) as are fibroelastomas. Malignant primary tumors of the heart, the majority of which are sarcomas, are more commonly right-sided but have been found in the LV (47–49).

Secondary involvement of the LV by malignancies may occur by direct invasion of an extracardiac mass or by hematogenous spread (Fig. 17.30). Myocardial involvement can be diagnosed by noting a change in the tissue characterization of a segment of myocardium and akinesis of the myocardium that has been infiltrated (99). If this occurs adjacent to a homogeneous extracardiac mass, tumor infiltration should be suspected. Tumor infiltration can progress rapidly, and extensive myocardial replacement by tumor can occur, leading to severe heart failure and arrhythmias (100–102).

AORTA/VALVES

The most common aortic mass is an atheroma. Atheromas occur with greatest frequency in the descending aorta and aortic arch and least commonly in the ascending aorta. Aortic atheromatous disease represents a spectrum

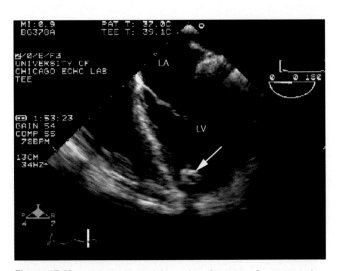

Figure 17.29. Midesophageal four-chamber view demonstrating a LV apical partially calcified thrombus (*arrow*).

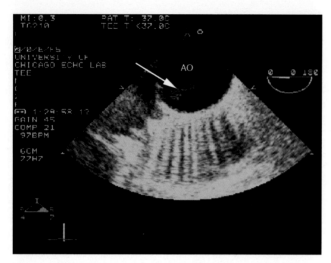

Figure 17.31. Short axis of the descending thoracic aorta (AO) showing a large protruding mobile atheroma (*arrow*).

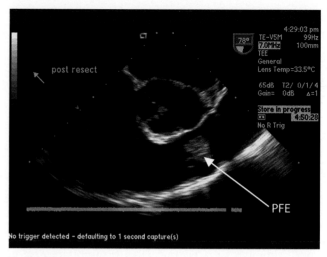

Figure 17.33. PFE attached to downstream side of the pulmonary valve. Mass moves independent of valve motion seen in RV inflow-outflow view.

of abnormality. Early atheromatous disease is defined by intimal thickening or minor plaque formation. Higher grade atheromas protrude into the aortic lumen. These plaques are heterogeneous and frequently have calcification. Atheromas typically involve a portion of the circumferential extent of the aorta, though in severe cases the aorta can be involved in its entire circumference. Large atheroma may have highly mobile protruding components that likely represent thrombus (Fig. 17.31). More extensive thrombus may be seen in aneurysmal segments of the thoracic aorta (Fig. 17.32).

Aortic plaques more than 4 to 5 mm in thickness or with mobile components are markers for significant embolic risk during cardiac surgery (103–107). Identification of the extent and location of atheroma on IO-TEE prior to aortic manipulation may help reduce perioperative stroke risk (15). Preliminary data using ultrasound-guided selection of the site for aortic cannulation and cross-clamping revealed the potential to reduce the risk

of perioperative stroke due to embolization of atherosclerotic debris (108,109). This is discussed more in the chapter on assessment of aortic disease.

Primary tumors of the aorta are rare. Secondary involvement of the aorta by tumor, although uncommon, has been reported. Primary lung malignancies often extend to invade local structures that may include the thoracic aorta. TEE has been used to help stage periaortic invasion of lung cancer in patients with a suspicion of aortic involvement by CT scanning (110). Aortic involvement by lung carcinoma may be confused with aortic pathology, such as intramural hematoma (111).

The most common benign tumor of the cardiac valves is papillary fibroelastoma (PFE). PFE are generally very small, round, mobile, pedunculated echodense masses, and the stalk is usually connected to the downstream side of the valve (Fig. 17.33). The aortic valve is most commonly involved, followed by the mitral, tricuspid, and pulmonary valves. Although PFE are often diagnosed incidentally, embolic phenomenon has been described.

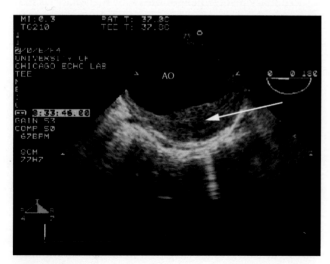

Figure 17.32. Dilated segment of the descending thoracic aorta (AO) with extensive thrombus (*arrow*).

KEY POINTS

■ TEE allows improved definition of cardiac mass size, shape, mobility, tissue characterization, location, attachment, and extent of myocardial involvement compared to the transthoracic examination.

■ IO-TEE can be invaluable in guiding the surgical approach for removal of an intracardiac mass, assessing the hemodynamic effects of a cardiac mass, and evaluating for residual mass and sequelae of mass removal on valvular and myocardial functions.

■ Knowledge of the normal structures, anatomic variants, and artifacts that can be confused with pathologic masses during a transesophageal examination is essential.

■ Most pathologic cardiac masses represent thrombus, infection, or tumor. Some of the rare conditions creating a mass effect include pericardial hematoma, pericardial cyst, bronchogenic cyst, hydatid cyst, hemangioma, AV nodal mesothelioma, and aneurysm of coronary artery or saphenous vein graft.

■ A reasonably secure diagnosis of a cardiac mass can usually be made by incorporating the location and appearance of the mass with associated echocardiographic findings and clinical data.

■ Cardiac involvement by malignancy is most commonly due to secondary or metastatic disease.

■ Primary cardiac tumors are uncommon and most (75%–80%) are benign. Of these, more than one half are myxomas.

■ The lack of malignant potential does not always indicate a "benign" clinical course, because nonmalignant intracavitary tumors may produce obstruction of blood flow. They may also partially dislodge, thus causing embolization.

REFERENCES

1. Mugge A, Daniel WG, Haverich A, et al. Diagnosis of noninfective cardiac mass lesions by two-dimensional echocardiography. Comparison of the transthoracic and transesophageal approaches. *Circulation* 1991;83:70–78.

2. Obeid AI, Marvasti M, Parker F, et al. Comparison of transthoracic and transesophageal echocardiography in diagnosis of left atrial-myxoma. *Am J Cardiol* 1989;63:1006–1008.

3. Alam M, Sun I. Transesophageal echocardiographic evaluation of left atrial mass lesions. *J Am Soc Echocardiogr* 1991;4: 323–330.

4. Leibowitz G, Keller NM, Daniel WG, et al. Transesophageal versus transthoracic echocardiography in the evaluation of right atrial tumors. *Am Heart J* 1995;130:1224–1227.

5. DeVille JB, Corley D, Jin BS, et al. Assessment of intracardiac masses by transesophageal echocardiography. *Tex Heart Inst J* 1995;22:134–137.

6. Shyu KG, Chen JJ, Cheng JJ, et al. Comparison of transthoracic and transesophageal echocardiography in the diagnosis of intracardiac tumors in adults. *J Clin Ultrasound* 1994;22:381–389.

7. Reeder GS, Khandheria BK, Seward JB, et al. Transesophageal echocardiography and cardiac masses. [See comments.] *Mayo Clin Proc* 1991;66:1101–1109.

8. Alam M, Sun I, Smith S. Transesophageal echocardiographic evaluation of right atrial mass lesions. *J Am Soc Echocardiogr* 1991;4:331–337.

9. Alam M, Rosman HS, Grullon C. Transesophageal echocardiography in evaluation of atrial masses. *Angiology* 1995;46: 123–128.

10. Koide Y, Mizoguchi T, Ishii K, et al. Intraoperative management for removal of tumor thrombus in the inferior vena cava or the right atrium with multiplane transesophageal echocardiography. *J Cardiovasc Surg* 1998;39:641–647.

11. Aru GM, Falchi S, Cardu G, et al. The role of transesophageal echocardiography in the monitoring of cardiac mass removal: a review of 17 cases. *J Card Surg* 1993;8:554–557.

12. Milano A, Dan M, Bortolotti U. Left atrial myxoma: excision guided by transesophageal cross-sectional echocardiography. *Int J Cardiol* 1990;27:125–127.

13. Borges AC, Witt C, Bartel T, et al. Preoperative two- and three-dimensional transesophageal echocardiographic assessment of heart tumors. *Ann Thorac Surg* 1996;61:1163–1167.

14. Borges AC, Bartel T, Mueller S, et al. Assessment of myxoma with dynamic three-dimensional echo-cadiography: a helpful new approach for the surgical management. *Am J Noninvasive Cardiol* 1994;8:313–316.

15. Task Force on Perioperative Transesophageal Echocardiography. Practice guidelines for perioperative transesophageal echocardiography. A report by the American Society of Anesthesiologists and the Society of Cardiovascular Anesthesiologists Task Force on Transesophageal Echocardiography. *Anesthesiology* 1996;84:986–1006.

16. Ofori CS, Sharma BN, Moore LC, et al. Disappearing cardiac masses—the importance of intraoperative transesophageal echocardiography. *J Heart Valve Dis* 1994;3:688–689.

17. Dujardin KS, Click RL, Oh JK. The role of intraoperative transesophageal echocardiography in patients undergoing cardiac mass removal. *J Am Soc Echocardiogr* 2000;13:1080–1083.

18. Brooker RF, Butterworth JF, Klopfenstein HS. Intraoperative diagnosis of left atrial-myxoma. *Anesth Analg* 1995;80:183–184.

19. Maslow A, Lowenstein E, Steriti J, et al. Left ventricular thrombi: intraoperative detection by transesophageal echocardiography and recognition of a source of post CABG embolic stroke: a case series. *Anesthesiology* 1998;89:1257–1262.

20. Leslie D, Hall TS, Goldstein S, et al. Mural left atrial thrombus: a hidden danger accompanying cardiac surgery. *J Card Surg* 1998;39:649–650.

21. Schuetz WH, Welz A, Heymer B. A symptomatic papillary fibroelastoma of the left-ventricle removed with the aid of transesophageal echocardiography. *Thorac Cardiovasc Surg* 1993;41:258–260.

22. Kawahito S, Kitahata H, Tanaka K, et al. Intraoperative management of a pediatric patient undergoing cardiac tumor resection with the aid of transesophageal and epicardial echocardiography. *Anesth Analg* 1999;88:1048–1050.

23. Mora F, Mindich BP, Guarino T, et al. Improved surgical approach to cardiac tumors with intraoperative two-dimensional echocardiography. *Chest* 1987;91:142–144.

24. Rousou JA, Tighe DA, Rifkin RD, et al. Echocardiography allows safer venous cannulation during excision of large right atrial masses. *Ann Thorac Surg* 1998;65:403–406.

25. Ralston L, Wasdahl W. Chiari's network. *Am J Med* 1958; 810–813.

26. Zema MJ, Temkin ML, Caccavano M. Echocardiographic appearance of the Chiari network. *J Clin Ultrasound* 1985;13: 671–614.

27. Werner JA, Cheitlin MD, Gross BW, et al. Echocardiographic appearance of the Chiari network: differentiation from right-heart pathology. *Circulation* 1981;63:1104–1109.

28. Goedde TA, Conetta D, Rumisek JD. Chiari network entrapment of thromboemboli: congenital inferior vena cava filter. *Ann Thorac Surg* 1990;49:317–318.

29. Goldschlager A, Goldschlager N, Brewster H, et al. Catheter entrapment in a Chiari network involving an atrial septal defect. *Chest* 1972;62:345–346.

30. Burke AP, Litovsky S, Virmani R. Lipomatous hypertrophy of the atrial septum presenting as a right atrial mass. *Am J Surg Pathol* 1996;20:678–685.

31. Ghods M, Lighty G, Ren J, et al. Lipomatous hypertrophy of the atrial septum. *Echocardiography* 1994;4:21–26.

32. Pochis WT, Saeian K, Sagar KB. Usefulness of transesophageal echocardiography in diagnosing lipomatous hypertrophy of the atrial septum with comparison to transthoracic echocardiography. *Am J Cardiol* 1992;70:396–398.

33. Fyke FE III, Tajik AJ, Edwards WD, et al. Diagnosis of lipomatous hypertrophy of the atrial septum by two-dimensional echocardiography. *J Am Coll Cardiol* 1983;1:1352–1357.

34. Saric M, Applebaum R, Culliford A, et al. Massive atrial septal lipomatous hypertrophy. *Echocardiography* 1999;16:833–834.

35. Shirani J, Roberts WC. Clinical, electrocardiographic and morphologic features of massive fatty deposits ("lipomatous hypertrophy") in the atrial septum. *J Am Coll Cardiol* 1993;22:226–238.

36. Olivares-Reyes A, Chan S, Lazar EJ, et al. Atrial septal aneurysm: a new classification in two hundred five adults. *J Am Soc Echocardiogr* 1997;10:644–656.

37. Schneider B, Hofmann T, Meinertz T, et al. Diagnostic value of transesophageal echocardiography in atrial septal aneurysm. *Int J Cardiac Imaging* 1992;8:143–152.

38. Pearson AC, Nagelhout D, Castello R, et al. Atrial septal aneurysm and stroke: a transesophageal echocardiographic study. *J Am Coll Cardiol* 1991;18:1223–1229.

39. Mugge A, Daniel WG, Angermann C, et al. Atrial septal aneurysm in adult patients. A multicenter study using transsthoracic and transesophageal echocardiography. [See comments.] *Circulation* 1995;91:2785–2792.

40. Veinot JP, Harrity PJ, Gentile F, et al. Anatomy of the normal left atrial appendage: a quantitative study of age-related changes in 500 autopsy hearts: implications for echocardiographic examination. *Circulation* 1997;96:3112–3115.

41. Vignon P, Spencer KT, Rambaud G, et al. Differential transesophageal echocardiographic diagnosis between linear artifacts and intraluminal flap of aortic dissection or disruption. *Chest* 2001;119:1778–1790.

42. Roberts WC. Primary and secondary neoplasms of the heart. *Am J Cardiol* 1997;80:671–682.

43. Abraham KP, Reddy V, Gattuso P. Neoplasms metastatic to the heart: review of 3314 consecutive autopsies. *Am J Cardiovasc Pathol* 1990;3:195–198.

44. Lam KY, Dickens P, Chan AC. Tumors of the heart. A 20-year experience with a review of 12,485 consecutive autopsies. *Arch Pathol Lab Med* 1993;117:1027–1031.

45. Sigman DB, Hasnain JU, Del Pizzo JJ, et al. Real-time transesophageal echocardiography for intraoperative surveillance of patients with renal cell carcinoma and vena caval extension undergoing radical nephrectomy. *J Urol* 1999;161:36–38.

46. Reynen K. Frequency of primary tumors of the heart. *Am J Cardiol* 1996;77:107.

47. Fenoglio JJ Jr, McAllister HA J, Ferrans VJ. Cardiac rhabdomyoma: a clinicopathologic and electron microscopic study. *Am J Cardiol* 1976;38:241–251.

48. Smythe JF, Dyck JD, Smallhorn JF, et al. Natural history of cardiac rhabdomyoma in infancy and childhood. [see comments]. *Am J Cardiol* 1990;66:1247–1249.

49. Burke AP, Virmani R. Cardiac rhabdomyoma: a clinicopathologic study. *Mod Pathol* 1991;4:70–74.

50. Goldman JH, Foster E. Transesophageal echocardiographic (TEE) evaluation of intracardiac and pericardial masses. *Cardiol Clin* 2000;18:849–860.

51. Pasierski TJ, Alton ME, Van Fossen DB, et al. Right atrial mobile thrombus: improved visualization by transesophageal echocardiography. *Am Heart J* 1992;123:802–803.

52. Nellessen U, Daniel WG, Matheis G, et al. Impending paradoxical embolism from atrial thrombus: correct diagnosis by transesophageal echocardiography and prevention by surgery. *J Am Coll Cardiol* 1985;5:1002–1004.

53. Burke A, Virmani R. More on cardiac myxomas. [letter; comment]. *N Engl J Med* 1996;335:1462–1463; discussion 1463–1464.

54. Markel ML, Waller BF, Armstrong WF. Cardiac myxoma. A review. *Medicine* 1987;66:114–125.

55. Smith ST, Hautamaki K, Lewis JW, et al. Transthoracic and transesophageal echocardiography in the diagnosis and surgical management of right atrial myxoma. *Chest* 1991;100:575–576.

56. Janigan DT, Husain A, Robinson NA. Cardiac angiosarcomas. A review and a case report. Cancer 1986;57:852–859.

57. Frohwein SC, Karalis DG, McQuillan JM, et al. Preoperative detection of pericardial angiosarcoma by transesophageal echocardiography. *Am Heart J* 1991;122:874–875.

58. Kullo IJ, Oh JK, Keeney GL, et al. Intracardiac leiomyomatosis-echocardiographic features. *Chest* 1999;115:587–591.

59. Podolsky LA, Jacobs LE, Ioli A, et al. TEE in the diagnosis of intravenous leiomyomatosis extending into the right atrium. *Am Heart J* 1993;125:1462–1464.

60. Tierney WM, Ehrlich CE, Bailey JC, et al. Intravenous leiomyomatosis of the uterus with extension into the heart. *Am J Med* 1980;69:471–475.

61. Sogani PC, Herr HW, Bains MS, et al. Renal cell carcinoma extending into inferior vena cava. *J Urol* 1983;130:660–663.

62. Skinner DG, Pritchett TR, Lieskovsky G, et al. Vena caval involvement by renal cell carcinoma. Surgical resection provides meaningful long-term survival. *Ann Surg* 1989;210:387–392; discussion 392–394.

63. Hatcher PA, Paulson DF, Anderson EE. Accuracy in staging of renal cell carcinoma involving vena cava. *Urology* 1992;39:27–30.

64. Basso LV, Gradman M, Finkelstein S, et al. Tricuspid-valve obstruction due to intravenous leiomyomatosis. *Clin Nucl Med* 1984;9:152–155.

65. Treiger BF, Humphrey LS, Peterson CV, et al. Transesophageal echocardiography in renal cell carcinoma: an accurate diagnostic technique for intracaval neoplastic extension. *J Urol* 1991;145:1138–1140.

66. Mizoguchi T, Koide Y, Ohara M, et al. Multiplane transesophageal echocardiographic guidance during resection of renal cell carcinoma extending into the inferior vena cava. *Anesth Analg* 1995;81:1102–1105.

67. Milne B, Cervenko FW, Morales A, et al. Massive intraoperative pulmonary tumor embolus from renal cell carcinoma. *Anesthesiology* 1981;54:253–255.

68. Allen G, Klingman R, Ferraris VA, et al. Transesophageal echocardiography in the surgical management of renal cell carcinoma with intracardiac extension. *J Cardiovasc Surg* 1991;32:833–836.

69. Katz ES, Rosenzweig BP, Rorman D, et al. Diagnosis of tumor embolus to the pulmonary artery by transesophageal echocardiography. *J Am Soc Echocardiogr* 1992;5:439–443.

70. O'Hara JF Jr, Sprung J, Whalley D, et al. Transesophageal echocardiography in monitoring of intrapulmonary embolism during inferior vena cava tumor resection. *J Cardiothorac Vasc Anesth* 1999;13:69–71.

71. Nixdorff U, Erbel R, Drexler M, et al. Detection of thromboembolus of the right pulmonary artery by transesophageal two-dimensional echocardiography. *Am J Cardiol* 1988;61:488–489.

72. Leibowitz D. Role of echocardiography in the diagnosis and treatment of acute pulmonary embolism. *J Am Soc Echocardiogr* 2001;14:921–926.

73. Rittoo D, Sutherland GR, Samuel L, et al. Role of transesophageal echocardiography in diagnosis and management of central pulmonary artery thromboembolism. *Am J Cardiol* 1993;71: 1115–1118.

74. Wittlich N, Erbel R, Eichler A, et al. Detection of central pulmonary artery thromboemboli by transesophageal echocardiography in patients with severe pulmonary embolism. *J Am Soc Echocardiogr* 1992;5:515–524.

75. Pruszczyk P, Torbicki A, Kuch-Wocial A, et al. Diagnostic value of transesophageal echocardiography in suspected haemodynamically significant pulmonary embolism. [See comments.] *Heart* 2001;85:628–634.

76. Pruszczyk P, Torbicki A, Pacho R, et al. Noninvasive diagnosis of suspected severe pulmonary embolism: transesophageal echocardiography vs spiral CT. [See comments.] *Chest* 1997;1 12:722–728.

77. Krivec B, Voga G, Zuran I, et al. Diagnosis and treatment of shock due to massive pulmonary embolism: approach with transesophageal echocardiography and intrapulmonary thrombolysis. [See comments.] *Chest* 1997;112:1310–1316.

78. Fagan LF, Castello R, Barner H, et al. Transesophageal echocardiographic diagnosis of recurrent right ventricular myxoma 2 years after excision of right atrial myxoma. *Am Heart J* 1990;120:1456–1458.

79. Waller BF, Fletcher RD, Roberts WC. Carcinoma of the lung causing pulmonary arterial stenosis. *Chest* 1981;79:589–591.

80. Nagasaka S, Taniguchi S, Kobayashi S, et al. Successful treatment of intraoperative pulmonary tumor embolism from renal cell carcinoma. *Heart Vessels* 1997;12:199–202.

81. Ernst G, Stollberger C, Abzieher F, et al. Morphology of the left atrial appendage. *Anat Rec* 1995;242:553–561.

82. Wrisley D, Giambartolomei A, Lee I, et al. Left atrial ball thrombus: review of clinical and echocardiographic manifestations with suggestions for management. *Am Heart J* 1991;121: 1784–1790.

83. Manning WJ, Silverman DI, Gordon SP, et al. Cardioversion from atrial fibrillation without prolonged anticoagulation with use of transesophageal echocardiography to exclude the presence of atrial thrombi. [See comments.] *N Engl J Med* 1993;328:750–755.

84. Klein AL, Grimm RA, Murray RD, et al. Use of transesophageal echocardiography to guide cardioversion in patients with atrial fibrillation. [See comments.] *N Engl J Med* 2001;344: 1411–1420.

85. Wood KA, Eisenberg SJ, Kalman JM, et al. Risk of thromboembolism in chronic atrial flutter. *Am J Cardiol* 1997;79:1043–1047.

86. Manning WJ, Weintraub RM, Waksmonski CA, et al. Accuracy of transesophageal echocardiography for identifying left atrial thrombi—a prospective, intraoperative study. *Ann Intern Med* 1995;123:817–822.

87. Aschenberg W, Schluter M, Kremer P, et al. Transesophageal two-dimensional echocardiography for the detection of left atrial appendage thrombus. *J Am Coll Cardiol* 1986;7: 163–166.

88. Mugge A, Kuhn H, Daniel WG. The role of transesophageal echocardiography in the detection of left atrial thrombi. *Echocardiography* 1993;10:405–417.

89. Heath D. Pathology of cardiac tumors. *Am J Cardiol* 1968;21: 315–327.

90. Feinglass NG, Reeder GS, Finck SJ, et al. Myxoma of the left atrial appendage mimicking thrombus during aortic valve replacement. *J Am Soc Echocardiogr* 1998;11:677–679.

91. St John Sutton MG, Mercier LA, Giuliani ER, et al. Atrial myxomas: a review of clinical experience in 40 patients. *Mayo Clin Proc* 1980;55:371–376.

92. Awad M, Dunn B, al Halees Z, et al. Intracardiac rhabdomyosarcoma: transesophageal echocardiographic findings and diagnosis. *J Am Soc Echocardiogr* 1992;5:199–202.

93. Weg IL, Mehra S, Azueta V, et al. Cardiac metastasis from adenocarcinoma of the lung. Echocardiographic-pathologic correlation. *Am J Med* 1986;80:108–112.

94. Onuigbo WI. Direct extension of cancer between pulmonary veins and the left atrium. *Chest* 1972;62:444–446.

95. Chen C, Koschyk D, Hamm C, et al. Usefulness of transesophageal echocardiography in identifying small left-ventricular apical thrombus. *J Am Coll Cardiol* 1993;21:208–215.

96. Parmley LF, Salley RK, Williams JP, et al. The clinical spectrum of cardiac fibroma with diagnostic and surgical considerations—noninvasive imaging enhances management. *Ann Thorac Surg* 1988;45:455–465.

97. Takahashi K, Imamura Y, Ochi T, et al. Echocardiographic demonstration of an asymptomatic patient with left-ventricular fibroma. *Am J Cardiol* 1984;53:981–982.

98. Wrisley D, Rosenberg J, Giambartolomei A, et al. Left ventricular myxoma discovered incidentally by echocardiography. *Am Heart J* 1991;121:1554–1555.

99. Lestuzzi C, Biasi S, Nicolosi GL, et al. Secondary neoplastic infiltration of the myocardium diagnosed by two-dimensional echocardiography in seven cases with anatomic confirmation. *J Am Coll Cardiol* 1987;9:439–445.

100. Lee PJ, Spencer KT. Pseudoaneurysm of the left ventricular free wall caused by tumor. *J Am Soc Echocardiogr* 1999;12:876–878.

101. Lynch M, Cobbs W, Miller RL, et al. Massive cardiac involvement by malignant lymphoma. *Cardiology* 1996;87:566–568.

102. Miyazaki T, Yoshida T, Mori H, et al. Intractable heart failure, conduction disturbances and myocardial infarction by massive myocardial invasion of malignant lymphoma. *J Am Coll Cardiol* 1985;6:937–941.

103. Tunick PA, Kronzon I. Atheromas of the thoracic aorta: clinical and therapeutic update. *J Am Coll Cardiol* 2000;35: 545–554.

104. Heinzlef O, Cohen A, Amarenco P. An update on aortic causes of ischemic stroke. *Curr Opin Neurol* 1997;10:64–72.

105. Blauth CI, Cosgrove DM, Webb BW, et al. Atheroembolism from the ascending aorta. An emerging problem in cardiac surgery. *J Thorac Cardiovasc Surg* 1992;103:1104–1111; discussion 1111–1112.

106. Davila-Roman VG, Barzilai B, Wareing TH, et al. Atherosclerosis of the ascending aorta. Prevalence and role as an independent predictor of cerebrovascular events in cardiac patients. *Stroke* 1994;25:2010–2016.

107. Katz ES, Tunick PA, Rusinek H, et al. Protruding aortic atheromas predict stroke in elderly patients undergoing cardiopulmonary bypass: experience with intraoperative

transesophageal echocardiography. *J Am Coll Cardiol* 1992; 20:70–77.

108. Ribakove GH, Katz ES, Galloway AC, et al. Surgical implications of transesophageal echocardiography to grade the atheromatous aortic arch. *Ann Thorac Surg* 1992;53:758–761; discussion 762–763.

109. Wareing TH, Davila-Roman VG, Barzilai B, et al. Management of the severely atherosclerotic ascending aorta during cardiac operations. A strategy for detection and treatment. *J Thorac Cardiovasc Surg* 1992;103:453–462.

110. Wang KY, Lin CY, Kuo-Tai J, et al. Use of transesophageal echocardiography for evaluation of resectability of lung cancer. *Acta Anaesthesiol Sin* 1994;32:255–260.

111. Draznin J, Spencer KT. Squamous cell carcinoma masquerading as a thoracic intramural hematoma. *Echocardiography* 2001;18:175–177.

QUESTIONS

1. Which of the following statements is false concerning neoplastic masses in the heart?
   A. Metastatic neoplasms are far more common than are primary tumors by a 20–30:1 ratio.
   B. Lung and breast tumors are two of the more common malignant tumors involving the heart.
   C. Melanomas have a predilection for metastasizing to the heart.
   D. Most secondary involvement of the heart by malignancy is myocardial.

2. Which of the following statements regarding primary tumors of the heart is false?
   A. Most primary cardiac tumors are benign.
   B. Cardiac lipomas are the most common benign primary cardiac tumor.
   C. Most primary malignant cardiac tumors are types of sarcoma.
   D. The most common location for a primary malignant tumor of the heart is the RA.

3. Which of the following statements regarding cardiac thrombi is true?
   A. Approximately 50% of cardiac thrombi in patients with atrial fibrillation are found in the RA.
   B. Detection of any irregularity on the wall of the LAA is highly suspicious for thrombus because the LAA is typically smooth walled.
   C. LV apical thrombi should be visualized in both systole and diastole, as well as in more than one view.
   D. TEE allows definitive distinction between cardiac thrombi and cardiac tumors.

Transesophageal Echocardiographic Evaluation for Noncardiac Surgery

K. Annette Mizuguchi ■ Carl Schwartz ■ Stanton K. Shernan ■ Andrew Maslow

Transesophageal echocardiography (TEE) is an established important diagnostic tool and monitor of cardiac performance in patients undergoing cardiac surgery (1–4). The role of TEE in the perioperative management of noncardiac surgical patients is increasingly being appreciated and has further been recognized by the addition of recommendations for intraoperative echocardiography in the most recent ACC/AHA/ASE guidelines for clinical application of echocardiography (5). This chapter will review the application and utility of TEE as a diagnostic rescue tool in patients experiencing significant intraoperative hemodynamic instability, as a monitor of cardiac performance, and as a tool to define cardiovascular pathology and guide interventions in the noncardiac surgical setting.

TEE AS A DIAGNOSTIC RESCUE TOOL

The role of TEE in critical emergency intraoperative settings is beneficial for establishing a diagnosis and directing definitive therapies in up to 80% of patients (6,7). Based on TEE analyses, almost a third of patients may have a change in medical therapy while 23% may have a change in surgical procedure (7). Intraoperative TEE was also helpful in defining the etiology of unexpected, intraoperative cardiac arrest in 19 of 22 noncardiac surgical patients (8). The TEE findings in these emergency settings included hypovolemia, pericardial tamponade, ventricular dysfunction, regional wall motion abnormalities, and intracardiac or intravascular thrombi.

Transthoracic echocardiography (TTE) can also be utilized in a rescue situation. However, in the emergency setting, acquisition of certain TTE imaging windows, that are dependent on patient positioning (e.g., parasternal and subcostal views), may be limited. Secondly, if the surgical procedure involves the chest or abdomen, probe placement may not be physically possible. Thirdly, when cardiopulmonary resuscitation is ongoing, TTE will require interruption of chest compressions to image the heart, whereas TEE does not. Lastly, mechanical ventilation, subcutaneous air, or emphysema may make image acquisition problematic. Therefore, in the perioperative setting, TEE may be more easily accessible and preferable (9).

When performing a TEE examination in the setting of a rescue situation, a thorough yet expeditious examination with an emphasis on determining all possible etiologies of hemodynamic compromise is required. Therefore, the examination must be focused and limited. Time permitting, obtaining the classical 20 views may be attempted, but initially the focus of the examination is to confirm or to find a diagnosis that may lead to a therapeutic intervention. All causes of potentially treatable major hemodynamic compromise need to be ruled out. Commonly encountered etiologies include myocardial ischemia, ventricular dysfunction, unrecognized hypovolemia, pulmonary embolus, aortic dissection, severe valvular disease, intracardiac masses or thrombi, pericardial effusion, and cardiac tamponade (Table 18.1). One limitation in using TEE in this setting is that in the absence of cardiac activity (i.e., asystole), it may be difficult to assess regional wall motion abnormalities. However, even episodic spontaneous rhythm may be sufficient for diagnosis of myocardial ischemia by TEE (10).

Unrecognized Hypovolemia

TEE can be used to estimate right and left ventricular preload and volume status by observing changes in ventricular end-diastolic area. In particular, TEE has a valuable role in assessing volume status in the face of apparent adequate fluid resuscitation suggested by

TABLE 18.1	Possible Causes of Hemodynamic Compromise Diagnosed with TEE
Myocardial ischemia, infarction	
Unanticipated hypovolemia	
Pericardial effusion, tamponade	
Pulmonary thrombus	
Intracardiac thrombus, mass or air	
Aortic dissection	
Acute valvular regurgitation	
Ventricular dysfunction	

more commonly used endpoints as central venous or pulmonary artery wedge pressure. Conventional pulmonary artery (PA) catheters measure pressure and not volume. Thus, while the pressure to volume relationship may be reasonably predictive in a compliant system, the relationship between left ventricular end-diastolic volume and right-sided PA pressures may not hold in the face of poor thoracic or lung compliance, positive airway pressure, vasoactive drugs, poor myocardial contractility, and mitral valve disease. A recent study retrospectively evaluated the role of TEE in optimizing resuscitation in 25 acutely injured patients who required TEE for persistent shock in the absence of ongoing surgical hemorrhage in the operating room and intensive care setting (11). Decreased left ventricular filling was diagnosed by TEE in 52% of these patients, despite a mean PA pressure of 19.5 mm Hg, and after the patients had received an average of 6.9 L of crystalloid and 14 units of blood products. This study supports previous reports showing that TEE assessment of left ventricular end-diastolic area is more accurate and clinically useful than estimates of preload based on hemodynamic data from a PA catheter (12,13). Therefore, in the face of ongoing, persistent hypotension, TEE can be used to efficiently and accurately diagnose hypovolemia or hypervolemia and may guide the subsequent management of such a patient.

Pulmonary Embolism

Although pulmonary angiography, spiral computer tomography, or ventilation-perfusion scintigraphy is used to diagnose pulmonary embolism (PE), these imaging techniques are not always possible or practical in the acutely, decompensated intraoperative patient. Therefore, TEE has been used as an alternative diagnostic tool (14). Direct visualization of a PA thrombus is consistent with an echocardiographic diagnosis of PE. In particular, the midesophageal ascending aortic short-axis view is useful for visualizing thromboembolism in the PA (Fig. 18.1). However, the interposition of the tracheobronchial tree between the esophagus and the aorta can make image acquisition difficult. In such cases, secondary signs suggestive of PE may be helpful. Signs consistent with acute right ventricular overload include right ventricular hypokinesis, right ventricular enlargement, flattening of the interventricular septum, and leftward bowing of the interatrial septum. Other signs suggestive of a PE include an underfilled and hyperdynamic left ventricle, dilated PA, increased peak velocity of tricuspid valve insufficiency, shortened pulmonary ejection acceleration time, or right ventricular dysfunction with sparing of the right ventricular apex (i.e., McConnell's sign) (15).

Recently, a retrospective study evaluated the diagnostic utility of TEE in 46 consecutive patients who underwent emergent pulmonary embolectomy (16). Presurgical TEE findings were compared with corresponding surgical

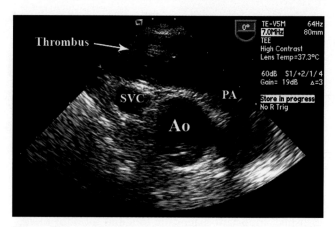

Figure 18.1. Midesophageal ascending aorta short-axis view showing a thrombus in the PA. PA, pulmonary artery; SVC, superior vena cava; Ao, ascending aorta.

findings to show that echocardiographic evidence for PE was correctly demonstrated in 46% of patients and that the sensitivity for diagnosing PE with intraoperative TEE within a particular PA location was 26% (range 17%–35%). Therefore, when a thrombus is seen within a particular location, it is highly suggestive of a pulmonary embolus. However, the absence of TEE evidence cannot exclude a pulmonary embolus. In addition, although right ventricular failure from pulmonary hypertension is consistent with pulmonary embolus, it can be precipitated by other causes of pulmonary hypertension.

Intracardiac Thrombi

TEE can visualize intracardiac thrombi or intracardiac air. In orthopedic surgery, emboli are released into circulation during the preparation and implantation of the prosthesis as a result of methylmethacrylate use (17–19). Such emboli have been associated with hemodynamic compromise ranging from decreases in blood pressure, increases in PA pressure, right and left ventricular regional wall motion abnormalities to frank cardiovascular collapse (20).

Venous air embolism, another source of hemodynamic compromise, can occur during any surgery where the surgical field is above the level of the heart. Neurosurgical procedures in the sitting position are notoriously associated with venous air embolism (21). When an embolic material or air is noted in the heart, it is important to remember to interrogate the interatrial septum for intracardiac shunts. There are numerous case reports where TEE was used to diagnose a culprit paradoxical embolus traversing the interatrial septum (22–24) (Fig. 18.2).

Pericardial Fluid

Rapid accumulation of pericardial fluid can lead to hemodynamic instability and eventual cardiac collapse. Acute accumulation of pericardial fluid in the noncardiac surgical setting can occur secondary to complications related

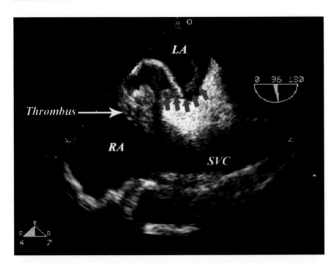

Figure 18.2. Midesophageal bicaval view showing intracardiac thrombus in the right atrium (RA). The small *blue arrows* note the thrombus traversing through a patent foramen ovale into the left atrium (LA) and the *large arrow* points to the thrombus in the RA. RA, right atrium; LA, left atrium; SVC, superior vena cava.

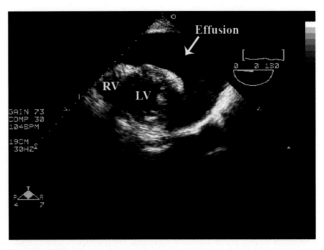

Figure 18.3. Transgastric short-axis view of the left ventricle showing a large posterior effusion. RV, right ventricle; LV, left ventricle.

to transvenous pacemaker or internal cardiac defibrillator lead extraction, electrophysiologic procedures (atrial ablation or mapping), transcatheter atrial septal defect closure, inferior vena cava (IVC) filter placement as well as laparoscopic or thoracoscopic procedures (25–28). Other disease states associated with pericardial effusion include malignancies, trauma, infection, inflammatory disease, radiation, aortic dissection, and postcardiothoracic surgery (29).

Echocardiographic features consistent with pericardial effusion and tamponade are noted in Table 18.2 (Fig. 18.3). Most of these features are readily diagnosed with TTE imaging as well as TEE. However, TEE may permit better visualization of intrapericardial clot and loculated pericardial effusions (29). In addition, access to optimal imaging windows may be limited by certain surgical procedures and by the presence of chest tubes and drains. Therefore, in the perioperative setting, TEE may be the diagnostic tool of choice.

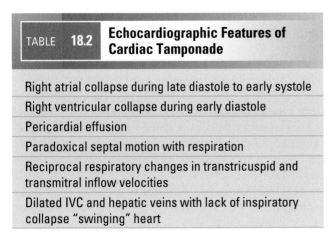

TABLE 18.2	Echocardiographic Features of Cardiac Tamponade
Right atrial collapse during late diastole to early systole	
Right ventricular collapse during early diastole	
Pericardial effusion	
Paradoxical septal motion with respiration	
Reciprocal respiratory changes in transtricuspid and transmitral inflow velocities	
Dilated IVC and hepatic veins with lack of inspiratory collapse "swinging" heart	

TEE AS A TOOL FOR MONITORING CARDIAC PERFORMANCE

Intraoperative TEE can be used in high-risk patients during nonemergency situations as a monitor to guide cardiac performance and prevent critical intraoperative events from evolving.

Myocardial Ischemia Monitoring

Intraoperative TEE monitoring is commonly indicated for early, preemptive detection of perioperative myocardial ischemia. Ischemic changes are diagnosed by detecting the presence of new segmental wall motion abnormalities (SWMA) characterized by persistent and significant decreased systolic wall thickening. However, diagnosis of wall motion abnormalities is limited by false-positives secondary to poor visualization of the endocardium (i.e., ultrasound "dropout" artifacts) and paradoxical or dyssynchronous septal motion secondary to bundle branch blocks, ventricular pacing, or postsurgical states. In addition, extracardiac compression of the inferior wall by ascites or abdominal contents may cause initial diastolic flattening followed by outward systolic bulging of the inferior wall that may mimic dyskinesis-associated ischemia or infarction. This "pseudodyskinesis" can be distinguished from true ischemia by evaluating inferior wall thickening. In pseudodyskinesis, the inferior wall is flattened in diastole, but unlike true ischemia, in systole, the inferior wall becomes round and thickens normally (30).

Although the reported specificity and negative predictive value of TEE for detecting myocardial ischemia are greater than 90%, the sensitivity and positive predictive value of TEE as an ischemia monitor are both less than 40% (31). This limitation may be due in part to the development of SWMA associated with myocardial stunning, hibernation, changes in loading conditions, metabolic changes, blood loss, or placement of an aortic cross clamp (32–36). Despite these shortcomings, TEE plays an important role as an ischemia monitor in high-risk patients. One study in vascular patients, demonstrated that new SWMA were noted with greater frequencies in supra-celiac aortic cross clamp placement (92%), compared to suprarenal (33%) and infrarenal cross clamp placement (0%) (36). Another study involving vascular surgery patients demonstrated that SWMA occur during aortic clamping or unclamping (37). This study noted that among patients with persistent SWMA changes, one had a nonfatal myocardial infarction and another had an intraoperative cardiac arrest and a fatal myocardial infarction. None of the patients in whom SWMA normalized suffered from any cardiac morbidity. Therefore, the authors concluded that intraoperative TEE monitoring allowed early recognition and treatment of cardiac dysfunction and therefore reduced the incidence and morbidity of perioperative cardiac complications (37).

Hemodynamic Monitoring

TEE monitoring can complement hemodynamic monitoring by providing real-time assessment of a patient's cardiac and volume status. This noncardiac surgical indication for intraoperative TEE has been demonstrated in a study of vascular surgical patients where supra-celiac aortic cross-clamping caused major increases in left ventricular end-systolic and end-diastolic areas, decreases in ejection fraction and SWMA while PA catheter or electrocardiogram data did not provide clues to these changes (36). In addition, TEE may provide useful data in situations where traditional PA catheter placement is problematic (i.e., critical aortic stenosis with left bundle branch block) or in the high-risk patient undergoing surgery including thoracotomies and certain plastic reconstructive procedures, which prohibit optimal electrocardiogram lead placement because the surgical incision covers the chest area.

The TEE transgastric midpapillary short-axis view is the most commonly used view to monitor myocardial ischemia as it allows assessment of the distribution of all three coronary arteries and rapid assessment of volume status. Limitations of TEE as a monitoring tool include its inability to continuously visualize structures and process the data into reliable numerical parameters, as well as the potential for user variability and suboptimal image acquisition.

TEE AS A CONFIRMATION TOOL

Intraoperative TEE can be used to direct surgical approach by allowing confirmation and subsequent detailed characterization of a patient's pathology or by more specifically confirming and guiding surgical techniques and interventions.

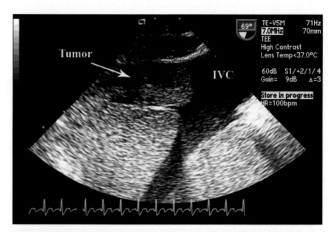

Figure 18.4. TEE view of renal cell tumor extending into IVC. IVC, inferior vena cava.

Defining Pathology

Intraoperative TEE can be useful for confirming a preoperative diagnosis and for providing a detailed characterization of the patient's pathology that can help direct the surgical approach and management. For example, intraoperative TEE can be used to assess the extent of tumor invasion or thrombus (38). In patients with pathology involving the superior vena cava (SVC), pulmonary vessels, pericardium, or aorta, TEE may contribute new information in up to 70% of patients when compared to computed tomography (39,40). Renal cell carcinoma frequently involves the cava. Up to 10% of patients with renal cell carcinoma present with extension into the IVC and 1% with further right atrial extension. Aggressive surgical resection of the tumor in the absence of metastatic disease improves survival in patients with IVC tumor or thrombus (41) (Fig. 18.4).

TEE has been used to assess the severity and etiology of pulmonary hypertension and integrity of the surgical anastomosis in thoracic surgical patients (42). Furthermore, echocardiographic visualization can prompt additional surgery if abnormalities in the pulmonary vascular anastomoses are noted (42,43). Therefore, TEE may be useful in evaluating disease progression and predicting a successful resection of a tumor or thrombus.

Guiding Surgical Intervention

TEE may be useful in assisting with cannula placement when cardiopulmonary bypass may be necessary to facilitate resection of tumors extending into the cava, or when deep hypothermic circulatory arrest may be required during resection of a giant intracranial aortic aneurysm (38,44) (Fig. 18.5). TEE can also be used to confirm appropriate deployment and function of endovascular aortic stents and intracardiac devices (45–47). The use of TEE to guide surgical interventions is considered as one of the Class I indications in the 2003 ACC/AHA/ASE guideline update for the clinical application of echocardiography (5).

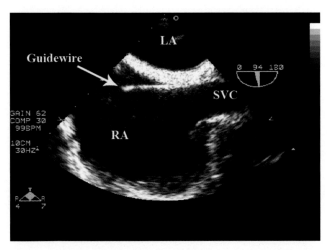

Figure 18.5. Midesophageal bicaval view showing guidewire for venous cannula placement in the SVC. SVC, superior vena cava; LA, left atrium; RA, right atrium.

CONCLUSIONS

Perioperative use of TEE in the noncardiac surgical setting has an important role in patient management. TEE is beneficial for the assessment of hemodynamic instability, as a complementary monitor in high-risk patients and as a tool to confirm cardiovascular pathology and guide surgical interventions. However, as with any tool, the risks and benefits need to be carefully evaluated. Although the complication rate from TEE placement is low, it is important to ascertain that each patient does not have pharyngeal, esophageal, or gastric pathology that will preclude its use (48). Increased availability of ultrasound technology and a rapidly growing number of trained personnel will significantly contribute to the expanding popularity and indications of TEE in the perioperative noncardiac surgical setting.

KEY POINTS

■ While TTE can be utilized in an emergency setting, acquisition of certain imaging windows, which are dependent on patient positioning, may be limited in the surgical patient. In addition, if the surgical procedure involves the chest or abdomen, TTE probe placement may not be feasible. Furthermore, when cardiopulmonary resuscitation is ongoing, TTE will require interruption of chest compressions to image the heart, whereas TEE does not. Lastly, mechanical ventilation, subcutaneous air, or emphysema may make TTE image acquisition problematic. Therefore, in the perioperative setting when an emergent ultrasound examination is requested, TEE may be more easily accessible and preferable.

■ When performing a TEE examination in the setting of a rescue situation, a thorough yet expeditious examination with an emphasis on determining all possible etiologies of hemodynamic compromise is required. Time permitting, obtaining the classical 20 views may be attempted, but initially an expeditious and focused examination is required to confirm or to find a diagnosis that may lead to a therapeutic intervention.

■ TEE in emergency intraoperative settings is useful for establishing a diagnosis and directing definitive therapies in up to 80% of patients. Based on TEE analyses, almost a third of patients may have a change in medical therapy while 23% may have a change in surgical procedure. Intraoperative TEE has also been shown to be helpful in defining the etiology of unexpected, intraoperative cardiac arrest in >85% of noncardiac surgical patients.

■ Commonly encountered etiologies of significant intraoperative hemodynamic instability diagnosed by echocardiography include myocardial ischemia, ventricular dysfunction, unrecognized hypovolemia, pulmonary embolus, aortic dissection, severe valvular disease, intracardiac masses or thrombi, pericardial effusion, and cardiac tamponade.

■ Intraoperative TEE can be used to assess the extent of tumor invasion or thrombus into the heart and great vessels. In patients with pathology involving the SVC, pulmonary vessels, pericardium, or aorta, TEE may contribute new information in up to 70% of patients when compared to computed tomography.

REFERENCES

1. Click RL, Abel MD, Schaff HV. Intraoperative transesophageal echocardiography: 5-year prospective review of impact on surgical management. *Mayo Clin Proc* 2000;75:241–247.
2. Couture P, Denault AY, McKenty S, et al. Impact of routine use of intraoperative transesophageal echocardiography during cardiac surgery. *Can J Anaesth* 2000;47:20–26.
3. Michel-Cherqui M, Ceddaha A, Liu N, et al. Assessment of systematic use of intraoperative transesophageal echocardiography during cardiac surgery in adults: a prospective study of 203 patients. *J Cardiothorac Vasc Anesth* 2000;14:45–50.
4. Sheikh KH, de Bruijn NP, Rankin JS, et al. The utility of transesophageal echocardiography and Doppler color flow imaging in patients undergoing cardiac valve surgery. *J Am Coll Cardiol* 1990;15:363–372.
5. Cheitlin MD, Armstrong WF, Aurigemma GP, et al. ACC/AHA/ASE 2003 guideline update for the clinical application of echocardiography—summary article: a report of the American College of Cardiology/American Heart Association Task Force on Practice Guidelines (ACC/AHA/ASE Committee to Update the 1997 Guidelines for the Clinical Application of Echocardiography). *J Am Coll Cardiol* 2003;42:954–970.

6. Brandt RR, Oh JK, Abel MD, et al. Role of emergency intraoperative transesophageal echocardiography. *J Am Soc Echocardiogr* 1998;11:972–977.

7. Suriani RJ, Cutrone A, Feierman D, et al. Intraoperative transesophageal echocardiography during liver transplantation. *J Cardiothorac Vasc Anesth* 1996;10:699–707.

8. Memtsoudis SG, Rosenberger P, Loffler M, et al. The usefulness of transesophageal echocardiography during intraoperative cardiac arrest in noncardiac surgery. *Anesth Analg* 2006;102:1653–1657.

9. Blaivas M. Transesophageal echocardiography during cardiopulmonary arrest in the emergency department. *Resuscitation* 2008;78:135–140.

10. van der Wouw PA, Koster RW, Delemarre BJ, et al. Diagnostic accuracy of transesophageal echocardiography during cardiopulmonary resuscitation. *J Am Coll Cardiol* 1997;30:780–783.

11. Burns JM, Sing RF, Mostafa G, et al. The role of transesophageal echocardiography in optimizing resuscitation in acutely injured patients. *J Trauma* 2005;59:36–40; discussion 2.

12. Cheung AT, Savino JS, Weiss SJ, et al. Echocardiographic and hemodynamic indexes of left ventricular preload in patients with normal and abnormal ventricular function. *Anesthesiology* 1994;81:376–387.

13. Bergquist BD, Bellows WH, Leung JM. Transesophageal echocardiography in myocardial revascularization: II. Influence on intraoperative decision making. *Anesth Analg* 1996;82:1139–1145.

14. Pruszczyk P, Torbicki A, Pacho R, et al. Noninvasive diagnosis of suspected severe pulmonary embolism: transesophageal echocardiography versus spiral CT. *Chest* 1997;112:722–728.

15. McConnell MV, Solomon SD, Rayan ME, et al. Regional right ventricular dysfunction detected by echocardiography in acute pulmonary embolism. *Am J Cardiol* 1996;78:469–473.

16. Rosenberger P, Shernan SK, Body SC, et al. Utility of intraoperative transesophageal echocardiography for diagnosis of pulmonary embolism. *Anesth Analg* 2004;99:12–16.

17. Ulrich C, Burri C, Worsdorfer O, et al. Intraoperative transesophageal two-dimensional echocardiography in total hip replacement. *Arch Orthop Trauma Surg* 1986;105:274–278.

18. Murphy P, Edelist G, Byrick RJ, et al. Relationship of fat embolism to haemodynamic and echocardiographic changes during cemented arthroplasty. *Can J Anaesth* 1997;44:1293–1300.

19. Koessler MJ, Fabiani R, Hamer H, et al. The clinical relevance of embolic events detected by transesophageal echocardiography during cemented total hip arthroplasty: a randomized clinical trial. *Anesth Analg* 2001;92:49–55.

20. Schlag G. Mechanisms of cardiopulmonary disturbances during total hip replacement. *Acta Orthop Belg* 1988;54:6–11.

21. Mirski MA, Lele AV, Fitzsimmons L, et al. Diagnosis and treatment of vascular air embolism. *Anesthesiology* 2007;106:164–177.

22. Barbour SI, Izban KF, Reyes CV, et al. Serpentine thrombus traversing the foramen ovale: paradoxical embolism shown by transesophageal echocardiography. *Ann Intern Med* 1996;125:111–113.

23. Burch TM, Davidson MF, Pereira SJ. Use of transesophageal echoardiography in the evaluation and surgical treatment of a patient with an aneurysmal interatrial septum and an intracardiac thrombus traversing a patent foramen ovale. *Anesth Analg* 2008;106:769–770.

24. Dorr M, Hummel A. Images in clinical medicine. Paradoxical embolism—thrombus in a patent foramen ovale. *N Engl J Med* 2007;357:2285.

25. Endo Y, O'Mara JE, Weiner S, et al. Clinical utility of intraprocedural transesophageal echocardiography during transvenous lead extraction. *J Am Soc Echocardiogr* 2008;21:861–867.

26. Farlo J, Thawgathurai D, Mikhail M, et al. Cardiac tamponade during laparoscopic Nissen fundoplication. *Eur J Anaesthesiol* 1998;15:246–247.

27. Hsin ST, Luk HN, Lin SM, et al. Detection of iatrogenic cardiac tamponade by transesophageal echocardiography during vena cava filter procedure. *Can J Anaesth* 2000;47:638–641.

28. Hosokawa K, Nakajima Y. An evaluation of acute cardiac tamponade by transesophageal echocardiography. *Anesth Analg* 2008;106:61–62.

29. Tsang TS, Barnes ME, Hayes SN, et al. Clinical and echocardiographic characteristics of significant pericardial effusions following cardiothoracic surgery and outcomes of echo-guided pericardiocentesis for management: Mayo Clinic experience, 1979 1998. *Chest* 1999;116:322–331.

30. Yosefy C, Levine RA, Picard MH, et al. Pseudodyskinesis of the inferior left ventricular wall: recognizing an echocardiographic mimic of myocardial infarction. *J Am Soc Echocardiogr* 2007;20:1374–1379.

31. Comunale ME, Body SC, Ley C, et al. The concordance of intraoperative left ventricular wall-motion abnormalities and electrocardiographic S-T segment changes: association with outcome after coronary revascularization. Multicenter Study of Perioperative Ischemia (McSPI) Research Group. *Anesthesiology* 1998;88:945–954.

32. Krupski WC, Layug EL, Reilly LM, et al. Comparison of cardiac morbidity rates between aortic and infrainguinal operations: two-year follow-up. Study of Perioperative Ischemia Research Group. *J Vasc Surg* 1993;18:609–615; discussion 15–17.

33. London MJ, Tubau JF, Wong MG, et al. The "natural history" of segmental wall motion abnormalities in patients undergoing noncardiac surgery. S.P.I. Research Group. *Anesthesiology* 1990;73:644–655.

34. Hauser AM, Gangadharan V, Ramos RG, et al. Sequence of mechanical, electrocardiographic and clinical effects of repeated coronary artery occlusion in human beings: echocardiographic observations during coronary angioplasty. *J Am Coll Cardiol* 1985;5:193–197.

35. Patel B, Kloner RA, Przyklenk K, et al. Postischemic myocardial "stunning": a clinically relevant phenomenon. *Ann Intern Med* 1988;108:626–628.

36. Roizen MF, Beaupre PN, Alpert RA, et al. Monitoring with two-dimensional transesophageal echocardiography. Comparison of myocardial function in patients undergoing supraceliac, suprarenal-infraceliac, or infrarenal aortic occlusion. *J Vasc Surg* 1984;1:300–305.

37. Gewertz BL, Kremser PC, Zarins CK, et al. Transesophageal echocardiographic monitoring of myocardial ischemia during vascular surgery. *J Vasc Surg* 1987;5:607–613.

38. Sigman DB, Hasnain JU, Del Pizzo JJ, et al. Real-time transesophageal echocardiography for intraoperative surveillance of patients with renal cell carcinoma and vena caval extension undergoing radical nephrectomy. *J Urol* 1999;161:36–38.

39. Ren WD, Nicolosi GL, Lestuzzi C, et al. Role of transesophageal echocardiography in evaluation of pulmonary venous obstruction by paracardiac neoplastic masses. *Am J Cardiol* 1992;70:1362–1366.

40. Lestuzzi C, Nicolosi GL, Mimo R, et al. Usefulness of transesophageal echocardiography in evaluation of paracardiac neoplastic masses. *Am J Cardiol* 1992;70:247–251.

41. Koide Y, Mizoguchi T, Ishii K, et al. Intraoperative management for removal of tumor thrombus in the inferior vena cava or the right atrium with multiplane transesophageal echocardiography. *J Cardiovasc Surg (Torino)* 1998;39:641–647.

42. Michel-Cherqui M, Brusset A, Liu N, et al. Intraoperative transesophageal echocardiographic assessment of vascular anastomoses in lung transplantation. A report on 18 cases. *Chest* 1997;111:1229–1235.

43. Hausmann D, Daniel WG, Mugge A, et al. Imaging of pulmonary artery and vein anastomoses by transesophageal echocardiography after lung transplantation. *Circulation* 1992;86:II251–II258.

44. Aebert H, Brawanski A, Philipp A, et al. Deep hypothermia and circulatory arrest for surgery of complex intracranial aneurysms. *Eur J Cardiothorac Surg* 1998;13:223–229.

45. Kleinman CS. Echocardiographic guidance of catheter-based treatments of atrial septal defect: transesophageal echocardiography remains the gold standard. *Pediatr Cardiol* 2005;26:128–134.

46. Moskowitz DM, Kahn RA, Konstadt SN, et al. Intraoperative transoesophageal echocardiography as an adjuvant to fluoroscopy during endovascular thoracic aortic repair. *Eur J Vasc Endovasc Surg* 1999;17:22–27.

47. Hellenbrand WE, Fahey JT, McGowan FX, et al. Transesophageal echocardiographic guidance of transcatheter closure of atrial septal defect. *Am J Cardiol* 1990;66:207–213.

48. Kallmeyer IJ, Collard CD, Fox JA, et al. The safety of intraoperative transesophageal echocardiography: a case series of 7200 cardiac surgical patients. *Anesth Analg* 2001;92:1126–1130.

QUESTIONS

1. Which of the following is an indirect echocardiographic sign of pulmonary embolism (PE)?
   A. Left ventricle enlargement
   B. Prolonged pulmonary ejection acceleration time
   C. Right ventricular hypokinesis with apical sparing
   D. Rightward bowing of the interatrial septum

2. Which of the following is least likely to account for the limited sensitivity and positive predictive value of transesophageal echocardiography (TEE) in detecting regional wall motion abnormalities as an indicator of ventricular ischemia in an emergency setting?
   A. Atrial pacing
   B. Hypovolemia
   C. Increased afterload
   D. Stunning

3. During an intraoperative cardiac arrest, in anticipating an etiology for hemodynamic instability, TEE is least likely to show evidence of a significant pericardial effusion during which of the following procedures?
   A. Atrial ablation
   B. Open cholecystectomy
   C. Thoracoscopic pulmonary wedge resection
   D. Transvenous pacemaker placement

CHAPTER 19

Ultrasound for Vascular Access

Rosemary N. Uzomba ■ Christopher A. Troianos

The perioperative availability of ultrasound (U/S) promotes use of this technology beyond examination of the heart and thoracic vessels. The recent popularity of ultrasound-guided peripheral nerve blockade and surgical applications that utilize ultrasound to examine abdominal and pelvic structures makes ultrasound readily available in the perioperative setting. This chapter reviews the use of ultrasound for vascular access, including central and peripheral venous access and arterial access. A review of the clinical need for perioperative vascular access is followed by a discussion regarding the technical issues associated with using ultrasound for vascular access, an evidence-based approach for routine use, training and service issues, and finally future directions.

INDICATIONS FOR VASCULAR ACCESS

Central Venous Access

Vascular access is indicated for hemodynamic monitoring and for administration of medications and fluids. Access to the larger veins that comprise the central circulation is necessary for the administration of fluids that are not appropriate for peripheral veins, placement of devices and catheters, and for monitoring pressures within the thorax. Placement of catheters into the central circulation requires specialized knowledge and skill and is associated with risks related to access and with maintenance. Complications associated with vascular access are generally caused by injury to structures that are in close proximity to the vessel intended for vascular access and may include arteries, nervous tissue, pleural structures, and thoracic duct (left neck). Vascular access complications that occur with placement of central venous catheters prior to surgery may not be fully appreciated by the clinicians caring for the patient in the perioperative setting, particularly for catheters placed by physicians not working in the perioperative arena. Anesthesiologists, critical care physicians, internists, pediatricians, radiologists, and surgeons, with varying levels of training, expertise, and recent experience, are permitted to place these catheters in a variety of clinical settings and among a varied patient population ranging from the newborn to elderly patient. It is important that all practitioners

utilize safe and effective vascular access techniques that minimize risks and allow for recognition of complications and management of the consequences of central venous catheter placement.

The central circulation may be accessed from a variety of entry points, including the internal or external jugular veins, subclavian (SC) veins, femoral veins, and upper extremity veins. The site chosen for central venous catheter placement depends on a variety of factors, including the experience of the operator, available sites (away from the operative field), expected duration of access, and whether other devices will need to be placed through the site. The right internal jugular vein (IJV) is generally preferred by anesthesiologists because of its accessibility during surgery, direct route into the right atrium, and predictable location. Patient anatomy is an important component of successful vascular access. Morbid obesity, shorter neck, previous surgery or radiation in the area of the vascular access, and patient positioning are all important factors that influence successful cannulation and risk of complications. The clinical setting of muscle paralysis, mechanical ventilation, massive blood loss, and coagulopathy that are not uncommon in the operating room may also negatively impact successful vascular access. Ultrasound guidance becomes particularly important in these settings of difficult access that predispose patients to increased risk to vascular access using a landmark (LM)-guided approach.

Arterial Access

Arterial access may also be obtained from a variety of sites, including the radial, brachial, axillary, femoral, and dorsalis pedis arteries. The preferred site depends on a variety of factors, including the experience of the operator, availability (away from the operative field), expected duration of access, and whether other devices will need to be placed through the site. The radial artery is generally preferred by anesthesiologists because of its accessibility, predictable location, low complication rate associated with its use, and because it is usually palpable among patients with normal pulsatile blood pressure. The radial artery is not the sole blood supply to the tissues perfused by this artery, unlike the axillary, brachial, and femoral arteries. Ultrasound can facilitate access of these arteries in the challenging settings of obesity, altered anatomy, low-perfusion states, nonpulsatile flow, and unsuccessful cannulation using a LM-guided approach. Ultrasound-guided arterial access is performed at the same locations as LM-guided approaches but also allows for use of nontraditional sites of entry because of vessel imaging.

Peripheral Access

Peripheral venous access typically occurs by direct visualization of veins within the dermis, limiting access to the more superficial veins. Ultrasound facilitates access to anatomically deeper veins that might otherwise not be appreciated with direct visualization. A study of emergency medicine physicians placing peripheral intravenous catheters in difficult-access patients using real-time ultrasonographic guidance was compared with traditional approaches using palpation and LM guidance. Successful cannulation was greater for the ultrasonographic group (97%) versus control (33%). The ultrasonographic group required less overall time (13 vs. 30 minutes, [95% CI 0.8–25.6]), less time to successful cannulation from first percutaneous puncture (4 vs. 15 minutes, [95% CI 8.2–19.4]), and fewer percutaneous punctures (1.7 vs. 3.7, [95% CI 1.27–2.82]) and had greater patient satisfaction (8.7 vs. 5.7, [95% CI 1.82–4.29]) than the traditional LM approach (1).

TECHNICAL CONSIDERATIONS

Types of U/S: 2D and Doppler

Two types of ultrasound are available in the clinical setting to aid in vascular access. These include two-dimensional (2D) gray-scale imaging and audible Doppler guidance. Ideally, the equipment should be readily available, easily transportable, and easy to use. Audible Doppler units are generally the most compact type of ultrasound technology and are commonly used as hand-held devices that can be positioned close to the chosen site of vascular access. These units produce a characteristic audible sound that identifies vascular structures according to the flow of blood through the vessel that lies beneath the sampling area. Information is provided through a sound amplifier and speaker. The lack of visual gray-scale imaging obviates the need for a video screen and thus lends to the smaller size of these units.

2D ultrasound provides gray-scale imaging of structures underlying the skin beneath the probe and allows for visualization of the anatomy and anatomic relation of the vessel intended for cannulation and other surrounding structures, including veins, arteries, and nerves. Paramount to successful use of ultrasound for vascular access is the acquisition of the requisite knowledge and skill for using a 2D imaging device to perform a three-dimensional (3D) task. Operators of ultrasound equipment must be trained to develop manual skills after a thorough

understanding of ultrasound principles that includes interpretation of the ultrasound images. Image resolution is directly related to the frequency of the transmitted ultrasound while penetration is inversely related to the frequency. Vascular structures are generally within a few centimeters the surface, and therefore higher frequency ultrasound is preferred because resolution is more desirable than penetration.

Types of Transducer Probes

Probes come in a variety of shapes and sizes depending on the manufacturer and their intended use (Fig. 19.1). Some have a larger square-shaped footprint, while others have smaller or more rectangular footprint. Some probes have a needle guide attached to the probe, which directs the cannulating needle into the imaging plane viewed on the screen (Fig. 19.2). The type of probe used will depend on operator experience, comfort, and dexterity as well as patient characteristics (e.g., pediatric patients require a probe with a smaller footprint).

Style of Probe Use: "Free hand" Versus Needle Guide

The style choice is particularly important for the beginner ultrasonographer who may not possess the necessary dexterity to position the target vessel in the center of the imaging screen, while simultaneously directing the needle toward the middle of the ultrasound probe. One study that evaluated ultrasound-guided cannulation of the IJV with and without a needle guide showed that use of a needle guide significantly enhanced cannulation success after first (68.9%–80.9%, p = 0.0054) and second (80.0%–93.1%, p = 0.0001) needle passes. Cumulative cannulation success by the seventh needle pass was 100%, regardless of technique. The needle guide specifically improved first-pass success among more junior operators

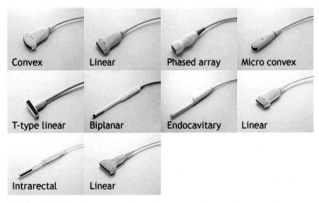

Figure 19.1. Types of Transducer Probes. Ultrasound transducer probes come in a variety of shapes and sizes depending on their manufacturer and intended use. The footprint can be small, wide, linear, or curvilinear. (From Soundvision Corporation, http://www.cvsales.com/cvs/PartsProbes/MindrayProbes.aspx, with permission.)

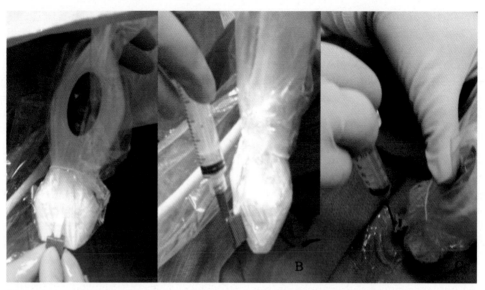

Figure 19.2. Ultrasound Probe with Needle Guide Attachment. **A:** Demonstrating the placement of the needle on notched section of probe. **B:** Syringed needle placed through the slot on the guide. **C:** Single operator ultrasound-guided central venous access.

(65.6%–79.8%, $p = 0.0144$) while arterial puncture averaged 4.2%, regardless of technique ($p > 0.05$) or operator ($p > 0.05$). On the other hand, the experienced operator may find the needle guide cumbersome choosing instead the "maneuverability" of the free hand style (Fig. 19.3).

Although the needle guide facilitated prompt cannulation with ultrasound in the novice operator, it offered no additional protection against arterial puncture. However, arterial puncture not only occurs from a misalignment between needle and imaging screen but may also occur

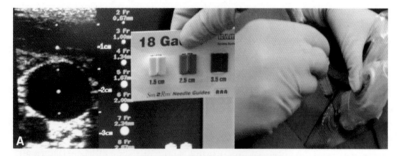

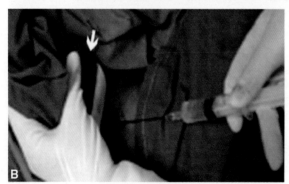

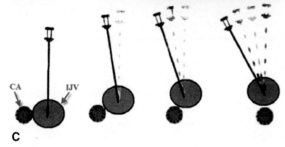

Figure 19.3. Needle-Guided versus "Free-Hand" Ultrasound-Guided Vascular Access. **A:** Needle-guided vascular access offers depth control. **B:** Free hand vascular access offers more maneuverability of needle angulation. **C:** Needle redirection based upon ultrasonically observed anatomic relationship of the internal jugular vein and carotid artery. (From Turba UC, Uflacker R, Hannegan C, et al. Anatomic relationship of the internal jugular vein and the common carotid artery applied to percutaneous transjugular procedures. *Cardiovasc Intervent Radiol* 2005;28[3]:303–306, with permission.)

due to a through-and-through puncture of the vein into a posteriorly positioned artery. This occurs because of a lack of needle depth control rather than needle direction (2). Needle depth is also an important consideration because the anatomy may change as the needle is advanced deeper within the site of vascular access. The ideal probe should have a guide that not only directs the needle to the center of the probe but also directs the needle at the appropriate angle beneath the probe (Fig. 19.4). This type of guide accounts for the limitation of using 2D ultrasound to perform the 3D task of vascular access.

Short Axis Versus Long Axis Versus "Oblique" Axis

Another technical consideration is whether to image the target vessel in its short axis (SAX) or its long axis (LAX) (Fig. 19.5). The advantage of the SAX view is that it allows for better visualization of surrounding structures, thereby directing the cannulating needle toward the target vessel and avoiding damage to surrounding structures. The advantage of the LAX view is that it allows for better identification of the needle tip, thereby avoiding advancement of the needle deeper than the target vessel. A study among clinicians with a variety of experience (fourth-year medical students, residents, attendings, and nurses) obtaining simulated vascular access using a gel

model, in LAX with linear versus curvilinear transducers, demonstrated a statistically significant difference in the number of surface breaks and redirects and the perceived difficulty but with no difference in time to cannulation. Novice ultrasound users found the curvilinear transducer easier to use for simulated vascular access in the LAX (3).

A prospective, randomized observational study of emergency medicine residents determined whether SAX or LAX ultrasound approach resulted in faster vascular access for novice ultrasound users (4). A synthetic skin arm model was used to note (a) time from skin break to vein cannulation, (b) number of skin breaks and needle redirections, and (c) a 10-point Likert scale denoting the difficulty of access perceived by the operators. The SAX approach yielded a cannulation time that was 112% faster as compared to the LAX approach. Moreover, the novice U/S users perceived that the SAX approach was slightly less difficult to master than the LAX. This observation reflects two important points. The operator's "hand-eye" coordination skill in aligning the ultrasound probe and needle is probably the most important variable influencing needle and target visibility. Secondly, SAX imaging enables the constant visualization of adjacent structures even when "hand-eye" coordination skills are not completely developed. LAX imaging requires greater "hand-eye" coordination.

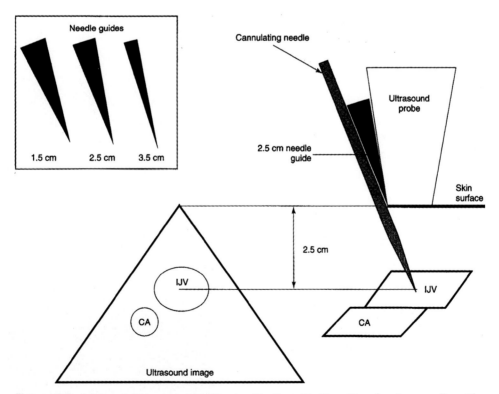

Figure 19.4. Schematic Demonstrating Varying Needle guide Sizes. Use of various needle guides to direct the cannulating needle to various depths, depending on the location of the target vessel beneath the skin. (From Troianos CA . Intraoperative monitoring. In: Troianos CA, ed. *Anesthesia for the Cardiac Patient*. New York: Mosby, 2002, with permission.)

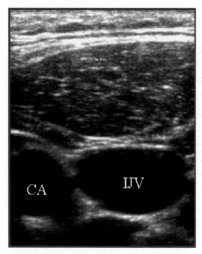 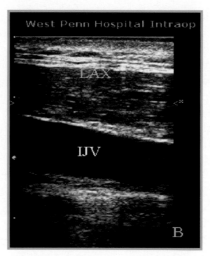 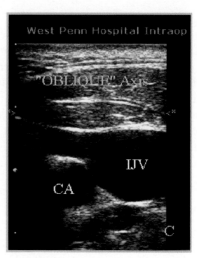

Figure 19.5. Ultrasound Imaging of Neck Vessels Via Three Different Axis Imaging Orientation. The IJV and CA can be imaged using several different axes planes. **Panel A** shows the vessels viewed on SAX—the advantage being the ability to view both vessels simultaneously. In **Panel B,** the ultrasound probe has been turned orthogonal to the image in panel A and shows the IJV in LAX. The LAX allows deeper structures to be seen at the expense of loss of visualization of the CA. **Panel C:** The "oblique" axis offers a compromise between the two views in **panels A** and **B** (see text). IJV, internal jugular vein; CA, carotid artery; SAX, short-axis plane; LAX, long-axis plane.

An alternative means for ultrasound-guided vascular access is to use an oblique axis rather than the traditional short-axis approach. This view allows better visualization of the needle shaft and tip but also offers the safety of imaging all relevant anatomically significant structures at the same time and in the same plane. This "halfway" orientation between the short and long axes of the vessel allows visualization of the needle as it enters the vessel, thus capitalizing on the strengths of the LAX while optimizing short-axis visualization of important structures during intravenous line placement (5).

Real Time Versus Site Marking U/S

Another important technical consideration is the use of ultrasound guidance in real time (during needle advancement) versus site marking with ultrasound guidance (before needle advancement). Site marking with ultrasound offers the appeal of not having to use the probe sterilely, which obviates the need for sterile coverings, ultrasound gels, and needle guides. Use of ultrasound as a vessel locator beneath the skin does not guide the needle into the vessel but merely becomes a LM-guided approach for vascular access. The IJV is identified by its ellipsoid shape and nonpulsatile, compressible features. The carotid artery (CA), in contrast, is round shaped, pulsatile, and noncompressible (Fig. 19.6). Precannulation skin marking with ultrasound shows no benefit to a LM-guided cannulation approach for cannulation success and complication rate (6). Sixty neonates and infants weighing less than 7.5 kg were randomly assigned to an ultrasound-guided skin-marking method (n = 27) versus real-time

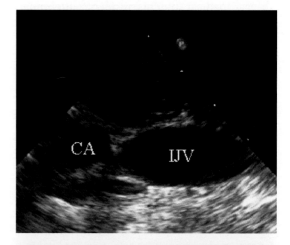

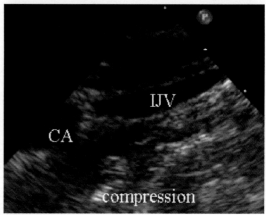

Figure 19.6. Ultrasound Demonstration of Compressibility of Vein. 2D SAX image demonstrating features that differentiate the IJV from the CA. The IJV is an ellipsoid-shaped vessel that is easily compressed and nonpulsatile.

ultrasound-assisted internal jugular venous catheterization (n = 33). Venous puncture was completed faster (p = 0.03), the time required to catheterize was shorter (p < 0.01), and fewer needle passes were needed in the real-time group, compared with the skin-marking group. Specifically, fewer than three attempts at puncture were made in 100% of patients in the real-time group versus 74% of patients in the skin-marking group (p < 0.01). A hematoma and an arterial puncture occurred in one patient each in the skin-marking group (7). The addition of skin marking to real-time ultrasound use does not improve success rates but does increase the time to successful cannulation (8).

ULTRASOUND-GUIDED CENTRAL VENOUS ACCESS

Evidence-Based Analysis for Ultrasound Use

Meta-analyses

Several meta-analyses touting the benefit of ultrasound-guided central venous catheter placement have been conducted (9–11). Supported, in part, by the Agency for Healthcare Research and Quality (AHRQ), Randolph et al. in the mid-1990s reviewed eight randomized, controlled trials published to that point. The data synthesis concluded that U/S guidance significantly decreased IJ and SC catheter placement failure, the number of attempts and the number of complications with a relative risk reduction (RRR) of 68%, 40%, and 78%, respectively, compared with the standard LM method (Table 19.1).

The Institute of Medicine published a report *"To Err is Human,"* in 1999, publicizing the frequent occurrence of medical error (12). In response, the AHRQ sponsored efforts to determine a list of best practices to improve patient safety. Part of the publication entitled *"Making Health Care Safer: A Critical Analysis of Patient Safety Practices"* lauded real-time U/S guidance during central line placement as one of the 11 patient safety practices with the

TABLE 19.1	RRRs Favoring Ultrasound-Guided CVC
Risk	**Relative Risk Reduction[a] (95% CI)**
Failed Catheter Placement	0.32 (0.18–0.55)
Catheter Placement Complications	0.22 (0.10–0.45)
First Attempt Catheter Placement	0.60 (0.45–0.79)

CI, confidence interval.

a Adapted from Randolph AG, Cook DJ Gonzales CA, et al. Ultrasound guidance for placement of central venous catheters: a meta-analysis of the literature. Crit Care Med 1996 24(12):2053–2058.

greatest strength of supporting evidence to improve patient care (13–15). The most favorable outcomes associated with U/S guidance were found amongst novice and inexperienced operators (13). A literature review conducted in 2002 by Keenan (10) concurred that despite the heterogeneity of the subgroups analyzed, ultrasound increases the successful placement of IJ catheters and decreases complications in the hands of less experienced operators.

The National Health Service in the United Kingdom established a "Special Health Authority," the National Institute for Health and Clinical Excellence (NICE). NICE's technology appraisal board is responsible for, in part, establishing evidence-based guidelines that demonstrate both clinical and cost-effectiveness. NICE issued guidance number 49 in 2002, which recommended that elective central venous cannulation (CVC) in adults and children be placed under U/S guidance (16). The recommendations came after a systematic review and economic evaluation by Calvert et al. (17) and a meta-analysis by Hind et al. (11). Hind analyzed 18 studies and found significant RRR of IJV cannulation in several measured outcomes: (a) 86% RRR for failed catheter placements, (b) 57% RRR of complications with catheter placement, and (c) 41% RRR of failure on first attempt. Additionally, fewer attempts overall were required to successfully cannulate, and significantly less time was needed. The economic model provided by Calvert indicated that monetary savings would be approximately £2,000 (~$3,200) for every 1,000 procedures preformed under U/S guidance.

Landmark Versus Ultrasound

The evidence for routine use of ultrasound is found among multiple articles (18–24) spanning a variety of disciplines that uniformly demonstrate the superiority of ultrasound-guided CVC over LM-guided techniques (Table 19.2). The LM method utilizes external anatomical structures to make inferences regarding the structures that lie beneath the dermis. Many approaches have been described to locate the IJV. The approach most often undertaken makes use of the sternocleidomastoid muscle and the clavicle (Fig. 19.7). The eponymed Sedillot's triangle is an area subtended by these structures. A needle placed at the apex of Sedillot's triangle and aimed toward the ipsilateral nipple should encounter the IJV 1.0 to 1.5 cm beneath the skin surface. The use of external LMs to gain access to the central venous system is considered a safe technique that can be executed with relative ease in experienced hands. Nevertheless, the failure rate can range from 7.0% to 19.4% (25) partly due to the inability of external LMs to precisely correlate with the location of the vessel (26). Furthermore, it was observed that successful cannulation via LM method diminished to ≤25% per attempt after six attempts. Additionally, there exists a strong direct correlation between the number of attempts and the incidence of complications.

Several quality-of-care issues are also associated with CVC, namely, patient comfort and delay of treatment. More needle advances, number of attempts, and prolonged

Outcome Metrics[a]	Ultrasound Group	LM Group
Overall Success Rate (%)	96.7–100	82–96
First Attempt Success Rate (%)	73–85.7	35.9–56.7
Arterial Puncture (%)	1.1–1.7	8.3–10.6

TABLE 19.2 Outcome Metrics: Ultrasound-Guided Versus LM-Guided CVC

[a] Ranges adapted from References 2, 11, 35, 41, and 43.

insertion times lead to increased patient anxiety and discomfort. A prolonged insertion time also delays appropriate monitoring and infusion of fluids/medications necessary to institute definitive care. These and other quality of care issues must be considered when choosing the appropriate method for central venous access.

Many studies have shown a clear advantage of U/S-guided CVC over LM-guided CVC. Troianos et al. (18) demonstrated that the overall success rate of CVC can be improved from 96% to 100% with the use of U/S. This may not seem significant until one considers the improved first attempt success rate (54%–73%), the decrease in number of attempts (2.8–1.4 attempts), decrease in time to cannulation (117–61 seconds), and a reduction in arterial punctures

(8.43%–1.39%). Similar success was demonstrated in a study of patients undergoing SC vein cannulation (27). The ultrasound group had fewer attempts, better patient compliance, and a zero incidence of pneumothorax while the incidence of pneumothorax in the LM group was 4.8%.

Anatomic Considerations

Variable location of IJV

There are many anatomic considerations that can be evaluated with the use of ultrasound that might otherwise remain illusory and unaddressed with a LM approach. The IJV is classically described as exiting the external jugular foramen at the base of the skull posterior to the internal carotid. The IJV assumes a more anterolateral position (in relation to the carotid) as it travels caudally. However, aberrant anatomy exists in the adult and pediatric populations. Denys and Uretsky (28) showed that the IJV was located anterolateral to the CA in 92%, more than 1 cm lateral to the carotid in 1%, medial to the carotid in 2%, and outside of the path predicted by LMs in 5.5% of patients studied. Most notably, the anatomy of the IJV was sufficiently aberrant to complicate access by "blind" LM method in approximately 8.5% of patients (25,28). This is the clear and intuitive advantage of U/S-guided CVC; that is, its ability to identify patients in whom the LM technique is *not* likely to be successful. Several studies (6,28,29) have demonstrated the variable locations of the IJV (Fig. 19.8).

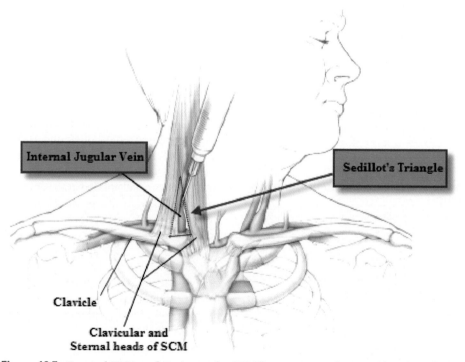

Figure 19.7. External LMs used to Access the IJV. There are several approaches described to access the IJV. The most common approach utilizes apex of Sedillot's triangle (see text). SCM, sternocleidomastoid muscle. (Modified from McGee DC, Gould MK. Preventing complications of central venous catheterization. *N Engl J Med* 2003;348:1123–1133, with permission.)

Medial   Lateral

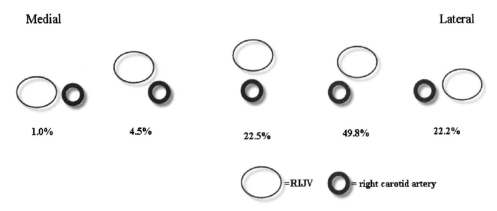

1.0%   4.5%   22.5%   49.8%   22.2%

⬭ =RIJV   ⬤ = right carotid artery

Figure 19.8. Variable Locations of the IJV. Schematic demonstrating the variable locations of the IJV in relation to the CA. The percentages indicate the proportion of patients with the various arrangements. More often, the IJV will be anterolateral and lateral to the CA. (Adapted from Gordon AC, Saliken JC, Johns D, et al. US-guided puncture of the IJV: complications and anatomic considerations. *J Vasc Interv Radiol* 1998;9[2]:333–338, with permission.)

Overlap of IJV and CA

The anatomic relation between the IJV and CA was elucidated by studies describing overlap of the two vessels (7,29,30). Sulek et al. (31,32) prospectively examined the effect of head position on the relative position of the CA and the IJV. The percent of overlap between the IJV and the CA increased as the head was rotated contralaterally from neutral (0 degree) to 40 to 80 degrees. Troianos et al. found more than 75% overlap among 54% of all patients whose head was rotated to the contralateral side (image plane positioned in the direction of the cannulating needle) (Fig. 19.9). Additionally, two thirds of older patients (age ≥ 60) had a more than 75% overlap of IJV-CA. Age was the only demographic that was associated with vessel overlap. Overlap portends the possibility of unintentional CA puncture or worse arterial cannulation with a large bore catheter. Routine U/S-guided CVC placement should involve "single wall" puncture of the anterior wall. The anterior wall of the vessel indents (partially compresses) as the needle approaches the vein. The compressive effect is released as the needle enters the vein (heralded by the aspiration of blood into the syringe) and the vessel's normal shape is resumed (Fig. 19.10). A low-pressured IJV may completely compress during needle advancement causing puncture of the anterior *and* posterior walls ("double wall puncture") without blood aspiration into the syringe (33,34). IJV-CA overlap increases the possibility of unintentional arterial puncture as the "margin of safety" decreases.

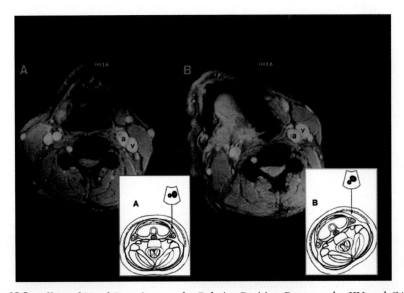

Figure 19.9. Effect of Head Rotation on the Relative Position Between the IJV and CA. MRI imaging demonstrating the effects of head rotation on the relative positions between the IJV and CA. The corresponding *insets* show the artistic rendition of MRI findings. **Panel A** shows the patient with the head in neutral position. **Panel B** shows the patient with the head turned toward the left side (see text). a, right CA; v, right IJV (with permission).

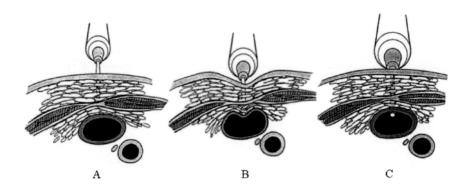

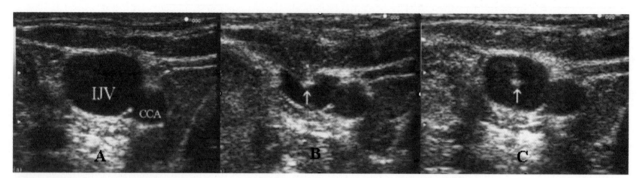

Figure 19.10. Compressive Affect of Needle Advancement on Central Vein. Schematic (**top panels**) and 2D ultrasound (**lower panels**) depict vein compression (**A,B**) with needle advancement. **C:** The vein resumes its normal shape once the vein has been entered. *Arrow* = needle. (From Phelan MP. A novel use of the endocavity (transvaginal) ultrasound probe: central venous access in the ED. *Am J Emerg Med* 2003;21[3]:220–222 and Oguzkurt L, Tercan F, Kara G, et al. US-guided placement of temporary IJV catheters: immediate technical success and complications in normal and high-risk patients. *Eur J Radiol* 2005;55[1]:125–129, with permission.)

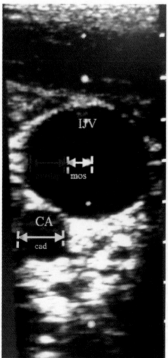

Figure 19.11. Margin of Safety with Internal Jugular Venous Cannulation. The "*margin of safety*," represented by the *white arrow*, is the distance between the midpoint of the IJV to the lateral border of the CA. This distance represents the zone where a "double wall" puncture of the IJV could occur and puncture of the CA would be avoided. The *red arrow* represents the "*overlap*" of the IJV and CA. It is the distance between the lateral border of the CA and the medial border of the IJV. The "*percent overlap*" is ratio of the overlap to the diameter of the CA, represented by the *yellow arrow*. The % overlap increases as the head rotates from a neutral position to the contralateral side. Mos, margin of safety; cad, carotid artery diameter. (Adapted from Wang R, Snoey ER, Clements RC, et al. Effect of head rotation on vascular anatomy of the neck: an ultrasound study. *J Emerg Med* 2006;31[3]:283–286, with permission.)

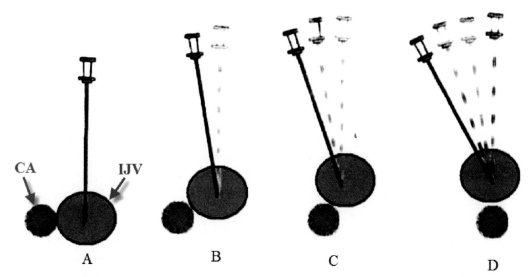

Figure 19.12. Sonographic Visualization of Vessels Improves Needle Redirection. Ultrasound visualization of IJV and CA allows safest angulation of the needle away from the artery. As the IJV goes from a lateral (**A**) to anterolateral (**B and C**) to an anterior (**D**) position in relation to the CA, the needle is redirected from 0 to 45 degrees away from the artery. (From Turba UC, Uflacker R, Hannegan C, et al. Anatomic relationship of the internal jugular vein and the common carotid artery applied to percutaneous transjugular procedures. *Cardiovasc Intervent Radiol* 2005;28[3]:303–306, with permission.)

Some authors describe the "margin of safety" as the distance between the *midpoint* of the IJV and the *lateral border* of the CA. This zone represents the area of nonoverlap between the IJV and CA (Fig. 19.11). The margin of safety decreases and the percent overlap increases from 29% to 42% to 72% as the head is turned to the contralateral side from 0 degree (neutral) to 45 to 90 degrees, respectively. These U/S findings may explain the mechanism of carotid artery puncture, allowing for the selection of the safest needle angulation, advancement, and redirection away from the artery, as visually guided with ultrasound (39) (Fig. 19.12).

Other anatomic variables

Rare vascular anomalies (e.g., double IJV) and anatomic variations of the IJV and surrounding tissues have been observed in 36% of patients in one study (36). U/S examination identifies the presence of the vein and anomalous features and provides an assessment of its patency, thus avoiding futile attempts at cannulation of an absent (2.5% of patients) or thrombosed vein (19) (Fig. 19.13). The size of the vein can also be ascertained. Denys et al. (19) observed a small fixed IJV among 3% of patients. A vein diameter of less than 7 mm (cross-sectional area <0.4 cm²) decreases the success rate of cannulation (37,38). These findings prompt early redirection to another site without wasting time and risking patient discomfort (30). There can be significant disparity in patency and size between the right IJV and the left IJV (right IJV usually larger than the left IJV) (Fig. 19.14) (38–41). Maneuvers that increase the size of the IJV thus potentially improve the success of cannulation, and include the Valsalva maneuver (Fig. 19.15) and the Trendelenburg position (39,42–44).

Liver compression may also increase IJV size in pediatric patients (19).

Complications

Regional anatomy is the most important factor considered when addressing for complications that occur during CVC (Table 19.3). The frequency of complications is variable according to the insertion site. Other mutables

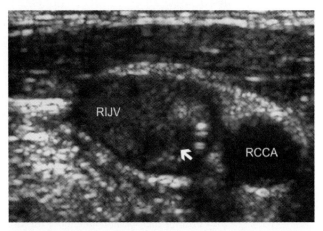

Figure 19.13. Thrombosed IJV. Sonographic image of thrombus (*arrow*) in RIJV. The vessel was unable to be compressed. RIJV, right internal jugular vein; RCCA, right common carotid. Note that the RIJV lies medial to the CA in this example. (From Karakitsos D, Labropoulos N, De Groot E, et al. Real-time ultrasound-guided catheterisation of the internal jugular vein: a prospective comparison with the landmark technique in critical care patients. *Crit Care* 2006;10[6]:R162, with permission.)

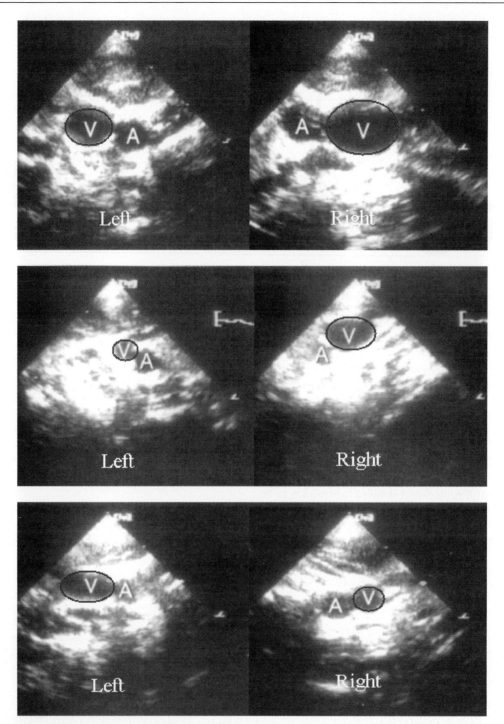

Figure 19.14. Right Versus Left IJV Size Disparity. **A:** 2D ultrasound images of CSA of the left and right IJVs in the same patient. In this patient, the CSA of the LIJV is less than RIJV. This is more often the case when there is a disparity in CSA between the two sides. **B:** In this patient, the CSA of the LIJV is less than 50% of the RIJV CSA. **C:** In this patient, the CSA of the LIJV is more than the RIJV. This is less often the case. In this patient, ultrasonographic imaging of the RIJV may prompt the operator to choose the LIJV for cannulation. A, artery; V, vein; CSA, cross-sectional area; LIJV, left internal jugular vein; RIJV, right internal jugular vein. (From Lobato EB, Sulek CA, Moody RL, et al. Cross-sectional area of the right and left internal jugular veins. *J Cardiothorac Vasc Anesth* 1999;13[2]:136–138, with permission.)

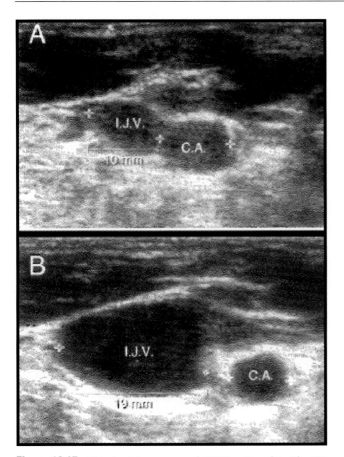

Figure 19.15. Valsalva Maneuver and IJV Size. **Panel A:** The IJV and CA are about equal in size. **Panel B** shows the same patient after a Valsalva. The IJV has almost doubled its size from 10 to 19 mm. IJV, internal jugular vein; CA, carotid artery. (From Gallieni M. Central venous catheterization of dialysis patients. *J Vasc Access* 2000;1:10–14, with permission.)

affecting complication rates are operator experience and patient specific variables (e.g., obesity, critically ill patients, emergency cases, presence of coagulopathy, etc.). Nevertheless, the incidence of major (e.g., vascular injury requiring repair) and minor (e.g., arterial puncture without significant hematoma) complications varies between 0.5% and 20% (13,25,45). This means, if 5 million CVC insertions occur annually (46), then 25,000 to 1 million patients per year may experience complications. CVC placement with U/S guidance decreases the relative risk of many complications.

Site of cannulation

The three most common complications associated with CVC placement (arterial puncture, hematoma, pneumothorax) are variable in their frequency of occurrence, partly due to the variable sites available for CVC placement. Puncture of the attendant artery may occur at the three most common insertion sites (IJV, SC, and femoral vein). The LM method is associated with an arterial puncture risk of 6.3% to 9.4%, 3.1% to 4.9%, and 9.0% to 15.0% for the IJV, SC, and femoral vein, respectively (18,19,46).

TABLE 19.3	Complications Associated with CVC
Vascular injury	
Arterial puncture/cannulation	
Hematoma	
Thrombosis/stenosis	
Arteriovenous fistula formation	
Pseudoaneurysm formation	
Cerebral vascular accident	
Neural injury	
Brachial plexus	
Cervical plexus	
Vagus nerve	
Phrenic nerve	
Cardiopulmonary injury	
Pneumothorax	
Hemothorax	
Chylothorax (thoracic duct injury)	
Venous air embolus	
Other	
Dysrhythmias	
Infection	

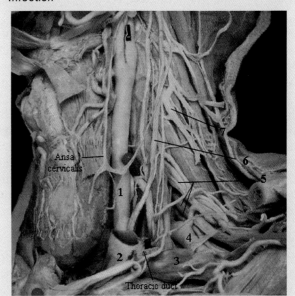

1. Carotid artery, left
2. Internal jugular vein, left (cut)
3. Subclavian vein, left
4. Subclavian artery, left
5. Brachial plexus
6. Vagus nerve
7. Cervical plexus

Adapted from McMinn RM, et al. Color Atlas of Human Anatomy. 3rd ed. London: Mosby-Wolfe, 1993:191, with permission.

TABLE 19.4 Complications by Site of CVC			
	Complications[a]		
Site	Arterial Puncture (%)	Pneumothorax (%)	Hematoma (%)
IJV	6.3–9.4	<0.1–0.2	<0.1–2.2
SCV	3.1–4.9	1.5–3.1	1.2–2.1
Fem	9.0–15.0	N/A	3.8 4.4

[a]Ranges adapted from References 2,11, and 30.
IJV, internal jugular vein; SCV, subclavian vein; Fem, femoral vein.

Similarly, Ruesch et al. (47) demonstrated a higher incidence of arterial puncture for the IJV versus the SC vein (SCV) during central venous access. Anatomically, the SC artery is more difficult to puncture because of its posterior position relative to the anterior scalene muscle and its superior and posterior courses relative to the SCV. In contrast, pneumothorax and hemothorax are more likely to occur during attempted SC versus IJV central venous access (1.5%–3.1% vs. <0.1%–0.2%) (18,19,46). Lastly, arterial puncture and hematoma formation occur with the greatest frequency via the femoral approach (18,19,46) (Table 19.4). U/S guidance during IJV cannulation decreases the incidence of arterial puncture, hematoma formation, and pneumothorax (48). U/S guidance may or may not reduce the complication rates associated with SC and femoral venous access. Some studies show no difference in complications between U/S- versus LM-guided access (45,49) while other studies demonstrate a reduced complication rate with U/S (27,34,35,50–52). The discrepancy may stem from the experience of the operator and the entry point for subclavian cannulation. Gualitieri et al. demonstrated that a more lateral approach to the SC vein affords the novice an improved safety margin and success rate, particularly when using U/S. This more lateral approach (at the lateral border of the first rib) actually accesses the axillary vein (Fig. 19.16).

Operator Experience

Many studies have examined the experience level of the operator with regard to the success rate of U/S-guided CVC placement, but there is variability in the definition of "experience." Some studies assign experience according to level of training (student, resident, fellow, attending) or a minimum number of successful CVC placements. Despite the variability in the definition of "experience," a consistent relationship exists between the less experienced operators and the complication rate. Less experienced operators require more cannulation attempts. Three or more attempts yield a *six-fold* increase in complications (45). A study designed to specifically address the success and complication rates of inexperienced operators using the LM- or U/S-guided technique showed an overwhelming advantage with the use of U/S over LM (50).

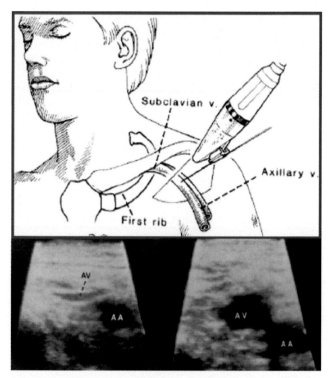

Figure 19.16. Lateral Approach to SC/Axillary Vein. The SC vein becomes the AV at the lateral border of the first rib (**top panel**). The AV is not encumbered by the clavicle and is therefore easier to access than the subclavin vein. The **bottom panels**: Note the relative position of the AV and AA. The axillary vein compresses with probe pressure while the artery does not. AV, axillary vein; AA, axillary artery. (From Gualtieri E, Deppe S, Sipperly M, et al. Subclavian venous catheterization: greater success for less experienced operators using ultrasound guidance. *Crit Care Med* 1995;23[4]:692–697, with permission.)

The success rate increased from 44% to 92% while the complication rate decreased from 41% to 4% with the use of U/S. After implementation of NICE guidance No. 49 in the United Kingdom, the reduction in complication rates was greater for inexperienced registrars (11.2%) than for experienced consultants (1.6%) (53). There appears to be a "leveling of the playing field" with regard to successful CVC when experienced and inexperienced operators use U/S. Augoustides et al. demonstrated a first attempt success rate for cannulation of the IJV with ultrasound guidance of 71% regardless of the experience level (2). An additional observation was the high arterial puncture rate (29.4%) among experienced operators. At first glance, this prospective observational study did not demonstrate a benefit to U/S guidance nor protection against arterial injury compared with LM-directed CVC for experienced operators. However, the small number of patients in the LM group and the fewer attempts made by attending physicians in the most challenging patients may have introduced selection bias. The plausible explanation offered by these authors suggested that residents perform most central venous access procedures in an academic department, while the attending only undertakes the most difficult CVC cannulation attempts (i.e. cases where there are anatomical difficulties or hematoma formation).

A selection propensity is thus introduced in favor of arterial puncture and against the more experienced operators.

Patient Variables

Patients at high risk for complications benefit most from ultrasound guidance. Variables such as obesity (54) and its attendant impediments (short thick neck, obscured external LMs) emphasize the value of U/S-guided CVC. Mansfield et al. noted that a body mass index greater than 30 resulted in a failure rate of 20.1%. Other high-risk variables include hemostasis disorders, uncooperative or unconscious patients, critically ill patients who may be hypovolemic, and patients who have had multiple catheter insertions. Oguzkurt prospectively reviewed 171 temporary IJV dialysis catheters placed sonographically by interventional radiologists in high-risk patients (27.7% with bleeding tendency, 10% poorly compliant, 2% obese, 37% previous catheters, and 21.3% bedside procedure because their medical condition was not suitable for transport to the radiology suite) (22). The success rate was 100%, with only seven complications among the 171 procedures. The carotid puncture rate was 1.8%, while oozing around the catheter, small hematoma formation, and pleural puncture without pneumothorax occurred at a rate of 1.4%, 0.4%, and 0.4%, respectively.

Karakitsos et al. (23) prospectively randomized 450 high-risk critical care patients to ultrasound-guided versus LM-guided CVC placement among operators with comparable experience levels. The rate of CA puncture, hematoma formation, hemothorax, and pneumothorax in the LM guide group was 10.6%, 8.4%, 1.7%, and 2.4%, respectively. This rate was significantly greater than the U/S-guided group, which boasted a CA puncture, hematoma, hemothorax, and pneumothorax rate of only 1.1%, 0.4%, 0%, and 0%, respectively. This underscores the value of ultrasound guidance in safeguarding against complications among high-risk patients. Critically ill hypovolemic patients (42) and coagulopathic patients (24) may also draw benefit from the utilization of U/S.

Ultrasound Use in Pediatric Patients

The vessels in pediatric patients are smaller and surrounding structures to be avoided are anatomically closer in these patients. Image depth, gain, and focus must be adjusted to strike a balance between overview and detail. The transducer probe must be of sufficient frequency to optimize penetration and resolution. Concerns with image resolution in the pediatric patient supercede the penetrance issue due to the superficial nature of the central veins.

The same maneuvers that affect IJV cannulation in adults (extreme head rotation, overzealous CA palpation with attendant IJV compression, etc.) also affect IJV cannulation in the pediatric population. Four percent of children younger than 6 months have unusually small IJVs (diameter <5 mm), which may decrease the likelihood of successful IJV cannulation (55,56). As in adults, the greatest advantage offered by U/S-guided CVC is the rapid identification of a vein that may be aberrantly positioned, absent, or thrombosed. This affords the operator ample opportunity to choose an alternate cannulation site, thus avoiding futile insertion attempts and the possibility of hematoma formation. A neck hematoma in the adult is usually an insignificant complication; however, a neck hematoma in a child, particularly a small infant, may collapse the vein to such a degree that successful cannulation necessitates search for an alternative CVC site.

The success rate and occurrence of complications of CVC depend on factors that include the age and size of the child, operator experience, and the presence of aberrant vasculature. Verghese and colleagues noted that percutaneous cannulation of the IJV in infants was technically more difficult and carried a higher risk of CA puncture than in older children and adults. They studied 95 infants undergoing cardiac surgery. The infants, who were less than 12 months old and weighed less than 10 kg, were randomized to LM- versus U/S-guided CVC. Pediatric anesthesia fellows were trained in the LM and ultrasonographic methods of CVC and were aided and supervised by attending pediatric cardiac anesthesiologists. The cannulation time, number of attempts, success rate, and number of CA punctures were recorded for each group. The success rate was 100% for the U/S group compared with only 77% for the LM group. The number of attempts and the time required for successful cannulation were significantly decreased in the U/S group. Most noteworthy was the percent of CA punctures in both groups: 25% using the LM method and 0% using the ultrasound. Other studies mirror the high success rate (94%–100%) and low CA puncture incidence (5%–6%) of U/S-guided CVC in pediatric patients (7,44,57). Grebenik offered critical review of some of these studies, specifically addressing the small sample sizes in studies that claimed ultrasound superiority over the LM method (58). Grebenik's own work investigated 124 infants and children, and demonstrated a higher success rate (89.2%) in the LM group as compared with the U/S group (80%). Their rate of CA puncture was also better in the LM group (6.2%) versus the ultrasound group (11.9%). Admittedly, the authors found the U/S probe "bulky" and the needle guide "cumbersome," suggesting that a smaller probe should be used for smaller patients ("small parts probe"). This study also emphasizes the point that less experienced operators derive the greatest benefit from U/S guidance. Hosokawa used a less cumbersome probe and relatively inexperienced anesthesia residents to achieve a 100% success rate with U/S-guided CVC.

Despite the limited number of studies in the pediatric literature, the existent studies provide overwhelming support to the advantageous nature of U/S-guided CVC placement in this population. A review by Leyvi et al. (59) noted that inexperienced operators had the greatest success when utilizing U/S for patients older than 1 year and more than 10 kg. The overall success in this age and weight group was 94.7% using U/S versus 75.9% with LM guidance. This study did not reach statistical significance among infants aged 3 to 6 months and weighing less than 10 kg. Given the limited studies among pediatric patients less than 3 months old, some have called into question the 2002 NICE guidelines recommending the use of U/S guidance as the preferred method for elective insertion of IJV catheters in children. The concern is that the NICE guidelines may tacitly condone the indefensibility of any CVC complications that occur sans U/S guidance. The NICE guidance, like any other guidelines, should not be considered a sanctioned manifesto but more as a purveyance of the most current information to aid medical personnel in the care of their patients. The medical personnel must astutely utilize the recommendations and not castigate unprincipled whimsy or unfounded bias. The question then becomes: if a tool is made widely available, is cost effective, and improves the success rate of an invasive procedure, should it become standard of care?

Ultrasound Use as Standard of Care?

The impediments to widespread implementation of U/S guidance for CVC placement are the purchase cost of the U/S machine, its availability, and the time and cost required to train operators. This belies the real limitation to widespread use: physician bias. It is likely that the most common use of U/S would be as a "rescue" device, only after several failed attempts with a LM-guided method. Biases remain despite literature resplendent with evidence touting its superiority over LM-guided techniques. Nearly 41% of 1,494 cardiac anesthesiologists in a recent survey responded that an U/S machine was always or almost always available for use during CVC placement, yet only 15% always/almost always used the machine. Of the 67% who never/almost never use U/S guidance, 45.7% cited "no apparent need" as the most common reason. Bailey astutely surmised that this perception is directly "at odds with the aim of patient safety" especially in light of the Institute of Medicine and the AHRQ's call for patient safety initiatives (14).

ULTRASOUND-GUIDED ARTERIAL ACCESS

Arterial access is conventionally obtained using external LMs and palpation techniques. A major concern of arterial cannulation is partial or complete occlusion (thrombus, hematoma, spasm, or dissection) causing gangrene, necrosis, and loss of limb or life. Clinicians are embracing the use of ultrasound for arterial access in an effort to assuage fears of arising complications. Ultrasonography can aid arterial access through various sites, including radial, brachial, axillary, and femoral.

Yeow et al. (60) performed 50 antegrade common femoral artery (CFA) punctures for selective superficial femoral artery (SFA) access under sonographic guidance. Access was indicated for vascular sheath insertion, balloon angioplasty, and for intra-arterial chemoinfusion therapy

to treat osteosarcoma. Antegrade CFA access requires needle puncture inferior to the inguinal ligament but superior to the CFA bifurcation to minimize the risk of unintentional external iliac artery puncture, which may lead to pelvic bleeding. A more distal SFA puncture is associated with an increased risk of pseudoaneurysm and arteriovenous fistula formation. A successful cannulation is thus defined as CFA puncture above its bifurcation and selective cannulation of the SFA. These investigators demonstrated a 96% success rate within an average procedure time of 3 minutes (±1 minute) and expressed their aversion to the "blind" palpation technique. The palpation method cannot ensure puncture within the safe zone of the CFA because of its variable length before bifurcation. Additionally, selective SFA cannulation is difficult. Sonographically the authors were able to provide 100% access to the CFA within its safety zone and recommended this method especially when antegrade CFA access is problematic.

The radial artery is the most frequently cannulated artery, but access may nevertheless be problematic even in experienced hands. Ultrasound can facilitate arterial access in settings that would be challenging with the external LM/palpation method. Patients with obesity, altered anatomy, low perfusion states, and multiple failed attempts are common challenging scenarios. Additional attempts may be prohibitive due to vasospasm, intimal dissection, or hematoma formation, when the pulse may not be palpable. Sandhu and Patel used ultrasonography as a rescue technique after several unsuccessful landmark guided radial artery cannulation attempts (61). SAX and LAX 2-D imaging and color Doppler were used to confirm pulsatile flow. The SAX view was used most commonly. The LAX image was useful when the entire length of the needle, catheter, and artery could be visualized in the same imaging plane (Fig. 19.17A–C). LAX imaging was possible when the diameter of the artery was of sufficient size to allow visualization of the needle tip piercing the arterial wall. The SAX was more useful when the artery was tortuous or constricted. The authors cannulated the radial artery in the mid forearm when the artery was not palpable more distally. The radial artery pulse is not palpable at the mid forearm due to its location posterior to the brachioradialis muscle. A benefit of mid forearm placement is the absence of adjacent nerves, thus allowing tolerance for needle redirection by the patient. U/S-guided radial artery catheterization was not only more successful in the mid forearm when the artery was not palpable more distally but provided an alternative to brachial or axillary artery cannulation (with their attendant risk of possible limb ischemia). Ultrasonography also improves the success rate of placing indwelling radial artery catheters in children (age 40 ± 33 months). Schwemmer randomized 30 children to palpation versus ultrasound and measured radial artery cross-sectional area. They demonstrated an overall success of 100%, first attempt success of 67%, and 1.3 ± 0.5 mean number of attempts. Comparatively, the palpation group had an overall success rate of 80%, a first

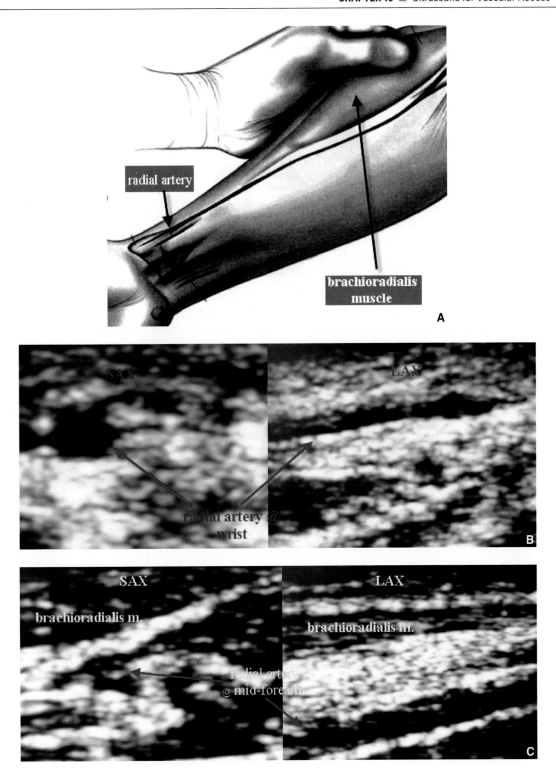

Figure 19.17. Ultrasound-Guided Radial Artery Access. **A:** Course of radial artery. The location of the radial artery is more superficial at the wrist and runs deep to the brachioradialis muscle at the mid-forearm. **B:** SAX and LAX ultrasound images of the radial artery at the wrist. **C:** Short and LAX ultrasound images of the radial artery at the mid-forearm. The radial artery is deep to the brachioradialis muscle.

attempt success rate of 20% with 2.3 ± 1.3 attempts of (62). Most revealing, dorsiflexion of the wrist significantly reduced the cross-sectional area of the artery by 19%. This is most important in pediatric patients, where any further compromise of an already diminutive radial artery may prohibit successful cannulation.

Although the amount of evidence supporting U/S-guided arterial access is not as abundant as that bolstering CVC, the utility of arterial access sonography is clear and plenary. It provides visualization of needle and catheter placement ensuring that the catheter is interarterial. U/S provides visual guidance when palpation is not helpful. Moreover, it allows for immediate recognition of complications (e.g., perivascular hematoma formation), unanticipated consequences (e.g., intimal dissection, thrombosis), and excessively small vessels (especially important among pediatric patients).

DEVELOPMENT OF ULTRASOUND VASCULAR ACCESS SERVICE

Training Issues

Current methods for training inexperienced operators include cadaver labs, synthetic models, and direct supervision in a controlled environment (63). Models that exist for training purposes may be cost-prohibitive. The ideal model for procedural training would provide simulation of a "real patient experience." The training would allow multiple attempts, availability, and be affordable with the goal of improving patient safety. A couple of factors must be considered during training. There is a rapid learning curve, and the experience of the operator may be misleading. A "novice" may have little experience in both placing CVC and U/S imaging. Novice may also refer to someone who is inexperienced with use of U/S but is a skilled proceduralist at CVC. The type and amount of training will vary for these two types of "novices."

Several subspecialties have developed policy statements addressing training and proficiency recommendations regarding the use of ultrasonography. The American College of Emergency Physicians (ACEP) requires development of both cognitive and psychomotor skills during training (64). The cognitive component includes didactics addressing (a) basic physics and principles, (b) knobology, (c) image acquisition, (d) identification and interpretation of artifacts, (e) identification of relevant anatomy and anatomic variants, and (f) use of videotaped and static images illustrating proper technique and pitfalls. The psychomotor component can be taught (a) within a laboratory setting utilizing cadaveric specimens or nonhuman tissue models such as Blue Phantom, chicken breast inserted with colored fluid-filled tubing or fluid-filled tubing in agar base; (b) with computer simulation; and (c) with hands-on proctored examinations on real patients. The number of examinations needed to become proficient is variable and

may in part depend on the physicians' specialty training. The Royal College of Radiology recommends 25 insertions. Sznajder considered more than 50 CVC insertions during the pre-U/S era as "skilled." Experience with U/S needed to attain proficiency should be less, approximately ten successful U/S-guided placements, largely due to the advantage of clear anatomical demarcation.

Cost Effectiveness

The economics of an ultrasound-guided vascular access service should consider the benefits of improved success, decreased complications, cost of purchasing and maintaining the equipment, and training of clinicians and other personnel associated with use of ultrasound in the clinical setting. The impediment to widespread implementation of U/S guidance for CVC placement most often cited is cost-effectiveness (65). Hind et al. conducted a cost-effectiveness analysis in the United Kingdom based on a conservative model (66). The economic evaluation considered capital cost of the equipment, maintenance, and depreciation. Additional costs not identified included training costs and opportunity costs (both lost and gained). An example of lost opportunity costs is equipment setup time. Opportunities gained include the reduction in operating room time wasted waiting for central line placement, reduction in complications, and potential litigation cost. Three of the five most common complications (CA puncture/cannulation, hemothorax, and pneumothorax) cited in the 2004 ASA closed claims analysis of injuries and liabilities related to CVC were related to vascular access and were thus possibly preventable with use of U/S. The payment for these closed claim case complications ranged from $1,280 to $527,000 (67). Death occurred in 31% of patients, and payment was made in 54% of patients who experienced CA puncture. The morbidity or mortality occurred as a result of stroke (31%), airway obstruction due to hematoma (25%), arterial repair (18%), or case cancellation (25%). Although severe complications have been reported with placement of an 18-gauge catheter into a CA, there were few claims for injury based on the frequency of carotid punctures (1.9%–9.4% depending on operator experience) in this review. The more serious complications associated with placement of the pulmonary artery catheter introducer sheath admonishes any *de rigueur* complacency with CVC access. Correct cannulation should therefore be routinely confirmed by either U/S, pressure waveform analysis, or both.

FUTURE DIRECTIONS

Three-Dimensional Guidance

One pitfall with U/S-guided CVC placement is that "a 2D tool is used to perform a 3D task." The learning curve associated with 2D U/S is contingent upon the operator understanding the significance of the anatomically obtained information (68). This learning process goes beyond mastering *technical* expertise but encompasses the development of *conceptual* expertise. A 3D image must be reconstructed from the 2D imagery of the anatomic structure of interest. An example would be through-and-through anterior to posterior wall puncture of the IJV, that is, "*double-wall puncture*," *venous transfixation or "overshoot."* SAX imaging of the IJV and CA displays the needle as a small dot as it approaches the U/S beam. In some instances, the needle is never imaged and there is only indirect evidence of needle advancement by vessel indentation or compression. The echogenicity thought to be the needle tip in the SAX view, may in fact, be the needle shaft, thereby increasing the likelihood of double wall puncture, and subsequent arterial puncture *despite* the use of U/S guidance. Viewing of the needle advancement is "out of plane" when using SAX imaging (Fig. 19.18). With LAX imaging the entire course of the needle, from shaft to tip, is "in plane" with the U/S beam (Fig. 19.19). There are advantages and disadvantages for each imaging plane. The advantages of the SAX plane are ease of use and increased successful CVC placement, especially for the novice (4). SAX imaging allows simultaneous visualization of both the arterial and venous structures. The disadvantage of SAX imaging is the inability to distinguish needle tip from shaft with the attendant risk of venous transfixation and possible CA puncture (especially in the

setting of IJV-CA overlap). LAX plane imaging allows for the entire needle course to be visualized but at the expense of the inability to view the artery and the vein. Chapman et al. describe a technique that improves visualization of the needle path by concurrently (Fig. 19.19). "rocking" the transducer into the path of the needle (69).

An evolving concept is the use of 3D imaging to reduce the pitfalls that beleaguer 2D (SAX or LAX) imaging while at the same time maintaining the advantages. French et al. (70) described their use of 3D static and real-time imaging during U/S-guided CVC placement. Three orthogonal (perpendicular) planes are simultaneously visualized: the SAX, the LAX, and the coronal plane. This coronal plane is called the "plan view" by the authors because it is similar to an architectural plan that shows building layouts from an overhead view (Fig. 19.20). A dot is used to mark the position of intersection amongst the three views (Fig. 19.21). The potential to improve accuracy of CVC is extraordinary since the dot can be steered to differing depths functioning as a target during needle insertion. The needle is imaged "in plane" and "out of plane" simultaneously, thus avoiding "overshoot." Moreover, potential topographical information such as intraluminal thrombi or intimal dissection could be elucidated in detail. As with most sonographic imaging modalities, 3D imaging has great potential for future use, but requires further investigational studies to define its significance (Fig. 19.22).

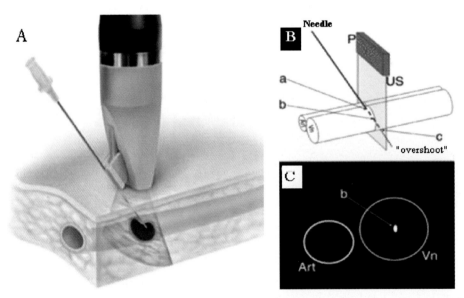

Figure 19.18. SAX Ultrasound Imaging of Vessel. **Panel A:** Both needle and vessel are imaged in SAX. Vessel indentation is often the only indirect evidence of needle advancement. **Panels B and C:** The needle crosses the U/S scanning beam orthogonally. That is, the needle is "out of [the U/S plane." The echogenic dot created may represent either the tip or shaft of the needle. As the needle advances, unintentional puncture of the vessel's posterior wall ("overshoot") may occur. Art, artery; Vn, vein; US, plane of the ultrasound beam; P, probe; a, needle enters anterior wall of vein; b, needle crosses plane of ultrasound beam; c, needle exits the posterior wall of vein-"oversoot"; US, ultrasound. (From French JL, Raine-Fenning NJ, et al. Pitfalls of ultrasound guided vascular access: the use of three/four-dimensional ultrasound. *Anaesthesia* 2008;63[8]:806–813, with permission.)

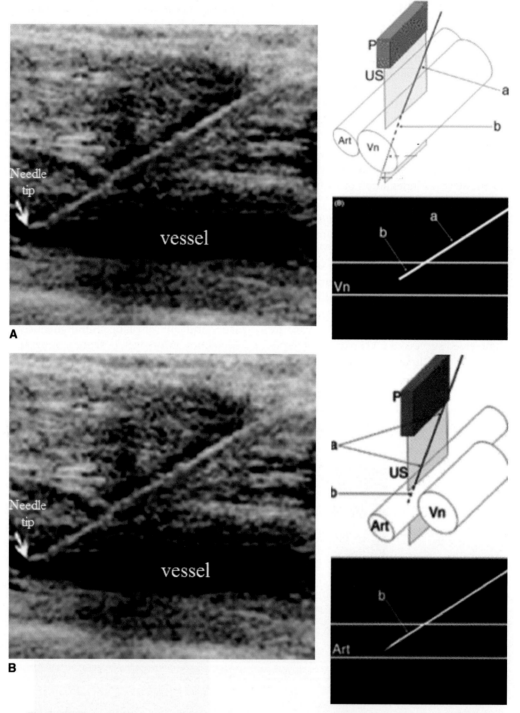

Figure 19.19. LAX Ultrasound Image of the Vessel. **A:** 2D LAX view of the vessel means that the needle will be "in plane" with the ultrasound beam. The entire length of the needle, from the shaft to the tip, is visualized. In this image, the vein is the vessel being accessed. Art, artery; Vn, vein; US, plane of the ultrasound beam; P, probe; a, needle shaft in the plane of the ultrasound beam; b, needle shaft inside the vein. **B:** The vessel visualized and unintentionally accessed is the artery. This is a pitfall in utilizing the LAX view. Art, artery; Vn, vein; US, plane of the ultrasound beam; P, probe; a, needle shaft in the plane of the ultrasound beam; b, needle shaft inside the artery. (From French JL, Raine-Fenning NJ, et al. Pitfalls of ultrasound guided vascular access: the use of three/four-dimensional ultrasound. *Anaesthesia* 2008;63[8]:806–813, with permission.)

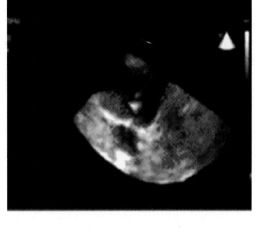

Figure 19.20. Three Orthogonal Planes used in Multiplanar Imaging. Multiplanar imaging allows for simultaneous visualization of the vessel in three orthogonal (perpendicular) planes. The transverse plane views the vessel on its SAX (i.e., the "x"-axis). The longitudinal plane views the vessel on its LAX (i.e., the "y"-axis). The coronal plane (i.e., the "z"-axis) of the vessel is termed the "plan" axis because of its resemblance to layout plans that view structures from overhead. (From French JL, Raine-Fenning NJ, et al. Pitfalls of ultrasound guided vascular access: the use of three/four-dimensional ultrasound. *Anaesthesia* 2008;63[8]:806–813, with permission.)

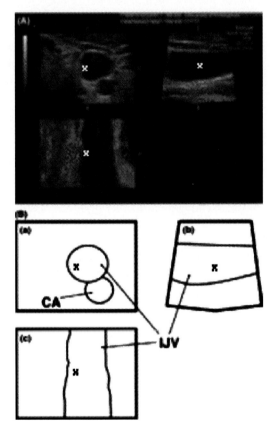

Figure 19.21. Mutltiplanar Imaging of the IJV. A multiplanar ultrasound image of the left IJV is obtained using a mechanically steered array transducer. The **top** images depict the screen images while the **bottom** illustrations are a reference diagram representing the three planes: (a) transverse, (b) longitudinal, and (c) "plan" view. The small "x" seen in all the views represents the steering marker. Simultaneous viewing of all three axes can occur and allows for venous access uncomplicated by arterial puncture. (From French JL, Raine-Fenning NJ, et al. Pitfalls of ultrasound guided vascular access: the use of three/four-dimensional ultrasound. *Anaesthesia* 2008;63[8]:806–813, with permission.)

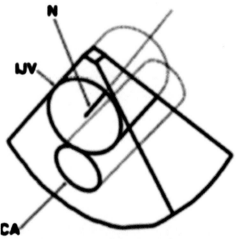

Figure 19.22. 3D Imaging of the IJV. 3D volumetric ultrasound imaging of right IJV using a matrix transducer. The cannulating needle is shown inside the vein. **Top** image = screen image, **bottom** image = reference diagram. (From French JL, Raine-Fenning NJ, et al. Pitfalls of ultrasound guided vascular access: the use of three/four-dimensional ultrasound. *Anaesthesia* 2008;63[8]:806–813, with permission.)

Development of Practice Guidelines

Many believe that U/S-guided CVC placement is rapidly becoming standard of care (15,53,71–73). The natural progression is development of guidances addressing standardization of nomenclature, application, quality assurance, training, and credentialing. The Joint Commission Public Policy Initiative published an executive summary recognizing that adherence to clinical guidelines effectively improves quality, reduces variation in care, and improves financial performance. The common thread is the improvement in patient safety.

Ultrasound guidelines for vascular access should mirror those of other ultrasonographic modalities. They should include (a) standardization of nomenclature (to encourage accurate multidisciplinary communication and conveyance of information), (b) description of the examination relevant to the practice of U/S-guided CVC placement, (c) description of the imaging planes used to identify needle and guidewire placement, d) guidance on adequate interpretation, and (e) documentation of the examination and findings (written and/or hard copy record of normal/variant/abnormal results). Equipment quality assurance would require periodic maintenance and cleaning after each patient encounter and appropriately scheduled calibration. Periodic quality review would serve not only as a tool for education and feedback to novice operators but as a monitoring tool for ongoing performance among credentialed operators.

Since U/S use is not the sole domain of any one specialty, the American Medical Association policy on ultrasound imaging privileging recommends "education standards be developed by the physician's respective specialty." ACEP suggests criteria for credentialing include an outlined training curriculum and continuous quality improvement process. This is the ultimate direction for those committed to patient safety.

KEY POINTS

- The increasing availability of ultrasound technology in the perioperative setting promotes the use of ultrasound beyond the intraoperative evaluation of the heart and great vessels.
- Ultrasound guidance can be used for central venous, arterial, and peripheral venous vascular access.
- Ultrasound guidance improves the success rate, reduces the time to cannulation, and reduces complications associated with central venous access in adults and pediatric patients.
- Ultrasonography of central vascular structures requires a high-frequency transducer probe to improve image resolution.

- A thorough understanding of the cognitive and technical skills necessary for performing ultrasound guidance vascular access is the key to improving patient care using this tool.
- SAX imaging allows for better visualization of surrounding structures whereas LAX imaging allows for better needle visualization along its entire course.
- Ultrasound-guided vascular access is especially beneficial in "high-risk" patients, for example, patients who are obese, coagulopathic, hypovolemic, or uncooperative or who have had multiple cannulations of the intended vessel.
- Ultrasound-guided vascular access provides its greatest benefit to novice operators.
- Anatomic considerations that are elucidated with ultrasound vascular access include vessel size, patency, and location in relation to the attendant artery.
- There is a steep learning curve for attaining the requisite skills to perform ultrasound-guided vascular access. Training should include didactic lectures as well as proctored "hands-on" experience.
- 3D ultrasonography of vascular structures can aid in the development of the *conceptual expertise* essential to accomplish central venous access.
- 3D vascular ultrasonography coalesces the advantages of SAX and LAX imaging averting the unintentional puncture of the attendant artery.
- The economics of an ultrasound-guided vascular access service should consider the benefits of improved success, decreased complications, cost of purchasing and maintenance of the equipment, and training of clinicians and other personnel associated with use of ultrasound in the clinical setting.
- The inclination of ultrasound-guided vascular access leans toward it becoming standard of care; therefore, the development of practice guidelines will be a future necessity.

ACKNOWLEDGMENTS

The authors would like to thank Robert K. Uzomba for his immense computer technical support and graphic design expertise.

REFERENCES

1. Costantino TG, Parikh AK, Satz WA, et al. Ultrasonography-guided peripheral intravenous access versus traditional approaches in patients with difficult intravenous access. *Ann Emerg Med* 2005;46(5):456–461.
2. Augoustides JG, Horak J, Ochroch AE, et al. A randomized controlled clinical trial of real-time needle-guided ultrasound for internal jugular venous cannulation in a large university anesthesia department. *J Cardiothorac Vasc Anesth* 2005;19(3):310–315.

3. Resnick JR, Cydulka R, Jones R. Comparison of two transducers for ultrasound-guided vascular access in long axis. *J Emerg Med* 2007;33(3):273–276.

4. Blaivas M, Brannam L, Fernandez E. Short-axis versus long-axis approaches for teaching ultrasound-guided vascular access on a new inanimate model. *Acad Emerg Med* 2003;10(12):1307–1311.

5. Phelan M, Hagerty D. The oblique view: an alternative approach for ultrasound-guided central line placement. *J Emerg Med* 2008. [Epub ahead of print]

6. Milling t, Holden C, Melniker L, et al. Randomized controlled trial of single operator vs. two-operator ultrasound guidance fo internal jugular central venous cannulation. *Acad Emerg Med* 2006;13(3):245–247.

7. Hosokawa K, Shime N, Kato Y, et al. A randomized trial of ultrasound image-based skin surface marking versus real-time ultrasound-guided internal jugular vein catheterization in infants. *Anesthesiology* 2007;107(5):720–724.

8. Resnick JR, Cydulka RK, Donato J, et al. Success of ultrasound-guided peripheral intravenous access with skin marking. *Acad Emerg Med* 2008;15(8):723–730. [Epub 2008 Jul 11]

9. Randolph AG, Cook DJ Gonzales CA, et al. Ultrasound guidance for placement of central venous catheters: a meta-analysis of the literature. *Crit Care Med* 1996;24(12):2053–2058.

10. Keenan SP. Use of ultrasound to place central lines. *J Crit Care* 2002;17(2):126–137.

11. Hind D, Calvert N, McWilliams R, et al. Ultrasonic locating devices for central venous cannulation: meta-analysis. *BMJ* 2003; 327(7411):361.

12. Institute of Medicine. *To Err is Human: Building a safer health system.* Washington, DC: National Academies Press, 2000.

13. Rothschild JM. Ultrasound guidance of central vein catheterization. Making health care safer: a critical analysis of patient safety practices. AHRQ publication. 2001:245–253.

14. Bailey PL, Glance LG, Eaton MP, et al. A survey of the use of ultrasound during central venous catheterization. *Anesth Analg* 2007;104:491–497.

15. Feller-Kopman D. Ultrasound-guided internal jugular access: a proposed standardized approach and implications for training and practice.*Chest* 2007;132(1):302–309.

16. National Institute for Clinical Excellence. NICE technology appraisal number 49: guidance on the use of ultrasound locating devices for placing central venous catheters. 2002.

17. Calvert N, Hind D, McWilliams RG, et al. The effectiveness and cost-effectiveness of ultrasound locating devices for central venous access: a systematic review and economic evaluation. *Health Technol Assess* 2003;7(12):1–84.

18. Troianos CA, Jobes DR, Ellison N. Ultrasound-guided cannulation of the internal jugular vein. A prospective, randomized study. *Anesth Analg* 1991;72(6):823–826.

19. Denys BG, Uretsky BF, Reddy PS. Ultrasound-assisted cannulation of the internal jugular vein—A prospective comparison to the external landmark guided technique. *Circulation* 1993;87:1557–1562.

20. Farrell J, Gellens M. Ultrasound-guided cannulation versus the landmark-guided technique for acute haemodialysis access. *Nephrol Dial Transplant* 1997;12(6):1234–1237.

21. Bansal R, Agarwal SK, Tiwari SC, et al. A prospective randomized study to compare ultrasound-guided with nonultrasound-guided double lumen internal jugular catheter insertion as a temporary hemodialysis access. *Ren Fail* 2005;27(5):561–564.

22. Oguzkurt L, Tercan F, Kara G, et al. US-guided placement of temporary internal jugular vein catheters: immediate technical success and complications in normal and high-risk patients. *Eur J Radiol* 2005;55(1):125–129.

23. Karakitsos D, Labropoulos N, De Groot E, et al. Real-time ultrasound-guided catheterisation of the internal jugular vein: a prospective comparison with the landmark technique in critical care patients. *Crit Care* 2006;10(6):R162.

24. Tercan F, Ozkan U, Oguzkurt L. US-guided placement of central vein catheters in patients with disorders of hemostasis. *Eur J Radiol* 2008;65(2):253–256.

25. Sznajder JI, Zveibil FR, Bitterman H, et al. Central vein catheterization: failure and complication rates by three percutaneous approaches. *Arch Intern Med* 1986;146:259–261.

26. Gallieni M. Central venous catheterization of dialysis patients. *J Vasc Access* 2000;1:10–14.

27. Orsi F, Grasso RF, Arnaldi P, et al. Ultrasound guided versus direct vein puncture in central venous port placement. *J Vasc Access* 2000;1(2):73–77.

28. Denys BG, Uretsky BF. Anatomical variations of internal jugular vein location: impact on central venous access. *Crit Care Med* 1991;19(12):1516–1519.

29. Troianos CA, Kuwik RJ, Pasqual JR, et al. Internal jugular vein and carotid artery anatomic relation as determined by ultrasonography. *Anesthesiology* 1996;85(1):43–48.

30. Gordon AC, Saliken JC, Johns D, et al. US-guided puncture of the internal jugular vein: complications and anatomic considerations. *J Vasc Interv Radiol* 1998;9(2):333–338.

31. Sulek CA, Gravenstein N, Blackshear RH, et al. Head rotation during internal jugular vein cannulation and the risk of carotid artery puncture. *Anesth Analg* 1996;82(1):125–128.

32. Wang R, Snoey ER, Clements RC, et al. Effect of head rotation on vascular anatomy of the neck: an ultrasound study. *J Emerg Med* 2006;31(3):283–286.

33. Ellison N, Jobes DR, Troianos CA. Internal Jugular cannulation. *Anesth Analg* 1994;78:198 [letter].

34. Docktor BL, Sadler DJ, Gray RR, et al. Radiologic placement of tunneled central catheters: rates of success and of immediate complications in a large series. *Am J Roentgenol* 1999;173(2):457–460.

35. Turba UC, Uflacker R, Hannegan C, et al. Anatomic relationship of the internal jugular vein and the common carotid artery applied to percutaneous transjugular procedures. *Cardiovasc Intervent Radiol* 2005;28(3):303–306.

36. Benter T, Teichgräber UK, Klühs L, et al. Anatomical variations in the internal jugular veins of cancer patients affecting central venous access. Anatomical variation of the internal jugular vein. *Ultraschall Med* 2001;22(1):23–26.

37. Mey U, Glasmacher A, Hahn C, et al. Evaluation of an ultrasound-guided technique for central venous access via the internal jugular vein in 493 patients. *Support Care Cancer* 2003;11(3): 148–155.

38. Lichtenstein D, Saifi R, Augarde R, et al. The internal jugular veins are asymmetric. Usefulness of ultrasound before catheterization. *Intensive Care Med* 2001;27:301–305.

39. Lobato EB, Sulek CA, Moody RL, et al. Cross-sectional area of the right and left internal jugular veins. *J Cardiothorac Vasc Anesth* 1999;13(2):136–138.

40. Khatri VP, Wagner-Sevy S, Espinosa MH, et al. The internal jugular vein maintains its regional anatomy and patency after carotid endarterectomy: a prospective study. *Ann Surg* 2001; 233(2):282–286.

41. Botha R, van Schoor AN, Boon JM, et al. Anatomical considerations of the anterior approach for central venous catheter placement. *Clin Anat* 2006;19(2):101–105.

42. Mallory DL, Shawker T, Evans RG, et al. Effects of clinical maneuvers on sonographically determined internal jugular vein size during venous cannulation. *Crit Care Med* 1990;18(11):1269–1273.

43. Armstrong PJ, Sutherland R, Scott DH. The effect of position and different manoeuvres on internal jugular vein diameter size. *Acta Anaesthesiol Scand* 1994;38:229–231.

44. Verghese ST, Nath A, Zenger D, et al. The effects of the simulated valalva maneuver, liver compression and/or trendelenburg position on the cross-sectional area of the internal jugular vein in infants and young children. *Anesth Analg* 2002;94:250–254.

45. Mansfield PF, Hohn DC, Fornage BD, et al. Complications and failures of subclavian-vein catheterization. *N Engl J Med* 1994;331:1735–1738.

46. McGee DC, Gould MK. Preventing complications of central venous catheterization. *N Engl J Med* 2003;348:1123–1133.

47. Ruesch S, Walder B, Tramer M. Complications of central venous catheters: internal jugular versus sbclavian access—A systematic review. *Crit Care Med* 2002;30(2):454–460.

48. Giacomini M, Iapichino G, Armani S, et al. How to avoid and manage a pneumothorax. *J Vasc Access* 2006;7(1):7–14.

49. Martin MJ, Husain FA, Piesman M, et al. Is routine ultrasound guidance for central line placement beneficial? A prospective analysis. *Curr Surg* 2004;61:71–74.

50. Gualtieri E, Deppe S, Sipperly M, et al. Subclavian venous catheterization: greater success for less experienced operators using ultrasound guidance. *Crit Care Med* 1995;23(4):692–697.

51. Sharma A, Bodenham R, Mallick A. Ultrasound-guided infraclavicular axillary vein cannulation for central venous access. *Br J Anaesth*. 2004;93(2):188–192.

52. Brooks AJ, Alfredson M, Pettigrew B, et al. Ultrasound-guided insertion of subclavian venous access ports. *Ann R Coll Surg Engl* 2005;87(1):25–27.

53. Wigemore TJ, Smythe JF Hacking MB, et al. Effect of the implementation of NICE guidelines for ultrasound guidance on the complication rates associated with central venous catheter placement in patients presenting for routine surgery in a tertiary referral centre. *Br J Anaesth* 2007;99(5):662–665.

54. Beaulieu Y, Marik PE.Bedside ultrasonography in the ICU: part 2. *Chest* 2005;128(3):1766–1781.

55. Leung J, Duffy M, Finckh A. Real-time ultrsonographically-guided internal jugular vein catheterization in the emergency department increases success rates and reduces complications: a randomized, prospective study. *Ann Emerg Med* 2006;48(5):540–547.

56. Verghese ST, McGill WA, Patel RI, et al. Ultrasound-guided internal jugular venous cannulation in infants: a prospective comparison with the traditional palpation method. *Anesthesiology* 1999;91(1):71–77.

57. Alderson PJ, Burrows FA, Stemp LI, et al. Use of ultrasound to evaluate internal jugular anatomy and to facilitate central venous cannulation in pediatric patients. *Br J Anaesth* 1993;70:145–148.

58. Grebenik CR, Boyce A, Sinclair ME, et al. NICE guidelines for central venous catheterization in children. Is the evidence base sufficient? *Br J Anaesth* 2004;92(6):827–830.

59. Leyvi G, Taylor DG, Reith E, et al. Utility of ultrasound-guided central venous cannulation in pediatric surgical patients: a clinical series. *Paediatr Anaesth* 2005;15(11):953–958.

60. Yeow KM, Toh CH, Wu CH, et al. Sonographically guided antegrade common femoral artery access. *J Ultrasound Med* 2002;21(12):1413–1416.

61. Sandhu NS, Patel B. Use of ultrasonography as a rescue technique for failed radial artery cannulation. *J Clin Anesth* 2006;18(2):138–141.

62. Schwemmer U, Arzet HA, Trautner H, et al. Ultrasound-guided arterial cannulation in infants improves success rate. *Eur J Anaesthesiol* 2006;23(6):476–480.

63. Ault MJ, Rosen BT, Ault B. The use of tissue models for vascular access training. Phase I of the procedural patient safety initiative. *J Gen Intern Med* 2006;21(5):514–517.

64. ACEP Policy Statements. *Emergency Ultrasound Guidelines*. Approved by the ACEP Board of Directors June 2001. American College of Emergency Physicians. www.acep.org

65. Atkinson P, Boyle A, Robinson S, et al. Should ultrasound guidance be used for central venous catheterisation in the emergency department? *Emerg Med J* 2005;22(3):158–164.

66. Calvert N, Hind D, McWilliams R, et al. Ultrasound for central venous cannulation: economic evaluation of cost-effectiveness. *Anaesthesia* 2004;59(11):1116–1120.

67. Domino KB, Bowdle TA, Posner KL, et al. Injuries and liability related to central vascular catheters. *Anesthesiology* 2004;100:1411–1418.

68. Riopelle JM, Ruiz DP, Hunt JP, et al. Circumferential adjustment of ultrasound probe position to determine the optimal approach to the internal jugular vein: a noninvasive geometric study in adults. *Anesth Analg* 2005;100:512–519.

69. Chapman GA, Johnson D, Bodenham AR. Visualisation of needle position using ultrasonography. *Anaesthesia* 2006;61(2):148–158.

70. French JL, Raine-Fenning NJ, Hardman JG, et al. Pitfalls of ultrasound guided vascular access: the use of three/four-dimensional ultrasound. *Anaesthesia* 2008;63(8):806–813.

71. Scott DH. It's NICE to see in the dark. *Br J Anaesth* 2003;90(3):269–272.

72. Abboud PA, Kendall JL. Ultrasound guidance for vascular access. *Emerg Med Clin North Am* 2004;22(3):749–773. Review.

73. Skippen P, Kissoon N. Ultrasound guidance for central vascular access in the pediatric emergency department. *Pediatr Emerg Care* 2007;23(3):203–207.

1. For vascular access ultrasonography, the transducer probe needs to be of
   A. high frequency, allowing for improved tissue penetration and improved image resolution
   B. low frequency, allowing for improved tissue penetration and improved image resolution
   C. high frequency, allowing for improved image resolution; tissue penetration is less important because of superficial depth of vascular structures
   D. low frequency, allowing for improved image resolution; tissue penetration is less important because of superficial depth of vascular structures

2. Which viewing axis is easiest for novice vascular ultrasound operators to use when attempting central venous access?
   A. SAX
   B. LAX
   C. Oblique access
   D. All of the above

3. True or False. Turning the head to the contralateral side improves the success and decreases the complication rate during internal jugular venous cannulation.

4. 3D ultrasound vascular access allows for all of the following *except*
   A. imaging of the vessel in the transverse, longitudinal, and coronal axes
   B. avoidance of venous transfixion with needle advancement
   C. intraluminal topography elucidation
   D. avoidance of complications

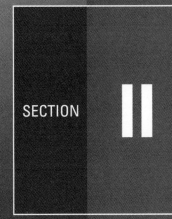

SECTION **II**

Echocardiography in the Critical Care Setting

CHAPTER 20

Overview and Relevance of Transesophageal Echocardiography in Critical Care Medicine

David T. Porembka ■ Nicolas Aeschlimann ■ Jose Diaz-Gomez

Echocardiography, and transesophageal echocardiography (TEE) in particular, is a vital diagnostic and monitoring imaging modality for the intensivist. The field of echocardiography spans several different applications, ranging from surface transthoracic echocardiography (TTE) and portable handheld echocardiography, to contrast echocardiography, stress echocardiography, and TEE, among others. Numerous investigations have proven the value of echocardiography, especially TEE, in the critically ill and injured patient, changing lives with the identification of both obvious and subtle cardiothoracic diseases. Because this powerful imaging tool is immediately available and portable, delays in diagnosis are uncommon; rather than echocardiography, TEE, specifically, should be (and is in some institutions) the standard of care and management in assisting the intensivist in the diagnosis of a variety of maladies. The effect of TEE technology is quite formidable, and numerous investigations have borne this out. The therapeutic effect of TEE ranges from 10% to 69%, with the majority of investigations falling into the 60% to 65% range. The diagnostic yield of TEE is far greater, approaching 78%. This introductory chapter will summarize the importance of echocardiography, its efficacy, and its high-yield imaging capability, particularly when compared with other imaging modalities, including TTE.

This chapter will review the clinical data revealing the importance of echocardiography and its efficacy, particularly TEE, in the critical care setting. Also, there will be special emphasis on the role of the critical care practitioner who embraces this powerful diagnostic and monitoring tool. The noninvasive cardiologist and the cardiovascular anesthesiologist are quite aware of its (echocardiography's) capabilities and its role in their practice, but they are not at the bedside in the intensive care setting when its need is required in a timely fashion. In addition, the intensivist has a keen perspective and a different mind set dealing with the critically ill and injured patient.

IMAGING ORIENTATION AND NOMENCLATURE

The standard anatomic views of cardiac structures are referred to in other chapters in this book, and have also been reported extensively elsewhere (1–6). Via the surface approach, the nomenclature for transducer location is described as parasternal, apical, subcostal, and suprasternal. The imaging planes are referred to as long axis, short axis, and four chamber. The associated reference points are apex, base, lateral, and medial (Figs. 20.1–20.5).

The core elements of a systematic TEE examination for interrogation of the following structures are

■ Left ventricle: internal dimensions and wall thickness, segmental wall motion abnormalities, overall systolic function (including estimation of ejection fraction), and diastolic filling.
■ Aortic valve and root: aortic root dimension and appearance, aortic valve anatomy, and evidence of regurgitation or stenosis.
■ Mitral valve and left atrium: mitral anatomy and motion, evidence of stenosis or regurgitation, and left atrial size.

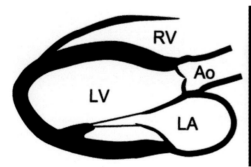
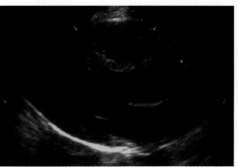

Figure 20.1. Parasternal long-axis view is shown. Ao, aorta; LA, left atrium; LV, left ventricle; RV, right ventricle. (Reproduced from Feigenbaum H, Armstrong WF, Ryan T, eds. *Feigenbaum's Echocardiography.* 6th ed. Baltimore, MD: Lippincott Williams & Wilkins, 2005, with permission.)

Figure 20.2. A: parasternal long-axis view is adjusted so that the scan plane is parallel to the long axis of the left ventricle (LV). In this plane, the proximal aorta (Ao) appears normal. **B:** plane is rotated slightly counterclockwise to better align with the long axis of the ascending aorta. By doing so, the true dimension of the aortic root is apparent. LA, left atrium; RV, right ventricle. (Reproduced from Feigenbaum H, Armstrong WF, Ryan T, eds. *Feigenbaum's Echocardiography.* 6th ed. Baltimore, MD: Lippincott Williams & Wilkins, 2005, with permission.)

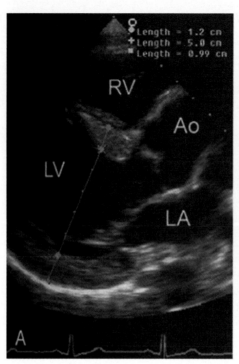
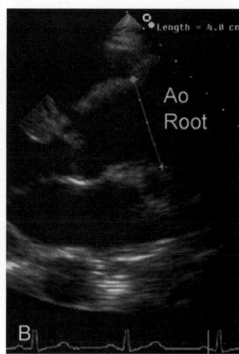

- Right heart: right ventricular size and systolic function (qualitative), right atrial size, valve anatomy and function, and estimated pulmonary artery pressure.
- Pericardium: evidence of thickening or effusion.

The imaging planes for TEE in the esophageal position are the four-chamber, two-chamber, and long-axis left ventricular. In the standard transgastric position, the planes are the short axis and the two chamber. In the deep transgastric (apical) position, there are two planes, four chamber and long axis. To complete the examination, the thoracic aorta is visualized in its entirety with the exception of the distal ascending aorta and arch vessels. The

views for the cardiac valves and chambers are referenced in Figures 20.6 to 20.9.

Invariably, the acoustic windows for TEE are greater than with the surface approach, but there are several significant limitations (7). TEE limitations include the following: underestimation of true cardiac volumes, the left ventricular apex may be foreshortened and masses and aneurysms missed, imaging of the superior or distal

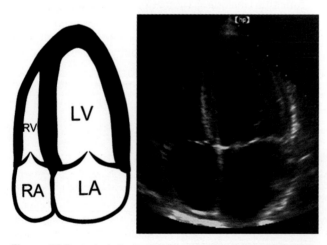

Figure 20.3. Apical four-chamber view is shown. RV, right ventricle; LV, left ventricle; RA, right atrium; LA, left atrium. (Reproduced from Feigenbaum H, Armstrong WF, Ryan T, eds. *Feigenbaum's Echocardiography.* 6th ed. Baltimore, MD: Lippincott Williams & Wilkins, 2005, with permission.)

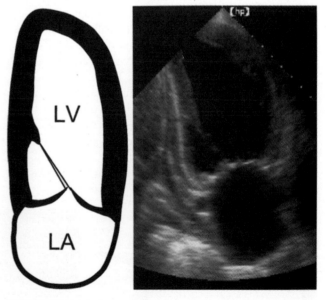

Figure 20.4. Apical two-chamber view is demonstrated. LV, left ventricle; LA, left atrium. (Reproduced from Feigenbaum H, Armstrong WF, Ryan T, eds. *Feigenbaum's Echocardiography.* 6th ed. Baltimore, MD: Lippincott Williams & Wilkins, 2005, with permission.)

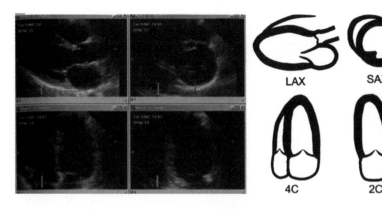

Figure 20.5. In a quad screen format, the four views most often included are the parasternal long- and short-axis and the apical four- and two-chamber views. LAX, long axis; SAX, short axis; 4C, four chamber; 2C, two chamber. (Reproduced from Feigenbaum H, Armstrong WF, Ryan T, eds. *Feigenbaum's Echocardiography*. 6th ed. Baltimore, MD: Lippincott Williams & Wilkins, 2005, with permission.)

ascending portion of the thoracic aorta is limited, and reverberation artifacts may at times be confusing to the examiner. Further, the arch vessels are not easily interrogated. In this latter situation, angiography, computed tomography angiography or magnetic resonance imaging are both helpful and complementary.

INDICATIONS AND CONTRAINDICATIONS

The indications depend on the patient, the disease state, the clinical setting (emergency department, critical care ward, cardiothoracic ward, operating room), and the operator's knowledge base and skill (Tables 20.1–20.4, Fig. 20.10) (8). Invariably, in the intensive care arena, the principal indications are usually the result of hemodynamic instability (shock), isolated or coexisting hypoxemia, myocardial ischemia or infarction, heart failure and associated complications, valvular abnormalities (native and prosthetic), cardiac masses, sources of embolism either from the cardiac chambers or the aorta, endocarditis, and pericardial disease, especially pericardial tamponade. The indications for echocardiography will vary depending on the surface approach or esophageal route, as one would expect. In the patient with difficult acoustic windows, the subcostal view might only be obtained to evaluate ventricular function. At times, there will be a crossover; in other

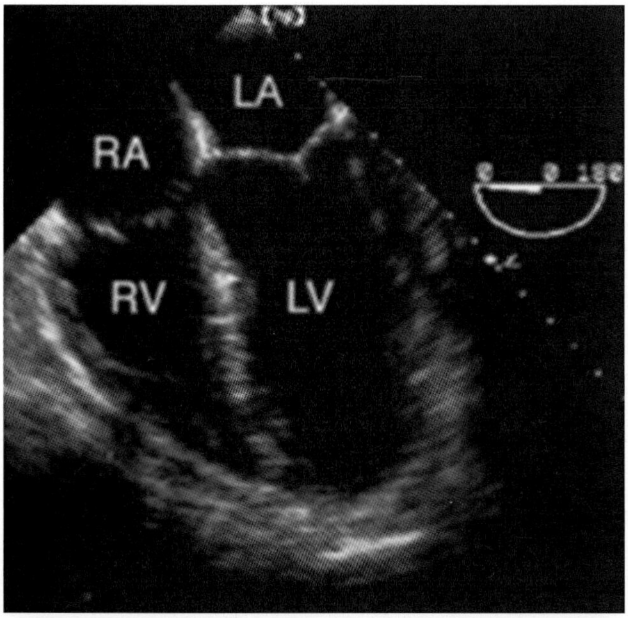

Figure 20.6. With the transducer positioned in the esophagus, a four-chamber view is illustrated. RA, right atrium; LA, left atrium; RV, right ventricle; LV, left ventricle. (Reproduced from Feigenbaum H, Armstrong WF, Ryan T, eds. *Feigenbaum's Echocardiography*. 6th ed. Baltimore, MD: Lippincott Williams & Wilkins, 2005, with permission.)

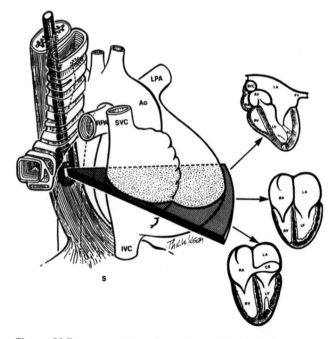

Figure 20.7. Three of the echocardiographic views that can be obtained with the horizontal probe in the mid-esophageal location. LPA, left pulmonary artery; Ao, aorta; RPA, right pulmonary artery; SVC, superior vena cava; IVC, inferior vena cava; S, stomach; LA, left atrium; PV, pulmonary vein; AV, aortic valve; LV, left ventricle; RV, right ventricle; RA, right atrium; CS, coronary sinus. (Reproduced from Feigenbaum H, Armstrong WF, Ryan T, eds. *Feigenbaum's Echocardiography*. 6th ed. Baltimore, MD: Lippincott Williams & Wilkins, 2005, with permission.)

Figure 20.8. Four of the short-axis views that can be obtained with the horizontal probe in the upper esophagus. LPA, left pulmonary artery; Ao, aorta; SVC, superior vena cava; RPA, right pulmonary artery; IVC, inferior vena cava; S, stomach; LA, left atrium; LUPV, left upper pulmonary vein; RUPV, right upper pulmonary vein; LAA, left atrial appendage; PV, pulmonary valve; RAA, right atrial appendage; LCA, left coronary artery; RCA, right coronary artery; FO, foramen ovale; RV, right ventricle; N, noncoronary cusp; R, right coronary cusp. (Reproduced from Feigenbaum H, Armstrong WF, Ryan T, eds. *Feigenbaum's Echocardiography.* 6th ed. Baltimore, MD: Lippincott Williams & Wilkins, 2005, with permission.)

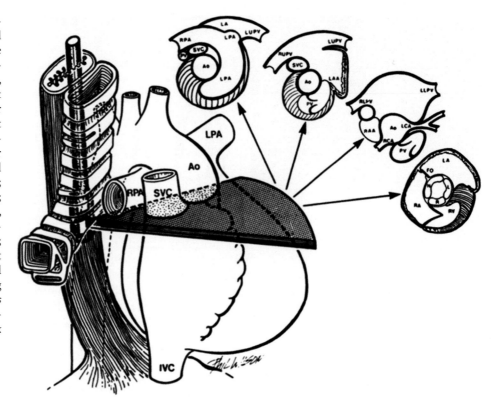

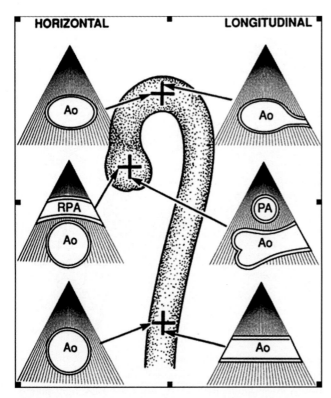

Figure 20.9. Various horizontal and longitudinal views of the aorta that can be obtained with transesophageal echocardiography. Ao, aorta; RPA, right pulmonary artery; PA, pulmonary artery. (Reproduced from Feigenbaum H, Armstrong WF, Ryan T, eds. *Feigenbaum's Echocardiography.* 6th ed. Baltimore, MD: Lippincott Williams & Wilkins, 2005, with permission.)

words, a physician may begin with TTE, then proceed immediately to TEE because of inadequate acoustic windows or inconclusive data. It is quite common, particularly in the surgical patient, to have dressings, tapes, or chest tubes interfering with the window of interrogation. Also, body habitus might present problems because of morbid obesity or severe chronic obstructive pulmonary disease. In addition, there may be the presence of a pneumothorax, which would greatly impair the acoustic window. Therefore, in these circumstances, it may be prudent to proceed immediately to a comprehensive TEE examination (7,9–30).

The contraindications to TEE are rather straightforward, especially when there is the possibility of esophageal disease (cancer, tear, penetrating injury, obstruction, or strictures) or recent gastric or esophageal surgery. In patients with upper gastrointestinal bleeding not diagnosed with endoscopy, the procedure should be avoided. Upper airway trauma and cervical neck injury are a concern, but careful manipulation of the soft tissue and anterior displacement of the mandible (while in neutral position) will allow access to the upper esophagus (Table 20.5) (1–3,5,6,24,31–41).

The TEE procedure itself is not without risk. Once the presence or absence of absolute contraindications has been considered, there must be careful consideration of the airway and oropharynx. If the patient has a potentially "full" stomach, there must be careful control of the airway. Otherwise, a "nothing by mouth" status of 6 hours is

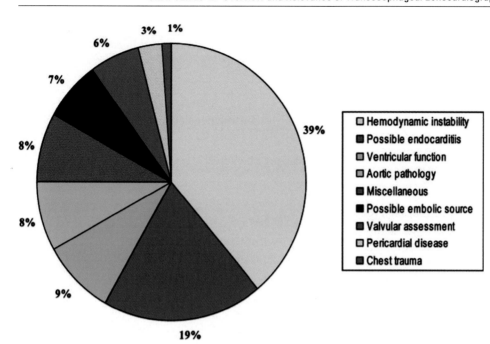

Figure 20.10. Indications for performing TEE for 2,508 studies in the ICU. (Reproduced from Huttemann E, Schelenz C, Kara F, et al. The use and safety of transoesophageal echocardiography in the general ICU: a minireview. *Acta Anaesthesiol Scand* 2004;48:827–836, with permission.)

Legend (pie chart):
- ☐ Hemodynamic instability
- ■ Possible endocarditis
- ☐ Ventricular function
- ☐ Aortic pathology
- ■ Miscellaneous
- ■ Possible embolic source
- ☐ Valvular assessment
- ☐ Pericardial disease
- ■ Chest trauma

TABLE 20.1 Admission Diagnosis

	No.	%
Admission after elective surgery	86	39.8
Multiple trauma	41	19.0
Traumatic brain injury	16	7.4
Intracranial hemorrhage	15	6.9
Acute abdomen (ileus, peritonitis, mesenteric infarction)	15	6.9
Infection, sepsis	13	6.0
Cerebral infarction	9	4.2
Subarachnoid hemorrhage	6	2.8
Necrotizing pancreatitis	6	2.8
Miscellaneous: anaphylactic shock, quadriplegia, Guillain-Barré syndrome, respiratory insufficiency, HELLP syndrome	6	2.8
Thoracic trauma	3	1.4
Total	216	100

HELLP syndrome, hemolysis, elevated liver enzymes, and low platelet count syndrome.
Adapted with permission from Huttemann E, Schelenz C, Kara F, et al. The use and safety of transoesophageal echocardiography in the general ICU: a minireview. Acta Anaesthesiol Scand *2004;48:827–836.*

TABLE 20.2 Diagnostic Findings

Main Diagnosis (Disease Mechanism Responsible for Clinical Condition)	No.	%
Hypovolemia	34	15.7
LVD and septic shock	33	15.3
LVD	26	12
RVD and septic shock	24	11.1
RVD	12	5.6
Pulmonary embolism	10	4.6
Valve dysfunction	10	4.6
Pericardial tamponade	8	3.7
Intracavity thrombi	8	3.7
Myocardial contusion	8	3.7
BVD and septic shock	7	3.2
BVD	3	1.4
Endocarditis (vegetations)	3	1.4
Miscellaneous		
Aortic dissection	1	0.5
Aortic rupture	1	0.5
Liver hematoma	1	0.5
Myocardial infarction	2	1
Total diagnostic impact	191	88.4

LVD, left ventricular dysfunction; RVD, right ventricular dysfunction; BVD, biventricular dysfunction.
Reproduced with permission from Huttemann E, Schelenz C, Kara F, et al. The use and safety of transoesophageal echocardiography in the general ICU: a minireview. Acta Anaesthesiol Scand *2004;48:827–836.*

warranted, keeping in mind that there are fair number of patients with physiologic "full stomach," such as in diabetes (gastric paresis). In these patients, the airway should be carefully assessed, and appropriate gastrointestinal precautions and medications should be used. Typically, the

TABLE 20.3	Example of How the Priority of Requested Echocardiographic Studies Might be Grouped

1. High diagnostic yield, emergency indications

    Hypotension—suspected pericardial tamponade

    Chest pain—suspected acute aortic dissection or acute myocardial infarction (nondiagnostic echocardiography)

    Heart failure—severe, unknown etiology

    Complications of endocarditis—new murmur, heart failure, prolonged PR interval

    Decompensated congenital heart disease

2. High diagnostic yield, nonemergency

    Cardiac murmur—stable patient with suspected significant valvular disease

    Clinical diagnosis of endocarditis—stable patient with definite clinical criteria for endocarditis

    Congestive heart failure—stable patient with new diagnosis of heart failure or change in clinical 1 status

    Suspected prosthetic valve dysfunction—currently stable patient with suspected valve dysfunction

    Congenital heart disease—patient with new diagnosis or previous surgery

    Coronary artery disease—stress echo for diagnosis or follow-up

    Chronic aortic root dilation

    Pulmonary heart disease or recurrent pulmonary emboli

3. High diagnostic yield but can be scheduled electively

    Known valvular heart disease—follow-up studies for ventricular size and systolic function with no interim change in clinical symptoms

    Preoperative assessment for elective surgery of patients with suspected cardiac dysfunction

    Baseline studies for cardiac surgery or valve replacement

    Source of embolus evaluation in patient <45 years of age or in patients with suspected cardiac disease

    Family history of inherited cardiac disease

    Suspected cardiac mass

    Hypertension

4. Moderate to low diagnostic yield

    Cardiac "source of embolus" in patient >45 years of age with no evidence of cardiac disease

    Screening examinations in arrhythmia patients, organ-transplant donors or recipients, or "routine" preoperative patients

Used with permission from Otto CM. Textbook of Clinical Echocardiography. 3rd ed. Philadelphia, PA: WB Saunders, 2004.

patient in question is quite ill and the airway should be secured or is already protected because of the patient's tenuous status. In the marginal patient who is delirious or uncooperative, sedation, then neuromuscular blockade, may be considered if sufficient sedation/analgesia is instilled. Usually, the risks associated with the placement of the TEE probe are hemodynamic aberrations, possible hypoxemia, and very rarely, esophageal tears. Only a few deaths may have been associated with the procedure, but it is an association and not a direct consequence. As with any procedures, risks must be balanced against the benefits, but obviously, this ratio is quite low, especially when vital information is obtained and acted on, particularly in the gravely ill patient, and therapeutic interventions are implemented (1,3–5,7,24,31–42).

EFFECT AND IMPORTANCE OF ECHOCARDIOGRAPHY

There are a variety of echocardiographic techniques available that span different levels of training, understanding, and expertise (Table 20.6) (8,10–16,20–23, 25–27,29,30,36,43). For the intensivist, surface echocardiography or TTE should be a viable option, but TEE is a necessity. The two questions that arise are, should portable echocardiography or handheld echocardiography be a required skill, and should a limited examination be sufficient to confirm or exclude a pathology? A third question that must be entertained is, which patients require a comprehensive TEE examination? This idea bridges the art of echocardiography and the field of intensive care

TABLE 20.4 Some Indications for TEE

Endocarditis with suspected paravalvular abscess

Suspected endocarditis when TTE nondiagnostic

Suspected prosthetic (especially mitral) valve dysfunction

Perioperative evaluation of MV anatomy and function before and after MV repair

Evaluation of posterior structures (e.g., interatrial baffle, sinus venosus ASD) in congenital heart disease

Suspected aortic dissection

Detection of left atrial thrombus (e.g., before catheter balloon mitral commissurotomy)

Search for cardiac "source of embolus" (including patent foramen ovale) in patients with an explained systemic embolic event

Whenever transthoracic images are nondiagnostic and echocardiography is indicated (e.g., LV function postcardiac surgery)

TTE, transthoracic echocardiography; MV, mitral valve; ASD, atrial septal defect; LV, left ventricular.
Used with permission from Otto CM. Textbook of Clinical Echocardiography. 3rd ed. Philadelphia, PA: WB Saunders, 2004.

medicine. Overall, information gained or excluded is 50% to 75% greater with TEE when compared with TTE (8,10–16,20–23,25–27,29,30,36,43).

The effect of TEE technology is quite formidable, and numerous investigations have borne this out. The therapeutic effect of TEE ranges from 10% to 69%, and the majority of investigations fall into the 60% to 65% range (Tables 20.7–20.9, Figs. 20.11–20.13) (8,10–16,20–23, 25–27,29,30,36,43). The diagnostic yield for TEE is far greater, reaching almost 78%. In searching the subset of patients with hemodynamic instability, the assistance of TEE is quite useful. Typically, the acoustic window is dramatically better with TEE because of the juxtaposition of the probe in the esophagus to the heart and extracardiac structures. As early as the study by Heidenreich et al. (17), one could easily determine the cause of hypotension. The majority of the cases are due to left ventricular systolic failure. A significant number of patients exhibit a hyperdynamic state. Other important causes identified are right ventricular systolic dysfunction, pericardial compression, and hypovolemia. This study corroborates with similar studies during this time period (8,20,22,23,25,29). In the investigation by Sohn et al. (29), the prominent pathology was global and regional involvement. This pathology is followed by valvular disease and then in equal distributions of infective endocarditis, pericardial tamponade, and aortic dissection. What is not so subtle is

TABLE 20.5 Complications of TEE in the Intensive Care Unit (21 Studies with n = 2,508 Examinations)

Category	Details	n
Airway	Displacement of tracheostomy tube (1), pulmonary aspiration during tracheal intubation before TEE (1)	2
Ventilation	Respiratory failure (1), transient hypoxia (4)	5
Circulation	Hypotension (15), hypertension (4), increases in pulmonary artery pressure (1)	20
Arrhythmias	Atrial flutter-fibrillation (5), VES (1)	6
Cardiac arrest	Circumstances not further specified (1) due to abruptly discontinued inotropic support but successful resuscitation not related to TEE study (1)	2
Seizures	Grand mal seizure (1)	1
Vomitus	(1)	1
Coughing	(7)	7
Oropharyngeal mucosal lesions	Superficial mucous lesion (1), self-terminating oral blood suffusion (15), oropharyngeal bleeding (1)	17
Removal of feeding tubes	Unintentional dislodgement of nasogastric or nasojejunal feeding tubes (21)	20
	Total	81 (3.5%)
	Excluding complications related to tube dislodgement	61 (2.6%)

VES, ventricular extrasystole.
In a total of 2,508 TEE examinations in the ICU, 81(3.5%) complications were described. If the dislodgement of feeding tubes is excluded—because the relevance is debatable and it remains unclear whether it has been systematically noted—61(2.6%) complications occurred.
Reproduced with permission from Huttemann E, Schelenz C, Kara F, et al. The use and safety of transoesophageal echocardiography in the general ICU: a minireview. Acta Anaesthesiol Scand 2004;48:827–836.

TABLE 20.6	Echocardiographic Modalities	
Modality	**Indications**	**Training**
Handheld ultrasound	Bedside evaluation by physician for pericardial effusion, LV global and regional function	Level 1 echo training
Intraoperative TEE	Evaluation of valve repair and other complex procedures	Anesthesiologists with training in echocardiography
Perioperative TEE	Evolution of the LV, RV performance limited views	Training in basic and comprehensive TEE examination
	Interrogation of the aorta and mitral valve	
	Pulmonary vein flow patterns for diastolic function	
	Identification of atrial and appendage clots	
Stress echo	Suspected or known coronary disease	Performance, risks, and interpretation of stress studies
	Myocardial viability	
	Valve and structural heart disease	
3D echo	Congenital heart disease	Image acquisition and analysis
	Rapid acquisition for LV regional function	
Contrast echo	Detection of patent foramen ovale LV endocardial detection, intracardiac shunt	Intravenous administration of contrast agents
Intravascular ultrasound	Degree of coronary narrowing and plaque morphology viewing	Interventional cardiology
Intracardiac echo	Interventional procedures (ASD closure)	Invasive cardiology training and experience
	EP	

LV, left ventricular; TEE, transesophageal echocardiography; RV, right ventricular; 3D, three-dimensional; ASD, atrial septal defect; EP, electrophysiology procedures.
Adapted with permission from Otto CM. Textbook of Clinical Echocardiography. 3rd ed. Philadelphia, PA: WB Saunders, 2004.

when a clinician suspects a pathology (prime indication) and does not detect it; there can be unsuspected findings. These unsuspected findings are described by Heidenreich et al. (17)—pericardial tamponade, right ventricular failure, severe mitral regurgitation, right atrial thrombus, an embolic source, or left ventricular outflow tract obstruction.

As stated earlier, the clinician may use information just from echocardiography rather than delay patient care for placement of a pulmonary artery catheter (PAC). Sometimes, in an emergent setting, anatomically, a PAC may not be easily placed or positioned. There may be chaos in trying to do so. In lieu of a PAC, Poelaert et al. (43) revealed that one can manipulate fluid replacement and vary inotropes or vasodilators with accuracy. In this study, data are helpful in 74% of the cases while suspected abnormalities are excluded (27%). Similarly, in comparing the two echocardiographic technologies (surface and esophageal), interventions such as catecholamine infusions, fluid augmentation, surgical interventions, antibiotics, and

beta-blockade are implemented more appropriately with TEE than TTE (150%). In relation to surgical interventions, they are fourfold higher in the TEE subgroup (8). When reviewing the effect in altering management, TEE is convincing (60% overall; medical alteration, 19%; surgical intervention, 29%) (20).

In a retrospective study of 308 patients, Colreavy et al. (13) reemphasized the importance of TEE in the critically ill. The indications for TEE are hypotension (40%), assessment of ventricular function (27%), pulmonary edema (5%), source of embolus (4%), interrogation of the aorta (4%), and miscellaneous (5%). In the former group, the root cause is identified in 67% of the cases, leading to a management change in a significant number of patients (31%). Surgery proceeds in 22% of these cases just from the data from the TEE, thus avoiding time-consuming additional tests. Overall, in this study, there was a 33% therapeutic benefit. The diagnostic yield approximates 55% (13). In the echocardiography study by Schmidlin et al. (26) (301 postoperative cardiac surgical patients),

45% of the patients exhibited a new diagnosis or a pathology was excluded. The indications in their study are typical in this setting: control of hemodynamic function, 34%; sudden hemodynamic deterioration, 29%; suspicion of pericardial tamponade, 9%; and miscellaneous, 14%. Consistently, there is a significant effect (73%) from the information obtained from imaging. Again, pharmacologic and fluid manipulation are accomplished in a significant number of cases (40%) (26).

A major use of echocardiography is, in extreme hemodynamic situations, to ascertain one important distinction: what is the cause of hypotension? Is it a myocardial issue, a low intravascular volume problem, or a pathology that is extracardiac or a combination of the above? The management is quite different in all of these cases. The clinician can immediately determine how to intervene by interrogating ventricular performance with echocardiography. It is not unusual to seek the "truth" without any invasive monitoring (PAC). Timing is crucial, and the information from PACs can be misleading (43). This is seen in the multiple-system trauma patient, a septic shock patient, or in a patient with a cardiac arrest situation (44–49). In a patient whose cardiac status is normal before the pathologic insult (either the myocardial performance is known from previous admissions or the patient is a young trauma individual with no presumed history of cardiovascular dysfunction), the dimensions in hypovolemia (systole and diastole) are decreased, with occasional systolic cavitary obliteration of the ventricle (44,50). Of note, the decrease in dimensions or area change can detect hypovolemia, regardless of whether there is a history of dilated ventricle (congestive heart failure) (50). It is not unusual in these situations (hypovolemia) and in hyperdynamic states of sepsis, systemic inflammatory response syndrome (SIRS), and liver failure, to find turbulence in the left ventricular outflow tract via color flow Doppler and observe inward movement of the distal anterior mitral valve leaflet in systole (51–53). Hypovolemia in a patient with normal left ventricular performance before the insult is easily determined by TEE and, as previously mentioned, in patients with poor systolic function. In hypertensive patients of long-standing history and in patients with left ventricular outflow tract obstruction, aortic stenosis, obstructive cardiomyopathy, and similar pathogeneses, the ventricle is presented with a pressure overload situation. These patients are at risk for hypotension once preload reaches a lower critical level (51–53). In patients with a volume overload situation, once the ventricle dilates, as in long-standing obstruction of critical aortic stenosis or in situations of severe aortic insufficiency, particularly in an acute event, the dimensions (volume) of the ventricle are extended, but in relative hypovolemia, even with large end-diastolic and end-systolic volumes, a decrease to a critical level may cause hypotension. Echocardiography, particularly TEE, easily detects these changes serially (51–53). Thus, the clinician can serially evaluate the improvement in dimen-

sions, the loss of turbulence via color flow Doppler, and the presence of left ventricular outflow tract obstruction while resuscitation is ongoing (44,50).

Another clinical scenario that echocardiography imparts a dramatic impact on is in the following clinical situation. For example, if a physician did have the availability of invasive monitoring and the following variables were present: low cardiac index of 1.1 L/min/m², a heart rate of 100 beats/min, a central venous pressure of 17 mm Hg, and a pulmonary artery occlusion pressure of 17 mm Hg, the patient could either have "relative" hypovolemia or poor myocardial performance. In this clinical scenario, it is not uncommon for the presence of left ventricular diastolic impairment to falsely elevate the pulmonary artery occlusion pressure. Without echocardiography, it would be difficult to judge the hemodynamic performance and "volume status," and treatments in these two clinical scenarios are significantly diverse. In addition, if the patient presents with acute lung injury requiring significant levels of mean airway pressure or elevated levels of positive end-expiratory pressure, the uncertainty is greater. It is also common in young trauma patients to exhibit worsening hemodynamics only until shock proceeds. In extreme hemodynamic situations with the existence of acidosis from lack of adequate organ perfusion and cellular dysfunction, myocardial performance, including systolic and diastolic dysfunction, is markedly impaired. Myocardial performance, especially contractility, can only be judged by the information from echocardiography (31,32,45,54–61). Also, patients with autonomic dysfunction and patients who may have beta blockade, for a variety reasons, may not present with tachycardia even though there is a known decrease in volume status (observation of actual blood loss), and its extent, evolution, and resolution are assessed by observing the dimensions (volume) and function of the ventricle (51–53).

To take it to another level (which has not been investigated sufficiently), is the addition of echocardiography as a formal initial diagnostic tool in the resuscitation of the critically ill beneficial or efficacious? Rivers et al. (62) suggest that early interventions in these patients in the emergency department by measuring central venous saturation (which is not the same as mixed venous saturation) as a guide to resuscitation would improve survival. Unfortunately, this is crude and physiologically global and peripheral. However, if the clinician would add echocardiography in a serial dynamic fashion, and early in the course of diagnosis and treatment, more corrective measures might be implemented.

In a review, Otero et al. (63) revealed the benefit of early goal-directed therapy in sepsis and refer to its use in other common pathologies, such as myocardial infarction and stroke. Unfortunately, none of these reports include bedside echocardiography, even the handheld device. Possessing this technology, it intuitively makes sense to have it available, and with appropriately trained personnel immediately at hand to use it in a judicious manner

TABLE 20.7	Analysis of 21 Studies on TEE in the ICU						
Author (Ref.)	Journal	Design	Year	Study Period (months)	TEE (n)	ICU Type (%)	Mortality
Alam (10)	*Prog Cardiovasc Dis*	R	1996	48	121	CICU	NA
Bruch et al. (11)	*Am J Cardiol*	R	2003	12	117	M (52) CT-SICU (48)	NA
Chenzbraun et al. (12)	*Clin Cardiol*	R	1994	39	113	CT-SICU (52) MICU (34) CCU (13)	NA
Colreavy et al. (13)	*Crit Care Med*	R	2002	48	308	MICU (68) CT-SICU (32)	38
Font et al. (14)	*Cleve Clin J Med*	R	1991	26	112	CICU	NA
Foster and Schiller (15)	*J Am Soc Echocardiogr*	R	1992	30	83	GICU (50) CCU (47) M (3)	NA
Harris et al. (16)	*Echocardiography*	R	1999	18	206	CICU	23
Heidenreich et al. (17)	*J Am Soc Echocardiogr*	P	1995	14	61	CICU	48
Huettemann et al. (18)	*Acta Anaesthesiol Scand*	R	2004	42	216	SICU	44
Hwang et al. (19)	*Chest*	R	1993	24	78	GICU (60) ER (40)	NA
Karski (36)	*Semin Cardiothorac Vasc Anesth*	R	2006	36	130	CICU	NA
Khoury (20)	*Am Heart J*	R	1994	41	77	SICU (48) CCU (24) MICU (19) NICU (7)	NA
McLean (21)	*Anaesth Intensive Care*	R	1998	24	53	GICU	NA
Oh et al. (22)	*Am J Cardiol*	R	1990	12	51	CCU (49) SICU (29.4) MICU (21.5)	NA
Pearson et al. (23)	*Am Heart J*	R	1990	10	62	CCU (49) CT-SICU (21) MICU (19) SICU (11)	NA
Poelaert et al. (43)	*Chest*	R	1995	7	103	GIGU	51
Puybasset et al. (25)	*Ann Fr Anesth Reanim*	P	1993	10	32	MICU (53) CT-SICU (34) SICU (13)	61
Schmidlin et al. (26)	*Crit Care Med*	R	2001	48	301	CT-SICU	22
Slama et al. (28)	*Intensive Care Med*	R	1996	18	61	MICU (52) CT-SICU (48)	39
Sohn et al. (29)	*Mayo Clin Proc*	R	1995	78	127	MICU (56) CT-SICU (44)	51
Vignon et al. (8)	*Chest*	R	1994	12	96	MICU (57) CT-SICU (43)	NA
Wake et al. (30)	*Can J Anaesth*	R	2001	36	130	CT-SICU	24

NS, pharmacologic treatment, fluid therapy; R, randomized; P, prospective; NA, not applicable. CICU, ICUs with a high proportion of coronary and/or cardiac surgical patients, but not further specified; CT-SICU, cardiothoracic-surgical ICU; MICU, medical ICU; SICU, surgical ICU; CCU, coronary care unit; GICU, general ICU (general adult ICU critical illness, trauma, major elective surgery); NICU, neurologic-neurosurgical ICU; ER, emergency room; M, miscellaneous.
[a]Uncooperativeness (2).
[b]Probe could not be advanced >30 cm (1).
[c]Probe could not be passed in one patient with a cervical fracture (1).
[d]Laryngoscopic guidance employed in 7%.

Patients Studies (% of ICU Admissions)	Ventilated Patients (%)	Feasibility	Complications (%)	Diagnostic	Overall Therapeutic	NS	Surgical
NA	22	98[a]	0	58	25	7	19
NA	NA	100	2	43	43	33	10
NA	65	NA[b]	7	45	26	8	18
4.2	99	99[c]	2	55	33	20	13
NA	40	NA	0	99	16	4	12
NA	NA	NA	0	77	32	13	19
NA	NA	NA	NA	47	32	19	13
NA	91	97[d]	5	97	61	41	20
6.6	98	100	6	88	69	63	6
NA	21	98[e]	0	85	NA	NA	26
NA	NA	NA	NA	42	NA	NA	NA
NA	47	100[f]	3	64	48	19	29
3.2	NA	100	NA	45	10	8	2
NA	59	98	4	59	NA	NA	24
NA	36	98[g]	5	44	NA	NA	8
11	56	NA	1	74	44	30	14
NA	100	100	0	78	NA	NA	NA
8.2	100	100	4	73	60	46	14
9.1	66	100	20	45	20	12	8
NA	81	98	2	52	NA	NA	21
NA	86	100	0	97	41	33	8
2.1	100	100	0	91	58	43	15

[e]Failed insertion (2).
[f]Difficult insertion (5).
[g]Failed insertion (patient with large aneurysm of the thoracic aorta compressing the esophagus) (1).
Number of patients in parentheses.
Adapted from Huttemann E, Schelenz C, Kara F, et al. The use and safety of transoesophageal echocardiography in the general ICU: a minireview. Acta Anaesthesiol Scand 2004;48:827–836.

TABLE 20.8	Population Characteristics and TEE Exams			
ASA/SCA Category		**I**	**II**	**III**
Total number of patients[a,b]	n = 214	89 (41)	67 (31)	58 (27)[a,b]
Age, mean years	57	57	58	57
Gender, male/female (n)	131/83	53/36	43/24	35/23
Patients with modified therapy after TEE	n = 86	53	21	12[a,b]
Percentage per category		60%	31%	21%
Age, mean years	60	61	60	52
Gender, male/female (n)	49/37	32/21	11/10	6/6
Patients without modified therapy after TEE	128	36	46	46[a,b]
Percentage per category		28%	36%	36%
Age, mean years	60	58	61	59
Gender, male/female (n)	81/47	19/17	33/13	29/17
Site of examinations				
OR	n = 155	44	57	54
RR	n = 4		3	1
SICU	n = 55	42	9	4[a,b]
No. of patients without modified therapy per site				
OR	n = 43	20	13	10[a,b]
RR	n = 3	2	1	
SICU	n = 40	31	7	2[a,b]
Total no. of modifications	n = 118	59	44	15[b,c]

ASA/SCA, American Society of Anesthesiologists/Society of Cardiovascular Anesthesiologists; OR, operating room; RR, recovery room; SICU, surgical intensive care unit.
[a]*p < 0.05 for category I versus II.*
[b]*p < 0.05 for category I versus III.*
[c]*p < 0.05 for category II versus III.*
Reproduced with permission from Denault AY, Couture P, McKenty S, et al. Perioperative use of transesophageal echocardiography by anesthesiologists: impact in noncardiac surgery and in the intensive care unit. Can J Anaesth 2002;49:287–293.

will no doubt make a significant impact. Nevertheless, this is implicated by Burns et al. (47) in an investigation of acutely ill trauma patients utilizing TEE. They show that approximately two thirds of their patients benefit from this technology by altering the management style. As one would expect, numerous patients with "acceptable" filling pressures (from the PAC) did in fact have inadequate filling. This reaffirms what is previously stated in acidotic conditions with impairment of ventricular performance and the lack of tissue oxygenation (47,64–67).

Common maladies in the intensive care setting are patients who exhibit sepsis, septic shock, and SIRS (68). Sepsis, bacteremia, and inflammation cause myocardial depression. It is one of those diseases that requires early and correct diagnosis, appropriate and timely interventions, the correct "amount" of fluid resuscitation, early use of the appropriate antibiotics, the implementation of the Acute Respiratory Distress Syndrome Network protocol when

acute lung injury ensues, and the implementation of inotropic/vasopressor support (27,46,48,56,58,60,61,69–75). The mechanism of the dysfunction is clearly not established, partly because dysfunction can be elicited by many different mechanisms, which can all affect disruption of myocardial mechanical function. In addition, the models of sepsis and bacteremia and inflammation may vary drastically in the sequence of coordinated immune response to the inflammatory or septic stimuli. A variety of patterns of cytokine expression affect the immune system and patterns of neurohumoral activation in response to the stress of sepsis or response. Stress-induced activation of the sympathetic nervous system and humoral responses to stress have a wide range of intensity that can be elicited. The fairly uniform response of the myocardium is volume or cardiac output and pressure work, as estimated by ventricular pressure, are impaired and myocardial contraction is compromised (27,46,48,55,58,60,61,69–75). At

TABLE 20.9	Summary of Surgical Modifications Related to the Use of TEE	
Hemodynamic instability in the ICU		
Tamponade leading to mediastinal exploration		8
Mitral regurgitation and myocardial ischemia after gynecological surgery leading to mitral valve replacement and coronary revascularization		1
Vascular surgery		
Aortic dissection associated with pericardial effusion leading to a femoral bypass before surgery		2
Absence of aortic dissection		2
Unsuspected atrial thrombus and severe mitral stenosis leading to thrombectomy and mitral valve replacement		1
Lung transplantation		
Right ventricular dysfunction leading to cardiopulmonary bypass		2
Air emboli leading to revision of vascular anastomosis		1
Neurosurgery		
Detection of patent foramen ovale before ramisectomy leading to surgical positional change		2
Total		**19**

Reproduced from Denault AY, Couture P, McKenty S, et al. Perioperative use of transesophageal echocardiography by anesthesiologists: impact in noncardiac surgery and in the intensive care unit. Can J Anaesth 2002;49:287–293, with permission.

times, diastolic function, assessed by ventricular relaxation and filling, is impaired (58,60,70,74,76–81). In addition to the dysfunction (systolic and diastolic) that occurs, there is a longer-term response of the ischemia/perfusion episodes and by numerous pharmacologic agents and heat stress and modified forms of polysaccharide. The myocardium develops protection after initial stress that during a second stress, the myocardium does not exhibit as much damage as does a nonprotected heart. Many agents can induce this protection, which has been termed *preconditioning*. Both early preconditioning (protection that is measurable minutes to hours after the initial stimuli) and late preconditioning (protection that is measurable in hours to days after the initial trigger or stimulus) are effective in protecting the heart from prolonged ischemia and reperfusion injury (27,46,48,55,56,58,60,61,69–75). Understanding the mechanisms of sepsis- /bacteremia-induced dysfunction and protection and whether that dysfunction and protection are the products of the same intracellular pathways is important in protecting the heart from a multitude of mechanism by which the myocardium maintains reserve capacity. Having echocardiography as a diagnostic and monitoring tool will improve understanding of this disease state and others.

There is a voluminous amount of literature and research concentrating on the myocardial effects of sepsis (55,56,61,69,72,73,75,82–84). It is no doubt difficult to mimic the human response in animal and cell-cultured models. Even similar species respond differently, depending on the type of septic-induced model (lipopolysaccharide, endotoxin, cecal ligation, and perforation). What is clear is this response may be paradoxic or opposite to intuitive thinking. Echocardiography is an extremely useful imaging device to assist in the management of these complex, yet paradoxic patients. In these complex and perplexing patients, the efficacy of TEE is observed. The

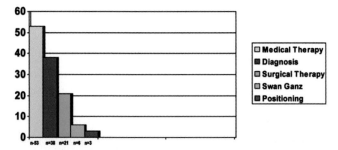

Figure 20.11. Distribution of the total number of modifications that are detailed according to category I–III indications for TEE. (Reproduced from Denault AY, Couture P, McKenty S, et al. Perioperative use of transesophageal echocardiography by anesthesiologists: impact in noncardiac surgery and in the intensive care unit. *Can J Anaesth* 2002;49: 287–293, with permission.)

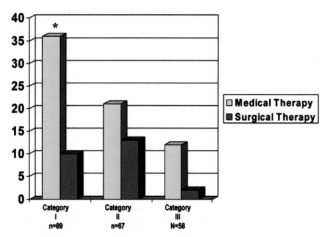

Figure 20.12. Medical and surgical effects according to indication category. *p < 0.001 for medical therapy in category I versus II and I versus III. (Reproduced from Denault AY, Couture P, McKenty S, et al. Perioperative use of transesophageal echocardiography by anesthesiologists: impact in noncardiac surgery and in the intensive care unit. *Can J Anaesth* 2002;49:287–293, with permission.)

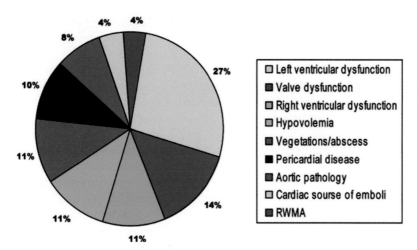

Figure 20.13. Diagnosis established by TEE in the ICU based on 2,508 studies. (Reproduced from Huttemann E, Schelenz C, Kara F, et al. The use and safety of transoesophageal echocardiography in the general ICU: a minireview. *Acta Anaesthesiol Scand* 2004;48:827–836, with permission.)

- ☐ Left ventricular dysfunction
- ■ Valve dysfunction
- ☐ Right ventricular dysfunction
- ☐ Hypovolemia
- ■ Vegetations/abscess
- ■ Pericardial disease
- ■ Aortic pathology
- ☐ Cardiac sourse of emboli
- ■ RWMA

unique difference in this study is evaluating prospectively the interpretations (training) of intensivists. In this study, ventricular function (right and left) and volume status are correctly identified by these practitioners (85).

One of the most controversial issues (hemodynamic manipulation) in intensive care medicine is what to do with patients who exhibit a hyperdynamic circulation (43,61,81,86). Globally, the effects (hyperdynamic circulation) on the myocardium are quite unique, and understanding its response may allow the clinician and the scientist to better appreciate the inflammatory and immune response of the human body to this disease and other diseases such as liver failure and the traumatic patient in shock. Echocardiography is the tool to evaluate this dynamic disease process. What are the end points of resuscitation utilizing echocardiography, volume or dimensions, systolic and diastolic functions? What is not known in any of these situations is when does it become an irreversible or a futile condition for which any heroic resources will not make a difference or lessen the severity?

In sepsis or SIRS, the physiologic effects on the heart are similar but yet dissimilar on the ventricle or atrium because of its inherent (premorbid) chamber physical properties (pressure/volume characteristics) or fluid dynamics. The left ventricle is used to high pressures on itself and, to a certain point, the chamber will thicken and then dilate or dilate from the overload situation. Commonly, in pressure overload clinical scenarios such as aortic stenosis, the former will occur, while in the increased volume overload return to the heart (aortic insufficiency), the chamber will thin and dilate. The resultant effects will obviously depend on timing and extent of these loading conditions. What may be novel in the inflammatory response is a paradoxic response between survivors and nonsurvivors. It seems that in survivors, there will be a Frank-Starling effect or what appears to be an increase in compliance of the left ventricle. However, this is true and not true. The left ventricle does dilate, but the compliance decreases. The extent is accentuated in survivors. In other words, at greater end-systolic and end-diastolic volumes or dimensions, the chance for survival is much enhanced (48). What seems paradoxic is that a decrease in the slope of isovolumetric/pressure line (an index of contractility

that is load independent) is associated with an increase in survival and a decrease in cardiac compliance (76).

The resultant effect will be a lower ejection fraction (which is load dependent) with high cardiac outputs, tachycardia, higher stroke volumes, and elevated mixed venous saturations. As the process ensues, hypotension will occur, impairment of cellular function will follow, and the global ventricular volume response to resuscitation and fluid will become ineffective (55,58,69,70). This compensatory survivor response must be short-lived (recognized early), and investigations reveal that in 48 to 72 hours, if there is no "normalization," the chance for survivor greatly diminishes. Persistent tachycardia is a marker of death (87). Several studies show the discontinuity of the heart rate in the presence of sepsis. There is an apparent sympathovagal imbalance and variability that is also observed in the pediatric population. Atrial dysrhythmias are common in the clinical presentation and the progression of sepsis. There is obvious atrial dysfunction, but it is not well studied as the ventricular response. TEE is an obvious diagnostic tool to interrogate this by evaluating atrial function and volume by reviewing the left atrial appendage flow characteristics in concert with analysis of ventricular function and volume, ventricular interaction of dependency, transmitral inflow velocities, and pulmonary venous flow patterns (70,88).

In sepsis or SIRS, the right ventricle responds similarly, but at some unknown end point, when the volume is exceedingly high, the compensatory response is no longer beneficial and mortality dramatically rises. This makes sense because, normally, the right ventricle does not handle high pressures or increased volumes because of the thinned, enveloped configuration. Possibly, an early cardiovascular response in sepsis is pulmonary artery hypertension. Of note, there is no known investigation primarily concentrating or evaluating this increase in pressure. However, this pulmonary artery hypertension appears to be associated with increased mortality, but no serial investigations have been completed. Also, no studies have either interrogated patients with preexisting pulmonary hypertension or heart failure who experience an inflammatory load. Echocardiography, especially TEE, would seem to be ideal for this type of study and of clinical utility (77,83).

In a clinical investigation by Poelaert et al. (43), based on transmitral inflow velocities and pulmonary venous flow patterns, patients with a decrease in transmitral inflow velocities and an abnormal pulmonary venous flow and a decrease in fractional area contraction are more likely to die as compared to two other subgroups. As expected, this pattern is particularly seen in the older patients.

This hyperdynamic circulatory response was earlier associated with a myocardial depressant factor and now is known for a variety of mediators, cytokines, and humoral factors that are all related and intertwined. It is also known that even ablating this hyperdynamic response with normalization of the circulating function will not lessen mortality but may even increase it. It is now known there is protective effect if exposed earlier to mediators/cytokines, and this septic-induced depression is reversible (55,56,69,72).

Early and accurate interventions may preclude the resultant affects of sepsis, inflammatory, and stress-related diseases. It is not known at what end point in this aggression to treat these patients, particularly hemodynamically. What is adequate volume replacement, which is key in the first response, to these patients? There must be an obvious end-diastolic volume to achieve, but it has yet to be characterized. Suffice it to say, continue fluid resuscitation as the patient responds. In the nonresponders, fluid replacement is important but probably to a lesser extent, and the addition of norepinephrine is efficacious. Hopefully, knowing the preexisting cardiac performance in these patients will assist in the determination of the pharmacologic interventions, fluid augmentation, and other modalities (79–81). It is intuitive that if the baseline cardiac function is poor, volume should be instilled judiciously and adjunct pharmacologic measures should be administered earlier and more aggressively. Echocardiography is a useful tool to initially identify and follow all of the hemodynamic variables. This diagnostic tool alone might suffice, but until further data are available, using it complementary with invasive monitoring is crucial and underlines the art of medicine, including echocardiography (44,55,56,69).

An obvious advantage of using echocardiography is real-time imaging and assessing various echocardiographic hemodynamic variables. Please refer to this supplement's section on hemodynamic assessment via echocardiography. Also, a reference for standards in Doppler is provided (89). In the critically ill, there are numerous loading conditions affecting measured indices via the PAC. The pulmonary occlusion pressure is inherently inaccurate, especially in these loading conditions, such as an increase in afterload, ventricular hypertrophy, aortic stenosis, and particularly clinical situations when inflammatory conditions are occurring. A decrease in left ventricular compliance is a common problem, but echocardiography can assess this abnormality via interrogation of the transmitral inflow velocities, tissue Doppler imaging, and patterns in the pulmonary venous flows (76,90). Identifying a patient with left ventricular diastolic dysfunction is a prognostic indicator in the cardiac surgical patient and patient with acute myocardial infarction (91). Septic patients are not

alone, but unfortunately, there are no investigations that identify this problem, alleviate the dysfunction acutely, and hence show improvement in clinical outcome.

Besides including septic shock or patients with SIRS, the management of other forms of shock should include echocardiography, particularly TEE. Shock is the inadequacy of cellular and tissue oxygen supply. There are different types of presentations, and sometimes they are multifactorial and perplexing. The intensive care clinician is quite familiar with these complex patterns, including the immunologic and biochemical features associated in inadequate perfusion states and cellular impairment. The benefit of TEE is to adequately identify the patterns and the response to treatments, including significant amount of fluid administration. Echocardiography provides acceptable estimates of most variables obtained from the PAC (e.g., cardiac output; right atrial pressure from the inferior vena caval dimensions and respiratory variations; systolic pulmonary artery pressure; left and right filling pressures; left and right ventricular dimensions or volumes; myocardial indices including ejection fraction, diastolic function, ischemic myocardium, and ventricular mass) (51–53).

Echocardiography can assess the response to fluid responsiveness that is crucial as a potential end point of resuscitation (60,86,92). As expected, surface technology is less efficacious than TEE. Again, assessing the dimensions or area is crucial. It appears that in comparison, areas are less reliable than dimensional change. Probably the best ventricular performance indices are the constructing of pressure–volume loops (which are load independent) (58,90,93). This a well-known method, as studied extensively by Suga and Sagawa (46,48,58,78–80,90,93–95). Pinsky et al. (79) show its clinical use and benefits. P:V loops allow an understanding of cellular dysfunction to act as a bridging mechanism that links the laboratory with the bedside (96). Understanding the basics of echocardiography and what it has to offer in a variety of critical care scenarios improves the clarity that may cloud the physiologic picture before its use (97,98).

Another significant important use for TEE is in atrial fibrillation. Frequently, atrial dysrhythmias occur in the intensive care unit (ICU), especially in postoperative cardiac surgical patients. TEE is a useful tool to diagnose a potential thrombus in the left atrium and appendage (99,100). There is proven efficacy of TEE-guided cardioversion of patients with atrial fibrillation at 6-month follow-up, particularly in patients when this rhythm disturbance is noted for lasting more than 48 hours (88,97,98).

TEE makes one of its greatest impacts in the identification of aortic diseases, which is well described in this supplement. Before TEE evolution, these disease processes were only speculated if ever considered. Much has been done revealing TEE's benefit and role in aortic trauma and its management, including the placement of aortic stents, the identification of the initial insult, and its progression and follow-up, as in aortic dissection and aneurysm (99–101). There is no question of the benefit of the ability to interrogate the aorta, especially in the hemodynamically unstable patient or in a multiple trauma patient who is complex and the pathologies are yet to be identified, particularly in the early trauma resuscitation and diagnosis (102,103). In some patients, in whom radiographic contrast agent institution is problematic, TEE reaches the forefront as a diagnostic tool. In this author's opinion, angiography is not the "gold standard" in the evaluation of aortic diseases, but this is far from uniform acceptance. Computed tomography is an ideal imaging method but is not without hazards and the need for transporting a patient who can succumb to previous unknown pathologies. Magnetic resonance imaging is the best imaging tool of the aorta but the same limitations are ever present. So, in the complex, unstable patient, TEE should be considered first and potentially complementary to the other imaging techniques (99).

Atherosclerosis of the aorta is a concern for the intensivist and the cardiac surgery physician, especially as a potential source of embolism (104,105). TEE is ideal for the diagnosis of this problem (105). Diagnosis of the potential for a central embolic event, such as stroke, has a significant effect on the morbidity and mortality of the patient (106). The aorta may be a nidus for peripheral system or multiple system disorders, even a source for sepsis. Not forgetting about the aorta may explain many issues to the intensivist from the early choice of imaging.

By reviewing the published data, TEE offers a convincing argument for its use. It is efficacious and proven safe. The review of the investigation by Huttemann et al. (18) reveals an in-house hospital mortality of 43.0%, which is not unexpected because, by nature, those requiring imaging are inherently critically ill. These patients are not always interrogated at admission or during the first 24 hours, when scoring systems invariably are completed. This cohort study shows an expected mortality of 10% to 16% (18). This is in concordance from previous investigations (22% to 61%) (17,21,25,26,28,29,43). Typically, as in our experience, this follows suit. When patients exhibit severe left ventricular dysfunction with shock (impaired tissue utilization including anaerobic metabolism), the mortality is quite higher than published proceedings. In patients with right ventricular failure and biventricular failure after cardiac procedures, again the mortality is exceedingly higher but not unexpected (91% and 63%, respectively). With isolated left ventricular dysfunction, the prognosis is immediate (44%), whereas hypovolemia (21%) and pericardial tamponade fare a better outcome (107). In patients who exhibit either pericardial or valvular disease, which are both alleviated by surgical intervention, the outcome is better overall (17,108). However, in patients who are in hyperdynamic condition, the outcome offers markedly worse results (17). Of interest, which has not been investigated well, if a patient who is in septic shock or who has liver failure and is exhibiting pulmonary hypertension yet not to the extent of failure, the mortality is exceedingly high, probably uniform. Having an intensivist at the bedside with this powerful diagnostic imaging may answer this issue with certainty and provide further insights into so many diseases.

The intensivist for obvious reasons should embrace TEE. TTE is a first imaging device that should be in consideration. Should surface echocardiography replace the stethoscope at the bedside to diagnose so many maladies? Should this tool be with the intensive care physician on the front line with the rapid response team, in the emergency department, and of course, in the intensive care arena? Numerous pathologies and problems, especially in the surgical arena, come to the intensivist with barely any workup or previous knowledge of any potential pathology that some may be subtle, hidden, and potentially catastrophic. Health care makes the case for limited and cost-saving measures (12,31–33,44,47). Reviewing the literature, echocardiography is significantly a cost-saving tool. It decreases morbidity and mortality and probably the length of ventilatory days, length of ICU days, and overall hospital days, but prospective analysis is the obvious next step, and intensive care physicians are an integral part of this equation. However, in investigation by Schmidlin et al. (26), there is a contrast in length of stay, ventilatory days, and mortality (26). This is explained that more gravely ill patients underwent a TEE examination, avoiding surface technology. The question arises as to where to get the training, the oversight, the compliance issues, and quality assurance with archival retrieval that is immediately available and secure (Table 20.10) (1,109,110).

TABLE 20.10	Summary of ACC/AHA Recommendations for Physicians in Echocardiography			
Level of Expertise	Duration (months)	No. of Studies Performed	Cumulative No. of Studies Interpreted	Annual Studies to Maintain Complete Competence
1	3	75	150	
2	6	150	300	300
3	12	300	750	500
Stress echo		100		100
TEE		50		25–50

TEE, transesophageal echocardiography.
Reproduced with permission from Otto CM. Textbook of Clinical Echocardiography. 3rd ed. Philadelphia, PA: WB Saunders, 2004.

KEY POINTS

■ Hemodynamic instability in the ICU is a class I indication for TEE.

■ TEE provides better acoustic windows than TTE in almost all mechanically ventilated patients.

■ TEE will generally lead to a change in management in greater than 50% of ICU patients when performed for hemodynamic instability.

■ TEE has better diagnostic performance characteristics than TTE for assessment of suspected infective endocarditis.

■ New certification examinations specifically testing knowledge of TEE in the noncardiac surgical setting signal the arrival of TEE as a mainstream diagnostic modality in critical care medicine.

■ Critical care medicine practitioners are well advised to develop skill in the basic principles of both TTE and TEE, since these techniques are likely to play an increasingly important role in the management of ICU patients in both cardiac and noncardiac intensive care units.

REFERENCES

1. Cheitlin MD, Armstrong WF, Aurigemma GP, et al. ACC/AHA/ASE 2003 guideline update for the clinical application of echocardiography: summary article. A report of the American College of Cardiology/American Heart Association Task Force on Practice Guidelines (ACC/AHA/ASE Committee to Update the 1997 Guidelines for the Clinical Application of Echocardiography). *Circulation* 2003;108:1146–1162.

2. Braunwald E, Zipes DP, Libby P, et al., eds. *Braunwald's Heart Disease: A Textbook of Cardiovascular Medicine.* 7th ed. Philadelphia: Elsevier Saunders, 2004.

3. Nanda NC, Domanski MJ, eds. *Atlas of Transesophageal Echocardiography.* 2nd ed. Baltimore, MD: Lippincott Williams & Wilkins, 2006.

4. Vannan MA, Lang RM, Rabowski H, et al., eds. *Atlas of Echocardiography.* Philadelphia, PA: Current Medicine, 2005.

5. Otto CM. *Textbook of Clinical Echocardiography.* 3rd ed. Philadelphia, PA: WB Saunders, 2004.

6. Feigenbaum H, Armstrong WF, Ryan T, eds. *Feigenbaum's Echocardiography.* 6th ed. Baltimore, MD: Lippincott Williams & Wilkins, 2005.

7. Weyman AE. The year in echocardiography. *J Am Coll Cardiol* 2006;47:856–863.

8. Vignon P, Mentec H, Terre S, et al. Diagnostic accuracy and therapeutic impact of transthoracic and transesophageal echocardiography in mechanically ventilated patients in the ICU. *Chest* 1994;106:1829–1834.

9. D'Cruz IA, ed. *Echocardiographic Anatomy: Understanding Normal and Abnormal Echocardiograms.* Stamford, CT: Appleton and Lange, 1996.

10. Alam M. Transesophageal echocardiography in critical care units: Henry Ford hospital experience and review of the literature. *Prog Cardiovasc Dis* 1996;38:315–328.

11. Bruch C, Comber M, Schmermund A, et al. Diagnostic usefulness and impact on management of transesophageal echocardiography in surgical intensive care units. *Am J Cardiol* 2003;91:510–513.

12. Chenzbraun A, Pinto FJ, Schnittger I. Transesophageal echocardiography in the intensive care unit: impact on diagnosis and decision-making. *Clin Cardiol* 1994;17:438–444.

13. Colreavy FB, Donovan K, Lee KY, et al. Transesophageal echocardiography in critically ill patients. *Crit Care Med* 2002;30:989–996.

14. Font VE, Obarski TP, Klein AL, et al. Trans-esophageal echocardiography in the critical care unit. *Cleve Clin J Med* 1991;58:315–322.

15. Foster E, Schiller NB. The role of trans-esophageal echocardiography in critical care: UCSF experience. *J Am Soc Echocardiogr* 1992;5:368–374.

16. Harris KM, Petrovic O, Davila-Roman VG, et al. Changing patterns of transesophageal echocardiography use in the intensive care unit. *Echocardiography* 1999;16:559–565.

17. Heidenreich PA, Stainback RF, Redberg RF, et al. Transesophageal echocardiography predicts mortality in critically ill patients with unexplained hypotension. *J Am Coll Cardiol* 1995;26:152–158.

18. Huttemann E, Schelenz C, Kara F, et al. The use and safety of transoesophageal echocardiography in the general ICU: a mini-review. *Acta Anaesthesiol Scand* 2004;48:827–836.

19. Hwang JJ, Shyu KG, Chen JJ, et al. Usefulness of transesophageal echocardiography in the treatment of critically ill patients. *Chest* 1993;104:861–866.

20. Khoury AF, Afridi I, Quinones MA, et al. Transesophageal echocardiography in critically ill patients: feasibility, safety, and impact on management. *Am Heart J* 1994;127:1363–1371.

21. McLean AS. Transoesophageal echocardiography in the intensive care unit. *Anaesth Intensive Care* 1998;26:22–25.

22. Oh JK, Seward JB, Khandheria BK, et al. Transesophageal echocardiography in critically ill patients. *Am J Cardiol* 1990;66:1492–1495.

23. Pearson AC, Castello R, Labovitz AJ. Safety and utility of transesophageal echocardiography in the critically ill patient. *Am Heart J* 1990;119:1083–1089.

24. Porembka DT. Transesophageal echocardiography. *Crit Care Clin* 1996;12:875–918.

25. Puybasset L, Saada M, Catoire P, et al. Contribution of transesophageal echocardiography in intensive care: A prospective assessment. *Ann Fr Anesth Reanim* 1993;12:17–21.

26. Schmidlin D, Schuepbach R, Bernard E, et al. Indications and impact of postoperative transesophageal echocardiography in cardiac surgical patients. *Crit Care Med* 2001;29:2143–2148.

27. Slama M, Maizel J. Echocardiographic measurement of ventricular function. *Curr Opin Crit Care* 2006;12:241–248.

28. Slama MA, Novara A, Van de Putte P, et al. Diagnostic and therapeutic implications of transesophageal echocardiography in medical ICU patients with unexplained shock, hypoxemia, or suspected endocarditis. *Intensive Care Med* 1996;22:916–922.

29. Sohn DW, Shin GJ, Oh JK, et al. Role of transesophageal echocardiography in hemodynamically unstable patients. *Mayo Clin Proc* 1995;70:925–931.

30. Wake PJ, Ali M, Carroll J, et al. Clinical and echocardiographic diagnoses disagree in patients with unexplained hemodynamic instability after cardiac surgery. *Can J Anaesth* 2001;48:778–783.

31. Beaulieu Y, Marik PE. Bedside ultrasonography in the ICU: Part 2. *Chest* 2005;128:1766–1781.

32. Beaulieu Y, Marik PE. Bedside ultrasonography in the ICU: Part 1. *Chest* 2005;128:881–895.
33. Brickner ME. Transesophageal echocardiography. *J Diagn Med Sonogr* 2005;21:309.
34. Harris KM, Li DY, L'Ecuyer P, et al. The prospective role of transesophageal echocardiography in the diagnosis and management of patients with suspected infective endocarditis. *Echocardiography* 2003;20:57–62.
35. Fuster V, Alexander RW, O'Rourke RA, et al., eds. *Hurst's the Heart*. 11th ed. New York: McGraw Hill Professional, 2004.
36. Karski JM. Transesophageal echocardiography in the intensive care unit. *Semin Cardiothorac Vasc Anesth* 2006;10:162–166.
37. Kronzon I, Tunick PA, eds. *Challenging Cases in Echocardiography*. Baltimore, MD: Lippincott Williams & Wilkins, 2005.
38. Mathew J, Chakib A, eds. *Clinical Manual and Review of Transesophageal Echocardiography*. New York: McGraw Hill, 2005.
39. Milani RV, Lavie CJ, Gilliland YE, et al. Overview of transesophageal echocardiography for the chest physician. *Chest* 2003;124:1081–1089.
40. Peterson GE, Brickner ME, Reimold SC. Transesophageal echocardiography: clinical indications and applications. *Circulation* 2003;107:2398–2402.
41. Price S, Nicol E, Gibson DG, et al. Echocardiography in the critically ill: current and potential roles. *Intensive Care Med* 2006;32:48–59.
42. Nowak M, Rosenberger P, Felbinger TW, et al. Perioperative echocardiography: basic principles. *Anaesthesist* 2006;55:337–361.
43. Poelaert JI, Trouerbach J, De Buyzere M, et al. Evaluation of transesophageal echocardiography as a diagnostic and therapeutic aid in a critical care setting. *Chest* 1995;107:774–779.
44. Axler O. Evaluation and management of shock. *Semin Respir Crit Care Med* 2006;27:230–240.
45. Bracco D, Dubois MJ. Hemodynamic support in septic shock: is restoring a normal blood pressure the right target? *Crit Care Med* 2005;33:2113–2115.
46. Burkhoff D, Mirsky I, Suga H. Assessment of systolic and diastolic ventricular properties via pressure-volume analysis: a guide for clinical, translational, and basic researchers. *Am J Physiol Heart Circ Physiol* 2005;289:H501–H512.
47. Burns JM, Sing RF, Mostafa G, et al. The role of transesophageal echocardiography in optimizing resuscitation in acutely injured patients. *J Trauma* 2005;59:36–40; discussion, 40–42.
48. Cesar S, Potocnik N, Stare V. Left ventricular end-diastolic pressure-volume relationship in septic rats with open thorax. *Comp Med* 2003;53:493–497.
49. Memtsoudis SG, Rosenberger P, Loffler M, et al. The usefulness of transesophageal echocardiography during intraoperative cardiac arrest in noncardiac surgery. *Anesth Analg* 2006;102:1653–1657.
50. Cheung AT, Savino JS, Weiss SJ, et al. Echocardiographic and hemodynamic indexes of left ventricular preload in patients with normal and abnormal ventricular function. *Anesthesiology* 1994;81:376–387.
51. Aboulhosn J, Child JS. Left ventricular outflow obstruction: subaortic stenosis, bicuspid aortic valve, supravalvar aortic stenosis, and coarctation of the aorta. *Circulation* 2006;114:2412–2422.
52. Mingo S, Benedicto A, Jimenez MC, et al. Dynamic left ventricular outflow tract obstruction secondary to catecholamine excess in a normal ventricle. *Int J Cardiol* 2006;112:393–396.
53. Araujo AQ, Arteaga E, Ianni BM, et al. Relationship between outflow obstruction and left ventricular functional impairment in hypertrophic cardiomyopathy: a Doppler echocardiographic study. *Echocardiography* 2006;23:734–740.
54. Duane PG, Colice GL. Impact of noninvasive studies to distinguish volume overload from ARDS in acutely ill patients with pulmonary edema: analysis of the medical literature from 1966 to 1998. *Chest* 2000;118:1709–1717.
55. Azevedo LC, Janiszewski M, Soriano FG, et al. Redox mechanisms of vascular cell dysfunction in sepsis. *Endocr Metab Immune Disord Drug Targets* 2006;6:159–164.
56. Barth E, Radermacher P, Thiemermann C, et al. Role of inducible nitric oxide synthase in the reduced responsiveness of the myocardium to catecholamines in a hyperdynamic, murine model of septic shock. *Crit Care Med* 2006;34:307–313.
57. Barbier C, Loubieres Y, Schmit C, et al. Respiratory changes in inferior vena cava diameter are helpful in predicting fluid responsiveness in ventilated septic patients. *Intensive Care Med* 2004;30:1740–1746.
58. Bombardini T. Myocardial contractility in the echo lab: molecular, cellular and pathophysiological basis. *Cardiovasc Ultrasound* 2005;3:27.
59. Joseph MX, Disney PJ, Da Costa R, et al. Transthoracic echocardiography to identify or exclude cardiac cause of shock. *Chest* 2004;126:1592–1597.
60. Marx G, Cope T, McCrossan L, et al. Assessing fluid responsiveness by stroke volume variation in mechanically ventilated patients with severe sepsis. *Eur J Anaesthesiol* 2004;21:132–138.
61. McDonough KH, Virag JI. Sepsis-induced myocardial dysfunction and myocardial protection from ischemia/reperfusion injury. *Front Biosci* 2006;11:23–32.
62. Rivers E, Nguyen B, Havstad S, et al. Early goal-directed therapy in the treatment of severe sepsis and septic shock. *N Engl J Med* 2001;345:1368–1377.
63. Otero RM, Nguyen HB, Huang DT, et al. Early goal-directed therapy in severe sepsis and septic shock revisited: concepts, controversies, and contemporary findings. *Chest* 2006;130:1579–1595.
64. Sugeng L, Mor-Avi V, Weinert L, et al. Quantitative assessment of left ventricular size and function: side-by-side comparison of real-time three-dimensional echocardiography and computed tomography with magnetic resonance reference. *Circulation* 2006;114:654–661.
65. Caiani EG, Corsi C, Sugeng L, et al. Improved quantification of left ventricular mass based on endocardial and epicardial surface detection with real time three dimensional echocardiography. *Heart* 2006;92:213–219.
66. Fukuda S, Hozumi T, Watanabe H, et al. Freehand three-dimensional echocardiography with rotational scanning for measurements of left ventricular volume and ejection fraction in patients with coronary artery disease. *Echocardiography* 2005;22:111–119.
67. Bezante GP, Rosa GM, Bruni R, et al. Improved assessment of left ventricular volumes and ejection fraction by contrast enhanced harmonic color doppler echocardiography. *Int J Cardiovasc Imaging* 2005;21:609–616.
68. Angus DC, Linde-Zwirble WT, Lidicker J, et al. Epidemiology of severe sepsis in the United States: analysis of incidence, outcome, and associated costs of care. *Crit Care Med* 2001;29:1303–1310.
69. Assreuy J. Nitric oxide and cardiovascular dysfunction in sepsis. *Endocr Metab Immune Disord Drug Targets* 2006;6:165–173.

70. Kumar A, Anel R, Bunnell E, et al. Pulmonary artery occlusion pressure and central venous pressure fail to predict ventricular filling volume, cardiac performance, or the response to volume infusion in normal subjects. *Crit Care Med* 2004;32:691–699.

71. Leone M, Boyle WA. Decreased vasopressin responsiveness in vasodilatory septic shock- like conditions. *Crit Care Med* 2006;34:1126–1130.

72. Martins PS, Brunialti MK, da Luz Fernandes M, et al. Bacterial recognition and induced cell activation in sepsis. *Endocr Metab Immune Disord Drug Targets* 2006;6:183–191.

73. Meldrum DR, Wang M, Tsai BM, et al. Intracellular signaling mechanisms of sex hormones in acute myocardial inflammation and injury. *Front Biosci* 2005;10:1835–1867.

74. Varpula M, Tallgren M, Saukkonen K, et al. Hemodynamic variables related to outcome in septic shock. *Intensive Care Med* 2005;31:1066–1071.

75. Wesche DE, Lomas-Neira JL, Perl M, et al. Leukocyte apoptosis and its significance in sepsis and shock. *J Leukoc Biol* 2005;78:325–337.

76. Groban L, Dolinski SY. Transesophageal echocardiographic evaluation of diastolic function. *Chest* 2005;128:3652–3663.

77. Kortgen A, Niederprum P, Bauer M. Implementation of an evidence-based "standard operating procedure" and outcome in septic shock. *Crit Care Med* 2006;34:943–949.

78. Pacher P, Mabley JG, Liaudet L, et al. Left ventricular pressure-volume relationship in a rat model of advanced aging-associated heart failure. *Am J Physiol Heart Circ Physiol* 2004;287:H2132–H2137.

79. Pinsky MR, Teboul JL. Assessment of indices of preload and volume responsiveness. *Curr Opin Crit Care* 2005;11:235–239.

80. Pinsky MR, Payen D, eds. *Protocolized Cardiovascular Management Based on Ventricular-Arterial Coupling.* New York: Springer-Verlag, 2005.

81. Poeze M, Solberg BC, Greve JW, et al. Monitoring global volume-related hemodynamic or regional variables after initial resuscitation: what is a better predictor of outcome in critically ill septic patients? *Crit Care Med* 2005;33:2494–2500.

82. Calder PC. n-3 fatty acids, inflammation, and immunity–relevance to postsurgical and critically ill patients. *Lipids* 2004;39:1147–1161.

83. Krishnagopalan S, Kumar A, Parrillo JE, et al. Myocardial dysfunction in the patient with sepsis. *Curr Opin Crit Care* 2002;8:376–388.

84. Young JD. The heart and circulation in severe sepsis. *Br J Anaesth* 2004;93:114–120.

85. Vieillard-Baron A, Charron C, Chergui K, et al. Bedside echocardiographic evaluation of hemodynamics in sepsis: is a qualitative evaluation sufficient? *Intensive Care Med* 2006;32:1547–1552.

86. Michard F, Alaya S, Zarka V, et al. Global end-diastolic volume as an indicator of cardiac preload in patients with septic shock. *Chest* 2003;124:1900–1908.

87. Marwick TH. Measurement of strain and strain rate by echocardiography: ready for prime time? *J Am Coll Cardiol* 2006;47:1313–1327.

88. Donal E, Yamada H, Leclercq C, et al. The left atrial appendage, a small, blind-ended structure: a review of its echocardiographic evaluation and its clinical role. *Chest* 2005;128:1853–1862.

89. Ommen SR, Nishimura RA, Appleton CP, et al. Clinical utility of doppler echocardiography and tissue Doppler imaging in the estimation of left ventricular filling pressures: a comparative simultaneous doppler catheterization study. *Circulation* 2000;102:1788–1794.

90. Jegger D, Jeanrenaud X, Nasratullah M, et al. Noninvasive doppler-derived myocardial performance index in rats with myocardial infarction: validation and correlation by conductance catheter. *Am J Physiol Heart Circ Physiol* 2006;290:H1540–H1548.

91. Moller JE, Pellikka PA, Hillis GS, et al. Prognostic importance of diastolic function and filling pressure in patients with acute myocardial infarction. *Circulation* 2006;114:438–444.

92. Michard F, Teboul JL. Predicting fluid responsiveness in ICU patients: a critical analysis of the evidence. *Chest* 2002;121:2000–2008.

93. Suga H. Cardiac energetics: from E(max) to pressure-volume area. *Clin Exp Pharmacol Physiol* 2003;30:580–585.

94. Gorcsan J III. Load-independent indices of left ventricular function using automated border detection. *Echocardiography* 1999;16:63–76.

95. Shoucri RM. Theoretical study of pressure-volume relation in left ventricle. *Am J Physiol* 1991;260:H282–H291.

96. Gorcsan J. Utility of hand-carried ultrasound for consultative cardiology. *Echocardiography* 2003;20:463–469.

97. Klein AL, Grimm RA, Jasper SE, et al. Efficacy of transesophageal echocardiography- guided cardioversion of patients with atrial fibrillation at 6 months: a randomized controlled trial. *Am Heart J* 2006;151:380–389.

98. Wyse DG. Pharmacologic approaches to rhythm versus rate control in atrial fibrillation: where are we now? *Int J Cardiol* 2006;110:301–312.

99. Elbehery S, Barrea C, Sluysmans T. Images in cardiology: traumatic left ventricular true aneurysm. Echocardiographic, MRI, and intraoperative images. *Heart* 2006;92:726.

100. Erbel R, Alfonso F, Boileau C, et al. Diagnosis and management of aortic dissection. *Eur Heart J* 2001;22:1642–1681.

101. Shiga T, Wajima Z, Apfel CC, et al. Diagnostic accuracy of transesophageal echocardiography, helical computed tomography, and magnetic resonance imaging for suspected thoracic aortic dissection: systematic review and meta-analysis. *Arch Intern Med* 2006;166:1350–1356.

102. Balm R, Hoornweg LL. Traumatic aortic ruptures. *J Cardiovasc Surg (Torino)* 2005;46:101–105.

103. Cinnella G, Dambrosio M, Brienza N, et al. Transesophageal echocardiography for diagnosis of traumatic aortic injury: An appraisal of the evidence. *J Trauma* 2004;57:1246–1255.

104. Jaffer FA, Libby P, Weissleder R. Molecular and cellular imaging of atherosclerosis: emerging applications. *J Am Coll Cardiol* 2006;47:1328–1338.

105. Kronzon I, Tunick PA. Aortic atherosclerotic disease and stroke. *Circulation* 2006;114:63–75.

106. Djaiani GN. Aortic arch atheroma: stroke reduction in cardiac surgical patients. *Semin Cardiothorac Vasc Anesth* 2006;10:143–157.

107. Reichert CL, Visser CA, Koolen JJ, et al. Transesophageal echocardiography in hypotensive patients after cardiac operations: comparison with hemodynamic parameters. *J Thorac Cardiovasc Surg* 1992;104:321–326.

108. Detaint D, Sundt TM, Nkomo VT, et al. Surgical correction of mitral regurgitation in the elderly: outcomes and recent improvements. *Circulation* 2006;114:265–272.

109. Quinones MA, Douglas PS, Foster E, et al. American College of Cardiology/American Heart Association clinical competence statement on echocardiography: a report of the American College of Cardiology/American Heart Association/American

College of Physicians. American Society of Internal Medicine Task Force on Clinical Competence. *Circulation* 2003;107: 1068–1089.

110. European Heart Rhythm Association, Heart Rhythm Society, Fuster V, et al. ACC/AHA/ ESC 2006 guidelines for the management of patients with atrial fibrillation: Executive summary. A report of the American College of Cardiology/American Heart Association Task Force on Practice Guidelines and the European Society of Cardiology Committee for Practice Guidelines (Writing Committee to Revise the 2001 Guidelines for the Management of Patients With Atrial Fibrillation). *J Am Coll Cardiol* 2006;48:854–906.

QUESTIONS

1. Which of the following are not usually well visualized with TEE?
   A. Ventricular septum
   B. Atrial septum
   C. Aortic arch vessels
   D. Descending aorta
   E. Ascending aorta

2. Which of the following is the commonest indication for TEE in the ICU setting?
   A. Hypotension
   B. Hypoxemia
   C. Suspected aortic dissection
   D. Assessment of myocardial infarction
   E. Assessment of pleural effusion

3. Which of the following is the best index of preload in the ICU?
   A. Ejection fraction
   B. Fractional area change
   C. End diastolic area
   D. End systolic area
   E. Pulmonary venous systolic velocity

4. In the complex, unstable patient with suspected loss of aortic integrity, which of the following is the best first choice investigation?
   A. Aortic MRI
   B. Aortic CT angiography
   C. On table TEE
   D. AP and lateral CXR
   E. Cardiac radionuclide scan

5. In TEE performed in the ICU, which of the following is the most common unsuspected diagnosis?
   A. Endocarditis
   B. Cardiac tamponade
   C. Liver hematoma
   D. Hypovolemia
   E. Aortic dissection

CHAPTER 21

Chest Wall Echocardiography in the Intensive Care Unit

Jason N. Katz ■ Nicolas Aeschlimann ■ Andrew D. Shaw

INTRODUCTION

Armed with a growing armamentarium of novel pharmacotherapies, diagnostic tools, and interventional devices, today's critical care physicians are better equipped than ever to handle maladies once considered universally fatal. At the same time, the patients who occupy these intensive care settings have evolved considerably, bringing with them greater comorbidities and hence greater risk for permanent sequelae of critical illness, including death. There is quite possibly no medical environment in which accurate and prompt diagnosis and therapy are as vitally important as in the intensive care unit (ICU), and clinicians are constantly searching for any demonstrable advantage in their battle against potentially fatal diseases.

One device that has shown considerable promise as a diagnostic and therapeutic tool for critical care clinicians is the transthoracic echocardiogram (TTE). This noninvasive imaging modality is particularly suitable for the intensive care environment because of its portability, its widespread availability, its accessibility, and its rapid diagnostic capabilities. Data derived from TTE imaging in the ICU can assist in the management of a variety of clinical conditions. It can be utilized for hemodynamic assessment, evaluation of valvular function and integrity, identification of global and focal myocardial dysfunction, differentiation of shock states, and investigation of unexplained hypoxemia, to name a few (Table 21.1).

In this chapter, we will discuss potential applications for transthoracic echocardiography in the ICU. Particular attention will focus on its use in obtaining noninvasively derived hemodynamic data, assessment of volume status, and physician guidance for the unstable, critically ill patient. While the image quality and technical superiority of transesophageal echocardiography over TTE are undeniable, the chest wall echocardiogram is considered by many to be the principal echocardiographic test for ICU clinicians.

BASIC IMAGING USING TRANSTHORACIC ECHOCARDIOGRAPHY

While the physics of TTE are beyond the scope of this chapter, a broad review of classic TTE images is an impor-

TABLE 21.1	Clinical Applications and Utility of Transthoracic Echocardiography in the ICU
Hemodynamic assessment	
Intracardiac pressures	
Volume status	
Cardiac output, SV	
PA pressure	
Valvular function and integrity	
Regurgitant valves	
Stenotic valves	
Sequelae of ischemia or infarction	
Infective endocarditis	
Iatrogenic or traumatic injury	
Mechanical valve thrombosis	
Pericardial disease	
Cardiac tamponade, pericardial effusion	
Constrictive pericarditis	
Ventricular function	
PE	
Intracardiac thrombus	
Intracardiac or intrapulmonary shunts	

tant prelude to a more focused discussion of disease states. In general, there are several long- and short-axis tomographic imaging planes acquired as part of the standard two-dimensional, chest wall echocardiographic examination. These include the parasternal views, the apical views, and the subcostal views.

For parasternal imaging, the transducer is placed in the left parasternal region, usually in the third or fourth intercostal space, ideally with the patient in a left lateral decubitus position. Here, long-axis views of the left ventricle (LV) may be displayed as a sagittal section of the heart. This view allows visualization of the aortic valve and aortic root, the left atrial cavity, the anterior

353

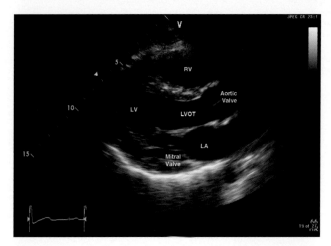

Figure 21.1. Parasternal long-axis view of the heart.

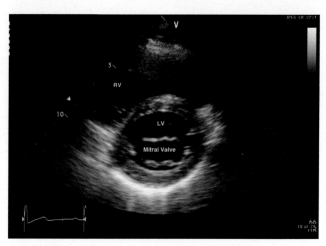

Figure 21.3. Parasternal short-axis view of the heart.

and posterior leaflets of the mitral valve (along with their chordal and papillary muscle attachments), the coronary sinus, the interventricular septum, and the LV outflow tract (LVOT) (Fig. 21.1). With slight clockwise rotation of the transducer and an inferomedial tilt, an inflow view of the right ventricle (RV) can be acquired. This particular view allows visualization of the right atrial (RA) cavity, the tricuspid valve, and the RV inflow (Fig. 21.2). With further clockwise rotation of the transducer, placing the ultrasound beam perpendicular to the plane of the LV long axis, a short-axis view of the LV may be seen. Additional angling of the transducer from cephalad to caudal allows cross-sectional imaging of various portions of the LV cavity, including short-axis views of the aortic valve, mitral valve, papillary muscles, and apex (Fig. 21.3).

Apical imaging can be obtained with the transducer placed near the patient's point of maximal impulse.

With counter-clockwise rotation of the ultrasound beam, the apical position will often provide desirable imaging of the heart's four chambers, atrioventricular valves, pulmonary veins, atrial septum, and aortic outflow tract (Fig. 21.4). This position also allows for ideal applications of Doppler echocardiographic technology.

Finally, the subcostal examination begins by placing the transducer in the epigastrium, slightly right of midline. With this view, evaluation of the hepatic vessels and inferior vena cava (IVC) is possible. Additional imaging of the cardiac chambers, valves, and pericardial space may be performed in the subcostal position and is often easier to obtain than in the apical or parasternal positions for patients with obstructive lung disease and those requiring positive-pressure ventilation (both of which can be distinct barriers to adequate sound transmission) (Fig. 21.5).

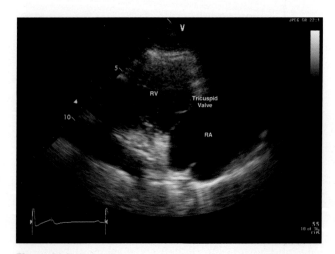

Figure 21.2. RV inflow.

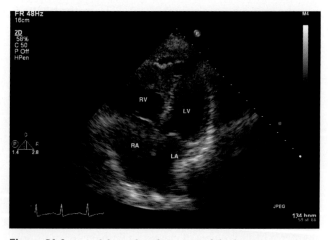

Figure 21.4 Apical four-chamber view of the heart.

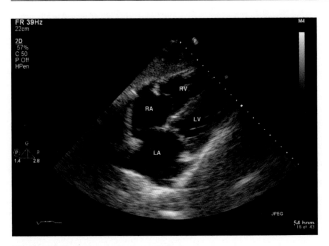

Figure 21.5. Subcostal view of the heart.

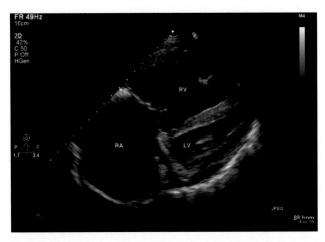

Figure 21.6. Echocardiographic evidence of RV pressure and volume overload.

HEMODYNAMIC ASSESSMENT OF THE CRITICALLY ILL PATIENT

Left Ventricular Function

An important component of any echocardiographic examination of the critically ill patient should include an assessment of LV systolic function. While many different measurements have been used and validated for quantifying ventricular function and performance, global function is most commonly assessed qualitatively by visual assessment and is often sufficient for the purposes of evaluating a patient in the ICU. For practical purposes, a heart with grossly preserved systolic function should demonstrate global thickening of the endocardium during contraction. In addition, in the parasternal long-axis view, the mitral apparatus of a normally contractile heart should descend toward the LV apex during systole.

While image quality can be challenging, particularly in patients mechanically ventilated, the application of harmonic imaging, and even chamber opacification with echo-contrast agents, can help improve endocardial border visualization. In a mechanically ventilated ICU cohort of patients, Vignon et al. (1) showed that TTE allowed adequate evaluation of global LV function in over three quarters of those imaged, emphasizing that even positive-pressure ventilation should not be a barrier to the noninvasive assessment of ventricular performance.

Right Ventricular Function

Many events can alter RV function in the critically ill patient. These include pulmonary embolism (PE), acute lung injury, positive-pressure ventilation, RV myocardial infarction (MI), global cardiomyopathies, tricuspid valve disease, and, in fact, any condition which acutely increases pulmonary vascular resistance and RV afterload. For qualitative assessment, the RV should be evaluated in multiple

tomographic planes. The RV is most often compared visually with the LV as this can provide substantial information about its size and function. One approach to this comparison involves measurements of both RV and LV end-diastolic areas. Several studies have suggested that a diastolic ventricular ratio of 0.6 to 1.0 signifies moderate RV dilatation, while a value ≥1.0 corresponds with severe RV enlargement (2,3). RV dilatation and dysfunction are also often accompanied by other findings easily identified by echocardiography, including RA enlargement, dilatation of the IVC, tricuspid regurgitation, and intraventricular septal flattening leading to "D-shaped" LV geometric distortion (4) (Fig. 21.6).

Furthermore, echocardiography can be used to assess and risk-stratify patients with acute PE based upon evidence of RV perturbations. This concept will be discussed in detail later in this chapter.

Stroke Volume and Cardiac Output

Assessment of intracardiac hemodynamics utilizes two-dimensional echocardiography and Doppler techniques. The accuracy of this noninvasive modality has been validated in comparison with invasively derived hemodynamic data through multiple studies (5,6).

Flow across any fixed orifice is equal to the product of the cross-sectional area (CSA) and the flow velocity. Because the flow velocity varies throughout each cardiac cycle, the summed Doppler-derived velocities are measured during routine echocardiographic examination in order to measure the total volume of flow during a given ejection period. This time velocity integral (TVI) is equal to the area enclosed by the baseline and Doppler spectrum, usually measured across the LVOT. Hence, stroke volume (SV) is equal to the CSA of the LVOT multiplied by the LVOT TVI (7).

Cardiac output is then obtained by multiplying the SV by the heart rate and cardiac index by dividing cardiac output by the patient's body surface area (see below).

$$\text{Flow rate} = \text{CSA} \times \text{flow velocity}$$

$$\text{Stroke volume} = \text{CSA} \times \text{LVOT TVI}$$

$$\text{Stroke volume} = \left(\frac{D}{2}\right)^2 \times \pi \times \text{LVOT TVI}$$

$$\text{Stroke volume} = D^2 \times 0.785 \times \text{LVOT TVI}$$

$$\text{CO} = (D^2 \times 0.785 \times \text{LVOT TVI}) \times \text{HR}$$

$$\text{CI} = \frac{\text{CO}}{\text{BSA}}$$

Intracardiac Filling Pressures and Volume Status

Effective estimations of cardiac filling pressures, in particular estimates of preload, are vital to the appropriate management of the critically ill patient. Transthoracic echocardiography is ideally suited to provide such pressure quantification and can be an extremely useful tool for the practicing intensivist.

By utilizing the Bernoulli equation ($\Delta P = 4V^2$), Doppler-derived blood-flow velocities can be converted to pressure gradients. Velocities measured across regurgitant valves can then be used to determine the pressure difference between two cardiac chambers. For instance, the peak tricuspid regurgitation velocity can be used to generate the pressure difference between the right atrium and RV; hence, the RV systolic pressure can be obtained by adding the estimated RA pressure to the calculated pressure difference. Similarly, the pulmonic regurgitation velocity, representing the diastolic pressure difference between the pulmonary artery (PA) and RV, can be used to derive the PA end-diastolic pressure when this pressure gradient is added to the RV end-diastolic pressure (often using the estimated RA pressure as a surrogate). In summary, commonly acquired pressures can be calculated as follows:

$$\text{RV systolic pressure} = \text{PA Systollic pressure}$$
$$= \text{RA} + [4 \times (\text{tricuspid regurg velocity})^2]$$

$$\text{PA end-diastolic pressure} = \text{RV end-diastolic pressure}$$
$$+ [4 \times (\text{pulmonic regurg velocity})^2] = \text{RA} + [4 \times (\text{pulm}$$
$$\text{LA pressure} = \text{SBP} - [4 \times (\text{mitral regurg velocity})^2]$$

$$\text{LVEDP} = \text{DBP} - [4 \times (\text{aortic regurg velocity})^2]$$

Other Doppler-derived criteria have shown promise in accurately estimating cardiac filling pressures. Nagueh et al. showed that the ratio of mitral E-wave to tissue Doppler Ea-wave (detected at the lateral mitral annulus) could reproducibly estimate LV end-diastolic pressure. These investigators found that the ratio, more accurate at extreme values, correlated well with pulmonary capillary wedge pressure (PCWP) values determined invasively. An E/Ea ratio of less than 8 sensitively correlated with

a normal PCWP, while values greater than 15 had high specificity for elevated PCWPs. Ratios between 8 and 15 had, however, much poorer sensitivity and specificity, and the impact of load-dependency on this formula remains a question to its widespread applicability (8).

Another means for assessing left atrial pressure (LAP) is through focused echocardiographic examination of transmitral (diastolic) inflow. It has been suggested that a normal transmitral inflow pattern may correlate with a LAP between 6 and 12 mm Hg, a pattern of impaired relaxation (grade I diastolic dysfunction) with a LAP between 8 and 14 mm Hg, a pseudonormal inflow pattern (grade II diastolic dysfunction) with a LAP between 15 and 22 mm Hg, and a restrictive pattern (grades III and IV diastolic dysfunction) with pressures exceeding 22 mm Hg. (Fig. 21.7) (9). Other potential echocardiographic clues to elevated left-sided pressures include dilated LV chamber size, bowing of the interatrial septum from left to right, and Doppler color-flow evidence of diastolic mitral regurgitation, to name a few.

Clues to circulating volume status can also be readily assessed by two-dimensional, chest wall echocardiography. Echocardiographic evidence of hypovolemia includes systolic obliteration of the LV cavity, a small IVC diameter, and marked IVC caliber variation with respiration (4). A dilated vena cava (diameter > 20 mm), in the absence of a normal inspiratory decrease (>50% of the IVC caliber with gentle sniff), often indicates an elevated RA pressure; though, this is less reliable in the patient receiving positive-pressure ventilation (10,11). On the other hand, a small, readily collapsible IVC reliably excludes an elevated RA pressure. Feissel et al. also evaluated the impact of IVC diameter variability on hemodynamic-response to volume loading. These investigators suggested, among a small cohort of mechanically ventilated patients with septic shock, that a ≥12% respiratory variability in IVC diameter could predict individuals who would respond to colloid challenge (increasing their cardiac output by at least 15%), with a positive predictive value of 93% and negative predictive value of 92% (12). The use of M-mode echocardiography can often help better define and quantify this collapsibility.

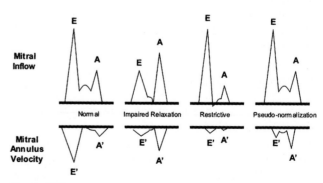

Figure 21.7. Patterns of diastolic dysfunction based upon transmitral inflow.

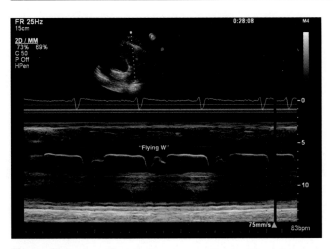

Figure 21.8 M-mode imaging in a patient with pulmonary hypertension.

Pulmonary Artery Pressures

Pulmonary hypertension is both a common cause and sequelae of critical illness in the ICU. Transthoracic echocardiography can provide relatively accurate and rapid determinations of PA pressures. Using the Bernoulli equation as described previously, both PA systolic and diastolic pressures can be calculated, as long as there is concomitant and sufficient tricuspid and pulmonic regurgitation, respectively. Other echocardiographic clues to elevated PA pressures include RV and RA chamber enlargement, a D-shaped LV cavity caused by a flattened interventricular septum, midsystolic closure of the pulmonic valve and loss of the atrial-wave deflection on M-mode ("flying W" pattern; Fig. 21.8), and atrial flow reversal in the hepatic vein due to both increased diastolic pressure and decreased compliance of the RV.

VALVULAR FUNCTION AND DISEASE

While a thorough discussion of echocardiographic evaluation of valvular heart disease is beyond the scope of this chapter, careful review of valvular function and integrity is, however, an important part of the echocardiographic examination in the ICU. In particular, several disease states deserve mention as key contributors to hemodynamic perturbations in the critically ill patient.

Valvular Stenosis

Aortic valve stenosis

Overt heart failure and cardiogenic shock are now uncommon presentations in patients with severe aortic stenosis. More commonly, patients will present for evaluation to their clinicians with slowly progressive angina or dyspnea rather than with a fulminant course. Aortic stenosis, however, can most certainly complicate the already unstable critically ill patient.

A normal aortic valve area (AVA) ranges between 3 and 4 cm². Severe AS, in the presence of preserved LV systolic function, can be defined by the presence of one or more of the following: (a) peak aortic valve velocity by continuous-wave Doppler of ≥400 cm/s, (b) mean aortic valve gradient of ≥50 mm Hg, and (c) AVA of less than 0.75 cm². If, however, LV function is impaired, both the peak aortic valve velocity and mean gradients may underestimate the degree of stenosis (13). Utilizing transthoracic echocardiography, the AVA can be calculated via the continuity equation, in which A1 = A2 × (V2/V1), where measurements are commonly taken at the aortic valve annulus (AVA = A1, aortic valve velocity = V1) and within the LVOT (LVOT area = A2, LVOT velocity = V2). Using Doppler principles, the AVA then can be determined by the following equation: AVA = π × (LVOT/2)² × LVOT TVI/AV TVI.

Echocardiographic clues to the etiology of aortic stenosis can also be identified through transthoracic imaging. In the parasternal long-axis view, the location of valve coaptation can be quite informative. Normally, a trileaflet valve will coapt in the center of the LVOT while a bicuspid valve typically has an eccentric (posterior) closure line. Additionally, leaflet thickening may be seen. In rheumatic AS, one will often see focal thickening of the free edges of a domed leaflet. On the other hand, in degenerative calcific AS, calcification typically progresses from the base of the leaflets to the tips. The parasternal short-axis plane can often provide important clues to the anatomy and morphology of the valve, including the number of leaflets and commissures.

Mitral Valve Stenosis

In the majority of cases, mitral valve stenosis results from rheumatic heart disease but can also be congenital in etiology or represent sequelae of infective endocarditis and progressive annular calcification (14,15). The goal of echocardiography for the patient with significant mitral stenosis is both to evaluate the valvular morphology and to assess the pathologic pressure gradient between the left atrium and LV. It is this gradient that can lead to the hemodynamic perturbations (elevated pulmonary pressures and pulmonary vascular resistance) and pulmonary edema that can result from untreated mitral stenosis. It should be noted that there are also many consequences of critical illness that can significantly exacerbate unknown MS—in fact, any situation that either increases transmitral flow (volume loading) or decreases diastolic filling time (e.g., tachycardia) can result in abrupt deterioration of an otherwise stable patient.

Application of Doppler techniques can help the astute intensivist in evaluating the patient with presumed mitral valve stenosis. A transmitral peak velocity greater than 100 cm/s suggests significant MS. Additionally, a transvalvular mean gradient greater than 12 mm Hg and a pressure half-time (time for transvalvular pressure to drop to half of its peak) greater than 220 mm Hg also can identify a severely stenotic mitral valve (13).

Valvular Insufficiency

Aortic Valve Regurgitation

While chronic aortic valve regurgitation is likely to complicate the course of many patients with critical illness, echocardiographic evaluation of acute aortic insufficiency (AI) is perhaps a more important determination during transthoracic imaging of the critically ill patient. The sudden increase in LV end-diastolic volume, coupled with insufficient ventricular adaptation, can result in the rapid development of pulmonary edema and even cardiogenic shock. Common etiologies of acute AI include infective endocarditis with valve destruction, abscess formation, aortic dissection, trauma, and iatrogenic injury (16).

The two-dimensional, chest wall echocardiogram is often sufficient to make the diagnosis of acute AI, though transesophageal echocardiography can be a useful adjunctive tool to more closely evaluate the structure and morphology of the valve and aortic root. Doppler criteria suggestive of severe AI include a pressure half-time less than 200 ms, holodiastolic flow reversal in the descending thoracic aorta, and a vena contracta width greater than 6 mm (13). Besides these noninvasive flow patterns, other findings which might suggest the need for definitive surgical therapy include the presence of perivalvular abscess, loss of valvular integrity due to flail leaflet or perforation, proximal aortic dissection, associated LV systolic dysfunction, and evidence of concomitant septal defects.

Mitral Valve Regurgitation

Similar to AI, acute mitral valve regurgitation results in sudden volume overload in cardiac chambers that have not had sufficient time to develop compensatory dilatation and hypertrophy. As a result, sudden increases in left atrial and LV volume can result in pulmonary vascular congestion, overt pulmonary edema, and even marked hemodynamic perturbations with cardiogenic shock. Hemodynamically significant MR can result from infective endocarditis with disruption of valvular integrity, traumatic and iatrogenic injuries, as well as acute ischemic dysfunction. Myocardial ischemia and infarction can cause the sudden onset of mitral insufficiency through two major mechanisms: (a) structural injury due to papillary muscle dysfunction and/or rupture (structural MR) and (b) indirect injury to the mitral valve apparatus with pathologic remodeling, leading to restricted mitral leaflet coaptation (functional MR). Hence, the evaluation of mitral valve disease is an important part of any echocardiographic examination in patients with recent MI who have evidence of hemodynamic instability.

Again, chest wall echocardiography is often the initial diagnostic procedure of choice when evaluating patients with suspected mitral valve regurgitation. Echocardiography should focus on the presence or absence of significant structural injury to the valve and supporting structures (e.g., chordae tendinae, papillary muscles). Other indicators of severe MR include systolic flow reversal in the pulmonary veins, an effective regurgitant orifice ≥ 40 mm^2, a regurgitant volume ≥ 60 mL, a regurgitant jet length greater than 4.4 cm and jet area greater than 40% of the left atrial chamber, and a vena contracta width greater than 0.50 cm, to name a few (13).

Mechanical Valve Thrombosis

The incidence of mechanical valve thrombosis ranges from 0.2% to 6% per year in those with aortic or mitral prostheses and as high as 13% in those with prosthetic tricuspid valves (17,18). When present, patients with thrombosis will often be critically ill with advanced hemodynamic deterioration. While traditional two-dimensional chest wall echocardiography is a useful initial study to help visualize the potentially abnormal valve and Doppler-derived data can assist in making the diagnosis, transesophageal echocardiography is the procedure of choice for evaluating the suspect valve. Acoustic shadowing and marked variability in Doppler flow among these unstable patients can significantly limit the diagnostic applicability of the chest wall echocardiogram. Nonetheless, vigilant echocardiographic examination of all prosthetic valves is prudent and necessary in the critically ill patient.

PULMONARY EMBOLISM

Multiple epidemiologic studies have suggested that there are anywhere from 55,000 to 600,000 patients diagnosed with acute PE in the United States alone each year, (19,20) and data from the largest international registry of these patients have indicated an in-hospital mortality rate of 7% (21). Furthermore, 3-month mortality rate for all patients who present to the hospital with PE is approximately 15% while concomitant hemodynamic instability increases the mortality numbers to nearly 50% (22). It is likely, however, that these figures grossly underestimate the true impact of this disease as autopsy data have suggested that as many as two thirds of all clinically significant pulmonary emboli are undiagnosed prior to death (23).

It is both the size of the embolus, as well as the presence or absence of preexisting cardiopulmonary disease, that determines its hemodynamic consequence. The increase in pulmonary vascular resistance and RV afterload, created by the space-occupying thrombus along with neurally and humorally mediated pulmonary vasoconstriction, results in increases in RV wall tension, impaired systolic function, RV dilatation, and elevated RV end-diastolic pressure and volume.

Despite an estimated 80% of patients with PE having normal systemic arterial pressures, it has been suggested that as much as 50% of these normotensive individuals have echocardiographic criteria suggestive of RV dysfunction; (24,25) furthermore, identification of RV dysfunction seems to identify a particularly high-risk cohort of patients at risk for greater short-term and long-term morbidity and mortality (26).

The two-dimensional, chest wall echocardiogram can be used to provide supportive evidence for acute PE. McConnell et al. (27) were among the first to analyze regional patterns of RV dysfunction in patients with and without acute PE. After retrospectively reviewing studies on 126 patients—a training cohort of 41 patients, followed by a validation cohort of 85 patients—they found that patients with acute PE seemed to have a distinct regional pattern of RV dysfunction, with akinesis of the mid–free wall, but preserved (and even hypercontractile) function at the RV apex. Postulated to be related to RV tethering against a hypercontractile RV, diminished RV wall stress at the apex, and localized RV free wall ischemia, "McConnell's sign" was suggested to have a positive predictive value of 71% and negative predictive value of 76% for identifying acute PE. However, more recent data have refuted these findings, calling into question the applicability of this echocardiographic finding (28).

Other investigators have attempted to identify more quantitative echocardiographic indices for PE diagnosis, including RV wall motion scores, the ratio of RV end-diastolic diameter to LV end-diastolic diameter, and pulmonary arterial diameter, to name a few. Table 21.2 shows other diagnostic values, which may indicate acute RV dysfunction from thromboembolic disease.

While transthoracic echocardiography can provide surrogate markers for acute PE (in the absence of identified thrombus-in-transit), and has been validated as a worthy risk-stratification tool, questions still remain about its utility in guiding therapy. Several studies have examined whether or not thrombolytic therapy, in eligible patient cohorts, can improve outcomes among patients with confirmed PE and echocardiographic-evidence of RV dysfunction. Perhaps the most discussed, randomized trial was performed by Konstantinides et al. (29).

Their study included PE patients with echocardiographically detected RV dysfunction, echo-defined pulmonary hypertension, or electrocardiographically determined RV strain. Patients were randomized to receive either heparin plus alteplase or heparin alone. Among the 256 randomized individuals, the authors found that the probability of 30-day event-free survival was significantly higher in the heparin-plus-alteplase group (p = 0.005); additionally, there was no statistically significant difference in major bleeding complications between the two groups (29). While this led the investigators to conclude that thrombolysis indications should be extended to those patients with submassive PE, others have pointed to significant design flaws, which limit their findings. In particular, the primary endpoint resulted almost entirely from the large number of patients in the anticoagulation-alone group who received secondary thrombolysis (so-called, escalation-of-therapy). This subjective, physician-guided decision allowed investigators to break the randomization code and hence added significant bias to the study results. Consequently, the role of thrombolytic therapy in patients with submassive PE remains uncertain.

PERICARDIAL DISEASE

Another important component to a thorough echocardiographic assessment in the critically ill patient involves a focused examination of the pericardial space. Pericardial fluid, in particular, is usually quite easily visualized by chest wall echocardiography. Most commonly, the parasternal long- and short-axis views, along with the apical views, can help identify the presence of a pericardial effusion. In mechanically ventilated patients and those with significant lung disease, in whom standard tomographic planes are suboptimal, the subcostal view can often provide adequate windows. For patients without any available transthoracic windows, transesophageal echocardiography can be a useful adjunctive diagnostic tool.

Most commonly, two processes resulting from pericardial disease need to be addressed during echocardiographic evaluation: cardiac tamponade and pericardial constriction. With pericardial effusions, the presence of symptoms usually correlates with the volume of fluid, the rate of accumulation, and the characteristics of the fluid. While the pericardial space can slowly accommodate up to 2 L of fluid without any hemodynamic or clinical sequelae, the unstretched pericardium can only accommodate 80 to 200 mL of rapidly developing fluid. Common causes of cardiac tamponade in the ICU are listed in Table 21.3.

Echocardiographically, there are numerous signs of clinically significant tamponade including RA diastolic collapse, RV early-diastolic collapse, left atrial diastolic collapse, an abnormal inspiratory increase in RV dimensions, respiratory variation of mitral (or tricuspid) inflow (suggested by a decrease on inspiration of the transmitral E-wave of >25% and a decrease in the tricuspid E wave of

TABLE 21.2	Echocardiographic Indices Suggestive of RV Dysfunction in Acute PE

Qualitative
RV hypokinesis
McConnell's sign
Paradoxical septal motion
Quantitative
RV:LV end-diastolic diameter > 1
RV:LV end-diastolic area > 0.6
RV end-diastolic diameter > 30 mm
PA systolic pressure > 30 mm Hg
Tricuspid regurgitant velocity > 2.8 m/s
PA mean pressure > 20 mm Hg
Right PA dilatation > 30 mm

TABLE 21.3	Potential Etiologies of Cardiac Tamponade in the ICU
Malignancy	
MI with free wall rupture	
Autoimmune disease	
Trauma	
Infection	
Postcardiac surgery	
Percutaneous coronary revascularization with perforation	

>40%), hepatic venous flow reversal, IVC plethora (failure to decrease the diameter by at least 50% with sniff), and LV pseudohypertrophy. While these criteria can assist the critical care physician in suggesting the presence of tamponade, it must be remembered that the condition remains, first and foremost, a clinical diagnosis. In addition to its diagnostic applicability, the chest wall echocardiogram can also help guide therapeutic, percutaneous pericardiocentesis. By determining the size, location, and depth of the effusion, needle guidance is possible with real-time sonography.

In the appropriate patient population, particularly those with recent cardiac surgery, pericardial constriction should also be considered in the critically ill patient. Constrictive pericarditis results from fibrous thickening of the pericardium resulting from chronic inflammation. Essentially, the heart is encased by a rigid pericardium, leading to a decrease in diastolic filling, an increase in intracardiac pressures, and a dissociation of intracardiac pressure from intrathoracic pressure. These elevated cardiac pressures and diminished diastolic filling can lead to an increase in venous (pulmonary and systemic) pressures with progressive signs and symptoms of predominantly right-heart failure. The most common etiologies of constriction include postsurgical, radiation therapy, idiopathic, and infection. Echocardiographic evidence of constriction includes flattening of the LV free wall, pericardial thickening, premature opening of the pulmonic valve (due to elevated RV end-diastolic pressures), septal bounce, IVC plethora, mitral inflow variability with inspiration (usually >25%), and an E-wave to tissue Doppler Ea-wave ratio ≥10 to 15, to name a few. The chest wall echocardiogram can also help to differentiate constrictive pericarditis from myocardial restriction. Unlike with constriction, the restrictive heart tends to have less (<10%) variability in mitral inflow with respiration, will commonly have RV systolic pressures greater than 55 mm Hg (usually <55 mm Hg with constriction), and have an RV-end diastolic pressure less than 1/3 of the systolic pressure. Additionally, pulmonary venous flow varies with inspiration in constriction but not with myocardial restriction.

MYOCARDIAL ISCHEMIA AND ITS COMPLICATIONS

Myocardial ischemia and infarction are another important cause and complication of ICU admission. Without prompt diagnosis and treatment, mechanical complications of acute MI are often fatal. The chest wall echocardiogram is a readily available and important tool for identifying myocardial ischemia or infarction, and its sequelae. In fact, it has been suggested that over 50% of patients with MI have nonspecific findings on initial ECG; while cardiac biomarkers (e.g., creatine kinase, CK-MB, and troponins) are quite useful in making the diagnosis, the sensitivity of these studies in the early periinfarction period is somewhat limited.

Immediately after ischemia or infarction, myocardial contractility diminishes. Regional wall motion abnormalities can often be readily identified by two-dimensional transthoracic echocardiography. Even in patients with classic ECG findings suggestive of acute MI, echocardiographic analysis can be an important risk-stratification tool in suggesting the amount of at-risk myocardium. Furthermore, after definitive therapy is provided, serial echocardiography can be useful in detecting the success of reperfusion therapy and the degree of myocardial viability.

The chest wall echocardiogram is also a vital tool for identifying potentially fatal complications of MI, including ventricular free wall rupture, papillary muscle rupture, aneurysm, intracardiac thrombus, cardiac tamponade, and ventricular septal defect. These entities should be considered, and evaluated echocardiographically, in any unstable patient who has recently been diagnosed with acute MI.

INTRACARDIAC AND INTRAPULMONARY SHUNTS

In the critically ill patient with paradoxical embolization or refractory hypoxemia, the presence of an intracardiac or intrapulmonary shunt must be excluded. Transthoracic echocardiography can play a vital role in the diagnostic evaluation of shunt physiology. Using agitated saline, contrast can be injected into the right side of the heart via an upper extremity vein. The normal appearance of contrast bubbles should be visualized in the superior vena cava, RA, RV, and PA. Because these bubbles are unable to pass through the pulmonary capillaries, no contrast should be seen on the left side of the heart. In the case of an intracardiac or intrapulmonary shunt, contrast will appear in the LA, LV, and aorta. Classic teaching suggests that an intracardiac communication should result in bubbles appearing in the left heart immediately after right-heart opacification (Fig. 21.9), while contrast in the left heart will be delayed three to five cardiac

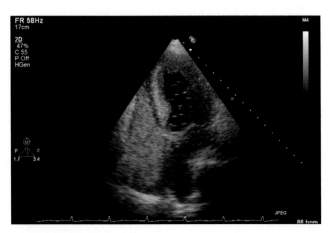

Figure 21.9. Saline microcavitation study showing evidence of intracardiac shunt.

cycles in cases of an intrapulmonary (e.g., pulmonary arteriovenous fistula) shunt (30). These microcavitation studies can markedly improve the detection rate for both intracardiac and intrapulmonary shunts. Even in cases of intracardiac communications, such as a patent foramen ovale, color-flow Doppler may be insufficient to make the diagnosis.

If an intracardiac shunt is suspected, both transthoracic and transesophageal echocardiographies can help further define the anatomic and structural nature of the defect. This is essential in anticipation of potential percutaneous or surgical repair. Echocardiography can also quantify the pulmonary-to-systemic shunt ratio (Qp/Qs) through spectral Doppler measurements. Similar to our previous discussion of SV calculations, both Qp and Qs can be calculated as follows:

$$Qp = RVOT\ TVI \times (RVOT\ diameter/2)^2 \times \pi$$

$$Qs = LOVT\ TVI \times (LVOT\ diameter/2)^2 \times \pi$$

A hemodynamically significant shunt is often defined as a Qp/Qs ratio greater than 2.

CONCLUSION

The chest wall echocardiogram can be a valuable diagnostic tool in the ICU; in particular, for the noninvasive cardiac evaluation of patients with hemodynamic instability. While technically superior imaging may often be obtained using a transesophageal approach, the wide availability, accessibility, and rapidity of the TTE make it an ideal imaging modality. It is particularly suited to provide vital hemodynamic, morphologic, and structural information for the critically ill patient, and it is quickly becoming a necessary component for the practice of critical care medicine.

REFERENCES

1. Vignon P, Chastagner C, Francois B, et al. Diagnostic ability of hand-held echocardiography in ventilated critically ill patients. *Crit Care* 2003;7:R84–R91.
2. Jardin F, Dubourg O, Bourdarias JP. Echocardiographic pattern of acute cor pulmonale. *Chest* 1997;111:209–217.
3. Vieillard-Baron A, Prin S, Chergui K, et al. Echo-Doppler demonstration of acute cor pulmonale at the bedside in the medical intensive care unit. *Am J Respir Crit Care Med* 2002;166:1310–1319.
4. Beauliu Y. Bedside echocardiography in the assessment of the critically ill. *Crit Care Med* 2007;35(Suppl.):S235–S249.
5. Currie PJ, Hagler DJ, Seward JB, et al. Instantaneous pressure gradient: a simultaneous Doppler and dual catheter correlative study. *J Am Coll Cardiol* 1986;7:800–806.
6. Currie PJ, Seward JB, Chan KL. Continuous wave Doppler determination of right ventricular pressure: a simultaneous Doppler-catheterization study in 127 patients. *J Am Coll Cardiol* 1985;6:750–756.
7. Oh JK, Seward JB, Tajik AJ. Hemodynamic assessment. In: Oh JK, Seward JB, Tajik AJ, eds. *The Echo Manual.* 2nd Ed. Philadelphia: Lippincott Williams & Wilkins, 1999:59–72.
8. Nagueh SF, Middleton KJ, Kopelen HA, et al. Doppler tissue imaging: a noninvasive technique for evaluation of left ventricular relaxation and estimation of filling pressures. *J Am Coll Cardiol* 1997;30:1527–1533.
9. Subramaniam B, Talmor D. Echocardiography for management of hypotension in the intensive care unit. *Crit Care Med* 2007;35(Suppl.):S401–S407.
10. Jue J, Chung W, Schiller NB. Does inferior vena cava size predict right atrial pressure in patients receiving mechanical ventilation? *J Am Soc Echocardiogr* 1992;5:613–619.
11. Jardin F, Vieillard-Baron A. Ultrasonographic examination of the venae cavae. *Intensive Care Med* 2006;32:203–206.
12. Feissel M, Michard F, Faller JP, et al. The respiratory variation in inferior vena cava diameter as a guide to fluid therapy. *Intensive Care Med* 2004;30:1834–1837.
13. Bonow RO, Carabello BA, Chatterjee K, et al. 2008 focused update incorporated into the ACC/AHA 2006 guidelines for the management of patients with valvular heart disease: a report of the American College of Cardiology/American Heart Association Task Force on Practice Guidelines (Writing Committee to revise the 1998 guidelines for the management of patients with valvular heart disease). Endorsed by the Society

of Cardiovascular Anesthesiologists, Society for Cardiovascular Angiography and Interventions, and Society of Thoracic Surgeons. *J Am Coll Cardiol* 2008;52:e1–e142.

14. Olson LJ, Subramanian R, Ackermann DM, et al. Surgical pathology of the mitral valve: a study of 712 cases spanning 21 years. *Mayo Clin Proc* 1987;62:22–34.

15. Horstkotte D, Niehues R, Strauer BE. Pathomorphological aspects, aetiology and natural history of acquired mitral valve stenosis. *Eur Heart J* 1991;12(Suppl. B):55–60.

16. Roberts WC, Ko JM, Moore TR, et al. Causes of pure aortic regurgitation in patients having isolated aortic valve replacement at a single US tertiary hospital (1993–2005). *Circulation* 2006;114:422–429.

17. Thorburn CW, Morgan JJ, Shanahan MX, et al. Long-term results of tricuspid valve replacement and the problem of the prosthetic valve thrombosis. *Am J Cardiol* 1983;51: 1128–1132.

18. Roudaut R, Labbe T, Lorient Roudaut MF, et al. Mechanical cardiac valve thrombosis: is fibrinolysis justified? *Circulation* 1992;86(Suppl. II):II-8–II-15.

19. Dalen JE, Alpert JS. Natural history of pulmonary embolism. *Prog Cardiovasc Dis* 1975;17:259–270.

20. Anderson FA, Wheeler B, Goldberg RJ, et al. A population-based perspective of the hospital incidence and case-fatality rates of deep vein thrombosis and pulmonary embolism. *Arch Intern Med* 1998;158:933–938.

21. Goldhaber SZ, Visani L, DeRosa M. Acute pulmonary embolism: clinical outcomes in the International Cooperative Pulmonary Embolism Registry (ICOPER). *Lancet* 1999;353: 1386–1389.

22. Rahimtoola A, Bergin JD. Acute pulmonary embolism: an update on diagnosis and management. *Curr Probl Cardiol* 2005;30:61–114.

23. Stein PD, Henry JW. Prevalence of acute pulmonary embolism among patients in a general hospital and at autopsy. *Chest* 1995;108:978–981.

24. Grifoni S, Olivotto I, Cecchini P, et al. Short-term clinical outcome of patients with acute pulmonary embolism, normal blood pressure, and echocardiographic right ventricular dysfunction. *Circulation* 2000;101:2817–2822.

25. Kasper W, Konstantinides S, Geibel A, et al. Prognostic significance of right ventricular afterload stress detected by echocardiography in patients with clinically suspected pulmonary embolism. *Heart* 1997;77:346–349.

26. Ribeiro A, Lindmarker P, Juhlin-Dannfelt A, et al. Echocardiography Doppler in pulmonary embolism: right ventricular dysfunction as a predictor of mortality rate. *Am Heart J* 1997;134:479–487.

27. McConnell MV, Solomon SD, Rayan ME, et al. Regional right ventricular dysfunction detected by echocardiography in acute pulmonary embolism. Am J Cardiol 1996;78:469–473.

28. Casazza F, Bongarzoni A, Capozi A, et al. Regional right ventricular dysfunction in acute pulmonary embolism and right ventricular infarction. *Eur J Echocardiogr* 2006;6:11–14.

29. Konstantinides S, Geibel A, Heusel G, et al. Heparin plus alteplase compared with heparin alone in patients with submassive pulmonary embolism. *N Engl J Med* 2002;347:1143–1150.

30. Oh JK, Seward JB, Tajik AJ. Contrast echocardiography. In: Oh JK, Seward JB, Tajik AJ, eds. *The Echo Manual*. 2nd Ed. Philadelphia: Lippincott Williams & Wilkins, 1999:245–256.

QUESTIONS

1. Intracardiac filling pressures can be estimated by echocardiography utilizing which equation/formula?
   A. La Place formula
   B. Bernoulli equation
   C. Continuity equation
   D. Proximal isovelocity surface area

2. Which of the following is most consistent with an echocardiographic diagnosis of constriction, as opposed to restriction?
   A. RV systolic pressure greater than 55 mm Hg
   B. RV end-diastolic pressure greater than 1/3 RV systolic pressure
   C. Mitral inflow variability with inspiration less than 10%
   D. Mitral E-wave to tissue Doppler E_A wave ratio less than 10

3. Which of the findings is not suggestive of elevated pulmonary pressures?
   A. Interventricular septal flattening with a "D-shaped" LV
   B. Flow reversal in the hepatic vein
   C. Elevated mitral E-wave to tissue Doppler E_A wave ratio
   D. Midsystolic closure of the pulmonic valve and atrial wave M-mode deflection ("flying W" pattern)

4. Which of the following is diagnostic of PE by chest wall echocardiography?
   A. IVC dilatation and impaired collapsibility
   B. RA enlargement
   C. McConnell's sign
   D. Thrombus-in-transit

CHAPTER 22

The Assessment of a Patient with Endocarditis

Christopher C.C. Hudson ■ Jordan K.C. Hudson ■ G. Burkhard Mackensen

INTRODUCTION

Infective endocarditis (IE), an infection of the endocardial surface of the heart, is a life-threatening medical condition associated with high morbidity and mortality (1). Despite being a well-recognized entity for over 100 years, the accurate diagnosis of IE remains very challenging, and tremendous costs are associated with both underdiagnosis and overdiagnosis (2,3). As early as 1885, William Osler spoke at the Goulstonian Lectures "Few diseases present greater difficulties in the way of diagnosis than malignant endocarditis, difficulties which in many cases are practically insurmountable" (4). Although much progress has been made since that time, there currently is no single investigation that can definitively establish the diagnosis of IE. The closest such tool is echocardiography, and it is for this reason that the 2008 American College of Cardiology/American Heart Association (ACC/AHA) guidelines for valvular heart disease consider echocardiography essential in diagnosis and management of IE (Table 22.1) (5,6). It is the hope of the authors that by the end of this chapter, a thorough understanding of IE and the invaluable role of transesophageal echocardiography (TEE) will be obtained.

EPIDEMIOLOGY AND RISK FACTORS

The generally accepted incidence of IE is 1.4 to 6.2 cases per 100,000 person-years (7–9). Men are more often affected than women (0.6:1 to 2.7:1 male:female ratio) and the incidence increases progressively with age, with a median age between 48 and 70 years (9). A wide variety of organisms can cause IE, but the two most common organisms are staphylococci (42.1%) and streptococci (29.6%) (10).

There are a number of risk factors for the development of IE. A recent population-based case-control study showed that poor dental hygiene, kidney disease, and diabetes mellitus were significantly associated with an increased incidence of IE (11). Other commonly accepted risk factors include intravenous drug use, HIV, structural heart disease (particularly mitral valve

TABLE 22.1	ACC/AHA Guidelines for TEE of IE
Class I: Evidence and/or general agreement that TEE should be performed	
1. Assess IE severity of valvular lesions in symptomatic patients if TTE is nondiagnostic	
2. Diagnosis of IE in patients with valvular heart disease and positive cultures if TTE is nondiagnostic	
3. Diagnosis of complications of IE that have potential impact on prognosis and management	
4. First-line modality to diagnose prosthetic valve endocarditis and assess for complications	
5. Preoperative evaluation in patients with known IE, unless TEE will delay urgent surgery	
6. Intraoperative management of patients undergoing valve surgery	
Class IIa: The weight of evidence or opinion favors the usefulness of TEE	
1. Diagnosis of possible IE in patients with persistent staphylococcal bacteremia without a known source	
Class IIb: The weight of evidence or opinion is less well established for the usefulness of TEE	
1. Diagnosis of possible IE in patients with nosocomial staphylococcal bacteremia	

Source: Bonow RO, Carabello BA, Chatterjee K, et al. 2008 focused update incorporated into the ACC/AHA 2006 guidelines for the management of patients with valvular heart disease: a report of the American College of Cardiology/American Heart Association Task Force on Practice Guidelines (Writing Committee to revise the 1998 guidelines for the management of patients with valvular heart disease). Endorsed by the Society of Cardiovascular Anesthesiologists, Society for Cardiovascular Angiography and Interventions, and Society of Thoracic Surgeons. J Am Coll Cardiol 2008;52(13):e1–e142.

TABLE 22.2	Proposed Modified Duke Criteria for the Diagnosis of IE

Diagnosis of IE

1. Pathological criteria
    a. Microorganisms demonstrated by culture or histological examination of a vegetation, a vegetation that has embolized, or an intracardiac abscess specimen; or
    b. Pathological lesions, vegetation, or intracardiac abscess confirmed by histological examination showing active endocarditis
2. Clinical criteria
    a. Two major criteria; or
    b. One major criterion and three minor criteria; or
    c. Five minor Criteria

Source: Li JS, Sexton DJ, Mick N, et al. Proposed modifications to the Duke criteria for the diagnosis of infective endocarditis. Clin Infect Dis 2000;30(4):633–638.

prolapse), prosthetic heart valves, and a history of IE (12–17). In regard to prosthetic heart valves, endocarditis develops in approximately 1% of patients at 12 months and 2% to 3% at 5 years time (18,19). Surprisingly, there is no difference in incidence of IE between mechanical and bioprosthetic valves.

DIAGNOSIS

As previously mentioned, the diagnosis of IE is extremely challenging for the clinician. As a result, there have been numerous schemes developed to diagnose IE (20–23). The most widely used criteria for assessing patients with suspected IE are the Duke Criteria (20). Proposed in 1994, this diagnostic tool integrates echocardiographic, laboratory, and physical findings and stratifies patients with suspected IE into the following three categories: (a) "definite" cases identified either clinically or pathologically (IE proved during surgery or at autopsy); (b) "possible" cases (not meeting the criteria for definite IE); and (c) "rejected" cases (no pathologic evidence of IE at surgery or autopsy, rapid resolution of the clinical picture, or firm alternative diagnosis. The Duke Criteria have been validated by several studies demonstrating robust sensitivity and specificity (24–27).

A major limitation of the original Duke Criteria was that it relied heavily on the use of transthoracic echocardiography (TTE) for the diagnosis. TEE has now been systemically evaluated in several trials demonstrating its superiority for detecting vegetations compared to TTE (2,28–31). TEE has both higher sensitivity and specificity versus TTE (93% and 96% vs. 63% and 95%) (30,31). The modified Duke Criteria were developed to address this obvious limitation (Tables 22.2 and 22.3) (21). TEE is now recommended as the first test in patients with prosthetic valves, rated at least "possible" IE by clinical criteria, and for complicated IE (i.e., paravalvular abscess). However, in

cases with low clinical suspicion or whenever TTE imaging is thought to be of good quality (e.g., in younger patients), it is considered reasonable to first perform a TTE (32).

ECHOCARDIOGRAPHY

Echocardiography is essential in the diagnosis and management of patients afflicted with infectious endocarditis (6). The echocardiographic findings can be divided into two essential components: (a) detection of an oscillating intracardiac mass or vegetation and (b) diagnosis of complications such as an annular abscess, partial dehiscence of a prosthetic valve, or new valvular regurgitation (33,34). In addition, echocardiography can be used as a prognostic tool in patients with IE (34,35). Lastly, there is an emerging role of the use of three-dimensional (3D) echocardiography in the diagnosis of IE (Fig. 22.1) (36).

Vegetation

Vegetations are the hallmark echocardiographic findings of IE. In general, vegetations appear as discrete, mobile, echo-dense masses that are typically adherent to the upstream surface of a valvular leaflet or the mural endocardium (Fig. 22.2) (34). It can sometimes be particularly challenging to distinguish a mass due to IE from other cardiac masses (i.e., thrombus, tumors, etc). Sanfilippo et al. summarized key echocardiographical findings to help distinguish true vegetation from a mimicking lesion (see Table 22.4) (34).

Complications Secondary to IE

There are several intracardiac complications that are commonly associated with IE and occur in over half of patients (37,38).

TABLE 22.3	Definitions for Criteria Used in the Proposed Modified Duke Criteria for the Diagnosis of IE

Major criteria

1. Positive blood cultures

   a. Two separate cultures for typical IE microorganisms: *Streptococcus viridians* or HACEK organism (*Hemophilus parainfluenzae, Hemophilus aphrophilus, Hemophilus paraphrophilus, Actinobacillus actinomycetemcomitans, Cardiobacterium hominis, Eikenella corrodens*, or *Kingella* species); or

   b. Persistently positive blood cultures of microorganisms consistent for IE; or

   c. Single positive blood culture for a *Coxiella* organism and/or Q fever

2. Positive echocardiographic findings

   a. Oscillating mass and/or vegetation; or

   b. Paravalvular abscess; or

   c. Dehiscence of a prosthetic valve

3. New valvular regurgitation

Minor criteria

1. Predisposition (history of IV drug use or congenital heart disease)

2. Fever of more than 38°C

3. Vascular phenomena (arterial emboli, pulmonary infarcts, intracranial hemorrhage, conjunctival hemorrhage, Janeway lesions)

4. Immunological phenomena (glomerulonephritis, Osler nodes, Roth spots) positive for rheumatoid factor

5. Positive blood culture that does not meet Major criteria

Source: Li JS, Sexton DJ, Mick N, et al. Proposed modifications to the Duke criteria for the diagnosis of infective endocarditis. Clin Infect Dis *2000;30(4):633–638.*

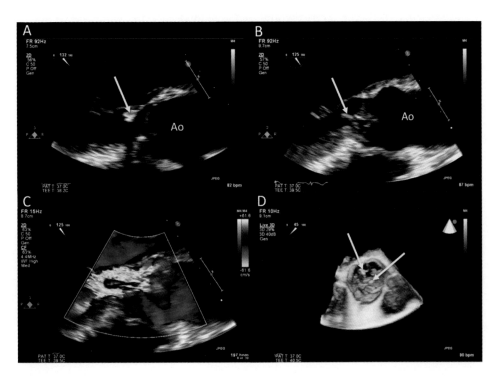

Figure 22.1. Midesophageal AV long-axis views demonstrating a case of severe endocarditis with large vegetations seen at both the noncoronary and left coronary cusps (**A,B**, *yellow arrows*) resulting in severe aortic regurgitation (**C**). The 3D image (**D**) confirms involvement of all three cusps in the IE. Ao, ascending aorta.

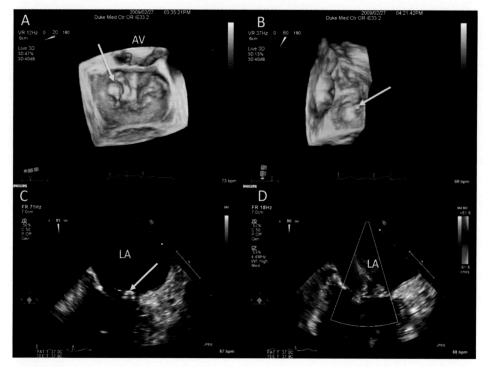

Figure 22.2. En face view of a mitral valve (**A**) with fungal endocarditis. The image was acquired with the live 3D zoom mode and is orientated in the surgical view with the AV at 12 o'clock. The vegetation is located close to the anterolateral commissure on the posterior mitral valve leaflet (**B**) and can also be clearly seen in the midesophageal two-chamber chamber view at 90 degrees (**C**). Color flow interrogation of the mitral valve demonstrates mild-moderate mitral regurgitation but no perforation of the leaflets (**D**). Vegetation identified by *arrows*. AV, aortic valve; LA, left atrium.

Valvular Regurgitation

It is very common to find varying degrees of regurgitation of the infected valves, particularly the aortic and mitral valves. There are several mechanisms for regurgitation: (a) perforation of the leaflet from abscess formation, (b) impairment of leaflet coaptation due to mobile, prolapsing vegetations, and (c) leaflet prolapse/flail secondary to structural weakness or rupture of supporting structures (39). A thorough examination of infected valves should be performed utilizing two-dimensional (2D) imaging and color-flow Doppler to evaluate severity.

Perivalvular Complications

Extension of the infection into surrounding tissues is an ominous sign. Present in approximately 30% of cases, the mortality ranges from 22% to 90% (28,40–42). Although

TABLE 22.4	Characteristics of Mass Likely and Unlikely to be Vegetation	
Characteristic	**Likely Vegetation**	**Unlikely Vegetation**
Texture	Gray scale and reflectance of myocardium	Reflectance of calcium or pericardium
Location	Upstream side of the valve in the path of the jet	Downstream side of the valve
Motion	Chaotic and orbiting	
Shape	Lobulated and amorphous; Stringy or hand-like strands; narrow attachment	

Source: Sanfilippo AJ, Picard MH, Newell JB, et al. Echocardiographic assessment of patients with infectious endocarditis: prediction of risk for complications. J Am Coll Cardiol 1991;18(5):1191–1199.

perivalvular complications can occur at any location, they are most commonly found in the proximity of the aortic valve (AV) and the annulus of prosthetic valves (43–45). With TEE, an abscess appears as an echolucent space or cavity.

Pseudoaneurysms and Intracardiac Fistulae

Pseudoaneurysms and intracardiac fistulae are rare complications of IE (29,46–48). Pseudoaneurysms result from weakening of the myocardium, caused by abscess. They commonly form in the area of the mitral-aortic intervalvular fibrosis (MAIVF), and their rupture can create a communication between the left atrium and ventricle (29,47). The boundaries of the MAIVF are the left half of the AV noncoronary cusp and the third of the AV left coronary cusp adjacent to the anterior mitral leaflet (48). Echocardiographic findings of this phenomenon are an echo-free cavity in the MAIVF region with evidence of flow and communication with color Doppler. Intracardiac fistulae have the same underlying pathophysiology, can be single or multiple, and generally originate from the aorta and communicate to the left or right atria (33,46). These can be identified using color flow Doppler looking for the presence of abnormal systolic jets into the left and right atria.

The Prognostic Utility of Echocardiography and IE

Echocardiography early in the course of IE has strong prognostic value (34,49,50). Sanfilippo et al. found the risk of adverse outcomes (i.e., death, embolization, need for surgery, heart failure, and inadequate response to antibiotics) positively correlated with increasing vegetation size and from this information developed a predictive scoring tool (see Table 22.5) (34). In multivariate analysis, they found the scoring system predicted complications with 70% sensitivity and 92% specificity in mitral valve endocarditis and with 76% sensitivity and 62% specificity in AV endocarditis.

Several studies have looked at the prognostic value of TEE and IE (49,50). Lancelloti et al. found that total length of vegetations on TEE was an independent risk factor for the development of systemic emboli and/or death (50). In a larger multicenter prospective European study, a similar result was found: vegetation length greater than 15 mm was an independent predictor of 1-year mortality (49). Other studies have shown that presence of mobile vegetation on TEE results in increased risk of embolism as well (51).

The Role of 3D Echocardiography

Real-time 3D echocardiography represents a novel clinical modality for the diagnosis and management of IE (36). A recent study showed that 3D TTE may improve the sensitivity of TTE in detecting endocarditis involving prosthetic valves (52). It may also be useful for assessing complications associated with endocarditis (53). It is important to remember that 3D echocardiography obeys the same physical laws of 2D ultrasound and therefore shares its limitations (36). Studies utilizing 3D TEE in the diagnosis of IE are very limited but suggest an incremental benefit when used in addition to 2D TEE (54,55).

SURGICAL INDICATIONS FOR INFECTIVE ENDOCARDITIS

Management of IE is incredibly complicated involving combinations of antimicrobial medications, anticoagulation, and surgery and is beyond the scope of this chapter (6). The benefits of surgery for the management of IE have not been studied in a randomized control trial due to the unacceptably high mortality without surgery (56–58). The 2008 ACC/AHA guidelines for valvular heart disease delineates separate surgical indications for native and prosthetic valves (see Table 22.6) (6). In general, surgical therapy is immediately indicated for patients with significant congestive heart failure or cardiogenic shock, with the caveat that the patient has a reasonable prospect of recovery. Hemodynamic status is the primary determinant of intraoperative mortality; thus, timing of surgery is crucial (5). Early intervention also increases the likelihood that the involved valve(s) can be repaired, thus avoiding the introduction of foreign prosthetic materials into an infected heart (6,59–61). In patients who have cerebrovascular complications secondary to IE, it is generally accepted that surgery should be delayed for at least 2 weeks because of the high risk for further neurologic deterioration (62).

TABLE 22.5	**Vegetation Risk Score for Complications**			
	Grade 1	**Grade 2**	**Grade 3**	**Grade 4**
Mobility	Fixed	Fixed base; free edge	Pedunculated	Prolapsing
Density	Calcified	Partially calcified	Denser than myocardium; not calcified	Equivalent to myocardium
Extent	Single	Multiple on single leaflet	Multiple leaflets	Extending extravalvularly

Source: Sanfilippo AJ, Picard MH, Newell JB, et al. Echocardiographic assessment of patients with infectious endocarditis: prediction of risk for complications. J Am Coll Cardiol 1991;18(5):1191–1199.

TABLE 22.6 Surgical Indications for Native and Prosthetic Valve Endocarditis

Native valves

1. Class I
    a. Acute IE with valvular stenosis or regurgitation in heart failure
    b. Acute IE with AR or MR with elevated LVEDP or LAP
    c. IE caused by a fungal or highly resistant organism
    d. IE complicated by heart block, annular/aortic abscess, or destructive lesion
2. Class IIa
    a. Patients with IE with recurrent emboli or persistent vegetation despite antibiotic treatment
3. Class IIb
    a. Patients with IE with mobile vegetations in excess of 10 mm

Prosthetic valves

1. Class I
    a. IE with associated heart failure
    b. IE with evidence of dehiscence
    c. IE with increasing valvular obstruction or regurgitation
    d. IE with complications (i.e., abscess)
2. Class IIa
    a. Persistent bacteremia or recurrent emboli despite antibiotics
    b. IE with recurrent infections
3. Class III
    a. Routine surgery not indicated for uncomplicated IE caused by first infection

AR, aortic regurgitation; MR, mitral regurgitation; LVEDP, left ventricular enddiastolic pressure; LAP, left atrial pressure.
Source: Bonow RO, Carabello BA, Chatterjee K, et al. 2008 focused update incorporated into the ACC/AHA 2006 guidelines for the management of patients with valvular heart disease: a report of the American College of Cardiology/American Heart Association Task Force on Practice Guidelines (Writing Committee to revise the 1998 guidelines for the management of patients with valvular heart disease). Endorsed by the Society of Cardiovascular Anesthesiologists, Society for Cardiovascular Angiography and Interventions, and Society of Thoracic Surgeons. J Am Coll Cardiol 2008;52(13):e1–e142.

INTRAOPERATIVE ASSESSMENT

TEE is extremely valuable intraoperatively. In the ACC/AHA/ASE 2003 Guideline Update for the Clinical Application of Echocardiography, there is a class I indication for intraoperative TEE in IE patients when preoperative testing was insufficient or extension to perivalvular tissue is suspected (63). At our institution, a thorough intraoperative TEE examination for a patient with IE includes (a) confirming the diagnosis, (b) looking for new vegetations, and (c) identifying complications secondary to IE (i.e., regurgitation, perforations, perivalvular extension and abscess, aneurysm, and fistula). Following disengagement from cardiopulmonary bypass, it is important to assess the adequacy of the surgical intervention. This includes the assessment of the valvular repair or replacement and closure of any fistulas. The perioperative echocardiographer also needs screen for any perivalvular leak as thorough documentation may avoid unnecessary confusion during follow-up about whether such leakage is due to a recurrent infection.

CONCLUSION

TEE is an essential modality for the diagnosis and management of patients with IE. TEE allows for accurate and definitive diagnosis of IE allowing for the initiation of appropriate treatments, antibiotics, and/or surgery in a timely manner. 3D echocardiography is an emerging technology and may provide further advances in the management of IE.

KEY POINTS

■ IE is an infection on the endocardial surface of the heart and is associated with high morbidity and mortality.
■ Risk factors for the development of IE include poor dental hygiene, kidney disease, diabetes mellitus, intravenous drug usage, HIV, structure heart disease, prosthetic heart valves, and history of IE.

- The modified Duke Criteria integrate echocardiographic, laboratory and physical findings and are sensitive and specific for the diagnosis of IE.
- Echocardiographic findings for IE include the presence of vegetations, valvular regurgitation, abscess, pseudoaneurysm, and intracardiac fistulae.
- Echocardiography has strong prognostic value for stratifying patients at risk for adverse outcomes.
- 3D TEE represents a novel clinical modality for the diagnosis and management of IE.
- Intraoperative TEE is extremely valuable and is a class I indication in IE patients. On examination, it is important to confirm diagnosis, look for new vegetations, identify associated complications, and assess surgical repair.

REFERENCES

1. Hill EE, Herijgers P, Claus P, et al. Infective endocarditis: changing epidemiology and predictors of 6-month mortality: a prospective cohort study. *Eur Heart J* 2007;28(2):196–203.
2. Heidenreich PA, Masoudi FA, Maini B, et al. Echocardiography in patients with suspected endocarditis: a cost-effectiveness analysis. *Am J Med* 1999;107(3):198–208.
3. Rosen AB, Fowler VG Jr, Corey GR, et al. Cost-effectiveness of transesophageal echocardiography to determine the duration of therapy for intravascular catheter-associated Staphylococcus aureus bacteremia. *Ann Intern Med* 1999;130(10):810–820.
4. Osler W. The Gulstonian lectures, on malignant endocarditis. *Br Med J* 1885;1(1262):467–470.
5. Alexiou C, Langley SM, Stafford H, et al. Surgical treatment of infective mitral valve endocarditis: predictors of early and late outcome. *J Heart Valve Dis* 2000;9(3):327–334.
6. Bonow RO, Carabello BA, Chatterjee K, et al. 2008 focused update incorporated into the ACC/AHA 2006 guidelines for the management of patients with valvular heart disease: a report of the American College of Cardiology/American Heart Association Task Force on Practice Guidelines (Writing Committee to revise the 1998 guidelines for the management of patients with valvular heart disease). Endorsed by the Society of Cardiovascular Anesthesiologists, Society for Cardiovascular Angiography and Interventions, and Society of Thoracic Surgeons. *J Am Coll Cardiol* 2008;52(13):e1–e142.
7. Berlin JA, Abrutyn E, Strom BL, et al. Incidence of infective endocarditis in the Delaware Valley, 1988–1990. *Am J Cardiol* 1995;76(12):933–936.
8. Hogevik H, Olaison L, Andersson R, et al. Epidemiologic aspects of infective endocarditis in an urban population. A 5-year prospective study. *Medicine (Baltimore)* 1995;74(6):324–339.
9. Tleyjeh IM, Abdel-Latif A, Rahbi H, et al. A systematic review of population-based studies of infective endocarditis. *Chest* 2007;132(3):1025–1035.
10. Fowler VG Jr, Miro JM, Hoen B, et al. Staphylococcus aureus endocarditis: a consequence of medical progress. *JAMA.* 2005;293(24):3012–3021.
11. Strom BL, Abrutyn E, Berlin JA, et al. Risk factors for infective endocarditis: oral hygiene and nondental exposures. *Circulation* 2000;102(23):2842–2848.
12. Carrel T, Schaffner A, Vogt P, et al. Endocarditis in intravenous drug addicts and HIV infected patients: possibilities and limitations of surgical treatment. *J Heart Valve Dis* 1993;2(2):140–147.
13. Chambers HF, Morris DL, Tauber MG, et al. Cocaine use and the risk for endocarditis in intravenous drug users. *Ann Intern Med* 1987;106(6):833–836.
14. Grover FL, Cohen DJ, Oprian C, et al. Determinants of the occurrence of and survival from prosthetic valve endocarditis. Experience of the Veterans Affairs Cooperative Study on Valvular Heart Disease. *J Thorac Cardiovasc Surg* 1994;108(2):207–214.
15. Manoff SB, Vlahov D, Herskowitz A, et al. Human immunodeficiency virus infection and infective endocarditis among injecting drug users. *Epidemiology* 1996;7(6):566–570.
16. McKinsey DS, Ratts TE, Bisno AL. Underlying cardiac lesions in adults with infective endocarditis. The changing spectrum. *Am J Med* 1987;82(4):681–688.
17. Tornos P, Sanz E, Permanyer-Miralda G, et al. Late prosthetic valve endocarditis. Immediate and long-term prognosis. *Chest* 1992;101(1):37–41.
18. Agnihotri AK, McGiffin DC, Galbraith AJ, et al. The prevalence of infective endocarditis after aortic valve replacement. *J Thorac Cardiovasc Surg* 1995;110(6):1708–1720; discussion 1704–1720.
19. Vlessis AA, Hovaguimian H, Jaggers J, et al. Infective endocarditis: ten-year review of medical and surgical therapy. *Ann Thorac Surg* 1996;61(4):1217–1222.
20. Durack DT, Lukes AS, Bright DK. New criteria for diagnosis of infective endocarditis: utilization of specific echocardiographic findings. Duke Endocarditis Service. *Am J Med* 1994;96(3):200–209.
21. Li JS, Sexton DJ, Mick N, et al. Proposed modifications to the Duke criteria for the diagnosis of infective endocarditis. *Clin Infect Dis* 2000;30(4):633–638.
22. Pelletier LL Jr, Petersdorf RG. Infective endocarditis: a review of 125 cases from the University of Washington Hospitals, 1963–72. *Medicine (Baltimore)* 1977;56(4):287–313.
23. Von Reyn CF, Levy BS, Arbeit RD, et al. Infective endocarditis: an analysis based on strict case definitions. *Ann Intern Med* 1981;94(4 Pt 1):505–518.
24. Bayer AS, Ward JI, Ginzton LE, et al. Evaluation of new clinical criteria for the diagnosis of infective endocarditis. *Am J Med* 1994;96(3):211–219.
25. Cecchi E, Parrini I, Chinaglia A, et al. New diagnostic criteria for infective endocarditis. A study of sensitivity and specificity. *Eur Heart J* 1997;18(7):1149–1156.
26. Hoen B, Beguinot I, Rabaud C, et al. The Duke criteria for diagnosing infective endocarditis are specific: analysis of 100 patients with acute fever or fever of unknown origin. *Clin Infect Dis* 1996;23(2):298–302.
27. Sandre RM, Shafran SD. Infective endocarditis: review of 135 cases over 9 years. *Clin Infect Dis* 1996;22(2):276–286.
28. Daniel WG, Mugge A, Martin RP, et al. Improvement in the diagnosis of abscesses associated with endocarditis by transesophageal echocardiography. *N Engl J Med* 1991;324(12):795–800.
29. Karalis DG, Bansal RC, Hauck AJ, et al. Transesophageal echocardiographic recognition of subaortic complications in

aortic valve endocarditis. Clinical and surgical implications. *Circulation* 1992;86(2):353–362.

30. Pedersen WR, Walker M, Olson JD, et al. Value of transesophageal echocardiography as an adjunct to transthoracic echocardiography in evaluation of native and prosthetic valve endocarditis. *Chest* 1991;100(2):351–356.

31. Shively BK, Gurule FT, Roldan CA, et al. Diagnostic value of transesophageal compared with transthoracic echocardiography in infective endocarditis. *J Am Coll Cardiol* 1991;18(2): 391–397.

32. Baddour LM, Wilson WR, Bayer AS, et al. Infective endocarditis: diagnosis, antimicrobial therapy, and management of complications: a statement for healthcare professionals from the Committee on Rheumatic Fever, Endocarditis, and Kawasaki Disease, Council on Cardiovascular Disease in the Young, and the Councils on Clinical Cardiology, Stroke, and Cardiovascular Surgery and Anesthesia, American Heart Association: endorsed by the Infectious Diseases Society of America. *Circulation* 2005;111(23):e394–e434.

33. Evangelista A, Gonzalez-Alujas MT. Echocardiography in infective endocarditis. *Heart* 2004;90(6):614–617.

34. Sanfilippo AJ, Picard MH, Newell JB, et al. Echocardiographic assessment of patients with infectious endocarditis: prediction of risk for complications. *J Am Coll Cardiol* 1991;18(5): 1191–1199.

35. Rohmann S, Erbel R, Darius H, et al. Prediction of rapid versus prolonged healing of infective endocarditis by monitoring vegetation size. *J Am Soc Echocardiogr* 1991;4(5): 465–474.

36. Jungwirth B, Mackensen GB. Real-time 3-dimensional echocardiography in the operating room. *Semin Cardiothorac Vasc Anesth* 2008;12(4):248–264.

37. Petitalot JP, Allal J, Poupet JY, et al. Cardiac insufficiency in infectious endocarditis. *Arch Mal Coeur Vaiss* 1985;78(4): 525–532.

38. Petitalot JP, Allal J, Thomas P, et al. Cardiac complications of infectious endocarditis. *Ann Med Interne (Paris)* 1985;136(7):539–546.

39. Waller BF, Howard J, Fess S. Pathology of mitral valve stenosis and pure mitral regurgitation—Part II. *Clin Cardiol* 1994;17(7): 395–402.

40. Arnett EN, Roberts WC. Prosthetic valve endocarditis: clinicopathologic analysis of 22 necropsy patients with comparison observations in 74 necropsy patients with active infective endocarditis involving natural left-sided cardiac valves. *Am J Cardiol* 1976;38(3):281–292.

41. Arnett EN, Roberts WC. Active infective endocarditis: a clinicopathologic analysis of 137 necropsy patients. *Curr Probl Cardiol* 1976;1(7):2–76.

42. Chan KL. Early clinical course and long-term outcome of patients with infective endocarditis complicated by perivalvular abscess. *CMAJ.* 2002;167(1):19–24.

43. Aguado JM, Gonzalez-Vilchez F, Martin-Duran R, et al. Perivalvular abscesses associated with endocarditis. Clinical features and diagnostic accuracy of two-dimensional echocardiography. *Chest* 1993;104(1):88–93.

44. Baumgartner FJ, Omari BO, Robertson JM, et al. Annular abscesses in surgical endocarditis: anatomic, clinical, and operative features. *Ann Thorac Surg* 2000;70(2):442–447.

45. Graupner C, Vilacosta I, SanRoman J, et al. Periannular extension of infective endocarditis. *J Am Coll Cardiol* 2002;39(7): 1204–1211.

46. Esen AM, Kucukoglu MS, Okcun B, et al. Transoesophageal echocardiographic diagnosis of aortico-left atrial fistula in aortic valve endocarditis. *Eur J Echocardiogr* 2003;4(3):221–222.

47. Agirbasli M, Fadel BM. Pseudoaneurysm of the mitral-aortic intervalvular fibrosa: a long-term complication of infective endocarditis. *Echocardiography* 1999;16(3):253–257.

48. Tak T. Pseudoaneurysm of mitral-aortic intervalvular fibrosa. *Clin Med Res* 2003;1(1):49–52.

49. Thuny F, Di Salvo G, Belliard O, et al. Risk of embolism and death in infective endocarditis: prognostic value of echocardiography: a prospective multicenter study. *Circulation* 2005; 112(1):69–75.

50. Lancellotti P, Galiuto L, Albert A, et al. Relative value of clinical and transesophageal echocardiographic variables for risk stratification in patients with infective endocarditis. *Clin Cardiol* 1998;21(8):572–578.

51. Di Salvo G, Habib G, Pergola V, et al. Echocardiography predicts embolic events in infective endocarditis. *J Am Coll Cardiol* 2001;37(4):1069–1076.

52. Kort S. Real-time 3-dimensional echocardiography for prosthetic valve endocarditis: initial experience. *J Am Soc Echocardiogr* 2006;19(2):130–139.

53. Horton CJ Jr, Nanda NC, Nekkanti R, et al. Prosthetic aortic valve abscess producing total right coronary artery occlusion: diagnosis by transesophageal three-dimensional echocardiography. *Echocardiography* 2002;19(5):395–398.

54. Kanzaki Y, Yoshida K, Hozumi T, et al. Evaluation of mitral valve lesions in patients with infective endocarditis by three-dimensional echocardiography. *J Cardiol* 1999;33(1):7–11.

55. Hansalia S, Biswas M, Dutta R, et al. The value of live/real time three-dimensional transesophageal echocardiography in the assessment of valvular vegetations. *Echocardiography* 2009;26(10):1264–1273.

56. Aksoy O, Sexton DJ, Wang A, et al. Early surgery in patients with infective endocarditis: a propensity score analysis. *Clin Infect Dis* 2007;44(3):364–372.

57. Durack DT. Evaluating and optimizing outcomes of surgery for endocarditis. *JAMA* 2003;290(24):3250–3251.

58. Vikram HR, Buenconsejo J, Hasbun R, et al. Impact of valve surgery on 6-month mortality in adults with complicated, left-sided native valve endocarditis: a propensity analysis. *JAMA* 2003;290(24):3207–3214.

59. Iung B, Rousseau-Paziaud J, Cormier B, et al. Contemporary results of mitral valve repair for infective endocarditis. *J Am Coll Cardiol* 2004;43(3):386–392.

60. Sternik L, Zehr KJ, Orszulak TA, et al. The advantage of repair of mitral valve in acute endocarditis. *J Heart Valve Dis* 2002;11(1):91–97; discussion 97–98.

61. Zegdi R, Debieche M, Latremouille C, et al. Long-term results of mitral valve repair in active endocarditis. *Circulation* 2005;111(19):2532–2536.

62. Eishi K, Kawazoe K, Kuriyama Y, et al. Surgical management of infective endocarditis associated with cerebral complications. Multi-center retrospective study in Japan. *J Thorac Cardiovasc Surg* 1995;110(6):1745–1755.

63. Cheitlin MD, Armstrong WF, Aurigemma GP, et al. ACC/AHA/ASE 2003 guideline update for the clinical application of echocardiography—summary article: a report of the American College of Cardiology/American Heart Association Task Force on Practice Guidelines (ACC/AHA/ASE Committee to Update the 1997 Guidelines for the Clinical Application of Echocardiography). *J Am Coll Cardiol* 2003;42(5):954–970.

QUESTIONS

1. All the following are MINOR criteria for infective endocarditis (IE) EXCEPT
   A. Fever greater than 38°C
   B. Oscillating mass
   C. Osler nodes
   D. Pulmonary infarct
   E. Janeway lesions

2. All the following are American College of Cardiology/American Heart Association (ACC/AHA) Class I transesophageal echocardiography (TEE) indications for IE EXCEPT
   A. Intraoperative management of patients undergoing valve surgery
   B. First-line modality to diagnosis IE involving prosthetic valves
   C. Diagnosis of complications associated with IE that affect management

D. Diagnosis of IE in patients with nosocomial staphylococcal bacteremia
E. Assessment of severity of valvular lesions if transthoracic echocardiography (TTE) is nondiagnostic

3. All the following are characteristic of vegetations EXCEPT
   A. Downstream of the valve
   B. Gray scale and reflectance of the myocardium
   C. Chaotic motion
   D. Orbiting motion
   E. Lobulated and amorphous

4. All the following are associated with endocarditis EXCEPT
   A. Vegetation
   B. Valvular regurgitation
   C. Pseudoaneurysm
   D. Mitral-pulmonic intervalvular fibrosis
   E. Abscess

CHAPTER 23

Rescue Echocardiography in the Critically Ill Patient

Stanton K. Shernan ■ Solomon Aronson

Category I applications of transesophageal echocardiography (TEE) include the role of "rescue TEE" for the evaluation of acute persistent and life-threatening hemodynamic disturbances in which ventricular function and its determinants are uncertain or have not responded to treatment. Category I indications are supported by the strongest evidence or expert opinion that TEE is useful in improving clinical outcomes (1). TEE is an effective diagnostic tool for determining the etiology and mechanism of significant, acute hemodynamic instability or hypoxemia in critically ill patients, and it can be used specifically to monitor cardiac performance, define cardiovascular pathology, and guide interventions (2).

The role of TEE in critical emergency settings is beneficial for establishing a diagnosis and directing definitive therapies in up to 80% of patients. Based on TEE analyses, almost a third of patients may have a change in medical therapy, while 23% may have a change in surgical procedure (3). TEE was shown to be helpful in defining the etiology of unexpected cardiac arrest in 19 of 22 patients (4). The TEE findings in these emergency settings included hypovolemia, pericardial tamponade, ventricular dysfunction, regional wall motion abnormalities, and intracardiac or intravascular thrombi. In 18 patients, TEE guided specific management beyond implementation of Advanced Cardiac Life Support protocols, including the addition of surgical procedures in 12 patients.

Although transthoracic echocardiography (TTE) can also be utilized in a rescue situation, in the emergency setting, the acquisition of TTE imaging windows that are dependent on patient positioning (e.g., parasternal and subcostal views) or in patients dependent upon mechanical ventilation may make image acquisition problematic. In addition, conventional TTE windows may not be accessible in the postoperative patient who has undergone thoracic or abdominal surgery. Furthermore, TTE imaging requires interruption of chest compressions during cardiopulmonary resuscitation, whereas acquisition of diagnostic TEE data can proceed without interference (5).

Category II indications are supported by weaker evidence and expert consensus (1). While TEE may be useful in improving clinical outcomes in these settings, absolute indications are less certain. A related Category II rescue indication for TEE includes augmented management of patients who need advanced hemodynamic monitoring.

Changes in management have been based upon confirming or invalidating a prior diagnosis, detection of new diagnoses, and acquisition of pertinent information acquired during periods of hemodynamic instability leading to changes in drug or goal-directed fluid therapy.

When performing a TEE examination in a rescue situation, the examination must be initially focused and limited. The focus of the examination should be directed toward confirming or finding a diagnosis that leads to therapeutic intervention. Nonetheless, if time permits, performing a comprehensive TEE examination should be attempted to determine the presence of unanticipated but possible related pathology. All causes of treatable hemodynamic compromise need to be ruled out. Commonly encountered etiologies include hypovolemia, pulmonary embolus, ventricular dysfunction, aortic dissection, severe valvular disease, intracardiac masses or thrombi, myocardial ischemia, pericardial effusion, and cardiac tamponade.

UNRECOGNIZED HYPOVOLEMIA

TEE can be used to estimate right (RV) and left ventricular (LV) preload and volume status by observing changes in ventricular end-diastolic area. TEE enables superior assessment of volume status in the face of active fluid resuscitation compared to central venous or pulmonary capillary wedge pressure. Conventional pulmonary artery catheters measure pressure and not volume. Thus, while the pressure to volume relationship may be reasonably predictive in a compliant system, the relationship between LV end-diastolic volume and right-sided pulmonary artery pressures may be less reliable in the face of reduced thoracic or lung compliance, positive airway pressure, vasoactive drugs, impaired myocardial contractility and mitral valve (MV) disease. A recent study retrospectively evaluated the role of TEE in optimizing resuscitation in 25 acutely injured patients who required TEE for persistent shock in the absence of ongoing surgical hemorrhage in the operating room and intensive care setting (6). Decreased LV filling was diagnosed by TEE in 52% of these patients despite a mean pulmonary artery pressure of 19.5 mm Hg and after the patients had received an average of 6.9 L of crystalloid and 14 units of blood products. This study supports previous reports showing that TEE assessment of LV end-diastolic area is more accurate and clinically useful than estimates of preload based on hemodynamic data from a pulmonary artery catheter (7). Therefore, in the face of ongoing, persistent hypotension, TEE can be used to efficiently and accurately diagnose hypovolemia or hypervolemia, and may guide the subsequent management of such a patient.

PULMONARY EMBOLISM

Although pulmonary angiography, spiral computer tomography, or ventilation-perfusion scintigraphy is used to diagnose pulmonary embolism (PE), these imaging techniques are not always possible or practical in the acutely, decompensated patient. Therefore, TEE has been used as an alternative diagnostic tool (8). Direct visualization of a pulmonary artery thrombus is consistent with an echocardiographic diagnosis of PE. In particular, the midesophageal ascending aortic short-axis view is useful for visualizing thromboembolism in the pulmonary artery (Fig. 23.1). However, the interposition of the tracheobronchial tree between the esophagus and the aorta can make image acquisition difficult. In such cases, secondary signs suggestive of a PE may be helpful including RV hypokinesis, RV enlargement, flattening of the interventricular septum, or leftward bowing of the interatrial septum (Fig. 23.2). Other echocardiographic signs sug-

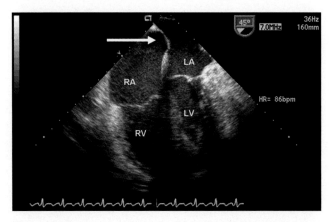

Figure 23.2. Transesophageal echocardiographic midesophageal four-chamber view demonstrating leftward bowing (*arrow*) of the interatrial septum in a patient with a pulmonary embolus. LA, left atrium; LV, left ventricle; RA, right atrium; RV, right ventricle.

gestive of a PE include an underfilled and hyperdynamic LV, dilated pulmonary artery, increased peak velocity of tricuspid valve insufficiency, shortened pulmonary ejection acceleration time, or RV dysfunction with sparing of its apex (i.e., McConnell's sign) (9).

Recently, a retrospective study evaluated the diagnostic utility of TEE in 46 consecutive patients who underwent emergent pulmonary embolectomy (10). Intraoperative, precardiopulmonary bypass (CPB) TEE findings were compared with corresponding surgical findings to show that echocardiographic evidence for PE was correctly demonstrated in 46% of patients, and that the sensitivity for diagnosing PE with intraoperative TEE within a particular pulmonary artery location was 26% (range 17%–35%). Therefore, when a thrombus is seen within a particular location, it is highly suggestive of a PE. However, the absence of TEE evidence cannot exclude a PE. In addition, although RV dysfunction from pulmonary hypertension is consistent with PE, it can be precipitated by other causes of pulmonary hypertension.

VENTRICULAR DYSFUNCTION

TEE is well suited to provide accurate evaluation of ventricular systolic function during hemodynamic instability. Among the many measures of global ventricular function, fractional area change (FAC) is relatively simple and can be obtained from the transgastric short-axis view. FAC is simply the proportion of diastolic area of the LV chamber in the midpapillary short-axis view that is reduced during systole:

$$\text{FAC\%} = [\text{end diastolic area} - \text{end systolic area}] \times 100/\text{end diastolic area}$$

Normal FAC is greater than 45%. While FAC is often estimated visually, the chamber circumference can be traced in both systole and diastole to provide objective measures of the areas for more accurate calculation. Since FAC is

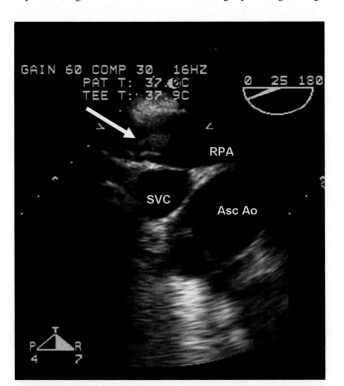

Figure 23.1. Transesophageal echocardiographic midesophageal ascending aorta short-axis view demonstrating a pulmonary embolus (*arrow*) in the right pulmonary artery (RPA). Asc Ao, ascending aorta; SVC, superior vena cava.

only measured in one plane, it may miss significant wall motion abnormalities located outside of the imaging sector and, therefore, may have limited accuracy in the assessment of overall ventricular function (11). Oblique planes of view may also reduce accuracy (12).

Ejection fraction (EF), which includes the volume change (stroke volume) of the whole ventricle rather than the area change of a single plane, is a more accurate measure of global ventricular function:

$$EF\% = [\text{end diastolic volume} - \text{end systolic volume}] \times 100/\text{end diastolic volume}$$

Normal EF is 55% to 75%. Generating accurate 3D volumes from 2D echocardiography can be a source of error. Therefore, geometric methods assume that the ventricle fits a stereotypical ellipsoidal shape. These include the single-plane ellipsoid method, cylinder-hemi-ellipsoid method, and area-length method, all of which estimate volume from diameter and length measurements in one or two planes. The geometric assumptions limit accuracy of EF, when segmental wall motion abnormalities or unusual ventricular shapes are present. In addition, if the plane in which the measurement is acquired does not include the true apex (i.e., a foreshortened view), then the LV volumes and EF will also be unreliable.

The modified Simpson method, also known as the disc summation method, is considered the best method for deriving ventricular volumes and EF. For this method, the endocardial border is traced in two orthogonal planes (e.g., midesophageal four-chamber and two-chamber views). Computer software then models the ventricle as a series of 20 or more stacked elliptical disks. The volume of each disk is then calculated from the thickness of the disk, the diameters of each ellipsoid disk, and all of summed volumes to yield the total ventricular volume. Cylindrical disks or rotating ellipsoid models can be generated from a single tomographic view but with reduced accuracy. The biplane disc summation method allows for variably shaped ventricles. It also can account for significant regional wall motion abnormalities but can still be limited by image quality or foreshortened views. To reduce foreshortening errors, the two views should not be combined if the chamber lengths differ by greater than 20%. It should be noted that neither FAC nor LVEF are pure indices of myocardial contractility as both are dependent upon loading conditions, especially at the extremes of preload and afterload.

AORTIC DISSECTION

TEE is useful for the diagnosis and classification of thoracic and abdominal aneurysms and dissections. An aneurysm of the aorta involves an increase in the luminal diameter of all three layers of the aorta. A pseudoaneurysm involves an interruption of the intima and media at the level of the aneurysmal sac and its communication with the native aorta.

Dissection of the aorta is a process in which the intima separates from the adventitial layer and is characterized by the presence of an intimal flap and false and true lumens (13). Aortic dissection can result from intimal rupture followed by cleavage formation and propagation of the dissection into the media, or from intramural hemorrhage and hematoma formation in the media subsequently followed by perforation of the intima. The presence of an intimal flap is the most characteristic feature of aortic dissection. The pathogenesis of dissection is complex. The medial degeneration tends to be more extensive in older individuals and in patients with hypertension, Marfan's syndrome, and bicuspid aortic valves (AV) (14). Aortic dissection is divided into acute and chronic types, depending on the duration of symptoms. Acute aortic dissection is present when the diagnosis is made within 2 weeks after the initial onset of symptoms, and chronic aortic dissection is present when the initial symptoms are more than 2 weeks duration. About one third of patients with aortic dissection fall into the chronic category. The most common site of initiation of aortic dissection is the ascending aorta (50%) followed by the aortic regions in the vicinity of the ligamentum arteriosum.

Anatomically, aortic dissection has been classified by two schemes. The DeBakey classification consists of the following three types: (a), both the ascending and the descending aorta are involved; (b) only the ascending aorta is involved; and (c), only the descending aorta is involved. The Stanford classification consists of the two types: type A, involving the ascending aorta regardless of the entry site location; and type B, involving the aorta distal to the origin of the left subclavian artery.

TEE may be particularly useful not only in diagnosing the location of the flap's origin and its extension, but also pathology including the potential for acute AV insufficiency (Fig. 23.3), involvement of the coronary ostia with an associated risk of myocardial ischemia, and a pericardial effusion.

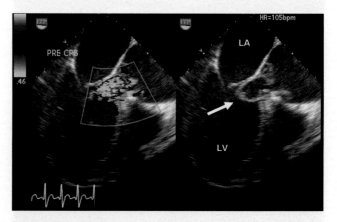

Figure 23.3. Transesophageal echocardiographic midesophageal long-axis view demonstrating an acute aortic dissection with the corresponding color flow Doppler jet of severe aortic insufficiency (**right**), and intimal flap (**left**: *arrow*) that involutes across the AV. LA, left atrium; LV, left ventricle; CPB, cardiopulmonary bypass.

SEVERE VALVULAR DISEASE

Critical aortic stenosis (AS) may be associated with acute hemodynamic compromise. The normal AV area is 2 to 4 cm². Calcific degeneration of the AV is the most common cause of AS, and it is characterized by restricted leaflet motion and calcification along the free edges of the leaflets. Patients with calcific degeneration usually become symptomatic over the age of 70 years. Rheumatic AS is more common in middle-aged immigrants from developing countries and often presents with thickened leaflet tips, which are calcified and fused at the commissures, producing a characteristic "doming" during systole. The orifice may become circular shaped. Rheumatic AS is almost always associated with rheumatic involvement of the MV. Congenital abnormalities of the AV (unicuspid, bicuspid, quadricuspid) may also be associated with AS. Bicuspid AV is the most common form, occurring in approximately 2% of the normal population. Symptoms usually occur in the fourth to sixth decades of life. The orifice is elliptical, rather than star shaped, and a calcified raphe is often present on one of the leaflets, giving the false impression of a tricuspid valve in diastole. Therefore, a bicuspid AV can only be reliably diagnosed in systole.

TEE examination of the insufficient MV should involve inspection of collateral structures in the heart that are altered as a result of the regurgitant process. Left atrial dilatation is commonly found in chronic mitral regurgitation (MR) of at least moderate severity but is not a feature of acute MR. Left to right bowing of the interatrial septum due to elevated left atrial pressure can often be appreciated in the midesophageal four-chamber view or the bicaval view. Signs of pulmonary hypertension, such as RV and atrial enlargement, often accompany progressive MR. A hypercontractile LV is a normal finding with severe MR. Spherical LV enlargement with eccentric hypertrophy is consistent with long-standing MR in which the compensatory processes of the ventricle are failing.

Papillary muscle rupture is occasionally a complication of myocardial infarction (MI) and, most frequently, affects the posteromedial muscle. It can result in severe bileaflet regurgitation involving the middle (A2/P2) and medial (A3/P3) scallops. The papillary muscle, chordae, and MV leaflet tips can often be seen flailing into and out of the left atrium.

MV endocarditis can affect native valves and result in regurgitation due to perforation, deformation, and destruction of the valve leaflets. Mitral stenosis is not usually observed. Commonly, vegetations arise on the upstream side of a valve, and in the case of the MV, they are usually seen in the left atrium (Fig. 23.4). The finding of MV endocarditis mandates a careful inspection of the other heart valves to rule out concurrent involvement. Leaflet perforation is identified by the appearance of one or more regurgitant jets that do not seem to arise from the coaptation line. A clue to this particular pathology is the presence of multiple convergence zones on color flow Doppler.

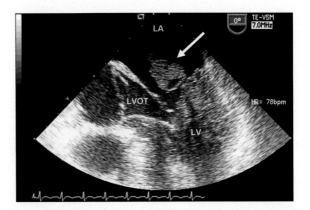

Figure 23.4. Transesophageal echocardiographic midesophageal five-chamber view demonstrating large vegetation (*arrow*) attached to the left atrial (LA) side of the posterior leaflet of the mitral valve. LV, left ventricle; LVOT, left ventricular outflow tract.

INTRACARDIAC THROMBI

TEE can visualize intracardiac thrombi or intracardiac air (Fig. 23.5). In orthopedic surgery, emboli are released into circulation during the preparation and implantation of the prosthesis when methylmethacrylate is used (15–17). Such emboli have been associated with hemodynamic compromise ranging from moderate decreases in systemic blood pressure, increases in pulmonary artery pressure, and limited RV and LV regional wall motion abnormalities to frank cardiovascular collapse (18).

Venous air embolism, another source of hemodynamic compromise, can occur during any procedure where the surgical field is above the level of the heart. Neurosurgical procedures in the sitting position are notoriously associated with venous air embolism (19). When embolic material or air is noted in the heart, it is important to interrogate the interatrial septum for intracardiac shunts. There are numerous case reports where TEE was used to diagnose a culprit paradoxical embolus traversing the interatrial septum (20).

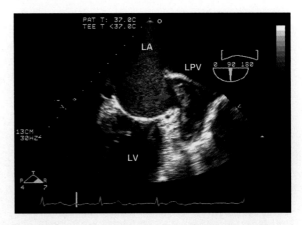

Figure 23.5. Transesophageal echocardiographic midesophageal two-chamber view demonstrating a large thrombus (*arrow*) in the left atrial appendage. LA, left atrium; LV, left ventricle; LPV, left pulmonary vein.

ISCHEMIA MONITORING

Ischemic changes detected by 2D echocardiography include new systolic wall motion abnormalities (SWMA) and decreased systolic wall thickening. Echocardiography is also useful for evaluating complications of myocardial ischemia including MI, congestive heart failure (CHF), valvular regurgitation, septal defects, thrombi, pericardial effusions, and ventricular free wall rupture. It should be noted that the sensitivity and positive predictive values for MI are less than 40%, possibly because not all ischemia results in MI (21). SWMA, for example, often overestimate the area of injury and may result from etiologies other than ischemia including myocardial stunning, hibernation, tethering, ventricular pacing as well as changes in loading conditions. The TEE transgastric midpapillary short-axis view is the most commonly used view to monitor myocardial ischemia as it allows assessment of the distribution of all three coronary arteries and rapid assessment of volume status. In the presence of asystole, episodic spontaneous rhythm may be sufficient for diagnosis of regional myocardial ischemia by TEE.

PERICARDIAL FLUID

Rapid accumulation of pericardial fluid can lead to hemodynamic instability and eventual cardiac collapse. Acute accumulation of pericardial fluid can cause severe hemodynamic instability and lead to cardiac tamponade (Fig. 23.6). A pericardial effusion can develop commonly post cardiac and aortic surgery, and secondary to complications related to transvenous pacemaker or internal cardiac defibrillator lead extraction, electrophysiologic procedures, transcatheter atrial septal defect closure, inferior vena cava filter placement as well as laparoscopic or thoracoscopic procedures. Other disease states associated with pericardial effusion include malignancies, trauma, infection, inflammatory disease, and radiation (22).

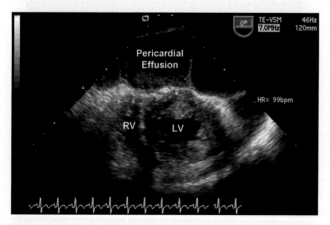

Figure 23.6. Transesophageal echocardiographic transgastric mid-short-axis view demonstrating a large pericardial effusion. LV, left ventricle; RV, right ventricle.

TABLE 23.1	Echocardiographic Findings Associated with Cardiac Tamponade
Early diastolic collapse of the RV
Early systolic right or left atrial inversion
Decreased right atrial or ventricular size
Abnormal ventricular septal motion
Respiratory variation in ventricular chamber size
Inferior vena cava plethora with blunted respiratory changes
Respiratory variation in atrial-ventricular valve, pulmonary venous, and hepatic vein Doppler flow-velocity profiles

Echocardiographic features consistent with pericardial effusion and tamponade are noted in Table 23.1. TEE may permit better visualization of intrapericardial clot and loculated pericardial effusions compared to TTE (23,24).

KEY POINTS

■ Category I applications of TEE include the role of "rescue TEE" for the evaluation of acute persistent and life-threatening hemodynamic disturbances in which ventricular function and its determinants are uncertain, or have not responded to treatment.

■ The role of TEE in critical emergency settings is beneficial for establishing a diagnosis and directing definitive therapies in up to 80% of patients. Based on TEE analyses, almost a third of patients may have a change in medical therapy, while 23% may have a change in surgical procedure.

■ Commonly encountered etiologies of acute hemodynamic compromise include hypovolemia, pulmonary embolus, ventricular dysfunction, aortic dissection, severe valvular disease, intracardiac masses or thrombi, myocardial ischemia, pericardial effusion, and cardiac tamponade.

REFERENCES

1. Practice Guidelines for Perioperative Transesophageal Echocardiography. A report by the American Society of Anesthesiologists and the Society of Cardiovascular Anesthesiologists Task Force on Transesophageal Echocardiography. *Anesthesiology* 1996;84:986–1006.

2. Brandt RR, Oh JK, Abel MD, et al. Role of emergency intraoperative transesophageal echocardiography. *J Am Soc Echocardiogr* 1998;11:972–977.

3. Suriani R, Cutrone A, Feierman D, et al. Intraoperative transesophageal echocardiography during liver transplantation. *J Cardiothorac Vasc Anesth* 1996;10:699–707.

4. Memtsoudis S, Rosenberger P, Noveva M, et al. Usefulness of transesophageal echocardiography during intraoperative cardiac arrest. *Anesth Analg* 2006;102:1653–1657.
5. Blaivas M. Transesophageal echocardiography during cardiopulmonary arrest in the emergency department. *Resuscitation* 2008;78:135–140.
6. Burns JM, Sing RF, Mostafa G, et al. The role of transesophageal echocardiography in optimizing resuscitation in acutely injured patients. *J Trauma* 2005;59:36–40.
7. Cheung AT, Savino JS, Weiss SJ, et al. Echocardiographic and hemodynamic indexes of left ventricular preload in patients with normal and abnormal ventricular function. *Anesthesiology* 1994;81:376–387.
8. Pruszczyk P, Torbicki A, Pacho R, et al. Noninvasive diagnosis of suspected severe pulmonary embolism: transesophageal echocardiography vs spiral CT. *Chest* 1997;112:722–728.
9. McConnell MV, Solomon SD, Rayan ME, et al. Regional right ventricular dysfunction detected by echocardiography in acute pulmonary embolism. *Am J Cardiol* 1996;78:469–473.
10. Rosenberger P, Shernan SK, Body SC, et al. Utility of intraoperative transesophageal echocardiography for diagnosis of pulmonary embolism. *Anesth Analg* 2004;99:12–16.
11. McGowan JH, Cleland JGF. Reliability of reporting left ventricular systolic function by echocardiography: a systematic review of 3 methods. *Am Heart J* 2003;146:388–397.
12. Cerqueira MD, Weissman NJ, Dilsizian V, et al. Standardized myocardial segmentation and nomenclature for tomographic imaging of the heart: a statement for healthcare professionals from the Cardiac Imaging Committee of the Council on Clinical Cardiology of the American Heart Association. *Circulation* 2002;105:539.
13. Willens HJ, Kessler KM. Transesophageal echocardiography in the diagnosis of diseases of the thoracic aorta: part 1. Aortic dissection, aortic intramural hematoma, and penetrating atherosclerotic ulcer of the aorta. *Chest* 1999;116:1772–1779.
14. Khan IA, Nair CK. Clinical, diagnostic, and management perspectives of aortic dissection. *Chest* 2002;122:311–328.
15. Ulrich C, Burri C, Worsdorfer O, et al. Intraoperative transesophageal two-dimensional echocardiography in total hip replacement. *Arch Orthop Trauma Surg* 1986;105:274–278.
16. Murphy P, Edelist G, Byrick RJ, et al. Relationship of fat embolism to haemodynamic and echocardiographic changes during cemented arthroplasty. *Can J Anaesth* 1997;44:1293–1300.
17. Koessler MJ, Fabiani R, Hamer H, et al. The clinical relevance of embolic events detected by transesophageal echocardiography during cemented total hip arthroplasty: a randomized clinical trial. *Anesth Analg* 2001;92:49–55.
18. Schlag G. Mechanisms of cardiopulmonary disturbances during total hip replacement. *Acta Orthop Belg* 1988;54:6–11.
19. Mirski MA, Lele AV, Fitzsimmons L, et al. Diagnosis and treatment of vascular air embolism. *Anesthesiology* 2007;106:164–177.
20. Dorr M, Hummel A. Images in clinical medicine. Paradoxical embolism—thrombus in a patent foramen ovale. *N Engl J Med* 2007;357:2285.
21. Comunale ME, Body SC, Ley C, et al. Multicenter Study of Perioperative Ischemia (McSPI) Research Group. The concordance of intraoperative left ventricular wall-motion abnormalities and electrocardiographic S-T segment changes. Association with outcome after coronary revascularization. *Anesthesiology* 1998;88:945–954.
22. Farlo J, Thawgathurai D, Mikhail M, et al. Cardiac tamponade during laparoscopic Nissen fundoplication. *Eur J Anaesthesiol* 1998;15:246–247.
23. Tsang T, Barnes M, Hayes S, et al. Clinical and echocardiographic characteristics of significant pericardial effusions following cardiothoracic surgery and outcomes of echo-guided pericardiocentesis for management: Mayo Clinic Experience, 1979–1988. *Chest* 1999;116:322–331.
24. Hosokawa K, Nakajima Y. An evaluation of acute cardiac tamponade by transesophageal echocardiography. *Anesth Analg* 2008;106:61–62.

QUESTIONS

1. Compared to transesophageal echocardiography (TEE), which of the following is a relative limitation of using transthoracic echocardiography (TTE) for perioperative rescue echocardiography in a hemodynamically compromised patient?
   A. Influence of intrathoracic air after thoracotomy or sternotomy on image quality
   B. Limited ability to access the chest or abdominal surface after surgery, to obtain imaging windows
   C. Need to interrupt chest compressions during cardiopulmonary resuscitation (CPR) to obtain images
   D. Need to obtain imaging windows that may require patient positioning (i.e., parasternal and subcostal views)
   E. All of the above
2. Secondary echocardiographic signs of acute pulmonary embolism (PE) include all of the following except
   A. Enlargement of the right ventricle (RV)
   B. Flattening of the interventricular septum
   C. Hypokinesis of the RV with apical sparing
   D. Rightward bowing of the interatrial septum
   E. Underfilled and hyperdynamic left ventricle (LV)
3. Which of the following is least likely to limit the use of segmental wall motion abnormalities as an echocardiographic sign of acute regional LV ischemia?
   A. Atrial pacing
   B. Changes in loading conditions
   C. Hibernation
   D. Myocardial stunning
   E. Tethering
4. Which of the following echocardiographic signs is most likely demonstrated in a patient with cardiac tamponade undergoing a rescue echocardiographic examination?
   A. Early diastolic collapse of the right atrium
   B. Early systolic collapse of the RV
   C. Dilated RV
   D. Inferior vena cava collapse
   E. Interventricular septal bounce

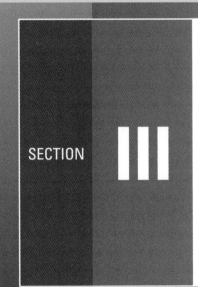

SECTION III

Advanced
Applications in
Perioperative
Echocardiography

CHAPTER 24

Epiaortic and Epicardial Imaging

James Richardson ■ Scott T. Reeves ■ Kathryn Glas

Intraoperative echocardiography made its debut in the form of epicardial ultrasound in the early 1970s (1). During the decade following, it was used for the evaluation of valvular anatomy and function during valve surgery and to assess left ventricular (LV) function during coronary artery bypass surgery (CABG). In the early 1980s, transesophageal echocardiography (TEE) was introduced to the operating room. After subsequent advances in TEE technology, epicardial techniques lost favor and were all but replaced by intraoperative TEE for the next 25 years. It has become evident in the past few years that there are still significant benefits to the use of epicardial imaging in the operative period, and its use has increased. Epiaortic ultrasound (EAU) has been utilized for superior visualization of the ascending aorta for more than 20 years, and recently guidelines for its use were published. The American Society of Echocardiography (ASE) and the Society of Cardiovascular Anesthesiologists (SCA) published the first guidelines for epicardial and epiaortic echocardiography examinations in 2007 and 2008, respectively (2–3). This chapter will review the rationale for performance of epicardial and epiaortic examinations (including outcome data related to their use), recommended images, technique for performance of these examinations, and guidelines for training.

EPICARDIAL IMAGING

Indications

Over the past 20 years, the use of TEE has become the mainstay in intraoperative echocardiography. It has allowed for more complete examinations of the heart and the aorta and does not involve an interruption of surgery to acquire images. Despite its dominance, the usefulness of TEE does have its limitations. On occasion, the TEE probe is difficult or impossible to pass into the esophagus or may be contraindicated due to a patient's anatomy, esophageal pathology (Zenker's diverticulum, stricture, cancer, or recent gastroesophageal surgery), or significant dysphagia or odynophagia. In these situations, the ability to perform an epicardial examination is essential, particularly in high-risk patients in whom imaging may improve their outcome (4). Another potential advantage to epicardial imaging is the opportunity

to obtain higher resolution images. In addition, anterior structures in the heart, such as the pulmonic valve, are potentially better visualized with an epicardial approach than with TEE.

Novel approaches to using epicardial echocardiography in the operating room are being investigated. During CABG surgery, target sites can be located using epicardial echocardiography. Flow through the grafts can also be determined to check for graft patency. Epicardial echocardiography has also been proposed as a quality assessment tool for the anastomosis site during CABG (5).

Imaging Guidelines

The published guidelines present seven epicardial echocardiographic imaging planes that are modified from standard transthoracic echocardiographic (TTE) views (2). The nomenclature for these modified views is consistent with the ASE recommended nomenclature for TTE (Figs. 24.1–24.7). The figures list both the epicardial imaging nomenclature and the corresponding TTE nomenclature. Image orientation discussions are based on normal

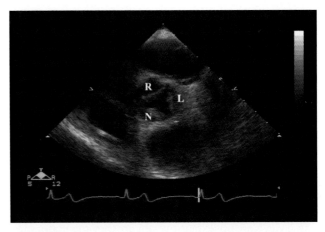

Figure 24.1. Epicardial AV SAX view (TTE parasternal AV SAX equivalent). When the orientation marker on the probe is oriented toward the patient's left shoulder, the image orientation below will be seen. As with TEE images, the commissure of the left and right leaflets is adjacent to the pulmonic valve, and the noncoronary cusp is adjacent to the intra-atrial septum. R, right coronary cusp of AV; L, left coronary cusp of AV; N, noncoronary cusp of AV.

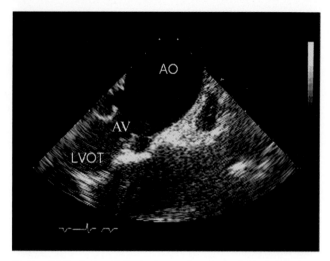

Figure 24.2. Epicardial AV LAX view (TTE suprasternal AV LAX equivalent). Doppler interrogation can be accomplished with this view, as can measurements of the annulus size. Ao, Ascending aorta; AV, aortic valve; LVOT, left ventricular outflow tract.

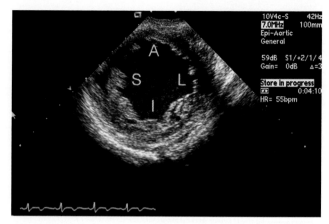

Figure 24.4. Epicardial LV SAX view (TTE parasternal LV mid-SAX equivalent). The probe is oriented toward the patient's left shoulder. A, Anterior wall; S, septal wall; I, inferior wall; L, lateral wall. To move from Figures 24.3 and 24.4, move the probe toward the LV apex. The posteromedial papillary muscle is adjacent to the "S." The RV can be seen by angling the probe toward the right without rotation. Excessive pressure from the probe can cause a regional wall motion artifact along the anterior wall, and potentially hypotension.

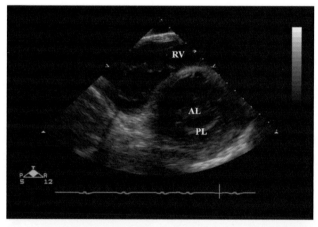

Figure 24.3. Epicardial LV basilar SAX view (TTE modified parasternal mitral valve basal SAX equivalent). The probe marker should be oriented toward the patient's left shoulder to obtain the image alignment shown below. The tricuspid valve is seen adjacent to the "RV." Note this image allows a view of the mitral valve that is similar to the surgical view. RV, Right ventricle; AL, Anterior leaflet, mitral valve; PL, Posterior leaflet, mitral valve.

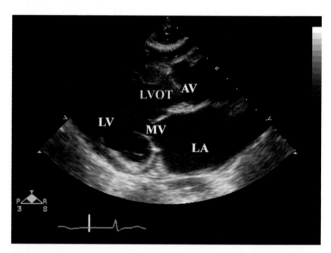

Figure 24.5. Epicardial LV LAX view (TTE parasternal LAX equivalent). To obtain this view, from Figure 24.4, rotate the probe toward the patient's right shoulder and adjust the angle superiorly. Measurements of the LV size and wall thickness can be obtained, as well as LA size. The mitral valve and AV can be assessed with CFD. AV, aortic valve; MV, mitral valve; LA, left atrium; LV, left ventricle (basilar portion); LVOT, left ventricular outflow tract.

cardiac anatomy; in patients with dextrocardia, the image would be reversed despite correct probe orientation. These views are not exhaustive nor are they mandatory for completion in each patient. They serve, however, to guide the echocardiographer through a complete examination (2D, color flow Doppler [CFD] and pulse wave Doppler [PWD]), where time and patient anatomy allow for their acquisition. In some cases, additional imaging planes may be required or desired to adequately address specific diagnostic questions.

EPIAORTIC IMAGING

Cerebral Dysfunction Following Cardiac Surgery

Stroke and cerebral vascular injury have been well established as complications following cardiac surgery (6–8) that result in significant morbidity and mortality. The presence and severity of atherosclerosis in the ascending aorta have been shown to be an independent predictor for stroke and embolic events in cardiac surgical patients

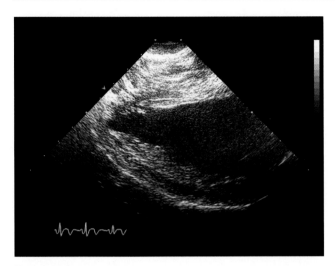

Figure 24.6. Epicardial two-chamber (TTE modified parasternal LAX equivalent). To obtain this image, rotate the probe approximately 90 degrees from Figure 24.4. Angulation superiorly will allow visualization of the LA and MV, angulation inferiorly will permit visualization of the mid and apical portions of the LV. The anterior wall is the closest to the probe in this image, and the inferior wall is the most posterior structure in this view.

(9–11). Therefore, over the last 20 years, there has been an effort to identify those patients with significant atheroma in the ascending aorta. Three intraoperative techniques have developed in the last two decades for the assessment of ascending aortic atherosclerosis: digital palpation, TEE, and EAU. Initially, digital palpation of the ascending aorta by the surgeons was the most common and preferred method. Later studies showed the superiority of TEE and

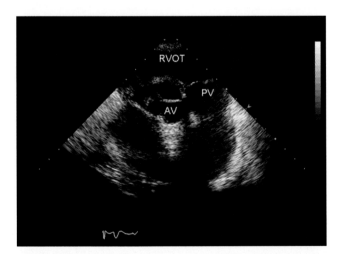

Figure 24.7. Epicardial RVOT view (TTE parasternal SAX equivalent). Place the probe gently on the RV surface to avoid excess compression. The orientation marker should be toward the left shoulder. By moving the probe toward the RV apex, both valves may be seen in the same image. It may be easier to move along the surface of the RV to view each valve individually than to view both simultaneously. Each valve can be assessed with color and spectral Doppler. AV, aortic valve; PV, Pulmonic valve.

EAU (12–15) over digital palpation. More recent studies have shown even superior sensitivity and accuracy with EAU compared to TEE (16,17). The current body of evidence supports EAU as the intraoperative diagnostic study of choice for evaluation of ascending aortic atheromatous lesions. Because of the prevalence of disease in the cardiac surgical population and the low risks of the procedure, some argue for routine EAU screening in all patients undergoing a cardiac surgical procedure requiring an open chest. However, to date, there are no conclusive studies that have proven that using EAU during cardiac surgery directly improves clinical outcomes, though one study suggests that the stroke rate may be reduced by altering surgical technique in response to findings on EAU (18). As such, the guidelines recommend epiaortic imaging for patients with risk factors for embolic stroke including old age, hypertension, unstable angina, chronic obstructive pulmonary disease, cerebrovascular disease, peripheral vascular disease, elevated creatinine levels, higher EuroSCOREs, and increased wall thickness of the descending aorta. As such, many patients presenting for cardiac surgery fall into this high-risk category.

Imaging Guidelines

The published guidelines present five EAU imaging planes that constitute what is considered a comprehensive examination (Figs. 24.8–24.10) (3). These views are not exhaustive nor are they mandatory for completion in each patient. The examination covers the length of the ascending aorta from the sinotubular junction to the takeoff of the innominate artery. The ascending aorta is divided into three segments: proximal, mid, and distal. Both the long-axis (LAX) (Fig. 24.8) and short-axis (SAX) (Fig. 24.9) views allow determination of these segments, although the LAX allows visualization of all three simultaneously in most patients. The proximal segment is defined as that portion of the ascending aorta beginning at the sinotubular junction and extending to the proximal wall of the right pulmonary artery (RPA). The mid segment is defined as that portion of the ascending aorta that is adjacent to the RPA. The distal segment is defined as that portion of the ascending aorta extending from the distal wall of the RPA to the innominate artery. Each segment should be analyzed separately in both the SAX and LAX views, and the diameter of each segment should be noted. In addition, each segment is divided into four areas: anterior, posterior, left, and right lateral walls. Therefore, a total of 12 areas can be described by the presence and severity of thickening of the aortic wall. Figure 24.10 contains three images: a phased array image (A) with two linear array images (B, C) from the same patient. Note a stand off is not needed for the phased array examination. Changing the depth of the image alters the width as well. Image B displays a total depth of 4 cm, with a close up view of the plaque and the option to see more of the width of the aorta, although the entire width is rarely seen in one screen with a phased

Long Axis View

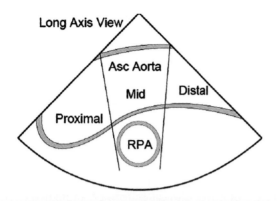

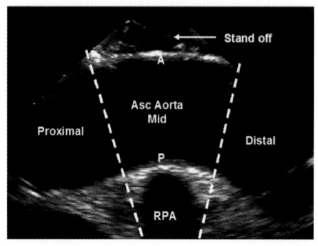

Figure 24.8. Epiaortic LAX view: phased array probe. The cartoon (**A**) and still image (**B**) LAX view are shown. The aorta can be divided into three segments for this examination. The proximal section is from the sinotubular junction to where the ascending aorta is adjacent to the RPA. The mid ascending aorta is that portion that is in continuity with the RPA. The distal ascending aorta extends from the distal RPA to the take off of the innominate artery. A standoff is necessary when using a phased array probe to ensure adequate visualization of the anterior surface of the aorta. Asc Aorta, ascending aorta; Mid, mid ascending aorta; A, anterior wall; P, posterior wall; RPA, right pulmonary artery.

array image. Image C is 6 cm; note the overall width of the image is less than in B.

Grading Systems

In order to objectively define the risks associated with aortic atheromatous disease, multiple methods of grading aortic atheromas have been described (Table 24.1) (19–22). These grading systems were developed for use in specific institutional studies, which used echocardiographic characteristics (aortic wall thickness, location of plaques, mobile or ulcerated component, etc.) to stratify and correlate degree of disease with embolic risk. No single grading system has been shown to be more accurate or precise than the others. Therefore, at this time, there is no standard method for grading aortic atheromatous disease. However, the studies that generated the various

Short Axis View

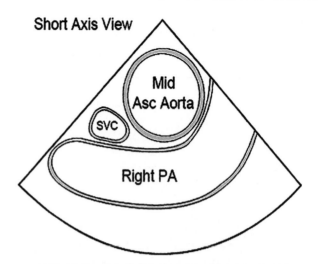

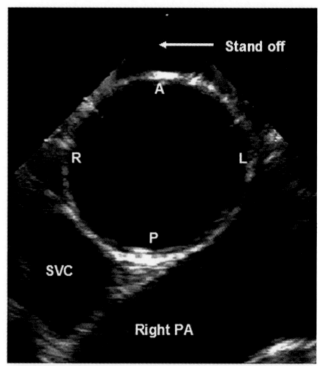

Figure 24.9. Epiaortic SAX view: phased array probe. The cartoon (**A**) and still image (**B**) are shown. If the probe marker cannot be easily identified due to the stand off, the probe should be rotated until the image in B is noted. The SVC should always be on the left side of the image. The SAX view is better for measuring plaque height and overall aortic size. SVC, superior vena cava; Right PA, right pulmonary artery; A, anterior wall; P, posterior wall; R, right lateral wall; L, left lateral wall.

grading systems do suggest that certain characteristics, including plaque height/thickness greater than 3 mm, a mobile component, or specific location in the ascending aorta, may indicate a higher risk of cerebrovascular injury (10). Further studies are necessary to determine the most appropriate grading system. However, for the purpose of comparing studies and outcomes, the development of a standard grading system is desirable and necessary.

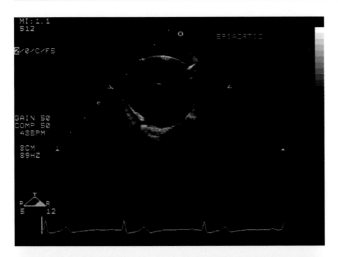

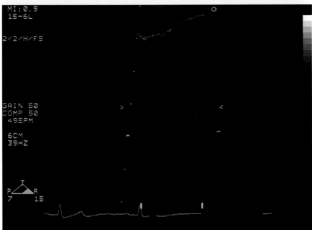

Figure 24.10. Epiaortic imaging: linear array probe. **A:** A phased array epiaortic image showing a plaque along the posterior wall to the left side of the screen. **B:** A linear array image with a total depth of 4 cm. Note the increased resolution of the plaque compared with images **A** or **C. C:** A linear array image from the same patient at 6 cm.

Implications for Surgical Management

Manipulation of the ascending aorta is routine in cardiac surgery and often unavoidable. In theory, manipulation of the ascending aorta during cardiac surgery that occurs as a result of aortic cannulation, clamping, decannulation, palpation, and "sandblasting" effect of cannula flow contributes to the dislodgement and embolization of ascending aorta and aortic arch atheroma. There is evidence supporting a correlation between the degree of aortic manipulation and the postoperative rate of cerebral vascular injury (23). As a result, surgical methods have been developed to avoid manipulation of the aorta when significant disease is identified. These techniques include the single cross clamp technique, off-pump coronary artery bypass grafting, circulatory arrest, use of proximal grafting devices, use of low turbulence cannulas, cannulas with deployable filters, axillary cannulation, and the "no touch" technique (10,24–28). One study showed that EAU examination led to a change in intraoperative surgical management in almost one third of CABG surgeries. However, in the same study, there was no difference in the number of transcranial Doppler-detected cerebral emboli before or after surgery (29). Another consideration is replacement of the ascending aorta. One study showed better outcomes

with replacement, though this technique has also been shown to increase mortality (30–31). There have been mixed results with these various techniques reported in the literature, with no clear advantage of one over the others. Further studies are required to determine which techniques are efficacious for the various degrees of disease.

TECHNIQUE

Epicardial and epiaortic imaging share a common probe-handling technique. A high frequency/resolution (>7 MHz) probe should be used for both examinations. The probe can be either phased array (Figs. 24.8 and 24.9) or linear array (Fig. 24.10), and some individuals are using the three-dimensional (3D) imaging matrix array probe for these applications. The probe must be placed in a saline- or acoustic gel-filled sterile sheath in order for it to be used in the surgical field. Some practitioners prefer the use of a second sheath for additional sterile precaution. When using a phased array probe, a standoff is recommended to improve near-field imaging. The probe operator holding the probe off the aortic surface may be able to simulate a standoff; however, results are better with an actual device. In order to optimize imaging

TABLE 24.1	Published Grading Systems for Aortic Atheroma Based on Echocardiograpic Appearance		
Reference	**Description of Grades**	**Patient Population**	**Outcome**
Katz et al. (19)	**I:** Normal to mild intimal thickening	Cardiac surgery	Stroke
	II: Severe intimal thickening without protruding atheroma		
	III: Atheroma protruding 5 mm into lumen		
	IV: Atheroma protruding 5 mm into lumen		
	V: Any thickness with mobile component or components		
Davila-Roman et al. (12)	**None:** No identifiable intimal thickening	CABG surgery[a]	Comparison TEE-EA
	Mild: 3.0 mm Intimal thickening without irregularities		
	Moderate: 3.0 mm Intimal thickening with diffuse irregularities and/or calcification		
	Severe: 5.0 mm Intimal thickening and one protruding debris or thrombus, calcification, or ulcerated plaque		
Ferrari et al. (20)	**I:** Plaque with a thickness ranging from 1 to 3.9 mm	Patients referred for TEE examination	Mortality, embolic events
	II: Plaque of 4 mm in thickness events		
	III: Any plaque, whatever its thickness, with an obvious mobile component (aortic debris)		
Trehan et al. (21)	**I:** Simple smooth-surfaced plaques, focal increase in echodensity, and thickening of intima extending <5 mm into the aortic lumen	CABG Surgery	Stroke, embolic events
	II: Marked irregularity of intimal surface, focal increase in echodensity, and thickening of adjoining intima with overlying shaggy echogenic material extending >5 mm into aortic lumen		
	III: Plaques with a mobile element		
Nohara et al. (22)	**I:** Normal or thickening of the intima extending <3 mm CABG surgery into the aortic lumen	CABG surgery	Stroke, embolic events
	II: Smooth-surfaced plaques and thickening of the intima extending 3 mm into the aortic lumen		
	III: Marked irregularity of the intimal surface and thickening of the intima extending 3 mm into the aortic lumen		
	IV: Plaque with a mobile element		

[a] *Atheroma grade was compared between biplane TEE and EAU in all patients studied.*
CABG, coronary artery bypass graft surgery; TEE, transesophageal echocardiography.

and enhance signal transmission, the mediastinal cavity is frequently filled with warmed sterile saline. In addition, the probe operator must be dressed in sterile gown and gloves, and he must observe sterile technique throughout the performance of the EAU imaging examination.

Each of these procedures requires two operators: the individual manipulating the probe and an individual to optimize and store the images. The probe is passed over the drape and placed into the sheath, taking care not to contaminate the sterile field. One of the two operators should be trained as an advanced echocardiographer as recommended in the ASE/SCA guidelines. The examination requires access to the heart or aorta, and involves an interruption of the surgical procedure in order to obtain the necessary images. This factor alone may have had the greatest influence in the preference of intraoperative TEE imaging rather than EAU. However, there are some important differences between epicardial/EAU and TEE that have contributed to the rebirth of the original intraoperative echocardiographic modality. Specifically, EAU and epicardial echocardiography should be considered in patients in whom the TEE probe is difficult or impossible to pass into the esophagus or may be contraindicated, or when improved visualization of anterior structures is necessary.

Epicardial Views

Epicardial imaging is similar to transthoracic imaging in that the probe is moved across the cardiac surface and angled or rotated in various directions to achieve the desired image. When first learning this technique, having a 3D heart model immediately available may assist in understanding the relationship of various structures to optimize probe movements and orientation. Note that the direction of the indicator marker on the probe is important when gathering and interpreting these images. It can be difficult to see the indicator marker through the sterile sheath, so it is suggested that the indicator be marked in some manner for easy identification during the examination. Failure to orient the probe correctly could lead to incorrect identification of the aortic valve (AV) leaflets or LV wall segments.

To obtain the epicardial AV SAX image (Fig. 24.1), place the probe on the proximal ascending aorta with the indicator marker toward the left shoulder. Rotate the probe clockwise 20 to 30 degrees to obtain the image shown. Note that anterior structures are closest to the probe so that the right coronary cusp is oriented at the top of the image. Continued rotation of the probe will develop the LAX view (Fig. 24.2). In this view, measurements of the annulus, left ventricular outflow tract (LVOT), and sinotubular junction diameters can be obtained. CFD can also allow evaluation of valvular regurgitation.

To obtain the epicardial LV basilar SAX view (Fig. 24.3), move the probe along the right ventricular (RV) apex until the basal LV and mitral valve are in view. The probe indicator should be oriented toward the patients left shoulder. In this image, the RV and tricuspid valves are the most anterior structures. Note the mitral valve view is similar to that seen by the surgeons during mitral valve procedures. The anterior leaflet is seen as the most anterior structure. Leaflet pathology can be identified, planimetry of valve area can be measured, and it is possible to partially assess directionality of CFD jets. RV free wall function and the tricuspid valve can also be assessed. The amount of pressure on the RV during this assessment should be minimized since excessive pressure can cause the RV to appear akinetic in the region directly beneath the probe.

The epicardial LV SAX (Fig. 24.4) view is inferior to the basilar view, necessitating movement of the probe toward the RV apex, frequently with inferior angulation of the probe. The probe should be angled toward the patient's left shoulder. The LV wall segments are reversed in the anterior-posterior axis from standard TEE views. However, if the probe is oriented correctly, the septal and lateral wall orientation is unchanged. Angling the probe to the patient's right should confirm visualization of the RV next to the septal wall. To obtain the epicardial LV LAX view (Fig. 24.5), the probe should be oriented toward the right shoulder and angled superiorly until the mitral valve and AV are in view. Angling the probe to the left should improve AV views, or toward the right to see the mitral valve better. In this view, the basilar LV can be seen, and measured if indicated. The mitral valve leaflets and subvalvular apparatus are visualized. CFD assessment allows determination of severity of mitral regurgitation and directionality of the regurgitant flow. The LVOT is well visualized for assessment of obstruction, narrowing or systolic anterior motion of the mitral valve leaflet. A small portion of the RV will also be seen anteriorly.

To obtain the epicardial two-chamber view (Fig. 24.6), the probe should be moved toward the LV surface and rotated further clockwise until the noted view is seen. Angulation of the probe superiorly will allow visualization of the MV and left atrial (LA) appendage. Angling the probe inferiorly should permit visualization of the mid LV and then apical LV. As in all other epicardial images, the anterior wall is closest to the probe and the inferior wall is the most posterior structure. A small or even normal sized LV can make this view more difficult to obtain. In addition, if the LV is positioned laterally in the thoracic cavity, it may be difficult to move the probe under the sternum to obtain the view.

The epicardial RV outflow tract view (Fig. 24.7) is obtained by placing the probe directly on the RV surface with the probe marker toward the left shoulder. In order to include the tricuspid and pulmonic valves, the probe needs to be moved along the RV surface toward the apex and angled toward the left shoulder. The pulmonic valve is seen in LAX, and Doppler modalities can be utilized to assess valvular stenosis or regurgitation, as well as to assess RV pressures. Angling the probe more superiorly allows Doppler assessment of the tricuspid valve. The seven views discussed above allow a comprehensive assessment of cardiac pathology. The examination can be individualized to add images for specific pathologies or limit views if there are patient or time constraints.

Epiaortic Views

Epiaortic views are obtained in the same manner as epicardial images. A standoff for a phased array probe is important for assessing the anterior wall of the ascending aorta. Each examination should be completed in the same order, and individual segments should be labeled on stored images to allow identification of the segments for creating a report. Each report should contain an indication of the highest grade of atherosclerosis as well as grading for the 12 individual segments of the ascending aorta, and separately for the aortic arch. The largest diameter of the ascending aorta, measured from intimal surface to intimal surface, should also be recorded. Many centers have found it helpful to also record changes in surgical management based on the examination results.

Epiaortic imaging should begin by placing the probe on the proximal ascending aorta and angling inferiorly and slightly lateral to visualize the AV in SAX. When moving the probe distally along the aortic surface, the aorta should be maintained in the middle of the image with the lateral walls seen when using a phased array probe. Initially this involves medial rotation and distal motion of the probe. At the level of the pulmonary artery, orientation of the aorta becomes more lateral and less superior and therefore requires angling of the probe laterally as it is moved distally. Once the aorta has been imaged in its entirety in SAX from the AV to the innominate takeoff, the probe can be rotated 90 degrees to assess the LAX views. Measurements of aortic diameter and plaque height should be obtained from the SAX views.

A comprehensive epicardial examination can be completed in 10 minutes while a comprehensive epiaortic examination can be completed in 5 minutes. As with all other echocardiographic examinations, images should be stored on analog or digital media, results should be discussed with the surgical team at completion of the examination, and a written report should be placed in the medical record within 24 hours.

KEY POINTS

- The seven recommended epicardial echocardiographic imaging planes include the (a) AV SAX; (b) AV LAX; (c) LV basilar SAX; (d) LV SAX; (e) LV LAX; (f) LV two-chamber; and (g) right ventricular outflow tract (RVOT) view.
- Published guidelines present five EAU imaging planes including (a) proximal ascending aorta SAX; (b) mid ascending aorta SAX; (c) distal ascending aorta SAX; (d) ascending aorta LAX; (e) aortic arch LAX.
- The current body of evidence supports EAU as the intraoperative diagnostic study of choice for evaluation of ascending aortic atheromatous lesions.
- Currently, there is no standard method for grading aortic atheromatous disease using EAU. However, the studies that generated the various grading systems do suggest that certain characteristics including plaque height/thickness greater than 3 mm, a mobile component, or specific location in the ascending aorta, may indicate a higher risk of cerebrovascular injury.

REFERENCES

1. Johnson ML, Holmes JH, Spangler RD, et al. Usefulness of echocardiography in patients undergoing mitral valve surgery. *J Thorac Cardiovasc Surg* 1972;64:922–934.
2. Reeves ST, Glas, KE, Holger E, et al. Council for Intraoperative Echocardiography of the American Society of Echocardiography. Guidelines for performing a comprehensive epicardial echocardiography examination: recommendations of the American Society of Echocardiography and the Society of Cardiovascular Anesthesiologists. *Anesth Analg* 2007;105(1):22–28.
3. Glas KE, Swaminathan M, Reeves ST, et al. Guidelines for the performance of a comprehensive intraoperative epiaortic ultrasonographic examination: recommendations of the American Society of Echocardiography and the Society of Cardiovascular Anesthesiologists; Endorsed by the Society of Thoracic Surgeons. *Anesth Analg* 2008;106(5):1376–1384.
4. Frenk VE, Shernan SK, Eltzschig HK. Epicardial echocardiography: diagnostic utility for evaluating aortic valve disease during coronary surgery. *J Clin Anesth* 2003;15:271–274.
5. Budde RPJ, Bakker PFA, Gründeman PF, et al. High-frequency epicardial ultrasound: review of a multipurpose intraoperative tool for coronary surgery. *Surg Endosc* 2008, doi:10.1007/s00464-008-0082-y.
6. van Dijk D, Keizer AMA, Diephuis JC, et al. Neurocognitive dysfunction after coronary artery bypass surgery: a systematic review. *J Thorac Cardiovasc Surg* 2000;120:632–629.
7. Selnes OA, Goldsborough MA, Borowicz LM, et al. Neurobehavioural sequelae of cardiopulmonary bypass. *Lancet* 1999;353:1601–1616.
8. Newman MF, Kirchner JL, Phillips-Bute B, et al. Longitudinal assessment of neurocognitive function after coronary-artery bypass surgery. *N Engl J Med* 2001;19:627–632.
9. Davila-Roman VG, Barzilai B, Wareing TH, et al. Atherosclerosis of the ascending aorta: prevalence and role as an independent predictor of cerebrovascular events in cardiac patients. *Stroke* 1994;25:2010–2016.
10. van der Linden J, Hadjinikolaou L, Bergman P, et al. Postoperative stroke in cardiac surgery is related to the location and extent of atherosclerotic disease in the ascending aorta. *J Am Coll Cardiol* 2001;38:131–135.
11. van der Linden, Bergman P, Hadjinikolaou L. The topography of aortic atherosclerosis enhances its precision as a predictor of stroke. *Ann Thorac Surg* 2007;83:2087–2092.
12. Davila-Roman VG, Phillips KJ, Daily BB, et al. Intraoperative transesophageal echocardiography and epiaortic ultrasound for assessment of atherosclerosis of the thoracic aorta. *J Am Coll Cardiol* 1996;28:942–947.
13. Bolotin G, Domany Y, De Perini L, et al. Use of intraoperative epiaortic ultrasonography to delineate aortic atheroma. *Chest* 2005;127:60–65.
14. Amarenco P, Cohen H, Tzourio C, et al. Atherosclerotic disease of the aortic arch and the risk of ischemic stroke. *N Engl J Med* 1994;331:1474–1479.
15. Royse C, Royse A, Blake D, et al. Screening the thoracic aorta for atheroma: a comparison of manual palpation, transesophageal and epiaortic ultrasonography. *Ann Thorac Cardiovasc Surg* 1998;4:347–350.
16. Suvarna S, Smith A, Stygall J, et al. An intraoperative assessment of the ascending aorta: a comparison of digital palpation, transesophageal echocardiography, and epiaortic ultrasonography. *J Cardiothorac Vasc Anesth* 2007;21:805–809.

17. Ibrahim KS, Vitale N, Tromsdal A, et al. Enhanced intra-operative grading of ascending aorta atheroma by epiaortic ultrasound versus echocardiography. *Int J Cardiol* 2008;128:218–223.

18. Hangler HB, Nagele G, Danzmayr M, et al. Modification of surgical technique for ascending aortic atherosclerosis: impact on stroke reduction in coronary artery bypass grafting. *J Thorac Cardiovas Surg* 2003;126:391–400.

19. Katz ES, Tunick PA, Rusinek H, et al. Protruding aortic atheromas predict stroke in elderly patients undergoing cardiopulmonary bypass: experience with intraoperative transesophageal echocardiography. *J Am Coll Cardiol* 1992;20:70–77.

20. Ferrari E, Vidal R, Cheavallier T, et al. Atherosclerosis of the thoracic aorta and aortic debris as a marker of poor prognosis: benefit of oral anticoagulants. *J Am Coll Cardiol* 1999;33:1317–1322.

21. Trehan N, Mishra M, Kasliwal RR, Mishra A. Reduced neurological injury during CABG in patients with mobile aortic atheromas: a five-year follow-up study. *Ann Thorac Surg* 2000;70:1558–1564.

22. Nohara H, Shida T, Mukohara N, et al. Ultrasonic plaque density of aortic atheroma and stroke in patients undergoing on-pump coronary bypass surgery. *Ann Thorac Cardiovasc Surg* 2004;10:235–240.

23. Kapetanakis EI, Stamou SC, Dullum MK, et al. The impact of aortic manipulation on neurologic outcomes after coronary artery bypass surgery: a risk-adjusted study. *Ann Thorac Surg* 2004;78:1564–1571.

24. Hogue CW, Palin CA, Arrowsmith JE. Cardiopulmonary bypass management and neurologic outcomes: an evidence-based appraisal of current practices. *Anesth Analg* 2006;103:21–37.

25. Royse AG, Royse CF, Ajani AE, et al. Reduced neuropsychological dysfunction using epiaortic echocardiography and the exclusive Y graft. *Ann Thorac Surg* 2000;69:1431–1438.

26. Hammon JW, Stump DA, Butterworth JF, et al. Single cross-clamp improves 6-month cognitive outcome in high-risk coronary bypass patients: the effect of reduced aortic manipulation. *J Thorac Cardiovasc Surg* 2006;131:114–121.

27. Sabik JF, Lytle BW, McCarthy PM, Cosgrove DM. Axillary artery: alternative site of arterial cannulation for patients with extensive aortic and peripheral vascular disease. *J Thorac Cardiovasc Surg* 1995;109:885–890.

28. Svensson LG, Blackstone EH, Rajeswaran J. Does the arterial cannulation site for circulatory arrest influence stroke risk? *Ann Thorac Surg* 2004;78:1274–1284.

29. Djaiani G, Ali M, Borger MA, et al. Epiaortic scanning modifies intraoperative surgical management but not cerebral embolic load during coronary artery bypass surgery. *Anesth Analg* 2008;106:1611–1618.

30. Rokkas CK, Kouchoukos NT. Surgical management of the severely atherosclerotic ascending aorta during cardiac operations. *Semin Thorac Cardiovasc Surg* 1998;10:240–246.

31. Kouchoukos NT, Wareing TH, Daily BB, et al. Management of the severely atherosclerotic aorta during cardiac operations. *J Card Surg* 1994;9:490–494.

QUESTIONS

1. Epicardial imaging is indicated for all of the following except
   A. In a patient in whom a TEE probe is impossible to pass into the esophagus
   B. In a patient with extensive esophageal pathology
   C. To better visualize posterior structures
   D. To obtain higher resolution images compared with TEE

2. Which of the following statements regarding the performance of a comprehensive epiaortic ultrasound (EAU) examination is incorrect?
   A. The examination includes the length of the ascending aorta from the sinotubular junction to the main pulmonary artery bifurcation
   B. The ascending aorta should be examined in three separate segments: proximal, mid, and distal
   C. The diameter of each ascending aortic segment should be noted
   D. Each segment of the ascending aorta is divided into the anterior, posterior, left and right lateral walls

3. Which of the following statements regarding proper epicardial or epiaortic probe-handling technique is correct?
   A. A low-frequency/resolution probe should always be used
   B. As long as the probe is placed in a sterile sheath, sterile gowns and gloves are not required by the probe operator
   C. Only linear arrays can be used for epicardial and epiaortic imaging
   D. The individual responsible for diagnostic interpretation of the epicardial and epiaortic images should be trained as an advanced echocardiographer as recommended in the ASE/SCA guidelines

CHAPTER 25

Assessment of Congenital Heart Disease in the Adult Patient

Isobel Russell ■ Elyse Foster ■ Kathryn Rouine-Rapp

Advances in cardiac surgery, anesthesia, intensive care, and diagnosis over the last 50 years have permitted survival of 85% of infants with congenital heart disease (CHD) into adulthood (2). Between 1985 and 2000, the prevalence of CHD in the general population increased among both children and adults such that since 1985 there have been more adults in the general population with CHD than children and nearly equal numbers of adults and children with severe CHD (3). The median age of all patients with CHD increased, and a majority (57%) of females were observed among adults with CHD. Although accurate statistics are lacking, the range of estimates of adults with CHD in the United States varies from 787,000 to 1.3 million (4,5). It is estimated that the number of patients with CHD reaching adulthood is approximately 16,000 per year in the United States alone (2). The Bethesda consensus report (2) suggests that these patients should receive care in regional centers for adult CHD, and the patients should keep their own copies of information on operations, cardiac catheterizations, and other diagnostic tests, such as echocardiograms in the form of a "health passport."

INDICATIONS

Indications for transesophageal echocardiography (TEE) in adult patients with CHD should follow established guidelines by the American Society of Anesthesiologists and the Society of Cardiovascular Anesthesiologists (SCA) (6) and the American College of Cardiology/American Heart Association Task Forces (7). It should be emphasized that a complete diagnosis of the congenital heart lesion should be defined prior to performance of intraoperative TEE. The lesion, coexisting pathology, hemodynamics, cardiac size, and function should be well delineated by cardiac catheterization, transthoracic echocardiography, TEE, cardiac magnetic resonance imaging, or multislice

computer tomography (8–11). Intraoperative TEE should not be used as a replacement for an inadequate preoperative evaluation.

Summaries from the two reports on the indications for intraoperative TEE for CHD include the following:

1. "Practice guidelines for perioperative TEE."
   Most cardiac defects requiring repair under cardiopulmonary bypass are a category 1 indication for intraoperative TEE, including precardiopulmonary and postcardiopulmonary imaging. Category 1 is defined as that being supported by the strongest evidence or expert opinion substantiating that TEE is useful in improving clinical outcomes (6).
2. "ACC/AHA guidelines for the clinical application of echocardiography."
   Monitoring and guidance during cardiothoracic procedures associated with the potential for residual shunts, valvular regurgitation, obstruction, or myocardial dysfunction are a class 1 indication, defined as conditions for which there is evidence and/or general agreement that a given procedure or treatment is useful and effective (7). This definition was developed under the indications for TEE in pediatric patients with CHD but is applicable to adolescents and adults with CHD.

Approach

Image orientation, nomenclature guidelines, and a comprehensive intraoperative echocardiographic examination should follow those suggested by the American Society of Echocardiography (ASE) (12) and ASE/SCA guidelines (13). Appropriate TEE views for evaluation of congenital heart lesions are described in Table 25.1 and Figure 25.1. Assessment of the connections of the various cardiac segments, atrial arrangement or situs, venoatrial, atrioventricular, and ventriculoarterial connections should be performed. Septal and valvular structures should then be evaluated, including assessment of flow velocities with Doppler echocardiography and assessment of strain rate with Doppler tissue imaging (14). In general, the approach for each lesion is to define the intracardiac anatomy and associated defects, assess the ventricular function, and evaluate any residual lesions (Table 25.2). Comprehensive reference atlases include

This chapter is, in large part, based on the following publication (1): Russell IA, Rouine-Rapp K, Stratmann G, et al. Congenital heart disease in the adult: a review with internet-accessible transesophageal echocardiography. Anesth Analg 2006;102:694–723.

TABLE 25.1	Congenital Heart Lesions—Appropriate TEE Views for Evaluation of Congenital Heart Lesions

Lesion	TEE Plane
Atrial septal defects	• ME four-chamber for ostium secundum and primum defects • ME bicaval for interatrial septum for sinus venosus defects and possible anomalous pulmonary veins
Ventricular septal defects	• ME four-chamber, LAX for perimembranous (Type 2), inlet (Type 3) and muscular (Type 4) VSDs, chamber sizes, presence of ventricular septal aneurysm • ME AV LAX, deep TG LAX views for evaluation of the aortic valve for insufficiency and herniation • ME RV inflow and outflow for PI
Atrioventricular septal defects	• ME four- and two-chamber for the bridging leaflets and their attachments, extent of intracardiac defects, size of septal defects, and extent of AV valve regurgitation
AS (valvular and subvalvular)	• Deep TG LAX for AS, insufficiency, and aortic root size • ME AV SAX evaluation of aortic valve morphology • ME four-chamber for LV hypertrophy and function assessment
Transposition of the great arteries	• ME four-chamber to evaluate AV valve regurgitation and baffle assessment after Senning/Mustard procedures • ME bicaval view additionally for caval junctions and pulmonary veins • TG mid SAX for ventricular function and SWMA • Deep TG LAX for ventriculoarterial connections and anastomoses after arterial switch
Tetralogy of Fallot	• ME AV LAX and deep TG LAX for definition of aortic override and obstruction of the RVOT and estimation of gradients • ME RV inflow-outflow for RVOT evaluation • ME four-chamber view for position and extension of VSD and other additional VSDs
Truncus arteriosus	• ME four-chamber view for VSD position and extent • ME AV SAX to evaluate truncal valve • ME AV LAX and deep TG LAX for evaluation of truncal insufficiency and determination of truncal anatomy
Patent ductus arteriosus	• Difficult to visualize by 2D TEE, but ductal flow can be visualized in the ME asc aortic SAX view by presence of abnormal continuous high-velocity aliased flow
Pulmonic valve stenosis	• ME RV inflow-outflow and deep TG LAX view for outflow tract evaluation and gradient estimation • ME asc aortic SAX for evaluation of pulmonic valve and MPA
Single ventricles	• ME four-chamber, two-chamber and deep TG LAX for atrioventricular morphology and atrioventricular and ventriculoarterial connections • ME bicaval view for evaluation of Glenn anastomosis

asc, ascending; AV, aortic valve; LAX, long axis; ME, midesophageal; RV, right ventricle; RVOT, right ventricular outflow tract; SAX, short axis; SWMA, segmental wall motion abnormality; TG, transgastric.

Pediatric Echocardiography, edited by N. Silverman (Williams and Wilkins), *Transesophageal Echocardiography in Congenital Heart Disease*, edited by O. Stumper and G. Sutherland (Little, Brown and Company), and *Congenital Heart Disease in Adults*, edited by J.K. Perloff and J.S. Child (W.B. Saunders).

CHD can be classified in several ways: according to the underlying physiology of either shunt; obstructive, regurgitant, and mixed lesions; according to the presence and absence of cyanosis; or according to the level of complexity of the lesion. For purposes of simplicity,

this chapter will organize the lesions according to level of complexity, with greater emphasis on the more common lesions.

SIMPLE LESIONS

Atrial Septal Defects

Atrial septal defects (ASDs) are one of the most common defects in the adult population, accounting for one fourth

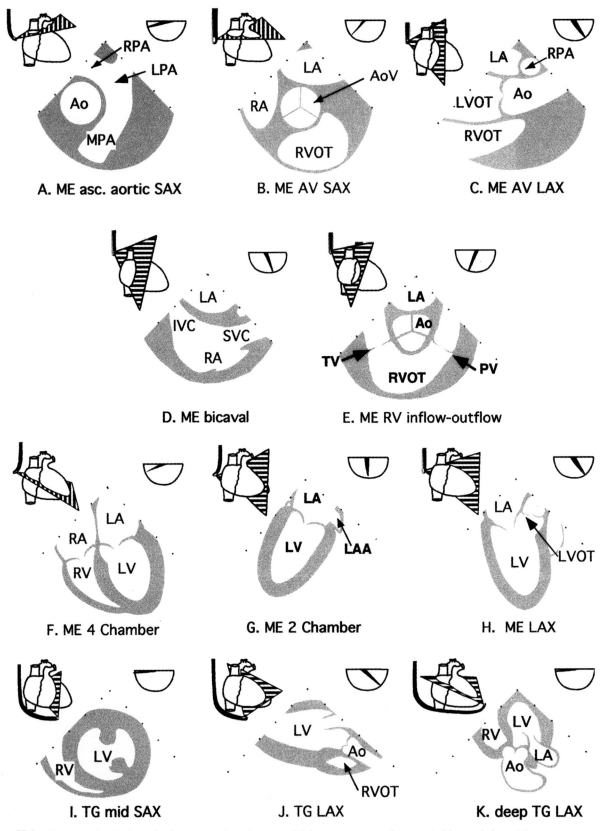

Figure 25.1. Cross-sectional views depicting imaging planes useful for assessment of congenital heart defects. The appropriate multiplane angle is indicated by the icon on the right adjacent to each view. The imaging plane is indicated by the schematic drawing of the heart on the **left**. Asc., ascending; Ao, aorta; AoV, aortic valve; IVC, inferior vena cava; LA, left atrium; LAA, left atrial appendage; LAX, long axis; LPA, left pulmonary artery; LV, left ventricle; LVOT, left ventricular outflow tract; ME, midesophageal; MPA, main pulmonary artery; RA, right atrium; RPA, right pulmonary artery; RV, right ventricle; RVOT, right ventricular outflow tract; SAX, short axis; SVC, superior vena cava; TG, transgastric; TV, tricuspid valve.

TABLE 25.2	**Indications for Primary Surgery, Common Postoperative Complications and Indications for Reoperation in CHD**		
Lesion	**Indication for Primary Repair**	**Post-Repair Complications**	**Indication for Reoperation**
Atrial septal defect	Qp:Qs ≥ 1.8:1 Paradoxical embolization	Atrial fibrillation, CVA[a]	Secundum: none Primum: MR
Ventricular septal defect	Qp:Qs ≥ 1.5:1	Patch leak Endocarditis[b] Progressive PHTN	Patch leak when Qp:Qs ≥ 1.5:1
Patent ductus arteriosus	Qp:Qs > 1.5:1	Persistent shunt Endoarteritis[b] Progressive PHTN	Persistent shunt
Atrioventricular canal defect	Qp:Qs > 1.5:1 Mitral regurgitation	Patch leak Endocarditis Progressive MR Atrial fibrillation Atrioventricular block	MR Patch leak
Anomalous pulmonary venous drainage	Qp:Qs > 1.5:1	Obstruction of the pulmonary veins	N/A
Tetralogy of Fallot	No previous repair	Patch leak Pulmonary insufficiency Residual PS Heart block Ventricular and atrial arrhythmias Sudden death Endocarditis	Hemodynamically significant PI or PS
Transposition of Great vessel	N/A	*Postatrial switch:* RV failure Tricuspid regurgitation Baffle obstruction Atrial arrhythmias Heart block Endocarditis *Postatrial switch:* Supravalvar AS (neopulmonic stenosis) Coronary artery stenosis	Significant baffle obstruction Progressive RV failure Tricuspid regurgitation
Ebstein's anomaly	Severe tricuspid regurgitation RV failure	Atrial arrhythmias Progressive TR	Severe TR
Tricuspid atresia	N/A	*Post-Fontan* Atrial arrhythmias Protein-losing enteropathy Ascites	Conduit obstruction
Aortic stenosis	AVA < 0.8 cm^2 in presence of symptoms	*Post-Valvotomy* Progressive AI or restenosis Ventricular arrhythmias Sudden death Endocarditis	Severe AS or AI in the presence of symptoms or LV dysfunction

(*continued*)

Lesion	Indication for Primary Repair	Post-Repair Complications	Indication for Reoperation
Subaortic stenosis	Gradient >30 mm Hg or the development of AI at a lower gradient	Progressive AI Restenosis Endocarditis	Severe AI or recurrent stenosis in the presence of symptoms
Pulmonary stenosis	Transpulmonary gradient >50 mm Hg Transpulmonary gradient <50 mm Hg with RV hypertrophy or symptoms	Restenosis Pulmonic valve insufficiency Endocarditis rare	Severe PS or PI in the presence of symptoms
Coarctation of aorta	Upper extremity HTN Transcoarctation gradient >25 mm Hg	Residual HTN Saccular aneurysm Dissecting aneurysm Circle of Willis aneurysm CVA Premature CAD AS/AI Endocarditis or endarteritis	Recurrent coarctation AS/AI (see above) CAD Saccular or dissecting aneurysm

aThese complications are most common when repair is performed at age >40.
bEndocarditis and endarteritis are likely only in the presence of persistent shunt.
Qp:Qs, pulmonary to systemic flow ratio; CVA, cerebrovascular accident; PHTN, pulmonary hypertension; MR, mitral regurgitation; PI, pulmonic valve insufficiency; PS, pulmonary stenosis; AS, aortic stenosis; TR, tricuspid regurgitation, RV, right ventricle; AVA, aortic valve area; CAD, coronary artery disease; HTN, hypertension.

to one third of all lesions, and occurring more commonly in women (15). There are four types of ASDs:

1. Ostium secundum defect (70%), which occurs in the midseptum region of the fossa ovalis. Varying degrees of mitral valve prolapse and mitral regurgitation (MR) can occur, but hemodynamically significant lesions are uncommon.
2. Ostium primum defect (15%–25%) is located in the inferior portion of the interatrial septum, near the atrioventricular valves. It also is considered a form of a partial atrioventricular canal defect (see below). Abnormalities of the atrioventricular valve can occur with a "cleft" anterior mitral valve and septal tricuspid valve (TV) leaflet with variable degrees of regurgitation.
3. Sinus venosus defect (10%) is usually superior and posterior in relation to the superior vena cava (SVC) (more frequently) and/or inferior vena cava (IVC). These defects frequently are associated with an anomalous drainage of one or more pulmonary veins into the right atrium (RA) or SVC (16).
4. Coronary sinus defects (extremely rare) occur between the left atrium (LA) and coronary sinus and can be associated with a persistent left SVC.

Imaging with intraoperative TEE is performed following the guidelines in Table 25.1 to confirm the presence, size, and location of the defect; degree of atrioventricular valve regurgitation; ventricular function; and associated anomalies, such as anomalous pulmonary veins (Fig. 25.2). Anomalous pulmonary veins may be difficult to diagnose

by TEE. Thus, pulmonary venous drainage should be documented preoperatively using transthoracic echocardiography or alternative imaging techniques such as cardiac magnetic resonance imaging or CT angiography. Postoperatively, TEE is used to detect residual shunts by color Doppler and contrast, to assess ventricular function, and to assess for pulmonary venous obstruction and valvular regurgitation. To evaluate for residual shunts, agitated saline contrast should be used because the microbubbles are readily apparent even when a very small number of microbubbles cross a defect (17). The method used is to vigorously agitate 0.5 to 1.0 mL of the patient's blood between two syringes filled to a total of 10 mL of saline (18). The agitated saline is injected intravenously; positive pressure is applied via the airway circuit (or a Valsalva maneuver) and then released suddenly to increase RA pressure. TEE images are observed for the presence of microbubbles in the left heart chambers. The site of the defect can often be identified by careful inspection guided by color flow Doppler or transit of the microbubbles.

A defect in the interatrial septum allows pulmonary venous return to pass from the left to the right atrium. Because this left-to-right shunt increases the venous return to the right ventricle (RV), the RV stroke volume and pulmonary blood flow are increased compared with the systemic blood flow. RV volume overload results. Indirect evidence of an atrial septal defect includes right-sided chamber enlargement and appearance of saline contrast in the left heart chambers as there is always a minor degree of right to left shunting. Color flow Doppler

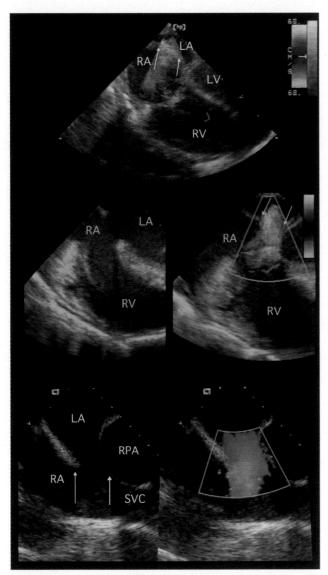

Figure 25.2. Atrial Septal Defects. **Top:** Secundum ASD (ME four-chamber view). **Middle:** Primum ASD (ME four-chamber view). **Bottom:** Sinus venosus ASD (ME bicaval view). *Arrows* indicate the defect in the atrial septum. Left-to-right shunting is demonstrated by blue color flow Doppler. LA, left atrium; LV, left ventricle; RA, right atrium; RV, right ventricle; RPA, right pulmonary artery; SVC, superior vena cava.

echocardiography can demonstrate flow across the atrial septum and detect mitral or tricuspid regurgitation.

Primary or patch closure of an atrial septal defect in childhood provides excellent operative results and nearly normal long-term survival in adults (19,20). Additionally, a recent retrospective study suggested improved 10-year survival in patients over the age of 40 years treated surgically (95%) compared with those treated medically (84%) (20). A prospective clinical trial (21) randomized adult patients with secundum ASDs with shunt ratios greater than 1.7:1 to surgical versus medical management, showing improved survival with surgical closure. However, late repair does not appear to reduce the incidence of

arrhythmias, which are generally related to preoperative atrial dilatation or postoperative incisional reentry (22). Operative patch closure is recommended if the degree of left-to-right shunting is sufficiently large to cause RA enlargement and RV enlargement, and if the defect cannot be closed percutaneously. Other indications for closure include paradoxical embolism and documented orthodeoxia-platypnea, a syndrome associated with intermittent right to left shunting in the absence of pulmonary hypertension (PHTN). Percutaneous closure with a variety of devices is now widely available and feasible for most ostium secundum defects. Sinus venosus, coronary sinus, and ostium primum ASDs still require surgical closure. In patients with ostium primum defects, surgical valve repair with or without annuloplasty may reduce the severity of the mitral and tricuspid regurgitation. If severe MR persists, valve re-repair or replacement is necessary.

Closure of an ASD in the presence of PHTN requires special consideration. According to the current guidelines, it may be considered when there is net left-to-right shunting and the pulmonary vascular resistance is less than 2/3 systemic, or if there has been demonstrated response to pulmonary vasodilator therapy. In these patients, careful monitoring of RV function following ASD closure is required and use of pulmonary vasodilators postoperatively may be required.

Ventricular Septal Defects

Ventricular septal defects (VSD) are the most common cardiac abnormality in infants and children (15). Adult patients with unoperated VSDs are encountered less frequently than those with ASD because large defects are usually closed surgically in childhood when there is evidence of congestive heart failure or PHTN. In infancy and childhood, defects have a high rate of spontaneous closure—90% of those that close do so by the time the child is 10 years of age.

VSDs can be classified by anatomic location into four types. Recently a revised classification scheme for VSDs was provided in guidelines from the AHA/ACC. Those four types of VSDs will be included parenthetically here (23).

1. Perimembranous VSDs (Type 2) are found in the membranous region of the septum and can extend into the muscular, inlet, or outlet regions. They account for 70% of VSDs. Part of the border is formed by fibrous continuity between the tricuspid and aortic valves (24).
2. Muscular VSDs (Type 4) account for 20% of VSDs, are surrounded by a muscular rim and located within the trabecular portion of the septum, or in the central or apical areas. Multiple defects can occur. Either two or three, or multiple small VSDs may occur in a defect known as "swiss cheese septum."
3. Doubly committed, subarterial or supracristal VSDs (Type 1) account for 5% of VSDs, are found just below the aortic and pulmonary valves, and can have

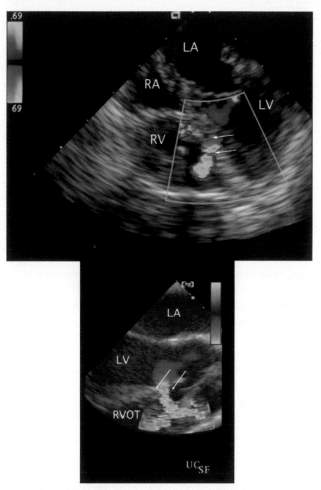

Figure 25.3. Ventricular Septal Defects. **Top:** Residual muscular VSD (Type 4) (ME four-chamber view) as indicated by the *arrows*, with color flow Doppler demonstrating the left-to-RV shunting. **Bottom:** Subarterial (doubly committed) VSD (Type 1) with color flow Doppler demonstrating the left-to-right-ventricular shunting into the RVOT. LA, left atrium; LV, left ventricle; RA, right atrium; RVOT, right ventricular outflow tract.

associated aortic cusp herniation and aortic regurgitation. Part of the border of this defect is formed by fibrous continuity between the aortic and pulmonary valves (24).

4. Inlet VSDs (Type 3) occur close to the atrioventricular valves in the posterior and inlet portions of the septum and account for 5% of VSDs.

TEE is particularly helpful in evaluation of these defects (Table 25.1). If the left-to-right shunt is large, the LA and left ventricle (LV) are dilated. RV dimension is normal unless there is PHTN. Preoperatively, TEE confirms the presence, size, and location of the defect as well as the degree of atrioventricular and aortic valve regurgitation (Fig. 25.3). In the presence of a perimembranous VSD (Type 2), the septal leaflet of the TV can become adherent to the defect; thus, tricuspid regurgitation may occur and can occasionally be severe. Hemodynamically significant aortic valve regurgitation is most common in the presence

of a subarterial VSD (Type 1) with herniation of the right coronary cusp. The peak velocity across the VSD can be used to estimate the RV systolic pressure and pulmonary artery systolic pressure (25). According to current guidelines, closure of a VSD is indicated when the pulmonary-to-systemic flow (Qp/Qs) is greater than or equal to 2.0 or if there is evidence of LV volume overload. Another indication is a history of endocarditis. In patient with PHTN, VSD closure should be considered if the net Qp/Qs is greater than 1.5 and the pulmonary vascular resistance is less than 2/3 systemic resistance but should not be performed if there is severe irreversible pulmonary vascular disease. Percutaneous closure is possible for many muscular VSD's (Type 4). However, most perimembranous (Type 2) and inlet (Type 3) VSD's require surgical closure. Postoperatively, TEE is used to detect residual shunts by color Doppler and contrast and to assess ventricular function, residual aortic or pulmonic insufficiency, and right ventricular outflow tract (RVOT) obstruction.

A VSD permits a left-to-right shunt to occur at the ventricular level. The physiologic consequences are determined by the size of the defect and the relative resistance of the systemic and pulmonary vascular beds. If the VSD is small and restricts blood flow, there is a large pressure difference between the LV and the RV in systole. If the VSD is large (nonrestrictive), there is no pressure difference between the LV and the RV, and the magnitude of the shunt depends on the ratio of pulmonary vascular resistance to systemic vascular resistance. If the pulmonary vascular resistance is lower than the systemic vascular resistance, the left-to-right shunt can be large. When the increased pulmonary blood flow returns to the LV, LV diastolic volume and stroke volume increase.

By the time the patient has reached adolescence or early adulthood, there is virtually no chance that the VSD will close spontaneously (Table 25.2). If the left-to-right shunt is large, congestive heart failure is likely. If a large VSD is associated with PHTN, the chance of the development of pulmonary vascular disease is high. In adults diagnosed with VSD, the overall 10-year survival after initial presentation is approximately 75%. Functional class greater than 1, cardiomegaly, and elevated pulmonary artery pressure (>50 mm Hg) are clinical predictors of an adverse prognosis (12).

Complete AV Septal Defect

In complete AV septal defect (AVSD), there is failure of the endocardial cushions to close the atrial and ventricular septa, affecting the complete formation of the mitral valve and TV. As a result, patients have a VSD, a primum ASD, and varying degrees of AV valve anatomic abnormalities and regurgitation. With large left-to-right shunts at the atrial and ventricular levels and systemic pressures in the RV because of the VSD, pulmonary vascular disease occurs very early. Most adults with uncorrected complete AVSD are cyanotic with increased pulmonary vascular resistance secondary to irreversible vascular changes (Eisenmenger's syndrome). These adults are not candidates for correction due to PHTN. When the repair has been performed in childhood, residual mitral or tricuspid regurgitation often remains.

TEE is useful for defining the type and extension of the septal defects (Table 25.1) and the morphology of the AV valve "bridging leaflets," which span the common orifice (26). TEE of an AVSD demonstrates complete absence of the crux of the heart, with both low atrial and high VSDs (Fig. 25.4). In the adult, color flow imaging and Doppler studies usually show regurgitation of both AV valves and evidence of pulmonary artery hypertension.

The lesions in these patients are usually corrected in infancy. The surgery consists of patch closure of the ASD and VSDs, and repair of the AV valves. The unoperated adult with a complete AVSD is rarely a candidate for a complete repair because of the frequent and early development of pulmonary vascular disease. However, these patients may be candidates for heart-lung transplantation or lung transplantation with intracardiac repair (Table 2.2). For the patient who has been corrected in infancy, the most common postoperative sequela is progressive mitral valve regurgitation owing to breakdown of the original repair. Other sequelae of the original surgery that may require late intervention include the presence of LV to RA shunts and progressive subaortic stenosis (AS). Patch leaks should be addressed if possible at the time of reoperation. Postoperatively, the adequacy of the valve repair and the subaortic resection should be evaluated.

Congenital Aortic Stenosis

The pathophysiology of congenital AS is similar to that of acquired AS. However, in congenital left ventricular outflow tract (LVOT) obstruction, the anatomic level of

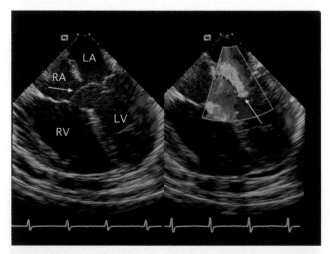

Figure 25.4. Atrioventricular Septal Defects. Atrioventricular septal defect (ME four-chamber view) demonstrating the anterior-bridging leaflet (*arrow*) and interatrial and interventricular defects. The right frame demonstrates color flow Doppler of the left-sided atrioventricular valve regurgitation (*arrow*). LA, left atrium; LV, left ventricle; RA, right atrium; RV, right ventricle.

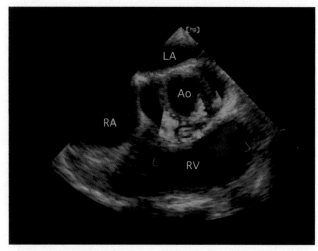

Figure 25.5. Bicuspid Aortic Valve. Bicuspid aortic valve (ME aortic valve SAX view) demonstrating the two cusps, instead of three, during systole. Ao, aortic valve; LA, left atrium; RA, right atrium; RV, right ventricle.

obstruction can be supravalvular or subvalvular whereas in acquired AS, it is usually valvular. Valvular AS is due to abnormal development of the commissures and subsequent valve malformation of a functionally bicuspid valve, occurring in 2% to 3% of the population (Fig. 25.5). Patients with the most severely malformed and stenotic valves may require intervention in infancy. Even with a less-restricted orifice, the disturbed flow through the valve causes progressive thickening and calcification and may eventually result in severe stenosis and varying degrees of valvular insufficiency that manifest later in life. In supravalvular AS, the narrowing is usually above the level of the sinuses of Valsalva. Therefore, the coronary arteries arise from the aorta proximal to the obstruction and are subjected to an elevated systolic pressure equal to that of the LV. The high pressures cause coronary artery dilatation and may accelerate atherosclerosis.

In the most common form of subaortic stenosis, there is a discrete membrane immediately below the aortic valve, resulting in a systolic jet that traumatizes the valve leaflets, leading to aortic regurgitation. There is frequent association of LVOT obstruction with coarctation of the aorta and also mitral valve abnormalities.

TEE is diagnostic in valvular AS with direct visualization of the valve leaflets by two-dimensional (2D) imaging and measurement of the pressure gradient across the LVOT by Doppler interrogation. The gradient is frequently underestimated due to poor alignment of the Doppler beam with the outflow tract. Associated lesions, especially aortic coarctation should be sought, and the severity of LV hypertrophy and dysfunction should also be assessed. TEE can also visualize a subaortic membrane or supravalvar stenosis. With discrete membranous subvalvular AS, progressive aortic regurgitation can occur. If severe, aortic valve replacement may be necessary.

After aortic valvotomy for severe stenosis during childhood, approximately one fourth of patients will need repeat surgery for recurrent stenosis or progressive aortic insufficiency (AI) in the next 25 years (Table 25.2) (27). Without surgical intervention, approximately one third of children with initial peak systolic gradients below 50 mm Hg and about 80% of those with initial gradients between 50 and 79 mm Hg will need surgery within 25 years (27). With symptomatic, hemodynamically significant valvular AS (i.e., an aortic valve area [AVA] < 0.8 cm²) and a flexible noncalcified valve, balloon valvotomy may have therapeutic success similar to that of operative valvotomy—even in young adults. However, when there is calcification or associated AI, valve replacement is required. An alternative is the Ross procedure, which involves placement of a homograft in the pulmonary valve position and the native pulmonary valve in the aortic position. The advantages of this innovative, although technically challenging, approach is that it obviates the need for anticoagulation without using bioprosthetic valves, which have an excessive rate of degeneration; however, it is not as advantageous in the adult because growth is not a major issue. In addition, 5 to 7 years following the Ross procedure, 50% of patients may develop neoaortic root dilation, and 30% may develop moderate tosevere neoaortic valve regurgitation and the need for reoperation (28).

Coarctation of the Aorta

In the most common form of aortic coarctation, there is narrowing immediately distal to the takeoff of the left subclavian artery or more commonly at the level of the insertion of the ligamentum arteriosus. The constriction may take the form of a shelf or a localized hourglass narrowing of the distal arch proximal to the ligamentum. It is difficult to visualize the actual site of the coarctation in the adult patient with TEE. However, color Doppler studies of the descending aorta may detect flow acceleration or turbulent jets (29). An associated bicuspid aortic valve can also be identified by TEE. Angiography or MRI is usually needed to define the site and extent of narrowing.

Arterial hypertension is usually present proximal to the aortic obstruction (Table 25.2). Repair should be undertaken when the coarctation is severe enough to cause proximal hypertension and the gradient across the coarctation is greater than or equal to 20 mm Hg. Many adult patients will have multiple collateral vessels seen on aortography or cardiac MR and atheromatous changes at the site of the coarctation, which can complicate surgery. If the gradient is less than 20 mm Hg and collaterals are present, repair is indicated. The choice of percutaneous or surgical repair in the adult with a native coarctation depends on a number of factors and should be carefully considered. In patients with discrete recoarctation, percutaneous intervention with stenting is generally preferred. Older pediatric age at the time of initial intervention is associated with a higher rate of reinterventions long-term (30). Aortic aneurysms can occur around the area of the coarctation or elsewhere in the aorta and in the branches of the circle of Willis (so-called berry aneurysms).

Pulmonic Valvular Stenosis

Although pulmonic valve stenosis is congenital in origin, it may be progressive. The obstruction to outflow puts an afterload burden on the RV, resulting in RV hypertrophy. Severe RV hypertrophy with increased systolic compression may compromise intramural coronary flow. Because of the increased RV myocardial oxygen demand, this situation can lead to subendocardial ischemia.

It is unusual to see an adult with severe valvular pulmonary stenosis (PS). Adult patients with valvular PS usually do well, but eventually RV failure can occur. In the adult, severe pulmonary valve stenosis, requiring intervention, is defined as a peak systolic gradient in excess of 60 mm Hg, although intervention may be recommended for lesser degrees of stenosis in the presence of symptoms. Surgical valvotomy has been an extremely successful operation for long-term relief of pulmonary valve obstruction. A recent natural history study of surgically treated severe (gradient ≥ 80 mm Hg) pulmonic stenosis demonstrated an excellent 25-year survival of 95%, equivalent to the normal population (Table 25.2) (31). In patients with severe valvular PS, percutaneous balloon valvuloplasty is the current treatment of choice and has replaced surgical valvotomy in patients with flexible valves. Following percutaneous balloon valvuloplasty, pulmonary valve regurgitation can occur in 25% of adult patients (32).

TEE demonstrates the stenotic, doming pulmonary valve and thickening of the free wall of the RV (Fig. 25.6). The orifice can range from a pinhole to several millimeters but is rarely critical in the adult. The pulmonary valve is best seen in the basal horizontal views where it is

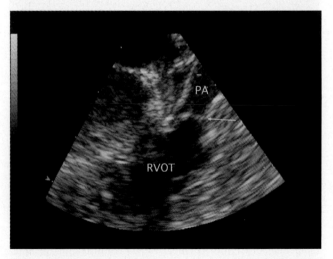

Figure 25.6. Pulmonic Valve Stenosis. Pulmonic valve stenosis (ME RV inflow-outflow view) demonstrating the doming stenotic valve (*arrow* points to the pulmonic valve). PA, pulmonic artery; RVOT, right ventricular outflow tract.

seen in long axis (LAX) (midesophageal [ME] asc aortic short axis [SAX] and RV inflow-outflow view) (Fig. 25.1; Table 25.1). Accurate measurements of the pressure gradient across the RVOT are possible with Doppler interrogation, usually from the trans-gastric (TG) view.

Patent Ductus Arteriosus

The patent ductus arteriosus (PDA), which accounts for 10% of cases of CHD, connects the proximal descending aorta with the pulmonary artery at its bifurcation. The magnitude of the left-to-right shunt depends on the size of the patent ductus and the pulmonaryvascular resistance-to-systemic vascular resistance ratio in a manner similar to that of the ventricular septal defect.

On 2D echocardiography, the ductus itself is rarely seen, but visualization of abnormal, continuous, high-velocity "aliased" flow within the main pulmonary artery MPA) near the left branch is seen on color flow Doppler imaging (33,34). Pulmonary artery systolic pressures can also be estimated (35).

The marked increase in pulmonary blood flow results in left-sided volume overload with an increase in the size of the LA, LV, ascending aorta, and aortic arch. The LV volume overload can result in congestive heart failure. Similar to a large VSD, the high pressure, high flow state can cause severe PHTN and Eisenmenger's syndrome as a result of pulmonary vascular disease.

PDA closure is indicated when there is net left-to-right shunting and evidence of LA and LV enlargement or prior endocarditis. However, it is reasonable to close small asymptomatic PDA's with a catheter-based approach. In the presence of pulmonary arterial hypertension, closure should only be considered in the presence of a net left-to-right shunt.

In the past, closure, by surgical ligation and division of the PDA, was performed to prevent the long-term danger of infective endarteritis. Today, options for closure of a PDA include transcatheter device or coil closure, open thoracotomy, and video-assisted thoracoscopic surgery. However, in many centers, the preferred alternative to surgical ligation in an adult is transcatheter closure (36–38) and surgery is only indicated if the ductus is too large for percutaneous device closure.

Coronary Artery Anomalies

Although coronary artery anomalies are rare, they should be considered in young patients (usually in the second or third decades of life) presenting with symptoms suggestive of ischemia, including exertional syncope or chest pain. The most common coronary anomalies seen in adults are anomalous origin of the left circumflex coronary artery from the right sinus of Valsalva, coronary to pulmonary artery fistulas, coronary cameral fistulas (fistulous connection between the coronary artery and the coronary chamber, usually RA or RV), and abnormal origin of the left coronary artery from the anterior sinus of Valsalva or the right coronary artery from the left posterior sinus of Valsalva.

COMPLEX LESIONS

Tetralogy of Fallot

Tetralogy of Fallot, the most common cyanotic defect after infancy, refers to a combination of four lesions consisting of

1. A VSD
2. Infundibular stenosis with or without valvular pulmonic stenosis
3. An aorta overriding the VSD
4. RV hypertrophy, which is a compensatory response to the other lesions

The RV obstruction and large VSD result in a high RV pressure that is similar to LV pressure. When the resistance due to the RV outflow obstruction is greater than systemic vascular resistance, there is a right-to-left shunt, arterial desaturation, and if severe, cyanosis. If the RV outflow obstruction is not severe, there may be little or no right-to-left shunt. The shunt may even be left-to-right, and the pulmonary valve and arteries may be normal or large. This lesion is sometimes referred to as "pink" or "acyanotic" tetralogy of Fallot. In tetralogy of Fallot, associated abnormalities include a right-sided aortic arch in about 25% of patients. In this anomaly, the aorta arches over the right mainstem bronchus, lies to the right of the trachea and esophagus, and descends on the right. Commonly, the first branch off the aorta is the left innominate artery (39). Other associated abnormalities include ASD in 10% (so-called Pentalogy of Fallot) and coronary anomalies in 10%. In adult patients with a perimembranous VSD (Type 2), there can be acquired hypertrophy of RV muscle bundles, resulting in dynamic outflow obstruction with pathophysiology similar to tetralogy of Fallot. This entity has been termed "double chambered RV."

TEE is particularly useful for defining the degree of aortic override, which is best seen in the longitudinal plane (Fig. 25.7). In patients with unrepaired tetralogy of Fallot, TEE demonstrates severe RV hypertrophy including the infundibulum usually with a thickened, malformed pulmonary valve. There is a large perimembranous VSD (Type 2) in the vicinity of the membranous septum with evidence of right-to-left shunting and a dilated overriding aorta. The gradient across the RVOT can be measured by spectral-Doppler. Most patients with tetralogy of Fallot have had palliative operations or corrective surgery by the time they are teenagers. Occasionally, a patient reaches adulthood without surgery. Sometimes patients present with only palliative systemic to pulmonary arterial shunts such as Blalock-Taussig shunt (subclavian to pulmonary artery), Potts' shunt (descending aorta to left pulmonary artery [LPA]),

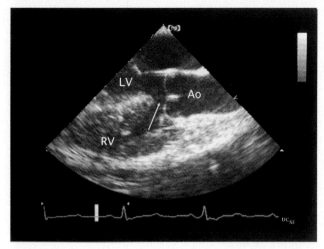

Figure 25.7. Tetralogy of Fallot. Tetralogy of Fallot (ME LAX view) showing the aortic override over the ventricular septum. The *arrow* points to the ventricular septal defect. Ao, aorta; LV, left ventricle; RV, right ventricle.

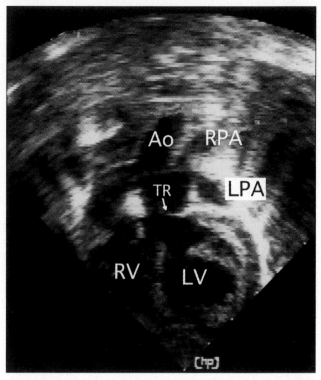

Figure 25.8. Truncus Arteriosus. Truncus arteriosus (deep TG LAX view, with apex of the heart displayed at the bottom) showing the biventricular origin of the large central vessel arising above the ventricular septal defect. The right and left pulmonary arteries (RPA, LPA) and the aorta (Ao) originate from the large common arterial trunk. TR, truncal vessel (Reproduced with slight modification from Muhiudeen IA, et al. Transesophageal TG echocardiography in infants and children. *J Am Soc Echocardiogr* 1995;8:231, with permission).

or Waterston's shunts (ascending aorta to right pulmonary artery [RPA]). Before surgical correction was possible, most patients died in the second decade of life.

Although it is an extremely successful operation, total intracardiac repair for tetralogy of Fallot has several potential significant postoperative residua, including residual RVOT obstruction, pulmonary valve regurgitation, peripheral pulmonary artery stenosis of one or both pulmonary arteries, ventricular septal patch leaks, and arrhythmias (Table 25.2). In the early and intermediate follow-up period, important residual RVOT obstruction appears to be the major source of morbidity and mortality. However, in the late follow-up period, patients in whom a transannular patch was required at the time of initial surgical repair to relieve outflow obstruction are at risk of developing pulmonary insufficiency with eventual RV failure owing to volume overload and ventricular arrhythmias, disability, and even death. Patients in this group who develop moderate to severe pulmonary insufficiency undergo pulmonary valve replacements as adults but without consistent improvement of RV systolic function postoperatively (40). Overall postoperative survival in patients with tetralogy of Fallot is about 90% at about 30 years after surgery (41).

Truncus Arteriosus

In truncus arteriosus, the embryonic truncus fails to divide into an aorta and a pulmonary artery, retaining the single semilunar valve and a VSD. The pulmonary, aortic, and coronary arteries thus arise from the single truncal root. Classification is based on the anatomic origin of the pulmonary arteries from the single trunk (42,43). The pulmonary trunk arises either separately from the common trunk and close to the truncal valve (Type I) or as separate vessels from the truncus (Types II and III).

In the unoperated child, TEE can demonstrate the presence of a single semilunar valve, the size of the VSD, and estimates of LV volume (Fig. 25.8). If the pulmonary arteries arise without stenosis from the truncus and the VSD is large, pulmonary blood flow will be markedly increased, volume overloading the LV, and causing heart failure and PHTN. Without surgery as an infant, the patient will not survive to adulthood. If the pulmonary arteries are stenotic at their origin, there will be a systolic ejection murmur and the pulmonary blood flow may be low, normal, or only mildly increased. Survival of the unoperated adult is the exception.

The truncus patient is usually managed surgically by closing the VSD and incorporating the semilunar valve on the left side as the aortic valve. A valved conduit is placed from the RV to the pulmonary artery. If the semilunar (truncal) valve is severely incompetent, valve replacement may be necessary. Depending on the severity of the pulmonary artery stenoses, varying techniques including surgical and balloon catheter techniques are used to relieve the obstruction. Residual obstruction to the pulmonary arteries, truncal valvular regurgitation, and obstruction of the conduit can be late complications, which may bring the adult patient to surgery. Patients with truncal valvular regurgitation are more likely to need truncal valve replacement at long-term follow-up (44). Pulmonary conduit replacement or revision is almost always needed and patients can present with conduit valve stenosis and/or insufficiency. Relief of RVOT construction at the site of the pulmonary conduit can be accomplished via percutaneous valve replacement with subsequent improved biventricular systolic function and increased exercise capacity in adults (45).

Transposition of the Great Arteries

Infants with transposition of the great arteries are born with the great arteries arising from the wrong ventricle. The aortic valve arises anteriorly from the RV, and the pulmonic valve posteriorly from the LV. Without cross-connections such as a patent foramen ovale, ASD, VSD, or PDA, this lesion is incompatible with life.

Infants with this condition rarely survive without intervention. With only rare exceptions, adults have had a palliative atrial switch procedure (such as the Mustard or Senning procedures), in which baffles were created to divert blood flow from the systemic veins to the LV and the pulmonary veins to the RV. Because the RV continues to serve the systemic circulation, it is subject to failure often with progressive tricuspid regurgitation. Patients with atrial switch operations are rarely candidates for reoperation. However, baffle leaks and baffle obstructions can now be addressed percutaneously. These patients may eventually come to transplant. Since the 1980s, an arterial switch operation, the Jatene procedure, has been performed to reconnect the great arteries to their proper ventricle, reconnect the coronary arteries to the new aortic location, and restore a "normal" circulation (Table 25.2). Late problems after the arterial switch surgery include dilatation of the neoaortic root, aortic regurgitation, supravalvar and branch PS. Ostial stenoses of the coronary arteries and myocardial ischemia have also been noted.

TEE evaluation with multiple planes, including contrast injection, should include baffle assessment after the Senning and Mustard procedure to evaluate potential baffle leaks or pulmonary venous obstruction by the intra-atrial baffle (Table 25.1). Evaluation of ventricular function is important because patients with an atrial switch procedure are at risk from failure of the systemic "right" ventricle. Patients with the arterial switch operation (Jatene procedure) can have coronary artery obstruction, atrial or ventricular patch leaks, aortic valvular regurgitation, and supravalvular obstruction at the site of the aortic and pulmonary artery anastomoses. Medical therapy to treat failure of the systemic RV includes afterload reduction with vasodilators, digoxin, and diuretics. Noninvasive and invasive studies may demonstrate the need for further surgical palliative procedures.

Physiologically Corrected Transposition (L-Transposition)

L-transposition is characterized by malposition of the great vessels and ventricular inversion, with the LV connected to the RA and pulmonary artery and the RV connected to the LA and aorta. Blood flow is physiologically correct, but an anatomic RV serves as the systemic ventricle. Most previously undiagnosed adults with this lesion usually have no associated cardiac defects. Corrected transposition is frequently discovered as a result of the physical findings due to associated congenital defects, such as VSD and subpulmonic valve stenosis. With no other abnormalities, this lesion may remain undetected until the patient presents with congestive heart failure or syncope, owing to complete heart block (24).

Without additional lesions, patients with corrected transposition may live to old age. The development of complete heart block is common and occurs at a rate of approximately 5% per year in adults. In the presence of severe accompanying lesions, surgical correction may be possible. The systemic ventricle, an anatomic RV, may show progressive failure requiring medical treatment. Adult patients with L-transposition rarely come to surgery. Patients previously operated upon for pulmonic stenosis may have conduit stenosis or valve failure. Tricuspid regurgitation may result from RV failure. However, TV replacement or repair is rarely beneficial.

TEE examination should include identification of ventricular morphology and function and associated lesions, such as VSD and pulmonary outflow tract obstruction.

Ebstein's Anomaly

In Ebstein's anomaly, the septal and posterior leaflets of the TV are dysplastic and displaced from the tricuspid annulus apically into the body of the RV (46–48). Thus, a portion of the RV is above the TV (the atrialized RV) and enlarges the true RA. Patients are diverse in presenting symptoms and severity of TV abnormality. The valve may be regurgitant, and if a patent foramen ovale or an ASD is present (80% of patients), there can be a large right-to-left shunt. These patients are cyanotic, are likely to present in infancy, and may have had palliative procedures with atrial septal defect closure. The presentation in adolescents or adults is more likely related to progressive tricuspid regurgitation and heart failure or arrhythmias than to cyanosis. Nevertheless, some patients with severe displacement of the TV can live normal lives with minimal symptoms.

TEE is diagnostic, with a normal basal attachment of the large redundant anterior leaflet and displaced immobile septal and posterior leaflets, demonstrating the morphology of the abnormal TV with a tricuspid regurgitant jet arising apically within the RV (Fig. 25.9). The RA and RV are enlarged.

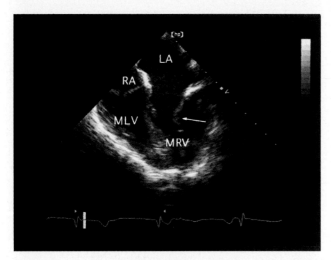

Figure 25.9. Corrected transposition with Ebstein deformity of the TV. Corrected transposition of the great arteries with the morphologic right ventricle (MRV) below the LA and the morphologic left ventricle (MLV) below the RA. The septal leaflet of the TV is inferiorly displaced well below the insertion of the mitral valve (ME four-chamber view). LA, left atrium; RA, right atrium.

Once the patient has survived childhood, the prognosis is favorable, even with severe displacement of the TV. If the tricuspid regurgitation is severe, then the ability to increase cardiac output may be diminished and the patient may have progressive limitation of activity with fatigability. Closure of an ASD and reconstruction of the TV with an annuloplasty or even replacement has been performed with success, although short- and long-term results after TV replacement can be suboptimal due to postoperative right heart failure and decreased cardiac output (49). Another approach is to do a Glenn operation (SVC to pulmonary artery cavopulmonary connection) (50) to partially unload the RV by diverting SVC flow directly to the RPA. Indications for tricuspid repair or replacement include symptoms and exercise intolerance, cyanosis, paradoxical embolization, or progressive cardiomegaly or RV dilatation. The indications for reoperation are similar. If atrial tachycardia is present with an anomalous atrioventricular conduction pathway, radiofrequency ablation of the AV pathway can successfully treat the paroxysmal atrial tachycardia.

Single Ventricle

A number of CHD lesions are included in the single ventricle category. Hypoplasia of either the RV or LV results in a single functional ventricle. This category includes hypoplastic left heart syndrome, double-inlet LV, and tricuspid atresia.

TEE evaluation should include multiple views to evaluate atrioventricular and ventriculoarterial connections,

and ventricular size and morphology. Adult patients with a single ventricle lesion may have a modified Blalock Taussig shunt, a Glenn anastomosis SVC to pulmonary artery cavopulmonary connection (50), or a Fontan connection (total caval to pulmonary connection) (51,52). Visualization of the Glenn anastomosis is not always possible by TEE, but it can sometimes be demonstrated using longitudinal planes.

The Fontan procedure includes a variety of surgical approaches that connect either the RA or the vena cavae directly to the pulmonary arteries, bypassing the RV. Pulmonary blood flow is propelled by the systemic venous pressure and negative inspiratory force, reducing the volume overload to the LV. TEE is particularly useful for evaluation of ventricular function and valvular regurgitation. The Glenn or Fontan procedure is usually performed in childhood, but occasionally adults are candidates for the procedure. Patients with the Fontan procedure can do well into the third and fourth decades. Successful pregnancies have been reported in these patients. The patients have an elevated systemic venous pressure and can have ascites and peripheral edema for months after surgery. Eventually these resolve, but later complications include chylous pleural effusions, protein-losing enteropathy, and eventual ventricular failure. Atrial tachyarrhythmias, especially in those patients where the RA is part of the connection to the pulmonary artery, can cause significant morbidity and mortality.

Adult patients with single-ventricle physiology may come to cardiac surgery for

1. Revision of previous Fontan or Glenn procedures
2. Primary Fontan or Glenn procedures
3. Revision of arteriopulmonary shunts
4. Transplantation

Dextrocardia and Dextroposition

In patients with dextrocardia and situs inversus, the vena cava, atria, ventricles, and great vessels are all reversed and, thus, connected appropriately. Frequently, there are associated congenital heart lesions, and the right lung may be hypoplastic.

CONCLUSIONS

In many medical centers, TEE is now the standard of care for intraoperative assessment of patients with CHD. In noncardiac surgery, TEE can be used to evaluate ventricular volume, function, underlying pathology, and to assess any residual lesions. TEE clearly has significant perioperative impact in the care of patients with CHD undergoing cardiac surgery, including confirmation, altered or new diagnoses along with revision of the surgical plan in as many as 5% to 7% of cases.

■ ASDs are one of the most common defects in the adult population. There are four types: ostium secundum defect (70%), ostium primum defect (15%–25%), sinus venosus defect (10%), and coronary sinus ASDs (<2%).

■ VSDs are the most common cardiac abnormality in infants and children and have a high rate of spontaneous closure. Primary closure is indicated for a Qp:Qs > 2:1 in the absence of Eisenmenger's physiology.

■ Atrioventricular septal defects include a VSD, an ASD, and varying degrees of AV valve regurgitation.

■ *Congenital AS*: The anatomic level of obstruction can be supravalvular, valvular, or subvalvular. AS is due to a malformed valve that is usually functionally bicuspid.

■ *Tetralogy of Fallot*, the most common cyanotic defect after infancy, consists of a VSD, infundibular stenosis with or without valvular pulmonic stenosis, an aorta overriding the VSD, and RV hypertrophy.

■ *Transposition of the Great Arteries*: The aortic valve arises from the RV, and the pulmonic valve arises from the LV.

■ *Physiologically Corrected Transposition (L-Transposition)*: Transposition consists of malposition of the great vessels and ventricular inversion, with the LV connected to the RA and pulmonary artery and the RV connected to the LA and aorta. VSD and pulmonic stenosis are the most common associated lesions. Complete heart block is frequent.

■ In *Ebstein's anomaly*, the leaflets of the TV are dysplastic and displaced from the tricuspid annulus apically into the body of the RV. Interatrial septal defects or patent foramen ovale is present in 50% of patients.

■ A number of CHD lesions comprise what is known as *single ventricles*, usually resulting in hypoplasia of the RV or LV.

REFERENCES

1. Russell IA, Rouine-Rapp K, Stratmann G, et al. Congenital heart disease in the adult: a review with internet-accessible transesophageal echocardiographic images. *Anesth Analg* 2006;102(3):694–723.

2. Care of the adult with congenital heart disease. Presented at 32nd Bethesda Conference, Bethesda, Maryland, October 2–3, 2000. *J Am Coll Cardiol* 2001;37:1161–1198.

3. Marelli AJ, Mackie AS, Ionescu-Ittu R, et al. Congenital heart disease in the general population: changing prevalence and age distribution. *Circulation* 2007;115(2):163–172.

4. Warnes CA, Liberthson R, et al. Task Force 1: the changing profile of congenital heart disease in adult life. *JACC* 2001;37(5):1170–1175.

5. Hoffman JIE, Kaplan S, Liberthson RR. Prevalence of congenital heart disease. *Am Heart J* 2004;147:425–439.

6. Thys D, Abel M, Bollen B, et al. Practice guidelines for perioperative transesophageal echocardiography. *Anesthesiology* 1996;84:986–1006.

7. Cheitlin M, Alpert J, Armstrong W, et al. ACC/AHA guidelines for the clinical application of echocardiography. A report of the American College of Cardiology/American Heart Association Task Force on Practice Guidelines (Committee on Clinical Application of Echocardiography). *Circulation* 1997;95:1686–1744.

8. Samyn MM. A review of the complementary information available with cardiac magnetic resonance imaging and multi-slice computed tomography (CT) during the study of congenital heart disease. *Int J Cardiovasc Imaging* 2004;20(6):569–578.

9. Child JS. Transthoracic and transesophageal echocardiographic imaging: anatomic and hemodynamic assessment. In: Perloff JK, Child JS, eds. *Congenital Heart Disease in Adults*. Philadelphia: W.B. Saunders, 1998:91–128.

10. Child JS, Marelli AJ. The application of transesophageal echocardiography in the adult with congenital heart disease. In: Maurer G, ed. *Transesophageal Echocardiography*. New York: McGraw-Hill, 1994:159–188.

11. Kaplan S, Adolph RJ. Pulmonary valve stenosis in adults. *Cardiovasc Clin* 1979;10:327–339.

12. Schiller NB, Maurer G, Ritter SB, et al. Transesophageal echocardiography. *J Am Soc Echocardiogr* 1989;2:354–357.

13. Shanewise JS, Cheung AT, Aronson S, et al. ASE/SCA guidelines for performing a comprehensive intraoperative multiplane transesophageal echocardiography examination: recommendations of the American Society of Echocardiography Council for Intraoperative Echocardiography and the Society of Cardiovascular Anesthesiologists Task Force for Certification in Perioperative Transesophageal Echocardiography. *Anesth Analg* 1999;89:870–884.

14. Abd El Rahman MY, Hui W, Dsebissowa F, et al. Comparison of the tissue Doppler-derived left ventricular Tei index to that obtained by pulse Doppler in patients with congenital and acquired heart disease. *Pediatr Cardiol* 2005;26(4):391–395.

15. Brickner ME, Hillis LD, Lange RA. Congenital heart disease in adults. *N Engl J Med* 2000;342(Pt 1):256–263; 342(5 Pt 2):334–342.

16. Maxted W, Finch A, Nanda NC, et al. Multiplane transesophageal echocardiographic detection of sinus venosus atrial septal defect. *Echocardiography* 1995;12:139–145.

17. Van Hare G, Silverman N. Contrast two-dimensional echocardiography in congenital heart disease: techniques, indications and clinical utility. *J Am Coll Cardiol* 1989;13:673–686.

18. Valdes-Cruz LM, Pieroni DR, Roland JM, et al. Recognition of residual postoperative shunts by contrast echocardiographic techniques. *Circulation* 1977;55:148–152.

19. Murphy JG, Gersh BJ, McGoon MD, et al. Long-term outcome after surgical repair of isolated atrial septal defect. Follow-up at 27 to 32 years. *N Engl J Med* 1990;323:1645–1650.

20. Konstantinides S, Geibel A, Olschewski M, et al. A comparison of surgical and medical therapy for atrial septal defect in adults. *N Engl J Med* 1995;333:469–473.

21. Attie F, Rosas M, Granados N, et al. Surgical treatment for secundum atrial septal defects in patients >40 years old.

A randomized clinical trial. *J Am Coll Cardiol* 2001;38: 2035–2042.

22. Gatzoulis MA, Freeman MA, Siu SC, et al. Atrial arrhythmia after surgical closure of atrial septal defects in adults. *N Engl J Med* 1999;340:839–846.

23. Warnes CA, Williams RG, Bashore TM, et al. ACC/AHA 2008 Guidelines for the Management of Adults With Congenital Heart Disease: a Report of the American College of Cardiology/ American Heart Association Task Force on Practice Guidelines (Writing Committee to Develop Guidelines on the Management of Adults With Congenital Heart Disease) Developed in Collaboration With the American Society of Echocardiography, Heart Rhythm Society, International Society for Adult Congenital Heart Disease, Society for Cardiovascular Angiography and Interventions, and Society of Thoracic Surgeons. *J Am Coll Cardiol* 2008;52:e143–e263.

24. Bédard E, Shore DF, Gatzoulis MA. Adult congenital heart disease: a 2008 Overview. *Br Med Bull* 2008;85:151–180.

25. Silbert DR, Brunson SC, Schiff R, et al. Determination of right ventricular pressure in the presence of a ventricular septal defect using continuous wave Doppler ultrasound. *J Am Coll Cardiol* 1986;8:379–384.

26. Rastelli G, Kirklin JW, Titus JL. Anatomic observations on complete form of persistent common atrioventricular canal with special reference to atrioventricular valves. *Mayo Clin Proc* 1966;41:296–308.

27. Keane JF, Driscoll DJ, Gersony WM, et al. Second natural history study of congenital heart defects. Results of treatment of patients with aortic valvar stenosis. *Circulation* 1993;87: I16–I27.

28. Frigiola A, Ranucci M, Carlucci C, et al. The Ross procedure in adults: long-term follow-up and echocardiographic changes leading to pulmonary autograft reoperation. *Ann Thorac Surg* 2008;86(2):482–489.

29. Simpson IA, Sahn DJ, Valdes-Cruz LM, et al. Color Doppler flow mapping in patients with coarctation of the aorta: new observations and improved evaluation with color flow diameter and proximal acceleration as predictors of severity. *Circulation* 1988;77:736–744.

30. Reich O, Tax P, Bartáková H, et al. Long-term (up to 20 years) results of percutaneous balloon angioplasty of recurrent aortic coarctation without use of stents. *Eur Heart J* 2008;29(16): 2042–2048.

31. Hayes CJ, Gersony WM, Driscoll DJ, et al. Second natural history study of congenital heart defects. Results of treatment of patients with pulmonary valvar stenosis. *Circulation* 1993;87:I28–I37.

32. Fawzy ME, Kinsara AJ, Stefadouros M, et al. Long-term outcome of mitral balloon valvotomy in pregnant women. *J Heart Valve Dis* 2001;10(2):153–157.

33. Mugge A, Daniel WG, Lichtlen PR. Imaging of patent ductus arteriosus by transesophageal color-coded Doppler echocardiography. *J Clin Ultrasound* 1991;19:128–129.

34. Takenaka K, Sakamoto T, Shiota T, et al. Diagnosis of patent ductus arteriosus in adults by biplane transesophageal color Doppler flow mapping. *Am J Cardiol* 1991;68:691–693.

35. Marx GR, Allen HD, Goldberg SJ. Doppler echocardiographic estimation of systolic pulmonary artery pressure in patients with aortic-pulmonary shunts. *J Am Coll Cardiol* 1986;7: 880–885.

36. Nezafati MH, Soltani G, Vedadian A. Video-assisted ductal closure with new modifications: minimally invasive, maximally effective, 1,300 cases. *Ann Thorac Surg* 2007;84(4):1343–1348.

37. Atiq M, Aslam N, Kazmi KA. Transcatheter closure of small-to-large patent ductus arteriosus with different devices: queries and challenges. *J Invasive Cardiol* 2007;19(7):295–298.

38. Rao PS. Summary and comparison of PDA closure methods. In: Rao PS, Kern MJ, eds. *Catheter Based Devices for the Treatment of Non-Coronary Cardiovascular Disease in Adults and Children*. Philadelphia: Lippincott Williams & Wilkins, 2003:219–228.

39. Knight L, Edwards JE. Right aortic arch. Types and associated cardiac anomalies. *Circulation* 1974;50(5):1047–1051.

40. Graham TP Jr. The year in congenital heart disease. *J Am Coll Cardiol* 2008;52(18):1492–1499.

41. Murphy JG, Gersh BJ, Mair DD, et al. Long-term outcome in patients undergoing surgical repair of tetralogy of Fallot. *N Engl J Med* 1993;329:593–599.

42. Calder L, Van Praagh R, Van Praagh S, et al. Truncus arteriosus communis: clinical, angiographic, and pathologic findings in 100 patients. *Am Heart J* 1976;92:23–38.

43. Collett RW, Edwards JE. Persistent truncus arteriosus: a classification according to anatomic types. *Surg Clin North Am* 1949;29:1245–1270.

44. Rajasinghe HA, McElhinney DB, Reddy VM, et al. Long-term follow-up of truncus arteriosus repaired in infancy: a 20-year experience. *J Thorac Cardiovasc Surg* 1997;113(5):869–878.

45. Coats L, Khambadkone S, Derrick G, et al. Physiological and clinical consequences of relief of right ventricular outflow tract obstruction late after repair of congenital heart defects. *Circulation* 2006;113(17):2037–2044.

46. Roberson DA, Silverman NH. Ebstein's anomaly: echocardiographic and clinical features in the fetus and neonate. *J Am Coll Cardiol* 1989;14:1300–1307.

47. Quaegebeur JM, Sreeram N, Fraser AG, et al. Surgery for Ebstein's anomaly: the clinical and echocardiographic evaluation of a new technique. *J Am Coll Cardiol* 1991;17:722–728.

48. Vargas-Barron J, Rijlaarsdam M, Romero-Cardenas A, et al. Transesophageal echocardiographic study of Ebstein's anomaly. *Echocardiography* 1995;12:253–261.

49. Iscan ZH, Vural KM, Bahar I, et al. What to expect after tricuspid valve replacement? Long-term results. *Eur J Cardiothorac Surg* 2007;32(2):296–300.

50. Trusler GA, Williams WG, Cohen AJ, et al. William Glenn lecture. The cavopulmonary shunt. Evolution of a concept. *Circulation* 1990;82:IV131–IV138.

51. Fyfe DA, Ritter SB, Snider AR, et al. Guidelines for transesophageal echocardiography in children. *J Am Soc Echocardiogr* 1992;5:640–644.

52. Stumper O, Sutherland GR, Geuskens R, et al. Transesophageal echocardiography in evaluation and management after a Fontan procedure. *J Am Coll Cardiol* 1991;17:1152–1160.

QUESTIONS

1. The most common atrial septal defect in the adult population is the
   A. primum
   B. secundum
   C. sinus venosus
   D. coronary sinus

2. Longitudinal plane imaging is extremely useful for which of the following lesions?
   A. Atrioventricular septal defect
   B. Secundum atrial septal defect
   C. Patent ductus arteriosus (PDA)
   D. Tetralogy of Fallot

3. After an arterial switch for transposition of the great arteries, all of the following can occur *except*
   A. Supravalvar aortic stenosis (AS)
   B. Left ventricular (LV) dysfunction
   C. Protein-losing enteropathy
   D. Coronary artery stenosis

Assessment of Perioperative Hemodynamics

CHAPTER 26

Nikolaos J. Skubas ■ Albert Perrino

Doppler echocardiography, typically in conjunction with 2D imaging, is used to perform a quantitative hemodynamic assessment (Table 26.1). The accuracy of Doppler-derived measurements has been validated in the cardiac catheterization laboratory (1–4) but remains dependent on the quality of the acquired data and thus on the skill and knowledge of the echocardiographer. Technical factors essential to acquiring accurate hemodynamic assessment data include obtaining near-parallel alignment of the ultrasound beam with the blood flow of interest, minimal interference from adjacent blood flows, and, for many calculations, precise 2D echocardiographic determination of the cross-sectional area (CSA) of the blood stream.

In comparison to transthoracic echocardiography (TTE) where the probe is easily positioned across the chest to interrogate the blood flow of interest, hemodynamic assessment with transesophageal echocardiography (TEE) is limited as the probe is confined within the esophagus. The introduction of the multiplane TEE probe represents a significant advance in hemodynamic assessment by allowing a far greater number of echocardiographic imaging planes from which blood flows may be interrogated. This chapter focuses on quantitative hemodynamic assessment using 2D and Doppler echocardiography. M-mode and 2D echocardiographic signs of hemodynamic abnormalities, determination of diastolic function with Doppler, and estimation of cardiac-filling pressures based on diastolic parameters are discussed in more detail in other chapters.

TABLE 26.1 Hemodynamic Data Obtainable with 2D and Doppler Echocardiography

Volumetric measurements
  SV
  CO
  Pulmonary-to-systemic flow ratio (Qp/Qs)
  RV and LV ejection fraction
Pressure gradients
  Maximum gradient
  Mean gradient
Valve area
  Stenotic valve area
  Regurgitant orifice area
Intracardiac and PA pressures
  RV systolic and diastolic pressure
  PASP
  PA mean pressure
  PADP
  LAP
  LVEDP
Ventricular dp/dt

DOPPLER MEASUREMENTS OF STROKE VOLUME AND CARDIAC OUTPUT

Calculation of Stroke Volume

The flow rate of a fluid through a fixed orifice is directly proportional to the product of its CSA and the mean velocity of the fluid within the orifice as given by the *hydraulic orifice formula* (Fig. 26.1):

$$\text{Flow rate (cm}^3/\text{s)} = \text{CSA (cm}^2) \times \text{flow velocity (cm/s)}$$

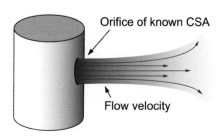

Flow rate (cm³/s) = CSA (cm²) x flow velocity (cm/s)

Figure 26.1. The Hydraulic Orifice Formula. The volumetric flow rate through an orifice is equal to the product of its CSA and the flow velocity through the orifice. If flow velocity is constant, so is flow rate; however, if flow velocity varies, so will flow rate.

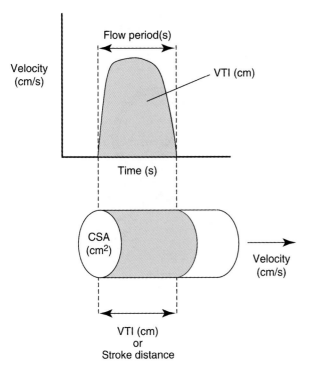

Figure 26.2. Doppler VTI and Stroke Distance. As flow in the heart and great vessels is pulsatile, blood flow velocity varies during the period of ejection (or filling), as shown by the Doppler velocity curve. The tracing of the Doppler velocity curve (VTI) is equivalent to the distance blood flow travels with one beat of the heart (stroke distance).

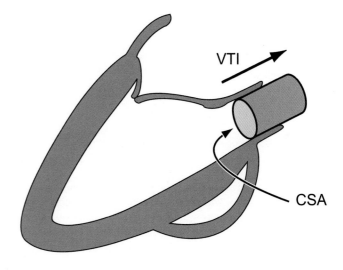

$$SV\ (cm^3) = CSA\ (cm^2) \times VTI\ (cm)$$

Figure 26.3. Doppler SV Calculation. The VTI of the Doppler velocity curve can be conceptualized as the length of a cylinder of blood (stroke distance) ejected through a CSA on one heartbeat. SV is calculated as the product of CSA and VTI.

The cardiovascular system is pulsatile; therefore, the velocity of instantaneous blood flow varies. The acceleration and deceleration of blood flow velocity during systole (ejection period) and diastole (filling period) provide distinct Doppler profiles for a given orifice (cardiac valve, vena cavae, pulmonary veins, pulmonary artery [PA], or aorta). The summation of the instantaneous flow rates over the entire flow period is called the *velocity-time integral* (VTI), or alternatively the *time-velocity integral* (TVI). Conceptually, for each cardiac cycle, the VTI is the distance that blood travels. The echocardiographer traces the Doppler velocity signal, and the VTI is then calculated by the ultrasound machine's analysis software (Fig. 26.2).

Stroke volume (SV) is calculated as the product of CSA and VTI (Fig. 26.3):

$$SV\ (cm^3) = CSA\ (cm^2) \times VTI\ (cm)$$

SV can be calculated from specific locations within the heart or great vessels by using the appropriate Doppler velocity signal to determine the VTI (referred to as stroke distance) at the same location that 2D imaging is used to determine CSA. In descending order of preference, the preferred sites for SV calculation are the left ventricular outflow tract (LVOT), the pulmonary annulus, and the mitral annulus. The VTI is usually measured with pulsed

wave Doppler, but continuous wave Doppler may also be utilized to determine the aortic valve (AV) VTI in the absence of subvalvular or supravalvular aortic obstruction. In the latter case, the velocity signals obtained by continuous and pulsed wave Doppler across the AV should be the same. If the CSA of the "orifice" to be measured is assumed to be circular, it can be calculated by using the formula for the area of a circle (of radius r) after measuring the orifice diameter (D) in cm:

$$CSA\ (cm^2) = \pi \times r^2 = \pi \times (D/2)^2 = 0.785 \times D^2$$

The Doppler method for determining SV at a particular site is predicated on the following (Table 26.2):

TABLE 26.2	**Assumptions for Accurate Doppler SV Calculations**

1.	Blood flow is laminar with a flat flow velocity profile.
2.	VTI measurement represents the average of several measurements: 3–5 measurements in normal sinus rhythm, 8–10 measurements in atrial fibrillation.
3.	VTI is measured with Doppler beam parallel to blood flow
4.	Measurements of VTI and CSA (i.e., diameter) are made at the same time and at the same anatomic location.
5.	CSA (i.e., diameter) measurement is accurate.

Normal LVOT Flow   Normal Aortic Flow   Post-Stenotic Flow

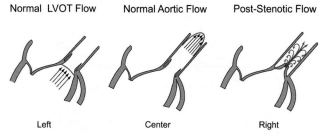

Left   Center   Right

Figure 26.4. Common flow patterns. **Left:** Acceleration of blood within the LVOT leads to laminar flow with a flat velocity profile. **Center:** Friction along the wall of the ascending aorta leads to laminar flow with a parabolic flow profile. **Right:** Aortic stenosis results in a narrow, high-velocity laminar jet originating from the stenotic orifice surrounded by turbulent flow.

First, blood flow is assumed to be laminar and the spatial flow velocity profile is assumed to be flat (i.e., all blood cells are moving in the same direction and at the same speed), as is generally the case in the left ventricular outflow tract (LVOT) (Fig. 26.4). A narrow band of velocities and a smooth spectral signal obtained with pulsed wave Doppler are evidence of laminar flow in the great vessels and across normal cardiac valves. A flat flow velocity profile can be demonstrated by showing uniform velocities while moving the pulsed wave Doppler sample volume from side to side within the flow of interest from two orthogonal views. When SV is calculated from blood flow in the LVOT, the sample volume should be placed 5 mm proximal to the AV. Correct position of the sample volume is verified by recording the closing click of the AV. Tracing of the VTI should be done at the outer edge of the modal velocity (i.e., the brightest portion of the spectral envelope) (5).

Second, the VTI used in calculating SV is assumed to represent the average VTI. Therefore, several measurements (3 to 5) taken throughout the respiratory cycle should be averaged for a patient in normal sinus rhythm, whereas between 8 and 10 measurements should be averaged for a patient in atrial fibrillation.

Third, the VTI is assumed to be recorded with the Doppler ultrasound beam parallel to the flow (i.e., intercept angle $\theta = 0$). In this case, velocities measured by Doppler are accurate based on a cosine $\theta° = 1$ in the Doppler equation (Fig. 26.5). However, as $\theta°$ increases from 20 to 60 degrees, the underestimation in the calculated Doppler velocity increases from 6% to 50% (Fig. 26.6). Small adjustments of the TEE probe transducer position and pulsed wave Doppler sample volume (or continuous wave Doppler beam) are necessary to obtain the highest velocity signal. Multiple imaging planes should be utilized when possible to confirm that the highest velocity signal is obtained. Listening to the quality of the audio broadcast of the Doppler signal in addition to observing the Doppler display guides optimal alignment of the ultrasound beam with the targeted flow of interest. The highest velocity signal obtained (clear, high-pitched audio signal) identifies the most parallel alignment of the Doppler beam with blood flow.

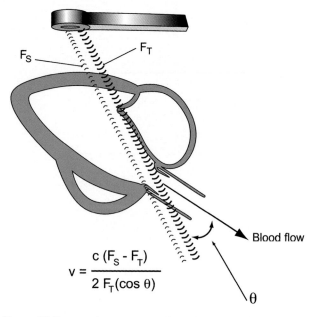

$$v = \frac{c\,(F_S - F_T)}{2\,F_T(\cos\theta)}$$

Figure 26.5. Doppler equation. Blood flow velocity (v) is calculated based on the Doppler shift, which is the change in frequency between transmitted (F_T) and backscattered (reflected from moving red blood cells, F_S) ultrasound. c, speed of sound in blood); θ, intercept angle between blood flow and interrogating Doppler ultrasound beam.

Fourth, CSA and VTI measurements are assumed to be made *at the same anatomic location*. CSA diameter is measured most accurately when the 2D ultrasound beam is perpendicular to blood flow velocity, while VTI is

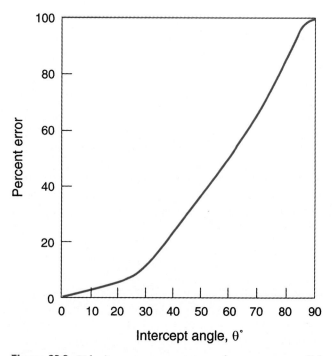

Figure 26.6. Velocity measurement error due to a nonparallel intercept angle. The percentage error in the velocity calculation using the Doppler equation markedly increases with large intercept angles between blood flow and Doppler ultrasound beam.

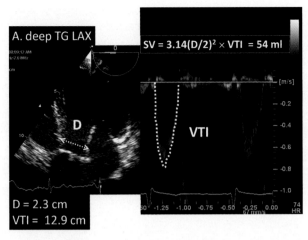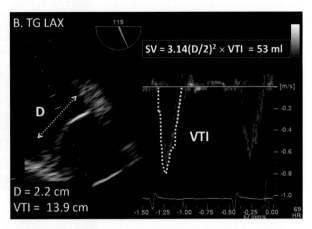

Figure 26.7. LVOT Doppler SV Calculation. **Panel A:** The diameter (D) of the LVOT is measured at midsystole, from the junction of AV cusp to the septal myocardium to the junction of AV cusp to the anterior mitral leaflet, in the deep transgastric long-axis view (deep TG LAX). In the same view, the VTI of the LVOT velocity is imaged with the pulsed wave Doppler sample volume placed just proximal to the AV. Notice the closing click of the AV. **Panel B:** Alternatively, D can be measured at midsystole in the transgastric long-axis view. In the same view, VTI of the LVOT velocity is imaged with the pulsed wave Doppler sample volume placed just proximal to the AV. Notice the closing click of the AV.

measured most accurately when the Doppler ultrasound beam is parallel to blood flow. Thus, 2D diameter measurements and Doppler velocity profiles are often not recorded from the same imaging plane. Nevertheless, every effort should be made to perform these measurements *at the same anatomic location* and *in close sequence* in order to minimize error in the calculated SV.

Fifth, the measured CSA is assumed to represent the average CSA during systole. Changes in CSA during the flow period, or deviations from an assumed circular geometry, are inherent problems in Doppler SV calculations. For these reasons, the ventricular outflow valves (aortic and pulmonic) are the most reliable sites for Doppler-derived SV measurements (6). Precise measurements of diameter are essential. In the case of an assumed circular orifice, a small error in diameter measurement will result in a large error in the calculated CSA due to the quadratic relationship between the radius and area of a circle (i.e., CSA = $\pi \times r^2$). To increase accuracy, multiple diameter measurements should be averaged prior to calculation of CSA. The use of high-frequency multiplane TEE probes for measuring diameters (or areas) undoubtedly increases the reliability of these measurements when compared to the use of lower-frequency monoplane or biplane TEE probes.

Calculation of Cardiac Output

Cardiac output (CO) can be estimated after determining a Doppler SV and measuring heart rate (HR) (7). Cardiac index (CI) is calculated by dividing CO by body surface area (BSA):

$$CO \text{ (L/min)} = SV \text{ (L)} \times HR \text{ (min}^{-1})$$

$$CI \text{ (L/min/m}^2) = CO \text{ (L/min)} / BSA \text{ (m}^2)$$

CO measurements performed with TEE, usually at the LVOT or AV in the absence of aortic regurgitation (AR), have been shown to correlate well with measurements made by thermodilution (8–13). Accurate estimation of CO depends on accurate determinations of the VTI and CSA, as previously discussed.

Calculation of LVOT Stroke Volume (Fig. 26.7)

The pulsed wave Doppler sample volume is placed in the LVOT just proximal to the AV (~5 mm), using either the transgastric long-axis or the deep transgastric long-axis view for determination of the VTI_{LVOT}. The LVOT diameter is best obtained from the midesophageal long-axis view of the AV, from the junction of the aortic leaflets with the anterior mitral leaflet posteriorly to the junction of the leaflet with the septal myocardium anteriorly, and the largest of three to five measurements should be taken.

Calculation of Transaortic Valve Stroke Volume (Fig. 26.8)

The *continuous wave* Doppler beam is directed through the AV in either the transgastric long-axis or the deep transgastric long-axis view for determination of the VTI_{AV}.

The CSA of the AV can be determined by one of two methods. Planimetry can be used to measure the area of the triangular-shaped AV orifice *during midsystole* from a cine of the midesophageal short-axis view of the AV (11). Alternatively, AV area can be calculated from a quick caliper cine-loop measurement of the length of the side (cm) of the equilateral opening of the valve *during midsystole* using the following formula

$$CSA_{AV} \text{ (cm}^2) = 0.433 \times (\text{side})^2$$

Figure 26.8. Transaortic valve Doppler SV Calculation. **A:** Planimetry of the CSA of AV orifice at midsystole from a cine-loop of the midesophageal short-axis view of AV (ME AV SAX). **B:** Alternatively, the length of a side (S) of the AV can be measured in midsystole and used to calculate the AVA. **C:** The velocity time integral (VTI_{AV}) can be measured with the continuous wave Doppler beam placed through the AV using a deep transgastric long-axis view (deep TG LAX). **D:** Alternatively, VTI_{AV} can be measured with continuous wave Doppler using a TG LAX view.

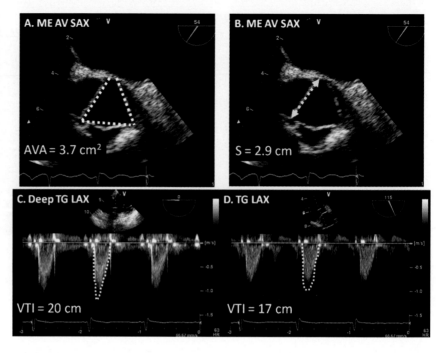

Several measurements may be made and then averaged in order to improve accuracy.

Calculation of Pulmonary Annulus Stroke Volume (Fig. 26.9)

The VTI of the main pulmonary annulus (VTI_{PA}) is recorded with the pulsed wave Doppler sample volume placed in the main PA using the upper esophageal aortic

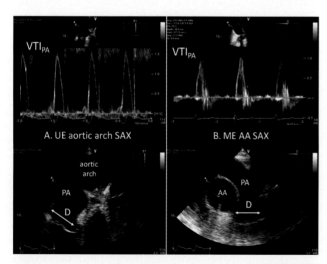

Figure 26.9. Pulmonary Annulus Doppler SV Calculation. **A:** VTI of PA (VTI_{PA}) is measured using pulsed wave Doppler with the sample volume in the main PA using the upper esophageal short-axis view of the aortic arch (UE aortic arch SAX). The diameter (D) of the main PA is measured from the same view at the same location. **B:** Alternatively, VTI_{PA} and diameter of the main PA are measured using the midesophageal short-axis view of the ascending aorta (ME AA SAX).

arch short-axis view (with the transducer rotated between 80 and 90 degrees) or the midesophageal short-axis view of the ascending aorta. The diameter of the main PA is measured from either view *at the same location* for determination of the CSA using the formula for the area of a circle:

$$CSA_{PA} \ (cm^2) = 0.785 \times D_{PA}{}^2$$

In either case, poor visualization and fluctuation in the diameter of the main PA during the cardiac cycle make SV measurement at this location more problematic than those obtained at the LVOT or AV (6).

Calculation of RVOT Stroke Volume (Fig. 26.10)

The right ventricular outflow tract (RVOT) may be visualized using a transgastric RV inflow-outflow view with the transducer rotated between 110 and 150 degrees and the probe turned to the right. The pulsed wave Doppler sample volume is placed in the RVOT just proximal to the pulmonic valve for determination of the VTI_{RVOT}. The diameter (cm) of the RVOT is best obtained from the same view *at the same location* for determination of CSA, using the formula for the area of a circle:

$$CSA_{RVOT} \ (cm^2) = 0.785 \times D_{RVOT}{}^2$$

Alternatively, the diameter of the RVOT can be measured from the upper esophageal short-axis view of the aortic arch.

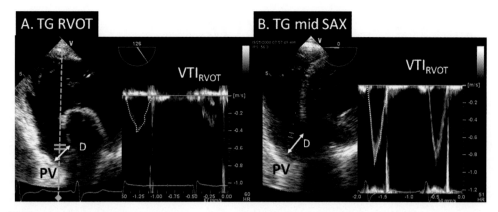

Figure 26.10. RVOT Doppler SV Calculation. **A:** VTI of RV outflow tract (VTI_{RVOT}) is measured using pulsed wave Doppler (dotted line) with the sample volume placed just proximal to the pulmonic valve (PV) from a transgastric RV inflow-outflow view (TG RVOT). (The imaging array is rotated to 130 degrees, and the probe is in a neutral or turned rightward). RVOT diameter (D) is measured at the same view. Notice the increased Doppler angle that results in decreased velocity and VTI. **B:** Alternate site for these measurements is the TG mid short-axis (SAX) view of the LV. (The transducer is advanced and turned until the RVOT and PV are imaged.)

Calculation of Transmitral Stroke Volume (Fig. 26.11)

The pulsed wave Doppler sample volume is placed at the level of the mitral annulus (not the mobile tips of the mitral valve leaflets), using the midesophageal four-chamber view for determination of the VTI_{MV}. Although the mitral valve orifice is elliptical, the assumption of a circular orifice is acceptable (5). The diameter of mitral annulus (D) should be measured from the base of the anterior to posterior leaflets during early to mid diastole, usually one frame after the leaflets begin to close following the initial opening:

$$CSA_{MV}\ (cm^2) = 0.785 \times D_{MV}\ /\ D_{MV}{}^2$$

The irregular semielliptical shape of the mitral valve orifice and the fluctuation in its size during diastole make SV measurement at this location less reliable than at the LVOT or AV (6).

DOPPLER MEASUREMENT OF PULMONARY-TO-SYSTEMIC FLOW RATIO (QP/QS) (FIG 26.12)

The ratio of pulmonic-to-systemic blood flow Qp/Qs usually indicates the magnitude of a shunt (e.g., atrial septal defect, ventricular septal defect [VSD], or patent pulmonary ductus arteriosus) and provides useful information for determining the need for or the timing of surgery. Qp/Qs can be calculated once the systemic SV (measured at the LVOT or AV) and pulmonic SV (measured at the PA or RVOT) have been determined (14):

$$Qp/Qs = SV_{PA}\ /SV_{LVOT}$$

Potential errors in the estimation of Qp/Qs are the same as for any Doppler determinations of SV. The possibility of compounding errors in the calculation of Qp/Qs with this formula should be kept in mind. For example, if SV_{PA} is overestimated and SV_{LVOT} is underestimated, then Qp/Qs may be significantly overestimated. This potential

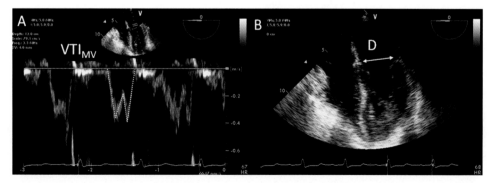

Figure 26.11. Transmitral Doppler SV Calculation. The diastolic VTI across the mitral valve (VTI_{MV}) is measured using pulsed wave Doppler with the sample volume placed within the mitral valve annulus using any midesophageal view of the mitral valve. **A:** VTI_{MV} measured in the midesophageal four-chamber view (ME 4C). **B:** The diameter (D) of mitral valve annulus is measured in ME 4C, from the base of the anterior and posterior leaflets during early to middiastole.

Qp/Qs

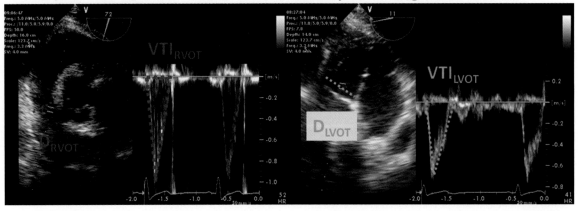

A. Deep TG RV long axis

B. Deep TG LV long axis

$$Qp = 0.785 \times D_{RVOT}^2 \times VTI_{RVOT} = 56 \text{ ml}$$ $$Qs = 0.785 \times D_{LVOT}^2 \times VTI_{LVOT} = 52 \text{ ml}$$

Figure 26.12. Qp/Qs Calculation. **A:** Pulmonary flow (Qp) is calculated using one of the RVOT views, here the transgastric mid short-axis (TG mid SAX) view of the LV. **B:** Systemic flow (Qs) is calculated using the deep TG LV long-axis (deep TG LAX) view. Diameters (D) and VTIs are measured at the same site. Here, Qp/Qs = 1.08, which is insignificant (no shunt).

propagation of errors will lead to a range in the confidence intervals for Qp/Qs, which is unacceptable to many clinicians using TEE. Furthermore, in the presence of significant AR Qp/Qs will be underestimated.

DOPPLER ASSESSMENT OF REGURGITATION

Regurgitant volume and fraction—Volumetric Method (Fig. 26.13)

Regurgitant volume (RV) is the volume of blood that flows backward through a regurgitant valve during one cardiac cycle. Conservation of mass dictates that SV deliv-

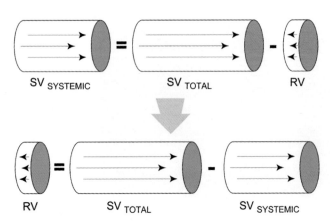

Figure 26.13. Volumetric method for calculation of RV. Conservation of mass dictates that RV must be equal to the difference between the total forward SV across the regurgitant valve (SV_{TOTAL}) and the systemically delivered SV ($SV_{SYSTEMIC}$).

ered to the systemic circulation ($SV_{SYSTEMIC}$) must equal the total forward SV across a regurgitant valve (SV_{TOTAL}) minus the RV:

$$SV_{SYSTEMIC} = SV_{TOTAL} - RV$$

Thus, RV can be calculated once SV_{TOTAL} and $SV_{SYSTEMIC}$ have been determined:

$$RV = SV_{TOTAL} - SV_{SYSTEMIC}$$

The regurgitant fraction (RF) for any valve is calculated as the ratio of RV to total forward flow across the regurgitant valve expressed as a percentage:

$$RF (\%) = (RV/SV_{TOTAL}) \times 100\%$$

Assessment of Mitral Regurgitation (Fig. 26.14)

In mitral regurgitation, the mitral inflow SV is SV_{TOTAL} and the LVOT SV is the $SV_{SYSTEMIC}$. The mitral valve RV is estimated by subtracting the LVOT SV from the mitral valve inflow SV (15):

$$RV_{MV} = SV_{MVI} - SV_{LVOT}$$
$$RF_{MV} (\%) = (RV_{MV}/SV_{MVI}) \times 100\%$$

This method of assessing mitral regurgitation is performed infrequently during TEE examinations as it is time consuming and there is a possibility of compounding errors while calculating Doppler SV, even more so for

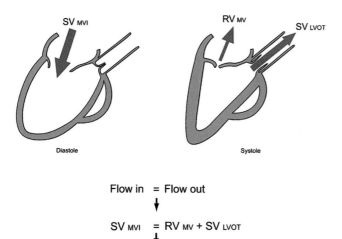

Flow in = Flow out

$$SV_{MVI} = RV_{MV} + SV_{LVOT}$$

$$RV_{MV} = SV_{MVI} - SV_{LVOT}$$

Figure 26.14. Assessment of Mitral RV using the Volumetric Method. Diastolic flow into the LV must equal forward systolic flow. Therefore, the mitral RV (RV_{MV}) must equal the difference between the mitral valve inflow SV (SV_{MVI}) and the LVOT SV (SV_{LVOT}).

the irregularly shaped mitral valve orifice (semielliptical) that fluctuates in size during diastole (6). Furthermore, this calculation is not accurate (and mitral RV will be underestimated) in the presence of significant AR, requiring an alternative site be used such as the RVOT.

Assessment of Aortic Regurgitation (Fig. 26.15)

In AR, SV_{TOTAL} is the LVOT forward SV and $SV_{SYSTEMIC}$ is the mitral valve inflow SV. Their difference, the aortic valve RV, can be estimated by subtracting the mitral valve

inflow SV from the LVOT forward SV. The aortic RF can be calculated subsequently (15):

$$RV_{AV} = SV_{LVOT} - SV_{MVI}$$

$$RF_{AV} \ (\%) = (RV_{AV}/SV_{LVOT}) \times 100\%$$

This method of assessing AR is also performed infrequently during TEE examinations due to the previously mentioned limitations. Furthermore, in the presence of significant mitral regurgitation, this calculation is not accurate, because the LV empties forward and backward, and aortic RV will be underestimated. In such cases, the RVOT should be used to estimate systemic SV.

Proximal Convergence Method

Blood flow accelerates as it approaches a narrow orifice (i.e., the regurgitant orifice in mitral regurgitation). The distribution of flow velocities takes on the form of multiple concentric shells that are shaped like hemispheres. All points on each hemispheric shell have the same velocity, hence the term proximal isovelocity surface area (PISA). Based on conservation of flow, the flow rate across each shell is the same as the flow rate across the narrow orifice (Fig. 26.16) (16,17). The closer to the orifice, the higher the velocity and the smaller the shell surface area. These isovelocity shells can be visualized with color flow imaging by adjusting the Nyquist limit. The aliasing velocity on the color flow map represents the instantaneous blood velocity or PISA of the displayed shell (Fig. 26.17). With mitral regurgitation, the regurgitant blood travels from the LV through the regurgitant mitral orifice into the left atrium (LA) in a direction toward the TEE transducer. As

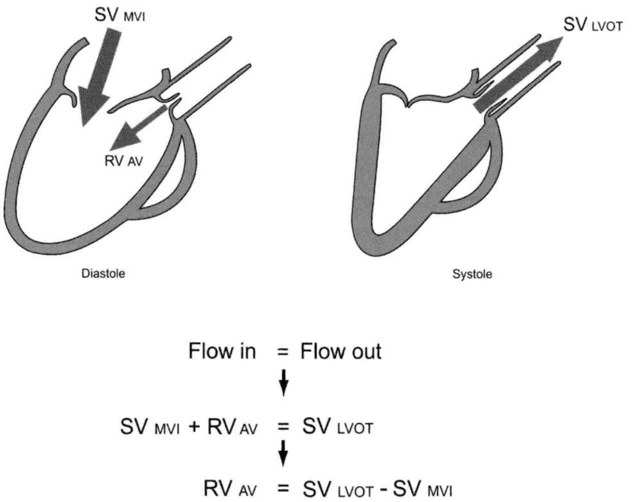

Flow in = Flow out

$$SV_{MVI} + RV_{AV} = SV_{LVOT}$$

$$RV_{AV} = SV_{LVOT} - SV_{MVI}$$

Figure 26.15. Assessment of Aortic RV Using the Volumetric Method. Diastolic flow into the LV must equal systolic flow out. Therefore, the aortic RV (RV_{AV}) must be equal to the difference between the LVOT SV (SV_{LVOT}) and the mitral valve inflow SV (SV_{MVI}).

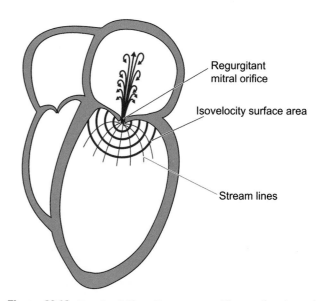

Figure 26.16. Proximal Flow Convergence. The acceleration of blood from within a large chamber toward a small orifice results in the formation of multiple concentric "isovelocity" shells with decreasing radius. In mitral regurgitation, these isovelocity shells occur in the LV.

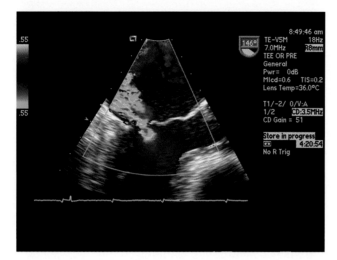

Figure 26.17. PISA by color flow imaging. These PISAs can be demonstrated with Doppler color flow imaging within the LV in the setting of mitral regurgitation.

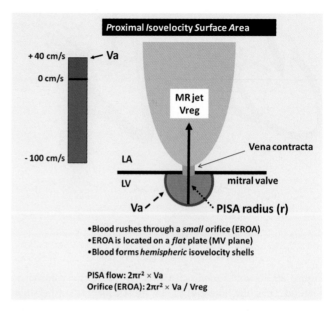

Figure 26.18. Proximal flow Convergence Method for Calculating EROA in Mitral Regurgitation (MR). Conservation of mass dictates that the PISA flow rate must equal the regurgitant flow rate across the mitral EROA. Va is the PISA velocity as imaged by shifting the color scale baseline upward (lowering the Nyquist limit in the direction of MR jet) and r is the PISA radius.

the positive aliasing velocity is reduced (e.g., from 70 to 40 cm/s) by shifting the baseline velocity upward, the transition from blue to red in the outermost PISA shell will occur farther from the regurgitant orifice resulting in a hemispheric shell with a larger radius (r). The instantaneous flow rate through a *hemispheric* PISA is equal to the product of the area of the PISA and the instantaneous velocity of blood at the PISA:

$$\text{PISA flow rate (mL/min)} = \text{PISA area (cm}^2)$$
$$\times \text{ blood velocity at PISA (cm/s)}$$

$$\text{PISA flow rate} = 2\pi \times r^2 \times \text{aliasing velocity}$$

$$\text{PISA flow rate} = 6.28 \times r^2 \times \text{aliasing velocity}$$

Since the flow rate across each of these isovelocity shells equals the flow rate through the regurgitant orifice, the PISA flow rate can be calculated as the product of the effective regurgitant orifice area (EROA) and the instantaneous regurgitant velocity (Fig. 26.18):

$$\text{PISA flow rate} = \text{regurgitant flow rate}$$

$$\text{PISA flow rate (mL/min)}$$
$$= \text{EROA (cm}^2) \times \text{regurgitant velocity (cm/s)}$$

The EROA is therefore calculated as the greatest PISA flow rate divided by the peak regurgitant velocity:

$$\text{EROA} = \text{PISA flow rate/regurgitant velocity}$$

$$\text{EROA (cm}^2) = (6.28 \times r^2 \times \text{aliasing velocity})/V_{RJ}$$

where r is in cm and the aliasing velocity and peak regurgitant jet velocity (peak V_{RJ}) are in cm/s.

The PISA approach is also useful to calculate RV. Just as forward SV is equal to the product of CSA and the forward

flow VTI, RV is equal to the product of EROA and VTI of the regurgitant jet (VTI_{RJ}):

$$\text{RV} = \text{EROA} \times \text{VTI}_{RJ}$$
$$= (6.28 \times r^2 \times \text{aliasing velocity}/V_{RJ}) \times \text{VTI}_{RJ}$$

As seen in this example for mitral regurgitation, the calculation of RV using the flow convergence method is dependent on obtaining four measurements (Fig. 26.19): the PISA radius and the aliasing velocity (using color-flow Doppler on the ventricular side of the mitral valve), and the peak velocity and VTI of the mitral regurgitant (MR) jet (using continuous wave Doppler on the LA aspect of the mitral valve).

The proximal convergence method (PISA) has been validated for assessing mitral regurgitation in many experimental and clinical studies (18,19). Advantages of the PISA method over other volumetric methods include the ability to make all necessary measurements from a single imaging window and the fact that flow rate is measured directly (not requiring the subtraction of one large quantity from another). Nevertheless, there are four potentially significant limitations to the proximal flow convergence method.

First, as the regurgitant orifice is not infinitely small, the hemispheric shape of a PISA is not maintained all the way to the orifice. Thus, the use of the standard formula may underestimate flow (20). Second, flow may be constrained by structures proximal to the regurgitant orifice such that the PISA is not a full hemisphere. Such a constraint results in flow overestimation if the standard formula is used. Most of this overestimation can be corrected

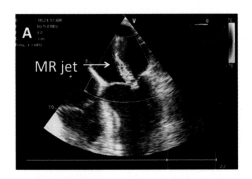

Va = 40 cm/s
r = 0.43 cm
V_{MR} = 5 m/s
VTI_{MR} = 170 cm

PISA flow = 46 cm³/s
EROA = PISA flow / MR vel
　　　 = 46 / 500 cm²
　　　 = 0.09 cm²
RV = 16 ml

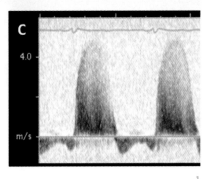

Figure 26.19. Data Necessary for Calculation of Mitral RV using the PISA Method. **A:** The MR jet is visualized using color Doppler imaging. **B:** After appropriate baseline shifting (upward, toward the direction of regurgitant blood), the PISA radius is measured from a cine-loop of the MR jet frozen during midsystole and the aliasing velocity noted. **C:** The peak velocity and VTI of the MR jet are measured from a continuous wave Doppler velocity tracing.

by incorporation of a funnel angle to better calculate the shape of the PISA (see the section "Continuity Equation" and Fig. 26.24) (21). Third, while it is generally easy to identify where the color Doppler changes from blue to red, it is often difficult to locate the exact center of the regurgitant orifice used to identify the origin of the PISA radius (22). As the radius is squared in the proximal flow convergence formula, a 10% error in radius measurement may lead to a 20% error in calculated flow rate and regurgitant orifice area. Fourth, the degree of regurgitation is not constant throughout systole in many patients, and determining regurgitant severity based on the maximal regurgitant orifice area may overestimate the actual hemodynamic impact of the regurgitant lesion (23). Color M-mode can help in verifying that PISA is holosystolic and in measuring the radius accurately. In spite of these limitations, the flow convergence method is a quantitative, relatively simple to perform method, applicable in a large number of patients with valvular regurgitation.

Simplified Proximal Convergence Method

A simplified proximal convergence method has been developed for estimating MR orifice area with only one measurement (24), based on the assumption that the pressure difference between the LV and LA is 100 mm Hg during systole (corresponding to a 5 m/s MR jet). With this assumption, if the aliasing velocity is set to *approximately* 40 cm/s and the radius of the nearest PISA (r) is measured, then the mitral EROA can be estimated as follows:

$$\text{EROA (cm}^2) = (6.28 \times r^2 \times 40)/500 = 0.5 \times r^2$$

$$\text{EROA} = r^2/2$$

In most instances, the results using the simplified method are similar to those determined using the standard proximal flow convergence method. Obviously, the error created by using the simplified method will increase as the pressure difference between the LV and LA differs from 100 mm Hg. Nevertheless, this error should not exceed 20% to 25% as long as the pressure difference between the LV and LA ranges between 64 and 144 mm Hg (corresponding to 4 and 6 m/s, respectively).

DOPPLER MEASUREMENT OF PRESSURE GRADIENTS

Blood flow velocities, measured using the Doppler principle, are used to assess the pressure gradient across an orifice (25,26).

The Bernoulli equation describes the relationship between the increase in the velocity of a fluid (i.e., blood) across an orifice (i.e., a stenotic valve) and the pressure gradient across that orifice (Fig. 26.20):

$$\Delta P = P_2 - P_1 = \frac{1}{2} \rho(V_2^2 - V_1^2) + \rho(dV/dt)ds + R(v)$$

where the first term describes convective acceleration (ρ = the density of the fluid, V_1 = the peak velocity of fluid proximal to the narrowed orifice, and V_2 = the peak velocity of fluid through the narrowed orifice), the second term describes flow acceleration, and the third term describes viscous friction.

Since pressure gradients are most often determined at peak flow, the effects of flow acceleration can be ignored. Furthermore, the effects of viscous friction are only

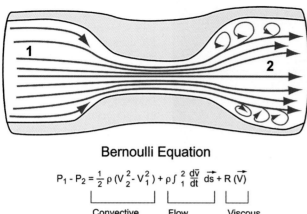

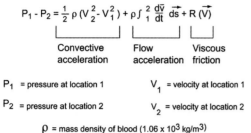

Bernoulli Equation

$$P_1 - P_2 = \frac{1}{2}\rho\,(V_2^2 - V_1^2) + \rho\int_1^2 \frac{d\vec{v}}{dt}\,\overrightarrow{ds} + R\,(\vec{V})$$

| Convective acceleration | Flow acceleration | Viscous friction |

P_1 = pressure at location 1 V_1 = velocity at location 1

P_2 = pressure at location 2 V_2 = velocity at location 2

ρ = mass density of blood (1.06×10^3 kg/m³)

Figure 26.20. The Bernoulli Equation. The Bernoulli equation describes the relationship between the increase in the velocity of a fluid across a narrowed orifice and the pressure gradient across that narrowed orifice.

significant in orifices with an area less than 0.25 cm² (27). Thus, in clinical echocardiography, the Bernoulli equation can be simplified by ignoring the effects of flow acceleration and viscous friction:

$$\Delta P = \frac{1}{2}\rho(V_2^2 - V_1^2)$$

Furthermore, since the distal blood flow velocity (V_2) is substantially greater than the proximal blood flow velocity (V_1) for most clinically significant lesions, the difference $V_2^2 - V_1^2$ can be approximated by V_2^2 alone. Thus, assuming the density of blood to be 1.06×10^3 kg/m³, the Bernoulli equation can be simplified even further:

$$\Delta P = 4V_2^2$$

where ΔP is the pressure gradient across the orifice in mm Hg and V_2 is the peak blood flow velocity across the orifice in m/s. The simplified Bernoulli equation is applicable to almost all pressure gradient calculations in clinical echocardiography except those circumstances where the simplifying assumptions are invalid. For example, in the setting of aortic stenosis and significant LVOT obstruction, the simplified Bernoulli equation would overestimate the AV pressure gradient because V_2^2 would overestimate $V_2^2 - V_1^2$.

Doppler echocardiography measures *instantaneous* blood flow velocities, and the simplified Bernoulli equation calculates *instantaneous* pressure gradients. The maximum instantaneous pressure gradient is, therefore, always associated with the maximum Doppler velocity. The mean pressure gradient is obtained by manually

tracing the Doppler-derived velocities over the entire flow period allowing the analysis package to calculate the mean pressure gradient (Fig. 26.21). Assuming the Doppler sample volume or beam is positioned correctly, both maximum and mean pressure gradients can be determined from low-velocity jets with either pulsed wave or continuous wave Doppler velocity signals using the calculation package built in the echocardiographic system. However, pulsed wave Doppler cannot reliably measure velocity ≥ 1.4 m/s. Consequently, it is common practice to use continuous wave Doppler when determining maximum and mean valvular pressure gradients, while keeping in mind that erroneous assumptions will be reached if the wrong flow signal is interrogated (i.e., in the case of coexisting LVOT obstruction and aortic stenosis).

The Doppler beam is positioned to interrogate the highest velocity jet; otherwise, the pressure gradient may be significantly underestimated. This is of most concern when measuring high-velocity jets due to valve stenosis or regurgitation. Often small adjustments in the TEE probe transducer position and the Doppler beam are necessary

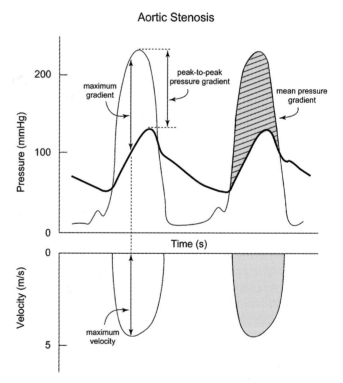

Figure 26.21. Maximum and Mean Pressure Gradients. As seen in this diagram of LV and systemic arterial pressure tracings (**top**) and the Doppler velocity spectrum (**bottom**) in aortic stenosis, the maximum instantaneous pressure gradient corresponds to the maximum Doppler velocity. The maximum AV instantaneous pressure gradient determined by Doppler is greater than the peak-to-peak hemodynamic gradient sometimes reported following cardiac catheterization. However, the mean pressure gradient determined by Doppler, the average of Doppler pressure gradients over the entire flow period (see *shaded area*), correlates well with the mean gradient determined by cardiac catheterization (see *hatched area*).

to obtain the highest-velocity signal. It is advisable to interrogate from multiple windows when possible so that the interrogating Doppler beam is aligned parallel with the blood flow of interest. Accuracy is improved by assessing multiple Doppler flow profiles, typically 3 to 5 for a regular rhythm and up to 10 for an irregular rhythm. Many studies have shown an excellent correlation with Doppler-derived pressure gradients using TEE and catheter-derived pressure gradients across mitral valve stenosis, various prosthetic valves, LVOT obstruction, and RVOT obstruction (2–4,28,29). Other times, TEE may be superior, as when determining the diastolic transmitral pressure gradient in mitral stenosis. The transmitral pressure gradient may be overestimated by cardiac catheterization if pulmonary capillary wedge pressure is used instead of direct left atrial pressure (LAP) measurement (30).

DOPPLER DETERMINATION OF VALVE AREA

Continuity Equation (Fig. 26.22)

The continuity equation is an expression of the principle of conservation of mass, which is most simply expressed as "flow in" equals "flow out". More specifically, the continuity equation states that stroke volume (SV_2) across a stenotic orifice is equal to the stroke volume (SV_1) proximal to the lesion. Thus, using the Doppler formula for SV, the area of a stenotic valve (CSA_2) can be calculated as follows:

$$SV_2 = SV_1$$
$$CSA_2 \times VTI_2 = CSA_1 \times VTI_1$$
$$CSA_2 = CSA_1 \times (VTI_1/VTI_2)$$

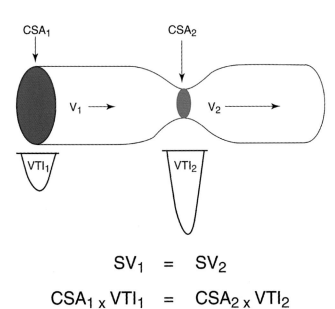

$$SV_1 = SV_2$$
$$CSA_1 \times VTI_1 = CSA_2 \times VTI_2$$

Figure 26.22. The Continuity Equation. SV proximal to a stenosis (SV_1) must equal SV across a stenosis (SV_2).

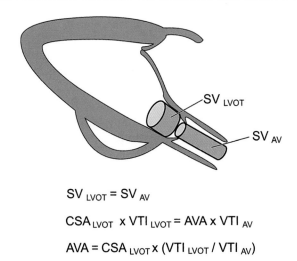

$$SV_{LVOT} = SV_{AV}$$
$$CSA_{LVOT} \times VTI_{LVOT} = AVA \times VTI_{AV}$$
$$AVA = CSA_{LVOT} \times (VTI_{LVOT} / VTI_{AV})$$

Figure 26.23. The Continuity Equation in Aortic Stenosis. SV across the LVOT must equal SV across the AV. VTI, velocity time integral.

The continuity equation is used in echocardiography to determine the area of a stenotic valve (i.e., aortic valve area [AVA] in aortic stenosis) or the EROA (i.e., in mitral regurgitation).

Continuity Equation in Aortic Stenosis (Fig. 26.23)

In aortic stenosis, SV across the AV must equal the SV across the LVOT. Thus, AVA may be calculated using the continuity equation as follows, with either TEE or multiplane TEE (31,32):

$$AVA = CSA_{LVOT} \times (VTI_{LVOT}/VTI_{AV})$$
$$AVA\,(cm^2) = 0.785 \times D_{LVOT}{}^2 \times (VTI_{LVOT}/VTI_{AV})$$

where D_{LVOT} (cm) is the LVOT diameter, VTI_{LVOT} (cm) is measured using pulsed wave Doppler, and VTI_{AV} (cm) is measured using continuous wave Doppler. Because the shapes of the VTI_{LVOT} and VTI_{AV} Doppler profiles are similar in aortic stenosis, the ratio of the maximum velocities (V_{LVOT}/V_{AV}) may be substituted for the ratio of the VTIs (VTI_{LVOT}/VTI_{AV}) without introducing significant error into the AVA calculation:

$$AVA\,(cm^2) = 0.785 \times D_{LVOT}{}^2 \times (V_{LVOT}/V_{AV})$$

The primary concern in determining AVA with the continuity equation using TEE is related to the possible underestimation of VTIs (or peak velocities) in the LVOT and/or AV due to suboptimal beam alignment.

Continuity Equation in Mitral Regurgitation (the Flow Convergence Method)

In mitral regurgitation, flow across the regurgitant mitral orifice (CSA_2) must equal flow at a PISA (CSA_1). The EROA for mitral regurgitation may be calculated using the continuity equation (as seen earlier in the section on the flow convergence method for calculation of RV) (16). This same technique has been used to quantify left-to-right atrial shunting after balloon mitral commissurotomy using TEE (33).

Continuity Equation in Mitral Stenosis (the Flow Convergence Method)

In mitral stenosis, flow at a PISA (CSA_1) must equal flow across the stenotic mitral valve orifice (CSA_2). Thus, the mitral valve area (MVA) may be calculated using the PISA method, as mentioned above in the mitral regurgitation section. As the PISA proximal to a stenotic mitral valve is most often not a full hemisphere, an angle correction factor is usually necessary (Fig. 26.24). The MVA is, thus, given by the following equation where r is the PISA radius, V_{MS} is the peak velocity of the mitral stenosis jet, and α is the angle between the mitral leaflets (17):

$$MVA(cm^2) = 6.28 \times r^2 \times (aliasing\ velocity/V_{MS}) \times (\alpha°/180°)$$

where r is in centimeters and the aliasing velocity and peak mitral stenosis jet velocity (V_{MS}) are in cm/s.

Pressure Half-time

The rate of decline in the pressure gradient across a diseased valve is related to the severity of the valvular abnormality (34). With valvular stenosis, a slower rate of decline indicates more severe stenosis (Fig. 26.25), whereas with valvular regurgitation a faster rate of decline indicates more severe regurgitation (Fig. 26.26). This rate of decline

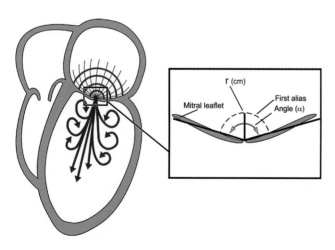

$$PISA = \frac{\alpha}{180} \times hemispheric\ area$$

Figure 26.24. PISA Correction in Mitral Stenosis. PISA is not a full hemisphere, and an angle correction is necessary to calculate MVA in mitral stenosis. r, PISA radius; α, angle between mitral valve leaflets.

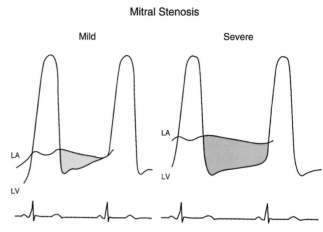

Figure 26.25. Rate of Pressure Decline Across a Stenotic Valve. In mitral stenosis, a slower rate of pressure decline indicates more severe stenosis.

in the pressure gradient across a valve can be described by the pressure half-time (PHT).

The PHT is defined as the time required for the peak pressure gradient to decline by 50% (Fig. 26.27) (35). Due to the fixed relationship between velocity and pressure gradient, the PHT will also be equal to the time required for the peak Doppler velocity to decline to a value of peak velocity/$\sqrt{2}$ (36,37). Furthermore, PHT is also proportional to the deceleration time (DT), which is defined as the time required for the deceleration slope to reach the zero velocity baseline (Fig. 26.28):

$$PHT\ (ms) = 0.29 \times DT\ (ms)$$

PHT is commonly used to estimate the MVA of stenotic native mitral valves using an empirically determined constant of 220 (36,38):

$$MVA\ (cm^2) = 220/PHT\ (ms)$$

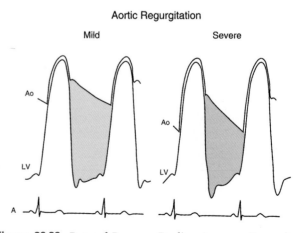

Figure 26.26. Rate of Pressure Decline Across a Regurgitant Valve. In AR, a faster rate of pressure decline indicates more severe regurgitation.

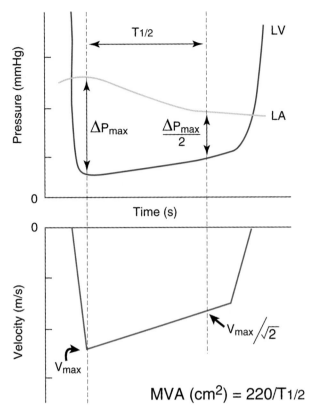

Figure 26.27. The PHT in Mitral Stenosis. The PHT is the time interval required for the pressure gradient to drop by half. On the Doppler velocity curve, it is the time interval required for the maximum velocity to drop to the maximum velocity/ $\sqrt{2}$. T1/2, pressure half-time; P, pressure; v, peak velocity.

$$MVA \ (cm^2) = 220/T_{1/2}$$

PHT is affected not only by MVA but also by the characteristics of the receiving chamber (LV for mitral stenosis). Impaired LV relaxation prolongs PHT (and may underestimate MVA), while concomitant AR or decreased LV compliance elevates LV diastolic pressure, decreases the diastolic transmitral pressure gradient, and shortens PHT (and may overestimate MVA). For the same reasons, PHT cannot be used for estimating the area of a normal mitral valve, as it is more dependent on LV compliance than valve area (39). The profile of the mitral inflow E wave is altered during atrioventricular block, making PHT an unreliable estimate of MVA. Following mitral valvuloplasty, the compliances of the LA and LV may be altered for several days, making the PHT method unreliable. Furthermore, PHT overestimates the area of normal prosthetic mitral valves.

Another common application of PHT is for the assessment of AR (40). The PHT of the AR Doppler velocity signal is significantly shorter (<250 ms) with severe AR due to the rapid equilibration of arterial diastolic pressure and LV diastolic pressure (41,42). It should be noted that PHT in AR is also dependent on LV size and compliance. The same aortic RV will result in a shorter PHT in acute AR compared to chronic AR due to the smaller size and lower compliance of the LV. The PHT will also be shortened by an increased systemic vascular resistance, which may lead to an overestimation of the severity of AR (43). Finally, in the presence of mitral regurgitation, PHT is unreliable in estimating the severity of AR.

DOPPLER DETERMINATION OF INTRACARDIAC PRESSURES

Estimation of intracardiac, PA, and aortic pressures can be estimated by combining a pressure gradient calculated by the Bernoulli equation, with a known or estimated pressure from a proximal or distal chamber (Table 26.3).

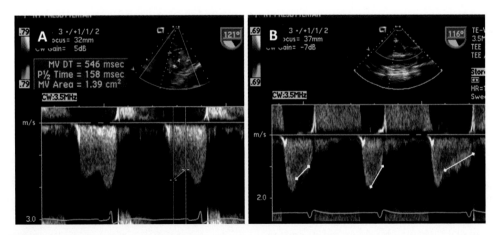

Figure 26.28. Deceleration Time. The DT is the time interval required for the doppler velocity curve to reach the zero baseline. **A:** The DT (as well as PHT) is measured using continuous wave Doppler from any midesophageal view of the mitral valve. **B:** When the slope is not a straight line, DT is measured from the longest slope. In irregular R-R intervals (i.e., atrial fibrillation), the measurement is performed from at least three to five beats and the average value is calculated.

TABLE 26.3	Estimation of Pulmonary and Intracardiac Pressures

Pressure	Equation
RVSP or PASP	(1) $RVSP = 4(v_{TR})^2 + RAP$
RVSP or PASP	(2) $RVSP = SBP - 4(v_{VSD})^2$
MPAP	(3) $MPAP = 4(v_{peakPR})^2 + RAP$
PADP	(4) $PADP = 4(v_{end\text{-}diastolic\ PR})^2 + RAP$
LAP	(5) $LAP = SBP - 4(v_{MR})^2$
LVEDP	(6) $LVEDP = DBP - 4(v_{end\text{-}diastolic\ AR})^2$
RAP	(7) $LAP = 4(V_{ASD}[or\ PFO])^2 + RAP$

Equations (1) and (2) are invalid in the presence of pulmonic stenosis or RVOT obstruction. Equations (2) and (5) are invalid in the presence of aortic stenosis or LVOT obstruction.
RVSP, right ventricular systolic pressure; PASP, pulmonary artery systolic pressure; MPAP, mean pulmonary artery pressure; PADP, pulmonary artery diastolic pressure; LAP, left atrial pressure; RAP, right atrial pressure; LVEDP, left ventricular end-diastolic pressure; v, peak velocity; TR, tricuspid regurgitation; PR, pulmonic regurgitation; MR, mitral regurgitation; AR, aortic regurgitation; SBP, systolic blood pressure; DBP, diastolic blood pressure; RVOT, right ventricular outflow tract; LVOT, left ventricular outflow tract; ASD, atrial septal defect; PFO, patent foramen ovale.

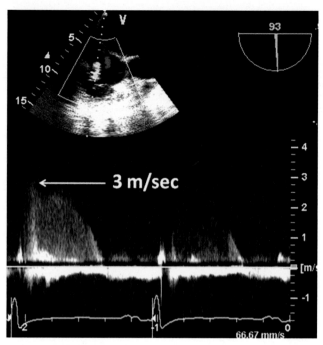

Figure 26.29. Measurement of TR Jet Velocity for Estimation of RVSP or PASP. The peak TR jet velocity can be obtained with continuous wave Doppler using TEE from the midesophageal four-chamber view, the midesophageal RV inflow-outflow view, or as seen in this example of a patient with pulmonary hypertension in a modified midesophageal bicaval view.

Estimation of RVSP (Fig. 26.29)

The right ventricular systolic pressure (RVSP) can be estimated by adding a known or estimated right atrial pressure (RAP) to the calculated RA-RV pressure gradient (44,45).

$$RVSP = \text{trans-tricuspid valve systolic gradient} + \text{RA pressure}$$

$$RVSP\ (mm\ Hg) = 4(v_{TR})^2 + RAP\ (mm\ Hg)$$

where the peak tricuspid regurgitant (TR) jet velocity (v_{TR}) is given in m/s.

The peak velocity of the TR jet is used to calculate the systolic pressure difference between the RV and RA using the simplified Bernoulli equation (46). The peak TR jet velocity can be obtained with continuous wave Doppler, from either the midesophageal RV inflow-outflow view, a modified midesophageal bicaval view, or the midesophageal four-chamber view.

If a direct measurement of RAP (or central venous pressure) is not available, it may be estimated in spontaneously breathing patients as seen in Table 26.4.

In patients with a VSD and a left-to-right shunt, the RVSP may be calculated by subtracting the LV-RV pressure difference from the systolic blood pressure, which is

a good estimate of left ventricular systolic pressure (LVSP) in most patients:

$$RVSP = \text{LV systolic pressure} - \text{VSD systolic gradient}$$

$$RVSP\ (mm\ Hg) = \text{systolic blood pressure}\ (mm\ Hg) - 4(V_{VSD})^2$$

where the peak velocity across the VSD (V_{VSD}) is given in m/s. In the presence of aortic stenosis or LVOT obstruction,

TABLE 26.4	Estimation of RAP		
Inferior Vena Cava Diameter	**Change with Negative Inspiration (i.e., sniff)**	**Estimated RAP (mm Hg)**	
Small (<1.5 cm)	Collapse	0–5	
Normal (1.5–2.5 cm)	Decrease by >50%	5–10	
Normal (1.5–2.5 cm)	Decrease by <50%	10–15	
Dilated (>2.5 cm)	Decrease by <50%	15–20	
Dilated (with dilated hepatic veins)	No change	>20	

systolic blood pressure will underestimate LVSP, and this formula is invalid.

Estimation of PASP

In the absence of pulmonic stenosis or RVOT obstruction, RVSP and pulmonary artery systolic pressure (PASP) are essentially identical, and PASP can be estimated using the RVSP formula (46):

$$PASP \text{ (mm Hg)} = RVSP \text{ (mm Hg)}$$
$$= 4(V_{TR})^2 + RAP \text{ (mm Hg)}$$

where the peak TR jet velocity (V_{TR}) is given in m/s.

Estimation of PADP (Fig. 26.30)

The late peak velocity of the pulmonic regurgitant (PR) jet can be used to calculate the diastolic pressure difference between the PA and RV at end-diastole using the simplified Bernoulli equation. The late peak PR jet velocity is obtained with continuous wave Doppler using multiplane TEE from a transgastric RV inflow-outflow view with the transducer rotated from 110 to 150 degrees and the probe turned to the left. Alternatively, it can be obtained from an upper esophageal short-axis view of the aortic arch or ascending aorta if the PR jet is visualized adequately. The pulmonary artery diastolic pressure (PADP) is estimated by adding a known or estimated RA pressure, which is assumed to be equal to RV diastolic pressure, to the calculated PA-RV pressure gradient during late diastole (47):

$$PADP = \text{trans-pulmonic late diastolic gradient}$$
$$+ RV \text{ diastolic pressure}$$
$$PADP \text{ (mm Hg)} = 4(V_{late\,PR})^2 + RAP \text{ (mm Hg)}$$

where the late peak velocity of the PR ($V_{late\,PR}$) is given in m/s.

Estimation of MPAP

The early peak velocity of the PR jet can be used to calculate the pressure difference between PA and RV in early diastole using the simplified Bernoulli equation. The early peak PR jet velocity is obtained as described in the prior section. The mean pulmonary artery pressure (MPAP) can be estimated by adding a known or estimated RA pressure, which approximates RV pressure during diastole, to the calculated PA-RV pressure gradient during early diastole (47):

$$MPAP = \text{trans-pulmonic early diastolic gradient}$$
$$+ RV \text{ diastolic pressure}$$
$$MPAP \text{ (mm Hg)} = 4(V_{peak\,PR})^2 + RAP \text{ (mm Hg)}$$

where the early peak velocity of the PR jet ($V_{early\,PR}$) is given in m/s.

Estimation of LAP (Fig. 26.31)

The peak velocity of the MR jet can be used to calculate the pressure difference between the LA and LV using the simplified Bernoulli equation. The peak MR jet velocity is obtained with continuous wave Doppler by TEE from

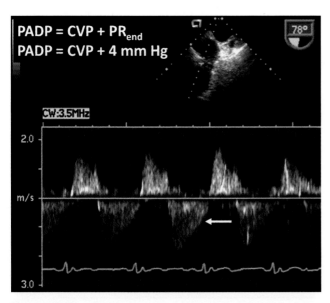

Figure 26.30. Estimation of PADP from the End-diastolic Velocity of the Pulmonic Regurgitation (PR) Jet. In the upper esophageal aortic arch short-axis view, the spectral display of PR is recorded with continuous wave Doppler. The late diastolic velocity (*arrow*) corresponds to the pressure gradient between the PA (in this example, ~4 mm Hg) and RV (the latter is approximated by the central venous pressure, CVP).

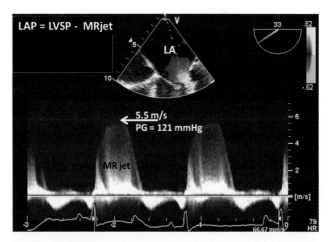

Figure 26.31. Measurement of Mitral Regurgitation (MR) Jet for Estimation of LAP. The peak MR jet velocity (*arrow*) is displayed with continuous wave Doppler in any of the midesophageal views of the mitral valve (here, midesophageal four-chamber view). LVSP, approximated by systolic arterial pressure (in the absence of aortic stenosis).

any midesophageal view of the mitral valve. The LAP can be estimated by subtracting the LA-LV pressure gradient from the LVSP (48,49):

$$LAP = LV \text{ systolic pressure} - \text{trans-mitral systolic gradient}$$

$$LAP \text{ (mm Hg)} = \text{systolic blood pressure (mm Hg)} - 4(V_{MR})^2$$

where the peak velocity of the MR (V_{MR}) is given in m/s. In the presence of aortic stenosis or LVOT obstruction, systolic blood pressure will underestimate LVSP and this formula is invalid.

Estimation of LVEDP (Fig. 26.32)

The peak end-diastolic velocity of the AR jet can be used to calculate the difference between the diastolic aortic pressure and the left ventricular end-diastolic pressure (LVEDP) using the simplified Bernoulli equation. The peak end-diastolic velocity of the AR jet is determined with the continuous wave Doppler beam placed through the AV from a transgastric long-axis or deep transgastric long-axis view. The LVEDP is estimated by subtracting the end-diastolic aortic-to-LV pressure gradient from the aortic diastolic pressure (49):

$$LVEDP = \text{aortic diastolic pressure} - \text{end-diastolic trans-aortic pressure gradient}$$

$$LVEDP \text{ (mm Hg)} = \text{diastolic blood pressure (mm Hg)} - 4(V_{end\,AR})^2$$

where the peak end-diastolic velocity of the AR jet ($V_{end\,AR}$) is given in m/s.

DOPPLER MEASUREMENT OF dp/dt

The rate of pressure increase within the LV during isovolumic contraction, LV dp/dt, is a measure of LV systolic function. As LAP does not change significantly during isovolumic contraction, changes in the velocity of the MR jet reflect changes in LV pressure. Thus, a continuous-wave Doppler interrogation of the MR jet can be used to determine LV dp/dt. LV dp/dt is calculated from the time interval between 1 and 3 m/s on the MR Doppler velocity profile using the simplified Bernoulli equation (Fig. 26.33). The following formula is used to calculate LV dp/dt:

$$LV \, dp/dt = [4 \times (3 \text{ m/s})^2 - 4 \times (1 \text{ m/s})^2]/dt$$

$$LV \, dp/dt = [36 - 4 \text{ mm Hg}]/dt$$

$$LV \, dp/dt = 32 \text{ mm Hg}/dt$$

where dt is the time interval in seconds for the MR jet velocity to increase from 1 to 3 m/s. Thus, a longer time interval indicates a reduced LV dp/dt and reduced systolic function. LV dp/dt is normally ≥ 1,200 mm Hg/s with

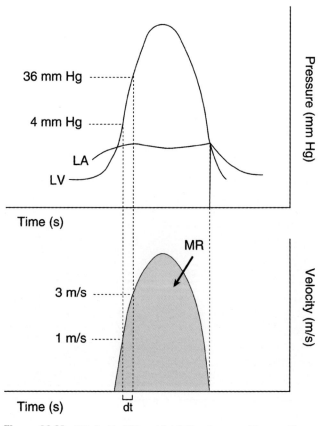

Figure 26.33. LV dp/dt. LV and LAP Tracings are Shown Along with the Corresponding Doppler Velocity Tracing for Mitral Regurgitation (as from a midesophageal view). dp/dt is calculated from the time interval it takes the MR jet to increase from 1 to 3 m/s. dp/dt, rate of pressure increase (in the LV) during isovolumic contraction.

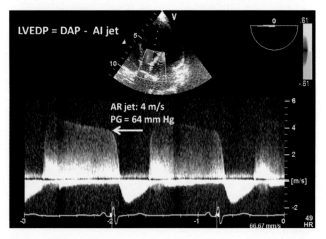

Figure 26.32. Measurement of the Late Peak Velocity of the Aortic Regurgitation (AI) Jet for Estimation of LVEDP. The peak end-diastolic velocity of the AI jet (*arrow*) is determined with the continuous wave Doppler beam placed through the AV from a transgastric long-axis or deep transgastric long-axis view (as in here). DAP, diastolic arterial pressure.

values less than 1,000 mm Hg/s corresponding to reduced LV systolic function. Doppler-derived LV dp/dt correlates well with catheter-derived LV dp/dt (50,51). Postoperative LV systolic function has been correlated with preoperative LV dp/dt in patients undergoing mitral valve surgery (52).

RV dp/dt can also be calculated from a continuous wave Doppler interrogation of the TR jet; however, the following formula is used:

$$RV\ dp/dt = [4 \times (2\ m/s)^2 - 4 \times (1\ m/s)^2]/dt$$

$$RV\ dp/dt = [16 - 4\ mm\ Hg]/dt$$

$$RV\ dp/dt = 12\ mm\ Hg/dt$$

where dt is the time interval in seconds for the MR jet to increase from 1 to 2 m/s.

KEY POINTS

- Doppler-derived measurements of blood flow velocities are the basis for quantitative estimation of hemodynamic parameters. Errors in measurement often can be attributed to poor alignment of the Doppler beam with blood flow or interrogation of neighboring blood flow.
- SV is calculated by obtaining the Doppler VTI and CSA from locations such as the LVOT and RVOT:

$$SV = CSA \times VTI$$

- Doppler-derived SVs can be used to determine CO, the pulmonary-to-systemic shunt ratio (Qp/Qs), and regurgitation volume.
- The proximal flow convergence method is used to determine regurgitant severity by calculation of the EROA:

$$EROA = (6.28 \times r^2 \times aliasing\ velocity)/V_{RJ}$$

- The flow convergence method is useful in evaluating regurgitation as it is quantitative, relatively simple to perform, and applicable in a large number of patients with valvular regurgitation.
- The continuity equation is useful for calculating AVA as flow through the LVOT must equal flow through the AV:

$$AVA = CSA_{LVOT} \times (VTI_{LVOT}/VTI_{AV})$$

- In valvular stenosis, a longer PHT indicates more severe stenosis, whereas with valvular regurgitation a shorter PHT indicates more severe regurgitation. The PHT can be used to estimate the MVA

of a stenotic native mitral valve using the following empirically derived formula:

$$MVA\ (cm^2) = 220/PHT\ (ms)$$

- Estimation of an intracardiac chamber and PA pressures is possible by combining a pressure gradient calculated from a Doppler velocity using the simplified Bernoulli equation with a known or estimated pressure from a proximal or distal chamber. Example:

$$RVSP\ (mm\ Hg) = 4(v_{TR})^2 + RAP\ (mm\ Hg)$$

REFERENCES

1. Callahan MJ, Tajik AJ, Su-Fan Q, et al. Validation of instantaneous pressure gradients measured by continuous wave Doppler in experimentally induced aortic stenosis. *Am J Cardiol* 1985;56:989–993.
2. Currie PJ, Seward JB, Chan KL. Continuous wave Doppler determination of right ventricular pressure: a simultaneous Doppler-catheterization study in 127 patients. *J Am Coll Cardiol* 1985;6:750–756.
3. Currie PJ, Hagler DJ, Seward JB, et al. Instantaneous pressure gradient: a simultaneous Doppler and dual catheter correlative study. *J Am Coll Cardiol* 1986;7:800–806.
4. Burstow DJ, Nishimura RA, Bailey KR, et al. Continuous wave Doppler echocardiographic measurement of prosthetic valve gradients: a simultaneous Doppler-catheter correlative study. *Circulation* 1989;80:504–514.
5. Quinones MA, Otto CM, Stoddard M, et al. Recommendations for the quantification of Doppler echocardiography: a report from the Doppler Quantification Task Force of the Nomenclature and Standards Committee of the American Society of Echocardiography. *J Am Soc Echocardiogr* 2002;15:167–184.
6. Stewart WJ, Jiang L, Mich R, et al. Variable effects of changes in flow rate through the aortic, pulmonary, and mitral valves on valve area and flow velocity; impact on quantitative Doppler flow calculations. *J Am Coll Cardiol* 1985; 6:653–662.
7. Zoghbi WA, Quinones MA. Determination of cardiac output by Doppler echocardiography: a critical appraisal. *Herz* 1986;11:258–268.
8. Savino JS, Troianos CA, Aukburg S, et al. Measurements of pulmonary blood flow with transesophageal two-dimensional and Doppler echocardiography. *Anesthesiology* 1991; 75: 445–451.
9. Muhiuden IA, Kuecherer HF, Lee E, et al. Intraoperative estimation of cardiac output by transesophageal pulsed Doppler echocardiography. *Anesthesiology* 1991;74:9–14.
10. Gorcsan III J, Diana P, Ball BS, et al. Intraoperative determination of cardiac output by transesophageal continuous wave Doppler. *Am Heart J* 1992;123:171–176.
11. Darmon PL, Hillel Z, Mogtader, et al. Cardiac output by transesophageal echocardiography using continuous-wave Doppler across the aortic valve. *Anesthesiology* 1994;80: 796–805.
12. Maslow AD, Haering J, Comunale M, et al. Measurement of cardiac output by pulsed wave Doppler of the right ventricular outflow tract. *Anesth Analg* 1996;83:466–471.

13. Perrino AC, Harris SN, Luther MA. Intraoperative determination of cardiac output using multiplane transesophageal echocardiography: a comparison to thermodilution. *Anesthesiology* 1998;89:350–357.

14. Valdes-Cruz LM, Horowitz S, Mesel E, et al. A pulsed Doppler echocardiographic method for calculating pulmonary and systemic blood flow in trial level shunts: validation studies in animals and initial human experience. *Circulation* 1984; 69:80–86.

15. Rokey R, Sterling LL, Zohgbi WA, et al. Determination of regurgitation fraction is isolated mitral or aortic regurgitation by pulsed Doppler two-dimensional echocardiography. *J Am Coll Cardiol* 1986;7:1273–1278.

16. Bargiggia GS, Tronconi L, Sahn DJ, et al. A new method for quantitation of mitral regurgitation based on color flow Doppler imaging of flow convergence proximal to regurgitant orifice. *Circulation* 1991;84:1481–1489.

17. Rodriguez L, Thomas, JD, Monterroso V, et al. Validation of the proximal flow convergence method: calculation of orifice area in patients with mitral stenosis. *Circulation* 1993; 88: 1157–1165.

18. Vandervoort PM, Rivera JM, Mele D, et al. Application of color Doppler flow mapping to calculate effective regurgitant orifice area. An in vitro study and initial clinical observations. *Circulation* 1993;88(3):1150–1156.

19. Flachskamph FA, Fireske R, Engelhard B, et al. Comparison of transesophageal Doppler methods with angiography for evaluation of the severity of mitral regurgitation. *J Am Soc Echocardiogr* 1998;11:882–892.

20. Rodriguez L, Anconina J, Flaschskampf FA, et al. Impact of finite orifice size on proximal flow convergence. Implications for Doppler quantification of valvular regurgitation. *Circ Res* 1992;70(5):923–930.

21. Pu M, Vandervoort P, Griffin BP, et al. Quantification of mitral regurgitation by the proximal convergence method using transesophageal echocardiography. Clinical validation of a geometric correction for proximal flow constraint. *Circulation* 1995;92(8):2169–2177.

22. Vandervoort PM, Thoreau DH, Rivera JM, et al. Automated flow rate calculations based on digital analysis of flow convergence proximal to regurgitant orifices. *J Am Coll Cardiol* 1993;22(2):535–541.

23. Schwammenthal E, Chen C, Benning F, et al. Dynamics of mitral regurgitant flow and orifice area. Physiologic application of the proximal flow convergence method: clinical data and experimental testing. *Circulation* 1994; 90(1):307–322.

24. Pu M, Prior DL, Fan X, et al. Calculation of mitral regurgitant orifice area with the use of the simplified proximal convergence method: initial clinical application. *J Am Soc Echocardiogr* 2001;14(3):180–185.

25. Hatle L, Angleson B. *Doppler Ultrasound in Cardiology: Physical Principles and Clinical Applications.* 2nd ed. Philadelphia: Lea & Febiger, 1985.

26. Nishimura RA, Miller FA Jr, Callahan MJ, et al. Doppler echocardiography: theory, instrumentation, technique, and application. Mayo Clin Proc 1985;60:321–343.

27. Perrino AC, Reeves ST. *A Practical Approach to Transesophageal Echocardiography.* 1st Ed. Philadelphia: Lippincott Williams & Wilkins, 2003.

28. Hatle L, Brubakk A, Tromsdal A, et al. Noninvasive assessment of pressure drop in mitral stenosis by Doppler ultrasound. *Br Heart J* 1978;40:131–140.

29. Teirstein PS, Yock PG, Popp RL. The accuracy of Doppler ultrasound measurements of pressure gradients across irregular, dual, and tunnel-like obstructions to blood flow. *Circulation* 1985;72:577–584.

30. Nishimura RA, Rihal CS, Tajik AJ, et al. Accurate measurement of the transmitral gradient in patients with mitral stenosis: a simultaneous catheterization and Doppler echocardiographic study. *J Am Coll Cardiol* 1994;24:152–158.

31. Skjaerpe T, Hegrenaese L, Hatle L. Noninvasive estimation of valve area in patients with aortic stenosis by Doppler ultrasound and two-dimensional echocardiography. *Circulation* 1985;72:810–818.

32. Blumberg FC, Pfeifer M, Holmer SR, et al. Quantification of aortic stenosis in mechanically ventilated patients using multiplane transesophageal Doppler echocardiography. *Chest* 1998;114:94–97.

33. Rittoo D, Sutherland GR, Shaw TR. Quantification of left-to-right atrial shunting defect size after balloon mitral commissurotomy using biplane transesophageal echocardiography, color flow Doppler mapping, and the principle of proximal flow convergence. *Circulation* 1993;87:1591–1603.

34. Nakatani S, Masuyama T, Kodama K, et al. Value and limitations of Doppler echocardiography in the quantification of stenotic mitral valve area: comparison of the pressure half-time and the continuity equation methods. *Circulation* 1988; 77:78–85.

35. Libanoff AJ, Rodbard S. Atrioventricular pressure half-time: measurement of mitral valve orifice area. *Circulation* 1968; 38:144–150.

36. Hatle L, Angelson B, Tromsdal A. Noninvasive assessment of atrioventricular pressure half-time by Doppler ultrasound. *Circulation* 1979;60:1096–1104.

37. Thomas JD, Weyman AE. Doppler mitral pressure half-time: a clinical tool in search of theoretical justification. *J Am Coll Cardiol* 1987;10:923–929.

38. Smith MD, Handshoe R, Handshoe S, et al. Comparative accuracy of two-dimensional echocardiography and Doppler pressure half-time methods in assessing severity of mitral stenosis in patients with and without prior commissurotomy. *Circulation* 1986;73:100–107

39. Sidebotham D, Merry A, Legget M. *Practical Perioperative Transesophageal Echocardiography.* 1st Ed. London: Butterworth-Heinemann, 2003.

40. Teague SM, Heinsimer JA, Anderson JL, et al. Quantification of aortic regurgitation utilizing continuous wave Doppler ultrasound. *J Am Coll Cardiol* 1986;8(3):592–599.

41. Samstad SO, Hegrenaes L, Skjaerpe T, et al. Half-time of the diastolic aortoventricular pressure difference by continuous wave Doppler ultrasound: a measure of the severity of aortic regurgitation? *Br Heart J* 1989;61:336–343.

42. Grayburn PA, Handshoe R, Smith MD, et al. Quantitative assessment of the hemodynamic consequences of aortic regurgitation by means of continuous wave Doppler recordings. *J Am Coll Cardiol* 1987;10:135–141.

43. Griffin BP, Flaschskampf FA, Reinold SC, et al. Relationship of aortic regurgitant velocity slope and pressure half-time to severity of aortic regurgitation under changing hemodynamic conditions. *Eur Heart J* 1994;15(5):681–685.

44. Come PC. Echocardiographic recognition of pulmonary arterial disease and determination of its cause. *Am J Med* 1988; 84:384–393.

45. Yock PG, Popp RL. Noninvasive estimation of right ventricular systolic pressure by Doppler ultrasound in patients with tricuspid regurgitation. *Circulation* 1984;70:657–662.

46. Chan KL, Currie PJ, Seward JB, et al. Comparison of three Doppler ultrasound methods in the prediction of pulmonary artery pressure. *J Am Coll Cardiol* 1987;9:549–554.

47. Lee RT, Lord CP, Plappert T, et al. Prospective Doppler echocardiographic evaluation of pulmonary artery diastolic pressure in the medical intensive care unit. *Am J Cardiol* 1989;64:1366–1377.

48. Gorcsan III J, Snow FR, Paulsen W, et al. Noninvasive estimation of left atrial pressure in patients with congestive heart failure and mitral regurgitation by Doppler echocardiography. *AM Heart J* 1991;121:858–863.

49. Nishimura RA, Tajik AJ. Determination of left-sided pressure gradients by utilizing Doppler aortic and mitral regurgitation signals: validation by simultaneous dual catheter and Doppler studies. *J Am Coll Cardiol* 1988;11:317–321.

50. Bargiggia GS, Bertucci C, Recusani F, et al. A new method for estimating left ventricular dp/dt by continuous wave Doppler echocardiography: validation studies at cardiac catheterization. *Circulation* 1989;80:1287–1292.

51. Chung NS, Nishimura RA, Holmes DR Jr, et al. Measurement of left ventricular dp/dt by simultaneous Doppler echocardiography and cardiac catheterization. *J Am Soc Echocardiogr* 1992;5:147–1452.

52. Leung DY, Griffin BP, Stewart WJ, et al. Left ventricular function after valve repair for chronic mitral regurgitation: predictive value of preoperative assessment of contractile reserve by exercise echocardiography. *J Am Coll Cardiol* 1996;28:1198–1205.

QUESTIONS

1. Which of the following statements concerning determination of SV using Doppler is *incorrect*?
   A. VTI and area should be determined at the same location.
   B. The spatial flow velocity profile should be flat.
   C. VTI should be determined with the ultrasound beam parallel to blood flow.
   D. VTI and area should both be determined during systole.

2. Which of the following statements regarding determination of mitral regurgitation severity using the proximal flow convergence method is *incorrect*?
   A. Because the regurgitant orifice is not infinitely small, the hemispheric shape of PISAs is not maintained all the way to the orifice and thus, flow underestimation may occur.
   B. Flow may be constrained by structures proximal to the regurgitant orifice such that PISAs are not full hemispheres leading to flow overestimation.
   C. It is often difficult to locate the exact center of the regurgitant orifice resulting in an error in the measured PISA radius.
   D. Results using the simplified method significantly overestimate mitral regurgitation severity compared with the standard method.

3. Which of the following statements related to the determination of aortic stenosis severity is *incorrect*?
   A. In the setting of aortic stenosis and significant LVOT obstruction (dynamic or fixed), the simplified Bernoulli equation will overestimate the AV pressure gradient.
   B. Mean gradients determined by Doppler have correlated well with those simultaneously measured by cardiac catheterization.
   C. The primary concern in determining AVA with the continuity equation using TEE is related to the possible underestimation of the area of the LVOT.
   D. Since the shapes of the VTI_{LVOT} and VTI_{AV} Doppler profiles are similar, the ratio of the maximum velocities (V_{LVOT}/V_{AV}) may be substituted for the ratio of the VTIs (VTI_{LVOT}/VTI_{AV}) in the continuity equation without introducing significant errors into the AVA calculation.

4. Which of the following statements concerning determination of MVA using the PHT method is *incorrect*?
   A. PHT cannot be used for estimating the area of a normal mitral valve as it is more dependent on LV compliance than the area of the valve.
   B. The PHT will be decreased by more than mild AR and therefore will overestimate MVA.
   C. Following mitral valvuloplasty, the compliances of the LA and LV may be altered for several days, making the PHT method unreliable.
   D. The PHT method underestimates the area of normal prosthetic mitral valves.

5. Which of the following statements regarding estimation of an intracardiac or pulmonary pressure is *incorrect*?
   A. Estimation of the PASP using an estimated (or measured) RAP and the peak velocity of the TR jet is not valid in the setting of RVOT obstruction.
   B. Estimation of RVSP from the systemic systolic blood pressure and the peak velocity across the VSD is not valid in the setting of significant AR.
   C. Estimations of LAP from the systemic systolic blood pressure and the peak velocity of the MR jet are not valid in the setting of significant LVOT obstruction.
   D. LVEDP can be estimated from the peak end-diastolic velocity of the AR jet and the systemic diastolic pressure.

CHAPTER 27

Assessment in Higher Risk Myocardial Revascularization and Complications of Ischemic Heart Disease

Kyungrok Kim ■ Robert M. Savage ■ Joseph Sabik ■ Bruce W. Lytle

HISTORICAL PERSPECTIVES

The first association between coronary artery disease and myocardial dysfunction was suggested in 1779 by Caleb Hillier Parry who described his autopsy findings of hardened "ossified" blockages in the coronary arteries and death associated with "syncope anginos" (1). It was 3 years later that William Heberden provided his classic description of the syndrome of pectoralis dolor as "a disagreeable sensation in the breast" associated with exertion (2). In 1856, Rudolf Virchow described the evolution of fibrous thickening in the arterial wall into arterial atheroma because of a reactive inflammatory process resulting in fibrotic proliferation cells (3). Since these early characterizations of coronary artery disease, remarkable advances have been made in our understanding of this disease process and its management. In 1910, Alexis Carrell performed the first aortocoronary bypass surgery in a dog, using a preserved carotid artery between the ascending aorta and left anterior descending (LAD) coronary artery (4). However, it was not until early 1958 that Longmire was credited with performing the first internal mammary to coronary artery anastomosis following a right coronary endarterectomy, which had "disintegrated" (5). As seen in Tables 27.1 and 27.2, the management of coronary artery disease has been driven by numerous factors and spans more than two centuries from initial scientific observations to the advanced direct surgical and percutaneous approaches to myocardial revascularization. While there may be a number of surgical teams credited with performing the first coronary artery bypass surgery, it was René Favaloro's report, in 1968, of 171 patients undergoing direct surgical myocardial revascularization that ushered in the modern era of coronary bypass surgery (Fig. 27.1) (6–8). Since that time, there have been number of milestones in the evolution of myocardial revascularization.

1. The introduction of myocardial protection strategies
2. Demonstration of long-term advantages of internal mammary artery (IMA) conduits
3. Advances in cardiovascular anesthetic management
4. Introduction of percutaneous approaches to revascularization
5. Introduction of intraoperative echocardiography (IOE) into patient management
6. Improved management of the complications of ischemic heart disease
7. Identification of the variables improving repeat coronary bypass surgery
8. Development of ventricular support devices
9. Development of ventricular reconstruction surgery

TABLE 27.1	History of Coronary Artery Disease and its Management	
Year	**Investigator**	**Milestone**
1770–1935		**Observations Considerations for Treatment**
1779	Caleb Hillier Parry	Discovered relation between angina and coronary ossification
1856	Rudolf Virchow	Described inflammatory process of atheroma development
1856	William Heberden	Characterized classic angina
1880	Langer	Described coronary collateral communications

(continued)

Year	Investigator	Milestone
1899	Francois-Franck	Described sympathetic innervation
1902	Kocher	Absence of angina in thyroidectomy patient
1910	**Alexis Carrell**	**Experimental aortocoronary bypass with preserved carotid artery**
1916	Jonnesco	Performed first cardiac sympathetectomy
1926	Boas	Subtotal thyroidectomy for treatment of angina
1929	Richardson and White	Series of patients undergoing ganglionic sympathetectomy
1930	Sussman	Performed cardiac irradiation for sympathetic denervation
1930s	Carrell and Lindberg	Developed primitive heart lung machine
1935–1953		**Indirect myocardial revascularization**
1930	**Claude S. Beck**	**Performed epicardial abrasion to increase collateral flow**
1934	Robertson	Ligated coronary sinus to redirect coronary flow
1937	O'Shaughnessy	Used omental flap to epicardium for revascularization
1937	John Gibbon Jr	Bypassed a dog's heart during PA occlusion
1938	Griffith and Bates	Direct implantation of blood vessels into myocardium
1946	**Arthur Vineberg**	**Reported internal mammary implants directly into myocardium**
1946	Beck	Arterialized coronary sinus
1951	Gordon Murray	Direct arterial repair and venous interposition homografts
1953	William Mustard	Carotid to coronary bypass
1953	**John Gibbon**	**First effective heart-lung bypass machinery**
1954–1966		**Early direct coronary artery bypass**
1954	Murray	First successful bypass on beating heart of a dog
1955	Melrose	Elective potassium-induced arrest
1957	**F. Mason Sones**	**First cineangiogram of coronary artery**
1958	**William Longmire**	**Grafted IMA to coronary vessel**
1958	Senning	Coronary endartectomy with plaque excision and graft
1960 (reported 1964)	Robert Goetz	IMA to right coronary anastomosis
1962 (reported 1974)	**David Sabiston**	**First saphenous vein CABG**
1964	Vasilii Kolesov	Performed internal mammary to LAD graft without CPB
1964 (reported 1973)	**Garrett and DeBakey**	**First successful saphenous vein bypass graft**
1966	Bailey	Gastroepiploic artery implantation into myocardium
1967-present		**Modern era of revascularization**
1967	**René Favaloro**	**First series of free SVG and end-to-side anastomosis**
1968	Dudley Johnson	Other saphenous vein grafting series
1970	René Favaloro	Double IMA grafts alone or in combination with SVG
1968	René Favaloro	Aortocoronary bypass for unstable angina and AMI
1968	René Favaloro	Combined CABG and valve replacement or aneurysmectomy
1973	Alan Carpentier	Free radial artery grafts
1974	**Gerald Buckberg**	**Myocardial protection strategies using cardioplegia**
1976–1986	**Floyd Loop**	**Reported survival benefit IMA-LAD graft**

Mueller RL, Rosengart TK, Isom W. The history of surgery for ischemic heart disease. Ann Thorac Surg 1997;63:869–878.

TABLE 27.2	Challenges with Guideline Indications for Myocardial Revascularization Using CABG and PCI

1. Rapid pace of technology
2. Time between scientific investigation and technology
3. Time difference in disease recurrence for CABG and PCI
4. Comparability of CABG-PCI study groups (selection bias, nonrandomized patient, and disease risk factors)
5. Randomized trials for degree of risk
6. Initial therapy studies include crossover success
7. Differences in definitions of restenosis in CABG and PCI
8. Secondary prevention in studies differs
9. High volume center studies not as relevant to low volume practices
10. Unique capabilities of Individual centers in CABG and PCI
11. Difficulties of informed consent

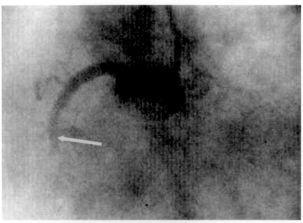
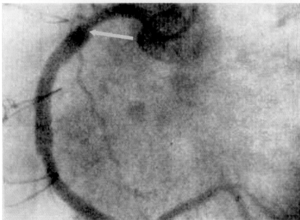

Figure 27.1. Rene Favaloro and Mason Sones of the Cleveland Clinic united as a team in demonstrating the feasibility of safely performing saphenous vein interposition and aortocoronary bypass grafts. In May of 1967, this angiogram demonstrated the intersegmental graft with end-to-end anastomoses. In December of 1968, Favaloro, Sones, and Effler summarized the advances in the first large series of 171 patients. (Reused from Favaloro RG. Landmarks in the development in coronary bypass surgery. *Circulation* 1998;98[5]:466–478, with permission.)

INDICATIONS FOR MYOCARDIAL REVASCULARIZATION

The American College of Cardiology recently revised their Guidelines for Coronary Artery Bypass Graft Surgery (CABG) (Table 27.3) (9). A number of factors created an evolution in the current indications for myocardial revascularization by traditional surgical CABG or percutaneous coronary intervention (PCI). The factors are related to patient selection, differences in institutional CABG and PCI capabilities, temporal differences in recurrence for CABG and PCI, accelerated pace of innovations affecting the scientific study relevancy, and the inherent difficulties in comparing CABG and PCI due to the inability to account for all of the definable and less definable outcome risks in randomized studies (9,10). While the pace may slow, physicians involved in the care of patients with coronary artery disease will need to stay current with the scientific literature and ongoing innovations in revascularization.

DEFINITION OF HIGHER RISKS IN PATIENTS UNDERGOING CORONARY ARTERY BYPASS GRAFT SURGERY

To assist patients in making an informed decision and enable the surgical team to develop optimal perioperative strategies, it is important to identify factors that may affect a patient's perioperative outcome. To identify risks of morbidity and mortality, patient- and disease-related features from patient's history, physical examination, or diagnostic evaluation are subjected to statistical analysis to determine the degree of correlation with adverse clinical events. Such risks are related to the severity and extent of ischemic heart disease or

TABLE 27.3	Indications for Coronary Artery Bypass Surgery

Classification of recommendations

Class I: Conditions for which there is evidence and/or general agreement that a procedure is beneficial and effective.

Class II: Conditions for which there is conflicting evidence and/or a divergence of opinion about the usefulness of a procedure treatment.

    IIa: Conflicting evidence but weight of evidence/opinion is in favor of benefit/efficacy.

    IIb: Conflicting evidence and benefit/efficacy are less well established by evidence/opinion.

Class III: Conditions for which there is evidence and/*or* general agreement that the procedure/treatment is *not* useful or effective.

Level of evidence

A: Data from multiple randomized trials or meta-analysis

B: Data from single randomized trial or nonrandomized studies

C: Consensus opinion of experts only or standard of care

Asymptomatic or mild angina

Class I

    1. Left main disease (A)

    2. Left main equivalent (A)

    3. Three-vessel disease, EF < 0.50 and/or large ischemic areas (C)

Class IIa

    Prox LAD Dz + 1 to 2-vessel disease (A)

Class IIb

    One-vessel or two-vessel Dz + large at-risk viable area (B)

Stable angina

Class I

    1. Left main Dz (A)

    2. Left main equivalent (A)

    3. Three-vessel Dz (benefit greater with LVEF < 0.50) (A)

    4. Two-vessel Dz with prox LAD stenosis + either EF < 0.50 or ischemia (A)

    5. One-vessel or two-vessel Dz (no prox LAD stenosis) + large at-risk area (B)

    6. Disabling angina on max med Rx and acceptable risk (B)

Class IIa

    1. Prox LAD Dz + one-vessel disease (A)

    2. Two-vessel or one-vessel Dz (no prox LAD Dz) mod viable ischemic area at-risk (B)

Class III (not recommended)

    1. One to two vessel Dz (no prox LAD Dz) symptoms not ischemia, < max med Rx, small ischemia viable area (B)

    2. Borderline coronary Dz (50%–60%) + no ischemia (B)

    3. Insignificant coronary Dz (<50%) (B)

Unstable angina (Non-STEMI)

Class I

    1. Left main stenosis (A)

    2. Left main equivalent (>70% prox LAD + prox LCx) (A)

    3. Active ischemia not responsive to med Rx + PCI not possible (B)

(*continued*)

TABLE 27.3	Indications for Coronary Artery Bypass Surgery (*Continued*)

Class IIa

1. Prox LAD Dz with one-vessel or two-vessel Dz (A)

Class IIb

One-vessel or two-vessel disease not involving the proximal LAD when PCI not possible/optimal (B)

Emergent/urgent CABG STEMI

Class I

1. Failed PCI + persistent pain or unstable hemodynamics + suitable Sx anatomy (B)
2. Persistent recurrent ischemia on max med Rx and suitable Sx anatomy + significant area at risk + not PCI candidates (B)
3. During surgery for VSD or ischemic MR (B)
4. Cardiogenic shock <36 hours of MI (age < 75) + ST elevation, LBBB, posterior MI + suitable Sx anatomy (A)
5. Life-threatening ventricular arrhythmias and left main Dz (>40%) or equivalent (B)

Class IIa

1. <6 to 12 MI + suitable anatomy not candidates or failed fibrinolysis/PCI (B)
2. CABG mortality elevated (<3 to 7 days MI); benefit CABG by risk-benefit (B)

Class III (not recommended)

1. Persistent angina + small area myocardium at-risk and stable hemodynamics (C)
2. Successful epicardial reperfusion + poor microvascular reperfusion (C)

Poor LV function

Class I

1. Left main Dz (B)
2. Left main equivalent (B)
3. Prox LAD Dz + two-vessel or three-vessel Dz (B)

Class IIa

Significant viable noncontracting revascularizable myocardium (B)

Class III (not recommended)

No evidence of ischemia or significant revascularizable viable myocardium (B)

Life threatening ventricular arrhythmias

Class 1

1. Left main stenosis (B)
2. Three vessel disease (B)

Class IIa

1. One to two vessel Dz causing the arrhythmias (B)
2. Prox LAD Dz + one to two vessel Dz (B)

Class III (not recommended)

VT with scar + no ischemia (B)

CABG after failed PCI

Class I

1. Ischemia or threatened occlusion with significant at-risk area (B)
2. Hemodynamic compromise (B)

Class IIa

1. Foreign body crucial anatomic position (C)
2. Unstable hemodynamics + impaired coagulation + no previous stemotomy (C)

(*continued*)

Class IIb
Unstable hemodynamics + impaired coagulation + previous sternotomy (C)
Class III
1. Absence of ischemia (C)
2. Inability to revascularize target anatomy or no-reflow state (C)
Previous CABG
Class I
1. Disabling angina with max med Rx or atypical angina with ischemia (B)
2. No patent grafts + left main Dz or equivalent/three vessel disease (B)
Class IIa
1. Bypassable distal vessel(s) with large area threatened myocardium (B)
2. Atherosclerotic LAD vein graft (Dz > 50%) or large at-risk areas (B)
Valve surgery at time of CABG
Class I
Severe AS 1 criteria for AVR (B)
Class IIa
1. Mod MR correction probably indicated (B)
2. Mod AS acceptable combined risks (B)
Class IIb
Mild AS if acceptable combined risk (C)
Arterial conduits
Class I
In all CABG, the LAD Dz should considered for left IMA graft (B)
Transmyocardial revascularization (laser)
Class IIa
Angina refractory to Rx 1 not candidates for PCI-CABG (A)

Adapted from Eagle KA, Guyton RA, Davidoff R, et al. ACC/AHA guidelines for coronary artery bypass graft surgery: a report of the American College of Cardiology/American Heart Association task force on practice guidelines (committee to revise the 1991 guidelines for coronary artery bypass graft surgery). J Am Coll Cardiol 1993;34:1262–1346.

other comorbid chronic disease processes. While many factors are associated with higher morbidity and mortality, it is typically only those commonly occurring that permit a statistical correlation with outcomes. From these studies, outcome prediction may be based on cumulative risks (9). While many of these risks are easily defined (Table 27.3), others are more difficult to define objectively. Yet, many of these issues have a significant impact on the patient's outcome. More difficult to define risks are

1. Availability of suitable bypass conduits
2. Diffuseness of distal coronary atherosclerosis (reducing distal coronary blood flow)
3. Presence of noncardiac atherosclerosis
4. Uncommon combinations of patient comorbidities (11,12)

Risk Factors and Mortality

There have been a number of studies evaluating the clinical variables associated with perioperative death (13–15). They are difficult to compare due to differences in the definitions of clinical or disease variables, clinical end points, institutional differences in clinical practices, and clinical outcomes. Jones et al. (16) combined the data from seven large studies to evaluate recurring factors that contribute to in-hospital mortality following CABG. This resulted in a clinical study population of more than 172,000 patients, enabling the identification of two levels of variables. Those variables having the strongest correlation with outcome included

1. Patient's age
2. Gender

3. Previous cardiac surgery
4. Operation urgency
5. Ventricular ejection fraction (EF)
6. Characterization of coronary anatomy (left main >50% stenosis, number of vessels with >70% stenosis)

Age, urgency of procedure, and reoperation were the variables most strongly correlated with mortality. There were other variables identified that influenced mortality, but they were not as strongly correlated (Table 27.4).

TABLE 27.4	**Coronary Artery Bypass Surgery Relative Mortality Risks**	
Risk Factor	**Relative Risk**	**Risk Score**
Core variables		
Age	Add 1.01–1.05	
	Per year > 50	
60–69		1.5
70–79		2.5
>80		6
Previous CABG	1.39–3.6	5
Urgency		
Elective	1	0
Urgent		
(required to stay in hospital)	1.2–3.5	2
Emergent		
(refractory compromise)	2–7.4	5
Salvage (ongoing CPR)	6.7–29	5
Sex	1.2–1.63 for female	
Female		
LV ejection fraction		
40%–60%	1	
<40%		2
30%–39%	1.6	
20%–29%	2.2	
<20%	4.1	
Left main stenosis		
50%–89%		1.5
>90%		2
Number of major coronaries >70%		
Three-vessel disease	1.5	1.5
Two-vessel disease	1.3	1.3
One-vessel disease	1	1
Influencing variables		
History of angina		
CHF		
Recent MI (<1 week)	1.5	1.5
PCI index		
Ventricular arrhythmia		
Mitral regurgitation		

(*continued*)

Risk Factor	Relative Risk	Risk Score
Comorbidities		
Diabetes	1	1
Cerebrovascular disease		
Peripheral vascular Dz	1.5	1.5
Renal dysfunction		
Hemodialysis	4	4
Creatinine >2.0	2	2
Other variables		
COPD		2
WBC > 12K		2.5
Total point score		**Mortality risk**
0–5		0.2%–0.7%
6–10		1%–3%
11–15		4%–11.5%
16–17		14.1%–18.7%
18		>23%

Trials that were initiated in the first decade of coronary bypass surgery demonstrated that patients with left main or triple vessel disease and abnormal left ventricular (LV) function had an improved long-term survival when coupled with an aggressive strategy of complete revascularization (17,18). Since then, there have been remarkable improvements in the management of this unique group of higher risk patients with the advent of myocardial protection strategies, integrated perioperative care, secondary prevention, use of arterial grafts, and the increased collective experience of the surgical community. This has led to a growing consensus, as outlined by the recent ACC guidelines for coronary artery bypass surgery, that left main equivalent or triple vessel disease combined with abnormal LV function is an indication for surgical revascularization (Table 27.2) (9). Despite recent improvements in the medical management of this group of patients, the yearly mortality remains at 12%, indicating that surgical management of this high-risk group is warranted (19). This strategy is further supported by an understanding that

1. Ischemia is the inciting event of death when these patients are treated medically.
2. Revascularization results in decreased incidence of ischemic-related sudden death.
3. The low mortality rate of patients, with poor LV function, undergoing CABG is 0.8% to 3.2% in experienced centers (11).

Allman et al. performed a meta-analysis of 24 studies, representing a total of 3,088 patients, with an average EF of 32%. They demonstrated that CABG to areas of viable myocardium reduced the mortality by 80% (20). Patients without areas of viable myocardium did not demonstrate a survival benefit, regardless of the severity of ventricular dysfunction. With 6% to 9% of patients over the age of 65 exhibiting ischemic cardiomyopathy, this higher risk population will continue to challenge the medical community to develop innovative strategies to meet this growing concern (21–23).

Risk Factors and Morbidity

Clinical studies have been performed evaluating those variables influencing the perioperative morbidity (Table 27.5) (24–27). Many have evaluated specific morbidities, including central nervous system dysfunction, cardiac morbidity (recurrence of angina, LV dysfunction, perioperative myocardial infarction [MI], and dysrhythmias), and renal dysfunction. Neurologic dysfunction following CABG surgery is considered in two broad categories. Type 1 deficits involve major focal neurologic deficits, stupor, and coma. Type 2 deficits are characterized as alterations in cognitive function. In a multicenter study involving 2,108 patients, Roach et al. (28) identified CNS dysfunction in 6% of patients, which was evenly distributed between Type 1 and Type 2 deficits. Predictors of both types of neurologic dysfunction included age >70 and a history of hypertension. Risk factors associated with Type 1 deficits included diabetes, use of an IABP, prior neurologic event, perioperative hypotension, use of an LV vent, and a history of unstable angina. Atheromatous disease involving the proximal ascending aorta, as detected by intraoperative echo (transesophageal echocardiography

TABLE 27.5	Coronary Artery Bypass Surgery Morbidity Risk Factors
Risk factor	
Patient	
Age	
Sex	
Cardiac-related factors	
Previous CABG	
Left main stenosis	
Triple vessel disease	
Recent MI (<1 week)	
Ejection fraction	
Urgency	
Comorbidities	
Obesity	
Diabetes	
Cerebrovascular disease	
Peripheral vascular Dz	
Renal dysfunction	
COPD	
WBC > 12k	

TABLE 27.6	Coronary Artery Bypass Surgery Cleveland Clinic Severity Score	
Age 65–74 y		1
Age 75 years or older		2
Weight ≤ 65 kg		1
Emergency		6
Severe LV dysfunction		3
Operative AV stenosis		1
Operative MV insufficiency		3
Prior cardiovascular surgery		2
Prior cardiac operation		3
Diabetes on medication		1
COPD on medication		2
Cerebrovascular		1
Serum creatinine l.6–1.8 mg		1
Serum creatinine >1.9 mg		4
Anemia (Hct ≤ 34%)		2
Maximum score		**31**

[TEE] and epivascular imaging), has also been closely associated with Type 1 neurologic events. Risk factors associated with Type 2 deficits include a history of previous CABG, congestive heart failure (CHF), peripheral vascular disease (PVDz), alcohol consumption, or dysrhythmias (28).

Renal dysfunction is a significant contributor to perioperative morbidity. Antunes et al., in 2004, evaluated 2,445 CABG patients for factors associated with the development of postoperative renal dysfunction (creatinine ≥2.1 mg/dL or increase of 0.9 mg/dL) (25). Renal dysfunction occurred in 5.6% of this patient population with a mortality of 8.8% compared to 0.1% for those without renal dysfunction. Risk factors associated with post-CABG renal dysfunction included age, preexisting renal dysfunction, bypass time, and angina class III/IV.

In looking at factors associated with a higher risk of death and postoperative morbidity, Higgins et al. (29) developed and validated a severity scoring system using measurable factors that defined a patient population at increased risk (Table 27.6) (Fig. 27.2A–C). This Cleveland Clinic Preoperative Cardiac Surgical Severity Score assigned points (from 1 to 6) for the factors most closely associated with mortality and morbidity (29). As the severity score index became greater than four, the incidence of morbidity and mortality markedly increased. The highest number of points was assigned to emergent surgery (6–8)

while serum creatinine greater than 1.9 mg/dL was given four points. Severe LV dysfunction, prior cardiac surgery, and mitral valve insufficiency were assigned three points each. In correlating the total severity score with morbidity and mortality outcomes, patients with a total score approximately four have a higher risk for postoperative morbidity and mortality when undergoing myocardial revascularization (29).

IMPORTANCE OF ISCHEMIC HEART DISEASE IN FUTURE HEALTH CARE DELIVERY

Despite recent advances in the management of ischemic heart disease, the National Center for Health Statistics and World Health Organization report that it remains the leading cause of death throughout the world and will remain so through the year 2020 (21,22). The factors behind these trends are related to the increased incidence of coronary artery disease and associated risk factors in aging patients (e.g., diabetes, hypertension, and obesity). The number of individuals over the age of 65 is expected to increase from 35 to 71 million by the year 2030 in the United States alone (Fig. 27.3) (23). Of individuals over the age of 65, greater than 65% have cardiovascular disease (Fig. 27.4) (21,30). This age group has an increasing incidence of atherosclerotic vascular disease. More alarming is the increasing incidence of these factors in younger generations, suggesting that the cardiovascular epidemic will continue for years to come. Consequently, we find

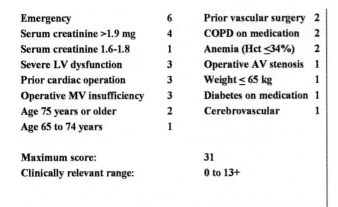

Emergency	6	Prior vascular surgery	2
Serum creatinine >1.9 mg	4	COPD on medication	2
Serum creatinine 1.6-1.8	1	Anemia (Hct ≤34%)	2
Severe LV dysfunction	3	Operative AV stenosis	1
Prior cardiac operation	3	Weight ≤ 65 kg	1
Operative MV insufficiency	3	Diabetes on medication	1
Age 75 years or older	2	Cerebrovascular	1
Age 65 to 74 years	1		

Maximum score: 31

Clinically relevant range: 0 to 13+

A

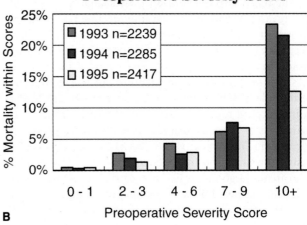

B

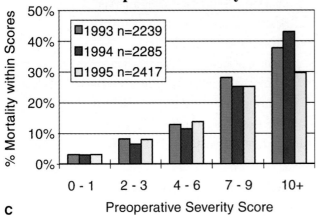

C

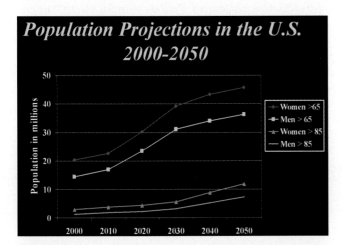

Figure 27.2. **A:** The Cleveland Clinic Severity Score was developed and validated in 1992 to predict those patients who were at risk for significant morbidity and mortality based on preoperative risk factors. **B,C:** Those patients with severity score of four represent a patient population at higher risk of developing significant perioperative morbidity and increased mortality.

ourselves in the midst of a growing cardiovascular pandemic in the United States and throughout the world, with ischemic heart disease constituting the major cause of significant cardiovascular morbidity and mortality (31). In addition, 80% of the elderly over 60 years old have at least one chronic disease and 50% have two chronic dis-

eases (22). In addition to these demographic trends, the number of percutaneous revascularizations will continue to increase. Patients with coronary artery disease are living longer. This has resulted in a surgical revascularization population that is older, has more diffuse coronary disease, has more frequent complications associated with chronic

Figure 27.3. The aging of the United States population. It is estimated by the Center for Health Statistics that there will be more than 52 million individuals over the age of 65 living in the United States.

Figure 27.4. Age and incidence of coronary artery disease in men and women. The Center for Disease Control and Prevention reports that there is an age-related increase in the incidence of coronary artery disease.

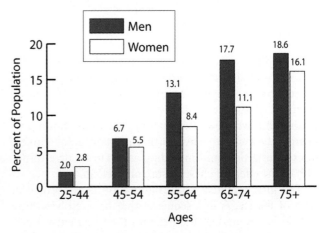

ischemic disease, and has a more frequent history of previous surgical interventions (PCI and CABG).

The morbidity and mortality associated with myocardial revascularization have steadily declined over the last 35 years (32). If we are to maintain this trend, it will be necessary to develop strategies for addressing those critical issues that guide the intraoperative decision-making process. The purpose of this chapter is to provide an overview of the role of IOE in the management of patients undergoing surgical revascularization of the myocardium. The principles of the intraoperative echo examination will be identified. The critical issues that must be addressed to insure the successful management of higher risk patients who are undergoing surgical myocardial revascularization will be examined, followed by outcome studies characterizing the effectiveness of such perioperative strategies. We will then focus on the complications of ischemic heart disease and their echocardiographic diagnosis and intraoperative management as guided by TEE. This discussion will conclude with an examination of future clinical applications of intraoperative TEE.

PRINCIPLES OF PERFORMING INTRAOPERATIVE ECHO EXAMINATION IN CABG SURGERY

The intraoperative echo examination for higher risk patients undergoing myocardial revascularization is guided by principles related to the unique demands of the environment and the potential for sudden changes in the patient's cardiovascular function (Table 27.7). Because of this potential for change in cardiovascular function throughout the procedure, complete diagnostic TEE examinations are performed at each of the progressive phases of the surgical procedure:

1. Pre-CPB
2. Pre-Sep from cardiopulmonary bypass (CPB)
3. Post-Sep CPB
4. Post–chest closure

In addition, should the patient encounter hemodynamic instability at any point during the course of the procedure, an overview is performed followed by a more "focused diagnostic examination" directed by the clinical course and overview examination. The examination following chest closure insures that grafts are not kinked, interrupting flow and impeding an accurate determination of the effect of chest closure on preload.

The intraoperative TEE examination is performed at each of the stages in a sequence that first resolves those critical issues guiding the patient's management yet recognizes the ongoing management of the patient and the need to document a complete examination for future comparison. To prevent significant midexam revelations from occurring, an abbreviated 60-second overview

TABLE 27.7 Principles of Intraoperative Echo Examination Higher Risk Coronary Artery Bypass Surgery

1. Addresses critical issues
2. Systematic examination
   • Organized by priority
   • Initial overview examination
   • Focused diagnostic examination
   • Comprehensive examination documented
3. Efficient
4. Severity assessment by weighted integration
5. Study results recorded and discussed with surgeon
6. Comprehensive digital study archived
7. Results compared to preoperative data
   • Variances addressed
   • Communicated with surgical team
   • Potential Rx alterations discussed with cardiologist
8. Qualified personnel trained and credentialed
9. IOE examination under CQI process
10. Equipment maintained and updated

examination may be performed followed by the remainder of the examination. In addition to the diagnostic issues that are already on the agenda, the abbreviated overview examination provides an up-to-date assessment of additional issues that might be addressed.

Because of the inherent difficulties in distinguishing degrees of degenerative calcification and fibrosis of the aorta and heart, subdued lighting in the OR reduces monitor glare, enabling a more accurate assessment of aortic arteriosclerosis, myocardial fibrosis, and calcification of cardiovascular structures. Periods without electrocautery interference during critical portions of the intraoperative examination also contribute to the acquisition of quality two-dimensional (2D) images and Doppler-derived hemodynamic data. Such an atmosphere permits the precise recognition of intricate structural abnormalities (vegetation, thrombi, right-to-left shunts), which may have potentially devastating consequences if missed. It also enables the acquisition of the quality of diagnostic information, which may confidently guide the pivotal surgical and hemodynamic decisions.

The conclusions of the TEE examination are communicated directly to the surgical team in addition to being documented in the patient's permanent medical record. Digital loops and images, which support the diagnostic conclusions and constitute the complete systematic examination, are achieved for future retrieval for comparison and reviewed under an organized continuous quality improvement (CQI) process.

Critical Issues in CABG Surgery Addressed by Intraoperative Echo (Tables 27.8A,B)

The purpose of the intraoperative echo is not to replace the patient's preoperation assessment but to confirm and refine it. Due to the clinical dynamic associated with ischemic heart disease, it is always possible that new ventricular or valve dysfunction may occur as a consequence of intervening ischemia or infarction. In addition to providing an ongoing method of monitoring the patients' cardiovascular function, IOE is used to address a number of critical issues that may influence the outcome of coronary bypass surgery. These critical issues include the diagnosis of previously unrecognized cardiovascular abnormalities requiring additional unplanned surgical intervention or altering the patient's anesthetic-hemodynamic management, development of the cannulation-perfusion strategy to prevent neurologic dysfunction, an assessment of the results of the surgical procedure and potential complications, and a final documentation of a comprehensive baseline study for future comparison. Each phase of the procedure has issues that are important to address depending on the extent of the patient's preoperative assessment. If there is a concern regarding the viability of a specific region of myocardium, a pre-CPB dobutamine stress test may be performed as discussed in "Assessment of Myocardial Viability" in Chapter 23 (33,34).

Intraoperative Monitoring

There are a number of determinants of cardiac function that may be monitored intraoperatively by TEE (Table 27.9A), including preload, diastolic function, contractility, regional myocardial function, valve function, and afterload. Compared with the hemodynamics and calculations derived from measurements obtained with the pulmonary artery (PA) thermodilution catheter, TEE provides a more direct physiologic assessment of each determinant of cardiac function (Table 27.9B). Hemodynamic instability is more often encountered in higher risk patients. It may be caused by hypovolemia, ventricular dysfunction, or low systemic vascular resistance. In these circumstances, the intraoperative echo provides a rapid method of assessing global (LV and right ventricle [RV]) ventricular function, preload, presence of segmental dysfunction indicating myocardial ischemia, and an indication of lower systemic vascular resistance (low MAP with hypercontractile LV).

The 2D echocardiography provides both qualitative and quantitative evaluation of systolic ventricular function. The midesophageal four-chamber (ME 4-chamber) and two-chamber (ME 2-chamber) views, the ME long-axis (ME LAX) view and transgastric short-axis (TG SAX) views (basal, midpapillary, and apical), and the TG LAX view allow assessment of global and regional ventricular functions. The 2D quantitative measures of LV systolic

function include ventricular dimensions, volume, stroke volume (SV), cardiac output (CO), EF, and regional wall motion abnormalities (RWMA). Left ventricular ejection fraction (LVEF) can be calculated from LV end-systolic volume (LVESV) and LV end-diastolic volume (LVEDV) as the ratio (LVEDV ? LVESV)/LVEDV. CO can be calculated using the area-length formula across a cardiac valve (most commonly the aortic valve): $CO = 0.785 \times LVOT\ D^2 \times LVOT_{VTI} \times HR$ (LVOT, left ventricular outflow tract; D, LVOT diameter; $LVOT_{VTI}$, velocity time integral [VTI], measured with Doppler spectrum across the aortic valve; and HR, heart rate). IOE determination of CO using TEE is helpful even when a PA catheter is used because the thermodilution technique is inaccurate in patients with significant tricuspid valve (TV) regurgitation (35).

TABLE 27.8A	Critical Issues in Higher Risk Coronary Artery Bypass Surgery

1. Intraoperative monitoring
2. Diagnosis of unrecognized abnormalities changing management
   - Unplanned surgical procedures
   - Anesthetic-hemodynamic management
3. Cannulation and perfusion strategy
4. Predict post-CPB complications
5. Surgical results and potential complications
   - Global and regional functions
     - Functioning bypass grafts
     - Inotropic support
     - Mechanical support (IABP or LVAD/RVAD ECMO)
   - Valve function
     - Ischemic MR
     - TR
     - AR (LV distension prior to separation)
   - Complications of cannulation
     - Aortic dissection
     - Plaque disruption
   - Complications of myocardial protection
     - Regional dysfunction (septal)
     - RV dysfunction
     - Coronary sinus trauma
6. Documentation of comprehensive study (future reference)
   - Global and regional (LV and RV) functions
   - Valve function
   - LA, RA, and shunt potential
   - Aorta (ascending, arch, and descending)

TABLE 27.8B Critical Surgical Decisions in Higher Risk Coronary Artery Bypass Surgery	
Impact of Echo on Surgical Decision Making	
Echo Finding	**Surgical Decisions**
Proximal aortic mobile atheroma	Off pump versus on CPB
	Alternative arterial cannulation (axillary, femoral)
	Identify cross-clamp site (epiaortic echo)
	Identify ascending aortic cannulation site
	Identify site for antegrade cardioplegia insertion
Calcified atheromatous aorta	Off-pump CABG
	All arterial grafts (IMA, gastroepiploic)
	Axillary cannulation
	Circulatory arrest
Significant aortic regurgitation	LV venting
	Direct coronary administration of cardioplegia
Demonstrable regional viability	Coronary bypass graft of anatomy suitable
Pre-CPB	Additional unplanned bypass grafts
New RWMA	Pre-CPB IABP, additional grafts, check angio
New valve dysfunction	Unplanned MVREP or MVR
	Unplanned AVR, TVREP, or TVR
Post-CPB new RWMA	Delayed wean from CPB, revision of grafts
	IABP
Postbypass global LV dysfunction	Return to CPB
	Additional grafts
	Graft revision
	IABP
	LVAD
Post-CPB localized aortic dissection	Localized repair
Post-CPB extensive Type I or II aortic dissection	Replace ascending aorta
Reduced celiac axis flow (metabolic acidosis)	Explore abdomen for gut ischemia
Mechanical complications of ischemic heart disease	
VSD, aneurysm, pseudoaneurysm	Repair of structural defect
LV or LA thrombus	Thrombus removal
Ischemic MR (ruptured papillary muscle)	MVR or MVRep

Preload

Preload has been indirectly assessed utilizing either the PA catheter (pulmonary artery occlusion pressure [PAOP], pulmonary artery end diastolic pressure [PAEDP]) or left atrial catheter (left atrial pressure [LAP]). Because preload recruitment is dependent upon end-diastolic volume (EDV), compliance of the ventricle is an integral component of normal systolic function. In circumstances of a noncompliant ventricular chamber, the LV end-diastolic pressure may not accurately reflect the volume of the LV. Clements et al. (36) reported on 14 patients undergoing surgery for abdominal aortic aneurysms in which TEE, PA catheterization, and portable radionuclide measurements of EDV were simultaneously determined. There was a very close correlation between the TEE (end-diastolic diameter [EDD] and area) and the accepted gold standard of radionuclide measurement of EDV. Interestingly, there was no correlation between PA catheter and the ultrasound or nuclear methods of preload assessment. Standard criteria for diagnosing hypovolemia include an EDD less than 25 mm, systolic obliteration of the LV cavity, and a LV end-diastolic area of less than 55 cm^2 (37).

TABLE 27.9A	Intraoperative Assessment of Cardiac Function	
Determinant	**TEE**	**PA Catheter**
Preload	Direct volume assessment	PAOP
	PW Doppler pulmonary veins	RVEDP
	Interatrial septum shift	CVP
Diastolic function	Inflow patterns	Indirect PAOP
	Tissue Doppler	
Global contractility	LV/RV 2D image	Cardiac output
	CO by volumetric flow	Stroke volume
Regional function	Systolic thickening	NA
	Contraction pattern	
Valve function	2D imaging of structure	cv wave
	CF Doppler assessment	
Afterload	Calculation regional wall stress	SVR calculation
	Tissue Doppler imaging	

TABLE 27.9B	Intraoperative TEE Assessment of Hemodynamic Instability					
	MAP	**LV EDD**	**RV EDD**	**RV Fx**	**LV Fx**	**RWMA**
Hypovolemia	Low	Decreased	Decreased	Variable	Systolic collapse	No
Low SVR	Low	Normal	Variable	Variable	Systolic collapse	No
Low SVR and ischemia	Low	Variable	Variable	Decreased with RCA ischemia	Variable depending on extent	Yes
LV ischemia	Low	Dilated	Increased with global LV dysfunction	RCA ischemia decreased	Variable	Yes
Increased RV afterload	Increased PAM	Dilated	Increased	Variable	Systolic collapse	No
RV ischemia	Variable	Decreased	Increased	Decreased	Systolic collapse	No; except distal RCA
Tamponade	Variable	Compressed LV with left-sided tamponade	Collapsed with right-sided tamponade	Variable	Systolic collapse	No

Diastolic Function

Diastole is the period between aortic valve closure and mitral valve closure and is divided into four phases:

1. Isovolumic relaxation
2. Early rapid diastolic filling
3. Diastasis
4. Late diastolic filling caused by atrial contraction

Ventricular relaxation may be assessed by the isovolumic relaxation time (IVRT), the rate of pressure decline (−dp/dt), and a time constant of relaxation (ô). Compliance is estimated by the early diastolic LV filling (E wave), deceleration time (DT), late diastolic LV filling (AM wave), E:A ratio, the AP wave (reversed) of LA contraction, the s wave of the systolic LA filling phase, and the d wave of the LA diastolic filling phase.

Diastolic dysfunction is often the earliest marker of ischemia and, in the more advanced stages, is predictive of a poorer long-term prognosis. The earliest stage of abnormal diastolic filling is impaired or abnormal relaxation with inverse E/A ratio less than 1.0. With progression of the disease, pseudonormalization of diastolic filling flow occurs as a result of impaired myocardial relaxation balanced by elevation of mean LA pressures. The diagnosis is confirmed by abnormal pulmonary venous flow or response to Valsalva maneuver. The restrictive filling pattern is the most advanced form of diastolic dysfunction. Bernard et al. evaluated the diastolic function in 52 consecutive CABG patients. Thirty percent of their study population had diastolic dysfunction, including patterns of abnormal relaxation (50%), pseudonormal (40%), and restrictive physiology (10%) (38). Patients with diastolic dysfunction more frequently required initial inotropic support with restrictive physiology (100%), pseudonormal (88%), and abnormal relaxation (75%). The need for inotropic support at 12 hours postoperative was similarly increased for these patterns at 100%, 75%, and 50% (38).

Contractility

Assessment of contractility may be performed using visual estimations of global LV function or more volumetric methods based on Simpson's formula. While gross detection of subtle changes in overall ventricular performance may be difficult, detection of more substantial alterations in function lies within the capabilities of trained echocardiographers. The LV may be assessed utilizing the ME 4- or 2-chamber views or the TG mid SAX or LAX views. The percentage of 2D area change between end-diastole (measure at the ECG R-wave) and end systole is estimated. Global LV function may be classified as normal (estimated EF > 50%), mild global LV dysfunction (estimated EF 30%–50%), moderate global LV dysfunction (estimated EF > 15%–30%), and severe global LV dysfunction (estimated EF < 15%). EF measurements represent the SV as a percentage of the EDV (EF = EDV ? ESV/EDV). If there are no regional wall motional abnormalities, simple LV diameters, measured at the mid PM level, may be used to estimate EF (EF = $EDD^2 - ESD^2/EDD^2$). The volumes may also be calculated utilizing the modified Simpson method whereby the length of the LV cavity and the diameter of individual discs are used to calculate and summate the volume in each of a series of discs comprising the LV cavity. With modern ultrasound platforms, these measurements may be either determined on-line (using the automated backscatter technique described above) or off-line. The LVEDV and LVESV are determined automatically, and the EF is calculated as in the formula expressed above.

Myocardial Ischemia

One of the earliest manifestations of myocardial ischemia occurring with coronary occlusion is reduction in systolic thickening of the myocardium supplied by the occluded artery. This is followed by increase in diastolic dysfunction and, about 45 seconds after, by the ST segment changes on surface ECG (39). Minutes later, if there is a large enough perfusion defect, global ventricular dysfunction develops and manifests as elevated filling pressures. The segmental wall motion is assessed by evaluating two variables: the wall thickening and the local change of radius (movement of the myocardium toward the center of the heart). Consequently, the assessment of new RWMA by

intraoperative TEE is a very sensitive marker to detect myocardial ischemia. However, there are other causes of wall motion abnormalities including ventricular pacing, interventricular conduction disturbances, alterations in afterload, ventricular systolic translocation, and tethering associated with adjacent wall motion abnormalities. Under normal conditions, there is marked wall thickening, usually greater than 30% increase in wall thickness during systole, whereas the decrease in radius is usually greater than 30% during systole. Mild hypokinesia corresponds with moderate wall thickening and a 10% to 30% decrease in the local radius while in severe hypokinesia there is only minimal wall thickening and a 0% to 10% decrease in the local radius. Akinesia is characterized by the absence of wall thickening and no change in the radius, and dyskinesia corresponds with thinning and a protruding of myocardial wall away from the heart center. Using radioactive microspheres and ultrasonic dimension crystals, Savage et al. (39) quantified transmural myocardial perfusion and compared it with the various degree of wall motion abnormalities. It was determined that hypokinesia was associated with 25% to 50% decrease in the transmural blood flow, while akinesia was related to a decrease of blood flow in three quarters of the wall thickness. With dyskinesia, there was 100% reduction in blood flow to a dyskinetic region of myocardium.

van Daele et al. (40) monitored 98 patients undergoing cardiac surgery with TEE, electrocardiogram, and the PA catheter. Myocardial ischemia was diagnosed in 14 of 98 patients based on the presence of wall motion abnormalities. Interestingly, in only 10 of these 14 patients were there electrocardiographic changes indicating ischemia. The PA catheter wedge pressure increased in the 14 patients by 3.5 mm Hg. This was an insignificant change in the wedge pressure compared with the baseline and only provided an overall sensitivity of 33% and a predictive value of 16%. Smith et al. (41) compared assessment of myocardial ischemia with the ECG versus transesophageal echo. The authors evaluated 50 patients undergoing myocardial revascularization surgery who were monitored with TEE and multilead ECG. They found that 24 of the patients had echocardiographic evidence of ischemia compared to only six by ECG. All the patients who had ECG evidence of ischemia had RWMA visible on TEE images, whereas there were numerous patients who had RWMA and did not have ECG changes indicating myocardial ischemia. In all cases, segmental wall motion abnormalities occurred before ECG changes. Three of the patients had myocardial infarction.

Afterload

While afterload may be estimated by calculation of systemic vascular resistance, it is more accurately characterized by determination of systolic wall stress. Systolic wall stress may be calculated using a combination of ultrasound and blood pressure measurements. Wall stress is represented by the Laplace formula, which expresses the direct proportionality between stress and systolic blood pressure and the LV end-diastolic diameter (LVEDD) and the inverse relation to the LV wall thickness (WTh). This relation is expressed in the simplified equation:

$$\text{Wall stress} = (P)\ (LVEDD)^2/(WTh)$$

where P, systolic pressure; WTh, wall thickness; and LVEDD, LV end-diastolic diameter.

Unplanned Surgical Intervention or Alteration of Hemodynamic Management

Because of the thoroughness of the preoperative assessment for patients undergoing surgical myocardial revascularization, it is unusual today to find significantly undiagnosed or underdiagnosed cardiovascular disease. However, in circumstances where there has been an intervening clinical event, such as a recent silent myocardial infarction or the patient being rushed for surgery, it is possible for such intraoperative revelations to lead to alterations in the surgical or anesthetic-hemodynamic management. In a retrospective analysis of 12,566 cardiac surgery patients, Eltzschig et al. reported that intraoperative CPB TEE examinations influenced surgical decision making in 9.2% of the cases. In the subset of 3,835 patients undergoing isolated CABG, surgical decisions were influenced by 6.9% of the TEE examinations (41a). In a separate retrospective analysis of 3,245 cardiac surgery patients, Click et al. (42) reported that intraoperative echo was utilized in 292 (9%) undergoing CABG surgery. In this patient subset, IOE was most commonly used to evaluate suspected valve abnormalities. The largest percentage (33%) of new pre-CPB findings occurred in the CABG subset of patients. Some patients were found to have less MR intraoperatively than their preoperative evaluation with the result that their mitral valve was not inspected. Mitral annular dilation caused by LV dilation and mitral apparatus dysfunction is the most common mechanism of mitral regurgitation (MR) in patients with ischemic heart disease. Remodeling leads to changes in the shape and size of the ventricle and may alter the structural integrity of the mitral valve apparatus. While ischemic MR may be either transient or chronic, it is clear that the hemodynamic perturbations of the anesthetic agents and effects of positive pressure ventilation may alter the severity of mitral or tricuspid regurgitation.

In a similar group of patients undergoing CABG with ischemic MR, Cohn et al. (43) reported that 90% were downgraded from moderate to less than mild to moderate MR by IOE examination (Fig. 27.5). Seven of the patients went from moderate MR to no MR intraoperatively and consequently did not receive a MVRep or mitral valve replacement (MVR). Postoperatively three out of seven patients returned to their original 3+ MR and 4 returned to moderate MR on their postoperative transthoracic echocardiography (TTE) (43).

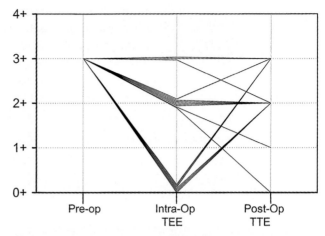

Figure 27.5. In a group of 18 patients with moderate (3+) ischemic MR undergoing CABG, Cohen et al. reported that seven were downgraded to no significant (0) MR by intraoperative TEE following induction of anesthesia. Postoperative transthoracic echo demonstrated that four of these patients had mild to moderate (2+) MR and three had returned to moderate (3+) MR (43).

Grewal et al. demonstrated that 51% of patients with MR improved by at least one MR severity grade when assessed under general anesthesia. The most significant changes occurred in patients with ischemic MR with normal MV leaflets (44). Bach et al. compared the severity of preoperative MR with the IOE, discovering that patients with structural valve leaflet abnormalities (flail) did not have a significant change in their severity assessment, whereas those with functional ischemic MR decreased significantly (45).

In a prospective study of 82 consecutive higher risk CABG patients performed at the Cleveland Clinic, there were a total of seven patients who underwent unplanned valve surgery. Two received an aortic valve replacement for underdiagnosed aortic stenosis, one patient had a pulmonic valve replacement for undiagnosed stenosis, and three patients underwent mitral valve repair procedures for MR of greater severity (>moderate) than the preoperative evaluation (Tables 27.10A,B) (38a). Consistent with the findings of Cohn, Grewal, and Bach, there were no cancellations of a planned mitral valve procedure because of a finding of less MR than was present preoperatively. Sheikh et al. (46) found a 2% incidence of CABG patients demonstrating greater MR leading to MV surgery. Interestingly they found 11% of their CABG patients had less MR than their preoperative evaluation and the MV procedure was cancelled. From a clinical perspective, if the variance in the OR is more than two grades less, the potential exists that the patient may have indolent ischemia at the time of the original examination. In these circumstances, if canceling the MV procedure is a consideration, altering the loading conditions with neosynephrine or challenging with a bolus of intravenous fluid may duplicate the MV dysfunction seen preoperatively as shown by Shiran et al. in a prospective trial of patients with ischemic MR (46a). Other undiagnosed findings that may lead to alterations

TABLE 27.10A Cleveland Clinic Higher Risk CABG Study Surgical Management Alterations					
	Pre-CPB	Pre-SEP CPB	Post-SEP CPBP	Post-CC	#PTS
MV repair	3	0	0	0	3
AO VR	2	0	0	0	2
PVR	1	0	0	0	1
LV vent	7	0	0	0	7

TABLE 27.10B Cleveland Clinic Higher Risk CABG Study Surgical Management Alterations					
	Pre-CPB	Pre-SEP CPB	Post-SEP CPBP	Post-CC	#PTS
Off-pump CABG	3	NA	NA	NA	3
Axillary cannulation	6	NA	NA	NA	6
Circulatory arrest	1	NA	NA	NA	1
GLOBAL DYSFX	6	25	37	37	37
RWMA	8	18	8	1	35
RV DYSFX	2	12	15	15	15
Diastolic DYSFX	13	5	12	15	15
UN-DX valve DZ	13	3	2	3	16
Under-DX valve	15	0	0	0	16

in the patient's surgical management include complications of ischemic heart disease. These include LV or left atrial (LA) thrombi, atrial fibrillation, pseudoaneurysms, ruptured papillary muscle, ischemic ventricular septal defects (VSD), and LV aneurysms.

Previous studies have demonstrated the ability of pre-CPB diagnostic IOE to alter the anesthetic management of patients undergoing CABG surgery. Couture et al. (47) utilized IOE in 624 patients undergoing CABG and found that it altered the anesthetic hemodynamic management in 53% of this population. Berquist et al. (48) evaluated the impact of IOE on the management of 75 patients undergoing CABG procedures. In 17% of patients, IOE was critical in the decision-making process and supportive in 43% with the management of ischemia and guidance of fluid administration being predominant (48). In our study of 82 consecutive CABG patients, global LV dysfunction was diagnosed in 37 (45%) patients and characterized as mild (18.5%), moderate (35%), or severe (59%). RV dysfunction was diagnosed in 15 (18%) patients with predominant moderate (47%) and severe (53%) dysfunction (38a). There were 35 patients with new or increased RWMA (42.6%) detected by IOE.

Electrocardiographic evidence of myocardial ischemia was noted in only seven patients, and in all patients, the electrocardiographic changes followed the regional wall motion changes. Postoperative persistence of the regional wall motion abnormality remained in three of these patients, and one of these three patients sustained a myocardial infarction documented by creatine kinase level and electrocardiogram. Intraoperative TEE demonstrated significant valve disease that had not been previously reported and led to alteration in the hemodynamic management in 32 patients (38a).

Cannulation and Perfusion Strategy to Prevent Neurologic Dysfunction

Neurologic dysfunction occurs in up to 30% to 80% of patients following coronary bypass surgery (26,49,50). It has been classified as either Type 1 (focal neurologic deficit) or Type 2 (cognitive dysfunction or encephalopathy). While both types may be associated with aortic atherosclerosis, Type 1 has the strongest correlation. Newman et al. also defined a higher risk population for developing perioperative CNS dysfunction (28,50). They reviewed

2,417 patients undergoing CABG surgery, looking for predictors and risk factors of perioperative neurologic events, such as a stroke, TIA, or coma (Table 27.11A). It was found that the predictors of the neurologic events included

1. Age over 65 years
2. Diabetes
3. Previous neurologic event
4. Previous cardiac surgery
5. Pulmonary disease
6. Unstable angina at the time of presentation

The more elderly and debilitated patients benefit most from cardiac surgery; yet, they sustain greater overall risk for morbidity and mortality after cardiac surgery.

In a multicentered study of more than 2,100 patients undergoing CABG, Roach et al. (28) reported an incidence of 3.1% Type 1 (focal cerebrovascular accident, transient ischemic attack [TIA], or persistent coma) and 3% Type 2 neurologic dysfunction (neurocognitive dysfunction or encephalopathy) (28). In addition to those factors associated with both types (increased age and hypertension), there were factors uniquely associated with Type 1 (previous neurologic deficit, perioperative hypotension, IABP, and ventricular venting) and Type 2 neurologic dysfunction (alcohol consumption, dysrhythmias, CHF, PVDz, and previous CABG).

TABLE 27.11A	Predictors of Neurologic Dysfunction	
Variable	**Type 1 Deficit Stupor Coma**	**Type 2 Cognitive**
Increased age >65–70	X	X
Proximal aortic atheroma	X (strongest)	
Hypertension	X	X
History of diabetes	X	
COPD	X	
Unstable angina	X	
Prior CNS event	X	
Periop hypotension	X	X
IABP	X	
LV venting	X	
Alcohol history		X
Dysrhythmia		X
Prior CABG		X
Peripheral vascular disease		X
Macroemboli	X	
Macroemboli and microperfusion		X

The strongest predictor of Type 1 neurologic dysfunction post-CABG remains the presence of significant atheroma in the proximal aorta. Currently the indications for epiaortic echo include the presence of atheroma (grade 3 or higher in the descending aorta), any palpable aortic atheroma or calcified aorta, age greater than 65 to 70 years, a history of previous neurologic event, history of coronary artery bypass grafting, presence of PVDz, and presenting with one or more risk factors for atherosclerosis (38a). If those factors reported by Newman and Roach in Table 27.11A (history of diabetes, COPD, unstable angina, prior CNS event, need for LV vent, prior CABG, and PVDz) are combined with current practices, it may assist in identifying patients at higher risk. The use of intraoperative echo (TEE and epiaortic imaging) in the higher risk population provides a strategy to reduce perioperative neurologic dysfunction (Table 27.11B).

TEE can image the descending aorta, arch, and proximal ascending aorta. The site of aortic cannulation is not visualized by TEE, necessitating epiaortic scanning. Importantly palpation of the aorta is not as accurate in assessing severity of atherosclerotic changes in the aorta. Wareing et al. (51) demonstrated that palpation alone was only able to identify 38% of protruding plaques in the aorta. The study population included 500 patients older than 50, undergoing cardiac surgery. The same findings were confirmed by Konstadt et al. (52). The authors demonstrated that palpation of the aorta by the surgeon missed 83% of aortic atheroma detected by TEE or epiaortic scanning. Davila-Roman et al. (53) showed that when compared with epiaortic scanning and TEE, palpation of the aorta significantly underestimates the presence and severity of arteriosclerosis.

Blauth et al. (54) analyzed the autopsies in 221 patients undergoing myocardial revascularization or valve operations. Complete autopsies were performed in 129 patients (58.4%) and limited to the chest and abdomen in the remainder. Embolic disease was identified in 69 patients (31.2%). Atheroemboli or abnormalities consistent with atheroemboli were identified in 48 patients (21.7%). Atheroembolic disease was found in the brain in 16.3% of patients; there was a high correlation of atheroemboli with severe atherosclerosis of the ascending aorta. Atheroembolic events occurred in 46 of 123 patients (37.4%) with severe disease of the ascending aorta but in only 2 of 98 patients (2%) without significant ascending aortic disease ($p < 0.0001$) (55). There was a direct correlation between age, severe atherosclerosis of the ascending aorta, and atheroemboli. Incremental risk factors for atheroembolic disease are PVDz and severe atherosclerosis of the ascending aorta.

Assessment of the Surgical Results

The purpose of the preseparation CPB examination is to assess the degree of recovery of cardiac function and exclude the potential for complications. Issues that are

TABLE 27.11B	Cannulation and Perfusion Strategy
Intraoperative Echo Finding	**Surgical Options**
Proximal ascending atheroma	Off-pump CABG
	Axillary or femoral cannulation
	Identify cross-clamp site or circulatory arrest
	Identify site for antegrade cardioplegia
	Identify site for proximal grafts or all IMA grafts
	Single cross clamp
	Higher perfusion pressures
Ascending and descending atheroma	Axillary cannulation only
	Potential morbidity with IABP
	Higher perfusion pressures
Calcified arteriosclerotic ascending aorta	Off-pump CABG
	Axillary cannulation and circulatory arrest
	Replace ascending aorta
	All arterial grafts
	TMR
	PCI accepting incomplete revascularization
≥Mild aortic regurgitation	Monitor for LV distension
	LV venting
	Consider intercoronary antegrade cardioplegia
	Retrograde cardioplegia more important
	Cooling of heart for added protection
Post-pump localized dissection	Localized repair
	Replace ascending aorta with circulatory arrest

clarified by the TEE examination prior to separation from cardiopulmonary bypass include

1. Assessment of the regional myocardial function in the perfusion beds of the bypassed coronary vessels
2. Detection of significant complications related to cannulation and myocardial protection strategy
3. Assessment of the valve function of valves
4. Guidance of the deairing process

TEE helps identify the optimal time to separate from cardiopulmonary bypass once the heart is completely deaired and ejecting effectively.

As soon as the cross clamp is removed, intraoperative echo may be utilized to evaluate potential distensibility of the LV caused by aortic regurgitation. Until the LVOT is pressurized and the heart is actively ejecting, there may not be complete coaptation of the aortic valve leaflets. If the heart is slow to initiate an intrinsic rhythm and eject on its own, placement of an LV vent may be indicated with significant aortic regurgitation. Intraoperative TEE

provides a reliable method for assessing micro-air that may be distributed to the cerebral circulation or coronary. When simultaneous recordings of intracranial Doppler and TEE visualizing the descending aorta are performed, detection of micro-air emboli in the cerebral circulation is simultaneous with micro-air visualization in the descending thoracic aorta (55). Strategies to prevent further embolization to the coronary arteries or cerebral circulation include increasing the aortic vent flow, emptying the heart, and increasing pump flow, in addition to lowering the head with Trendelenburg positioning so that micro-air will accumulate at the ventricular apex more readily permitting needle aspiration. If waves of micro-air cycle are with the ventilator, ventilation may be transiently disrupted until it clears. Air may also collect at the dome of the LA adjacent to the aortic sinotubular junction or in the left atrial appendage (LAA). Micro-air may be visualized in the proximal right or left main coronary arteries. If this happens, the perfusion pressure can be increased to hasten passage of the micro-air through the circulation.

Aortic Dissection

Aortic dissection is a recognized complication of aortic cannulation and is readily identified by the post-CPB TEE or epicardial imaging. While most cannulation-related dissections are self-limiting, if not detected intraoperatively, they can present catastrophic challenges. Significant ulcerated plaques or ascending aortic disease may lead to the use of alternative cannulation sites.

Post-CPB LV Dysfunction

LV dysfunction following myocardial revascularization is usually associated with pre-CPB LV dysfunction and higher stages of diastolic dysfunction. Poor LV function post-CPB may be predicted by the pre-CPB IOE examination's assessment of diastolic and systolic parameters of LV function in addition to the completeness of myocardial revascularization and length of time spent on the heart-lung machine. Small changes in regional wall function may be indicative of alterations in coronary blood flow to the perfusion bed of the grafted vessels. Micro-air bubbles do cause RWMA, usually in the more superiorly originating right coronary artery.

Valve Dysfunction

Transiently, ischemic MR may occur in the periods preceding and following separation from cardiopulmonary bypass. After a period of equilibration, if the severity of MR persists, standard methods of severity assessment are utilized to direct the surgical decision-making process. If improvement of the underlying ventricular function, regional wall motion, or structural integrity of the MV apparatus is unlikely to improve, returning to CPB and repair or replacement of the MV may be indicated.

Prior to separation from cardiopulmonary bypass, more significant levels of aortic regurgitation may be noted until the heart is completely filled and ejecting. If the heart remains in asystole or is bradycardic with an inability to capture with pacing, the ventricle may distend. Ventricular distension may further contribute to post-CPB LV dysfunction.

Other Applications

IOE may be used to determine the need for or direct the placement of mechanical support device placement such as intra-aortic balloon pump (IABP) or left ventricular assist device (LVAD) (56). When a balloon is placed intraoperatively, the placement wire must be visualized in the aorta to prevent the development of an iatrogenic aortic dissection. Also, correct position of the balloon in the aorta (tip of the balloon below the left subclavian artery) can be verified with TEE.

Outcome Studies Neurologic Dysfunction

Duda et al. (57) compared 195 consecutive CABG patients evaluated by intraoperative surface aortic ultrasonography with 164 control patients in whom the ascending aorta was assessed by inspection and palpation only. Findings from the epiaortic echo led to a modification of the cannulation and perfusion strategy in 19 (10%) patients with hypothermic fibrillatory arrest with no cross-clamping of the aorta and LV venting in 14 patients, modification in the aortic cannulation site or single cross-clamping in three patients, and modification in placement of proximal anastomoses or all arterial grafts in two patients. No strokes occurred in this group and three patients died, yielding an operative mortality rate of 2.6%. In those patients in whom cannulation and perfusion strategy was guided by palpation of the aorta only, there were five strokes (3.0%), and six patients died (3.6%) with stroke contributing to the cause of death in one patient (57). They concluded that IOE (TEE and epivascular imaging) reduced the stroke rate in CABG compared with inspection and palpation of the aorta alone.

Kouchoukos et al. (58) evaluated intraoperative epiaortic detection and treatment of the severely atherosclerotic ascending aorta, which included epiaortic imaging and resection, and graft replacement of the involved segment using hypothermic ischemic arrest. Forty-seven CABG patients had resection and graft replacement of the ascending aorta. It was associated with lower mortality and stroke rates than those that were observed in patients with moderate or severe atherosclerosis in whom only minor modifications in technique were made to avoid embolization of atheroma.

Wareing et al. evaluated 1,200 of 1,334 consecutive patients (>65 years old) with epiaortic scanning of the aorta. Coronary artery disease was present in 88% of the patients, and moderate and severe atherosclerosis of the ascending aorta was found in 19.3% of the patients (51). Strategies for the prevention of perioperative neurologic dysfunction included alteration of the site of arterial cannulation, proximal graft anastomosis, antegrade cardioplegia administration, and replacement of the ascending aorta. There were 33 patients out of 1,200 who had carotid disease. They underwent combined carotid and cardiac surgery. 1,200 patients had 4% 30-day mortality; the stroke rate was 1.6% (51). Type 1 neurologic dysfunction was correlated with the degree of atherosclerosis in the ascending aorta. Interestingly, those patients who underwent replacement of the ascending aorta had no strokes. The stroke rates were higher for 111 patients with moderate or severe ascending aortic disease who had only minor interventions (6.3%) and for 16 patients with severe carotid artery disease who did not have carotid endarterectomy.

Davila-Roman et al. (53) performed epiaortic scanning on 1,200 patients undergoing heart surgery and demonstrated ascending aorta atherosclerosis in 19.3% of patients. Predictors of ascending aorta atherosclerosis were smoking, diffuse coronary disease, and increased age (>50 years old). Patients with neurologic dysfunction were more likely to have significant atherosclerosis in the ascending aorta. In a separate report of epiaortic scanning in 472 patients undergoing on-pump coronary artery bypass grafting surgery following CPB, new lesions in the aorta were found in 3.4% of patients (53). Of the 10 patients with mobile or intramural disruptions post-bypass, 60% were at the site of aortic cross-clamp application and 40% at the point of cannulation of the ascending aorta. Interestingly, atheroma less than 3 mm were associated with a 0.8% incidence of new lesions postbypass, whereas in patients with atheromas 3 to 4 mm (11.8%) and greater than 4 mm (33%) neurologic deficits correlated with the presence of atherosclerosis and new aortic lesions postbypass (53). Evidence from these studies suggest that TEE and epiaortic echocardiography predict stroke rate and help to stratify patient risk for adverse neurologic events in the perioperative period.

Using TEE, Hartman et al. (59) examined the descending aorta of 189 patients undergoing elective CABG surgery. As seen in Table 27.11C, they graded the severity of atheromatous disease as Grade 1 normal (mild intimal thickening), grade 2 (severe thickening <3 mm), grade 3 (atheroma 3–5 mm), grade 4 (protruding atheroma greater than 5 mm), and grade 5 (mobile atheroma). Nine of the 189 patients had stroke within 1 week of surgery. Patients with grade 1 or 2 atheromatous disease on TEE of their descending aorta had no strokes, whereas grade 3 had 5.5%, grade 4 had 10.5%, and grade 5 had 45.5% incidence of stroke. The one-week stroke rate was 5.5% (2/36), 10.5% (2/19), and 45.5% (5/11) for grades 3, 4, and 5 (59–62). For 6-month outcome, advancing aortic atheroma grade was a predictor of stroke (59–62). Atheromatous disease of the descending aorta was a strong predictor of stroke and death after CABG (59–62).

In the higher risk CABG population study performed at the Cleveland Clinic, epiaortic scanning was performed if the descending aorta demonstrated approximately grade 3 in the descending aorta on TEE or the patient was in the high-risk group (38a). If there were mobile plaques in the descending aorta and protruding plaques in the ascending aorta, axillary cannulation was performed. If the aorta was calcified with protruding plaques, axillary cannulation was utilized with circulatory arrest or the patient underwent off-pump coronary bypass. The changes in

cannulation and profusion strategy in the 82 consecutive patients based on echocardiographic examination included three patients who received coronary bypass surgery off pump because of the presence of significant protruding atheroma in the ascending aorta. There were six patients who had axillary cannulation because of concomitant protruding plaques in the descending aorta and ascending aorta (38a). One of these patients underwent circulatory arrest because of the coexistence of a calcified aorta that would preclude cross-clamp. When this study population was compared with a similar high-risk group of patients, without having intraoperative TEE, it was found that the incidence of stroke was three times greater than those patients in whom the cannulation site was based solely on palpation of the ascending aorta (3.8% vs. 1.2%). Epiaortic echocardiography helps to develop the cannulation and perfusion strategy, helps to make an educated decision regarding the need for circulatory arrest or femoral or axillary cannulation, and also guides the need for higher perfusion pressures during cardiopulmonary bypass. It also helps to determine the best location for the placement of the aortic cross clamp, the need for off-pump CABG, and to localize the best site for the proximal coronary graft and cardioplegia cannula.

Leung et al. (63) continuously monitored 50 patients undergoing elective CABG surgery with continuous TEE, ECG, and hemodynamic measurements during the pre-CPB, post-CPB, and 4 hours postoperatively (63). TEE and ECG evidence of ischemia were characterized during each of the periods and were associated with adverse clinical outcomes (postoperative myocardial infarction, ventricular failure, and cardiac death). Myocardial ischemia detected by TEE was predictive of poor outcome with 6 of 18 patients demonstrating ischemia by TEE having adverse cardiac outcomes compared with none of the 32 without such evidence (63). Seventy-six percent of the TEE ischemic episodes occurred without acute change in HR, BP, or PA pressure. It was concluded that the incidence of ECG and TEE ischemia was highest in the postbypass period, and postbypass RWMA were related to postoperative myocardial infarction, ventricular failure, and cardiac death.

Mishra et al. (64) have reported on the value of TEE in 5,016 patients (3,660 CABG patients). Pre-CPB TEE demonstrated findings that helped or modified the surgical plan in 993 of 3,660 CABG patients (27.13%). They reported 3,217 TEE-guided anesthetic-hemodynamic interventions in 944 CABG patients (25.79%) (64). Postbypass TEE identified the need for graft revision in 29 patients (0.8%) and the need for IABP in 29 patients (0.8%). Overall, 38.78% of patients benefited from pre-CPB and 39.16% from post-CPB use of TEE with an alteration of management in 26.7% of CABG patients as compared to 12.5% of those undergoing valve surgery (64).

Eltzschig et al. retrospectively evaluated the impact of pre- and post-CPB TEE on surgical decisions in 12,566 consecutive patients undergoing cardiac surgery (41a). In

TABLE 27.11C	Grading of Aortic Atheroma and Risk of Stroke	

Grade	Stroke	Definition
1	0%	Normal or mild aortic thickening
2	0%	Severe aortic thickening
3	5.6%	Protruding atheroma less than 5 mm in width
4	10.5%	Protruding atheroma over 5 mm in width
5	45.5%	Mobile atheroma

the subset of 3,835 patients undergoing isolated CABG, surgical decisions were influenced by 5.4% of the pre-CPB and 1.5% of the post-CPB TEE examinations. Newly identified pre-CPB TEE findings resulted in the addition of MV/AV procedure (3.3%) and cancellation of surgery (0.1%). Post-CPB TEE results identified the need for graft revision in 0.8% of the cases.

Couture et al. (47) evaluated the use of IOE in 851 patients; 624 (73.3%) of the patients were undergoing CABG. TEE was used to modify therapy in 10% of isolated CABG patients (higher in repeat and MIDCAB) and included four patients who returned to CPB for revision of their bypass grafts, additional valve procedure, ventricular aneurysm resection, LVAD, and detection of micro-air. The clinical impact was higher (39%) in patients undergoing combined CABG and valve procedures compared to isolated CABG (10%). There were unplanned surgical interventions in 30% of the study population and confirmation of the preoperative diagnosis in 34%. The anesthetic-hemodynamic management was altered in 53% of patients including treatment of hypovolemia, myocardial ischemia, and global dysfunction. Interestingly, evaluation of the aorta for atheroma and potential alteration of cannulation and perfusion strategy was not a part of this study (54).

Berquist et al. (48) performed intraoperative TEE in 75 patients undergoing CABG. There were 584 interventions: TEE was most important in 17%, contributed to guidance of fluid administration in 30%, and guided anti-ischemic therapy in 21%. TEE was found to direct critical surgical intervention in 3% of patients (48). Overall, 17% of all interventions were predominantly guided by IOE. The use of TEE and epiaortic imaging for guidance of the cannulation and perfusion strategy was not part of this study. Deutch et al. (65) evaluated 50 consecutive non-risk stratified patients undergoing CABG surgery and found that it was dispensable in 33 patients (66%), informative (22%), valuable (8%), and essential (4%). This included

two patients who had graft occlusion detected post-CPB by new RWMA. Benson and Cahalan (66) provided a projected cost savings of $300 per patient if routinely used in patients undergoing myocardial revascularization. A similar cost benefit analysis by Fanshawe et al. revealed a saving of $230 per patient undergoing cardiac surgery (66a).

In the higher risk Cleveland Clinic study involving 82 consecutive patients, there were 16 (19.5%) patients with undiagnosed valve disease and 16 patients with underdiagnosed valve disease (38a). This led to the adjustment of the anesthetic-hemodynamic management in 34% of the study population. Major alterations in the surgical management of patients occurred in 33% of patients, including performing CABG off-CPB (three patients), axillary cannulation (six patients), circulatory arrest (one patient), rush to bypass (two patients), return to CPB (four patients), and reopening the chest (two patients). Additional valve procedures were precipitated by intraoperative TEE findings in six patients, including mitral valve repair, aortic valve replacement, and pulmonic valve replacement. A transmitral pulmonary vein LV vent was placed in seven patients due to the finding of significant aortic regurgitation. When the higher risk study group, whose management was guided by intraoperative TEE and epivascular imaging, was compared with a similar group that did not receive routine intraoperative echo the outcomes noted in Table 27.12 were obtained. The incidence of hospital deaths, CNS morbidity, and cardiac morbidity were three times greater in those patients who did not receive IOE.

There are a variety of studies that provide a similar analysis of the frequency with which intraoperative echo altered the intraoperative management of patients undergoing CABG surgery. Click et al. (42) reported that only 8% of their patients undergoing CABG received IOE. Thirty-three percent of these patients had new findings pre-CPB and 8% post-CPB. The majority of these patients

TABLE 27.12	Cleveland Clinic Higher Risk CABG Study Intraoperative Echo Versus No Intraoperative Echo Comparison		
Patient and Outcome Variables	No Intraoperative TEE	Diagnostic Intraoperative TEE at Each Stage
Age	64.8	68.4
Number of patients	397	82
Average CCF severity score	5.9	6.1
In-hospital mortality	18 (3.8%)	1 (1.2%)[a]
Perioperative MI	14 (3.5%)	1 (1.2%)[a]
Focal neurologic deficit	18 (3.8%)	1 (1.2%)[a]

[a]Study was not a randomized comparison but relied on retrospective data comparison of similar high-risk patients undergoing CABG surgery during period of study.

were those in whom valve function was to be assessed intraoperatively. No mention was made in this study regarding the risk stratification of their CABG patient population or the cannulation and perfusion strategy guidance by intraoperative echo. Sheikh et al. (46) demonstrated that 2% of patients undergoing CABG had more significant MR than expected.

With the exceptions of the Mishra and the Eltzschig studies, these studies would seem to indicate that IOE may not have a similar impact on the clinical management as the Cleveland Clinic study. Or do they? The remarkable studies referred to above were performed in leading cardiac centers and are extremely valuable contributions to our understanding of the potential impact of intraoperative echo. However, the information that they provide does not apply directly to the prospective Cleveland Clinic study, which was performed by a surgical team utilizing intraoperative echo as a "gold standard" (38a). It is consistently used as a reliable guide in many of the surgical and anesthetic-hemodynamic decisions related to cannulation and myocardial protection, myocardial viability, valve dysfunction, need for off-pump CABG, and mechanical support (LVAD or IABP). The study reported by Click et al. (42) was a retrospective review that included mostly those CABG patients who required an intraoperative assessment of valve dysfunction. In addition, the risk stratification of patients undergoing CABG receiving intraoperative echo was not part of their retrospective analysis. The study reported by Berquist et al. (48) similarly did not include risk stratification or detection of aortic atheroma for modification of the cannulation and perfusion strategy.

For IOE to have an influential impact on patient management and outcome, a number of requirements must be met. These include

1. The need for reliably performed and interpreted intraoperative examination
2. Accurate communication of the information to the surgical and anesthetic-hemodynamic management team
3. A correct understanding of the information in conjunction with the patient preoperative evaluation
4. The correct choice of therapeutic intervention
5. Accurate execution of the surgical intervention

Because of institutional and individual variations in the use of information derived from the intraoperative TEE, it is difficult to accurately compare such decision making and outcome impact data. Ultimately, as our patient population ages and develops greater comorbidity, the perioperative team managing patients undergoing myocardial revascularization will require management strategies that more accurately guide the decision-making process and improve the outcome of our patients.

COMPLICATIONS OF ISCHEMIC HEART DISEASE

There are a number of complications of ischemic heart disease that are seen throughout the perioperative period. Complications that are commonly seen include atrial fibrillation, ischemic MR, rupture of the ventricular septum, LV aneurysm, ventricular pseudo-aneurysm, RV infarction, and LV thrombus (Table 27.13).

TABLE 27.13	Complications of Ischemic Heart Disease Intraoperative Echocardiographic Assessment	
Complication	**Pre-CPB IOE**	**Post-CPB IOE**
Atrial fibrillation	LA or LAA thrombi	Residual LAA thrombi or ligation-flow
LAA thrombus	Spontaneous contrast	Spontaneous contrast
	LAA PW Doppler velocities	LAA PW Doppler velocities
	Increased thrombus <20–30 cm/s	Increased thrombus <20–30 cm/s
	Increased thrombus >5.0 cm	Increased thrombus >5.0 cm^2
	Determine cause LAE	PV Doppler velocities
	MV inflow PW Doppler	LV/RV global-regional Fx
	Pulmonary vein PW Doppler	Cannulation-perfusion complications
	LVH	Document comprehensive examination
Ischemic MR	Severity of MR	Success of MVRep or MVR
	Mechanism of MR (I, IIIb, and/or II)	Post-MVRep SAM
	Annulus diameter (ME 4, LAX, Comm)	Residual second mechanism MR

(continued)

Complication	Pre-CPB IOE	Post-CPB IOE
	Height PMVL:AMVL	RV/LV global-regional Fx
	Coaptation-septal distance	Bypass graft Fx
	Ventricularization of coaptation	Pulmonary HTN reversal
		Document comprehensive examination
LV aneurysm	Location and size of aneurysm	LV/RV global and regional Fx
	Presence of mural thrombus	Bypass graft function
	Interference with MV apparatus	Need for IABP or LVAD
	Interpapillary distance	Pulmonary HTN
	Global and regional LV and RV Fx	MR—2nd to resection
	Tricuspid regurgitation	Ischemic
	LA size, LAA thrombi/contrast	Interpapillary distance
	Diastolic function assessment	Complications cannulation-perfusion
	Cannulation perfusion strategy	Residual thrombus
	Suitability of aorta for IABP	Document comprehensive examination
	Necessity for LVAD support	
	Shunt, AR, RVfx, TR	
Pseudoaneurysm	Location and number of communications	Residual communication
	Pseudoaneurysm flow volume	LV/RV global and regional Fx
	Viability of adjacent myocardium	Mitral or tricuspid regurgitation—2nd to resection
	Global-regional LV/RV Fx	
	Ischemic MR	• Ischemic MR
	Cannulation and perfusion strategy	Interpapillary distance
	Aortic or tricuspid regurgitation	Complications cannulation-perfusion
	Necessity for LVAD support	LV/RV global and regional Fx
	• Shunt, AR, apical thrombi	Pulmonary HTN
	• Aortic atheroma	Document comprehensive examination
VSD	Number, size, and location(s)	Residual VSD flow
	Calculate shunt flow	Residual communication
	LV/RV global-regional Fx	LV/RV global and regional Fx
	Adjacent myocardial viability	Mitral or tricuspid regurgitation—2nd to resection
		• Ischemic MR
		Interpapillary distance
		Complications cannulation-perfusion
		Pulmonary HTN
		Document comprehensive examination
RV infarction	RV global and regional Fx	RV global and regional Fx
	Tricuspid regurgitation	Tricuspid regurgitation
	Pulmonary HTN	Complications cannulation-perfusion
	Hepatic congestion-plethora	Pulmonary HTN
	Shunt potential	LV filling, global and regional Fx
	LV global and regional Fx	Need IABP or RVAD (ECMO) support
	• Inferior and septal segmental Fx	Document comprehensive examination

Atrial Fibrillation

Postoperative atrial fibrillation in CABG surgery occurs in up to 40% of patients and is associated with a significant morbidity (67). Dogan et al. evaluated patients undergoing coronary artery bypass with TEE to determine if there are identifiable risk factors for atrial fibrillation (68). Univariate predictors of atrial fibrillation include advanced age, low ejection fraction, enlargement of left atrium, increased P-wave dispersion, and proBrain natriuretic peptide (68). Because the entire LA is poorly visualized by TEE, the LAA area serves as a marker for LA enlargement. Patients who are in atrial fibrillation at the time of surgery undergo interventions to interrupt the macroreentry or micro-reentry circuit. In patients with paroxysmal atrial fibrillation and without LA enlargement, pulmonary vein isolation is usually performed using radiofrequency ablation. In patients with enlarged left atria, a macro-reentry circuit may emerge. Such patients often require a more comprehensive approach, including the classic Maze operation in addition to pulmonary vein isolation. Atrial fibrillation, secondary to ischemic heart disease, may be associated with LA enlargement and stagnant blood flow in the LAA. For patients undergoing CABG, as seen in Table 27.13, the goal is to determine the propensity for developing atrial fibrillation postoperatively. Because TEE cannot visualize the entire LA consistently, it is difficult to obtain a consistent diameter measurement. Despite these limitations, a LA diameter in the anterior-posterior plane (ME 2-chamber) with a LA diameter greater than 40 cm or indexed area measurement of greater than 2.0 cm/m^2, reduced LAA outflow velocities, presence of spontaneous contrast or thrombi may suggest the need for ligation of the LAA. For patients in atrial fibrillation scheduled for pulmonary vein isolation or Maze, additional measurements also include the LA/RA diameter and circumference as well as PV Doppler velocities are documented for comparison to post-CPB findings. The pulmonary vein PW Doppler velocities are documented for future comparison with suspected pulmonary vein stenosis though more commonly associated with percutaneous ablation procedures. Reduced LAA contractility in patients with atrial fibrillation (AF) has been associated with thrombus formation. LAA function, represented by PW Doppler measurement of LAA outflow velocity, is an important predictor for thrombus formation in patients with nonrheumatic atrial fibrillation. The extent of blood stasis and propensity for thrombus can be assessed during TEE by measurement of the peak PW Doppler velocity of outflow from the LAA. Spontaneous echocardiographic contrast, a swirling pattern of increased blood echogenicity, may be detected by TEE in the left atrium in patients with AF and is associated with blood stasis and a pro-thrombotic state. SEC is associated with an increased risk of systemic thromboembolic events. LA thrombi are associated with a larger LAA, and

decreased LAA outflow velocities (<20–30 cm/s), and a higher prevalence of severe spontaneous LA contrast (69). Interestingly, patients with atrial fibrillation less than 2 weeks have peak ejection velocities of 40 cm/s compared to 10 cm/s for those in atrial fibrillation greater than 2 weeks. Both spontaneous contrast and LA thrombi are associated with reduced outflow velocities of 18 versus 33 cm/s and 10 versus 22 cm/s (69). LAA thrombi were also associated with larger LAA area (5.4 vs. 3.9 cm^2). In patients with spontaneous contrast, reduced peak outflow velocities, and increased LAA area, ligation of the LAA may be considered.

Ischemic Mitral Regurgitation

For a more comprehensive discussion, please refer to Chapters 25, 27, and 28. By definition, ischemic MR is due to myocardial ischemia or infarction with structurally normal valvular leaflets and chordae (70,71). It occurs in 10% to 50% of the cases of myocardial infarction (70,71). However, ischemic MR may also be associated with transient ischemia. The intraoperative echo examination in patients with ischemic MR focuses on determining the mechanism of MV dysfunction in addition to its severity (Table 27.13). There are a number of different mechanisms of ischemic MR (72,73). Included among these mechanisms are papillary muscle rupture (Type II mechanism), apical tethering associated with ischemic cardiomyopathy (symmetrical bileaflet Type IIIb), posterior wall infarcts (asymmetrical posterior mitral valve leaflet [PMVL] Type IIIb), and transient ischemia leading to global dysfunction (central MR, symmetrical Type IIIb) or posterior or anterolateral wall motion abnormality with asymmetrical restriction of the mitral apparatus (asymmetrical IIIb) (74). There are a number of different mechanisms responsible for ischemic MR, including ventricular remodeling leading to a dilated spherical-shaped heart (eccentric remodeling) and/or global dysfunction of the LV with distending of the mitral apparatus and the tethering effect; in these patients, tenting of the mitral valve by the secondary chordae is seen. The risk factors for ischemic MR include an inferior and posterior myocardial infarction causing posterior leaflet restriction and LV dysfunction. The severity of MR depends on LV function; if regurgitation is secondary to a spherical LV remodeling, there is tethering of both mitral leaflets and this tends to produce a central jet of regurgitation (Fig. 27.6). Posterior, inferior, or posterolateral myocardial infarction can produce MR whose mechanism is related to an isolated restriction of the posterior leaflet and an override of the anterior leaflet with a posteriorly directed jet. It is important to keep in mind the influence of LV afterload and the color Doppler gain setting when judging and grading MR. The patients, who have trivial MR, are routinely given a pressor agent to see if this maneuver increases the mitral insufficiency. Intraoperative echo should be utilized to

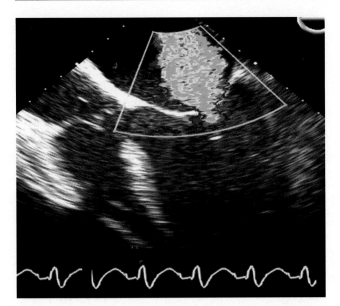

Figure 27.6. Patients with an ischemic cardiomyopathy may develop eccentric remodeling. The development of a more spherically shaped ventricle results in a subvalvular apparatus that symmetrically restricts the anterior mitral valve leaflet (AMVL) and PMVL equally, resulting in a central regurgitant jet.

confirm the presence of MR; however, it should not be used to determine whether a mitral valve repair needs to be performed when the patient has documented significant MR. If, however, there is no MR in the preoperative evaluation and one finds greater than 2 to 3+ MR, these patients will routinely undergo mitral valve annuloplasty or, depending on what the structural abnormality is, other types of repair.

Papillary muscle rupture, an extreme subset of ischemic MR, occurs in 1% of patients with acute myocardial infarction (Fig. 27.7) (75). It is seen 6 to 12 times more frequently in patients with infarcts involving the mid and apical inferior and posterior segments due to the single coronary artery perfusing the posteromedial papillary muscle (75). In contrast, the anterolateral papillary muscle is supplied by a dual blood supply from the circumflex (anterolateral obtuse marginal branch) and LAD (diagonal branch). If there is complete rupture, it usually involves both, because the posteromedial papillary muscle provides chordae to both the medial halves of the anterior and posterior mitral valve leaflets. Patients with ruptured papillary muscles develop the acute onset of pulmonary edema due to severe regurgitation into a noncompliant left atrium. Prior to the era of aggressive surgical management of these patients, the mortality approached 50% (70,71,73,75).

An acute infarct of the tip of the papillary muscle may also lead to an elongation or "ribboning" of the tip of the papillary muscle, which results in elongation of the overall tensile apparatus. This may result in a small focal prolapse of either the anterior or posterior MV leaflet. It is distinguished from that associated with myxomatous degeneration by its association with coronary disease, a small regional wall motion abnormality, or focal fibrosis of the tip of the papillary muscle head (75).

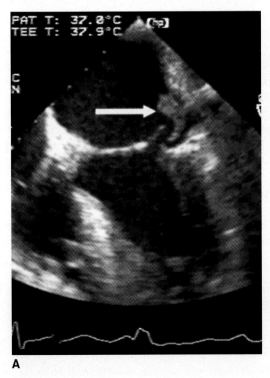

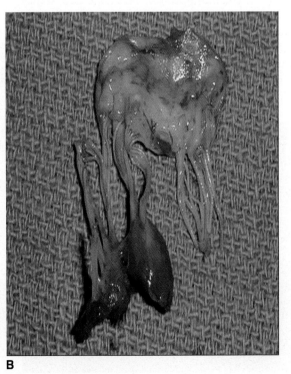

A   **B**

Figure 27.7. Rupture of an ischemic papillary muscle is a rare complication of ischemic heart disease. When it occurs, it most frequently involves the posteromedial papillary muscle due to its solitary blood supply from the posterolateral branch of the circumflex coronary artery as illustrated in this TEE 2D image (**A**) and anatomic specimen (**B**).

LV Aneurysm

Aneurysms of the LV are associated with transmural myocardial infarction and commonly occur in regions of the heart not usually provided with collateralized blood flow. Loop et al. (76) reported a series of patients with true aneurysms and found only 3% to be posterior (inferolateral). In contrast, in a report characterizing 65 consecutive autopsies of true aneurysms, 15 (23%) involved only the posterior wall (inferolateral) (69,70,75–77). Because such infarcts usually involve the posteromedial papillary muscle, the difference may be due to a more fulminate course leading to cardiogenic shock. In autopsy series, Roeske et al. (77) demonstrated an increased likelihood of permission for autopsy in circumstances of more rapid progression of cardiogenic shock. Massive inferoposterior myocardial infarctions are more frequently fatal than extensive anterior infarctions, and patients do not live long enough for aneurysm formation.

Despite their more frequent occurrence in the anteroapical and anteroseptal regions of the heart, they may be seen in the posterobasal (inferolateral basal) and inferoapical segments (Fig. 27.8). An anteroapical aneurysm is an example of mechanical complications following an anterior myocardial infarction in which there is actual thinning of the myocardium and scar formation in the apical region of the LV. It tends to occur in the transmural myocardial infarction and may be associated with the presence of apical thrombus. The apical aneurysm is commonly associated with LAD disease and anterior myocardial infarction (78). The intraoperative TEE examination may be used to guide the resection of the aneurysm. Depending on the size and location of the aneurysm, the ventricle may undergo significant reconstruction. It is important to maintain the various anatomic relations of the components of the mitral apparatus. To guide this process the relation of the aneurysm to the papillary muscles, size of the mitral annulus, interpapillary muscle distance, and regional function adjacent to the aneurysm are important considerations when determining the success of resection of the aneurysm. The echocardiographic characteristics of ventricular aneurysms include thin wall of the myocardium and a very wide neck to the aneurysm as opposed to a pseudoaneurysm, in which the narrowest portion or the aneurysm is at its neck. Usually there is dyskinetic motion of the aneurysmal wall and there may be a thrombus over that dyskinetic region inside the LV. If there is a thrombus present, the apex is hard, and there is no segmented wall motion abnormality, consideration should be given to an eosinophilic syndrome. Also, patients who develop posterobasal (inferolateral basal) aneurysm are prone to develop a thrombus in the aneurysm. Maneuvers that may increase sensitivity of the echocardiography in detecting LV thrombi include the use of echo contrast or B-mode imaging, the use of the highest transducer frequency, focused imaging of the region of interest, and color Doppler imaging.

Pseudoaneurysms

Clinically, pseudoaneurysms usually occur in patients who have ongoing or recurrent angina and hypotension, following a myocardial infarction. Signs of cardiac tamponade may or may not be present. It may be associated with or without cardiac tamponade. Postmyocardial infarction LV pseudoaneurysms occur when the LV rupture is contained by an overlying adherent pericardium (78). Ischemic pseudoaneurysms more frequently occur in the inferior and inferolateral segments of the LV due to the solitary coronary blood supply frequently seen in this region of the heart. Figure 27.9 illustrates a rupture of the inferior myocardium with associated pericardial effusion and thrombus. As seen in Table 27.13, the intraoperative echo examination in patients with pseudoaneurysms provides the surgical team with insight into the viability of the myocardium adjacent to the ventricular rupture. Such would permit a decision to either repair or patch the defect.

Ventricular Septal Defect

Ischemic rupture of the ventricular septum occurs in 1% to 3% of acute myocardial infarctions being evenly distributed between anterior and inferior septal ruptures (70,71,78). Figure 27.10 shows an example of a ventricular septum defect after posterior infarction. The risk factors for developing postinfarction VSD include old age, female gender, previous myocardial infarction, history of hypertension, and presentation 3 to 6 days post-MI (79). There may be single or multiple defects in the ventricular septum and usually is associated with RV dilatation and PA hypertension. The short-term survival of ischemic VSDs is reported within a very wide range between 42% and 75% (79,80). The intraoperative echo examination in

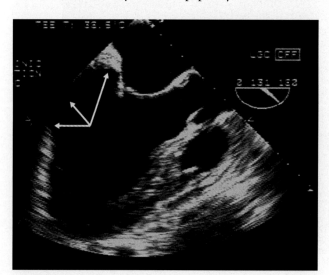

Figure 27.8. Posterobasal Aneurysm. Aneurysms of the LV are associated with transmural infarcts in regions of the heart that are not well collateralized.

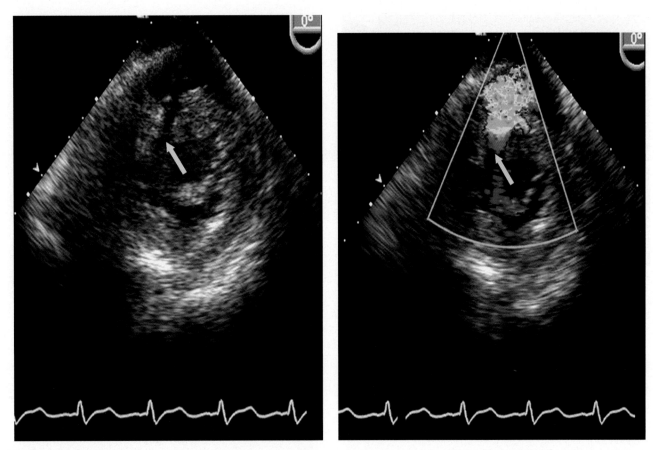

Figure 27.9. Pseudoaneurysm. Postmyocardial infarction LV pseudoaneurysms occur when the ventricular rupture is contained by overlying adherent pericardium.

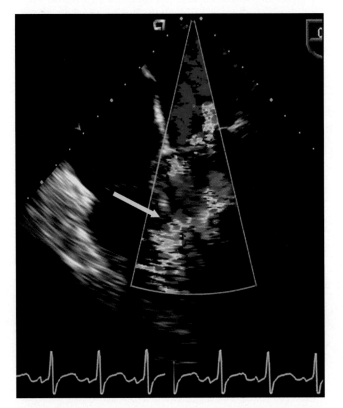

Figure 27.10. Ischemic VSDs occur in 1% to 3% of infarctions (usually within 7 days) and account for 5% of all postinfarction deaths.

patients with an ischemic VSD, is valuable in confirming the number, location, and size of the interventricular communications (Table 27.13). In addition to issues addressed in patients undergoing CABG surgery, determining the viability of myocardium adjacent to the VSD provides the surgical team with an understanding of the extent of the repair and propensity for additional necrotic myocardium, which may undermine the repair.

RV Infarction

RV infarction (Fig. 27.11) occurs in 30% of patients with inferior wall infarction and 25% of patients with posterior wall infarction, and it is associated with lesions in the right coronary artery (81). RV infarction may be associated with pulmonary hypertension and, depending on the degree of involvement of the LV, may result in a dilated LV cavity, which may cause MR. Echocardiographic signs of RV infarct include RV dilatation, decreased function (may be segmental), decreased TV annular motion, bowing of interatrial septum (R to L), and increased RA (81). Because RV infarcts are commonly associated with infarcts of the inferior LV, an understanding of the global and regional functions provides the perioperative team with a better understanding of potential issues that will manifest in the perioperative period. If the patient has LV dysfunction

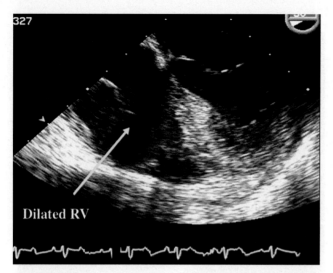

Figure 27.11. RV infarcts occur in 30% of inferior wall myocardial infarcts. Depending on the degree of LV dysfunction, pulmonary hypertension, and RV ischemia or infarction, the clinical manifestations may vary.

leading to pulmonary hypertension, the increased RV afterload will accelerate development of RV dysfunction, tricuspid regurgitation, and hepatic congestion.

FUTURE APPLICATIONS (TABLE 27.14)

While we have made great advances in the intraoperative management of our patients, with the increasingly older population with associated comorbidities, our health care system will be challenged as never before. To meet this challenge in a way that permits us to continue to provide the level of care that is demanded by the public, we will need to provide wiser and more efficient health care to either avoid the costly perioperative complications or recognize those patients who would not benefit from costly medical interventions. Michael Porter of the Harvard Business School understands that innovation is the one affordable solution of the future. Advances that are already in practice in the echocardiography laboratory may provide solutions to many of the most pressing concerns, including the intraoperative assessment of myocardial viability, monitoring of myocardial protection, prevention of neurologic dysfunction, more accurate assessment of renal perfusion, and the prediction of the long-term patency of bypass grafts.

Myocardial Viability

Accurate prediction of myocardial viability following revascularization is important in the higher risk patient for three reasons:

1. It is a predictor of long-term outcome.
2. Additional "wasted" time on cardiopulmonary bypass is required for unnecessary coronary grafts to nonviable tissue.
3. An accurate assessment of postbypass ventricular function is helpful.

Afridi et al. (82) reported on 318 patients undergoing revascularization with severe LV dysfunction and demonstrated that the presence of contractile reserve by dobutamine stress testing was a reliable predictor of survivability following surgical revascularization During the past decade, stress echocardiography has emerged as a safe and sensitive method for the detection of coronary artery disease, and it has been used to provide data for risk stratification during the perioperative period (20,82). The response of regional

TABLE 27.14	Future Applications of Intraoperative Echo	
Concern	**Current**	**Future**
Type 1 neurologic dysfunction	Palpation of aorta and inconsistent epiaortic scanning	Consistent epivascular scanning and intervention
Type 2 neurologic dysfunction	Palpation of aorta	Epivascular scanning
	TEE-guided micro-air clearance	Transcranial Doppler
Myocardial viability	Preoperative MRI, nuclear or dobutamine stress, spect scan	Intraoperative dobutamine stress test and contrast perfusion
Renal perfusion	Urine output	Renal ultrasound-guided intervention
Myocardial protection	Retrograde pressures	Contrast demonstration of myocardial plegia flow
	Appearance of retrograde blood	
	Antegrade resistance	
Prediction of long-term graft patency	RWMA or ischemia	Graft Doppler flow velocities and resistances
		Contrast perfusion intensity and washout

LV function to dobutamine is useful to characterize myocardium. In the therapeutic dose range, (5–20 μg/kg/min) CO is augmented by an increase in ventricular contractility, HR, and SV, and a β2-mediated decrease in systemic vascular resistance. Contractility increases at higher doses (20–40 μg/kg/min). Normal resting wall motion and the development of hyperdynamic function with increasing doses of dobutamine are hallmarks of normally perfused myocardium. The development of new wall motion abnormalities or the worsening of baseline systolic dysfunction with escalating doses of dobutamine increases myocardial ischemia. Contractile reserve, on the other hand, is consistent with viability and characterized by baseline wall motion abnormalities that improve with low-dose dobutamine (83,84). When such a low-dose augmentation of function is followed by progressive systolic dysfunction with higher doses (biphasic response), the accuracy of predicting postoperative cardiac morbidity or changes in regional function after revascularization is enhanced (82). Regional segments that remain akinetic (or dyskinetic) despite dobutamine infusion are nonviable. Dobutamine stress echocardiography has a high sensitivity (85%) and specificity (88%) when compared to angiography in patients with recent myocardial infarction (82).

Aronson et al. (85) performed intraoperative low-dose dobutamine stress echocardiography in 40 patients scheduled for elective CABG surgery for regional wall motion evaluation at four stages: baseline (after induction and intubation), with administration of low-dose dobutamine before cardiopulmonary bypass, after separation from cardiopulmonary bypass (early), and after administration of protamine (late). They analyzed 560 segments for 40 patients corresponding to these stages. Changes in myocardial function following low-dose dobutamine were highly predictive for early ($p < 0.0001$) and late ($p < 0.0001$) changes in myocardial function from baseline regional scores (86). It was also found that the positive predictive value of improved regional wall motion after CABG did not vary with LVEF, a history of myocardial infarction, or beta-blocker use. This study demonstrated the potential value of intraoperative dobutamine stress echocardiography to fine-tune the placement of grafts in patients in whom a decision has been made to proceed with CABG surgery without preoperative viability testing (Fig. 27.12). When combined with myocardial contrast perfusion imaging, this will permit the identification of hypoperfused regions prior to the patient's leaving the operating room (Fig. 27.13).

A second emerging imaging technique involves real-time myocardial contrast perfusion imaging (RTMCI). The intravenous injection of microbubbles (<10 μm) with the ability to cross the pulmonary circulation allows

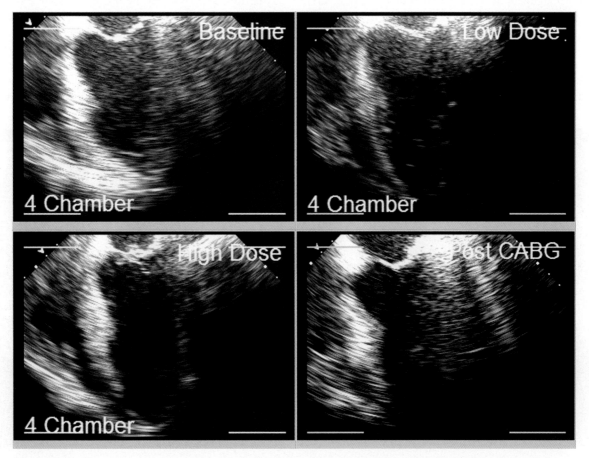

Figure 27.12. Intraoperative dobutamine stress echocardiography may provide an efficient strategy for determining myocardial viability in higher risk patients undergoing surgical revascularization.

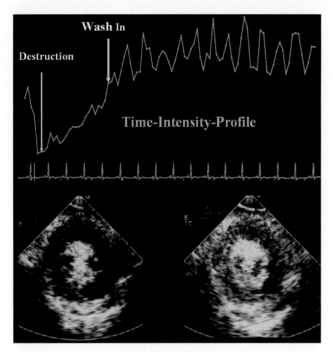

Figure 27.13. Intraoperative MCE may provide an opportunity to verify immediate and long-term graft patency by assessing various MCE parameters. These include baseline perfusion, wash-in flow rate, flow, and degree of collateralization.

real-time imaging of the microvascular blood flow to various regions of the heart (87). This imaging modality can be combined with dobutamine stress to simultaneously assess myocardial wall motion and perfusion. Several recent studies have demonstrated the role of RTMCI in detecting myocardial viability in acute myocardial infarct patients (88, 89, 90) with favorable results.

Main et al. specifically evaluated the in patients with a recent myocardial infarction and residual wall motion abnormalities within the distribution of the infarct-related artery, whether normal perfusion by myocardial contrast echocardiography (MCE) would accurately predict recovery of segmental left ventricular (LV) function (91). The investigators reported that normal or patchy perfusion predicted segmental recovery of function with SENSITIVITY of 77%, SPECIFICITY of 83%, positive predictive VALUE of 90%, negative predictive VALUE of 63%, and overall ACCURACY of 79%. Additionally, 90% of perfused segments improved, while the majority of nonperfused segments remained unchanged. Although utility of RTMCI has yet to be evaluated specifically for CABG patients in the intraoperative setting, above studies indicate the potential that the accurate identification of hypoperfused regions prior to the patient's leaving the operating room will become the standard of care.

Cardioplegia Administration

To demonstrate the ability of intraoperative contrast echocardiography to accurately predict antegrade cardioplegia distribution in patients undergoing CABG procedures, Aronson et al. (92) recorded intraoperative TEE images of the RV free wall, apex, and intraventricular septum. This was done before and following the injection of 4 cc of contrast into antegrade and retrograde cardioplegic catheters during cardioplegia delivery. When the observed cardioplegia distribution (by myocardial contrast echocardiography [MCE]) was compared with the predicted cardioplegia distribution, it was shown that antegrade cardioplegia delivery was distributed to the RV

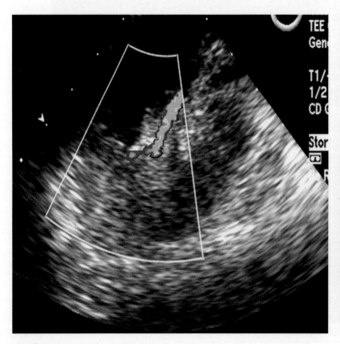

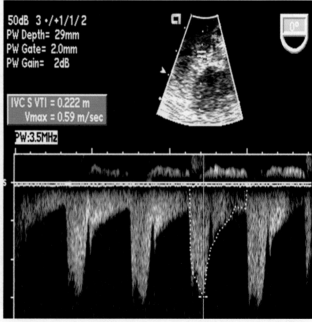

Figure 27.14. Intraoperative monitoring of renal perfusion, utilizing PW Doppler, may provide a means of assessing optimal renal perfusion pressure and response to pharmacologic interventions perioperative renal function.

in 31% of patients, despite 100% occlusion of the right coronary artery (93). Interestingly retrograde cardioplegia delivery to the RV occurred only 20% of the time (92). This study demonstrated the potential for MCE to guide the intraoperative administration of cardioplegia in the higher risk patient in whom myocardial protection may determine the success or failure of the patient's surgical intervention.

End Organ Perfusion

Renal Perfusion

Despite the many advances in nephrology and renal ultrasound, the intraoperative assessment of renal perfusion continues to rely on the historic indicator of urine output. Given the increased complexity of patients with chronic hypertension and diffuse noncoronary atherosclerosis, we will need to consider methods to continuously assess renal blood flow to initiate therapeutic measures in low-flow states (Fig. 27.14). Garwood et al. (94) performed renal ultrasound utilizing intraoperative TEE. They obtained Doppler-derived indices of renal blood flow (pulsatility index and resistive index) by obtaining 2D images of renal parenchyma and Doppler measurement of intrarenal arterial blood flow during IMA dissection before and after a 20-minute infusion of 2 μg/kg/min dopamine. Following infusion of dopamine, they demonstrated an increased velocity of systolic, diastolic, and mean renal blood flow velocity indicating an increase in renal blood flow from baseline (94). The pulsatility and resistive index decreased indicating a reduction in renal vascular resistance. This study clearly demonstrated the potential to utilize intraoperative TEE to acquire 2D images of the kidney and monitor renal arterial Doppler velocities during cardiac surgery. By providing a guide during such interventions, MAP and pump, flow may be optimized while on CPB. In addition, renal perfusion may be assessed following the initiation of dopamine or other vasoactive medications.

Transcranial Doppler and CNS Function

The utility of transcranial Doppler (TCD) in preventing Type II brain injury during CABG was demonstrated by Edmonds et al. in their retrospective study of 332 patients (95). TCD was utilized to detect cerebral hypoperfusion characterized by a decline in middle cerebral artery blood flow velocity to <20% of pre-incision baseline. When compared to the control group, those that received intervention (pharmacologic increase in MAP or increase in pump flow) had a reduction of type II injury (3.0% expected vs. 0.3% observed, P < .001).

Intraoperative TCD monitoring has also been used to detect microembolic phenomena during various stages of coronary artery bypass grafting. To determine the relation between transcranial Doppler and early neuropsychologic deficits, Sylivris et al. (96) correlated MRI findings with microembolic numbers during the bypass period in 41 consecutive patients undergoing coronary bypass grafting. Transcranial Doppler monitoring confirmed that most microemboli occurred during cardiopulmonary bypass and demonstrated a correlation between early neuropsychological deficit post-CABG with total microembolic load during bypass (86). This study indicates the potential that transcranial Doppler may some day be used to routinely monitor the intraoperative detection of microemboli during surgical manipulation of the aorta and events related to cannulation and perfusion strategy.

KEY POINTS

- Despite the many remarkable advances in the management of patients with coronary artery disease, ischemic heart disease remains the leading cause of death in the United States and the world. It is projected to remain so at least through 2020.
- The concept of myocardial revascularization has gone through a number of evolutionary phases from initial observations detailing the coronary anatomy and microvasculature to early experimental coronary artery bypass, early attempts at indirect and direct myocardial revascularization, the modern era of surgical coronary artery bypass relying on arterial conduits, and PCIs.
- Patient decisions regarding the mode of revascularization are driven by multiple factors, including the scientific body of evidence comparing surgical and percutaneous revascularization, the public's perception equating the most recent technology with better care, the patient's innate desire to avoid traditional surgery, and variation of institutional capabilities in surgical and percutaneous revascularization.
- Because of the rapid evolution of myocardial revascularization technology and the numbers of ongoing trials comparing the different approaches, the physicians responsible for patients' perioperative care need to stay abreast of the scientific information and latest innovations that serve as the basis for our patients' decisions.
- There are inherent difficulties in established indication guidelines for surgical and percutaneous revascularization. For example:
  - Randomized trials comparing these approaches are lengthy due to the different time intervals for recurrent disease requiring repeat revascularization for CABG (8–10 years) compared to PCI (1–5 years).
  - Trials are overpowered with lower risk patients with a low incidence of hard outcomes (death, MI, or stroke).

■ The ongoing evolution of new developments in both approaches to revascularization translates into the results of randomized trials always lagging behind the current generation of technology.

■ Difficulties in having comparable patient groups in randomized trials comparing revascularization approaches due to the many definable and indefinable risk factors that impact patient outcome.

■ Factors contributing to higher patient risk in myocardial revascularization include those factors related to a characterization of their manifestations of ischemic heart disease and the patients overall health. While some risk factors are easily defined and more readily subjected to statistical correlation with outcome (EF, number of coronary arteries involved, history of diabetes, etc.), others are more difficult to define but often are extremely important in determining the patient's eventual outcome (suitable conduits, diffuseness of distal disease, and collateral coronary flow).

■ Definable cardiovascular risk factors include age, ventricular function, number and location of coronary disease, PVDz, disease emergent operation, diabetes (insulin and non–insulin dependent) degree of aortic atherosclerosis, and the presence of structural complications of ischemic heart disease (MR, aneurysms, VSD, and pseudoaneurysm). Among the cardiac risk factors that are more difficult to define are degree of collateral, distal coronary flow, diffuseness of coronary disease, availability and quality of conduits, extent of non-coronary atherosclerosis, institutional experience, and operator dependent risks.

■ In addition to providing an ongoing method of monitoring the patient's cardiovascular function, IOE is used to address a number of critical issues that may influence the outcome of the coronary bypass surgery. These critical issues include the development of the cannulation-perfusion strategy to prevent neurologic dysfunction, the diagnosis of previously unrecognized cardiovascular abnormalities requiring surgical intervention or alteration of the patient's anesthetic-hemodynamic management, an assessment of the surgical procedure, and a final documentation of a comprehensive baseline study for future comparison.

■ Future daily applications of intraoperative echo in the higher risk coronary bypass patient may include intraoperative viability assessment, assessment of the effectiveness of cardioplegia administration, monitoring of renal perfusion and CNS embolic load, and an immediate prediction of long-term graft survival by coronary flow characterization.

REFERENCES

1. Parry CH. *An Inquiry into the Symptoms and Causes of the Syncope Anginosa Commonly Called Angina Pectoris, Illustrated by Dissections.* Bath: R. Cruttwell; London: Cadell and Davis, 1799.
2. Heberden W. *Commentaries on the History and Cure of Diseases.* News-gate: London: T. Payne, 1802. Pectoris dolor in Chapter 70:362–368.
3. Schoen FJ, Padera RF Jr. Cardiac surgical pathology. In: Cohn LH, Edmunds LH Jr, eds. *Cardiac Surgery in the Adult.* New York: McGraw-Hill, 2003:119–185.
4. Carrell A. On the experimental surgery of the thoracic aorta and the heart. *Ann Surg* 1910;52:83.
5. Shumacker HB Jr. *The Evolution of Cardiac Surgery.* Bloomington: Indiana University Press, 1992.
6. Favaloro RG. Saphenous vein autograft replacement of severe segmental coronary artery occlusion: operative technique. *Ann Thorac Surg* 1968;5:334.
7. Effler DB, Favaloro RG, Groves LK. Coronary artery surgery utilizing saphenous vein graft techniques. Clinical experience with 224 operations. *J Thorac Cardiovasc Surg* 1970;59(1):147–154.
8. Favaloro RG, Effler DB, Groves LK, et al. Direct myocardial revascularization with saphenous vein autograft. Clinical experience in 100 cases. *Dis Chest* 1969;56(4):279–283.
9. Eagle KA, Guyton RA, Davidoff R, et al. ACC/AHA 2004 guideline update for coronary artery bypass graft surgery: a report of the American College of Cardiology/American Heart Association Task Force on Practice Guidelines (Committee to Update the 1999 Guidelines for Coronary Artery Bypass Graft Surgery). *Circulation* 2004;110(14):e340–437.
10. Sundt TM III, Gersh BJ, Smith HC. Indications for coronary revascularization. In: Cohn LH, Edmunds LH Jr, eds. *Cardiac Surgery in the Adult.* New York: McGraw-Hill;2003:541–559.
11. Lytle BW. The role of coronary revascularization in the treatment of ischemic cardiomyopathy. *Ann Thorac Surg* 2003;75:S2–S5.
12. Lytle BW. Coronary artery reoperations. In: Cohn LH, Edmunds LH Jr, eds. *Cardiac Surgery in the Adult.* New York: McGraw-Hill, 2003:659–679.
13. Herlitz J, Brandrup G, Haglid M, et al. Death, mode of death, morbidity, and rehospitalization after coronary artery bypass grafting in relation to occurrence of and time since a previous myocardial infarction. *Thorac Cardiovasc Surg* 1997;45(3):109–113.
14. Tu JV, Sykora K, Naylor CD. Steering Committee of the Cardiac Care Network of Ontario. Assessing the outcomes of coronary artery bypass graft surgery: how many risk factors are enough? *J Am Coll Cardiol* 1997;30:1317–1323.
15. Hannan EL, Kilburn H, O'Donnell JF, et al. Adult open heart surgery in New York State: an analysis of risk factors and hospital mortality rates. *JAMA* 1990;264:2768–2774.
16. Jones RH, Hannan EL, Hammermeister KE, et al., for the Working Group Panel on the Cooperative CABG Database Project. Identification of preoperative variables needed for risk adjustment of short-term mortality after coronary artery bypass graft surgery. *J Am Coll Cardiol* 1996;28:1478–1487.
17. The VA Cooperative Study Group. Eighteen-year follow-up in the Veterans Affairs Cooperative Study of coronary artery bypass surgery for stable angina. *Circulation* 1992;86:121–130.
18. Alderman EL, Bourassa MG, Cohen LS, et al. Ten year follow-up of survival and myocardial infarction in the randomized Coronary Artery Surgery Study. *Circulation* 1990;82:1629–1646.

19. Uretsky BF, Thygesen K, Armstrong PW, et al. Acute coronary findings at autopsy in heart failure patients with sudden death. Results from the assessment of treatment with lisinopril and survival (ATLAS) trial. *Circulation* 2000;102:611–616.

20. Allman KC, Shaw LJ, Hachamovitch R, et al. Myocardial viability testing and impact of revascularization on prognosis in patients with coronary artery disease and left ventricular dysfunction: a meta-analysis. *J Am Coll Cardiol* 2002;39:1151–1158.

21. Kozak LJ, Lees KA, DeFrances CJ. Annual summary with detailed diagnosis and procedure data: National Hospital Discharge Survey, 2003. *Vital and Health Statistics Series 13*. May 2006;(160):1–206.

22. Pearson TA, Smith SC, Poole-Wilson P. Cardiovascular specialty societies and the emerging global burden of cardiovascular disease: a call to action. *Circulation* 1998;97:602–604.

23. Center for Disease Control and Prevention. Public health and aging: trends in aging—United States and worldwide. *JAMA* 2003:289(11):1371–1373.

24. Frye RL, Kronmal R, Schaff HV, et al., for the participants in the Coronary Artery Surgery Study. Stroke in coronary artery bypass graft surgery: an analysis of the CASS experience. *Int J Cardiol* 1992;36:213–221.

25. Antunes PE, Prieto D, Ferrão de Oliveira J, Antunes MJ. Renal dysfunction after myocardial revascularization. *Eur J Cardiothorac Surg* April 2004;25(4):597–604.

26. Gardner TJ, Horneffer PJ, Manolio TA, et al. Stroke following coronary artery bypass grafting: a ten-year study. *Ann Thorac Surg* 1985;40:574–581.

27. Mangano DT. Cardiovascular morbidity and CABG surgery—a perspective: epidemiology, costs, and potential therapeutic solutions. *J Card Surg* 1995;10:366–368.

28. Roach GW, Kanchuger M, Mangano CM, et al., for the Multicenter Study of Perioperative Ischemia Research Group and the Ischemia Research and Education Foundation Investigators. Adverse cerebral outcomes after coronary bypass surgery. *N Engl J Med* 1996;335:1857–1863.

29. Higgins T, Estafanous FG, Loop FD, et al. Stratification of morbidity and mortality by preoperative risk factors in coronary artery bypass patients. *JAMA* 1992;267:2344–2348.

30. US Census Bureau. US Population Estimates by Age, Sex, Race, and Hispanic Origin: 1990 to 1999. Washington, DC: US Census Bureau, April 11, 2000

31. Bonow RO, Smaha LA, Smith SC, et al. World Heart Day 2002: the international burden of cardiovascular disease: responding to the emerging global epidemic. *Circulation* 2002;106(13):1602–1605.

32. Ferguson BT, Hammill BG, Peterson ED, et al. A decade of change—risk profiles and outcomes for isolated coronary artery bypass grafting procedures, 1990–1999: a report from the STS National Database Committee and the Duke Clinical Research Institute. *Ann Thorac Surg* 2002;73:480–489.

33. Marwick TH. Use of standard imaging techniques for prediction of post revascularization functional recovery in patients with heart failure. *J Cardiac Failure* 1999;5:334–346.

34. Bonow RO. Myocardial viability and prognosis in patients with ischemic left ventricular dysfunction. *J Am Coll Cardiol* 2002;39:1159–1162.

35. Rafferty T, Durkin M, Hines RL, et al. The relationship between "normal" transesophageal color-flow Doppler-defined tricuspid regurgitation and thermodilution right ventricular ejection fraction measurements. *J Cardiothorac Vasc Anesth* 1993;7(2):167–174.

36. Clements FM, Harpole DH, Quill T, et al. Estimation of left ventricular volume and ejection fraction by two-dimensional transesophageal echocardiography: comparison of short axis imaging and simultaneous radionuclide angiography. *Br J Anaesth* 1990;64:331.

37. Sohn DW, Shin GJ, Oh JK, et al. Role of transesophageal echocardiography in hemodynamically unstable patients. *Mayo Clinic Proc* 1995;70(10):925–931.

38. Bernard F, Denault A, Babin D, Goyer C, Couture P, Couturier A, Buithieu J. Diastolic dysfunction is predictive of difficult weaning from cardiopulmonary bypass. *Anesth Analg* 2001 Feb;92(2):291–298.

38a. Savage RM, Lytle BW, Aronson S, et al. Intraoperative echocardiography is indicated in high-risk coronary artery bypass grafting. *Ann Thorac Surg* 1997;64:368–373.

39. Savage RM, Guth B, White F, et al. Correlation of regional myocardial blood flow and function with myocardial infarct size during acute ischemia in the conscious pig. *Circulation* 1981;64:284–290.

40. van Daele ME, Sutherland GR, Mitchell MM, et al. Do changes in pulmonary capillary wedge pressure adequately reflect myocardial ischemia during anesthesia? A correlative preoperative hemodynamic, electrocardiographic, and transesophageal echocardiographic study. *Circulation* 1990;81(3):865–871.

41. Smith JS, Cahalan MK, Benefiel DJ, et al. Intraoperative detection of myocardial ischemia in high-risk patients: electrocardiography versus two-dimensional transesophageal echocardiography. *Circulation* 1985;72(5):1015–1021.

41a. Eltzschig HK, Rosenberger P, Löffler M, Fox JA, Aranki SF, Shernan SK. Impact of intraoperative transesophageal echocardiography on surgical decisions in 12,566 patients undergoing cardiac surgery. *Ann Thorac Surg* 2008 Mar;85(3):845–852.

42. Click RL, Abel MD, Schaff HV. Intraoperative transesophageal echocardiography: 5-year prospective review of impact on surgical management. *Mayo Clin Proc* 2000;75(3):241–247.

43. Cohn LH, Rizzo RJ, Adams DH, et al. The effect of pathophysiology on the surgical treatment of ischemic mitral regurgitation: operative and late risks of repair versus replacement. *Eur J Cardiothorac Surg* 1995;9:568–574.

44. Grewal KS, Malkowski MJ, Piracha AR, et al. Effect of general anesthesia on the severity of mitral regurgitation by transesophageal echocardiography. *Am J Cardiol* 2000 Jan 15;85(2):199–203.

45. Bach DS, Deeb GM, Bolling SF. Accuracy of intraoperative transesophageal echocardiography for estimating the severity of functional mitral regurgitation. *Am J Cardiol* 1995;76(7):508–512.

46. Sheikh KH, de Bruijn NP, Rankin JS, et al. The utility of transesophageal echocardiography and Doppler color flow imaging in patients undergoing cardiac valve surgery. *J Am Coll Cardiol* 1990;15:363–372.

46a. Shiran A, Merdler A, Ismir E, et al. Intraoperative transesophageal echocardiography using a quantitative dynamic loading test for the evaluation of ischemic mitral regurgitation. *J Am Soc Echocardiogr* 2007 Jun;20(6):690–697.

47. Couture P, Denault AY, McKenty S, et al. Impact of routine use of intraoperative transesophageal echocardiography during cardiac surgery. *Can J Anesth* 2000;47:20–26.

48. Bergquist BD, Bellows WH, Leung JM. Transesophageal echocardiography in myocardial revascularization: II. Influence on intraoperative decision making. *Anesth Analg* 1996;82:1139–1145.

49. Murkin JM, Martzke JS, Buchan AM. A randomized study of the influence of perfusion technique and pH management

strategy in 316 patients undergoing coronary artery bypass surgery. II. Neurologic and cognitive outcomes. *J Thorac Cardiovasc Surg* 1995;110(2):349–362.

50. Newman MF, Wolman R, Kanchuger M, et al. Multicenter preoperative stroke risk index for patients undergoing coronary artery bypass graft surgery. Multicenter Study of Perioperative Ischemia (McSPI) Research Group. *Circulation* 1996;94(9 Suppl.):II74–II80.

51. Wareing TH, Davila-Roman VG, Daily BB, et al. Strategy for the reduction of stroke incidence in cardiac surgical patients. *Ann Thorac Surg* 1993;55(6):1400–1407; discussion 1407–1408.

52. Konstadt SN, Reich DL, Quintana C, et al. The ascending aorta: how much does transesophageal echocardiography see? *Anesth Analg* 1994;78:240–244.

53. Davila-Roman VG, Barzilai B, Wareing TH, et al. Atherosclerosis of the ascending aorta. Prevalence and role as an independent predictor of cerebrovascular events in cardiac patients. *Stroke* 1994;25(10):2010–2016.

54. Blauth CI, Cosgrove DM, Webb BW, et al. Atheroembolism from the ascending aorta. An emerging problem in cardiac surgery. *J Thorac Cardiovasc Surg* 1992;103(6):1104–1111; discussion 1111–1112.

55. Abu-Omar Y, Balacumaraswami L, Pigott DW, et al. Solid and gaseous cerebral microembolization during off-pump, on-pump, and open cardiac surgery procedures. *J Thorac Cardiovasc Surg* 2004;127(6):1759–1765.

56. Scalia GM, McCarthy PM, Savage RM, et al. Clinical utility of echocardiography in the management of implantable ventricular assist devices. *J Am Soc Echocardiogr* 2000;13(8):754–763.

57. Duda AM, Letwin LB, Sutter FP, et al. Does routine use of aortic ultrasonography decrease the stroke rate in coronary artery bypass surgery? *J Vasc Surg* 1995;21:98–107.

58. Kouchoukos NT, Wareing TH, Daily BB, et al. Management of the severely atherosclerotic aorta during cardiac operations. *J Cardiac Surg* 1994;9(5):490–494.

59. Hartman GS, Yao FS, Bruefach M III, et al. Severity of aortic atheromatous disease diagnosed by transesophageal echocardiography predicts stroke and other outcomes associated with coronary artery surgery: a prospective study. *Anesth Analg* 1996;83(4):701–708.

60. Katz ES, Tunick PA, Rusinek H, et al. Protruding aortic atheroma predicts stroke in elderly patients undergoing cardiopulmonary bypass; experience with intraoperative transesophageal echocardiography. *J Am Coll Cardiol* 1992;20:70–77.

61. Ribakove GH, Katz ES, Galloway AC, et al. Surgical implications of transesophageal echocardiography to grade the atheromatous aortic arch. *Ann Thorac Surg* 1992;53:758–763.

62. Tunick PA, Perez JL, Kronzon I. Protruding atheromas in the thoracic aorta and systemic embolization. *Ann Intern Med* 1991;115:423–427.

63. Leung JM, O'Kelly B, Browner WS, et al. Prognostic importance of post bypass regional wall motion abnormalities in patients undergoing coronary artery bypass surgery. *Anesthesiology* 1989;71:16.

64. Mishra M, Chauhan R, Sharma KK, et al. Real-time intraoperative transesophageal echocardiography—how useful? Experience of 5,016 cases. *J Cardiothorac Vasc Anesth* 1998;12(6):625–632.

65. Deutsch J II, Curtius JM, Leischik R, et al. Diagnostic value of transesophageal echocardiography in cardiac surgery. *Thorac Cardiovasc Surg* 1991;39:199–204.

66. Benson MJ, Cahalan MK. Cost-benefit analysis of transesophageal echocardiography in cardiac surgery. *Echocardiography* 1995;12:171–183.

66a. Fanshawe M, Ellis C. Habib S et al. A retrospective analysis of the costs and benefits related to alterations in cardiac surgery from routine intraoperative transesophageal echocardiography. *Anesth Analg* 2002 Oct;95(4):824–827.

67. Cox JL. A perspective of postoperative atrial fibrillation in cardiac operations. *Ann Thorac Surg* 1993;56:405–409.

68. Dogan SM, Buyukates M, Kandemir O, et al. Predictors of atrial fibrillation after coronary artery bypass surgery. *Coron Artery Dis* 2007 Aug;18(5):327–331.

69. Rubin DN, Katz SE, Riley MF, et al. Evaluation of left atrial appendage anatomy and function in recent-onset atrial fibrillation by transesophageal echocardiography. *Am J Cardiol* 1996;8(7):774–778.

70. Agnihotri AK, Madsen JC, Daggett WM Jr. Surgical treatment of complications of acute myocardial infarction: postinfarction ventricular septal defect and free wall rupture. In: Cohn LH, Edmunds LH Jr, eds. *Cardiac Surgery in the Adult.* New York: McGraw-Hill, 2003:681–714.

71. Reeder GS. Identification and treatment of complications of myocardial infarction, *Mayo Clin Proc* 1995;70:880–884.

72. Gillinov AM, Wierup PN, Blackstone EH, et al. Is repair preferable to replacement for ischemic mitral regurgitation? *J Thorac Cardiovasc Surg* 2001;122:1125.

73. Barbour DJ, Roberts WC. Rupture of a left ventricular papillary muscle during acute myocardial infarction: analysis of 22 necropsy patients. *J Am Coll Cardiol* 1986; 8(3):558.

74. Carpentier A. Cardiac valve surgery: the French correction. *J Thorac Cardiovasc Surg* 1983;86:323.

75. Gorman RC, Gorman JH III, Edmunds LH Jr. Ischemic mitral regurgitation. In: Cohn LH, Edmunds LH Jr, eds. *Cardiac Surgery in the Adult.* New York: McGraw-Hill, 2003:751–769.

76. Loop FD, Effler DB, Webster JS, et al. Posterior ventricular aneurysms: etiologic factors and results of surgical treatment. *N Engl J Med* 1973;288:237–233.

77. Roeske WR, Savage RM, O'Rourke R, et al. Clinicopathologic correlation in patients after myocardial infarction. *Circulation* 1981;63:36–45.

78. Brown, SL, Gropler RJ, Harris KM, et al. Distinguishing left ventricular aneurysm from pseudoaneurysm: a review of the literature. *Chest* 1997;111:1403–1409.

79. Kitamura S, Mendez A, Kay JH. Ventricular septal defect following myocardial infarction: experience with surgical repair through a left ventriculotomy and review of the literature. *J Thorac Cardiovasc Surg* 1971;61:186.

80. Lundberg S, Sodestrom J. Perforation of the interventricular septum in myocardial infarction: a study based on autopsy material. *Acta Med Scand* 1962;172:413.

81. Zehender MK, Kauder ES, Schonthaler M, et al. Right ventricular infarction as an independent predictor of prognosis after acute inferior myocardial infarction. *N Engl J Med* 1993;328:981–988.

82. Afridi I, Grayburn PA, Panza JA, et al. Myocardial viability during dobutamine echocardiography predicts survival in patients with coronary artery disease and severe left ventricular systolic dysfunction. *J Am Coll Cardiol* 1998;32:921–926.

83. Seeberger MD, Skarvan K, Buser P, et al. Dobutamine stress echocardiography to detect inducible demand ischemia in anesthetized patients with coronary artery disease. *Anesthesiology* 1998;88(5):1233–1239.

84. Leung JM, Bellows WH, Pastor D. Does intraoperative evaluation of left ventricular contractile reserve predict myocardial viability? A clinical study using dobutamine stress echocardiography in patients undergoing coronary artery bypass graft surgery. *Anesth Analg* 2004;99:647–654.

85. Aronson S, Dupont F, Savage R, et al. Changes in regional myocardial function after coronary artery bypass graft surgery are predicted by intraoperative low-dose dobutamine echocardiography. *Anesthesiology* 2000;93(3):685–692.

86. Edmonds HL Jr, Rodriguez RA, Audenaert SM, et al. The role of neuromonitoring in cardiovascular surgery. *J Cardiothorac Vasc Anesth* 1996;10:15–23.

87. Elhendy A, Porter TR. Assessment of myocardial perfusion with real-time myocardial contrast echocardiography: methodology and clinical applications. *J Nucl Cardiol.* 2005 Sep-Oct;12(5):582–590. Review.

88. Balcells E, Powers ER, Lepper W, et al. Detection of myocardial viability by contrast echocardiography in acute infarction predicts recovery of resting function and contractile reserve. *J Am Coll Cardiol.* 2003 Mar 5;41(5):827–833.

89. Janardhanan R, Moon JC, Pennell DJ, Senior R. Myocardial contrast echocardiography accurately reflects transmurality of myocardial necrosis and predicts contractile reserve after acute myocardial infarction. *Am Heart J.* 2005 Feb;149(2):355–362.

90. Abe Y. Muro T, Sakanoue Y, et al. Intravenous myocardial contrast echocardiography predicts regional and global left ventricular remodelling after acute myocardial infarction: comparison with low dose dobutamine stress echocardiography. *Heart.* 2005 Dec;91(12):1578–1583. Epub 2005 Mar 29.

91. Main MI, Magalski A, Chee NK, et al. Full-motion pulse inversion power Doppler contrast echocardiography differentiates stunning from necrosis and predicts recovery of left ventricular function after acute myocardial infarction. *J Am Coll Cardiol.* 2001 Nov 1;38(5):1390–1394.

92. Aronson S, Jacobsohn E, Savage R, et al. The influence of collateral flow on the antegrade and retrograde distribution of cardioplegia in patients with an occluded right coronary artery. *Anesthesiology* 1998;89(5):1099–1107.

93. Mueller RL, Rosengart TK, Isom W. The history of surgery for ischemic heart disease. *Ann Thorac Surg* 1997;63:869–878.

94. Garwood S, Davis E, Harris SN. Intraoperative transesophageal ultrasonography can measure renal blood flow. *J Cardiothorac Vasc Anesth* 2001;15(1):65–71.

95. Edmonds, HL Jr. Protective effect of neuromonitoring during cardiac surgery. *Ann N Y Acad Sci.* 2005 Aug;1053:12–19.

96. Sylivris S, Levi C, Matalanis G, et al. Pattern and significance of cerebral microemboli during coronary artery bypass grafting. *Ann Thorac Surg* 1998;66(5):1674–1678.

QUESTIONS

1. Which of the following factors are the strongest predictors of death following coronary bypass surgery?
   A. Increased age, emergency surgery, reoperation
   B. Increased age, hypertension, LV ejection fraction (EF)
   C. Emergency surgery, EF, LAD disease
   D. Female gender, EF, left main stenosis
   E. Renal dysfunction, left main disease, EF

2. Which of the following uses of intraoperative echo findings is most likely to impact patient mortality following CABG in the higher risk patient?
   A. Moderate MR with central jet direction
   B. Grade V atheroma in ascending aorta
   C. Moderate tricuspid regurgitation
   D. Pre-CPB anteroseptal dyskinesia
   E. Mitral inflow e wave deceleration time (DT) of 150 ms

3. Based on current projections by the National Center for Health Statistics and the U.S. Census Bureau, the number of individuals over the age of 65 with clinically significant coronary artery disease in the year 2020 will be what?
   A. 5,000,000
   B. 1,500,000
   C. 750,000
   D. 250,000
   E. 500,000

4. Myocardial protection strategies for patients with mild to moderate aortic regurgitation include which of the following?
   A. LV venting
   B. Direct intercoronary cardioplegia
   C. Retrograde cardioplegia
   D. Antegrade cardioplegia
   E. Aortic valve replacement

5. Patients with an ischemic cardiomyopathy and mitral regurgitation (MR) may have which of the following mechanisms of mitral valve dysfunction?
   A. Type I
   B. Type II
   C. Type IIIa
   D. Asymmetrical Type IIIb
   E. Symmetrical Type IIIb

CHAPTER 28

Assessment of the Mitral Valve in Ischemic Heart Disease

Matthew L. Williams ■ Christopher F. Sulzer ■ Donald D. Glower ■ Carmelo Milano ■ Solomon Aronson

Ischemic mitral regurgitation (IMR) is mitral regurgitation (MR) caused by acute or chronic ischemia or infarction. Acute IMR is caused by either myocardial dysfunction or rarely by infarction and subsequent rupture of a papillary muscle, while chronic IMR is caused by infarction that leads to either leaflet restriction, annular dilation, or both. IMR is associated with an unfavorable prognosis for both medical and surgical treatment. It has been reported that up to 41% of coronary artery bypass-grafting (CABG) candidates may also have chronic ischemic mitral insufficiency (1). When the severity of IMR necessitates CABG and mitral valve (MV) repair or replacement, this combined procedure has significantly increased in-hospital mortality relative to CABG alone (2).

Intraoperative management of IMR remains a challenge and intraoperative transesophageal echocardiography (TEE) may significantly improve intraoperative decision making and patient outcome (3). This chapter discusses the anatomic and physiologic principles of IMR and reviews the use of TEE in the diagnosis of this condition (4,5).

SCIENTIFIC PRINCIPLES

Prevalence and Outcome

IMR is present in 7% to 31% of patients undergoing coronary angiography (6,7). In a series of 140 patients with mitral insufficiency, 26% had IMR (8), with other reported causes of MR in that series being 41% myxomatous degeneration, 17% rheumatic valvular disease, 12% endocarditis, and 2% congenital pathology (Fig. 28.1). The same group reported that among 755 patients who had undergone a primary operation for MR (9), the total operative mortality rate was 4%, whereas the mortality rate in the group of patients with combined repair and CABG was 6.6%. Analysis of 150 consecutive patients with IMR undergoing either repair (63%) or replacement has been reported to result in different long-term outcome based on the underlying pathophysiology, rather than the type of procedure (10). The predictor of worse long-term survival (repair of functional IMR) indicates that pathophysiologic mechanisms may be the major determinants of survival rather than the type of surgical intervention (10). Retrospective analysis of 1,292 patients at the Cleveland Clinic over a 5-year period revealed an overall incidence of IMR of 6.5%, of which 40% had valve prolapse

and 60% had restrictive leaflet motion due to regional or global left ventricular (LV) dilatation (11). Forty-two percent of the patients had rheumatic valvular disease; 44% had degenerative valvular disease; and 6% had endocarditis or congenital valve malformation. A mean follow-up (3 ± 1.6 years) interval after repair revealed a superior survival in the patients with valve leaflet prolapse (96%) (Figs. 28.2–28.4) versus 48% for those with restricted valvular motion (11,12). In absolute terms, the long-term survival for patients who undergo surgery to correct IMR is lower than those who have surgery to correct degenerative MR (56% vs. 84% in one recent series). But when preoperative risk factors are controlled, long-term survival showed no significant difference. Thus, it appears that patient factors determine long-term outcome, rather than the surgery in isolation (13).

The reported in-hospital mortality rate for isolated CABG is 3%, whereas isolated MV procedures carry a reported in-hospital mortality rate of 2.5% to 6.2%. (14,15). Combined MV surgery and CABG is associated with a reported in-hospital mortality rate of 7% to 20% (2,14–16), with advanced age of the patients (≥80 years) being described as an independent risk factor leading to increased in-hospital mortality (19.6% vs. 12.2% in younger patients) as well as congestive heart failure (CHF), acute onset of ischemia requiring intensive care,

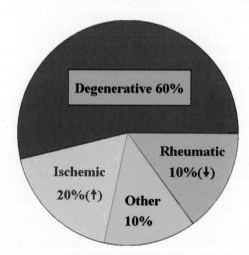

Figure 28.1. Prevalence of MV Disease. Ischemic etiology is increasing while rheumatic etiology is decreasing in the U.S. population.

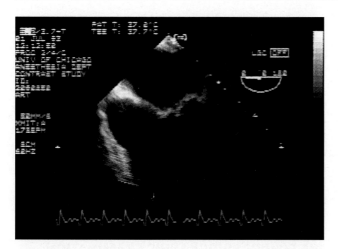

Figure 28.2. Prolapsed Posterior Leaflet of the MV. Magnified view of LA and coapted MV leaflets forming a chevron shape.

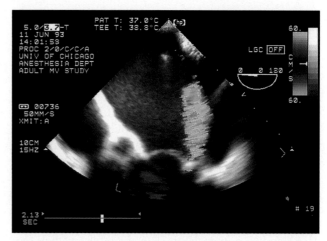

Figure 28.4. A posteriorly displaced regurgitant jet in a patient with a prolapsed anterior valve leaflet. Note the aliasing of the color hues, demonstrating high-velocity flow.

LV end-diastolic pressure greater than 15 mm Hg, and New York Heart Association class IV (2,5).

It has been demonstrated that MV regurgitation of even mild or moderate severity predicts adverse outcomes following isolated CABG procedures (17). While most agree that severe chronic ischemic MR should be corrected at the time of CABG, controversy remains as to the optimal therapy for mild or moderate ischemic MR. Authors have reported that CABG alone is sufficient therapy for patients with chronic ischemic MR (18). The group from the Cleveland Clinic, in a retrospective analysis, reported that the addition of annuloplasty to revascularization added little benefit in patients with 3+/4+ IMR (19). Others argue that intervention on the valve provides incremental benefit over CABG alone (20).

Long-term results of surgery for chronic IMR have been mixed in published reports, with long-term recurrence rates of at least moderate MR ranging from 28% to 11% (13,21).

It has been stated that ring annuloplasty is an "annular solution to a ventricular problem" and there are surgeons

who advocate alternative approaches to correct ischemic MR. Notably, investigators have attempted to restore the normal ventricular shape to decrease papillary muscle tethering and leaflet restriction by performing an intraventricular "pexy" (22). In addition, Kron et al. (23) have surgically translocated the papillary muscle to alleviate leaflet restriction. Despite favorable reports from these authors, these alternative techniques to restore competency in IMR have not gained widespread application.

Anatomy

The MV is a complex structure consisting of two leaflets (posterior and anterior), chordae tendinae (primary, secondary, and tertiary), and the papillary muscles (anterolateral [AL] and posteromedial [PM]).

The posterior leaflet consists of three scallops: medial, middle, and lateral. The corresponding portions of the anterior leaflet are medial, middle, and lateral thirds. The chordae consist of connective tissue (mainly collagen bundles) and extend from the head of each papillary muscle to the nearest half of each leaflet.

The primary chordae attach to the tip of the leaflet, the secondary chordae attach to the mid-portion of the leaflet, and the tertiary chordae attach to the base of the leaflet or mitral annulus. These tertiary chordae form a posterior chordal structure that has a stabilizing function. Interruption of the tertiary chordae due to ischemic/necrotic rupture in the corresponding myocardial zone (including papillary muscle) will have a significant impact on the maintenance of normal LV geometry and ventricular function. The number of papillary muscle heads varies from one to five.

The blood supply to the posterior papillary muscle is provided by one vessel (either right coronary artery or left circumflex artery) in 63% of the patients and two vessels in 37% (24). The anterior papillary muscle had a double-vessel blood supply (obtuse marginal and diagonal) in 71%

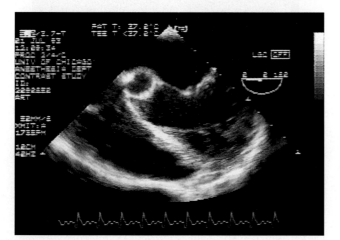

Figure 28.3. Classic chevron shape of coapted MV leaflets in a long-axis view. The posterior leaflet prolapses into the LA.

and single-vessel supply in 29%. In a study that included 20 patients monitored by TEE during coronary surgery, selective coronary graft injections of sonicated albumin microbubbles were performed to assess graft patency and papillary muscle perfusion. It was demonstrated that in the subgroup of 10 patients with an old inferior myocardial infarction (MI), MR was present only among those six with a single blood supply rather than a double blood supply.

The most commonly used nomenclature system is the Carpentier classification, where the posterior MV leaflet is divided into P1, P2, and P3 (lateral, middle, and medial) scallops (25). The anterior leaflet (comprising 60%–70% of the MV area and 30% of the annular circumference) is also divided similarly in the Carpentier classification into A1, A2, and A3 nomenclature (lateral, middle, medial) segments. The American Society of Echocardiography and the SCA incorporate the anatomic classification represented by the Carpentier scheme. MV regurgitation may be caused by malfunctioning of any component of the MV apparatus. Chronic regurgitation leads to dilatation of the left atrium (LA) and the annulus, which loses its physiologic ellipsoid shape during systole. The resulting circular annulus portends poor leaflet coaptation and MR. Increased LA dimension suggests an advanced degree of MR, although smaller dimensions do not exclude severe insufficiency.

Mechanism

The most commonly utilized classification scheme for MR is that of Carpentier. The classification of MV insufficiency proposed by Alain Carpentier included a description as follows: Type I: pure dilatation of the annulus, leaflet motion normal, leaflet perforation may be present; Type II: leaflet prolapse due to chordal rupture or elongation or papillary muscle rupture or elongation; and Type III: restricted leaflet motion due to papillary muscle dysfunction in conjunction with LV dysfunction.

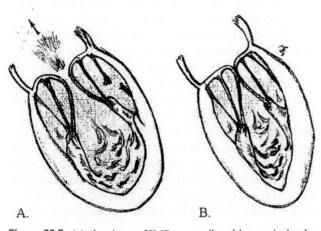

Figure 28.5. Mechanisms of IMR are attributable to apical tethering of the LV resulting in restricted MV leaflet motion and poor leaflet coaptation. The annulus is apically displaced due to chordae tendinae retaining their length constant between the tips of the leaflets and the papillary muscles (**A**). The normal MV apparatus is demonstrated (**B**).

Type III dysfunction can be further subcategorized into IIIa: restriction that occurs in diastole (not seen in ischemic MR); and IIIb: systolic tethering (26). Chronic IMR is a complex process that involves a combination of (a) annular dilatation plus flattening and (b) displacement of papillary muscles because of changes in function and geometry of the LV (Fig. 28.5). The final result is a MV that shows a combination of Carpentier's class I (dilated annulus) and class IIIb (restricted leaflets tenting into the LV) mechanisms of MR (27). The rare situation of acute ischemic IMR as a result of rupture of an infarcted papillary muscle represents Type II dysfunction.

THE ECHOCARDIOGRAPHIC EXAMINATION

The two-dimensional (2D) TEE examination of MV regurgitation before cardiopulmonary bypass (CPB) should provide information on the severity of MR, the origin and direction of the regurgitant jets, the degree of MV apparatus deformation, the LV geometry and dysfunction, and finally the hemodynamic impact (Figs. 28.6–28.9).

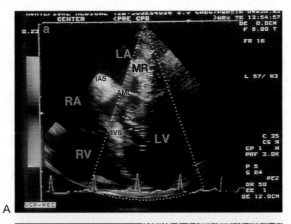

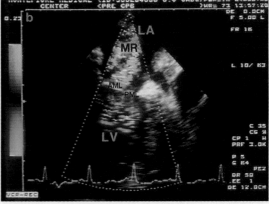

Figure 28.6. Color Doppler imaging shows mild to moderate MR in the three-chamber view (**A**) originating from the site of the posteromedial commissure in the two-chamber view (**B**). MR, mitral regurgitation; LA, left atrium; RA, right atrium; LV, left ventricle; RV, right ventricle; IAS, interatrial septum; IVS, interventricular septum; AML, anterior mitral leaflet; PML, posterior mitral leaflet.

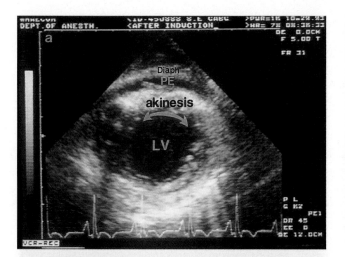

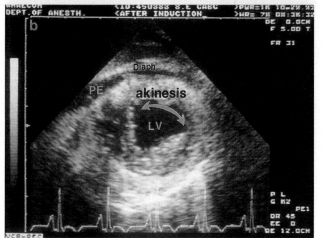

Figure 28.7. SAX view of the LV in the transverse scan at end-diastole (**A**) and end-systole (**B**). *Arrow* shows akinetic inferior septum (IS), inferior (I), inferoposterior (IP), and posterolateral segments of the LV. Diaph, diaphragm; PE, pericardial effusion.

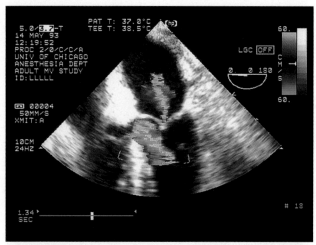

Figure 28.9. Central regurgitant jet in a patient with diffuse coronary disease. This type of jet is seen in patients with bileaflet restricted mobility or with either restricted or excessive mobility of both MV leaflets.

It is important to know that intraoperative TEE assessment tends to downgrade the evaluation of MR severity (28). General anesthesia, hemodilution, temperature, and the use of vasoactive drugs influence the hemodynamic variables that determine the severity of MR during surgery. These factors can affect preload, afterload, heart rate, and rhythm, which significantly influence the degree of MR at a given time (Fig. 28.10). Discordance between angiographic and echocardiographic evidence of mitral insufficiency may involve patients with unstable hemodynamics during angiography and those with high LV end-diastolic pressures whose disease has been palliated with thrombolytic therapy (6). Finally, mechanical

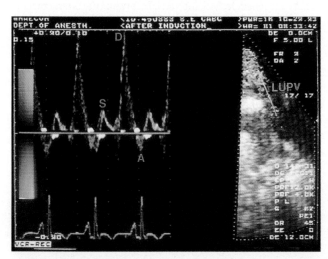

Figure 28.8. Decreased left pulmonary venous systolic flow (PVSF) compared with diastolic flow in the pulsed-wave mode. Negative velocity (A) is seen just after the D wave. S, peak pulmonary venous systolic filling; D, peak pulmonary venous diastolic filling; LUPV, left upper pulmonary vein.

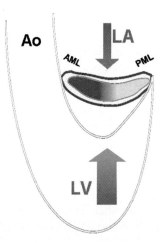

Figure 28.10. The saddle-shaped MV requires greater force to move the leaflets cephalad than caudad. IMR also may occur when the pressure gradient between the LV and the LA during early systole is low due to increased LA end-diastolic pressure, or diminished LV early-systolic pressure. AML, anterior mitral leaflet; PML, posterior mitral leaflet; LA, left atrium; LV, left ventricle; Ao, aorta.

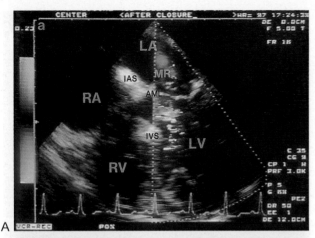

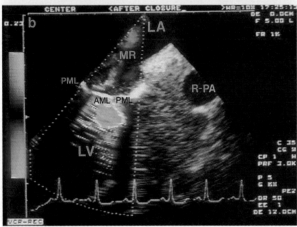

Figure 28.11. Color Doppler imaging shows trivial MR in the three-chamber view (**A**) originating from the site of the postero-medial commissure in the two-chamber view (**B**). MR, mitral regurgitation; LA, left atrium; RA, right atrium; RV, right ventricle; LV, left ventricle; IAS, interatrial septum; IVS, interventricular septum; AML, anterior mitral leaflet; PML, posterior mitral leaflet; R-PA, right pulmonary artery.

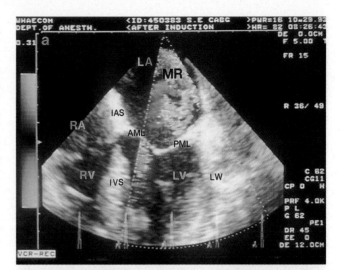

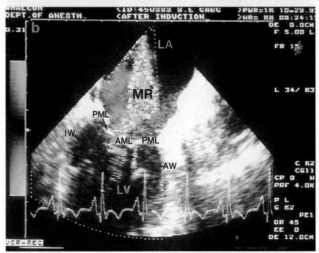

Figure 28.12. Color Doppler imaging shows severe MR originating from the posteromedial commissure in the three-chamber view (**A**) and the two-chamber view (**B**). MR, mitral regurgitation; LA, left atrium; RA, right atrium; RV, right ventricle; LV, left ventricle; IAS, interatrial septum; IVS, interventricular septum; AML, anterior mitral leaflet; PML, posterior mitral leaflet; LW, lateral wall; AW, anterior wall; IW, inferior wall.

LV unloading with an intra-aortic balloon pump may lead to underestimation of IMR severity. The use of phenylephrine (pure α agonist) may help increase the patient's blood pressures to preoperative values and unmask the true severity of MV regurgitation.

Interrogation of the MV apparatus in multiple planes before using color Doppler is useful to visualize and diagnose the mechanism of injury causing insufficiency (Figs. 28.11–28.14). Tomographic images of all components of the MV apparatus should be obtained and recorded, recognizing that 2D and Doppler determination of leaflet dysfunction and jet direction correctly diagnoses the mechanism of disease in up to 85% of patients (12) (Fig. 28.15).

Standard color Doppler imaging provides a semiquantitative assessment of the MR severity using jet geometry and multiple views of the regurgitant area. It is a highly sensitive method to detect even mild degrees of ischemic MR, and the measurement of the area of the regurgitation

jet has been widely used to evaluate the amount of the regurgitation (29). When interrogating the MV with color flow Doppler (CFD), using jet area, vena contracta, and proximal isovelocity surface area (PISA) will better define the severity of the lesion. The vena contracta width is particularly useful in the presence of an extremely eccentric jet (30).

One unique advantage of echocardiography is that it can accurately quantify the severity of MR. Using the PISA method and various volumetric methods, quantitative measures including regurgitant volume (RVol), regurgitant fraction (RF), and effective regurgitant orifice area (EROA) can be calculated (30). Performed correctly, these parameters are considered most accurate because they are objective. However, these measurements must be performed carefully by experienced echocardiographers.

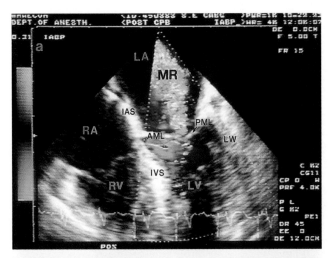

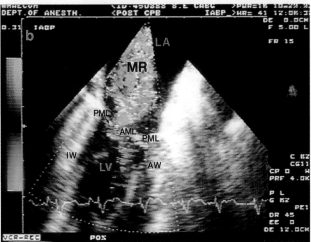

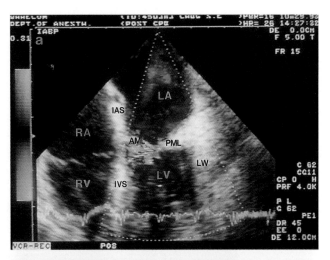

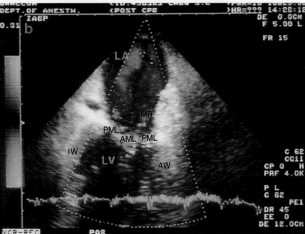

Figure 28.13. After revascularization, color Doppler imaging continues to show severe MR originating from the site of posteromedial commissure in the four-chamber view (**A**) and the two-chamber view (**B**) after initial weaning from the bypass. MR, mitral regurgitation; LA, left atrium; RA, right atrium; RV, right ventricle; LV, left ventricle; IAS, interatrial septum; IVS, interventricular septum; AML, anterior mitral leaflet; PML, posterior mitral leaflet; LW, lateral wall; AW, anterior wall; IW, inferior wall.

Figure 28.14. Color Doppler imaging shows trivial MR in the four-chamber view (**A**) and the two-chamber view (**B**) after annuloplasty. MR, mitral regurgitation; LA, left atrium; RA, right atrium; RV, right ventricle; LV, left ventricle; AML, anterior mitral leaflet; PML, posterior mitral leaflet; IAS, interatrial septum; IVS, interventricular septum; LW, lateral wall; AW, anterior wall; IW, inferior wall.

For example, the PISA signal must not impinge on a chamber wall in order to retain accuracy (30). Limitations of the PISA method are well recognized (31), being more accurate for central than eccentric regurgitant jets, and more accurate for a circular than a noncircular orifice.

The EROA is a measure of the severity of the lesion while the RVol is a measure of the volume overload; therefore, the former is not only independent of hemodynamic conditions but also a predictor of prognosis (30). Current guidelines recommend thresholds to define severe MR as an RVol ≥ 60 mL and an EROA ≥ 40 mm² (30). For ischemic MR, however, adverse outcomes are associated with lower values for these parameters suggesting that 30 mL for RVol and 20 mm² for EROA should be the preferred thresholds of severity (32).

RF volume can be indirectly measured as a difference between stroke volume (SV) through the MV (SVmv) and a nonregurgitant reference valve, such as the aortic valve (AV) (SVav). Further calculation of the RF (RFmv = SVmv − SVav/SVmv) can grade MR severity, where 30% to 50% is considered moderate. Limitations of this method include assumption that the left ventricular outflow tract (LVOT) and AV orifice and mitral annulus are circular, aortic regurgitation is absent, and no ventricular septal defect is present. Furthermore, the calculation error is squared if the LVOT or MV annulus area is not measured accurately.

Doppler interrogation of the pulmonary veins has produced insights into hemodynamics. This evaluation is a standard part of the normal TEE examination and usually includes pulse Doppler of the left upper pulmonary vein (LUPV). Normal pulmonary venous flow is antegrade during both ventricular systole and diastole (ventricular systolic component dominates), with slight retrograde

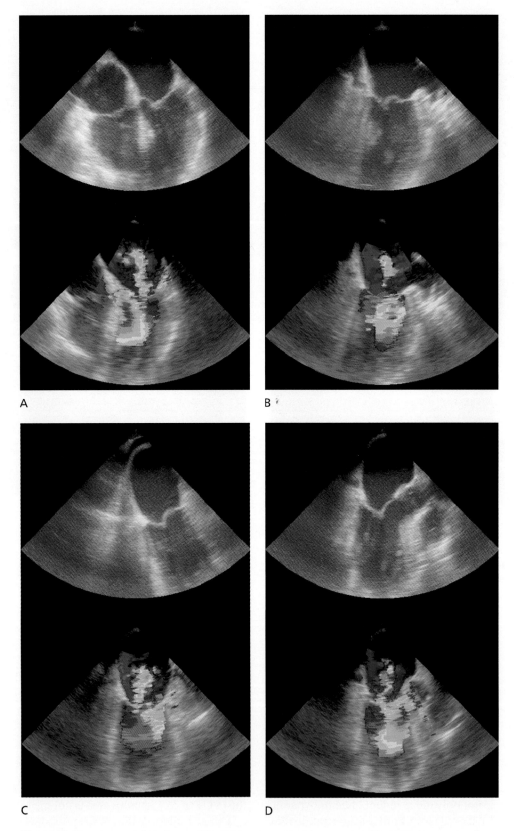

Figure 28.15. Tomographic planes of the MV apparatus with corresponding CFD images are demonstrated. There are ME four-chamber view (**A**), ME commissural view (**B**), ME two-chamber view (**C**), ME long-axis view (**D**), and transgastric short-axis view (TG SAX)(**E**).

(Continued)

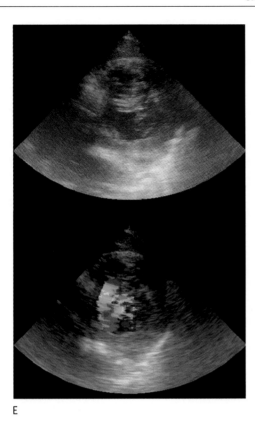

E

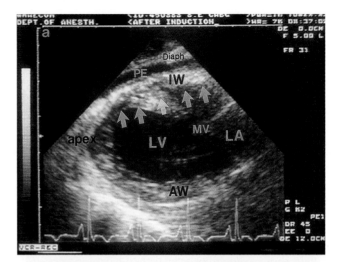

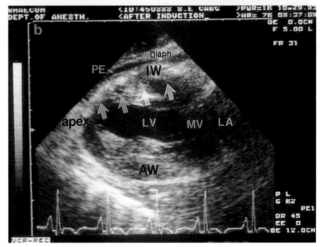

Figure 28.15. (*Continued*). The central regurgitant jet is visualized in all views. The TG SAX CFD image may suggest the anatomic location of the jet regarding the posterior leaflet scallops. Of note, complete analysis of the severity of the regurgitant jet requires evaluation of the PISA and pulmonary vein flow pattern.

Figure 28.17. Long-axis view of the LV in the longitudinal scan at end-diastole (**A**) and end-systole (**B**). *Arrows* show akinetic apical, middle, and basal-inferior segments of the LV. LA, left atrium; LV, left ventricle; MV, mitral valve; AW, anterior wall; IW, inferior wall; PE, pericardial effusion; Diaph, diaphragm.

flow during atrial systole (Figs. 28.8 and 28.16). The presence of systolic flow reversal in the pulmonary vein has been shown to be 93% sensitive and 100% specific for detecting severe mitral insufficiency (33).

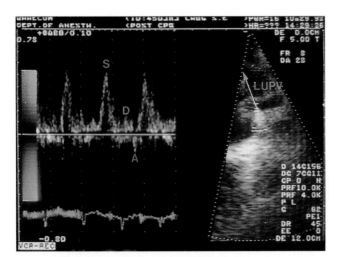

Figure 28.16. Normalization of left PVSF in pulsed-wave mode after annuloplasty. LUPV, left upper pulmonary vein; S, peak pulmonary venous systolic filling; D, peak pulmonary diastolic filling; A, negative velocity seen just before the S wave.

To evaluate the characteristics of the LV, it is necessary to evaluate the ventricular volumes, the sphericity index, the ejection fraction, the diastolic function, and the distribution of wall motion abnormalities (Figs. 28.7 and 28.17). Annular dimensions, coaptation depth, and tenting area are the most important parameters to describe the degree of MV apparatus deformation (Fig. 28.18). The coaptation depth and tenting area are positively related to the severity of LV dysfunction and remodeling (34). A tenting area of 6 cm² or more usually indicates grade 3 or higher MR (35). Recently, tenting volume derived from real-time three-dimensional echocardiography has been demonstrated to be a better novel index of MV remodeling than tenting area (36). Tenting volumes take into account all geometric components of tethering and tenting and may be a geometric parameter of IMR severity more helpful than other 2D parameters (36). Moreover, tenting volume presents sequential change during systolic phase very similar to a biphasic change of EROA,

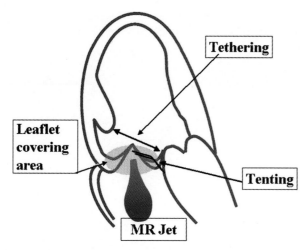

Figure 28.18. Echocardiography-derived indices to assess IMR include tethering (the distance between the posteromedial papillary muscle and the anterior annulus), tenting height (the distance of the MV leaflet from the tip to the hinge point of restrictive motion), leaflet covering area, and MV regurgitant jet area. MR, mitral regurgitation.

and the extent of these dynamic changes is influenced by LV systolic function (36). These findings suggest that the dynamic systolic change of EROA may be mainly determined by that of tenting volume (36). Thus, these parameters can be considered a mirror of the status of the LV and the degree of MR.

PROCEDURE EVALUATION

When evaluating mitral annuloplasty procedures, two important complications to consider are the creation of functional stenosis as well as dynamic obstruction of the LVOT, as both are possible following downsized annuloplasty.

In patients requiring ring annuloplasty, the valve area can be assessed with planimetric measurements. Pulse wave (PW) or continuous-wave Doppler measurement of flow velocity can be used to obtain the pressure half-time ($t_{1/2}$) or (PHT) of diastolic flow, which can be used to calculate the effective valve area as follows:

$$\text{Mitral valve area (cm}^2) = 220/t_{1/2}$$

The normal range of PHT is 50 to 70 milliseconds. Tachycardia, prolonged PR interval, and aortic insufficiency may alter its measurement. Of note, the MV area is approximately 1 cm^2 when the PHT is 220 milliseconds, so MV area is equal to $220/t_{1/2}$.

Echocardiographic evidence of systolic anterior motion (SAM) of the mitral leaflets in the presence of normal septal thickness is associated with the high-velocity flow disturbance seen in dynamic obstruction

of the LVOT. With a rigid Carpentier-Edwards ring for annuloplasty, the risk of the LVOT obstruction is 4.5% to 17%. LV dilation and septal dysfunction occur commonly in ischemic cardiomyopathy and IMR. In our experience, these elements prevent dynamic outflow tract obstruction and SAM is very unusual after undersizing annuloplasty for IMR.

Experimental research of ring annuloplasty in an animal model indicated that its implantation can reliably prevent delayed leaflet coaptation, which occurs after acute LV ischemia. Preischemic implantation of both the Duran and the Physio rings facilitated timely coaptation after induction of ischemia (37).

Preischemic implantation of either ring also preserved papillary-annular distances, which invariably tended to increase after the induction of ischemia in the control group (38). In a chronic ischemia animal model, reduction of MR was achieved by restoring tethering geometry toward normal by plication of the infarct region. Myocardial bulging was reduced without muscle excision or CPB. Immediately and up to 2 months after plication, mitral insufficiency was reduced (trace to mild) as tethering distance decreased (39).

In this experiment, implantation of a ring before induction of ischemia not only prevented delayed coaptation and preserved tethering distance as above but also prevented disturbances in the geometry of both MV leaflets (40). Neither flexible nor semirigid mitral annuloplasty rings appear to affect global or basal regional LV systolic function (40). It has been shown that rigid fixation of the mitral annulus does not result in regional systolic dysfunction at the base of the LV (41). A recent report of how mitral annular area and intercommissural and anteroseptal dimensions change throughout the cardiac cycle in a sheep model has demonstrated that a flexible Tailor partial ring preserves physiologic mitral annular folding dynamics (42).

Dilated cardiomyopathy with functional mitral insufficiency required repair of MR in 59% in a reported series of 49 patients, with 75% of the patients having an ischemic etiology (43). The importance of MV coaptation depth (MVCD), which is defined as the distance between the annulus and the coaptation point of the leaflets and is equivalent to the Mayo term *coaptation height*, was emphasized. As compared with healthy individuals with an average distance of 4.1 mm, the cardiomyopathic patients with an MVCD of less than 10 mm had postoperative functional MR of 1.2 degrees. If preoperative MVCD was greater than 11 mm, it led to an average postrepaired MR degree of 2.5. In this series, late survival was similar in both repair and replacement groups, with functional class also similar in those who survived (73%) at a mean follow-up period of 24 months.

It has been suggested that surgeons be more aggressive and not ignore substantial degrees of IMR at the time of CABG (44,45). Whether to perform a simple ring annuloplasty or a more reliable chordal-preserving mitral valve replacement (MVR) remains a challenging question. In one recent report, patients who underwent mitral repair (although not as ill as those who required MVR) had survival rates similar to those of the MVR group (43). However, other studies indicate that CABG/mitral replacement leads to worse survival than CABG/mitral repair when preoperative factors are controlled (46).

Valve repair with a downsized annuloplasty ring, in order to enhance coaptation, works satisfactorily in most cases of functional IMR, but the surgeon must pay attention to the interpretation of the associated mechanism and direction of the regurgitation. Simple ring annuloplasty is usually sufficient if Carpentier type I pathology is present, but it is not a universal remedy in cases of type III restricted systolic leaflet motion. There is growing evidence that recurrent MR may be less in IMR if a rigid, undersized, complete annuloplasty ring is used to obtain predictable reduction in the septal-free wall diameter of the MV (13,21,47–50).

In summary, ischemic mitral insufficiency carries a worse prognosis than MR from other causes (6,7,11). The use of TEE enables the assessment of valvular function in real time so that surgical plans and techniques can be adopted.

KEY POINTS

■ Up to 41% of CABG candidates have some degree of chronic ischemic mitral insufficiency.

■ The decision to intervene on the MV in patients undergoing CABG with less than severe MR is controversial.

■ Significant residual MR after revascularization is associated with increased immediate postoperative and long-term morbidity and mortality.

■ Combined MV surgery and CABG is associated with a reported in-hospital mortality rate of 7% to 20%, and this is increased with mitral replacement (45).

■ The intraoperative severity assessment of residual MR is further complicated by hemodynamic changes related to the effect of general anesthesia and is often underestimated.

■ Intraoperative TEE evaluation is critical in order to determine the mechanism of MR and guide a strategy for repair, and to gauge the effectiveness of the procedure.

■ Valve repair with a downsized annuloplasty ring, in order to enhance coaptation, works satisfactorily in most cases of functional IMR.

REFERENCES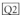

1. Izhar U, Daly R, Dearani J, et al. Mitral valve replacement or repair after previous coronary artery bypass grafting. *Circulation* 1999;100(Suppl. II):84–89.

2. Alexander K, Anstrom K, Muhlbaier L, et al. Outcomes of cardiac surgery in patients age ≥80 years: results from the national cardiovascular network. *J Am Coll Cardiol* 2000;35:731–738.

3. Grewal K, Malkowski M, Piracha A, et al. Effect of general anesthesia on the severity of mitral regurgitation by transesophageal echocardiography. *Am J Cardiol* 2000;85:199–203.

4. Shanewise J, Cheung A, Aronson S, et al. ASE/SCA guidelines for performing a comprehensive intraoperative multiplane transesophageal echocardiography examination: recommendations of the American Society of Echocardiography Council for intraoperative echocardiography and the Society of Cardiovascular Anesthesiologists Task Force for certification in perioperative transesophageal echocardiography. *J Am Soc Echocardiogr* 1999;12:884–900.

5. Miller J, Lambert A, Shapiro W, et al. The adequacy of basic intraoperative transesophageal echocardiography performed by experienced anesthesiologists. *Anesth Analg* 2001;92:1103–1110.

6. Sheikh KH, Bengtson JR, Rankin JS, et al. Intraoperative transesophageal Doppler color flow imaging used to guide patient selection and operative treatment of ischemic mitral regurgitation. *Circulation* 1991;84:594–604.

7. Hickey M, Smith L, Muhlbaier L, et al. Current prognosis of ischemic mitral regurgitation. Implications for future management. *Circulation* 1988;78(Suppl. I):51–59.

8. Cohn L, Kowalker W, Bhatia S, et al. Comparative morbidity of mitral valve repair versus replacement for mitral regurgitation with and without coronary artery disease. *Ann Thorac Surg* 1988;45:284–290.

9. Cohn L, Kowalker W, Bhatia S, et al. Comparative morbidity of mitral valve repair versus replacement for mitral regurgitation with and without coronary artery disease. 1988. Updated in 1995. *Ann Thorac Surg* 1995;60:1452–1453.

10. Cohn L, Rizzo R, Adams D, et al. The effect of pathophysiology on the surgical treatment of ischemic mitral regurgitation: operative and late risks of repair versus replacement. *Eur J Cardiothorac Surg* 1995;9:568–574.

11. Hendren W, Nemec J, Lytle B, et al. Mitral valve repair for ischemic mitral insufficiency. *Ann Thorac Surg* 1991;52:1246–1251.

12. Stewart W, Currie P, Salcedo E, et al. Evaluation of mitral leaflet motion by echocardiography and jet direction by Doppler color flow mapping to determine the mechanism of mitral regurgitation. *J Am Coll Cardiol* 1992;20:1353–1361.

13. Glower DD, Tuttle RH, Shaw LK, et al. Patient survival characteristics after routine mitral valve repair for ischemic mitral regurgitation. *J Thorac Cardiovasc Surg* 2005;129(4):860–868.

14. Ferguson T, Dziuban F, Edwards F, et al. STS National Database: current changes and challenges for the new millennium. *Ann Thorac Surg* 2000;69:680–691.

15. Andrade I, Cartier R, Panisi P, et al. Factors influencing early and late survival in patients with combined mitral valve replacement and myocardial revascularization and in those with isolated replacement. *Ann Thorac Surg* 1987;44:607–613.

16. Lytle B, Cosgrove D, Gill C, et al. Mitral valve replacement combined with myocardial revascularization: early and late results for 300 patients, 1970 to 1983. *Circulation* 1987;44:1179–1190.

17. Schroder JN, Williams ML, Hata JA, et al. Impact of mitral valve regurgitation evaluated by intraoperative transesophageal echocardiography on long-term outcomes after coronary artery bypass grafting. *Circulation* 2005;112(9 Suppl.): I293–I298.

18. Tolis GA Jr, Korkolis DP, Kopf GS, et al. Revascularization alone (without mitral valve repair) suffices in patients with advanced ischemic cardiomyopathy and mild-to-moderate mitral regurgitation. *Ann Thorac Surg* 2002;74(5):1476–1480.

19. Mihaljevic T, Lam BK, Rajeswaran J, et al. Impact of mitral valve annuloplasty combined with revascularization in patients with functional ischemic mitral regurgitation. *J Am Coll Cardiol* 2007;49(22):2191–2201.

20. Braun J, van de Veire NR, Klautz RJ, et al. Restrictive mitral annuloplasty cures ischemic mitral regurgitation and heart failure. *Ann Thorac Surg* 2008;85(2):430–436.

21. McGee EC, Gillinov AM, Blackstone EH, et al. Recurrent mitral regurgitation after annuloplasty for functional ischemic mitral regurgitation. *J Thorac Cardiovasc Surg* 2004;128(6): 916–924.

22. Menicanti L, DiDonato M, Frigiola A, et al. RESTORE Group. Ischemic mitral regurgitation: intraventricular papillary muscle imbrication without mitral ring during left ventricular restoration. *J Thorac Cardiovasc Surg* 2002;123:1041–1050.

23. Kron IL, Green GR, Cope JT. Surgical relocation of the posterior papillary muscle in chronic ischemic mitral regurgitation. *Ann Thorac Surg* 2002;74:600–601.

24. Voci P, Bilotta F, Caretta Q, et al. Papillary muscle perfusion pattern. A hypothesis for ischemic papillary muscle dysfunction. *Circulation* 1995;91(6):1714–1718.

25. Bollen B, Luo H, Oury J, et al. A systematic approach to intraoperative transesophageal echocardiographic evaluation of the mitral valve apparatus with anatomic correlation. *J Cardiothorac Vasc Anesth* 2000;14(3):330–338.

26. Carpentier A. Cardiac valve surgery—the "French correction." *J Thorac Cardiovasc Surg* 1983;86:323–337.

27. Gorman JH III, Ryan LP, Gorman RC. Pathophysiology of ischemic mitral insufficiency: does repair make a difference? *Heart Fail Rev* 2006;11:219–229.

28. Aklog L, Filsoufi F, Flores K, et al. Does coronary artery bypass grafting alone correct moderate ischemic mitral regurgitation? *Circulation* 2001;104(Suppl. 1):68–75.

29. Spain MG, Smith MD, Grayburn PA, et al. Quantitative assessment of mitral regurgitation by Doppler color flow imaging: angiographic and hemodynamic correlations. *J Am Coll Cardiol* 1989;13:585–590.

30. Zoghbi WA, Enriquez-Sarano M, Foster E, et al. Recommendations for evaluation of the severity of native valvular regurgitation with two-dimensional and Doppler echocardiography. *J Am Soc Echocardiogr* 2003;16:777–802.

31. Simpson IA, Shiota T, Gharib M, et al. Current status of flow convergence for clinical applications: is it a leaning tower of "PISA"? *J Am Coll Cardiol* 1996;27:504–509.

32. Grigioni F, Enriquez-Sarano M, Zehr KJ, et al. Ischemic mitral regurgitation: long-term outcome and prognostic implications with quantitative Doppler assessment. *Circulation* 2001;103: 1759–1764.

33. Lai LP, Shyu KG, Chen JJ, et al. Usefulness of pulmonary venous flow pattern and maximal mosaic jet area detected by transesophageal echocardiography in assessing the severity of mitral regurgitation. *Am J Cardiol* 1993;72:1310–1313.

34. Agricola E, Oppizzi M, Maisano F, et al. Echocardiographic classification of chronic ischemic mitral regurgitation caused by restricted motion according to tethering pattern. *Eur J Echocardiogr* 2004;5:326–334.

35. Yiu SF, Enriquez-Sarano M, Tribouilloy C, et al. Determinants of the degree of functional mitral regurgitation in patients with systolic left ventricular dysfunction: a quantitative clinical study. *Circulation* 2000;102:1400–1406.

36. Song JM, Fukuda S, Kihara T, et al. Value of mitral valve tenting volume determined by real-time three-dimensional echocardiography in patients with functional mitral regurgitation. *Am J Cardiol* 2006;98:1088–1093.

37. Timek T, Glasson JR, Dagum P, et al. Ring annuloplasty prevents delayed leaflet coaptation and mitral regurgitation during acute left ventricular ischemia. *J Thorac Cardiovasc Surg* 2000;119: 774–783.

38. Dagum P, Timek TA, Green GR, et al. Coordinate-free analysis of mitral valve dynamics in normal and ischemic hearts. *Circulation* 2000;102:III62–III69.

39. Liel-Cohen N, Guerrero JL, Otsuji Y, et al. Design of a new surgical approach for ventricular remodeling to relieve ischemic mitral regurgitation: insights from 3-dimensional echocardiography. *Circulation* 2000;101:2756–2763.

40. Lai DT, Timek TA, Dagum P, et al. The effects of ring annuloplasty on mitral leaflet geometry during acute left ventricular ischemia. *J Thorac Cardiovasc Surg* 2000;120:966–975.

41. Green GR, Dagum P, Glasson JR, et al. Semirigid or flexible mitral annuloplasty rings do not affect global or basal regional left ventricular systolic function. *Circulation* 1998;98:II128–II135; discussion II135–II136.

42. Dagum P, Timek T, Green GR, et al. Three-dimensional geometric comparison of partial and complete flexible mitral annuloplasty rings. *J Thorac Cardiovasc Surg* 2001;122: 665–673.

43. Calafiore AM, Gallina S, Di Mauro M, et al. Mitral valve procedure in dilated cardiomyopathy: repair or replacement? *Ann Thorac Surg* 2001;71:1146–1152; discussion 1152–1153.

44. Miller DC. Ischemic mitral regurgitation redux—to repair or to replace? *J Thorac Cardiovasc Surg* 2001;122:1059–1062.

45. Duarte I, Shen Y, MacDonald M, et al. Treatment of moderate regurgitation and coronary disease by coronary bypass alone: late results. *Ann Thorac Surg* 1999;68:426–430.

46. Milano CA, Daneshmand MA, Rankin JS, et al. Survival prognosis and surgical management of ischemic mitral regurgitation. *Ann Thorac Surg* 2008;86(3):735–744.

47. Filsoufi F, Castillo JG, Rahmanian PB, et al. Remodeling annuloplasty using a prosthetic ring designed for correcting type-iiib ischemic mitral regurgitation. *Revista Espanola De Cardiologia* 2007;60(11):1151–1158.

48. Timek TA, Lai DT, Liang D, et al. Effects of paracommissural septal-lateral annular cinching on acute ischemic mitral regurgitation. *Circulation* 2004;110(11 Suppl. 1):II79–II84.

49. Timek T, Lai D, Dagum P, et al. Mitral annular dynamics during rapid atrial pacing. *Surgery* 2000;128:361–367.

50. Gillinov A, Wierup P, Blackstone E, et al. Is repair preferable to replacement for ischemic mitral regurgitation? *J Thorac Cardiovasc Surg* 2001;122:1125–1141.

QUESTIONS

1. Among the following underlying causes of IMR, which carries the most promising 5-year prognosis after mitral valve (MV) surgery?
   A. MV dilation
   B. Restrictive anterior leaflet motion
   C. Ruptured papillary muscle

2. The least likely cause of IMR is
   A. infarction of the posterior medial papillary muscle due to single coronary blood supply
   B. ventricular regional wall motion abnormality without anterior mitral annular dilation
   C. early versus late systolic mitral leaflet loitering

3. Which of the following best explains why MV ring annuloplasty reduces the severity of IMR?
   A. It modifies the anterior displacement of the posterior mitral leaflet (PML) and posterior medial papillary muscle.
   B. It reduces radial displacement of the anterior and posterior papillary muscles.
   C. It reduces annular diameter.
   D. All of the above.

CHAPTER 29

Surgical Considerations in Mitral and Tricuspid Valve Surgery

A. Marc Gillinov ■ Erik A.K. Beyer ■ Gonzalo Gonzalez-Stawinski ■ Tomislav Mihaljevic

PRIMARY MITRAL VALVE DISEASE

The most common cause of mitral regurgitation in North America is degenerative mitral valve (MV) disease (1–4). In recent surgical series, myxomatous degeneration of the MV accounted for more than 50% of the cases (5). Rheumatic heart disease, though rare in industrialized nations, is still a frequent cause of mitral regurgitation and stenosis, requiring surgical correction in developing countries (4). Mitral regurgitation caused by coronary artery disease, termed ischemic mitral regurgitation, is increasingly common. Of patients evaluated for surgery for coronary artery disease, approximately one third will have some degree of mitral regurgitation (6). Infective endocarditis remains a problem and is the etiology of pure mitral regurgitation in 2% to 8% of patients presenting for surgical correction of mitral regurgitation (7). Severe endocarditic mitral regurgitation is related to ruptured chordae and/or leaflet perforation (8). Other diseases that can affect the MV include idiopathic calcification of the mitral annulus; systemic diseases, such as Marfan's and Ehlers-Danlos syndromes; and hypertrophic cardiomyopathy.

Preoperative evaluation of MV pathology is performed with transthoracic echo. Doppler echocardiography is the primary tool for assessing MV disease. It identifies the morphologic lesions, the degree of mitral regurgitation/stenosis, and quantifies ventricular function. During MV surgery, transesophageal echocardiography (TEE) is essential. It allows identification of the lesion and mechanisms of MV dysfunction (Tables 29.1 and 29.2). It also determines whether the valve is regurgitant, stenotic, or a combination of both. TEE is valuable in determining the likelihood of repair versus replacement. Intraoperative TEE delineates dynamic abnormalities related to valve opening and closing. It also characterizes leaflet abnormalities and regurgitant jet size and duration. Characteristics of the regurgitant jet help clarify the nature of the MV dysfunction. Usually, leaflet flail directs the regurgitant jet in the opposite direction of the flail segment, whereas restricted leaflets generally cause jets on the ipsilateral side of the pathologic segment. TEE, therefore, guides the surgeon's approach to reestablish effective coaptation in regurgitant valves and to improve opening in stenotic ones (9). Echocardiography is also necessary to assess the other valves and quantify ventricular function. Finally, TEE assesses the results of surgical intervention. Late durability of MV repair in degenerative disease is enhanced by TEE (10). Technical errors at surgery are identified accurately in the operating room, thereby allowing immediate correction.

PROSTHETIC MITRAL DISEASE

Since the first prosthetic heart valve was placed in 1960, millions of valves have been implanted. Although most patients do well following MV replacement, they are subject to a variety of complications (11,12). These complications include prosthetic valve endocarditis (PVE), periprosthetic leak, structural valve degeneration (SVD), valve thrombosis, and thromboembolism. PVE most frequently occurs in the first several months postoperatively, with an early incidence of up to 2% (13). The incidence then decreases to 0.17% to 1% per patient per year (14). Periprosthetic leaks occur when the seal between the sewing ring and the host tissue is inadequate. The incidence of periprosthetic leaks ranges between 0.3% and 2.2% per year (15,16). Structural failure related to valve design or material selection is rare with currently available mechanical valves. However, bioprosthetic valves have limited durability due to SVD (17).

TRICUSPID VALVE

Tricuspid regurgitation (TR) is most commonly caused by volume overload attributable to chronic left-sided valvular lesions (Table 29.3). Right ventricular and atrial volume overload causes annular dilatation and TR. About 10% to 50% of patients with severe MV dysfunction have significant TR (18). Functional TR is frequently accompanied by pulmonary hypertension and right ventricular dilatation and dysfunction (19). Organic involvement of the tricuspid valve (TV) by rheumatic disease can also result in TR. Another major etiology of TR is endocarditis. Endocarditis of the TV is prevalent in IV drug abusers and in patients with chronic indwelling venous catheters. Other less common causes of TR include fibrosis secondary to carcinoid disease and degenerative disease.

TABLE 29.1	Mitral Regurgitation: Etiology and Pathologic Changes
Etiologies	**Pathologic Changes**
Degenerative or myxomatous	Asymmetric dilatation of the posterior two thirds of the mitral annulus, resulting in posterior leaflet prolapse Chordae elongation or rupture
Rheumatic heart disease	Annular dilatation at the posteromedial commissure. Leaflet shortening Cleft obliteration and scallop fusion
Ischemic mitral regurgitation	Alterations in ventricular and papillary muscle geometry, with tethering of mitral leaflets resulting in failure of leaflet coaptation Unruptured/infarcted papillary muscle, causing papillary muscle elongation Ruptured papillary muscle resultant leaflet flail
Infective endocarditis	Infective valvular vegetations commonly on the atrial aspect of the leaflet at the line of valve closure Tissue necrosis, thus leaflet ulceration/perforation Annular abscesses Annular fistulae
Idiopathic calcification of the annulus	Calcification involving the hinge point of the leaflets, commonly involving the posterior leaflet
Connective tissue disorders (e.g., Marfan's syndrome and Ehlers-Danlos syndrome)	Excessive elongation of the papillary muscles Billowing and redundant leaflets

STRUCTURE AND ANATOMY

Mitral Valve

The components of the MV include the annulus, leaflets, chordae, and papillary muscles. A review of the anatomic and functional aspects as they pertain to MV surgery will be presented. The mitral annulus is composed of

muscular and fibrous tissue that anchors the base of the MV leaflets (20,21). The annular ring extends between the endocardium of the left atrium and the endocardium of the left ventricle and incorporates within its boundaries the valve tissue itself. In an average adult, the orifice area of the MV at the level of the annulus is approximately 6.5 cm² for women and 8 cm² for men (22). Diastolic and systolic annulus sizes differ by 23% to 40% (23). The annulus

TABLE 29.2	Mitral Stenosis: Etiology and Pathologic Changes
Etiologies	**Pathologic Changes**
Rheumatic heart disease (most common)	Leaflet thickening and fibrosis Commissural fusion Chordal fusion and shortening
Massive mitral annular calcification	Restrictive leaflet motion from invasive calcification disease
Congenital mitral stenosis	Congenital slit-like orifice in line of a mitral valve
Infective endocarditis	Large vegetations obstructing the mitral orifice
Inborn errors in metabolism (e.g., Fabry's disease, Hurler-Scheie syndrome)	Polysaccharide deposits within the valve structure, leading to leaflet thickening and eventual fibrosis
Cor triatriatum (rare)	Abnormal subdivision of the left atrium, partially obstructing the outflow of the pulmonary veins to the mitral orifice

TABLE 29.3	Tricuspid Valve Disease: Etiology and Pathologic Changes
Etiologies	**Pathologic Changes**
Functional regurgitation	Asymmetric annular dilatation universally involving the anterior and posterior leaflets
Rheumatic	Leaflet thickening and fibrosis Commissural fusion (commonly the anteroseptal commissural) Chordal fusion and shortening
Endocarditis	Vegetations usually on the atrial side of the valves
Carcinoid	Endocardial fibrous thickening on the ventricular surface of the valve

itself is extremely dynamic and changes in size, shape, and position throughout the cardiac cycle. During diastole, the annulus moves outward with the posterior wall of the left ventricle, allowing the shape of the annulus to become more circular (22).

Leaflets

The MV has two leaflets: the anterior and posterior. The anterior leaflet is triangular and the posterior leaflet is rectangular. The length of the basal attachments of the posterior leaflet is 0.5 cm longer than the basal attachment of the anterior leaflet (22). The posterior leaflet edge has multiple indentations or clefts, which are connected by fan-like cords. The commissures separate the anterior and posterior leaflets. Commissural cusps (leaflets) are also present and can vary in size with the posterior commissural cusp being more prominent. During diastole, the combined surface area of the two leaflets is 1.5 to 2 times the surface area of the functional mitral orifice. During systole, the anterior leaflet alone could cover the mitral orifice.

The Chords

The chordae are tendinous, string-like structures connecting the valvular tissue to the papillary muscles or the myocardium. The chords do not stretch more than 10% under physiologic conditions. They vary in length from approximately 3 to 0.2 cm from the valvular to the ventricular insertion (20). Chords arise as single projections from the ventricle and then divide in succession until attaching to the valve as small chords. The chords insert into the papillary muscle in a semicircular fashion. Chords, arising from the lowest portion of the papillary muscle, are known as strut chords because they support the central portion of the leaflets. Chords are further divided anatomically into marginal, intermediate, and basal chords based on their attachment to the ventricular surface of the leaflets in a plane perpendicular to the edge of the valve

leaflet. Marginal or first-order chordae attach to the edge of the valve leaflet and thereby prevent eversion of the free margin of the valve. The intermediate or second-order ("strut") chordae attach to the midsection/rough zone of the ventricular aspect of the leaflet and prevent billowing or doming of the cusp. Finally, the basal, or third-order chordae, which represent the largest chords morphologically, insert at the annulus and help maintain ventricular geometry (22).

Papillary Muscles

There are two distinct papillary muscles arising from the free wall of the left ventricle. The anterolateral papillary muscle is single and usually larger than the posteromedial muscle. It is located posterior and to the left in the left ventricle. The posteromedial papillary muscle is U-shaped and located near the septal border of the posterior wall. It can have two or more subheads. The posteromedial papillary muscle usually derives its blood supply from the right coronary artery, whereas the anterolateral papillary muscle has dual blood supply from the left anterior descending and circumflex coronary arteries (24). Therefore, the posterior papillary muscle is more susceptible to ischemic insults, which can directly affect valvular competence.

Tricuspid Valve

The TV is composed of an annulus, leaflets, chordae, and papillary muscles. The TV does not have a well-formed collagenous annulus. The normal annulus circumference is 10 cm in women and 11.2 cm in men (25). The atrioventricular groove folds into the TV leaflets. There are three leaflets of the TV that are named based on their anatomic locations: anterior, posterior, and septal. The leaflets are separated at the commissures and are tethered by chordae tendinae. The anterior leaflet is usually the longest, measuring on average 2.2 cm in length. The posterior leaflet typically has two or three scallops separated by cleft or indentations at its free edge (26). Chordae arise from three papillary muscles and consist of five different types: the fan shaped, rough zone, basal, free edge, and deep (26). On average, there are 25 chordae to the TV.

PATHOLOGY

Mitral Valve

Degenerative or Myxomatous Disease of the Mitral Valve

Dilatation of the mitral annulus is a major factor in mitral insufficiency caused by degenerative disease. It is the sole cause of mitral insufficiency in 15% of degenerative cases (27). The dilatation is asymmetric, causing the anterior to posterior diameter to become greater than the transverse diameter. Dilatation affects primarily the posterior two thirds of the annulus, which corresponds to the area of the posterior leaflet.

The most commonly encountered lesion in degenerative MV disease is posterior chordal rupture (5). Prolapse of the posterior leaflet because of elongated or ruptured chords is the cause of mitral regurgitation in the majority of cases (4). Of degenerative MVs operated on in one surgical series, 41% had ruptured posterior chords, 30% had elongated chords, and 10% had ruptured anterior chords (27). Other features of myxomatous MVs found on echocardiogram include billowing and redundant leaflets. Leaflet involvement may be localized (fibroelastic deficiency) or generalized (Barlow's disease). In 16% of patients, annular and leaflet calcification is seen in myxomatous disease of the MV. Prolapse of the MV leaflets is generally present in myxomatous MV disease. Intraoperative TEE determines the site of leaflet involvement and, therefore, dictates techniques of repair.

Left ventricular outflow tract obstruction (LVOTO) caused by abnormal systolic anterior motion (SAM) of the anterior leaflet of the MV occurs in 4% to 10% of patients having MV repair for myxomatous disease (28). Intraoperative TEE is essential in diagnosing this complication following repair. TEE can also help determine valvular pathology that would lend to the potential for SAM and thereby guide surgical decision making. Excess valvular tissue and septal hypertrophy are associated with a higher risk of LVOTO. A posterior leaflet with a significant redundant central portion pushes the anterior leaflet against the septum after correction of the mitral regurgitation (3). Therefore, a sliding leaflet repair is applied to floppy valves with large posterior leaflets in order to restore a more normal ratio of the anterior to posterior leaflet surface area. The incidence of SAM has been reduced in several recent surgical series to as low as 0% to 2% (28).

Rheumatic Disease of the Mitral Valve

Rheumatic MV disease remains a surgical challenge because of the progressive nature of its pathology and the young patient population affected. It is not repaired as frequently as degenerative disease. Rheumatic MV disease can result in stenosis, regurgitation, or a combination of the two.

The cardinal anatomic changes of MV stenosis are leaflet thickening and fibrosis, commissural fusion, and chordal fusion and shortening (29). Chordae tendinae can become shortened to the point that they appear to insert directly into the papillary muscle. As the disease progresses, a stenosed, slit-like orifice, termed "fishmouth," is produced. Surgical candidates for valve repair or replacement have valve areas less than 1.4 cm^2.

Isolated MV regurgitation secondary to rheumatic valvular disease is the result of leaflet shortening caused by scarring. Often the posterior leaflet is affected when the clefts are obliterated and the scallops become fused. In long-standing regurgitation, the leaflet free margin becomes thickened and folded in the direction of regurgitant flow. However, rheumatic mitral regurgitation is more often associated with valve stenosis caused by commissural fusion. Leaflet and annular calcification are also seen in long-standing rheumatic heart disease. This is readily seen on TEE as echo-dense areas. Also, annular dilatation in rheumatic disease is asymmetric and is often greatest toward the posteromedial commissure (30).

Intraoperative TEE helps establish repairability or the need for valve replacement in rheumatic heart disease. Some centers report a 65% repair rate for rheumatic mitral disease (31). For mitral stenosis, commissurotomy and valve debridement are often used. Generally, it is unnecessary to place an annuloplasty ring following a commissurotomy. However, when a central leak is observed and when the annulus is dilated, as shown by a circular rather than an oval shape, an annuloplasty ring should be considered. The ability to repair a stenotic rheumatic MV rests on the thickness of the valve leaflets and the presence of chordae tendinae. Patients with anterior leaflet and chordal pliability should be considered for repair (32). A regurgitant rheumatic MV should likewise be considered for repair if there is annular dilatation and the leaflets are thickened but mobile and the chords are thickened and elongated. Severe commissural fusion and subvalvular fibrosis are contraindications to repair (32).

Ischemic Disease of the Mitral Valve

Ischemic MV disease represents approximately 11% to 27% of patients undergoing surgery for MV disease. Compared to other etiologies of MV disease, surgery for ischemic MV disease is associated with higher mortality rates, ranging between 5% and 208% (33). This is clearly related to the underlying cause of mitral regurgitation—coronary artery disease.

Ischemic MV disease lacks a widely accepted classification scheme. This makes comparing studies difficult. For our purposes, ischemic MV disease will be divided into the three categories based on the mechanisms causing regurgitation. These categories include functional, infarcted but unruptured papillary muscle, and ruptured papillary muscle (34).

The most common cause of regurgitation in ischemic disease is functional. In a recent review by Gillinov, 76% of patients undergoing surgery for ischemic mitral regurgitation had functional impairment. In these patients, the leaflets and subvalvular apparatus appear morphologically normal at echo and upon direct inspection. The cause of regurgitation is failure of leaflet coaptation during ventricular systole. This produces a regurgitant jet on echo that is usually central but can be eccentric or complex (34).

The mechanism of functional ischemic mitral regurgitation is complex. Changes in annular, ventricular, and papillary muscle geometry and function appear to all contribute. The primary pathology involves alterations in ventricular and papillary muscle geometry that produce a tethering effect on the mitral leaflets. There is considerable debate whether annular dilatation is an important component of functional ischemic mitral regurgitation.

Patients in the functional group are amenable to treatment by annuloplasty alone. An undersized, rigid, complete annuloplasty produces excellent results in this subgroup of patients. The rationale for this is that by reducing annular size, the leaflet contact area is increased and thereby compensates for papillary muscle and left ventricular wall dyskinesis (33). Furthermore, this may result in ventricular remodeling over time (35).

The next most common subgroup of ischemic mitral regurgitation is the infarcted or elongated papillary muscle. On echo, the valve leaflet prolapses secondary to the elongated papillary muscle. Repair techniques can be performed for this process and include shortening of the papillary muscles. However, the tendency by most surgeons is to replace rather than repair the valve (33).

The least prevalent subgroup of ischemic mitral regurgitation is papillary muscle rupture. This is usually an acute and catastrophic event that presents differently from papillary muscle infarction without rupture. This usually occurs 2 to 7 days after MI and without urgent surgery; 50% to 75% of these patients die (36). Echo findings of a ruptured papillary muscle include a flail leaflet, which is easily visualized (37). Surgical repair by papillary muscle reimplantation or by resecting the prolapsing portion of the posterior leaflet is feasible. As is seen with infarcted papillary muscles, surgeons more often opt to replace the valve in these situations.

Preoperative and postoperative echo are essential when evaluating ischemic mitral regurgitation. The cause of regurgitation in ischemic disease must be determined preoperatively in order to assess repairability. Echocardiography can also identify crucial components of MV dysfunction that further guide therapy.

Endocarditis

Valve dysfunction as a result of bacterial endocarditis is an uncommon form of MV disease. In one large surgical series, only 3.4% of MV procedures were related to bacterial endocarditis (38). TEE plays a major role in the diagnosis and management of MV endocarditis. Echocardiographic features of bacterial endocarditis that suggest a need for surgical intervention include vegetation, perforation, annular abscess with sinus and fistula formation, and, less commonly, ruptured chords and papillary muscles (39). Most cases of acute endocarditis can be repaired, and early valve repair is recommended (40). Postoperative TEE is essential in order to determine the adequacy of repair.

Vegetations appear as echo-dense masses with irregular margins attached to the leaflet. They are most commonly found attached to the atrial side aspect of the MV leaflets and are related to the lines of valve closure. Vegetations can vary in size, where TEE resolution easily reaches 2 to 3 mm in diameter. Vegetation removal or partial leaflet resection is performed when isolated lesions are identified.

Tissue necrosis as a result of the infectious process can cause destruction of the MV leaflet. Ulcerations at the edge of the mitral leaflets and perforations of the body of the leaflets are manifestations of this process. Valvular regurgitation results and is demonstrated by TEE. Pericardial patches are used to repair perforations if the surrounding MV tissue is well preserved and the subvalvular apparatus is intact. Local progression of the infection into the annular tissue can produce an annular abscess. Though annular abscesses are uncommon, they may spread into the atrium, ventricle, and pericardial space. Mitral annular abscesses represent a great challenge to the surgeon. Thorough debridement of the abscess cavity is essential and repair undertaken with a pericardial patch (41). Fistulae also arise from abscess cavities and these are visible on TEE. The fistulae should be delineated carefully because this dictates the surgical approach to closing them (42).

Prosthetic Dysfunction

TEE allows superb visualization of prosthetic valves in the mitral position. Origins of prosthetic valve dysfunction and paraprosthetic pathology can be detailed with TEE. Structural valve dysfunction, paravalvular leaks, endocarditis, and thrombus are complications of prosthetic valves that often require surgical attention.

Prosthetic valves are predisposed to structural dysfunction and outright failure. Failure of a bioprosthesis is usually related to leaflet fracture with subsequent regurgitation. On TEE, this presents as an eccentric regurgitant jet (43). Mechanical prosthetic valves are more durable than bioprostheses but are nonetheless subject to structural dysfunction. A severe regurgitant jet noted on TEE is indicative of occluder dysfunction.

Paravalvular regurgitation is the result of an incomplete seal of the sewing ring and annulus. This typically occurs as a result of a failed suture line or an infectious process. Immediately following surgery, a small amount of paravalvular leak is common and tends to resolve over time as the suture line heals. However, identification of a large paravalvular leak on the postoperative TEE requires surgical intervention. A new paravalvular leak occurring months after surgery should alert the surgeon to the possibility of an infectious process.

PVE is a serious complication associated with prosthetic MVs. Vegetations, identified on echocardiogram, are pathognomonic of PVE and typically occur on the atrial side of the mitral prosthesis. TEE demonstrates vegetations in 80% of PVE cases (44). Bulky vegetations may interfere with opening and closure of mechanical prosthesis, causing either stenosis or regurgitation. Paravalvular abscesses are more common in patients with PVE than with native valve endocarditis and are seen as areas of low echodensity adjacent to the sewing ring of the prosthesis. Furthermore, progression of the infection may cause partial or complete dehiscence of the valve and result in paraprosthetic regurgitation. Surgical therapy is directed at radical debridement of infected tissue with reconstruction of cardiac structures with biologic materials (45).

Mechanical prostheses are prone to thrombus formation. TEE allows excellent visualization of thrombus on prosthetic MVs. Thrombi can occur on the sewing cuff, as well as on the occluder mechanism. On TEE, transvalvular gradients are increased when thrombus occludes the valve orifice. Regurgitation can also develop if the thrombus prevents complete closure of the valve leaflets.

Tricuspid Valve

Rheumatic Disease of Tricuspid Valve

Rheumatic fever is the most common cause of organic TR worldwide. Endocarditis of the TV is becoming increasingly prevalent in industrialized nations, secondary to drug abuse and chronically hospitalized patients with long-term central venous catheters. In the United States, the most common etiology of TR is related to annular dilatation, often referred to as functional TR.

Functional Tricuspid Regurgitation

Functional TR is related to increases in pulmonary artery pressure, caused by left ventricular failure or pulmonary vascular or interstitial disease. Diseases of the left-sided heart valves are frequently the cause of functional TR. Ten to fifty percent of patients with severe MV dysfunction have significant TR (46). Therefore, the TV should be evaluated thoroughly during echocardiographic evaluation of the MV.

In functional TR, the valve leaflets are normal but the annulus is dilated. Annular dilatation is asymmetric and develops at the portion of the annulus that corresponds to the anterior and posterior leaflets.

Early and late clinical outcomes are adversely affected when functional tricuspid insufficiency is left untreated. Therefore, it is important to address these lesions and aggressively treat them (47). Moderate-to-severe TR is easily visualized on TEE and should be surgically corrected. Common surgical repair techniques used to address TR

are the suture annuloplasty, such as the Kay or DeVega method, and placement of either a rigid or flexible annuloplasty ring. The annuloplasty ring remodels the annulus, decreases tension on the suture lines, increases leaflet coaptation, and prevents recurrent annular dilatation (48).

Following TV repair, TEE is essential so that the repair may be evaluated. Following tricuspid annuloplasty, residual TR of 2+ or more is associated with late tricuspid reoperation (49).

Rheumatic Disease of the Tricuspid Valve

Rheumatic postinflammatory scarring can result in combined tricuspid stenosis and regurgitation. Rheumatic TV disease is rarely an isolated lesion and as with rheumatic mitral disease, it is more common in the developing world. Echocardiographic evaluation of tricuspid rheumatic disease reveals leaflet thickening, commissural fusion, and chordal thickening. Anteroseptal commissural fusion is commonly pronounced. Coaptation of the TV leaflets is often incomplete, resulting in TR (50). In distinction to MV disease, secondary annular calcification is rare in TV disease. Symptomatic patients with rheumatic TV disease are usually managed by replacing the valve.

Endocarditis of the Tricuspid Valve

Tricuspid endocarditis has been increasing in frequency over the last two decades, primarily because of increased IV drug abuse and more liberal use of long-term indwelling venous catheters. Primary infection accounts for only 1% of all bacterial infective endocarditis (51). Vegetations, which usually appear on the atrial side of the TV, are the hallmark of infective TV endocarditis. On TEE, they appear as sessile or pedunculated echodensities attached to the valve surface or margins (50). Unlike mitral endocarditis, annular abscess is a rare complication of tricuspid endocarditis. Again, TEE is critical in determining the cause of tricuspid insufficiency and in guiding surgical correction. Surgical options for tricuspid endocarditis range from excising the valve to replacement. A recent study suggests that if the infectious process is limited to one leaflet, surgical excision with suture annuloplasty provides excellent results (52).

Carcinoid Disease of the Tricuspid Valve

Carcinoid heart disease occurs in patients with carcinoid tumors of the gastrointestinal tract that have metastasized to the liver and with carcinoid tumors in other sites that drain directly into the systemic venous circulation. The valvular lesions associated with carcinoid syndrome are usually limited to the right side of the heart. The predominant valve abnormality is TR. Patients with carcinoid heart disease present with right heart failure. TV lesions consist of endocardial fibrous thickening occurring on the ventricular aspect of the TV. TEE reveals leaflet thickening and chordal fusion (50). Surgical management of carcinoid TV disease relies mainly on replacing the diseased valve once symptoms become evident or echocardiographic evidence of right heart failure is revealed (53).

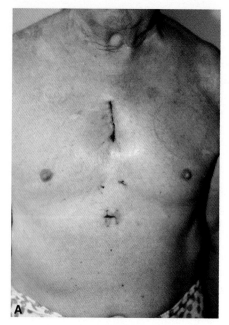
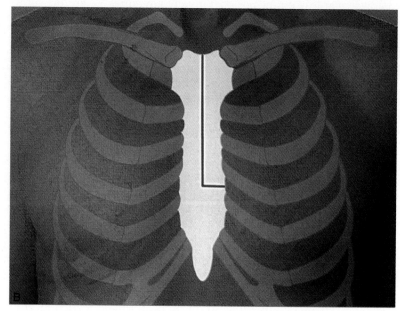

Figure 29.1. A: Healed skin incision of a patient who has undergone a hemisternotomy through a miniexposure. **B:** Typical hemisternotomy to access the MV.

SURGICAL MANAGEMENT OF MITRAL VALVE DISEASE

In the current era, the main objective of surgeons operating on patients with MV disease is to correct the pathology at hand to provide relief of signs and symptoms of the disease. The choice of intervention is dictated by the pathology. While in the past most patients were treated with valve replacement, presently every effort is made to preserve the MV apparatus. This results in the preservation of ventricular geometry, which is critical for ventricular function, while at the same time rendering patients anticoagulation-free. Every attempt should be made to conserve the MV; techniques for its repair are described in the following section.

SURGICAL PROCEDURES FOR MITRAL VALVE REGURGITATION

Operative Approach

For isolated MV disease, our approach of choice is a minimally invasive, right chest approach. This may entail a right minithoracotomy or an endoscopic, robotically assisted procedure (Fig. 29.1A,B). For the right minithoracotomy approach, the patient is positioned supine with the right arm distracted from the body (Fig 29.2). A 6- to 8-cm incision is created in the right 4th intercostal space, and the chest is entered after deflating the right lung. Cannulation for cardiopulmonary bypass is accomplished with echocardiographic guidance and Seldinger technique. A femoral venous cannula is advanced into the right atrium (RA) and superior vena cava, while arterial

return is achieved via a femoral arterial cannula. The aorta is occluded with a transthoracic cross-clamp, and the heart is arrested with both antegrade and retrograde cardioplegia.

The least invasive approach to the MV is a totally endoscopic procedure that entails application of the surgical robot. With the endoscopic robotic approach, five ports (each 1 cm or smaller) are placed on the right chest (Fig. 29.3). The ports are for the three robotic arms, a camera, and a working port through which sutures are handed to the surgeon. Echocardiographic imaging is essential for both cannulation and myocardial protection. Using echocardiographic guidance, a retrograde cardiople

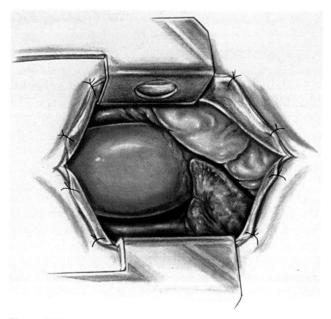

Figure 29.2. Exposure provided by hemisternotomy.

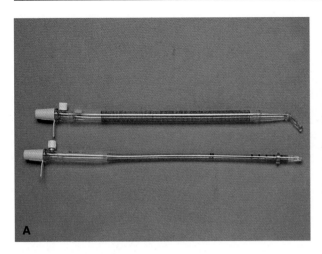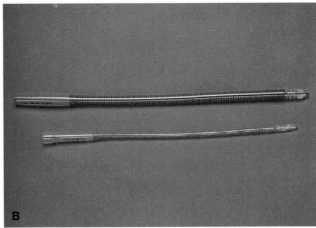

Figure 29.3. A: Comparison of size of standard adult aortic cannula and pediatric aortic cannula. **B:** Comparison of size of standard adult venous cannula and pediatric venous cannula.

gia catheter is placed from the internal jugular vein into the coronary sinus. Femoral venous and arterial cannulation is carried out as for the minithoracotomy approach. After establishing cardiopulmonary bypass, the endoclamp balloon is positioned in the ascending aorta. The balloon is inflated with echo visualization, occluding the aorta. Antegrade cardioplegia is delivered through the balloon catheter, while retrograde cardioplegia is delivered through the coronary sinus.

Because these right chest approaches entail peripheral cannulation, they are not suitable in patients with peripheral vascular disease or small femoral arteries. In addition, the endoclamp balloon cannot be used in patients with ascending aorta dimension greater than 38 mm. Finally, aortic regurgitation that is more than moderate in severity is a relative contraindication to a right chest approach to the MV.

With the patient cannulated and on CPB, the left atrium is approached via a standard lateral left atriotomy. Excellent exposure to the MV is facilitated with a MV retractor. The choice of surgical procedure is guided by complementary information provided by the pre-cardiopulmonary bypass echocardiogram (Table 29.4) and direct surgical inspection of the anatomy of the MV.

RING ANNULOPLASTY

Ischemic mitral regurgitation from annular dilatation and leaflet restriction from papillary-chordal tethering are best treated by an annuloplasty ring. Once access and exposure

TABLE 29.4	Surgically Relevant Echocardiographic Information in Mitral Valve Disease
Echocardiographic Parameter	**Relevant Surgical Information**
Annular diameter	Annular dilatation may be solely correctable with an annuloplasty ring
Direction of the regurgitant jet	Central jets correlate with functional regurgitation and thus ischemic annular dilatation Anterior jets correlate with posterior leaflet prolapse Posterior jets correlate with anterior leaflet prolapse
Anatomy of the leaflets	Flail leaflets can be evaluated, aiding in planning the type of repair (i.e., quadrangular resection for posterior leaflet flail versus choral transfer for anterior leaflet prolapse) Restricted leaflet motion and calcium deposition suggest the need for potential valve replacement in stenosis Leaflet vegetation or perforations secondary to endocarditis, which might require resection
Calcification of the annulus	Aids in planning intraoperative annular debridement
Shunts	Unsuspected septal defects, or fistulas, complicating abscess, requiring repair
Left atrial thrombus	Concomitant thrombectomy
Ventricular dimensions and function	Prognostic indicator

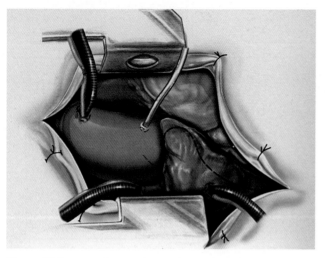

Figure 29.4. Typical cannulation for cardiopulmonary bypass through a ministernotomy. The dotted line on the RA represents the location of a future incision.

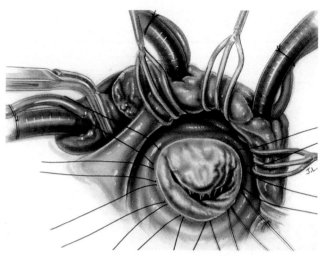

Figure 29.5. Annuloplasty ring sutures are placed on the posterior MV annulus for subsequent repair.

to the MV are gained the valve is carefully inspected for any concomitant pathology. Ring selection is done by measuring the anterior MV leaflet area. In general, a complete rigid or semi-rigid ring is favored.

TRIANGULAR RESECTION AND ANNULOPLASTY RING FOR POSTERIOR LEAFLET PROLAPSE OR FLAIL

The most common use of a triangular resection is a prolapsed middle scallop of the posterior leaflet, resulting from chordal rupture or elongation. A triangular resection is accomplished by initially identifying the margins of resection, and surrounding the normal chordae with silk ties. The flail scallop and its associated chordae are sharply resected with an 11-blade (Fig. 29.4). The defect is repaired primarily with running suture, and an annuloplasty band is placed. If primary repair of the remaining scallops is judged to result in excessive tension, then posterior advancement flaps are created by an incision along the posterior annulus towards each commissure for the final repair. Because we believe that longevity of the repair depends on the support of the surrounding annulus, every patient receives an annuloplasty ring.

CHORDAL TRANSFER FOR RUPTURED OR ELONGATED SEGMENT OF THE

Anterior Leaflet

Similar to posterior leaflet prolapse, anterior leaflet prolapse is caused by chordal elongation or rupture. However, because the anterior leaflet is attached to the

aortic valve annulus, repair of the anterior leaflet cannot be performed by segmental resection and annular plication. Thus, chordal transfer, or "flip over," was designed to treat patients with anterior leaflet flail. The principle behind this procedure lies in transposing a scallop, and its associated chordae, from the posterior leaflet onto the segment of diseased anterior leaflet.

Following MV exposure, the flailing segment of the anterior leaflet is isolated. Using nerve hooks, the portion of posterior leaflet to be transferred with its associated chordae is identified. The margin chordae of the area selected are encircled with silks. Two 5-0 Ethibonds are placed through the free edge of the selected area and the prolapsing segment. The area of posterior leaflet is resected, and each suture is tied, resulting in the approximation of the chordae to the prolapsing segment (Fig. 29.5) Additional sutures are placed onto the transfer to complete the repair. The remaining defect in the posterior leaflet is repaired with an annuloplasty ring for support as previously described.

Alternatively, anterior leaflet prolapse can be corrected by creation of artificial chordae. Durability of these chordae, which are constructed from polytetrafluoroethylene (PTFE), is excellent.

SURGICAL PROCEDURES FOR MITRAL VALVE STENOSIS

Mitral Valve Replacement

For MV replacement, there are two types of valves: bioprosthetic and mechanical valves. While superb durability has been reported with mechanical valves, patients receiving them require lifelong anticoagulation to prevent thromboembolic events. Thus, an attractive

TABLE 29.5	Surgically Relevant Echocardiographic Information in Tricuspid Valve Disease
Echocardiographic Parameter	**Relevant Surgical Information**
Annular diameter	Functional tricuspid regurgitation: valves are normal but dilated annulus. Findings would allow its repair rather than replacement
Anatomy of the leaflets	Leaflet thickening, commissural fusion, and chordal thickening suggest rheumatic or carcinoid valve disease and the need for replacement Valve vegetations (pedunculated or sessile echodensities) suggest endocarditis and the need for replacement
Right ventricular function	Right ventricular failure in a patient with carcinoid and valve disease suggests the need for valve replacement

alternative is a bioprosthetic valve. While these valves protect the patient from the untoward effects of anticoagulation, they are flawed by their lack of durability. However, in patients over the age of 70, structural deterioration is rare. Furthermore, results from clinical trials suggest that bovine pericardial MVs have a better long-term durability when compared with their porcine counterparts.

Despite good attempts to establish guidelines to help surgeons in choosing the right valve for the right patient, valve selection must be individualized for each patient. It depends on weighing the disadvantages of anticoagulation-related complications associated with mechanical valves against the disadvantages of decreased longevity of the bioprosthetic valves. Thus, mechanical valves are placed in young patients lacking contraindications to anticoagulation or in patients who already take anticoagulants. Alternatively, in older patients (>70), or in patients in whom anticoagulation is contraindicated, a bioprosthetic valve is the valve of choice.

To replace the MV, we use the same approach as previously described, unless other pathology (i.e., coronary artery disease or endocarditis) precludes this technique. The diseased MV should be debrided of all calcium deposits and fibrous material. It is essential to preserve the mitral leaflets and chordae tendinae to preserve ventricular function when replacing the MV. Debridement restores leaflet flexibility and allows insertion of an artificial valve. When inserting a mechanical valve, it is essential to ensure that the remaining MV leaflets or chordae do not obstruct, or become caught in, the valve mechanism, preventing proper valve function.

Selection of the appropriate size valve is facilitated by using commercially available sizers. To insert the valve, sutures are initially placed through the valve annulus and then the sewing ring. Our preference is to use pledges with our valve sutures placed on the atrial side of the annulus to avoid interfering with valve function. Once the valve is seated in the annulus, the sutures are tied. As with repairs, the replaced valve is tested both directly and with echocardiography.

SURGICAL MANAGEMENT OF TRICUSPID VALVE DISEASE

Surgical Therapy for Functional Tricuspid Valve Disease

The surgical approach for functional TV disease can be performed as above. Functional TR is seldom the only indication for operation. Again, as with MV disease, the surgical plan for management of TV dysfunction is guided by the findings of the intraoperative echocardiographic examination, as well as direct inspection of the TV (Table 29.5). Thus, commonly, functional tricuspid insufficiency is repaired with an additional surgical procedure. Key to this procedure is the fact that it can be performed as the last part of a case without the use of an aortic cross-clamp. Regardless, the TV is approached through a lateral right atriotomy. A MV retractor can be used to aid exposure. Once tricuspid insufficiency is confirmed, a valve sizer is used to determine ring size (Fig. 29.6). The commissures of the sizer should equal the extreme attachments of the septal

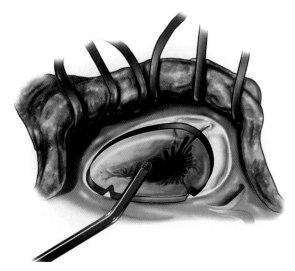

Figure 29.6. Measuring the septal area in a case depicting function TV insufficiency.

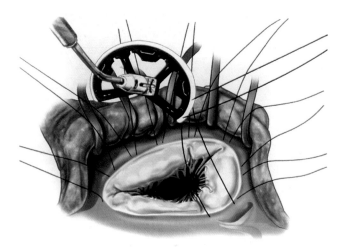

Figure 29.7. With the annuloplasty ring sutures in place, each individual suture is threaded through an annuloplasty ring.

leaflet. For patients with TR, the chosen ring should be one to two sizes smaller than the measured distance. The first suture is placed along the anterior leaflet just above the anterior/septal commissure.

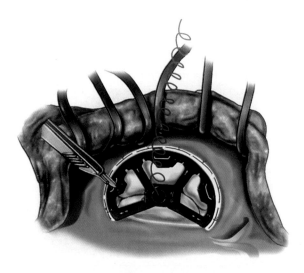

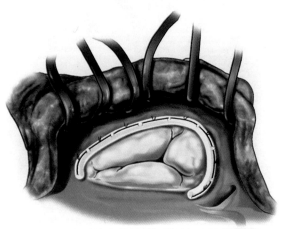

Figure 29.8. **A:** After each suture is tied, the ring is uncoupled from its holder. **B:** Completed TV repair with an annuloplasty ring

Suture placement continues clockwise until the medial aspect of the coronary sinus, approximately half-way across the septal leaflet. After completing the annular sutures, the stitches are placed through the annuloplasty ring (Fig. 29.7). Sutures are tied, the repair is tested, and the atriotomy is closed with a permanent running suture (Fig. 29.8). Intraoperative echocardiography is used to confirm the adequacy of repair.

TRICUSPID VALVE REPLACEMENT

Surgical replacement of the TV is reserved for rheumatic TV disease with its accompanying stenosis, TV endocarditis, and carcinoid-linked TV disease. Common to these etiologies is valve destruction not amenable to repair.

For all the previous entities, the leaflets are excised, and the orifice of the valve is measured with valve sizers. With the appropriate valve, selected valve sutures are placed around the tricuspid annulus and then through the valve. Similar to all other techniques, the atriotomy is closed with a running suture and TEE confirms the adequacy of the repair.

KEY POINTS

■ Prolapse of the posterior leaflet secondary to elongated or ruptured chords is the most common cause of mitral regurgitation in degenerative disease of the MV.

■ SAM may occur following repair of a degenerative MV and is caused by a tall posterior leaflet, displacing the anterior leaflet toward the septum during systole.

■ Patients with rheumatic MV disease who should be considered for repair are those with anterior leaflet and chordal pliability.

■ The most common cause of mitral regurgitation in ischemic disease is failure of leaflet coaptation during ventricular systole.

■ In patients with bacterial endocarditis, vegetations, leaflet perforation, annular abscess, and ruptured chords or papillary muscles found on TEE suggest the need for surgical intervention.

■ Periprosthetic valve regurgitation is the result of an incomplete seal of the sewing ring and annulus caused by either a failed suture line (early) or an infectious process.

■ Clinical outcomes are adversely affected when moderate-to-severe functional TR is not corrected surgically.

■ TV endocarditis is increasing in frequency secondary to the increased use of long-term venous catheters and the rise in IV drug abuse.

REFERENCES

1. Cosgrove DM. Mitral valve repair in patients with elongated chordae tendineae. *J Card Surg* 1989;4:247–253.
2. Reul RM, Cohn LH. Mitral valve reconstruction for mitral insufficiency. *Prog Cardiovasc Dis* 1997;39:567–599.
3. David TE, Armstrong S, Sun Z, et al. Late results of mitral valve repair for mitral regurgitation due to degenerative disease. *Ann Thorac Surg* 1993;56:7–14.
4. Olson LJ, Subramanian R, Ackerman DM, et al. Surgical pathology of the mitral valve: a study of 712 cases spanning 21 years. *Mayo Clin Proc* 1987;62:22–34.
5. Gillinov AM, Cosgrove DM. Mitral valve repair. *Oper Tech Thor Cardiovasc Surg* 1998;3:95–108.
6. Fenster MS, Feldman MD. Mitral regurgitation: an overview. *Curr Prob Cardiol* 1995;20:193–228.
7. Waller BF, Morrow AG, Maron BJ, et al. Etiology of clinically isolated, severe, chronic, pure mitral regurgitation: analysis of 97 patients over 30 years of age having mitral valve replacement. *Am Heart J* 1982;104:276–288.
8. Buchbinder NA, Roberts WC. Left-sided valvular active infective endocarditis. A study of forty-five necropsy patients. *Am J Med* 1972;53:20–35.
9. Stewart WJ, Salcedo EE. Echocardiography in patients undergoing mitral valve surgery. *Semin Thorac Cardiovasc Surg* 1989;1:194–202.
10. Gillinov AM, Cosgrove DM, Blackstone EH, et al. Durability of mitral valve repair for degenerative disease. *J Thorac Cardiovasc Surg* 1998;116:734–743.
11. Roberts WC. Complications of cardiac valve replacement: characteristic abnormalities of prostheses pertaining to any or specific site. *Am Heart J* 1982;103:113–122.
12. Zabalgoitia M. Echocardiographic assessment of prosthetic heart valves. *Curr Probl Cardiol* 2000;25(3):157–218.
13. Calderwood SB, Swinski LA, Waternaux CM, et al. Risk factors for the development of PVE. *Circulation* 1985;72:31–37.
14. Rutledge R, Kim BJ, Applebaum RE. Actuarial analysis of the risk of prosthetic valve endocarditis in 1598 patients with mechanical and bioprosthetic valves. *Arch Surg* 1985;120:469–472.
15. Czer LS, Chaux A, Matloff JM, et al. Ten-year experience with the St. Jude Medical valve for primary valve replacement. *J Thorac Cardiovasc Surg* 1990;100:44–54.
16. Copeland JG III, Sethi GK. Four-year experience with the CarboMedics valve: the North American experience. North American team of clinical investigators for the CarboMedics prosthetic heart valve. *Ann Thorac Surg* 1994;58:630–637.
17. Fann JI, Burdon TA. Are the indications for tissue valves different in 2001 and how do we communicate these changes to our cardiology colleagues? *Curr Opin Cardiol* 2001;16(2):126–135.
18. Breyer RH, McClenathan JH, Michaelis LL, et al. Tricuspid regurgitation: a comparison of nonoperative management, tricuspid annuloplasty, and tricuspid valve replacement. *J Thorac Cardiovasc Surg* 1976;72:867–874.
19. Carpentier A, Deloche A, Hanania G, et al. Surgical management of acquired tricuspid valve disease. *J Thorac Cardiovasc Surg* 1974;67:53–56.
20. Davila JC, Palmer TE. The mitral valve: anatomy and pathology for the surgeon. *Arch Surg* 1962;84:38–62.
21. Silverman ME, Hurst JW. The mitral complex: interaction of the anatomy, physiology, and pathology of the mitral annulus, mitral valve leaflets, chordae tendineae, and papillary muscles. *Am Heart J* 1968;76:399–418.
22. van Rijk-Zwikker GL, Delemarre BJ, Huysmans HA. Mitral valve anatomy and morphology: relevance to mitral valve replacement and valve reconstruction. *J Card Surg* 1994;9(2 Suppl.):255–261.
23. Ormiston JA, Shah PM, Tei C, et al. Size and motion of the mitral valve annulus in man. II. Abnormalities in mitral valve prolapse. *Circulation* 1982;65:713–719.
24. Voci P, Bilotta F, Caretta Q, et al. Papillary muscle perfusion pattern: hypothesis for ischemic papillary muscle dysfunction. *Circulation* 1995;91:1714–1718.
25. Kitzman DW, Scholz DG, Hagen PT, et al. Age-related changes in normal human hearts during the first 10 decades of life. Part II (Maturity): a quantitative anatomic study of 765 specimens from subjects 20 to 99 years old. *Mayo Clin Proc* 1988;63(2):137–146.
26. Silver MD, Lam JH, Ranganathan N, et al. Morphology of the human tricuspid valve. *Circulation* 1971;43:333–348.
27. Loop FD, Cosgrove DM, Stewart WJ. Mitral valve repair for mitral insufficiency. *Eur Heart J* 1991;12(Suppl. B):30–33.
28. Gillinov AM, Cosgrove DM III. Modified sliding leaflet technique for repair of the mitral valve. *Ann Thorac Surg* 1999;68:2356–2357.
29. Spencer FC. A plea for early, open mitral commissurotomy. *Am Heart J* 1978;95:668–670.
30. Galloway AC, Colvin SB, Baumann FG, et al. Current concepts of mitral valve reconstruction for mitral insufficiency. *Circulation* 1988;78:1087–1098.
31. Duran CM, Gometza B, De Vol EB. Valve repair in rheumatic mitral disease. *Circulation* 1991;84(Suppl. 5):III125–III132.
32. Yau TM, El-Ghoneimi YA, Armstrong S, et al. Mitral valve repair and replacement for rheumatic disease. *J Thorac Cardiovasc Surg* 2000;119:53–60.
33. Oury JH, Cleveland JC, Duran CG, et al. Ischemic mitral valve disease: classification and systemic approach to management. *J Card Surg* 1994;9(Suppl. 2):262–273.
34. Gillinov AM, Wierup PN, Blackstone EH, et al. Is repair preferable to replacement for ischemic mitral regurgitation? *J Thorac Cardiovasc Surg* 2001;122:1125–1141.
35. Bolling SF, Pagani FD, Deeb GM, et al. Intermediate-term outcome of mitral reconstruction in cardiomyopathy. *J Thorac Cardiovasc Surg* 1998;115:381–388.
36. Kishon Y, Oh JK, Schaff HV, et al. Mitral valve operation in postinfarction rupture of a papillary muscle: immediate results and long-term follow-up of 22 patients. *Mayo Clin Proc* 1992;67:1023–1030.
37. Moursi MH, Bhatnagar SK, Vilacosta I, et al. Transesophageal echocardiographic assessment of papillary muscle rupture. *Circulation* 1996;94:1003–1009.
38. Hendren WG, Morris AS, Rosenkranz E, et al. Mitral valve repair for bacterial endocarditis. *J Thorac Cardiovasc Surg* 1992;103:124–129.
39. Bayer AS, Bolger A, Taubert K, et al. Diagnosis and management of infective endocarditis and its complications. *Circulation* 1998;98:2936–2948.
40. Dreyfus G, Serref A, Jebara V, et al. Valve repair in acute endocarditis. *Ann Thorac Surg* 1990;49:706–713.
41. David TE, Bos J, Christakis GT, et al. Heart valve operations in patients with active infective endocarditis. *Ann Thorac Surg* 1990;49:701–705.

42. Ryan EW, Bolger A. TEE in the evaluation of infective endocarditis. *Card Clin* 2000;18:773–787.

43. Zabalgoitia M, Herrera CJ, Chaundhry FA, et al. Improvement in the diagnosis of bioprosthetic valve dysfunction by TEE. *J Heart Valve Dis* 1993;2:595.

44. Shulz R, Werener GS, Fuchs JB, et al. Clinical outcome and echocardiographic findings of native and prosthetic valve endocarditis in the 1990s. *Eur Heart J* 1996;17:281–288.

45. Lytle BW, Priest BP, Taylor PC, et al. Surgical treatment of prosthetic valve endocarditis. *J Thorac Cardiovasc Surg* 1996;111:198–207.

46. Gillinov AM, Cosgrove DM. Tricuspid valve repair for functional TR. *Op Tech Thor CV Surg* 1998;3(2):134–139.

47. Frater R. Tricuspid insufficiency. *J Thorac Cardiovasc Surg* 2001;122:427–429.

48. Gatti G, Maffei G, Lusa AM, et al. Tricuspid valve repair with the Cosgrove-Edwards annuloplasty system: early clinic and echocardiographic results. *Ann Thor Surg* 2001;72:764–767.

49. Kuwaki K, Morishita K, Tsukamoto M, et al. Tricuspid valve surgery for functional tricuspid valve regurgitation associated with left-sided valvular disease. *Eur J Cardiothorac Surg* 2001;20:577–582.

50. Blaustein AS, Ramanathan A. Tricuspid valve disease. Clinical evaluation, physiopathology, and management. *Cardiol Clin* 1998;16:551–572.

51. Chan P, Ogilby JD, Segal B. Tricuspid valve endocarditis. *Am Heart J* 1989;117:1140–1146.

52. Carozza A, Renzulli A, DeFeo M, et al. Tricuspid repair for infective endocarditis: clinical and echocardiographic results. *Tex Heart Inst J* 2001;28:96–101.

53. Connolly HM, Schaff HV, Mullany CJ, et al. Surgical management of left-sided carcinoid heart disease. *Circulation* 2001;104(12 Suppl.):I36–I40.

QUESTIONS

1. What is the direction of the regurgitant jet on Doppler TEE for prolapse of the posterior mitral valve (MV) leaflet?
   A. Posterior
   B. Lateral
   C. Anterior
   D. Central
   E. Distal

2. The most common cause of tricuspid regurgitation (TR) in the United States is
   A. a carcinoid tumor
   B. rheumatic disease
   C. Ehlers-Danlos syndrome
   D. functional secondary to mitral dysfunction
   E. endocarditis

3. Third-order chordae of the MV
   A. prevent billowing of the leaflets
   B. attach to the free margin of the leaflet
   C. arise from the lowest portion of the papillary muscle

D. are the smallest chords morphologically
E. insert into the annulus and maintain ventricular geometry

4. The most commonly encountered lesion in degenerative MV disease is
   A. restricted motion of the anterior leaflet
   B. prolapse of the posterior leaflet
   C. prolapse of the anterior leaflet
   D. restricted motion of the posterior leaflet
   E. annular calcification

5. Systolic anterior motion (SAM) occurs in what percentage of patients following MV repair for myxomatous disease?
   A. 5%
   B. 15%
   C. 20%
   D. 30%
   E. 45%

CHAPTER 30

Surgical Considerations and Assessment in Nonischemic Mitral Valve Surgery

Douglas C. Shook ■ Michael Essandoh ■ Robert M. Savage ■ William J. Stewart

HISTORICAL PERSPECTIVES

Over the last three decades, there have been great advances in mitral valve (MV) surgery closely affiliated with innovations in the intraoperative applications of echocardiography. In 1972, Johnson et al. reported the first use of echocardiography in MV surgery by demonstrating a successful open mitral commissurotomy using epicardial m-mode (1). Frazin, Talano, and Stephanides subsequently demonstrated the ability to accurately measure valve size and flow velocities using a transducer passed into the esophagus on a thin cable (2). In the late 1970s, Hisanga et al. placed a two-dimensional (2D) ultrasound transducer prototype on a flexible gastroscope (3). Kremer, Hanrath, Roizen et al. first reported the intraoperative use of transesophageal echocardiography for monitoring patients undergoing abdominal aortic aneurysm resections in 1982 (4,5). Goldman et al. demonstrated the potential intraoperative impact of echocardiography by detecting mitral regurgitation (MR), utilizing contrast-enhanced epicardial imaging in valve surgery (6). Takamoto et al. demonstrated the use of real-time color flow (CF) mapping during valve surgery (7).

IMPORTANCE OF INTRAOPERATIVE ECHOCARDIOGRAPHY (IOE) IN MV SURGERY

Early use of intraoperative guidance during mitral valve repairs (MVRep) surgery using Doppler CF mapping was reported by Stewart et al. (8). Since then, its use in guiding the intraoperative management of patients undergoing MV surgery has continued to expand. Intraoperative echocardiography (IOE) has demonstrated a unique ability to yield new diagnostic information impacting the surgical and hemodynamic management of patients in MV surgery (9–13). Based on such scientific evidence and expert opinion, the American College of Cardiology (ACC) and the American Heart Association (AHA) classified MVRep and mitral valve replacement (MVR) as Class I and IIA indications for IOE (14). The ability of IOE to impact the outcome of surgical

procedures involving the MV has established it as a universal diagnostic and monitoring standard of care for the intraoperative management of patients undergoing MV surgery (15–20).

IMPORTANCE OF INTRAOPERATIVE ECHOCARDIOGRAPY (IOE) MV ASSESSMENT IN THE FUTURE OF CARDIOTHORACIC ANESTHESIA

Consequently, there is a growing demand for clinicians with an experienced understanding of the echocardiographic assessment of the MV and its use in the intraoperative decision-making process (14). Because of the increasing numbers of patients projected to undergo surgical interventions for MV dysfunction over the next 20 years, this demand will continue (21–25). These projections are based on our aging population (Fig. 30.1), the high incidence of significant MV disease in the elderly, and the large percentage of patients having surgery within 10 years of their initial diagnosis of MV dysfunction (26–29) (Figs. 30.2 and 30.3). Because of the many advantages that MVRep offers the patient, an expanding number of cardiac centers are developing a successful experience with MVRep in all etiologies (30–32). With this increasing

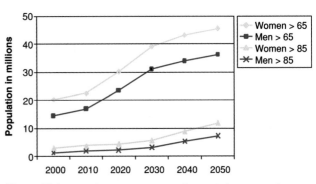

Figure 30.1. Population projections forecast the aging of America. By the year 2030, the United States Census Bureau estimates that 20% of individuals living in the United States will be over the age of 65.

	Age (years)					p value for trend	Frequency adjusted to 2000 US adult population
	18-44	45-54	55-64	65-74	≥75		
Participants (n)	4351	696	1240	3879	1745	..	209 128 094
Male, n (%)	1959 (45%)	258 (37%)	415 (33%)	1586 (41%)	826 (47%)	..	100 994 367 (48%)
Mitral regurgitation (n=449)	23, 0·5% (0·3-0·8)	1, 0·1% (0-0·8)	12, 1·0% (0·5-1·8)	250, 6·4% (5·7-7·3)	163, 9·3% (8·1-10·9)	<0·0001	1·7% (1·5-1·9)
Mitral stenosis (n=15)	0, 0% (0-0·1)	1, 0·1% (0-0·8)	3, 0·2% (0·1-0·7)	7, 0·2% (0·1-0·4)	4, 0·2% (0·1-0·6)	0·006	0·1% (0·02-0·2)
Aortic regurgitation (n=90)	10, 0·2% (0·1-0·4)	1, 0·1% (0-0·8)	8, 0·7% (0·3-1·3)	37, 1·0% (0·7-1·3)	34, 2·0% (1·4-2·7)	<0·0001	0·5% (0·3-0·6)
Aortic stenosis (n=102)	1, 0·02% (0-0·1)	1, 0·1% (0-0·8)	2, 0·2% (0·6-1·9)	50, 1·3% (1·0-1·7)	48, 2·8% (2·1-3·7)	<0·0001	0·4% (0·3-0·5)
Any valve disease							
Overall (n=615)	31, 0·7% (0·5-1·0)	3, 0·4% (0·1-1·3)	23, 1·9% (1·2-2·8)	328, 8·5% (7·6-9·4)	230, 13·2% (11·7-15·0)	<0·0001	2·5% (2·2-2·7)
Women (n=356)	19, 0·8% (0·5-1·3)	1, 0·2% (0·01-1·3)	13, 1·6% (0·9-2·7)	208, 9·1% (8·0-10·4)	115, 12·6% (10·6-15·0)	<0·0001	2·4% (2·1-2·8)
Men (n=259)	12, 0·6% (0·3-1·1)	2, 0·8% (0·1-2·8)	10, 2·4% (1·2-4·4)	120, 7·6% (6·3-9·0)	115, 14·0% (11·7-16·6)	<0·0001	2·5% (2·1-2·9)

Prevalence data are n, % (95% CI). Percentages are rounded to one decimal place.

A

Figure 30.2A. From National Heart, Lung, & Blood Institute (NHLBI) population-based database studies to obtain from the general population who had been assessed prospectively with echocardiography. (Nkomo VT, Gardin JM, Skelton TN, Gottdiener JS, Scott CG, Enriquez-Sarano M. Burden of valvular heart diseases: a population-based study. *Lancet* 2006; 368: 1005–1011.) (105)

Figure 30.2B. Prevalence of Valve Disease by Age; From NHLBI population-based database of general population assessed prospectively with echocardiography. (Nkomo VT, Gardin JM, Skelton TN, Gottdiener JS, Scott CG, Enriquez-Sarano M. Burdenof valvular heart diseases: a population-based study. *Lancet* 2006; 368: 1005–1011.) (105)

probability of successful MVRep, the ACC and AHA Task Force on Practice Guidelines for the Management of Patients with valvular heart disease have recommended earlier surgical referral for patients with MV dysfunction who are candidates with a high probability of successful MVRep (33). Currently, the Society of Thoracic Surgeons STS database reports that only 33% of isolated MV procedures from reporting cardiac surgery programs are MVReps (34). This is in contrast to the 90% incidence of MVRep reported by some cardiac centers experienced with MVRep (Fig. 30.4) (30–32). If the number of advanced MVRep procedures is to grow, it will require an increased availability of echocardiographic expertise throughout for the duration of such surgical procedures (14,33).

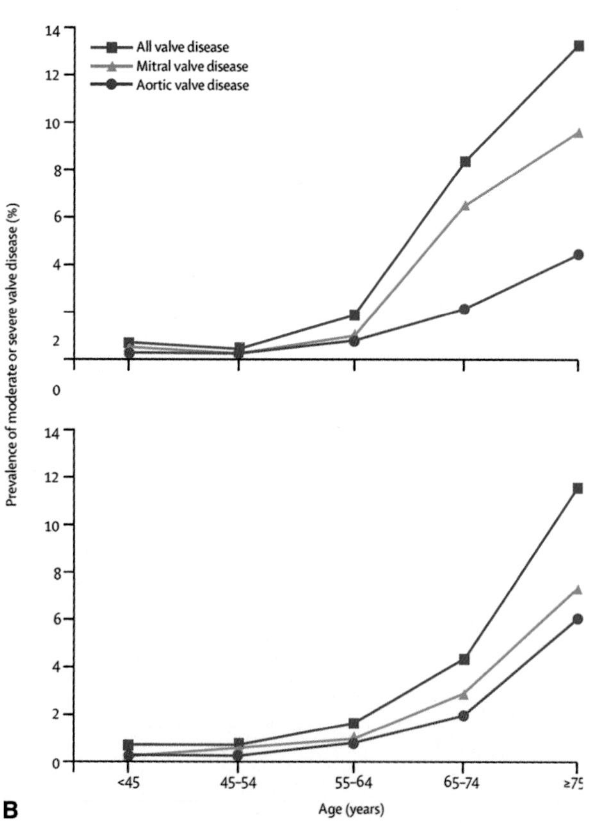

INTRAOPERATIVE ECHOCARDIOGRAPHY AND CRITICAL ISSUES IN MV SURGERY

For patients scheduled for elective MV surgery, the purpose of the IOE exam is not to replace the preoperative diagnostic evaluation but to confirm the severity of MV dysfunction, refine an understanding of its mechanism, and ensure the surgical results (Table 30.1). However, there are some unusual scenarios where decisions to perform, or not perform, MV surgery are made following the results of the IOE exam.

1. The first of these involves patients with preoperative mild-moderate MR or mitral stenosis (MS) undergoing another cardiac surgical procedure and confirmation of a decision to avoid MV surgery is desired. In these circumstances, customary monitors are placed, prior to induction, to better understand the patient's baseline hemodynamics. During the intraoperative assessment, hemodynamics similar to those recorded at a preoperative echocardiographic exam or just prior to induction are reproduced.

2. The second such scenario is significant MV dysfunction that was either undiagnosed or is more severe than was determined by the preoperative evaluation. When the MR is of surgical severity, adding a mitral procedure is

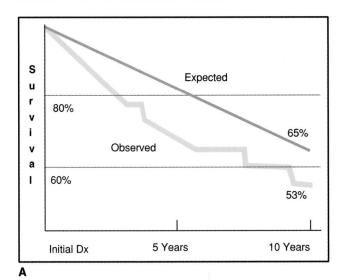

A

Figure 30.3A. Enriquez-Sariano et al. compared the cardiac morbidity and long-term survival at 5 and 10 years in patients diagnosed with flail MV leaflet to normal survival for age. Schaff HV, Orszulak TA, et al. Valve repair improves the outcome of surgery for mitral regurgitation: a multivariate analysis. Circulation. 1995;91:1022–1028. (105a)

EVENT	OVERALL POPULATION			
	NO. OF EVENTS	5-YEAR RATE	10-YEAR RATE	LINEAR-IZED YEARLY RATE
				percent
Death from any cause	45	28±4	43±7	6.3
Death from cardiac cause	31	21±4	33±7	4.3
Congestive heart failure	55	30±4	63±8	8.2
Chronic atrial fibrillation†	13	8±3	30±12	2.2
Thromboembolism	13	12±3	12±3	1.9
Hemorrhage	3	1±1	3±2	0.4
Endocarditis	10	5±2	8±3	1.5
Mitral-valve surgery	143	57±3	82±4	20.0
Mitral-valve surgery or death	188	69±3	90±3	26.3

Outcome in subgroups of patients

B

Figure 30.3B. Ling et al. and Enriquez-Sariano et al. have demonstrated that a high percentage of patients with structural MR either expire or have surgery within 10 years of their initial diagnosis. Timing of MV surgery. *Br Heart J* 28:79–85, Jan.

often a good idea, as long as it does not prohibitively increase the surgical risk-to-benefit ratio.

3. The final situation is finding MR that is significantly less than expected or absent. When findings of the precardiopulmonary bypass (pre-CPB) IOE suggest a change in the operative plan, considerable thought must be given to the reasons for this discrepancy. However, intraoperative conditions may underestimate the amount of MR present under "street conditions" that have led to the well-established plan to perform MV surgery. We often challenge such patients by increasing preload and afterload (volume loading and phenylephrine) to see if

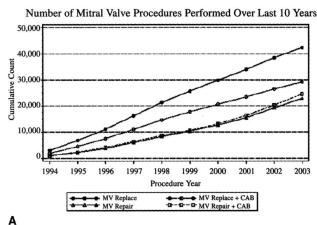

A

Figure 30.4A. The 2003 Executive Summary of the Society of Thoracic Surgeons documents the continued growth of MV surgery. More than 30% of all MV surgeries since 1994 involved a reconstructive approach to MV dysfunction (34). The percentage of MVRep versus replacements continues to increase.

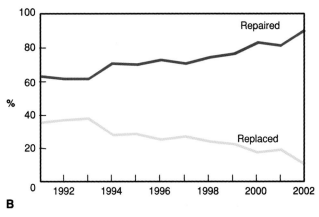

B

Figure 30.4B. The percentage of MVRep procedures performed in patients undergoing isolated MV surgery at the Cleveland Clinic has consistently increased since 1995.

the underrepresentation of MR might be a transient or misleading issue. When the operative mission is changed substantially, it is helpful to contact the consultative clinicians who have been involved in the long-term management of the patient. These are also situations where it is advisable to use the most quantitative assessments of severity, such as those recommended by the ASE Nomenclature and Standards Committee Task Force on Native Valve Regurgitation (35).

Because MVRep is the preferred treatment for MV dysfunction of all etiologies, every patient is considered a potential candidate for repair. The most significant surgical issues, which the initial intraoperative exam assists in resolving include

1. The probability of successful MVRep
2. The necessity to perform other surgical interventions related to the patient's secondary, associated, or coexisting cardiovascular dysfunction
3. The assessment of the results of the surgical procedure

TABLE 30.1	IOE Exam and Critical Issues in MV Surgery

1. Confirm and refine preoperative assessment
   - Confirm MV dysfunction and severity
   - Determine repairability of valve
     - Refine pathoanatomy and mechanism
     - Explain variances
2. Determine the need for unplanned surgical intervention
   - Secondary pathophysiology
   - Associated abnormality
   - Unrelated process
3. Determine cardiac dysfunction impacting management
   - Secondary pathophysiology
   - Dysfunction associated with primary etiology
   - Coexisting dysfunction
4. Cannulation and perfusion strategy
5. Address surgical procedure–specific issues
6. Predict complications
7. Assess surgical results
   - Initial and ongoing patient management
   - Results of surgery
   - Complications

assistance with the postcardiopulmonary bypass (post-CPB) assessment of the repair and, if necessary, determining the mechanism(s) of an initially unsuccessful MVRep or other potential post-CPB complications. However, even with the experienced surgeon, the IOE exam serves as a final pre-intervention diagnostic screen for previously undiagnosed but significant valve or other cardiac dysfunction.

The decision to perform additional surgical interventions is made during the pre-CPB evaluation for significant secondary pathophysiology and associated or coexisting cardiovascular disease. Chaliki et al. discovered that in 1,265 patients undergoing MV surgery, 146 (12%) had new pre-CPB findings that altered their intraoperative management (38). Sheikh et al. evaluated 154 consecutive patients who had IOE assessment in conjunction with a valve operation. The IOE yielded unsuspected findings prior to CPB that either modified or changed the planned operation in 19% of patients (39). Other important issues that the IOE exam addresses include the cannulation perfusion and myocardial protection strategy, specific surgical procedure–related issues (i.e., need for sliding annuloplasty), determination of the probability of certain post-CPB complications, and assessment of the results of surgical intervention. The information provided from the systematic IOE exam provides the intraoperative team with an up-to-date road map, which will guide the surgical decision-making process and direct the hemodynamic management of the patient throughout the operation (40).

ORGANIZATION OF CHAPTER

IOE has become an integral part of the comprehensive management of the patient undergoing MV surgery. As we will see, it has a direct influence on the intraoperative decision-making process for the surgical and hemodynamic management of the patient. It has a lasting impact on long-term outcome. The majority of patients having MV surgery are customarily scheduled following a thorough and extensive evaluation. Consequently, the intraoperative focus shifts from one of exhaustive assessment of severity of MV dysfunction to those essential issues that will impact the course of the surgical intervention and, ultimately, patient outcome. These issues include an understanding of the mechanism(s) of MV dysfunction, the potential repairability of the valve, and the patient's intraoperative management. Consequently, we will emphasize the technique of the intraoperative exam used for developing a three-dimensional (3D) understanding of the etiology and mechanics causing dysfunction of the MVAp. This chapter will provide an understanding of how the intraoperative transesophageal echocardiography (TEE) exam is incorporated into the daily management of patients undergoing MV surgery. It will focus on those aspects of the intraoperative exam that permit an accurate and efficient assessment of the critical

The surgeon's ability to repair the MV is determined by a number of factors, including the underlying etiology, the structural integrity of the anatomic components of the mitral valve apparatus (MVAp), and the mechanism of dysfunction caused by the underlying pathologic process (36,37). The surgeon's strategy for repair or replacement is a result of examination of the anatomy of the MVAp in correlation with the functional assessment of the MVAp provided by the IOE exam. The direct inspection of the MVAp includes an evaluation of the left atrium (size and secondary regurgitant lesions), annulus (secondary jet lesions, degree dilatation, scarring, and deformity), valve leaflets (thickness, motion, and coaptation), chordae (redundancy, thickness, and presence of fusion or rupture), papillary muscle (elongation, infarct, or rupture), and the free wall of the left ventricle (LV). From this information, the surgeon establishes the most effective line of attack, incorporating a variety of MVRep techniques or replacing the valve.

For the surgeon less experienced in MVRep surgery, the IOE exam contributes to an accelerated learning curve by enabling surgeons to immediately compare the findings of their direct inspection with those of the echocardiography examination. The more accomplished surgeon has developed repair strategies based on surgical experience in conjunction with IOE. The echocardiographer provides greater

issues that must be addressed for patients undergoing MV surgery. To reinforce the fundamental considerations in the chapter, a summary of "Key Concepts" is provided at the beginning and a brief review at the conclusion. An overview of the surgical anatomy of the MVAp and the TEE imaging planes used in intraoperative assessment is provided. We will then concentrate on the efficient approach to the systematic echocardiographic exam for patients undergoing MV surgery including evaluation of MV pathology, secondary pathophysiology, and associated or coexisting cardiovascular disease. Finally, we concentrate on additional details required from the intraoperative examination to ensure the successful outcome of patients undergoing the wide range of MV surgical interventions.

KEY CONCEPTS

■ The MVAp is a complex structure consisting of the fibrous cardiac skeleton, saddle-shaped mitral annulus, MV leaflets, chordae, papillary muscles, and ventricular wall complex. Pathologic processes that lead to structural damage to the anatomic integrity of the components of the MVAp may result in MV dysfunction.

■ The purpose of the IOE exam is to confirm and refine the patient's preoperative assessment as issues that are critical to their intraoperative management are resolved.

■ MVRep is the treatment of choice for MV dysfunction resulting from all etiologies because of its superior long-term survival, preservation of ventricular function, and greater freedom from thromboembolism, endocarditis, and anticoagulant-related complications.

■ For patients scheduled for elective MV surgery, the most significant surgical issues that the IOE exam assists in resolving include the repairability of the MVAp, the necessity to perform other surgical interventions, and the post-CPB assessment of the surgical procedure and complications.

■ The feasibility of MVRep is guided by the real-time assessment of the MVAp and the mechanism of dysfunction by the IOE exam, in conjunction with the surgeon's direct inspection of the MVAp.

■ The IOE exam is performed according to the unique demands of the cardiac surgical environment, with the pre-CPB and post-CPB exams organized by priority to ensure that critical issues are addressed should the patient require the initiation of CPB.

■ The pre-CPB IOE exam determines the severity and anatomic mechanism of MV dysfunction, in addition to assessing secondary or associated pathophysiology, cannulation-perfusion strategy, the potential for post-CPB complications, and providing an ongoing assessment of cardiac function.

■ The post-CPB IOE exam provides a quality assurance safety net with immediate assessment of the surgical

procedure and diagnosis of complications related to the surgery or disease process.

■ The IOE exam relies upon integrated methods of severity assessment that may be efficiently performed in a multitasking environment. The methods included here are those recommended by the American Society of Echocardiography's (ASEs) Task Force on Native Valvular Regurgitation. They have been validated by accepted standards to ensure their ability to reliably guide the intraoperative decision-making process.

■ The severity of MV dysfunction is evaluated intraoperatively by the integration of multiple 2D and Doppler parameters. The reliance on any one method of assessing severity is weighted by dependability of the specific data acquired and the quantitative reliability of a particular technique. Such an integrated approach minimizes the individual measurement error inherent to each.

■ Color flow Doppler (CFD) is a method to screen for severe MV dysfunction. Its use as a stand-alone method of severity assessment to guide the intraoperative decision-making process is not recommended (35).

■ The 3D echocardiographic exam of the MV complements a complete 2D exam.

MITRAL VALVE APPARATUS

Normal Anatomy of the Mitral Valve Apparatus

The MVAp is the anatomical term describing the structures associated with MV function. It consists of the fibrous skeleton of the heart, the mitral annulus, mitral leaflets, mitral chordae, and the papillary muscle–ventricular wall complex (Fig. 30.5) (41–45). This complex structure is

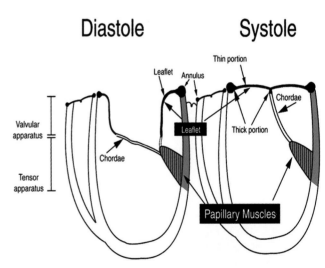

Figure 30.5. The MV is composed of five distinct anatomic structures including the mitral annulus, valve leaflets, chordae, papillary muscles, and ventricular wall. Dysfunction of any one of these structures will eventually interfere with the effective coaptation of the valve leaflets with associated valve regurgitation and its associated sequelae.

comprised of the tensor apparatus (fibrous annulus, left ventricular myocardium from the fibrous MV annulus to the base of papillary muscle insertion, the papillary muscles, and the chordae) and the valvular apparatus (valve leaflets). Maintenance of the continuity of the tensor and valvular apparatus is essential for normal ventricular and MV functions (41,42).

Fibrous Skeleton

The fibrous skeleton of the heart is formed by the three U-shaped cords of the aortic annulus and their extensions, forming the right trigone, left trigone, and a smaller fibrous structure from the right aortic coronary cusp to the root of the pulmonary artery (42,44,46). This skeleton plays a primary function in structural support of the heart. The U-shaped cords of the aortic annulus merge to form the right and left fibrous trigone (46). A fibrous skeleton extends between the aortic and mitral annulus and is referred to as the intervalvular fibrosa (44–46).

Mitral Annulus

Fibrous tissue extends from the left and right atrioventricular orifices, forming the annulus of the mitral and tricuspid valves (41,43,47,48). The mitral annulus serves as a transition between the left atrium, mitral leaflets, and LV. The base of the anterior mitral valve leaflet (AMVL) is closely associated with the left trigone, intertrigonal space, and right trigone area (Fig. 30.6) (44). The fibrous mitral annulus is an ellipsoidal, 3D, saddle-shaped structure that thins posteriorly where it is more prone to dila-

tation in pathologic conditions (Fig. 30.7A–C) (48). The resulting increased tension on the posterior valve leaflet at its thinnest region contributes to the 60% incidence of chordal tears in the P2 region. The annulus is saddle shaped during systole but changes to a circular shape in diastole (Fig. 30.7B) (36). The anterior mitral annulus is more rigid. It undergoes less change in shape during the cardiac cycle and is less prone to dilation (47,48). The U-shaped minor axis of the ellipsoid annulus is best visualized and measured in the midesophageal long-axis (LAX) imaging plane, whereas the U-shaped major axis is best visualized and measured in the ME commissural imaging plane (Fig. 30.7D). Accordingly, prolapse of valve leaflets (extension above the plane of the mitral annulus) is more accurately assessed in the midesophageal long-axis imaging plane due to its more basal position of the annulus compared to the commissural imaging plane (41,46,48).

Mitral Valve Leaflets

Morphologically, the MV has two leaflets referred to as the anterior and posterior leaflets (AMVL and PMVL). The mitral leaflets are attached to the fibrous annulus and to the free wall of the ventricle via papillary muscles and the primary edge and secondary midvalve chordae (43–45). The AMVL is triangular in shape and attached to the fibrous body at the left coronary cusp and anterior half of the noncoronary cusp of the aortic valve. The AMVL comprises about 55% to 60% of the total MV area and about 30% of the annular circumference (42,43). The posterior leaflet comprises 40% to 45% of the MV area and attaches to the mitral annulus posteriorly (Fig. 30.8) (41,42). As the heart normally lies in the chest cavity, the PMVL height (length) is usually less than

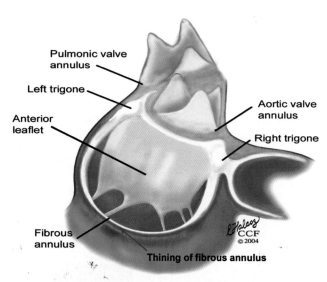

Figure 30.6. The fibrous skeleton of the heart is formed by the three U-shaped cords of the aortic annulus and by extensions forming the right trigone, left trigone, and a smaller fibrous structure from the right aortic coronary cusp to the root of the pulmonary artery. The skeleton provides a rigid structural foundation for the valves and chambers of the heart. The anterior leaflet attaches to the fibrous skeleton at the rigid intervalvular fibrosa, giving it less flexibility. The fibrous tissue of the mitral annulus thins posteriorly (*blue arrow*).

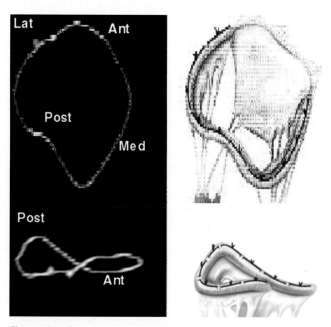

Figure 30.7A. 3D shape of MV annulus and with a 3D annuloplasty ring.

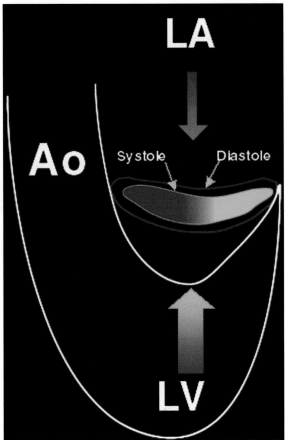

Figure 30.7B. During systole, the circular annulus circumferentially narrows, becoming a 3D saddle-shaped annulus. This effectively decreases the size of the MV orifice. Fibrosis or calcification of the annulus interferes with its mobility and effectively increases the area requiring leaflet apposition to prevent regurgitant flow.

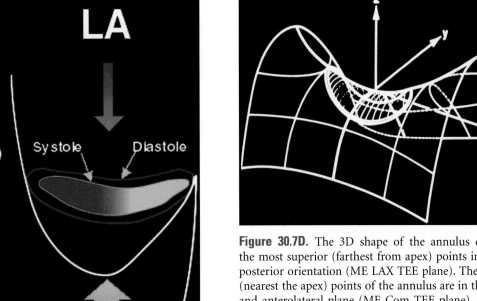

Figure 30.7D. The 3D shape of the annulus demonstrating the most superior (farthest from apex) points in the anterior-posterior orientation (ME LAX TEE plane). The most inferior (nearest the apex) points of the annulus are in the inferoseptal and anterolateral plane (ME Com TEE plane). Using the ME Com imaging plane will result in lower specificity in the diagnosis of MV prolapse or excessive leaflet motion.

the height of the AMVL (Fig. 30.9). During systole, the leaflets come together along a "line of coaptation," which extends anteriorly to the anterolateral commissure (ALC) and posteriorly to the posteromedial commissure (PMC) (Fig. 30.10). During diastole, the middle of the leaflet initially moves toward the ventricle followed by opening of the valve at the leaflet edges (44,48) (Fig. 30.11). The middle of the leaflet opens before the commissures. Once the leaflet extends fully, it may flutter and drift upward until the atrial contraction. The surface of each leaflet is divided into a rough zone (coapting surface where

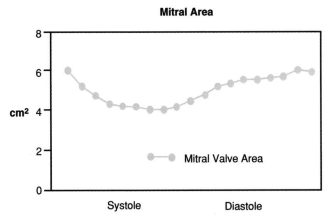

Figure 30.7C. The fibrous mitral annulus is an ellipsoidal saddle-shaped structure, which thins posteriorly where it is more prone to dilatation in pathologic conditions. During systole, the annulus decreases in size and becomes saddle shaped. In diastole, it changes to a circular shape. The anterior mitral annulus is more rigid and has minimal change in shape during the cardiac cycle.

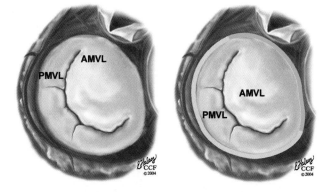

Figure 30.8. The MV has two leaflets referred to as the anterior and posterior leaflets (AMVL and PMVL). The mitral leaflets are circumferentially attached to the fibrous annulus. The AMVL is attached to the same fibrous body as the left coronary cusp (*blue arrow*). The AMVL comprises about 55% to 60% of the total MV surface area and about 30% to 40% of the annular circumference. The posterior leaflet comprises 40% to 45% of the MV area and 60% to 70% of the circumference as it attaches to the mitral annulus posteriorly.

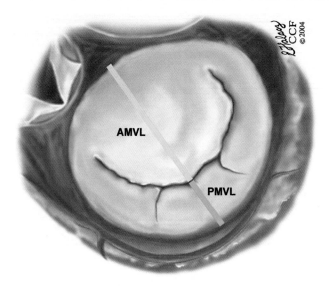

Figure 30.9. The MV has two leaflets referred to as the anterior and posterior leaflets (AMVL and PMVL). As the heart normally lies in the chest cavity, the PMVL height (length) is usually less than the height of the AMVL.

primary chords attach), clear zone (midportion of leaflet, secondary chordae attachments), and basal zone (leaflet attachment to the annulus and insertion of posterior tertiary chordae) (49). The basal two thirds of each leaflet is smoother than the distal third. The combined surface area of the mitral leaflets is twice that of the mitral orifice. This permits large areas of coaptation with a normal 3 to 5 mm of residual leaflet apposition distal to the point of coaptation (43–45). This line of coaptation between the two leaflets is semicircular and influences the segments of the valve leaflets, which are visualized in the standard imaging planes (Fig. 30.12). There is a range of mitral commissural orientations due to variation in the degree of annular size and rotation of the heart caused by individual anatomic variations and enlargement of cardiac chambers. Consequently, the commissure may be oriented more clockwise in some individuals, explaining the variability of segmental mitral anatomy visualized at the same transducer

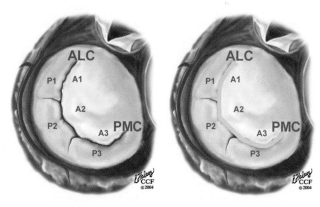

Figure 30.10. During systole, the leaflets come together along a "line of coaptation," which extends anteriorly to the ALC and posteriorly to the PMC.

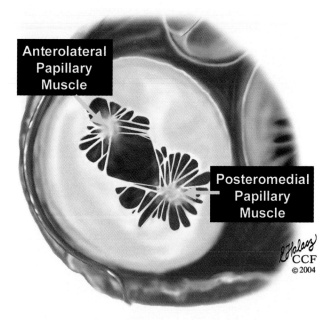

Figure 30.11. During diastole, the middle of the leaflet moves toward the ventricle with opening of the valve at the leaflet edges. The middle of the leaflet opens before the commissures. Once the leaflet extends fully, it may loiter until atrial contraction.

rotation in different patients (Fig. 30.13). The posterior MV leaflet typically consists of three scallops that are separated by prominently distinct indentations called clefts (Fig. 30.14). These scallops are referred to as lateral, middle, and medial. The lateral scallop is closest to the left atrial appendage (43,45). The anterior leaflet, for purely descriptive purposes, is segmented into the corresponding lateral, middle, and medial thirds.

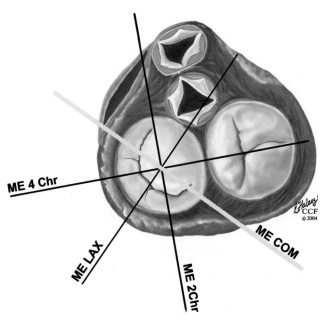

Figure 30.12. The line of coaptation between the two leaflets is semicircular, and the orientation of the commissure determines the segments of the valve leaflets that are visualized in the standard imaging planes.

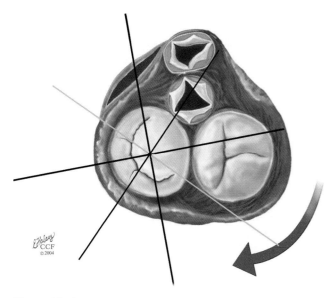

Figure 30.13. There is a range of mitral commissural shapes and orientations due to variation in annular size and rotation of the heart. This may be caused by individual anatomic variations and/or by enlargement of chambers that rotate the orientation of the commissure. Because of the fibrous skeleton, the orientation between the MV and aortic valve is consistent.

Chordae Tendinae

Chordae are fibrous attachments extending from the leaflet to the papillary muscles and posterior ventricular wall. During systole, the papillary muscles contract and keep the chordae taut, preventing prolapse of the leaflets into the left atrium. The spaces between the chordae also serve as secondary orifices between the left atrium and LV (41,43). With rheumatic fusion of the chordae, subvalvular narrowing of the ventricular inflow may be more pronounced than that caused by leaflet fusion (45). Up to 120 chordae attach to the undersurface and edge of the MV leaflets and annulus (Fig. 30.15). They are classified as *primary chordae* (extending from the PM to the leaflet edge), *secondary chordae* (extending from the PM to the mid-undersurface belly of the leaflet at the junction of the rough and clear zone), and *tertiary chordae* (extending from the posterior ventricular wall to the base of leaflet or annulus) (49). There are usually two dominant anterior secondary chordae that are referred to as strut or stabilizing, chordae, that attach to the medial and lateral halves of the AMVL (49,50). Interruption of these secondary stabilizing or posterior tertiary chordae may result in deterioration of ventricular function.

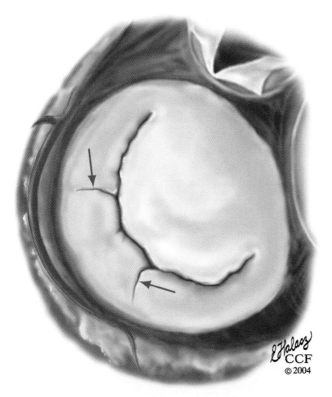

Figure 30.14. The posterior MV leaflet consists of three scallops that are separated by prominently distinct indentations called clefts (*red arrows*). These scallops are referred to as the (antero) lateral, middle, and (postero) medial. The (antero) lateral scallop is closest to the left atrial appendage. The anterior leaflet, for purely descriptive purposes, is segmented into the corresponding lateral, middle, and medial thirds.

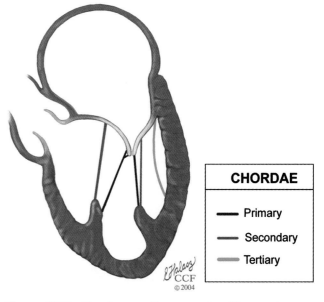

CHORDAE

— Primary
— Secondary
— Tertiary

Figure 30.15. Chordae are fibrous tendon-like attachments extending from the leaflet to the papillary muscles and posterior ventricular wall. During systole, the papillary muscles contract and keep the chordae taut, thereby preventing prolapse of the leaflets into the left atrium. Tandler and Quain classified chordae as first, second, and third order. The first order attach to the leaflet edges adjacent to the commissure. Secondary rough zone chordae insert 8 mm from the free margin. There are two dominant secondary chordae (strut or stay chordae) going to the medial and lateral halves of the AMVL. Third order basal chordae only extend to the base of the PMVL and maintain annular ventricular relation during the cardiac cycle.

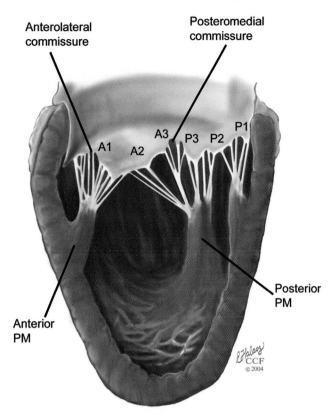

Figure 30.16. Originating from the anterolateral and poster-omedial walls of the LV (between the middle and apical segments) are the two papillary muscles called by their segmental ventricular origin: ALPM and PMPM. These papillary muscles run parallel to the adjacent ventricular wall. The larger ALPM usually has one or two heads whereas the smaller PLPM may have two or three. Chordal tendons from the head of each papillary muscle attach to both of the MV leaflets. The chordae that arise from the anterolateral PM extend to the lateral halves of the posterior and anterior MV leaflets. Consequently, the ALPM and PMPM subtend and support their respective commissure (49).

Papillary Muscles

Originating from the anterolateral and posteromedial walls of the LV (between the middle and apical segments) are the two papillary muscles named due to their ventricular origin, *anterolateral papillary muscle* (ALPM) and *posteromedial papillary muscles* (PMPMs) (Fig. 30.16) (41–43,49). These papillary muscles run parallel to the adjacent ventricular wall. The larger ALPM usually has one or two heads, whereas the smaller *posterolateral papillary muscle* (PLPM) may have two or three. Chordal tendons from the head of each papillary muscle attach to both of the MV leaflets. The chordae that arise from the anterolateral PM extend to the anterolateral halves of the posterior and anterior MV leaflets (Fig. 30.17). Consequently, the ALPM and PMPM subtend and support their respective commissure (49). The ALPM muscle is perfused by blood from the left anterior descending coronary artery and circumflex, whereas the PMPM is supplied by a posterior descending branch from a right dominant right coronary artery (RCA) or left dominant circumflex coronary artery (51). Consequently, isolated papillary muscle infarct or rupture of the PMPM is more common than a rupture of the ALPM.

Left Ventricle

The ALPM and PMPMs are inserted into the anterolateral and posteroinferior segments of the LV in the region near the interface between the middle and apical thirds of the ventricular chamber (41,44,51). The mechanical tensor function of the MVAp is maintained through the continuity that the ventricular walls provide in connecting the papillary muscles with the MV annulus (41). If there is scarring in the anterolateral or posteromedial free walls of the LV, this may result in traction on the MV annulus and deformity throughout the cardiac cycle. This may lead to restriction of the PMVL during systole, with a resulting override of the AMVL and a posteriorly directed regurgitant jet.

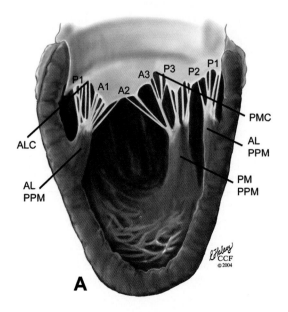

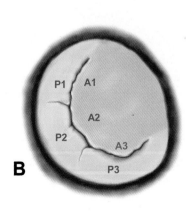

Figure 30.17. A: The posterior mitral valve leaflet (PMVL) and its supporting chordae are illustrated in *blue*. The AMVL and its supporting chordae are shown in *beige*. The ALPM provides chordae to the lateral half of the PMVL and the lateral half of the AMVL. The PMPM provides chordae to the medial half of the PMVL and the medial half of the AMVL. **B:** The PMVL and its three scallops are illustrated in *blue* coloration. The AMVL and its three segments are illustrated in *beige*.

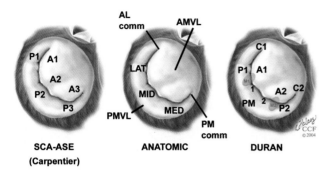

Nomenclature of the Mitral Valve Apparatus

There are three segmental nomenclatures commonly employed to describe the anatomy of the MVAp: the ASE-SCA (Carpentier), the anatomic, and the Duran (Fig. 30.18). The ASE Nomenclature and Standards Committee and the Society of Cardiovascular Anesthesiologists (SCA) adopted the Carpentier system for standardizing the segmental leaflet nomenclature (52). The Duran nomenclature system is an extremely valuable contribution to our understanding of the MVAp because it is established on the chordal attachments between the papillary muscles and the valve leaflet segments (43).

The ASE-SCA nomenclature (Carpentier) defines the three scallops of the posterior leaflet as P1 (lateral), P2 (middle), and P3 (medial) (Figs. 30.18 and 30.19). The P1 (lateral) scallop is adjacent to the ALC and is closest to the left atrial appendage. The P3 scallop is adjacent to the PMC (52). This nomenclature defines the three corresponding areas of the anterior leaflet and A1 (opposite P1), A2 (opposite P2), and A3 (opposite P3).

With the anatomic nomenclature (Fig. 30.18), the posterior leaflet consists of three scallops: lateral (antero), middle, and medial (postero), as described above (52). The (antero) lateral scallop is closest to the left atrial appendage. The anterior leaflet, for purely descriptive purposes, is divided into the corresponding lateral, middle, and medial thirds. The ALPM provides chordae to the lateral halves of the AMVL and PMVL (53). Consequently, the middle scallop of the posterior leaflet and middle segment of the anterior leaflet receive chordae from both papillary muscles (Figs. 30.17–30.19).

Figure 30.18. There are three segmental nomenclatures used to describe the anatomy of the MVAp: the ASE-SCA (Carpentier), the anatomic, and the Duran. The ASE Nomenclature and Standards Committee of the ASE and the SCA adopted the Carpentier system for standardizing the segmental leaflet nomenclature. The Duran nomenclature is an extremely valuable contribution to our understanding of the MVAp because it is established on the chordal distribution between the papillary muscles and the valve leaflet segments.

SCA-ASE standardized nomenclature: P, PMVL segments (P1, lateral scallop; P2, middle scallop; P3, medial scallop). A, AMVL segments (A1, lateral segment; A2, middle segment; A3, medial segment). Papillary muscles, commissures use anatomic descriptors (PMPM, posteromedial papillary muscle; ALPM, anterolateral papillary muscle; PMC, posteromedial commissure; ALC, anterolateral commissure).

Duran nomenclature: P, PMVL ([P1, lateral scallop; PM, middle scallop; PM1, lateral portion of middle scallop receiving chordae from the ALPM [M1]; PM2, medial portion of middle scallop receiving chordae from the PMPM [M2]]). The ALC is referred to as C1 and the PMC is C2.

ASE/SCA Terminology
(per Carpentier)

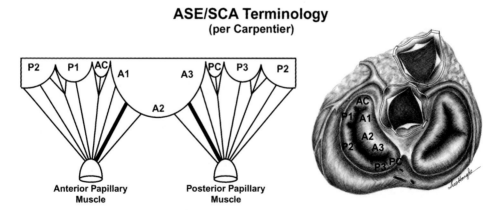

Figure 30.19. The SCA-ASE nomenclature (Carpentier) defines the three scallops of the posterior leaflet as P1 (lateral), P2 (middle), and P3 (medial). The P1 (lateral) scallop is adjacent to the ALC and is closest to the left atrial appendage. The P3 scallop is adjacent to the PMC. This nomenclature defines the three corresponding areas of the anterior leaflet and A1 (opposite P1), A2 (opposite P2), and A3 (opposite P3). Originating from the anterolateral and posteromedial walls of the LV (between the middle and apical segments) are the two papillary muscles called by their segmental ventricular origin, ALPM and PMPM. These papillary muscles run parallel to the adjacent ventricular wall. The larger ALPM usually has one or two heads, whereas the smaller PLPM may have two or three. Chordal tendons from the head of each papillary muscle attach to both of the MV leaflets. The chordae that arise from the anterolateral PM extend to the lateral halves of the posterior and anterior MV leaflets. The ALPM and PMPM subtend and support their respective commissural leaflets (49).

Duran Terminology

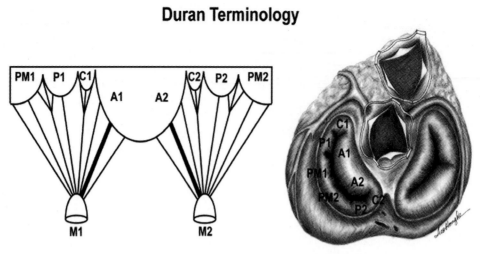

Figure 30.20. The Duran nomenclature system is based on the chordal distribution and refers to the three scallops of the posterior leaflet as P1 (lateral and closest to the left atrial appendage), PM (middle), and P2 (medial and adjacent to the PMC) (53). The middle scallop (PM) is further subdivided into the PM1 and PM2, corresponding to the portion of the middle scallop that receives chordae from the anterolateral (M1) and posteromedial (M2) papillary muscles. The anterior leaflet is divided into two areas, A1 and A2, corresponding to the areas subtended by the corresponding chordal attachments from the anterolateral (M1) and posteromedial (M2) papillary muscles. In addition, the two commissural leaflets of the valve are defined as C1 (anterolateral, between A1 and P1) and C2 (posteromedial, between A2 and P2) receiving chordae from M1 and M2, respectively.

The Duran nomenclature system is based on the chordal distribution and refers to the three scallops of the posterior leaflet as P1 (lateral and closest to the left atrial appendage), PM (middle), and P2 (medial and adjacent to the PMC) (Figs. 30.17–30.20) (53). The middle scallop (PM) is further subdivided into the PM1 and PM2, corresponding to the portion of the middle scallop that receives chordae from the anterolateral (M1) and posteromedial (M2) papillary muscles. The anterior leaflet is divided into two areas, A1 and A2, corresponding to the areas subtended by the corresponding chordal attachments from the anterolateral (M1) and posteromedial (M2) papillary muscles (53). In addition, the two commissural leaflets of the valve are defined as C1 (anterolateral, between A1 and P1) and C2 (posteromedial, between A2 and P2).

CORRELATION WITH IMAGING PLANES: THE 2D EXAMINATION OF THE MITRAL VALVE

The goal of the 2D echocardiographic exam of the MVAp is to develop a 3D understanding of the anatomy and mechanism of MV dysfunction. While 3D transesophageal echocardiography is being utilized more and more to evaluate MV dysfunction (Fig. 30.21), such an understanding is routinely available through a cognitive reconstruction of 3D anatomy utilizing multiplane 2D TEE imaging. The posterior and superior location of the midesophagus in relation to the adjacent blood-filled left atrium and MV annulus enables detailed 360 degrees

imaging of the MV leaflets and apparatus utilizing a 2D multiplane transducer (Fig. 30.22). If the rotational axis of the transducer is positioned in the center of the AMVL, it enables up to 360 degrees imaging of the MV leaflets and an understanding of the 3D structure of the MVAp (Fig. 30.23).

The MV may be examined utilizing up to ten or more variations of six of the recommended ASE-SCA imaging planes frequently used in evaluating the MVAp (Table 30.2). The primary ASE-SCA image planes to evaluate the MV

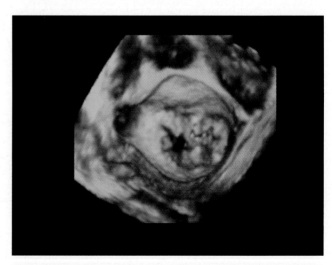

Figure 30.21. 3D visualization of a P2 flail leaflet with multiple ruptured chords (view for the left atrium, also know as the "surgeon's view" of the MV).

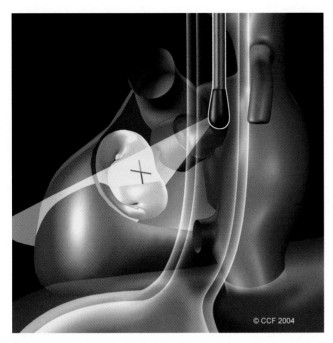

Figure 30.22. The posterior and superior location of the midesophagus in relation to the adjacent blood-filled left atrium and MV annulus enable ideal detailed 360 degrees imaging of the MV leaflets and apparatus utilizing a 2D multiplane transducer.

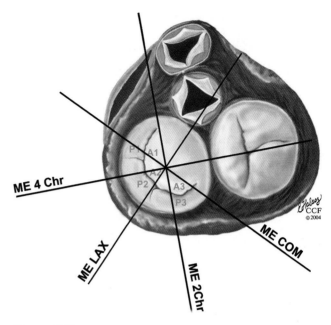

Figure 30.23. If the rotational axis of the transducer is positioned in the center of the AMVL, it enables 360 degrees imaging of the MV leaflets and an understanding of the 3D structure of the MVAp.

include the midesophageal four-chamber (ME 4 Chr MV), midesophageal commissural (ME Com MV), midesophageal two-chamber (ME 2 Chr MV), midesophageal LAX (ME LAX MV), transgastric short-axis (TG SAX MV), and transgastric two-chamber (TG 2 Chr MV) planes. These image planes are obtained by manipulations of the TEE probe including advancing or withdrawing, turning right (clockwise) and left (counterclockwise), rotating the

transducer angulations forward or backward, and flexing the probe to the right or left (Fig. 30.24).

The following section lists the standard imaging planes and their variations in the sequence in which they are commonly utilized in the evaluation of the MVAp. The probe manipulation required to obtain an image plane, which is a variation of the "ASE-SCA recommended cross-sectional view," is included with the description of the

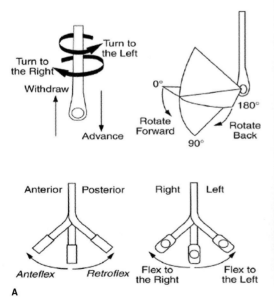

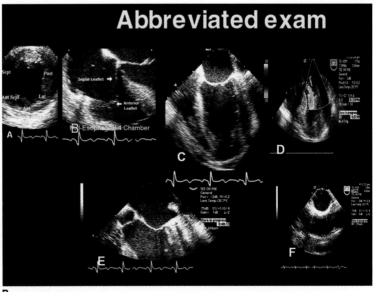

Figure 30.24. Standard image planes and their variations are obtained by manipulations of the TEE probe, including advancing or withdrawing, turning right (clockwise) and left (counterclockwise), rotating the transducer angulations forward or back, and flexing the probe to the right or left.

TABLE 30.2	Correlation of Image Plane and Cardiac Anatomy		
Imaging Plane Nomenclature	**Probe Depth (cm)**	**Transducer Angle (Degrees)**	**Probe Maneuver**
ME 5 Chr MV	28	0–15	Withdraw
ME 4 Chr MV	30	0–15	Probe insertion
LE 4 Chr MV	30	0–15	Advance
ME Com MV	30	45–70	Rotate transducer angle forward
ME Com right MV	30	45–70	Turn right (clockwise)

3D Imaging Plane View	2D Anatomic Imaging Plane	Corresponding Segmental Anatomy

(*continued*)

TABLE 30.2	Correlation of Image Plane and Cardiac Anatomy (*Continued*)			
ME Com left MV	30	45–70	Turn left (counterclockwise)
ME 2 Chr MV	30	80–110	Rotate transducer angle forward
ME LAX MV	30	110–150	Rotate transducer angle forward
TG SAX$_B$	35	0–5	Advance probe, rotate transducer angle forward
TG 2 Chr	35	70–90	Rotate transducer angle forward

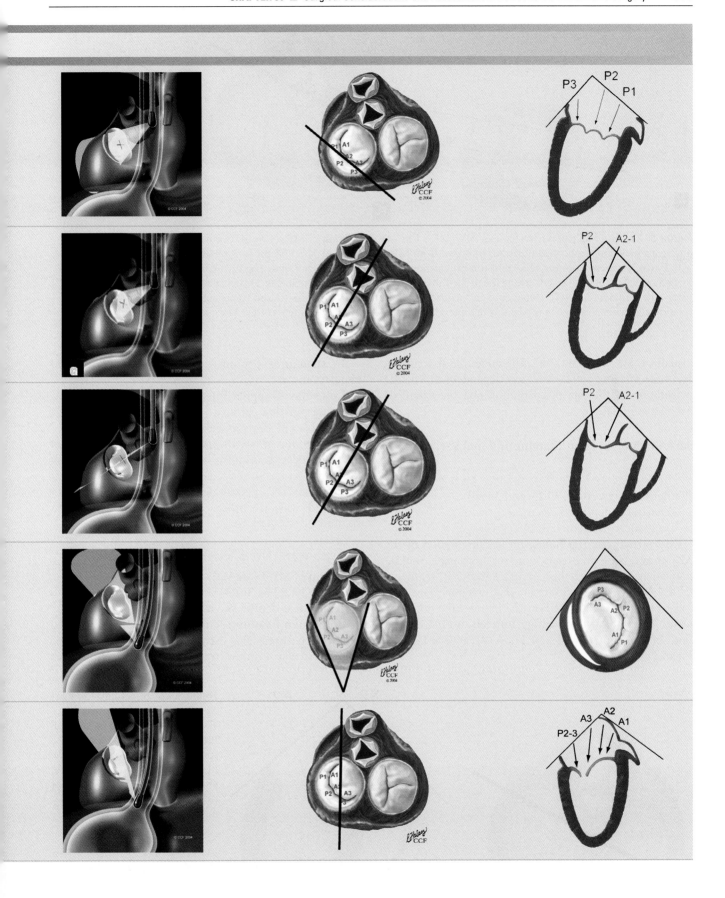

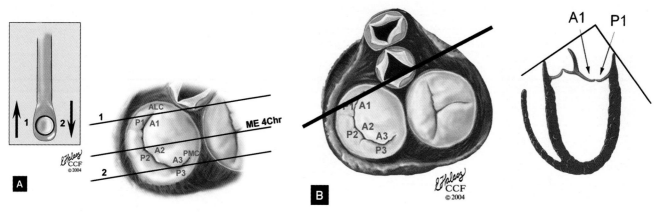

Figure 30.25. Midesophageal five-chamber MV (ME 5 Chr MV). Variation of ME 4 Chr MV; transducer depth: 30 cm; probe manipulation: withdraw from ME 4 Chr MV. **A:** The TEE probe is slowly withdrawn 1 to 2 cm from the ME 4 Chr imaging plane to obtain the ME 5 Chr view. The LE 4 Chr imaging plane is obtained by advancing the probe 1 to 2 cm from the ME 4 Chr plane. **B:** This imaging plane cuts through the LVOT. Depending on the orientation of the MV commissure and transducer rotation angle, the 2D plane may pass through the A1 segment, ALC, and P1 segments of the MV.

visualized MV anatomy (52). The anatomic description for these imaging planes is always dependent on the 3D orientation of the line of coaptation and the extent of probe manipulation.

Midesophageal Four-Chamber MV and Variations

Midesophageal Four-Chamber MV (ME 4 Chr MV)

(Table 30.2; Figs. 30.23, 30.25, and 30.26)
  Transducer depth: 30 cm
  Transducer rotation: 0 to 15 degrees
  MV structures: Depending on the orientation of the MV commissure and transducer rotation angle, the 2D plane may cut through the A2 and P2 and/or P1 segments of the MV. On the monitor in this imaging plane, the anterior leaflet is displayed on the left and the posterior leaflet on the right. Proceeding from left to right are the body of A2, coaptation of A2/P2 or A1P1, and the body of P2 and/or P1.

LV structures: Septum and lateral walls and anterior papillary muscle.
  Color flow Doppler: Interrogation for MR and severity using maximal jet area (MJA), vena contracta (VC), proximal isovelocity surface area (PISA).
  Continuous wave Doppler: MR—spectral Doppler intensity, peak transmitral velocity, determine V_{MR} for PISA; MS—transmitral gradient, pressure half-time, deceleration time (DT), determine peak V_{MS} for PISA.
  Pulsed wave Doppler: MR—E or A dominance, volumetric calculations.

Midesophageal Five-Chamber MV (ME 5 Chr MV)

Variation of ME 4 Chr MV
  (Table 30.2; Fig. 30.25)
  Transducer depth: 28 cm.
  Probe manipulation: Withdraw from ME 4 Chr MV.
  MV structures: This imaging plane cuts through the left ventricular outflow tract (LVOT). Depending on

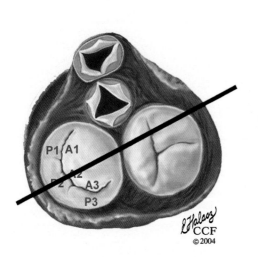

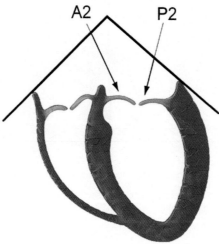

Figure 30.26. Midesophageal four-chamber MV (ME 4 Chr MV). The 2D plane may pass through the A2 segment, middle commissure, and the P2 scallop of the MV. The height of the P2 and A2 may be measured in this plane for comparison with the ME LAX MV measurements.

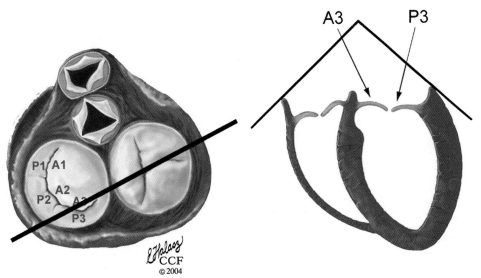

Figure 30.27. Lower-esophageal four-chamber MV (LE 4 Chr MV). Variation of ME 4 Chr transducer depth: 32 cm; probe manipulation: advance depending on the orientation of the MV commissure and transducer rotation angle. The 2D plane may pass through the A3 segment, PMC, and the P3 scallop of the MV.

the orientation of the MV commissure and transducer rotation angle, the 2D plane may cut through the A1 segment, ALC, and P1 segments of the MV. On the monitor in this imaging plane, the anterior leaflet is displayed on the left and the posterior leaflet on the right. Proceeding from left to right are A1, ALC, and P1.

LV structures: LVOT, anterior septum, anterolateral wall.

Lower-Esophageal Four-Chamber MV (LE 4 Chr MV)

Variation of ME 4 Chr
(Table 30.2; Figs. 30.25 and 30.27)
Transducer depth: 32 cm.
Probe manipulation: Advance from ME 4 Chr MV.
MV structures: Depending on the orientation of the MV commissure and transducer rotation angle, the 2D plane may cut through the A3 segment, PMC, and the P3 scallop of the MV. On the monitor in this imaging plane, the anterior leaflet is displayed on the left and the posterior leaflet on the right. Proceeding from left to right are A3, PMC, and P3.

LV structures: Inferoseptum, inferolateral wall.

Diagnostic value of the ME 4 Chr views: Withdrawing the probe between the ME 4 Chr to the ME 5 Chr and then to the LE 4 Chr with 2D and CFD imaging (aliasing velocity set at 50–55 cm/s) every segment of the AMVL and PMVL may be evaluated for degree of thickness, characterization of systolic and diastolic leaflet motion (excessive, normal, or restricted), and the integrity of the chordae (primary and secondary), exact point of origin of regurgitant flow (proximal flow convergence, PFC visualized below plane of valve connecting to the VC zone), or restricted stenotic antegrade flow (PFC initiating above the annular plane and continuing through a funnel-shaped valve). If there is excessive regurgitant flow, for purposes of mechanism determination, the aliasing velocity scale is increased toward 70 cm/s. If there are central and parallel regurgitant jets noted in adjacent imaging planes, where the PFC

and VC of only one are visualized, it is likely that these jets result from a similar mechanism, such as bileaflet tethering or symmetrical bileaflet prolapse. If two distinct jets are identified in the same or adjacent imaging planes and are crossing or directed in different directions, it is likely that these regurgitant jets represent two separate and distinct mechanisms of MR.

Continuous wave Doppler (CWD) through the mitral inflow or regurgitant orifice may be utilized to interrogate either a diastolic flow gradient or systolic regurgitation, utilizing the strength of the spectral envelope as indirect evidence of severity of MR. If the continuity equation is to be used for determination of MVA in the setting of MS, CWD interrogation is performed using five or more cycles if the patient is in atrial fibrillation. The MV inflow time-velocity integral (TVI) is measured using planimetry and entered.

Midesophageal Commissural MV and Variations

Midesophageal Commissural MV (ME Com MV)

(Table 30.2; Figs. 30.23 and 30.28)
Transducer depth: 30 cm.
Transducer rotation: 45 to 70 degrees.
MV structures: Depending on the orientation of the MV commissure and transducer rotation angle, the 2D plane may cut through the P3 scallop, the PMC, tip or body of A2, ALC, and the P1 segments of the MV. On the monitor (from left to right) are P3, PMC, A2, ALC, and P1. The annular plane drawn between the MV annulus on the left of the screen and the MV annulus on the right usually represents the most inferior (closest to the apex) aspects of the saddle-shaped annulus. A plane drawn between these points consequently may overcall MV prolapse.
MV annulus: Major axis.
LV structures: Anterior and posterior papillary muscles.
Color flow Doppler: Visualize MR from the PMC to the ALC.

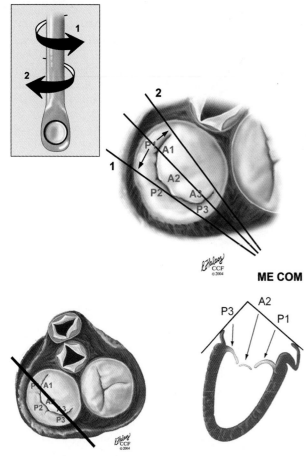

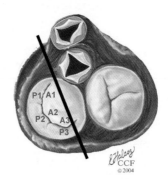

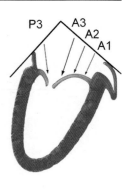

Figure 30.29. Midesophageal commissural right MV (probe turned right) (ME Com$_R$ MV). Variation of ME Com; transducer depth: 30 cm; probe manipulation: turn left or counterclockwise; transducer rotation: 45 to 70 degrees. Depending on the orientation of the MV commissure and transducer rotation angle, the 2D plane may pass through the P3, A3, A2, and A1 segments.

Figure 30.28. Midesophageal commissural MV (ME Com MV). Transducer depth: 30 cm; transducer rotation: 45 to 70 degrees. **A:** The ME Com MV is obtained by rotating the transducer forward to 45–70 degrees. Turning the probe to the right (clockwise) and to the left (counterclockwise) enables visualization of the variations of this imaging plane. **B:** Depending on the orientation of the MV commissure and transducer rotation angle, the 2D plane may cut through the P3 scallop, the PMC, tip of A2, ALC, and the P1 segments of the MV.

MV structures: Depending on the orientation of the MV commissure and transducer rotation angle, the 2D plane may cut through the P3, P2, and P1 scallops. The commissure may not be visualized except during diastole. On the monitor (proceeding from left to right) are P3, P2, and P1.

Diagnostic value of the ME Com MV views: 2D imaging at this imaging plane and its associated right (clockwise) probe turn followed by a left (counterclockwise) turn enable visualization of every segment of the AMVL and PMVL in addition to CFD interrogation of the posteromedial, midcommissure, and ALC. The P1 scallop of the PMVL is on the right and protrudes from the anterolateral mitral annulus. The P3 scallop protrudes from the inferoposterior mitral annulus. The center of the AMVL (tip of A2) is seen centrally between P1 and P3 during cardiac cycle.

The ME Com imaging plane represents the long axis of the elliptically shaped MV annulus. Because the inferoseptal and anterolateral annulus in the ME Com

Midesophageal Commissural Right MV (ME Com$_R$ MV)

Variation of ME Com MV
  (Table 30.2; Figs. 30.28 and 30.29)
  Transducer depth: 30 cm.
  Transducer rotation: 45 to 70 degrees.
  Probe manipulation: Turn right or clockwise.
  MV structures: Depending on the orientation of the MV commissure and transducer rotation angle, the 2D plane may cut through the P3 scallop, the PMC, the A3 segment, the A2 segment, and the A1 segment. On the monitor (proceeding from left to right) are P3, the PMC, A3, A2, and A1.

Midesophageal Commissural Left MV (ME Com$_L$ MV)

Variation of ME Com MV
  (Table 30.2; Figs. 30.28 and 30.30)
  Transducer depth: 30 cm.
  Transducer rotation: 45 to 70 degrees.
  Probe manipulation: Turn left or counterclockwise.

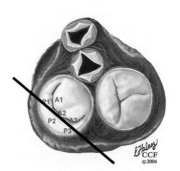

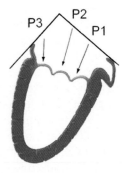

Figure 30.30. Midesophageal commissural left MV (probe turned left) (ME Com$_L$ MV): variation of ME Com; transducer depth: 30 cm; probe manipulation: turn left or counterclockwise; transducer rotation: 45 to 70 degrees. Depending on the orientation of the MV commissure and transducer rotation angle, the 2D plane may pass through the P3, P2, and P1 scallops.

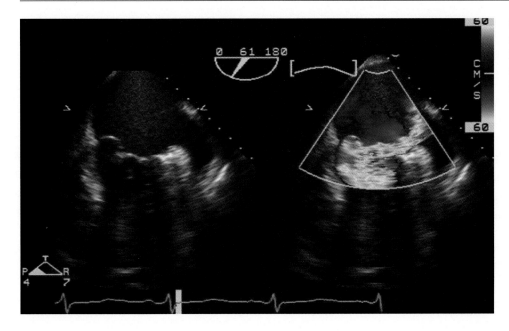

Figure 30.31. Midesophageal commissural right MV with a P3 prolapse seen on the **left** and an anterolateral directed regurgitant jet.

imaging plane represents the lowest (closest to the apex) points of the saddle-shaped annulus, caution is taken in diagnosing excessive leaflet excursion above the plane of the annulus.

From the ME Com MV imaging plane, the probe is turned to the right (clockwise) and the AMVL is visualized proceeding A3–2–1 in a left-to-right order. Depending on the orientation of the MV commissure, the P3 scallop of the PMVL may be visualized to the left (Fig. 30.31). From the ME Com MV imaging plane, the probe is turned to the left

or counterclockwise. The PMVL is visualized. The P3 scallop protrudes from the left inferoposterior annulus and the P1 scallop of the PMVL protrudes from the right anterolateral annulus. The commissure is not visualized. With a flail middle (P2) scallop of the PMVL, the flail segment may be seen above the middle (A2) portion of the AMVL like a hooded cobra raising its head (Fig. 30.32A, B). When CF imaging is utilized to determine the mechanism, the regurgitant jet appeared to be "confined" by the cobra's head. In the standard ME Com MV plane, the major axis of the MV

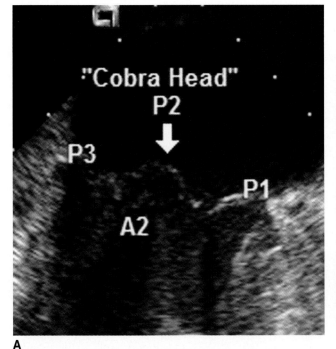

A

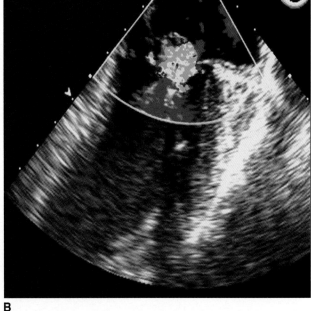

B

Figure 30.32. With a flail middle (P2) scallop of the PMVL, the flail segment may be seen rising above the middle (A2) portion of the AMVL like a hooded cobra raising its head. The anteriorly directed jet may be well confined by the P2 flail or prolapse.

annulus may be measured. A prolapsing or flail P1 or P3 segments may also be visualized in this imaging plane. As the probe is rotated to the right (clockwise), the imaging plane cuts through the A1–2–3 AMVL segments. This plane may also pass through the apex of the PMC. If there is an isolated P3 segmental flail, it will be visualized in this plane with the regurgitant jet directed anteriorly away from the flail segment. In addition, if there is a perforation or congenital cleft of the AMVL, with CFD, this maneuver will reveal the unusual regurgitant jet. In addition, the anterolateral and inferoseptal walls of the LV may be visualized. Scarring of these regions of the LV may result in annular retraction or leaflet restriction. This imaging plane may demonstrate both the ALPM and PMPM. In addition, this plane permits evaluation of the LV portion of the tensor apparatus associated with the papillary muscle and annular continuity.

Midesophageal Two-Chamber MV and Variations

Midesophageal Two-Chamber MV (ME 2 Chr MV)

(Table 30.2; Fig. 30.33)
Transducer depth: 30 cm.
Transducer rotation: 80 to 110 degrees.
Probe manipulation: Midline.
MV structures: Depending on the orientation of the MV commissure and transducer rotation angle, the 2D plane may cut through the P3 scallop; the PMC; and the A3, A2, and A1 segments. On the monitor (proceeding from left to right) are P3, PMC, A3 (tip), A2 (body), and A1 (body).
LV structures: Anterior and inferior walls and posterior papillary muscle.

Midesophageal Two-Chamber Right MV (ME 2 Chr_R MV)

Variation of ME 2 Chr MV
(Fig. 30.34)
Transducer depth: 30 cm.
Transducer rotation: (80–110 degrees).
Probe manipulation: Turn right (clockwise).
MV structures: Depending on the orientation of the MV commissure and transducer rotation angle, the 2D plane may cut through the P3 scallop, the apex of the PMC, the A3 segment, and the base of the A2 segment. On the monitor (proceeding from left to right) are P3, PMC, A3, and A2.

Midesophageal Two-Chamber Left MV (ME 2 Chr_L MV)

Variation of ME 2 Chr MV
(Figs. 30.33 and 30.35)
Transducer depth: 30 cm.
Transducer rotation: 80 to 110 degrees .
Probe manipulation: Turn left or counterclockwise.
MV structures: Depending on the orientation of the MV commissure and transducer rotation angle, the 2D plane may cut through the P3, P2, and P1 scallops. The commissure may not be visualized except during diastole. On the monitor (proceeding from left to right) are P3, P2, and P1.

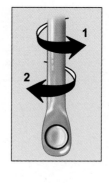
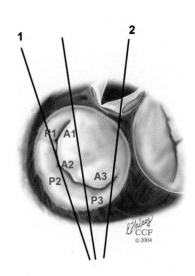

ME 2Chr

A

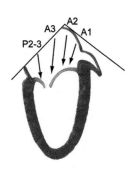

B

Figure 30.33. Midesophageal two-chamber MV (ME 2 Chr MV). Transducer depth: 30 cm; probe manipulation: midline; transducer rotation: 80 to 110 degrees. **A:** The ME 2 Chr imaging plane is obtained by rotating the transducer forward to 80–110 degrees. Variations of this plan are obtained by turning the probe to the right and left. **B:** Depending on the orientation of the MV commissure and transducer rotation angle, the 2D plane may cut through the P3 scallop, the PMC, the A3 segment, the A2 segment, and the A1 segment.

Diagnostic value of the ME 2 Chr views: This imaging plane is utilized for evaluating excessive motion of the P3 segment (flail or prolapse). With CF interrogation, it will demonstrate a regurgitant jet directed anteriorly. With an A3 flail, an inferoposteriorly directed jet will be visualized. The left atrial appendage is consistently visualized in this plane where left atrial appendage (LAA) appendage thrombi or spontaneous contrast may be visualized. Because of the parallel orientation of LAA flow with pulsed wave (PW) Doppler cursor, this is an ideal plane for interrogating the velocity of LAA systolic flow. In patients with LAA velocities below 50 cm/s, there is a propensity to form thrombi in the appendage. The PMPM and inferior wall of the LV may be evaluated in this imaging plane for infarcted scar with retraction of the inferior wall and annular retraction, which may result in an "override" of the A3 segment. Examination

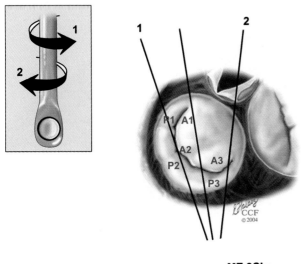

ME 2Chr

A

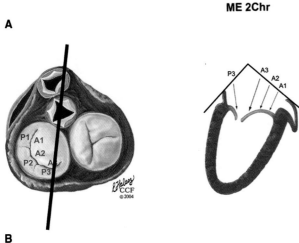

B

Figure 30.34. Midesophageal two-chamber right MV (turned right) (ME 2 Chr$_R$ MV). Variation of ME 2 Chr MV; transducer depth: 30 cm; transducer rotation: 80 to 110 degrees; probe manipulation: turn right (clockwise). Depending on the orientation of the MV commissure and transducer rotation angle, the 2D plane may cut through the P3 scallop, the apex of the PMC, the A3 segment, and base of the A2 segment.

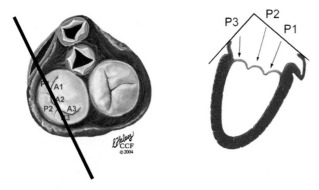

Figure 30.35. Midesophageal two chamber left MV (turned left) (ME 2 Chr$_L$ MV). Variation of ME 2 Chr MV; transducer depth: 30 cm. Probe manipulation: turn left or counterclockwise; transducer rotation: 80 to 110 degrees. Depending on the orientation of the MV commissure and transducer rotation angle, the 2D plane may cut through the P3, P2, and P1 scallops. The commissure may not be visualized except during diastole.

of the PMPM may demonstrate calcification or scarring, which is usually associated with coronary disease. Such scarring may lead to a restriction of the medial segments of the AMVL or PMVL. Occasionally, an infarcted papillary muscle may lead to elongation of the chordal attachment to the papillary muscle and associated segmental leaflet prolapse of one of the medial segments. The PMPM is usually perfused by a single branch from the left circumflex or RCA.

Midesophageal Long-Axis MV and Variations

Midesophageal Long-Axis MV (ME LAX MV)

(Table 30.2; Fig. 30.36)
   Transducer depth: 30 cm.
   Transducer rotation: 110 to 150 degrees.

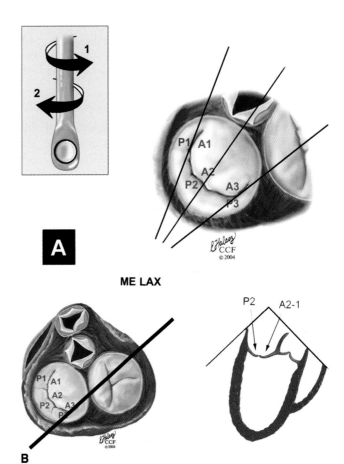

Figure 30.36. Midesophageal long-axis MV (ME LAX MV). Transducer depth: 30 cm; transducer rotation: 110 to 150 degrees. **A:** The ME LAX MV imaging plane is obtained by rotating the transducer forward to 110–150 degrees. Variations of this plan are obtained by turning the probe to the right and left. **B:** Depending on the orientation of the MV commissure and transducer rotation angle, the 2D plane passes through the minor axis of the MV annulus and aortic valve. The 2D plane may cut through the P2 scallop, the midcommissure, and through the A2 segment. Height of the PMVL, AMVL, and C-sept is measured in this plane and compared to the ME 4 Chr MV measurements. This plane demonstrates the most superior aspects of the MV annulus.

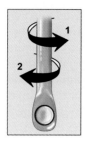

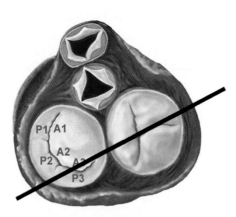

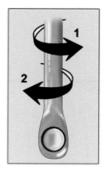

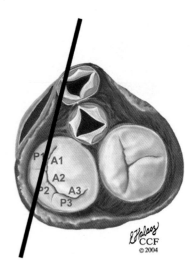

Figure 30.37. Midesophageal long-axis right MV (probe turned right) MV ME LAXR MV. Variation ME LAX MV; transducer depth: 30 cm; probe manipulation: turn right clockwise; transducer rotation: 110 to 150 degrees. Depending on the orientation of the MV commissure, transducer rotation angle, and extent of probe manipulation, the 2D plane may cut through the P2 scallop, the PMC, and P3 scallops. The commissure may not be visualized except during diastole.

MV structures: Depending on the orientation of the MV commissure and transducer rotation angle, the 2D plane passes through the minor axis of the MV annulus and aortic valve. The 2D plane may cut through the P2 scallop, the midcommissure, and through the A2 segment. On the monitor (proceeding from left to right) are P2, the midcommissure, and the A2 segment of the MV. The aortic valve is seen on the right of the screen. The MV annulus to the left of the screen and to the right—adjacent to the aortic valve—are the most superior (farthest from the apex) aspects of the annulus. A plane drawn between these points provides a more specific reference for diagnosing MV prolapse.

MV annulus: Minor axis.

LV structures: Anteroseptal and inferolateral walls. Typically, no papillary muscle is seen in this view.

Midesophageal Long-Axis Right MV (ME LAX_R MV)

Variation ME LAX MV

(Fig. 30.37)

Transducer depth: 30 cm.

Transducer rotation: 110 to 150 degrees.

Probe manipulation: Turn right or clockwise

MV structures: Depending on the orientation of the MV commissure, transducer rotation angle, and extent of probe manipulation, the 2D plane may cut through the P2 scallop, the PMC, and P3 scallop. The commissure may not be visualized except during diastole. On the monitor (proceeding from left to right) are P2, possibly the PMC, and P3.

Midesophageal Long-Axis Left MV (ME LAX_L MV)

Variation ME LAX MV

(Fig. 30.38)

Transducer depth: 30 cm.

Transducer rotation: 110 to 150 degrees.

Probe manipulation: Turn left or counterclockwise.

Figure 30.38. Midesophageal long-axis left MV (ME LAXL MV). Variation ME LAX MV; transducer depth: 30 cm; probe manipulation: turn left or counterclockwise; transducer rotation; 110 to 150 degrees. Depending on the orientation of the MV commissure, transducer rotation angle, and extent of probe manipulation, the 2D plane may cut through the P2 scallop, the ALC, and P1 scallops. The commissure may not be visualized except during diastole.

MV structures: Depending on the orientation of the MV commissure, transducer rotation angle, and extent of probe manipulation, the 2D plane may cut through the P2 scallop, the ALC, and the P1 scallop. The commissure may not be visualized except during diastole. On the monitor (proceeding from left to right) are P2, possibly the ALC, and P1.

Diagnostic value of the ME LAX MV views: Because P2 is the most frequent flail or prolapsing segment of all the valve segments/scallops, this imaging plane will commonly demonstrate a flail P2 scallop with its characteristic anteriorly directed jet. In addition, measurements of the height of the PMVL, AMVL, C-sept distance, and minor MV annular diameter may be made in this view. With rightward (clockwise) turning of the probe from the ME LAX imaging plane, the imaging plane is directed toward the PMC. MR from the PMC may be visualized at this point. Again, depending on the orientation of the mitral commissure, as the probe is rotated toward the PMC, it will initially pass through the medial aspect of the P2 scallop, the PMC, and the A3 segment of the AMVL. The visualized image (from left to right) will show the medial portion of the P2 scallop, the PMC, and the A3 segment of the AMVL. As the imaging plane passes through the apex of the PMC, the medial aspect of the P2 and P3 scallops will be visualized from left to right on the monitor screen. If there is a flail segment of the A3 or the P3 scallop, it will be visualized by this maneuver.

From the ME LAX imaging plane, the TEE probe is turned to the left (counterclockwise). This manipulation of the probe passes the imaging plane toward the ALC.

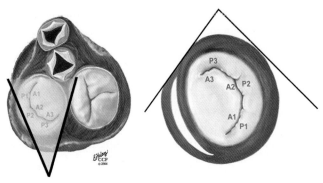

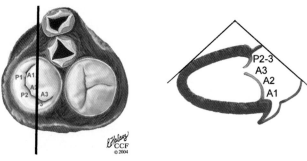

Figure 30.39. Transgastric basal short axis (TG SAXB). Transducer depth: 35 cm; transducer rotation: 0 to 5 degrees. In this imaging plane, the AMVL (A1–2–3, bottom to top) is visualized on the **left** and the PMVL (P1–2–3, bottom to top) is visualized on the **right**. The clear space to the left of the AMVL edge and toward the bottom of the screen is the LVOT, which is shaded in *gray*. Systolic turbulence in this area suggests SAM with LVOTO.

Figure 30.40. Transgastric two chamber (TG 2 Chr). Transducer depth: 35 cm; transducer rotation 70 to 90 degrees. This image is similar to the ME 2 Chr imaging plane except that the ventricle is horizontally oriented. Depending on the orientation of the MV commissure and transducer rotation angle, the 2D plane may cut through the P3 scallop, the PMC, the A3 segment, the A2 segment, and the A1 segment.

If there is an anterolateral commissural regurgitant jet, it will be visualized at this point. Depending on the orientation of the mitral commissure, as the probe is rotated toward the ALC, it will initially pass through the lateral aspect of the P2 scallop, the ALC, and the A1 segment of the AMVL. The visualized image (from left to right) will show the lateral P2 scallop, the ALC, the A1 segment, and the LVOT or aortic valve. As the imaging plane passes through the apex of the ALC, the lateral aspect of the P2 scallop and the P1 scallop will be visualized going left to right on the monitor screen.

Transgastric Basal Short Axis (TG SAXB)

(Table 30.2; Fig. 30.39)
 Transducer depth: 35 cm.
 Transducer rotation: 0 to 5 degrees.
 MV structures: In this imaging plane, the AMVL (A1–2–3, bottom to top) is visualized on the left and the PMVL (P1–2–3, bottom to top) is visualized on the right. The clear space to the left of the AMVL edge and toward the bottom of the screen is the LVOT.
 Diagnostic value of the TG SAX_B view: From the TG basal SAX, the competency of the MV may be evaluated for localization and determination of potential mechanism. With prolapsing segments, the may be an "echo-free" space adjacent to the line of coaptation with subsequent MR originating from the site of redundant leaflets. With MS, this imaging may be used to planimeter the valve or subvalvular apparatus. Because there may be more subvalvular stenosis in rheumatic MS, care should be taken to determine the level of most significant stenosis.

Transgastric Two Chamber (TG 2 Chr)

(Table 30.2; Fig. 30.40)
 Transducer depth: 35 cm.
 Transducer rotation: 70 to 90 degrees.

MV structures: This image is similar to the ME 2 Chr imaging plane except that the ventricle is horizontally oriented. Depending on the orientation of the MV commissure and transducer rotation angle, the 2D plane may cut through the P3 scallop, the PMC, and the A3, A2, and A1 segments. On the monitor (proceeding from top to bottom) are P3, PMC, A3, A2, and A1.

Diagnostic value of the TG 2 Chr view: The TG 2 Chr is a useful imaging plane for evaluating the subvalvular apparatus in patients with rheumatic MS or MR. Looking for the associated anatomic findings of chordal fusion, loss of interchordal spaces, degree of calcification, and leaflet motion with color may demonstrate more significant subvalvular stenosis than valvular.

Intraoperative Examination Approach

Principles of Intraoperative Examination (Table 30.3)

The principles of the IOE examination for patients undergoing MV surgery are guided by the unique demands of the cardiac surgery environment. By the very nature of this atmosphere, the IOE exam is performed in a sequence that first resolves the issues guiding patient management. Yet, it also acknowledges the more comprehensive aspects of active patient management and the need to provide digitally archived documentation of the patient's complete examination for future comparison. While these may appear to be conflicting objectives, eventually every echocardiographer incorporates both into the daily routine of an efficiently organized IOE exam with which they feel comfortable. To accomplish these goals (Table 30.4), the systematic IOE exam may be structured into a priority ordered exam and a more general comprehensive exam (54). To prevent significant midexam revelations from occurring and reordering priorities, the priority ordered exam is initiated by a brief abbreviated overview exam

TABLE 30.3	Principles of Intraoperative Echo Exam in MV Surgery

1. Addresses critical issues of MV surgery (Table 30.1)
2. Systematic examination
   - Organized by priority
   - Initial overview exam (patient management and exam organization)
   - Focused diagnostic exam (priority issues)
   - Comprehensive exam documented
3. Efficient (critical issues and comprehensive exam in prebypass period)
4. Severity by weighted integration 2D imaging and Doppler
5. Study results discussed with surgeon and documented in record
6. Comprehensive digital study achieved
7. Compares results with pre-OR data and addresses variances
   - Variance explained to extent possible
   - Communicated with surgical team
   - Communicated with patient's primary physician
8. IOE exam under continuous quality improvement (CQI) process
9. Training and hospital credentialing of qualified personnel
10. Equipment maintained and updated

followed by the more complete focused diagnostic exam. In addition to the diagnostic issues that are already on the agenda, the abbreviated overview exam provides an up-to-date assessment of additional issues that must be addressed. It also recognizes the important role of IOE in the ongoing management of the patient and, if necessary,

TABLE 30.4	Systematic Intraoperative Echo Exam in MV Surgery

Systematic IOE exam components

- Priority ordered examination
  - Abbreviated overview examination
    - Rapid assessment of cardiac function (patient management)
    - Diagnostic screen for organizing focused study
  - Focused diagnostic examination
- General comprehensive examination
- Remaining ASE-SCA

Stages of IOE exam in MV surgery

- Precardiopulmonary bypass (pre-CPB)
- Postcardiopulmonary bypass (post-CPB)
  - Preseparation CPB (pre-sep CPB)
  - Postseparation CPB (post-CPB)

permits the immediate adjustment of the patient's hemodynamic management while the remainder of the IOE exam takes place.

To ensure that the examination is conducted efficiently, the methods that are used in assessing the severity of MV dysfunction are those that are more easily performed in a multitasking environment. As recommended by the ASE Nomenclature and Standards Committee and Task Force on Valvular Regurgitation, the assessment of the severity of MV dysfunction and its secondary pathophysiology integrates both the structural and Doppler parameters of severity weighted by the quality of data obtained and quantitative reliability (35). Severity is graded as mild, moderate, and severe, using terms such as "mild-to-moderate" or "moderate-to-severe" to characterize intermediate levels of severity (35). The term *trace regurgitation* is used to describe that which is barely detected. For MS, the terms mild, moderate, and severe are also used.

Subdued lighting (reduced monitor glare) and periods without electrocautery interference during critical portions of the intraoperative exam contribute to collecting quality 2D images and Doppler-derived hemodynamic data. Such an atmosphere permits the precise recognition of intricate structural abnormalities (vegetation, thrombi, right-to-left shunts) that may have potentially devastating consequences if missed. It also enables the acquisition of the quality of diagnostic information that may confidently guide the pivotal surgical and hemodynamic decisions.

For organization purposes, the examination may be structured into two distinct phases: pre-CPB and post-CPB. The post-CPB incorporates an abbreviated preseparation bypass (pre-sep CPB) exam. Each of the phases has critical issues that are addressed during the progression of the procedure (Tables 30.5 and 30.6A,B). For patients undergoing MV surgery, a priority directed exam might be performed at each of these phases of the surgical procedure. If the patient encounters hemodynamic instability at any point during the course of the procedure, an abbreviated overview exam is performed followed by a more focused diagnostic exam directed by the clinical course or as revealed during the abbreviated overview exam. If the patient's course is not entirely smooth, an examination following chest closure may direct clinical intervention or provide assurance.

For each stage of the surgical procedure, the abbreviated overview exam is followed by the focused diagnostic exam in addressing issues pertaining to that stage of the surgery (Table 30.4). With resolution of the critical issues and digital storage of corresponding, the patient's comprehensive examination is completed by filling in any portions that were not performed during the focused diagnostic exam.

Conclusions of the systematic examination are communicated directly with the surgical team in addition to being documented in the patient's permanent medical record. The digital loops and images supporting the diagnostic conclusions and comprehensive exam are

TABLE 30.5	The Pre-CPB Exam

1. Confirm and refine preoperative assessment
   - Confirm MV dysfunction and severity
   - Determine repairability of valve
     - Refine pathoanatomy and mechanism
     - Explain variances
2. Determine the need for unplanned surgical intervention
   - Secondary pathophysiology
     - LV dysfunction
     - Increased LA or LAA thrombi
     - Pulmonary hypertension
     - Right ventricle (RV) dysfunction
     - Tricuspid regurgitation
     - Right to left shunt (PFO, ASD)
     - Hepatic congestion
   - Associated abnormality
     - Associated congenital anomalies
       - Cleft MV and primum ASD
     - Similar pathologic process
       - Ventricular dysfunction
       - Valve dysfunction
         - Acquired: rheumatic valve
         - Degenerative: myxomatous or calcific disease
         - Endocarditis
       - Vascular disorder
     - Unrelated process
       - Primary aortic valve stenosis or regurgitation
3. Cannulation and perfusion strategy
4. Addresses surgical procedure–specific issues
5. Predict complications
   - Inability to repair
     - Documented risks
       - SAM and LVOTO: PMVL height, C-sept distance
       - Dilated annulus, MACa^{2+}, >3 segments
       - Central MR jet
       - Rheumatic
       - Multiple mechanisms of valve dysfunction
       - Myxomatous and ischemic
       - Mitral stenosis
       - Endocarditis involving fibrous skeleton or annulus
     - Endocarditis
   - LVOT obstruction (MVRep or MVR)
   - Mitral annular calcification
     - Pseudoaneurysm
     - Perivalvular regurgitation
   - Ventricular dysfunction
   - Coagulopathy (hepatic congestion)

TABLE 30.6A	Preseparation (Pre-Sep) CPB Examination

Abbreviated Preseparation Exam

- Abbreviated assessment of cardiovascular function
  - Cardiac performance
  - Initial screen for complications
    - Cannulation and perfusion related
      - Check for dissection or intramural hematoma
    - Pre-CPB protruding plaques still present?
    - Procedure-related complications
    - New or secondary pathophysiology
- Initial assessment of MV surgery
  - Persistent MR or residual or new MS
  - Significant procedure-related complications (not improved by time)
    - Suture dehiscence
    - Leaflet damage
    - Pseudoaneurysm (slide related)
    - MV stenosis
    - Pseudoaneurysm
    - Left circumflex obstruction
    - Iatrogenic shunt: ASD, aorta to LA fistula
    - SAM and LVOT obstruction
    - Significant perivalvular regurgitation
    - Mechanical leaflet malfunction
    - LVOT strut obstruction
    - Midventricular disruption
    - Ring dehiscence
    - Significant perivalvular fistula
    - LA avulsion
- Monitor micro-air clearance
- Assess ventricular function and optimal
  - Time for separation CPB
- Secondary pathophysiology
  - Pulmonary hypertension
  - RV dysfunction or TR
- Complications of cannulation and perfusion
  - Aortic dissection or intramural hematoma
  - Micro-air or atheromatous emboli
    - Myocardial ischemia

Intraoperative Echocardiography Examination and Outcomes

Precardiopulmonary Bypass (Pre-CPB IOE)

Critical issues of the pre-CPB exam (Table 30.5)

archived for future retrieval. To ensure ongoing success of a valve surgery program, intraoperative TEE exams are reviewed under an organized continuous quality improvement (CQI) process, as recommended by the Intraoperative Council of the ASE (29).

The decision to proceed with surgical intervention is established by the progression of a patient's clinical symptomatology and objective assessment of severity of MV dysfunction and its secondary effects (14). The pre-CPB

TABLE 30.6B	Postseparation (Post-Sep) CPB Examination

- Assess cardiovascular function
- Diagnose complications and mechanisms
  - MV repair
    - Incomplete repair
      - Primary mechanism
        - Residual prolapse
        - Residual annular dilatation
      - Secondary mechanisms
        - Repaired P2 with type IIIb (asymmetric)
        - New ischemic MR
        - Commissural regurgitation
  - Technique related
    - Suture dehiscence
    - Interscallop malcoaptation
    - Overshortening leaflet
    - Leaflet damage
    - Pseudoaneurysm (slide-related)
    - MV stenosis
    - Pseudoaneurysm
    - Aortic valve incompetence
    - Circumflex coronary obstruction
    - Iatrogenic shunt: ASD, aorta to LA fistula
    - SAM and LVOT obstruction
  - MV replacement
    - Perivalvular regurgitation
    - Mechanical leaflet malfunction
    - LVOT strut obstruction
    - Midventricular disruption
    - Ring dehiscence Both MVRep and MVR
    - Perivalvular fistula
    - Pseudoaneurysm
    - LA avulsion
- Assess ventricular function
- Secondary pathophysiology
  - Pulmonary hypertension
  - RV dysfunction
- Complications of cannulation and perfusion
  - Aortic dissection or intramural hematoma
  - Micro-air emboli
    - Segmental ischemia
    - CNS dysfunction
  - Emboli (atheroma related)
    - Infarcted or ischemic intestine
    - Stroke
    - Renal infarct

Doppler exam (35,55,56). Determining the severity of MR relies on established Doppler parameters, including CF Doppler maximum jet area (CF Doppler MJA) mapping, CF Doppler VC diameter (57–59), PW Doppler interrogation of the pulmonary veins (57,60–62), and PFC determination of the "peak" regurgitant orifice area (ROA) (63–67). Should there be significant discrepancies, more extensive volumetric quantitative techniques are used.

Assessment of MS similarly incorporates 2D imaging and the Doppler exam. The 2D echocardiography incorporates a functional assessment of the MVAp, possibly utilizing the splitability index, and planimetry from the basal TG SAX imaging plane (55,68–70). As with the assessment of MR, CF Doppler provides a reliable screening assessment for MS (71). Noting transmitral diastolic PFC through the MV directs the exam to more quantitative methods of MS assessment. Additional quantitative methods include Doppler determination of the mean pressure gradient across the MV, use of the PISA to determine MV area, and pressure half-time and/or DT to estimate MV area (68–71). The continuity equation incorporates both PW and CWD techniques and is reasonably reliable as long as the reference valve is not regurgitant (55).

With the surgical team's understanding of the etiology, mechanism, and severity of dysfunction, feasibility of a successful valve repair is better recognized. The mechanism and underlying pathologic process directly affect the patient's long-term prognosis (29,53,55,56,72).

Other issues resolved by the pre-CPB exam include

1. Evaluating the presence and severity of significant secondary or coexisting cardiovascular disease that would alter the patient's surgical management.
2. Establishing the optimal cannulation-perfusion and myocardial protection strategy.
3. Assessing cardiac function to determine the optimal intraoperative hemodynamic management of the patient.
4. Assessing the probability for potential post-CPB complications related to the patient's MV surgery or use of CPB (aortic regurgitation, aortic dissection, and intramural hematoma).

The assessment of secondary physiology focuses on determining the presence of an increased LA pressure, pulmonary hypertension, secondary right ventricle (RV) dysfunction with dilatation, and/or enlargement of the tricuspid valve annulus. With MV dysfunction, there may be increased left atrial pressure with chronic dilatation of the chamber. In acute MR, the LA does not have time to dilate and the LA pressures are elevated more acutely with the onset of pulmonary congestion and hypertension. Utilizing pulse wave Doppler (PWD) interrogation of the pulmonary veins, the LA pressure may be estimated. If there is blunting of the S wave in all pulmonary veins, an elevation of LA pressure (>15 mm Hg) is usually present (55–57). In chronic MR, the left atrium may dilate to greater than 70 mm (56,57). With persistent elevations of LA pressure, the patient may develop fixed pulmonary hypertension

exam verifies the need for MV surgery by defining the mechanism of MV dysfunction and its severity. Determining the mechanism of MR is accomplished by integrating the 2D structural exam of the MVAp with the color

with RV dysfunction, eventually causing RV dilatation, and enlargement of the tricuspid annulus, leading to tricuspid valve regurgitation in up to 25% of patients having MV surgery (73). Right atrial pressure may be elevated leading to chronic hepatic congestion (diagnosed by a lack of respiratory variation in hepatic vein diameter).

Notwithstanding the many valuable and recognized contributions that IOE has made to the patient undergoing valvular heart surgery, the ability to identify patients who are at a higher risk for postoperative stroke and neurocognitive dysfunction continues to have a daily impact on the management of these patients. This is not only a devastating complication that impacts patient morbidity and mortality, but it significantly increases the costs associated with valvular heart surgery. The cannulation and perfusion strategy is directed by the IOE assessment of the proximal ascending and descending aorta. Epiaortic scanning should be performed if

1. Protruding plaques are seen in the descending aorta
2. Plaques are palpated at the anticipated site of cannulation or cross-clamping
3. The patient has significant risk factors for aortic atheroma (74)

Significant aortic regurgitation may identify patients at risk for ventricular distension or ineffective antegrade cardioplegia administration, which may direct an alternative protection strategy, such as direct interostial administration of antegrade cardioplegia or more heavily weighted dependence on retrograde cardioplegia administration. As the cross-clamp is released prior to reinstitution of a rhythm, cardiac distension may indicate the need for a vent through the pulmonary vein (75).

The Pre-CPB IOE Exam and Outcome Studies (Table 30.5)

IOE has been effectively utilized in guiding MVRep surgery since it was initially reported in 1986, using epicardial imaging with CFD determination of the mechanism of dysfunction (8). Not only has the IOE exam helped the individual patient, but it has also shortened the learning curves of cardiac surgeons and served as a catalyst to hasten the evolutionary development of MVRep. In 1998, Gillinov et al. reported on 1,072 patients who had successful MVRep surgery performed between 1985 and 1997 (76). The study included a subset of patients who had not received IOE guidance. In comparing those patients who received IOE compared with those who did not, the long-term durability was 98% compared to 92% (76). Following the initial surgical procedure, there was a preponderance of late failures that occurred within the first year (Figs. 30.41 and 30.42).

New Clinical Information

The pre-CPB IOE exam provides incremental information that impacts the surgical management of patients undergoing MV surgery. Michel-Cherqui et al. reported

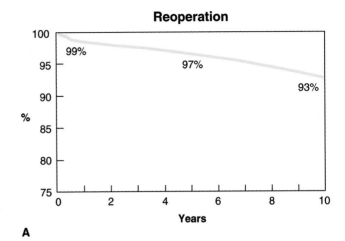

A

Figure 30.41A. Of 1,072 patients undergoing successful MVRep between 1985 and 1997, the long-term durability at 10 years was 93%.

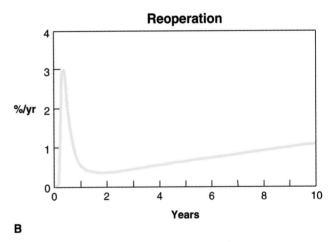

B

Figure 30.41B. Hazard curves for reoperation following successful MVRep. Though reoperations are an infrequent event, the first year is time of highest incidence.

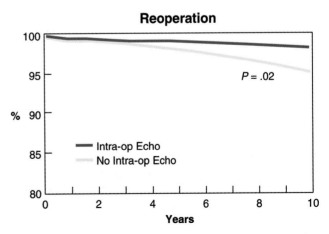

Figure 30.42. The patients who did not have intraoperative echo had a trend for lower long-term durability (92%) compared to those who received intraoperative guidance with TEE and/or epicardial echo (98%, $p < 0.02$) (77).

the results of 203 consecutive cardiac surgery patients and found a 17% incidence of IOE changing the preoperative diagnosis (77). Chaliki et al. found a 12% incidence of new findings influencing the intraoperative management of their patients (38). Lytle et al. reported that IOE discovered previously undiagnosed MV dysfunction requiring MVRep in 5% of 82 consecutive higher-risk patients undergoing myocardial revascularization (18).

Determine Mechanism and Probability of Repair

The IOE exam provides the surgeon with information enabling a more directed inspection of the mitral apparatus. In 1992, Stewart et al. reported the Cleveland Clinic's initial experience with 286 patients undergoing MVRep (78). In those patients who received IOE guidance, the surgical diagnosis of mechanism and location was compared with the results of the pre-CPB exam. The IOE exam diagnosed the localized mechanisms most accurately with posterior-leaflet prolapse or flail (93%), anterior-leaflet prolapse or flail (94%), and restricted leaflet motion or rheumatic thickening (91%). It correctly diagnosed papillary muscle elongation or rupture in 75%, ventricular and annular dilatation in 72%, leaflet perforation in 62%, and bileaflet prolapse or flail in 44%. Of the 5% of patients who had more than one mechanism, the IOE was only able to diagnose both mechanisms in 38%, and one of the two mechanisms in 92%. Overall, the accuracy for diagnosing mechanisms was 85% (33). In a similar study, Foster et al. reported the high accuracy of utilizing a more regimented systematic IOE exam, reporting agreement between the TEE and surgical localizations of mechanisms in 96% of native MV segments or scallops (224 of 234 segments or scallops, $p < 0.0001$) and 88% of perivalvular prosthetic regurgitant segments ($p < 0.001$) (79). Lambert et al. reported on the ability of a consistent systematic examination to accurately determine the location and mechanism of MV dysfunction (compared with surgical inspection) in 96% compared with 70% in an IOE exam that was not systematically performed (80). Omran et al. prospectively evaluated 170 consecutive patients undergoing MVRep with a systematic segmental examination of the MVAp. They found that IOE accurately identified abnormal segments in 90% to 97% of patients (81). Segments that were most accurately identified as abnormal were P2 (97%) and least accurately identified were A3 (90%). The accuracy of correctly localizing to AMVL and PMVL was 95% and 100%, respectively (81). In 1999, Caldarera et al. discovered that IOE provided accurate anatomic measurements of the anteroposterior diameter of the mitral annulus compared with surgical inspection (82). A measured diameter greater than 35 mm in the ME 4 Chr imaging plane was indicative of annular dilatation at the time of surgery requiring annuloplasty. In 1999, Enriquez-Sarano et al. compared the ability of IOE to accurately diagnose the etiology and mechanism of MV dysfunction in patients undergoing MVRep surgery with transthoracic echocardiography (TTE) (29). They found that IOE provided a superior ability to diagnose the correct etiology

(99% vs. 95%) and mechanism of dysfunction (99% vs. 94%). The IOE exam was also more accurate in diagnosing MV prolapse (99% vs. 95%) and flail segments (99% vs. 83%, $p < 0.001$). The IOE exam was able to predict, on the basis of accurately diagnosing etiology and mechanism, those patients who were most likely to have a successful MVRep ($p < 0.001$) and a higher 5-year survival ($p < 0.001$) (29). Similar studies have consistently demonstrated the diagnostic capabilities of the IOE exam to accurately provide the surgical team with the information that will enable them to correlate their surgical findings in determining the optimal surgical strategy for repair or replacement of the valve.

Variances with Preoperative MV Dysfunction Severity

Despite numerous reports demonstrating the ability to accurately determine the underlying anatomy and mechanism of dysfunction, there have been recognized discrepancies between the preoperative (both TEE and TTE) and intraoperative assessment of severity in some patients. Grewal et al. compared preoperative TEE with the IOE exam performed under general anesthesia to determine the unloading effect on the severity of MR. The severity of MR was assessed using CFD, MJA, and vena contracta jet diameter (VCJD) (84). They found 22 of the 43 patients (51%) improved by at least one MR severity grade when assessed under general anesthesia. They found the most significant changes occurred in patients with functional MR (normal MV leaflets) (83). However, patients with structural leaflet dysfunction (flail) demonstrated little if any change in the MR severity. Bach et al. also compared the severity of preoperative TEE with the IOE using similar parameters of severity assessment (84). They determined that patients with structural valve leaflet abnormalities (flail) did not have a significant change in their severity assessment whereas those with functional MR showed a decrease in MR severity ($p < 0.001$) (84).

In a report of 1,265 patients undergoing MV surgery in 1999, Chaliki et al. reported a total of 96 patients in whom the pre-CPB IOE exam found no significant structural or functional abnormality of the mitral apparatus (38). Based on this finding, the decision was made not to surgically inspect the valve in 95 of these patients. In patients with ischemic MR undergoing myocardial revascularization, Cohn et al. reported on patients undergoing myocardial revascularization with moderate preoperative MR. Ninety percent of these patients were downgraded to 0–2 by the IOE exam (20). Seven of the patients went from moderate MR to no MR intraoperatively and did not receive an MVRep or MVR. Postoperatively, three out of seven patients returned to their original 3+ MR, and four returned to 2+ MR on their postoperative TTE (20).

When explaining variances between the preoperative assessment and the intraoperative exam, as Thomas and many others have taught us, there are physical principles of ultrasound, which we use daily that contribute to the variance in our intraoperative assessment (29,57). The size of the maximum CF Doppler jet area (MJA) is determined by a number of considerations, including the ROA and the systolic LV-LA gradient. Other factors include the eccentricity of the regurgitant jet and settings used on the ultrasound platform (power, transducer receiver gain, frequency of the transducer—higher-frequency transducers causes greater Doppler shift, wall filter, pulse repetition frequency, color scale or Nyquist limit, and depth of the scan sector—affecting pulse repetition frequency). Because of the closer proximity of the TEE transducer to the heart, higher frequencies can be used, causing a more pronounced jet area because of the relative lack of tissue attenuation at the imaging distance for TEE. By having the CF Doppler scale higher than what may have been used in the preoperative assessment, the MJA will be comparatively reduced.

From a clinical perspective, if the variance in the operating room (OR) is more than two grades less, the possibility always exists that the patient may have had indolent ischemia at the time of the original exam. In these circumstances, if canceling the MV procedure is a consideration, altering the loading conditions with neosynephrine or challenging with a bolus of intravenous fluid may duplicate the MV dysfunction seen preoperatively, especially in patients with functional MR. It is always a good idea to consult other colleagues who may provide insight into the patient's clinical course or incorporate more quantitative methods that may not be utilized on a routine basis in an intraoperative practice (18,62,63).

In MV disease that chronically elevates the pulmonary artery pressures, leading to RV dysfunction and dilatation, the tricuspid annulus will eventually dilate. The need for tricuspid valve repair in patients undergoing MV surgery is reported to be approximately 25% and is indicated in the presence of greater than moderate TR (73). Almost all of these procedures are tricuspid valve repairs.

Predicting Complications

In an era of minimally invasive and other cutting-edge approaches to MV disease, the potential for difficulties keeps everyone vigilant. Such challenges do not become complications unless they remain undetected and adversely affect the patient. IOE clearly provides a safety net mechanism, enabling us to identify problems at a time when they may be more readily corrected. The pre-CPB exam has also been used to anticipate complications following MVRep and MVR (Table 30.5). Such complications are directly related to the surgical procedure, the patient's underlying disease process, or the use of CPB. Unsuccessful MVRep is classified as either immediate or late. Late failures occur after the patient's initial OR experience. Causes of immediate failure may be secondary to an extensively diseased valve, calcification, segmental involvement making the valve more difficult to repair, systolic anterior motion (SAM) of the MV with associated left ventricular outflow tract obstruction (LVOTO), suture dehiscence, development of ischemic MR, and incomplete repair. Many of these causes may be detected by the pre-CPB IOE with a prediction of the difficulty of repair, raising the index of

suspicion during the post pump evaluation. Marwick et al. reported on the factors associated with immediate failure during the initial MVRep procedure (85). Of 26 patients requiring second CPB runs for persistent MR, the causes were determined to be LVOTO (38%), suture dehiscence (23%), and "incomplete repair" (38%) (85). Agricola et al. reported on 255 consecutive patients undergoing MVRep for MR receiving a quadrilateral resection (86). Twenty-one patients had significant residual MR related to

1. Residual cleft, provoking interscallop malcoaptation
2. Residual prolapse of the anterior or posterior leaflets
3. Residual annular dilation
4. Left ventricular outflow obstruction
5. Suture dehiscence (64)

Omran et al. evaluated 170 consecutive patients undergoing MVRep, with 9% of patients receiving an MVR due to persistent significant MR (81). Using univariant and multivariant analysis, predictors of unsuccessful repair (or predicting the need for MVR) were

1. MV annulus > 5.0 cm
2. Mitral annular calcification (MAC)
3. Central MR jet
4. ≥3 segments/scallops with prolapse or flail

By allocating one point for each of these factors, if the score was 0, 1, or greater than 1, the observed risk was 0%, 10%, or 36% (81), respectively.

Systolic Anterior Motion with LVOT Obstruction (LVOTO)

SAM with LVOTO and an associated posteriorly directed jet has been reported in up to 16% of patients undergoing MVRep for myxomatous MV dysfunction (85,87,88). More recent experiences place the incidence under 1% to 2% of MVReps (37). When SAM with LVOTO occurs, inotropic agents and vasodilators (including vasodilating inhalation agents) should be discontinued. If the administration of volume and pressor agents does not reverse the process, further repair may be required, such as a sliding annuloplasty, which reduces the height of the PMVL. This will move the coaptation point further away from the LVOT reducing the probability of SAM. In 1988, Schiavone et al. reported a small series of 12 patients with postrepair SAM and LVOTO with a rigid ring (87). Of those patients who left the OR with persistent SAM and LVOTO, the severity of LVOTO had, in fact, diminished in follow-up at 27 months. However, when provoked with amyl nitrate, a significant gradient returned and was associated with significant MR (87). Lee et al. reported on a similar group of 14 patients, developing postrepair SAM and LVOTO (88). They determined that these patients had common features of reduced pre-CPB coaptation to septal (C-sept) distances (2.65 cm) and PMVL systolic heights of 1.9 cm (Figs. 30.43A, B and 30.44) (88). Carpentier developed the sliding annuloplasty in 1988 as a potential solution

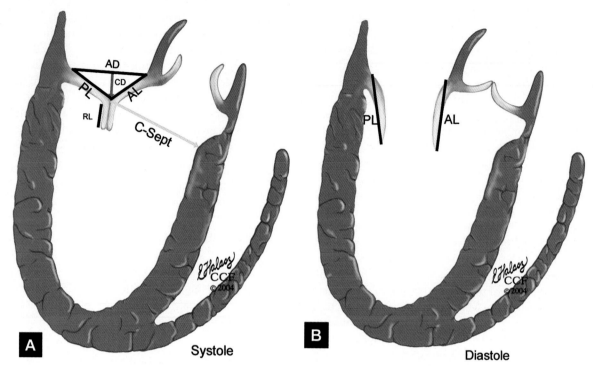

Figure 30.43A,B. Lee et al. (88) and Maslow et al. (92) have demonstrated in two separate studies that SAM with LVOTO may be predicted by a tall PMVL (>1.9) (88), PMVL/AMVL height less than 1.0 (93), a coaptation point to septal distance (C-sept) of less than 2.53 (88)–2.65 cm (92). Others have suggested an AMVL height of greater than 3.0 with reduced C-sept and an anteriorly displaced AL papillary muscle as other predictors. Measurements obtained in patients undergoing MVRep from the ME 4 Chr MV and ME LAX MV include the height of the PMVL (PL) and AMVL (AL), residual coaptated leaflet (RL), distance between superior plane of the annulus and coaptation point, the diastolic length of the AMVL and PMVL, and septal thickness in diastole.

to these issues (89). Cosgrove et al. reported that a sliding annuloplasty is performed on patients with a PMVL height of greater than 1.5 cm (Fig. 30.45) (90,91). Maslow et al. evaluated patients undergoing MVRep for myxomatous MV disease in an attempt to identify echocardiographic predictors of LVOTO associated with SAM of the anterior leaflet of the MV (92). Using intraoperative TEE and the ME 4 Chr imaging plane the lengths of the coapted AMVL and PMVL leaflets, the distance from the coaptation point to the septum (C-sept), annular diameters, and left ventricular internal diameter (LVID) at end systole were measured in 33 patients undergoing MVRep. Eleven patients developed significant SAM with LVOTO after MVRep. They had smaller AL/PL ratios (0.99 vs. 1.95, $p < 0.0001$) and C-sept distances (2.53 vs. 3.01 cm, $p = 0.012$) prior to pre-CPB compared to those who did not develop LVOTO with SAM (92). These findings were consistent with studies demonstrating that SAM with LVOTO following MVRep surgery is associated with anterior malposition of the point of coaptation. This study lends further support to the strategy of reducing posterior leaflet height to prevent post-MVRep LVOTO (89–91). From these studies an AMVL:PMVL ratio less than 1.0, PMVL height greater than 1.5 cm, and a small systolic LVOT diameter (C-septal distance < 2.6 cm) would indicate a higher risk MVRep patient population for developing post-CPB SAM and

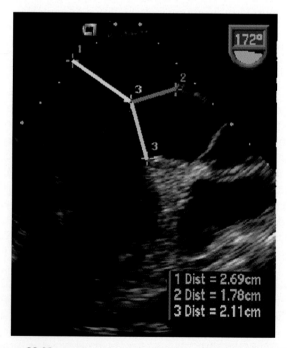

Figure 30.44. Predictors of post-MVRep SAM and LVOTO. AMVL:PMVL ratio less than 1.0, PMVL height greater than 1.5 cm, and a small systolic LVOT diameter (C-septal distance < 2.6 cm) would indicate a higher-risk MVRep patient population for developing post-CPB SAM and LVOTO (90–92).

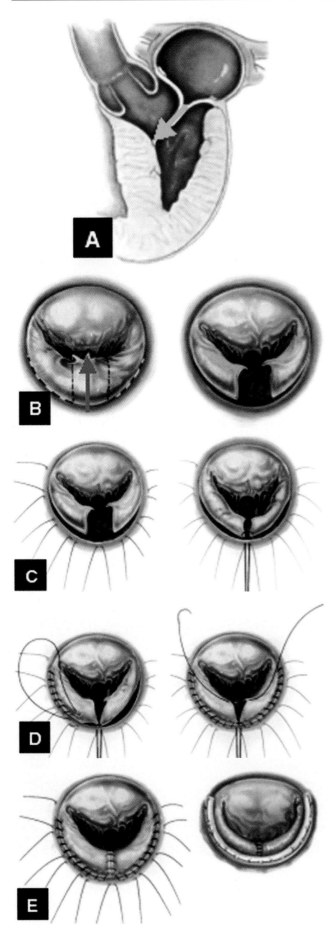

Figure 30.45. **A:** To prevent SAM of the MV with LV outflow tract obstruction (LVOTO), a sliding annuloplasty is performed. **B:** A quadrilateral resection of the P2 scallop with detachment of the PMVL from the annulus is performed. **C:** The posterior free edge of the respected P1 and P2 interface is anchored to the posterior annulus. **D:** The PMVL is reattached to the MV annulus posteriorly. **E:** A Cosgrove ring is used to reinforce the annuloplasty and prevent future annular dilatation. The procedure effectively increases the coaptation to septal distance (C-sept) (*blue* →). The coaptation distance is moved posteriorly, the height of the PMVL is reduced, and the distance between the septum and the coaptation point is increased.

LVOTO and the potential need for a posterior MV complete or modified sliding annuloplasty.

Periannular Annular Disruption

Other complications of MV surgery that may be predicted by the pre-CPB exam include post-CPB pseudoaneurysms (93,94). Patients with severe MAC in whom posterior annular debridement is required are at an increased risk. Demonstrating MAC pre-CPB and consulting with the surgeon regarding the extent of resection alert the team to the potential of pseudoaneurysm or annular disruption. Feindel reported a series of 54 patients with extensive MAC. When calcium was debrided and a new mitral annulus was created by suturing a strip of pericardium onto the endocardium with annular reconstruction, the 5-year survival was 73% (93).

LV Dysfunction

Post-CPB LV dysfunction may accompany MVRep. The greatest predictor of post-CPB LV dysfunction is preexisting LV function (95,96). The pre-CPB exam may also provide a quantitative indication for the need of post-CPB inotropic support. Patients with a pattern of restrictive diastolic dysfunction are at an increased risk for post-CPB dysfunction. Isada et al. reported the use of the CWD interrogation of the MR jet and estimation of LV and RV dP/dt (Fig. 30.46). A dP/dt less than 800 was found to be predictive of the need for post-CPB support (96).

Cannulation-Perfusion and Myocardial Protection Strategy

Davila-Roman et al. evaluated the relationship between the incidence of perioperative stroke and the presence of ascending aortic atheroma by examining 1,200 consecutive patients over the age of 50 with epiaortic echocardiography scanning (97). They determined that the incidence of stroke was almost eight times greater in patients with greater than 3 to 5 mm plaques in the ascending aorta. They demonstrated in a subsequent study, in an older group of patients, that the incidence of stroke was 33% in those patients with plaques in the ascending aorta greater than 4 mm (98). Wareing et al. also demonstrated that the surgical practice of performing epiaortic echocardiography scanning only when plaques were palpated missed 38% of plaques at the site of aortic cannulation or cross-clamp (99). Roach et al.,

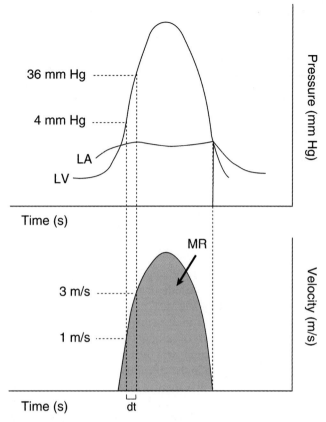

Figure 30.46. CWD interrogation of the MR jet and estimation of LV and LV dP/dt is calculated by determining the time required for the spectral envelope velocity to increase from 1 to 3 m/s, corresponding to an increase in the systolic LV-LA gradient from 4 to 36 mm Hg (gradient = $4V^2$). Isada et al. reported that a dP/dt less than 800 was associated with the need for post-CPB support (97).

in a large multicentered study involving over 2,100 patients, demonstrated a similar incidence of palpated atheroma documented by epivascular echocardiography, in addition to a strong association between atheromatous disease in the ascending aorta and postoperative focal neurological deficits (100). Subsequent studies by Konstadt et al. have demonstrated a similar incidence of missed or underestimated plaques by palpation techniques (101). Patients with identified risk factors—age over 65 years, diabetes, neurologic history, previous coronary artery bypass graft (CABG), and pulmonary disease—for atheromatous disease or demonstrable protruding plaques should receive epiaortic scanning to identify uncompromised areas for cannulation and cross-clamping (74).

Post-CPB Exam and Outcomes

Preseparation CPB abbreviated exam

For purposes of this discussion, the abbreviated exam prior to separation from CPB is included as part of the post-CPB exam, because it is functionally contiguous. This abbreviated exam serves as a safety net to immediately detect any significant complications that could adversely affect patients if they are prematurely weaned from CPB.

A rapidly performed abbreviated overview exam is followed by a more complete evaluation of the surgical intervention and potential complications associated with the procedure and use of CPB. Important issues that are clarified by the IOE exam prior to separation from CPB include

1. Detection of significant complications (aortic dissection, new segmental wall motion abnormality)
2. Optimizing the patient's cardiac performance
3. Assessing the function of other valves
4. Guidance of the de-airing process (microbubbles may be entrapped in the pulmonary circulation, atria, and ventricles during an open cardiac surgical procedure)
5. Identifying the optimal time to separate from CPB (the heart is completely de-aired and ejecting effectively)

As soon as the cross-clamp is removed, IOE may be utilized to evaluate the potential distensibility of the LV caused by aortic regurgitation. Even though the patient may not have had aortic regurgitation pre-CPB, until the LVOT is pressurized and the heart is actively ejecting, there may not be complete coaptation of the aortic valve leaflets. If the heart is slow to initiate an intrinsic rhythm and eject on its own, placement of an LV vent may be warranted.

As the heart starts to eject, it is always tempting to diagnose the results of the valve repair or replacement. However, unless there is an obvious structural problem, the final verdict should wait until the heart has recovered and hemodynamics are optimized. Initial significant regurgitant jets may resolve following MVRep, and perivalvular regurgitation may be absent post-CPB after protamine has been administered in patients undergoing MVR (102–104). A rapid abbreviated examination may be performed to initially evaluate left ventricular function, TR, MR, aortic regurgitation, and the descending aorta for evidence of complications related to cannulation and perfusion while on CPB.

The passage of micro-air bubbles may also be visualized (Fig. 30.47). The IOE is a reliable monitor for micro-air

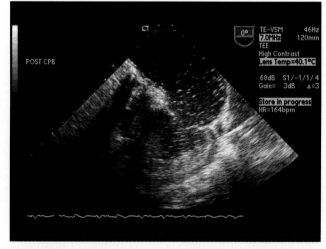

Figure 30.47. Micro-air detection. TEE detects the presence of significant amounts of micro-air bubbles that normally collect at the apex, LAA, and dome of the LA. Air emboli are more frequently seen in open cardiac procedures such as MV surgery.

that may be distributed to the cerebral circulation. When simultaneous recordings of intracranial Doppler and TEE visualizing the descending aorta are performed, detection of micro-air emboli in the cerebral circulation is simultaneous with micro-air visualization in the descending thoracic aorta. Strategies to prevent further embolization to the coronary arteries or cerebral circulation include

1. Having the perfusionist increase aortic vent flow accordingly
2. Emptying the heart
3. Increasing pump flow and lowering the head with Trendelenburg positioning so that micro-air will accumulate at the ventricular apex and can be aspirated

If waves of air are noticed that cycle with the ventilator, ventilation may be transiently interrupted until the micro-air clears. Air may also collect at the dome of the LA adjacent to the aortic sinotubular junction or in the left atrial appendage. Micro-air may be visualized in the proximal right or left main coronary arteries. If this occurs, the perfusion pressure may be increased to hasten passage of the micro-air through the circulation.

As the heart starts to more actively contract and the hemodynamics are optimized, assessment of the MV surgical intervention takes on more meaningful long-term significance. However, in addition to focusing on the surgical results, abbreviated IOE exams may avert the full effects of unfortunate complications. A rapidly performed abbreviated exam will detect complications, such as cannulation-related aortic dissections (Fig. 30.48). Functional assessments of left and right ventricle, tricuspid and aortic valves, the aorta proximal and distal to the cannulation site, and the interatrial septum (if a minimally invasive approach to the MV was utilized) will provide guidance for the optimal time of weaning from CPB.

Post-CPB Clinical Issues (Tables 30.6A, B, 30.13, and 30.14)

The post-CPB is an extension of the evaluation prior to separation from CPB. Following separation from CPB, overall cardiac performance may be assessed by an abbreviated overview examination (cardiac function and evaluation of cannulation-related complications) followed by an evaluation of the MV surgical procedure. In determining the success of the MVRep or MVR, a rapid 3D screening for MR or MS is easily performed with CF Doppler (aliasing velocity set at 50–60 cm/s). Because of the MVRep technique, persistent MR is in a different location and requires a complete 3D exam of the MV. If significant (> mild) MR is seen by the initial CF Doppler screen (using MJA), a more quantitative method, such as a simplified PISA estimate of peak ROA (scale set to 40 cm/s, ROA = $r^2/2$ assessment) or VC, is performed (Fig. 30.49). Use of CF Doppler MJA alone may be misleading. While the MJA may appear to be significant, color m-mode (CMM) may indicate an MR jet of brief duration (<50% systole) indicating MR of less significance. The duration of the CF jet by CMM or evaluating the severity of MR using more quantitative parameters, such as PISA (peak) ROA or VC, may clarify the significance of the jet. As previously discussed, permitting a period for the heart to fully recover, before making a final decision of MR severity, will filter out those patients who may develop transient ischemic MR post-MVRep related to myocardial ischemia encountered to some degree in all patients on CPB. If significant diastolic PFC is found, a transvalvular gradient is performed using CWD. If the mean gradient is greater than 6 to 8 mm Hg at a heart rate of 80 + 10 bpm, consideration should be given to a second pump run to further repair the MV or MVR.

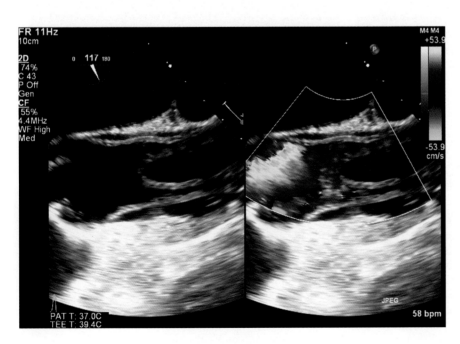

Figure 30.48. Post-CPB aortic dissection. A rapidly performed abbreviated exam will detect complications such as cannulation-related aortic dissections. To make certain that the finding is not an artifact, the pre-CPB documentation of the aortic anatomy is helpful for comparison.

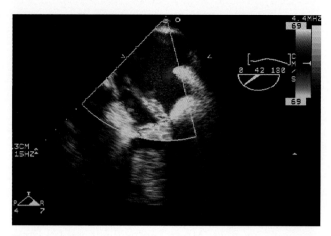

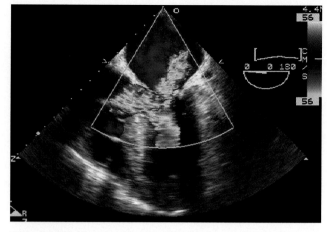

Figure 30.49. Regurgitation following MVRep is initially detected using CF Doppler. However, more quantitative methods (simplified PISA, VC, systolic reversal PV) are recommended for determining the grade of severity.

Figure 30.50. Post-MVRep SAM with LVOTO. Turbulence in the LVOT is a posteriorly directed MR jet characteristic for SAM with LVOTO.

Post-CPB Complications

Complications following MVRep or replacement, though infrequently encountered, include

1. Residual MR
2. Residual or new MS
3. SAM or prosthetic strut protrusion with LVOTO
4. Left or right ventricular dysfunction
5. Circumflex coronary "kinking" or occlusion from annuloplasty or valve ring suture
6. Pseudoaneurysm formation at site of debridement of MAC
7. Shunts-related endocarditis
8. Air embolism

9. Aortic regurgitation secondary to suture placement on the anterior mitral annulus or annular distortion
10. Complications related to cannulation and perfusion

Some of these complications could be potentially devastating. However, if recognized while the patient is in the operating room with the chest open, surgical intervention may prevent adverse impact on the patient's long-term course.

Mechanisms of persistent dysfunction following MVRep include SAM with LVOTO and a posterior jet of MR (Fig. 30.50), new or residual stenosis (Fig. 30.51), persistent primary mechanisms of MR, leaflet cleft or over-shortening associated with PMVL resection (Fig. 30.52), anterior-leaflet override after a quadralateral resection of

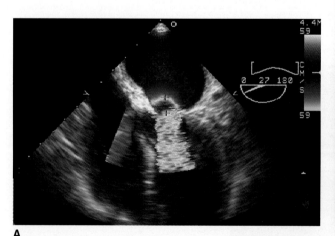

A   **B**

Figure 30.51. Post-MVRep stenosis. Usually stenosis following MV reconstruction is associated with attempts to repair rheumatic disease with pure MS or combined MS and MR. However, cases of stenosis have been associated with repair of myxomatous MV disease using a smaller sized annuloplasty ring. **A:** Usually stenosis following MV reconstruction is associated with attempts to repair rheumatic disease with pure MS or combined MS and MR. **B:** CWD will provide an estimation of the transvalvular gradient, the first sign of stenosis. Gradients are heart rate dependent, so a significant gradient should take the patient's heart rate into account. The presence of PFC is usually the first indication of a significant gradient. PT$_{1/2}$ is not a reliable method of assessing MV area postvalvuloplasty due to compliance alterations changing the constant used in the calculation. MVA using the continuity equation (using TVI), the Gorlin calculation, is more reliable.

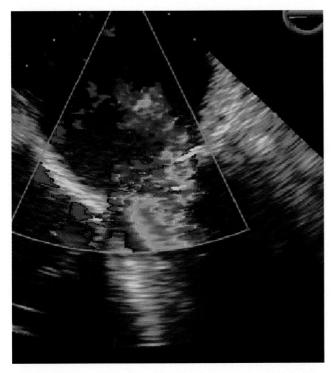

Figure 30.52. A leaflet cleft at the site of the quadralateral resection or overshortening of the PMVL may result in incomplete apposition and a posteriorly directed regurgitant jet.

the PMVL, suture dehiscence, perivalvular MR following MVRep or MVR (Fig. 30.53), and new ischemic MR associated with transient postbypass ischemia. In patients receiving prosthetic valves, perivalvular MR is more frequent in patients with annular calcification and has been associated with reoperations. In each of these circumstances, the post-CPB IOE exam provided crucial

identification of the mechanisms for the failed repair and directed their successful correction. In addition, with complete or incomplete chordal sparing techniques with MVR, the subvalvular apparatus may become entangled in the mechanical prosthesis apparatus, preventing complete leaflet closure (106).

Factors that may accentuate SAM and LVOTO with associated posteriorly directed MR include hypovolemia, excessive afterload reduction (vasodilators or anesthetic agents), and hyperdynamic ventricular function (increased sympathetic tone or inotropic agents). If the SAM persists following hemodynamic intervention with pressors and volume loading, the surgeon may elect to raise the height of coaptation by performing a sliding annuloplasty or other technique to reduce the height of the posterior MV leaflet (Fig. 30.45A,B). This effectively moves the mitral coaptation point further from the interventricular septum, thereby increasing the effective systolic diameter of the LVOT. In some circumstances, further attempts at valve repair are unsuccessful and valve replacement is necessary.

Other rare complications related to the MV procedure include ventricular septal defects following septal myectomy for correction of MR associated with SAM and myxomatous disease (Fig. 30.54), circumflex coronary occlusion with suture ligation or kinking during the placement of the prosthetic valve or annuloplasty ring (Fig. 30.55A, B), pseudoaneurysm following debridement of annular calcium (Fig. 30.56A–E), aortic regurgitation due to the anchoring trigonal suture for the annuloplasty ring engaging the left coronary cusp or distorting the aortic valve annulus, and aortic dissections related to aortic decannulation. Various post-CPB shunts have been detected by IOE at the site of the atrial septal surgical approach, as well as between the

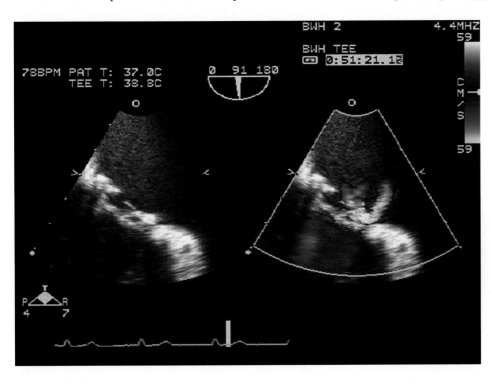

Figure 30.53. MR noted both within the annular ring and perivalvular (outside the ring). Based on the rotational plane, the leak is likely near the A1 annulus. It improved with protamine administration but did not resolve.

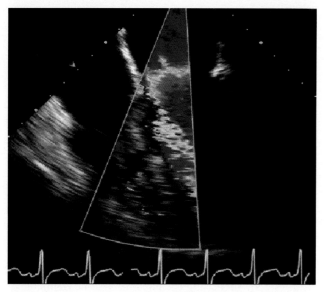

Figure 30.54. A ventricular septal defect (VSD) is an extremely rare complication of MVRep and is associated with the need to perform a septal myectomy in addition to primary reconstruction of the MVAp. Whenever a septal myectomy has been performed, great care is taken to closely interrogate the interventricular septum for a possible septal defect.

LA and aorta (Fig. 30.57A,B). All of these complications may be diagnosed by IOE while the chest is still open, if the index of suspicion is raised to a level where these concerns are routinely incorporated into the post-CPB examination.

Post-CPB Outcomes

Post-CPB complications following MV surgery include those related to the MV procedure and those related to cardiac surgery with CPB in general. The need for second pump runs following MVRep varies widely from 2% to 8%, and is dependent on the underlying etiology and mechanism of dysfunction in addition to the aggressiveness of attempted repairs (54,107). Fix et al. reported that patients requiring a second pump run do not incur

additional morbidity or mortality, including increased inotrope use, prolonged ventilation, bleeding, and intensive care/hospital length of stay (108).

The success rate for mitral repair is dependent upon the underlying pathoanatomy and mechanism of dysfunction. In patients at the Cleveland Clinic with myxomatous disease, second pump runs are required in less than 3% to 5% of patients (54,85,107). In this circumstance, IOE provides crucial information regarding the mechanisms for the failed repair. There have been a number of studies that have evaluated the causes of unsuccessful MVRep. Agricola et al. reported on the mechanisms of failed MVRep in 255 consecutive patients undergoing MVRep who received a quadrilateral resection of the PMVL (86). Mechanisms of failed MVRep were detected by IOE in 21 patients requiring re-repair. Post-CPB determined the exact mechanism of immediate failure determined using IOE; the mechanisms included

1. Residual cleft provoking interscallop malcoaptation (9 patients)
2. Residual prolapse of the anterior (1 patient) or posterior leaflets (4 patients)
3. Residual annular dilation (3 patients)
4. Left ventricular outflow obstruction (2 patients)
5. Suture dehiscence (2 patients)

In 20 of 21 patients, IOE guided the repair with resolution of the residual MR. The one patient who required MVR had persistent SAM with LVOTO despite the performance of a sliding annuloplasty. SAM occurs most commonly in patients with extremely redundant myxomatous valves with tall PMVL and AMVL as well as hypertrophied ventricles with hyperdynamic function. SAM with LVOTO has occurred more frequently with rigid annuloplasty systems (86). Understanding the factors associated with SAM and LVOTO has provided for a more aggressive approach to this potential complication with the more frequent use of a sliding annuloplasty during the initial repair with a lowered 1% to 2% incidence of post-MVRep SAM and LVOTO (54,107,109). Gillinov et al. reported

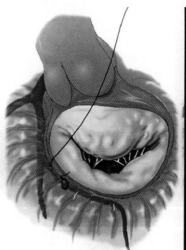

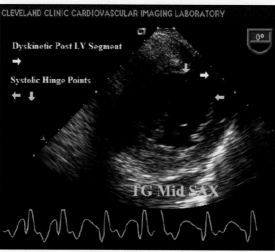

Figure 30.55. Occlusion of the left circumflex coronary artery (adjacent to the P1–P2 interface) by suture ligation or kinking of the vessel with placement of the annuloplasty ring or prosthetic MV. This occlusion results in the development of a new or significantly more severe wall motion abnormality. With kinking of the vessel, the wall motion abnormality may be intermittent.

130%

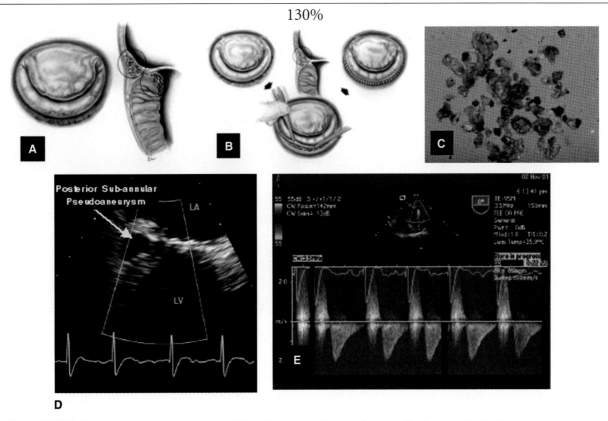

Figure 30.56A–E. A: MAC limits annular mobility during systole, thereby contributing to MR. **B,C:** Extensive debridement may be necessary and is associated with subannular aneurysms and pseudoaneurysm. Because the posterior annulus region is difficult to visualize in the open chest, intraoperative echo is important in establishing the diagnosis during the initial procedure. This patient required extensive debridement due to MAC while undergoing an MVRep. **D:** A subannular pouch was detected 20 minutes later and normal images of this area were visualized. **E:** PW Doppler documented the timing of the flow in and out of the pseudoaneurysm. The patient's subannular region was reinforced with pericardium, and he was weaned from CPB uneventfully and successfully discharged from the hospital.

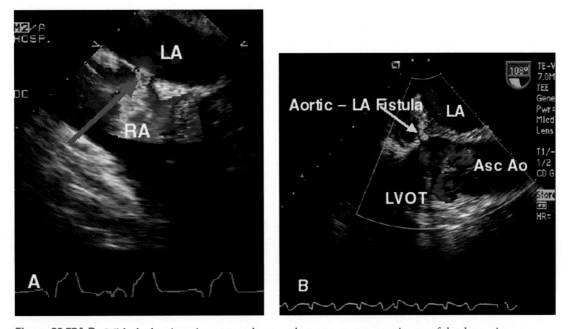

Figure 30.57A,B. With the less invasive approaches to valve surgery, exposure is one of the determining factors influencing the success of the surgical procedure. The post-CPB examination closely examines for potential complications related to exposure.

that even with predictors of LVOTO, more than 90% of degenerative MVs can be repaired successfully by employing a sliding repair to reduce the risk of SAM when the leaflet is greater than 1.5 cm long (91,92). If patients have a sigmoid-shaped superior septum, as is commonly seen in elderly patients, a septal myectomy or MVR may be required (90). Close evaluation for a post-CPB ventricular septal defect (VSD) is warranted in patients having a septal myomectomy performed. Understanding the factors precipitating SAM with LVOTO also enables the hemodynamic management of these patients to be anticipated and weaning the patient from CPB with adequate volume in the heart-lung machine to better ensure the ability to reverse mild LVOTO should it occur. Milas et al. have reported on the successful use of A-V sequential pacing in the successful management of SAM with LVOTO (110).

Gatti et al. performed IOE on 108 consecutive patients who underwent MVRep for degenerative MV dysfunction with MR. Eleven patients had residual MR with a CFD MJA of $\geq 2.0\,cm^2$ (111). They reported the successful use of the Alferi edge-to-edge technique improving the amount of MR without taking down the original MVRep. Exactly how much residual MR is acceptable? Fix et al. evaluated 76 out of 530 consecutive patients undergoing MVRep (1987–1989) in whom there was persistent 1^+ or 2^+ MR and discovered that there were no significant differences in posthospital mortality, thromboembolic events, hospitalizations for heart failure, or functional class (108). Kawano et al. used IOE in MVRep of 72 patients. They found residual MR with a grade of greater than $1+$ in five patients. One required immediate MVR, and rapid progression of MR was noted in the other three (15). Saiki et al. evaluated 42 patients who underwent MVRep for MR to determine the ability of post-CPB IOE (CFD MJA $\leq 2.0\,cm^2$) to predict late outcomes. Patients with trivial MR continued to have trivial MR with no progression ($p < 0.001$) (112).

Mitral Stenosis

Muratori et al. reported on 119 patients undergoing MVRep for predominant MR and reported a 0.8% incidence of newly acquired MS determined by transmitral gradient (87). CWD is a routine part of the post-CPB exam in MVRep and MVR in order to provide a baseline documentation of the patient's gradient. Post-CPB MS is usually associated with attempted repair of patients with rheumatic MV disease. New MS is an infrequent complication following MVRep. Following repair for nonrheumatic MR, a significant mean gradient (>4–6 mm Hg) is rare unless an edge-to-edge Alferi repair or commissural oversew is performed for a commissural prolapse or flail (107). In these circumstances, the mean gradient and heart rate are recorded and the valve area is planimetered using TG or epicardial imaging for accuracy (Fig. 30.58). Umana et al. and Privitera et al. reported on the transvalvular gradients following Alferi "bow-tie" repairs in patients with ischemic MR (113,114). Similar to pros-

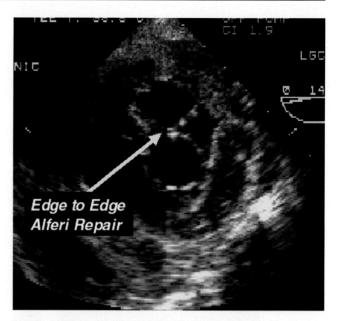

Figure 30.58. Following an MVRep utilizing an edge-to-edge "Alferi" repair technique, the transvalvular gradient and area of the double orifice are obtained to confirm that there is no significant stenosis (mean gradient >6–8 mm Hg at a heart rate of 80 bpm, planimetered area >2.5 cm^2).

thetic valves, patients following MVRep may have mildly elevated transvalvular mean gradients (<4–6 mm Hg). Significant gradients following MVRep, however, have been reported in nonrheumatic valves (115). Due to differences in immediate post-CPB diastolic function of the left-sided chambers, the pressure half-time method for determining MV area cannot be accurately relied upon.

Micro-Air and LV Function

In open cardiotomy procedures involving the MV, air is always an issue. Accepting the eventuality of such issues, despite the best attempts of de-airing, many surgical teams will flood the surgical mediastinal wound with CO_2 diffused through a surgical sponge to prevent a "jet wash" effect. Tingleff et al. evaluated 15 patients undergoing open cardiotomy operations (116). All had micro-air originating in the pulmonary veins. Twelve of the 15 patients had new episodes of micro-air up to 28 minutes after termination of CPB (116). Secknus et al. evaluated the use of IOE in minimally invasive MV surgery in 52 patients. Intracardiac air was seen transiently in all patients and was associated with new LV dysfunction in 22 (20%) patients. A statistically significant difference ($p < 0.001$) was noted with a decreased incidence of LV dysfunction in those patients who had no micro-air boluses after weaning from CPB (117).

Aortic Dissection

Varghese et al. reported on the IOE detection of an aortic dissection by the post-CPB IOE on a patient undergoing MVR (118). While most cannulation-related dissections are self-limiting, if not detected intraoperatively they can present catastrophic challenges. Significant ulcerated plaques or ascending aortic disease may lead to the use of alternative cannulation sites.

Post-CPB LV Dysfunction

LV dysfunction following MVRep is usually associated with pre-CPB LV dysfunction. LV dysfunction, however, may also be related to the repair procedure with an open cardiac chamber. Procedure-related LV dysfunction post-CPB may be caused by micro-air embolization to the coronary perfusion bed, the effects of the CPB duration and adequacy of myocardial protection, or related to left circumflex coronary artery obstruction. Ischemia in the perfusion bed of the circumflex coronary artery may be caused by complete obstruction due to suture ensnarement near the lateral scallop of the PMVL as the annuloplasty or prosthetic valve ring is sutured in place (Fig. 30.55A,B). Kinking of the circumflex has also been reported when extensive resection of a redundant PMVL. Tavilla et al. reported a case of a damaged circumflex coronary artery associated with a sliding annuloplasty repair, emphasizing the ability of a routine post-CPB assessment to rapidly detect new wall motion abnormalities (119). While compromise of the coronary circulation is a rare complication of MVRep, three such encounters over the last 12 years have been recognized by abbreviated overview assessments during the pre-SEP CPB exam or shortly after weaning from CPB. In all patients, the left circumflex was grafted with recovery of regional function without electrocardiographic or enzyme changes. Micro-air bubbles can cause regional wall motion abnormalities, usually in the more anterior originating right coronary artery. In 1990, Obarski et al. reviewed 224 patients undergoing either MVRep or replacement over a 24-month period and determined that 5.4% may have postoperative regional dysfunction related to micro-air embolization (120). Care is taken to adequately de-air the pulmonary circulation and pockets where air accumulates (ventricular apex, LAA, and dome of the LA).

Annular Disruption Following Surgical Debridement

Patients who present with extensive posterior MAC or periannular abscess requiring extensive debridement are at increased risk of periprosthetic or periannuloplasty ring fistula or pseudoaneurysm formation. With extensive subvalvular debridement, surgical reinforcement with pericardium is sometimes used. Fistulas or pseudoaneurysms between the LV and LA may also develop in patients with periannular abscesses (94,121) (Fig. 30.56A–E). In 1998, Genoni et al. reported on two dissections of the left atrium during MVRep. The dissections were intraoperatively detected by TEE imaging and successfully managed without perioperative morbidity (121).

Iatrogenic Shunts and Fistulas

Surgical exposure for minimally invasive MV surgery is an important determinant of successful repair of the valve. In the initial experience with such devices, iatrogenic

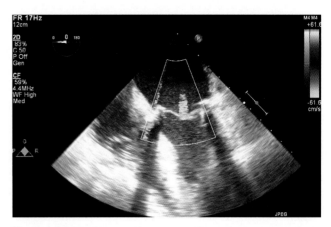

Figure 30.59. All bioprosthetic valves have insignificant amounts of regurgitation up to mild (1+) within the sewing ring and are usually central in origin and direction.

complications were encountered that were recognized by the IOE exam prior to separation from CPB. With recognition of these unusual findings, surgical intervention—while the patient was still cannulated—permitted their immediate resolution.

Perivalvular MR Following MVR

Perivalvular MR has an increased incidence in patients with MAC and reoperation, and it is associated with postoperative hemolysis. Though hemolysis is significantly decreased by comparison in MVRep, it can occur. Morehead et al. reported the results of IOE in 27 patients undergoing MVR with IOE, utilizing CFD to detect intravalvular and perivalvular MR. Before the administration of protamine, a total of 55 jets were detected (102). The CF Doppler regurgitation by MJA decreased an average of 70% ($p < 0.0001$) by quantitative methods of assessment. Mitral and mechanical valves each had more jets and overall greater MJA when compared to aortic and tissue valves. With certain bioprosthetic MV prostheses, it is not unusual to see mild (1–2+) central MR initially (Fig. 30.59). Ionescu et al. evaluated IOE in 300 patients undergoing MVR. With projections of cost savings from the complications that IOE diagnosed, they determined that extending routine IOE use to patients undergoing MVR provided a cost savings of $109 per patient (122).

Systematic IOE Examination in MV Surgery

Priority directed exam

The systematic examination in MV surgery is performed in an efficiently organized manner that will resolve those issues that guide intraoperative anesthetic-hemodynamic and surgical management of the patient, as well as document a comprehensive examination for future reference. As previously discussed, the systematic IOE examination in MV surgery is structured into a "priority directed exam" (abbreviated overview and focused diagnostic exam) and the more general comprehensive exam. Most pre-CPB exams are possible within a 10- to 15-minute period. Regardless of what name we attach to a portion of the exam, experienced intraoperative echocardiographers develop an organized sequence with which they are comfortable that enables them to

1. Overview the cardiovascular anatomy and function and organize the patient's exam
2. Resolve these critical issues in the sequence of the examination and
3. Document a comprehensive TEE examination for future comparison

While it is always tempting to jump directly to the most impressive findings from the patient's preoperative evaluation, the previously mentioned studies provide evidence suggesting that there are instances where all current significant findings were not included in the results of the patient's preoperative evaluation. It is the abbreviated examination that permits the focused examination to proceed unimpeded, without the concern of last-minute revelations just before or after proceeding onto CPB. The abbreviated exam is followed by a focused and subsequent comprehensive IOE exam that is digitally stored for documentation and future reference (Table 30.4).

Abbreviated Overview Exam (Table 30.7A; Fig. 30.24) (II)

The purpose of the abbreviated overview exam in patients undergoing MV surgery is to develop a complete understanding of the likely significant findings of the final exam from the outset. Because of the anatomic relation between the TEE probe position in the stomach and esophagus, every cardiac structure may be assessed utilizing 0 to 15 degrees transducer angulation for transverse imaging. If abnormalities, such as mobile protruding atheroma or significant aortic regurgitation, are discovered, it is possible to mobilize equipment and personnel for an epiaortic examination and include a more thorough examination of the aortic valve. Once the TEE probe has been inserted, the following one-minute exam sequence may be performed in which 2D and color Doppler assessment of the anatomy and function of all chambers, valves, and major thoracic vascular structures is obtained and digitally stored:

1. The TEE probe is advanced to the TG SAX imaging plane at a depth of approximately 40 cm. Using 2D imaging and storage of a representative digital loop, the global LV and RV functions are assessed.
2. For screening purposes only, CFD is initiated in a wide sector scan with an aliasing velocity at approximately 55 cm/s. This will result in a frame rate of 10 to 20 Hz, which is not reliable for detailed diagnostic evaluation. The TEE probe is slowly withdrawn with slight clockwise turning. By slightly advancing and withdrawing the TEE probe (2 cm) back and forth over the coaptation plane of the tricuspid valve, the valve structure and presence of abnormal regurgitation or turbulent transvalvular flow are noted and a representative digital loop is stored.

3. The TEE probe is slowly turned counterclockwise to the left and withdrawn to obtain a focused color Doppler view of the ME 4 Chr. Again, by slowly advancing and withdrawing the TEE probe (2 cm) back and forth over the coaptation plane of the MV, the structure and presence of abnormal regurgitation or stenosis is noted and a representative digital loop is stored.
4. The TEE probe is turned slightly clockwise and withdrawn until the ME 5 Chr is obtained with visualization of the LVOT and aortic valve. Again, by slowly advancing and withdrawing the TEE probe (2–3 cm) back and forth over the coaptation plane of the aortic valve and LVOT, the presence of abnormal regurgitation or turbulent systolic flow is noted and a representative digital loop is stored.
5. The TEE probe is slightly withdrawn (2 cm) from the ME 5 Chr to visualize the aortic root and presence of atheroma or pathology. A representative digital loop is stored in the ME Asc Aortic SAX.
6. The TEE probe is turned counterclockwise and the Desc Aorta SAX and LAX imaging plane is obtained. The entire descending aorta from the celiac axis to the arch and origins of the left subclavian, common carotid, and innominate may be visualized with 2D and color. "Running" the descending thoracic aorta pre-CPB has proven valuable for detecting persistent patent ductus arteriosus in adults (Fig. 30.60). A representative

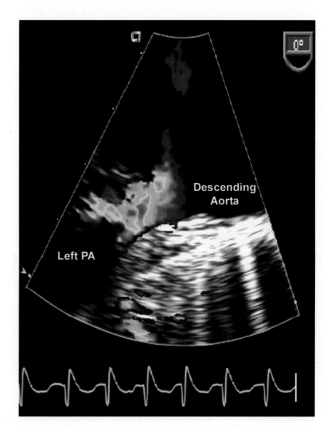

Figure 30.60. Evaluating the aorta for the rare patent ductus arteriosus may prevent interruption of strategies for cannulation and perfusion.

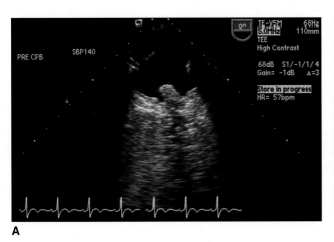
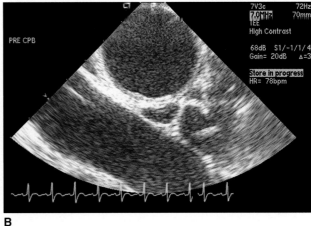

Figure 30.61. Epicardial scanning in patients with significant risk factors of developing atheroma or the finding of protruding plaques (**A**) in the descending thoracic aorta warrants (**B**) epiaortic scanning of the cannulation and cross-clamp sites.

digital loop of any significant atheroma is stored. If the atheroma is greater than 3 mm, epiaortic imaging is routinely performed (Fig. 30.61A–D).

In each of these rapid succession of imaging planes, the probe is advanced and withdrawn looking for evidence of valve regurgitation or transvalvular turbulence suggestive of stenosis. The ascending and descending thoracic aortas are evaluated for atheroma that would suggest the need for epicardial imaging. The results of this brief overview examination will serve as a guide for the organization of the remainder or the intraoperative examination.

Focused Diagnostic IOE Exam in MV Surgery (Table 30.7B)

Experienced echocardiographers develop a natural sequence with which they feel most comfortable over time. The focused diagnostic exam sequence suggested here is guided by the rare necessity to initiate CPB sooner than anticipated or to return to CPB during the post-CPB exam. The posterior and superior location of the midesophagus in relation to the MV annulus and the central rotational axis of the transducer, which may be positioned in the center of the AMVL, enable ideal imaging of the MVAp. With the possibility of 360 degrees imaging of the MVAp at any depth with the multiplane transducer, it is possible to understand the 3D anatomy of the MV anatomy and mechanism(s) of dysfunction. The anatomic progression of the depth of TEE probe insertion and transducer angulation permit an efficient and orderly progression with minimal probe or transducer manipulation.

As illustrated in Table 30.2, the MVAp is examined utilizing up to 12 or more variations of the six recommended ASE/SCA cross-section imaging views at the midesophageal (ME 4 chamber MV, ME commissural MV, ME 2 chamber MV, and ME LAX MV) and TG imaging (TG basal SAX MV and TG 2 Chr MV) probe depths. A 3D "feel" for the mitral apparatus anatomy is developed by advancing or withdrawing the TEE probe 2 to 3 cm (subtle anteflexing or retroflexing produces similar images) or by turning the TEE probe left (counterclockwise) and right (clockwise) from the standard midesophageal

TABLE **30.7A**	Priority-Ordered Intraoperative Exam: Abbreviated Overview TEE Examination in MV Surgery			
Standard Imaging Plane	**Probe Turn**	**Depth (cm)**	**CF Doppler Screen**	**Structures Examined**
Transgastric SAX 2D		40		LV and RV Fx
ME 4 Chr TV	Right	35	X	RV Fx TR
ME 4 Chr MV	Left	30	X	LV Fx MR MS
UE 5 Chr AoV	Central	28	X	LV Fx
UE LAX	Central	26		Aortic root
Desc Th Ao SAX	Left	40–20		Desc thoracic aorta

TABLE 30.7B Priority Ordered Intraoperative Exam Focused Diagnostic Exam

ASE/SCA Standard Imaging Plane [a]Variation	Probe Turn Right = Clockwise Left = Counterclockwise	Angle Rotation (in Degrees)	Probe Depth (in cm)	Chambers LV Segments	Valve Segments	CF Doppler	CW Doppler	Pulse Wave Doppler
1 ME 4 Chr	Midline	0–15	30	RA, RV, LA LV Septal and lateral	A2 P1–2	MR MS AR LVOT obstruction	MR TVI MS PT$_{1/2}$ MS DT MS gradient (peak and mean)	
2 ME 5 Chr[a]	Midline	0–15	28	RA, RV, LA LV, LVOT Anteroseptal and post	A1 P1 ALC	MR MS AR LVOT obstruction	MR TVI MS PT$_{1/2}$ MS DT MS gradient (peak and Mean) LVOTO AR/AS	LUPV LLPV PW Doppler AR
3 LE 4 Chr[a]	Midline	0–15	30	RA, RV, LA, LV Inferior-septal Posterolateral	A3 P3 PMC	MR MS	MR TVI MS PT$_{1/2}$ MS DT MS gradient (peak and mean)	
4 ME Comm	Midline	45–70	30	LA LV Anterolateral Inferior-septal	P1 ALC A2 PMC P3	MR MS	MR TVI MS PT$_{1/2}$ MS DT MS gradient (peak and mean)	
5 ME Comm right[a]	Right	45–70	30	LA LV Aortic valve Inferior-septal anterior-anteroseptal	A1 A2 A3	MR MS	MR TVI MS PT$_{1/2}$ MS DT MS gradient (peak and mean)	
6 ME Comm left[a]	Left	45–70	30	LA LV Inferior-lateral	P1–2 P2 P2–3	MR MS	MR TVI MS PT$_{1/2}$ MS DT MS gradient (peak and mean)	

7 ME 2 Chr	Midline	90	30	LA; LV; Inferior and septal; Anterolateral	A1A2A3; P3; PMC	MR MS	MR TVI; $MS\ PT_{1/2}$; MS DT; MS gradient (peak and mean)	
8 ME 2 Chr right	Right	90	30	LA; LV; Inferior-anteroseptal; LVOT	A1A2A3; PMC; P3	MR MS; AR AS; LVOT obst	N/A	
9 ME 2 Chr left	Left	90	30	LA; LV; Inferior-lateral	P3; P2	MR MS	N/A	
10 ME LAX	Midline	130	30	LA; LV; Anteroseptal posterior; LVOT; Aorta	A2; P2; MidCom	MR MS; AR AS; LVOT obst	MR TVI; $MS\ PT_{1/2}$; MS DT; MS gradient (peak and mean)	
11 ME LAX right[a]	Right	130	30	LA; LV; Anterior; Posterior-lateral	P3; PMC; P2–3	MR MS	MR TVI; $MS\ PT_{1/2}$; MS DT; MS gradient (peak and mean)	
12 ME LAX left[a]	Left	130	30	LA; LV; Posterior; Inferior-septal	A1–2; ALC; P1–2	MR MS	MR TVI; $MS\ PT_{1/2}$; MS DT; MS gradient (peak and mean)	
13 Bicaval	Right from MELAX	130	28	LA, RA, IAS; Fossa Ovalis; PFO; SVC, IVC, Cor sinus	N/A	PFO; Cor sinus	N/A	PW Doppler
14 RUPV and RLPV (bicaval)	Right	135	128–135	LA, RA, IAS; RU PV, RLPV; SVC, IVC, Cor sinus	N/A	RUPV; RLPV	PV gradient in lung TP	Severe MR has systolic reversal
15 TG SAX basal	Midline	0	32–35	LV (anterior, lateral, posterior, inferior, septal segments); RV	A1–2–3; ALC; P1–2–3; PLC	N/A	N/A	
16 TB 2 Chr	Midline	70–90	85	LV anterior and inferior wall; Subvalvular apparatus	A2 P1–2	MS MR; Subvalvular MS identification	N/A	

imaging planes. At every image plane 2D, CFD, CWD, and PWD are performed. To orient the imaging field and to permit more efficient digital storage for the comprehensive examination, 2D and CFD digital images are stored at initial depths that permit the visualization of the apex (in ME image planes) and the entire LV and RV in the TG SAX image planes. Should the need arise to initiate CPB, global and regional ventricular may be examined from the stored images and for future reference. Valve structures are examined in detail during the focused diagnostic exam by using the focusing or zoom option. This permits the visualization and storage of 2D and CFD images with better image and CF detail due to the increased magnification, as well as resolution and Doppler interrogation advantages related to increased pulse repetition frequency. 2D and Doppler (CFD, CWD, and PWD) interrogation of the MV and adjacent structures (pulmonary veins, tricuspid valve, and hepatic veins) are digitally stored at each image plane prior to advancing in the sequence to the next imaging plane.

General Comprehensive Exam

At the conclusion of the more focused diagnostic IOE exam, an account is taken with regard to the important diagnostic issues that need to be addressed, as well as the review of the cardiac valves, chambers, and aorta that are an important part of the comprehensive evaluation. Depending on which of the recommended standard imaging planes were omitted from the abbreviated focused diagnostic IOE exam, upon its completion the missing cross-sectional image views are obtained to complete the study.

PATHOLOGY

Consistent with the principles of the IOE examination, evaluation of the patient undergoing MV surgery is to refine the understanding of the underlying etiology, pathologic changes in the anatomic structure of the apparatus, and mechanism of dysfunction. Compared to transthoracic echocardiography, the intraoperative TEE has an improved imaging capability to accomplish this and more accurately determines the functional anatomy and mechanism of dysfunction (91).

Mitral Regurgitation

Etiology and Mechanisms of Mitral Regurgitation (Tables 30.8–30.10)

Etiologies

The etiologies of MR may be classified by either their acuity of onset or underlying etiology. The former classifies the etiology as being either acute or chronic. The latter classifies MR according to the acute or chronic pathologic

process. Due to the reduced incidence of rheumatic MV disease in the United States and the increasing age of the patient population, the most common cause of both acute and chronic MR is myxomatous degeneration (123–127). In fact, degenerative MR has become the predominant valvular abnormality involving the MV. Acute causes of MR are more commonly related to acute or chronic diseases, including myxomatous degeneration of the MV with associated chordal rupture. Other more common causes of acute MR include endocarditis, ischemic heart disease (with or without PM rupture), and traumatic disruption of the MVAp.

The chronic causes of MR include myxomatous degeneration of the MV, MAC, rheumatic valve disease, endocarditis, global LV dysfunction, hypertrophic obstructive cardiomyopathy (HOCM), radiation-induced fibrosis and scarring, degenerative connective tissue disorders, and congenital abnormalities (cleft MV, parachute MV) (125). Some patients simply have a normal sized MV in a small heart and resulting mismatch.

Myxomatous degeneration

Myxomatous degeneration is the most frequent cause of MR in the United States, occurring in 4% to 5% of the population. It has also been referred to as a "floppy MV," billowing mitral leaflet syndrome, MV prolapse, and fibroelastic disorder. Of those patients with MV prolapse, only 10% to 15% develop progressive MR (123). A very small number of patients progress to surgical MR.

Carpentier distinguishes Barlow's syndrome (MV prolapse) from the entity fibroelastic deficiency. Barlow's syndrome is characterized as occurring in middle-aged individuals and associated with excess tissue with myxoid degeneration. Fibroelastic deficiency is characterized as occurring more frequently in the elderly and is associated with leaflet thickening in the region of prolapse, with the remaining tissue being translucent and thinner than normal. Moderate annular dilatation is associated with fibroelastic deficiency (128).

In patients with myxomatous degeneration, there is annular thickening and dilatation, which is associated with infiltration of acid mucopolysaccharide material and architectural disorganization of elastin and collagen.

The clinical presentation of MV dysfunction in these patients is usually associated with annular dilatation and elongation of the primary chordae with associated chordal rupture. Patients with myxomatous degeneration may present with endocarditis, which leads to the potential for multiple mechanisms of valve dysfunction.

Eight hundred and thirty-three Omstead county residents, who were diagnosed with MV prolapse between 1989 and 1998, were followed for a 10-year period (129). The most frequent risk factors for cardiac death were moderate-to-severe MR and lowered ejection fraction. Secondary risk factors included left atrial enlargement, atrial fibrillation, and age ≥50. Patients with greater than moderate MR and decreased ejection fraction (<50%)

TABLE 30.8	**Acute and Chronic MR: Etiology and Pathology**	
Chronicity	**Etiology**	**Pathologic Anatomy**
Acute		
	Myxomatous	Ruptured chordae with segmental flail, endocarditis
Ischemia	Ischemic	Acute infarct of papillary muscle
		PM tethering or rupture
		Transient global dysfunction tethering
Inflammatory	Endocarditis	Leaflet perforation, vegetation obstructing closure, ruptured chordae, destruction of fibrous skeleton and annulus, associated with previous MV or AoV dysfunction or endocarditis
	Rheumatic fever	Thickening of leaflets, chordal elongation and prolapse of AMVL, enlarged annulus, active myocarditis with CHF
Other	Trauma	Ruptured papillary muscle, ruptured chordae, leaflet tear annular distortion
	Prosthetic	Sewing ring dehiscence, mechanical leaflet stuck open, endocarditis and bioprosthetic leaflet destruction
Chronic		
Degenerative	Myxomatous	Annular enlargement eventually in all redundant leaflets with abnormal connective tissue thinning of chordae
	Mitral annular Ca^{2+}	Posterior annulus Ca^{2+} deposition in granular or coalesced form creating subannular Ca^{2+} bars; extends into base of leaflets, causing immobilization; also deposited in annulus, decreasing mobility and systolic coaptation area
	Osteogenesis imperfecta	Chordal elongation and rupture
Ischemia	Dilated ischemic CM	Spherical remodeling with apical tethering of MVAp tethering
	Segmental infarct	PM infarct with tip elongation and segmental medial prolapse, inf-post infarct and restricted PM with decreased systolic annular motion
	Acute or chronic	Chronic LV remodeling and restrictive physiology; rapid development CHF and central and/or posterior MR due to restriction PMVL and apical tethering
Inflammatory	Rheumatic	Chronic fibrosis and Ca^{2+} of leaflets, chordae, PM, and annulus; commissural fusion with fish-mouth deformity (type IIIa mechanism MR)
	Postradiation	Fibrosis of leaflets, annulus, and subvalvular apparatus with calcific degeneration leads to incomplete coaptation; associated constrictive disease
	Rheumatoid arthritis	Rheumatic nodules on leaflets
	Systemic lupus	Liebman sacks endocarditis at base valve and into subvalvular apparatus
	Atrial myxoma	Large myxoma may obstruct MV inflow
	Sarcoidosis	Papillary muscle granulomas may cause retraction
Congenital	Cleft MV leaflet	Usually AMVL associated with endocardial cushion defects, endocardial fibroelastosis, anomalous origin of coronary artery
	Parachute MV	Absence of papillary muscle, endocardial fibroelastosis
	Disproportional LV	LV cavity small for body size with resulting redundancy of MVAp structures

534 SECTION III ■ Advanced Applications in Perioperative Echocardiography

TABLE 30.9	Etiology and Structural Alteration in the MVAp				
Etiology	**Annulus**	**MV Leaflets**	**Chordae**	**Papillary Muscles**	**Inf-Post and Antero-Lat LV**
Myxomatous degeneration	Enlargement	Redundant, thickened, prolapse	Elongated: propensity to rupture	Chordal attachment: tendency to rupture	Minimal effect
Ischemic MR	Retracted with scarring with decreased systolic narrowing and decreased apposition	Spherical LV causes tethering of both leaflets and tetted AMVL by secondary chordae	Attachment to papillary muscle head vulnerable with PM infarct	Solitary blood supply PMPM rupture or infarct with elongation or retraction	Scarred infarct leads to retraction of PMPM with asymmetrical restricted PMVL/ AMVL override
					Ischemic CM apical tethering
Rheumatic valve disease	Acute annular dilatation	Acute AMVL prolapse in children	Acute elongation and rupture	Inflammation with attachment elongation	Acute myocarditis with CHF and tethering
	Chronic fibrosis with Ca²⁺ decreases systolic narrowing of MV commissure and malcoaptation of MV leaflets	Chronic fibrosis and Ca²⁺ from leaflet edges toward base, comm fusion			Chronic myocarditis and underfilling with decreased systolic fx and restrictive physiology
Dilated cardiomyopathy	Annular dilatation associated with acute or chronic myocarditis post ant	Tenting of AMVL by secondary chordal tethering and bileaflet tethering	Eccentric remodeling increases tension middle post annulus leads to ruptured primary chordae to middle scallop	Spherical ventricle causes tensor apparatus to tether leaflet closure	Diminished LV function increases systolic area or MV annulus with apical tethering
	Diminished systolic mobility and malcoaptation				
Endocarditis	Abscess invading fibrous skeleton and annulus	Leaflet perforations and vegetations	Destruction of chordae with rupture	Active infection of PM and myocardium leads to PM scarring	Active myocarditis
Mitral annular calcification	Ca²⁺ of annulus with reduced systolic narrowing of MV annula and malcoaptation of MV leaflets	Ca²⁺ from leaflet bases toward tips	Calcific degeneration with rupture	Calcific degeneration of PM tips leads to rupture of chordal attachment	Ca²⁺ extends into subannular tissue; may have Ca²⁺ bars interfering with coaptation or MV inflow
Postradiation	Accelerated degeneration with fibrosis, retraction, and diminished mobility, malcoaptation of leaflets	Thickening and fibrosis with accelerated degeneration and Ca²⁺; decreased apposition	Fibrosis and decreased structural integrity prone to rupture	Fibrosis of PM tips with scarring causes retraction MV leaflets in systole with variable tethering	Diastolic dysfunction with constrictive pericarditis; direct and indirect systolic dysfunction

TABLE 30.10 MV Apparatus: Pathology, Mechanism, and Surgical Technique

Leaflet Motion and Carpentier Classification	MV Leaflets Motion	Annulus	PMVL Height ≥1.5	MR Jet Origin	MR Jet Direction	Leaflet Surgery	Annular Surgery
Type 1 (associated with IIIb)	AMVL normal PMVL normal Symmetric	Dilated	1.6	Length of commissure	Central origin	None	Ring annuloplasty
	AMVL normal PMVL normal Symmetric	Normal	1.3	Leaflet body	Eccentric	Pericardial patch	Ring annuloplasty
Type II Excessive	Bileaflet prolapse Symmetric	Dilated	2.2	Point of incomplete coaptation	Central	PMVL quad resect	Ring annuloplasty slide
	Prolapse/flail PMVL Asymmetric	Dilated	2.0	P2	Anterior	P2 quad resect	Ring annuloplasty slide
	Prolapse asymmetric/flail A2	Dilated	1.4	A2	Posterior	Chordal transfer PMVL quad resection	Ring annuloplasty
	Commissural prolapse Asymmetric	Dilated	1.4	A3, P3	Commissural	Suture commissure	Ring annuloplasty
Type IIIa Systolic/diastolic restricted	Rheumatic Symmetrical bileaflet restriction	Retracted, Ca²⁺	1.0	Entire commissure	Central	Open commissurotomy debridement	Ring annuloplasty
Type IIIb							
Systolic restriction	PMVL restriction Inf-post infarct Asymmetric	Retracted Inf-Post	1.5	P2–3	Posterior (AMVL override)	None	Ring annuloplasty
Type IIIb (associated with Type I spherical ventricle apical tethering)	AMVL and PMVL Restriction symmetric	Dilated	1.4	Along entire commissure	Central	None	Ring annuloplasty

The surgical strategy is developed by the surgeon's correlation of their direct inspection of the anatomic components of the MV apparatus with the findings of the intraoperative examination. The real-time assessment of the mechanism of dysfunction directs the surgeon to a closer inspection of segmental anatomy.
Adapted from Stewart WJ. Intraoperative echocardiography In: Topol E, ed. Topol's Textbook of Cardiovascular Medicine. Baltimore, MA: Lippincott, 2002.

experienced a 10-year mortality of 45% with a yearly cardiovascular morbidity of over 6% per year. Mills et al. examined the mechanical properties of myxomatous MV leaflets and chordae and found they were more extensible than normal.

Ischemic mitral regurgitation

By definition, ischemic MR is functional MR caused by coronary artery disease and may be transient or chronic due to a previous myocardial infarction. Transient ischemia results in global or regional dysfunction with the potential of either apical tethering with the production of a central jet of MR. A regional abnormality (such as posterolateral dyskinesia) may result in dysfunction of the myocardium and papillary muscle subtending the posteromedial scallop (P3). This may result in uncoordinated coaptation with the opposing AMVL and transiently result in a posterior-directed jet or central jet related to apical tethering (130).

Endocarditis

Endocarditis involving the left-sided valve structures usually involves the aortic valve. If endocarditis involves the MV, it usually implies the coexistence of underlying degenerative or rheumatic valve disease. The most common organisms involved in MV endocarditis are *Streptococcus* (*S.viridans* and *S.bovis*) and *Staphylococcus* (*S.aureus* or *S.epidermis*) (131). Muehrcke et al. characterized pathologic abnormalities, including the presence of vegetations, leaflet perforation, chordal rupture, and abscess formation (132). In MV endocarditis, the mechanism is usually associated with a preexisting underlying mechanism. Typical MV pathology associated with endocarditis includes leaflet perforation and obstructing vegetations that may interfere with antegrade flow into the LV. Compared with TTE, TEE has a much higher resolution and is therefore usually performed when endocarditis is suspected. Karp reported that up to 18% of cases with multiple valve endocarditis involve the aortic and MVs (131). The lesion on the MV may be secondary to an aortic regurgitant jet lesion of the AMVL with the appearance of a windsock.

Rheumatic mitral regurgitation

Rheumatic MV disease with predominant regurgitation has many features that distinguish it from those associated with pure rheumatic stenosis. The regurgitant form is associated with less calcification of the valve leaflets and subvalvular apparatus. There is diffuse thickening and fibrosis of the leaflets, resulting in restriction in systole and diastole (Carpentier type IIIa). Acute rheumatic valvulitis is infrequently seen in the United States. It is associated with fibrosis of the valve leaflets with prolapse of the AMVL causing predominant regurgitation (133). Other forms of the disease are amenable to surgical repair (134–138).

Primary pathophysiology

Acute MR results in a sudden volume overload of the LV. Due to the increased preload, the LV may actually become hypercontractile with much of the stroke volume proceeding into a noncompliant LA during systole. Because both the LA and LV are not as compliant as in a chronic disease process, patients rapidly develop pulmonary congestion, pulmonary hypertension, and eventually RV dysfunction with dilatation and tricuspid regurgitation. The amount of volume that is ejected into the left atrium is dependent upon the size of the systolic regurgitant orifice, the systolic pressure gradient between the LV and LA, and the systolic ejection time (inversely proportional to heart rate). With severe MR or a noncompliant left atrium, as the LA pressure progressively increases, the pressure differential between the LV and LA rapidly tapers at the end of systole, resulting in a "v wave cutoff sign" on CWD (Fig. 30.62).

In chronic MR, the LA has time to become more compliant, resulting in extremely large LA chamber sizes. Because the amount of regurgitant volume may be greater than 50%, the forward stroke volume is diminished. Eventually, the LV may fail with end-diastolic diameters (EDD) greater than 70 mm (55). With chronic MR, the LV may initially compensate for the added diastolic loading and ejection into a compliance chamber with hyperdynamic performance. However, if the loading conditions continue, the ventricle will eventually fail. In chronic MR, the effects of persistent volume overload of the LV may be tolerated for years; however, the ventricle eventually

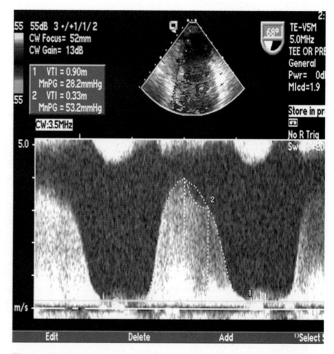

Figure 30.62. With severe MR or a noncompliant left atrium, as the LAP progressively increases, the pressure differential between the LV and LA rapidly tapers at the end of systole resulting in a "v wave cutoff sign" on CWD.

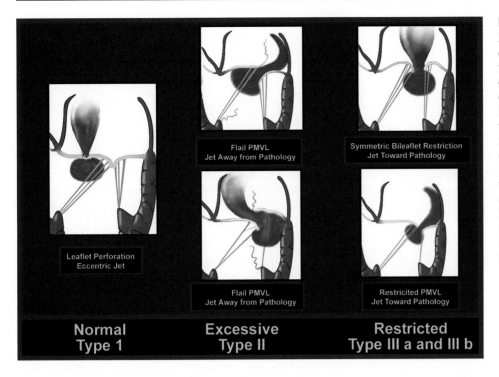

Figure 30.63. Mechanisms of MV dysfunction. MR is produced by pathologic changes in the structural integrity of the one or more of the components of the MVAp that ultimately interferes with apposition of the valve leaflets. Normal apposition is prevented by mechanisms of dysfunction that are related to (i) normal leaflet motion (type I) with annular dilatation or a cleft or perforated leaflet, (ii) excessive leaflet motion (type II), and (iii) restricted leaflet motion in systole and diastole (IIIa) and restricted in just systole (IIIb) perforation.

begins to develop eccentric hypertrophy with the development of a spherically shaped and dilated ventricle, with an increased annular-apical distance, resulting in apical tethering of the mitral leaflets and a secondary mechanism of additional MR.

Mechanisms of Mitral Regurgitation (Fig. 30.63; Tables 30.9–30.11)

MV apparatus and mechanism of mitral regurgitation (Table 30.9)

As previously discussed, the MVAp consists of five unique anatomic structures that work in concert as they function to prevent the retrograde flow of blood into the left atrium in systole and permit antegrade flow into the LV during diastole. The MVAp also helps maintain the functional integrity of the ventricle throughout the cardiac cycle. The range of etiologies of MV dysfunction produces pathognomonic changes in the structural integrity of one or more of the components of the MVAp (42,133,134). Apposition of the valve leaflets is an intricately choreographed process requiring each of the structures to work in concert to get the valve leaflets to the precise plane of apposition at the same time in the cardiac cycle. Significant regurgitation signals a failure of this integrated process. While on the surface, this would appear to occur because of excessive or restricted leaflet motion or annular dilatation, it is ultimately an expression of the abnormal structure and function of one or more of the components of the MVAp. The structural distortions include

1. Annular dilatation or lack of mobility
2. Leaflet redundancy or retraction
3. Chordal shortening, elongation, and rupture

4. Papillary muscle shortening, elongation, and rupture
5. Ventricular dilatation (apical tethering) or segmental abnormalities (transient dysfunction or scarring) (42,44,139)

In 1971, Carpentier characterized the mechanisms of MV dysfunction established on the principle that "function follows form." He recognized leaflet coaptation as the final manifestation of the structural integrity and function of the individual components. This led to the physiologic classification of MR based on the extent of systolic and diastolic excursion of the valve leaflets (126).

Type I: Normal Leaflet Motion (Fig. 30.63)

MR that involves a type I mechanism (normal leaflet motion) may be associated with a dilated annulus frequently caused by myxomatous degeneration or the posterior annular dilatation associated with chronic congestive heart failure or coronary artery disease. A type I mechanism of MR may also be seen in patients having endocarditis with leaflet perforations or a congenital cleft. The congenital cleft is frequently associated with endocardial cushion defects (140).

Type II: Excessive Leaflet Motion (Fig. 30.63)

Because the annulosa fibrosa thins out in the region adjacent to the base of the P2 scallop, dilatation is frequently seen in this location with increasing tension being applied to the chordae at that point. With myxomatous degeneration, these chordae are abnormal and frequently rupture, resulting in a flail P2 segment that is the most frequent of all segmental leaflet abnormalities and the easiest to

TABLE 30.11   MV Apparatus: Pathology, Mechanism, and Choice of Surgical Technique

	1	2	3	4	5	6	7	8	9	10
	Myx Deg					Ischemic MR			Mitral Annular Ca²⁺	Endocarditis
	Bileaflet Pro P3A3	Flail P3	Flail A2	Flail P2-Pro A1–2–3 P1+3	Flail P2 Bileaflet Pro	Infarcted Inf-Post PM Seg and PMPM	Ischemic CM	Ruptured Postero-medial	Mild PMVL Restriction	Perforated AMVL A2
Annulus	Dil	Dil	Dil	No	Dil	No	Yes	No	Sev Ca²⁺	No
P1	NI	NI	NI	Pro	Pro	NI	Rest	NI	Rest	NI
P2 Lat	NI	NI	NI	FI	FI	Rest	Rest	NI	Rest	NI
P2 Med	NI	NI	NI	FI	FI	Rest	Rest	FI	Rest	NI
P3	Pro	FI	NI	Pro	Pro	Rest	Rest	FI	Rest	NI
A1	NI	NI	NI	Pro	Pro	NI	Rest	NI	NI	NI
A2 Lat	NI	NI	FI	Pro	Pro	NI	Rest	NI	NI	NI
A2 Med	NI	NI	FI	Pro	Pro	NI	Rest	FI	NI	NI
A3	Pro	NI	NI	Pro	Pro	Pro	Rest	FI	NI	NI
PMVL height	2.2	2.2	1.3	2.0	1.2	1.4	1.1	1.2	1.0	1.3
Chordae										
P1	NI	NI	NI	EI	EI	NI	Rest	NI	NI	NI
P2 Lat	NI	NI	NI	Rupt	Rupt	NI	Rest	NI	NI	NI
P2 Med	NI	NI	NI	Rupt	Rupt	NI	Rest	PM rupt	NI	NI
P3	EI	EI	NI	EI	EI	EI	Rest	PM rupt	NI	NI
A1	NI	NI	NI	EI	EI	NI	Rest	NI	NI	NI
A2 Lat	NI	NI	FI	EI	EI	NI	Rest	NI	NI	NI
A2 Med	NI	NI	FI	EI	EI	Ovr	Rest	PM rupt	NI	NI

Component	1	2	3	4	5	6	7	8	9
A3	EI	NI	EI	EI	Rest	Exc	Exc	NI	NI
ALPM	NI	NI	NI	NI	Teth	NI	NI	NI	NI
PMPM	NI	NI	NI	NI	Teth	Ret	Rupt head	PM rupt	NI
Global LV	NI	NI	NI	NI	Sph	±Dil	Hyperdyn	NI	NI
Inf-Post LV	NI	NI	NI	NI		Akin			NI
Scar	Hypo	Akin		NI		NI			
Ant-Lat LV	NI	NI	NI	NI	Hypo	NI	NI	NI	NI
Leaflet motion	Exc	Exc	Exc	Exc	Restr	Restr	Exc	Exc	Restr
MR origin	PMC	P3	PMC	P2	ALC to PMC	P2–3	Medial half	A1–2–3	A2
MR direction	Cen Com	Ant Lat	Ant	1. Ant / 2. Cen	Cent	Post	DiffusLat	Post	Ant
Motion symmetrical	Sym	Asy	Asy	Asy	Sym	Asy	Asy	Asy	Sym
AnnPlast ring	Yes	Yes	Yes	Yes	Yes	Yes	Yes	Yes	No
Slide	Yes Mod	Yes Mod	Yes Mod	Yes	No	No	No	No	No
Quad	No	Mod	Yes	Yes	No	No	No	No	No
Com Sut	Yes	±	Yes	No	No	No	±	No	No
Chor transfer	±	Yes	No	No	No	Yes	No	No	No
Patch	No	No	No	No	No	No	No	No	Yes
Other	GortxCh				Alferi repair		PM Rea or MVR		AnnDeb

The intraoperative exam of the MV involves a detailed assessment of the individual components of the MVAp including the annulus (dilation, Ca²⁺, fibrosis), MV leaflets (thickness and motion), chordae (lengthy, thickness, fusion, and rupture), the papillary muscles (scarring, Ca²⁺, elongation, retraction, rupture), and the LV complex (global function, inferoposterior and anterolateral segmental function). CF Doppler is used to characterize the mechanism. Regurgitant jets are characterized by their severity, origin, and direction of the jet. Excessive motion of a segment produces a MR jet directed opposite the leaflet (unless the opposing leaflet has a similar degree of excessive motion). Symmetrical excessive or restricted leaflet motion produces a central jet. An asymmetrical segmental restriction is characterized by the MR jet being directed toward that segment from a "relative override" of the opposing leaflet segment. The surgical technique and probability of repair are determined by the etiology and the mechanism(s) of MR. Flail or prolapse of P2 is the most common presentation of myxomatous disease due to thinning of the fibrous annulus and localized annular dilatation.

In the examples above, every component of the MVAp has been evaluated. Surgical options are included to illustrate how the IOE exam is incorporated into the decision-making process. All valve repairs usually incorporate an annuloplasty ring for additional support to prevent future annular dilatation seen in myxomatous degeneration and LV dysfunction. The five surgical techniques most commonly used in MVRep include (a) an annuloplasty ring, (b) quadralateral resection, (c) sliding annuloplasty, (d) chordal transfer, or (e) commissural suture. Other techniques include the Alferi edge-to-edge suture, gortex chordae, and AMVL resection or plication.

Fl, flail; Pro, prolapse; Asy, asymmetrical; Sym, symmetrical; PM rupt, papillary muscle rupture; PM Rea, PM reattachment; Gotx Ch, gortex chordae; Sec Ca²⁺, severe Ca²⁺; NI, normal; Exc, excessive leaflet motion; Restr, restricted leaflet motion; Hyperdyn, hyperdynamic; Akin, akinetic segment.

repair. Elongated chordae may lead to prolapse of the MV leaflet or a flail leaflet with the leaflet tip pointing toward the top of the atrium (47).

Type III: Restricted Leaflet Motion (Fig. 30.63)

Type III is divided into IIIa (systolic and diastolic restriction) and IIIb (systolic restriction). Type IIIa is usually seen with rheumatic valve disease or extensive MAC, which extends into the leaflet tips with restricted excursion both systole and diastole. Type IIIb is seen clinically in patients with eccentric hypertrophy with spherically shaped ventricles with associated apical tethering of the mitral apparatus. IIIb abnormalities may or may not be associated with annular dilatation. Because of incomplete coaptation, the jet originates centrally and, if there is symmetrical tethering, is centrally directed. With rheumatic disease, the feasibility of repair is the lowest of all etiologies (137).

Intraoperative Echocardiography and Mechanisms of MVAp Dysfunction

In patients with MR, the 2D intraoperative exam is used to characterize the individual components of the MVAp (with a segment-by-segment analysis) and to evaluate how they function in concert with other related components. Added to the 2D echocardiographic exam is the CFD evaluation of the regurgitant jet, which is characterized by some of the following properties: location of origin, direction, and severity.

The direction of the regurgitant jet and its eccentricity may be predicted on the basis of leaflet excursion and the symmetrical excursion of the opposing leaflet segment. The presence of asymmetrical (unopposed) leaflet excursion (i.e., flail PMVL) results in a regurgitant jet away from the anatomic defect, whereas symmetrical opposing leaflet excursion (i.e., bileaflet prolapse) produces a central regurgitant jet. If both leaflets have similar "normal" motion (type I as with annular dilatation), excessive motion (type II as with bileaflet prolapse), or restricted motion (type IIIa rheumatic or IIIb apical tethering), the MR jet will be central.

Type I: Normal Leaflet Motion (Fig. 30.63)

Annular dilatation alone results in a lack of leaflet coaptation. Depending on the symmetry of the leaflet motion, the jet may either be central (symmetrical leaflet motion) or slightly posteriorly directed (mild PMVL restriction). With endocarditis, the leaflet motion remains normal; however, endocarditis may result in leaflet perforation or invasion of the cardiac skeleton. Endocarditis may also produce an eccentrically directed jet depending on the extent of leaflet involvement.

Type II: Excessive Leaflet Motion (Fig. 30.63)

With asymmetrical excessive leaflet motion, the regurgitant flow is directed away from the leaflet with excessive motion. With myxomatous disease, patients will frequently

have underlying bileaflet prolapse (with an associated central MR jet) and acutely ruptured primary chordae to the PMVL, producing an anteriorly directed jet. The patient may have two distinct jet directions, including a central jet associated with the underlying bileaflet prolapse and an anterior jet associated with the flail segment.

Type III Restricted Leaflet Motion (Fig. 30.63)

Because of incomplete coaptation, the regurgitant jet originates centrally and, if there is symmetrical tethering, is centrally directed. With asymmetric restricted leaflet motion, there may be an "override" of the opposing leaflet, and the jet is directed toward the abnormal leaflet. This is seen in posterior wall infarcts with unilateral retraction of the leaflet by a scarred papillary muscle or ventricular wall segment (132).

Comparison of IOE Exam and Direct Surgical Inspection (Tables 30.10 and 30.11)

Unlike the IOE exam, which evaluates the MVAp in a dynamic state, the surgical examination includes a direct inspection and determination of the passive mobility of the individual MVAp components. The characterization of leaflet motion by the surgeon and echocardiographer is similar but functionally distinct. The surgeon utilizes nerve hooks and passive extent of motion of the leaflet edge, whereas the echocardiographer characterizes the motion of the entire leaflet throughout the cardiac cycle. The echocardiographer is able to evaluate excursion of any portion of the leaflet above the annular plane. The surgeon evaluates the structure of the components of the MVAp and the range of motion of the valve leaflets. The surgeon may "fill up the heart" to demonstrate regions of the valve that do not passively coapt. The correlation of both evaluations results in a more accurate assessment of the mechanism of MV pathophysiology. In the end, it is the merging of the perspectives that each provides that leads to the final understanding of the mechanism or mechanisms of dysfunction and the choice of surgical techniques to be incorporated into the surgical strategy (30).

Surgical Technique and IOE Characterization (Tables 30.10 and 30.11)

The choice of surgical technique and repair strategy is based upon the etiology, the structural integrity of each component of the MVAp, and the underlying mechanism of inadequate leaflet coaptation (Table 30.10) (36,37,54,56,76,79,90). With myxomatous disease, there are five repair techniques that are most commonly employed:

1. Annuloplasty ring (almost all repairs) (76)
2. Quadrilateral resection (central or modified with segmental prolapse or flail PMVL)
3. Sliding annuloplasty (excessive length of PMVL > 1.5 cm)
4. Commissural suture (commissural flail or prolapse)
5. Chordal transfer (flip-over technique)

Other techniques used for this and other processes include

1. The Alferi edge-to-edge repair
2. Gortex chordae
3. Chordal shortening (decreased freedom from reoperation)
4. Resection or plication (excessively long AMVL)
5. AMVL extension (for tenting due to apical tethering of secondary chordae)
6. Leaflet debridement (rheumatic or endocarditis)
7. External posterior wall patching between the lower segments and annulus (141)
8. Posterior inflatable baffle to offset tethering of dilated heart (142)
9. Cutting of secondary chordae for apical tethering with tenting of AMVL (143)

If there is excessive leaflet motion of the center P2 scallop, a standard technique for repair includes a quadrilateral resection of the involved segment. If however, there is excessive leaflet motion of the center of the AMVL with a posteriorly directed jet, a chordal transfer may be performed. Degenerative disease is associated with eventual annular dilatation. Gillinov et al. reported that long-term durability was diminished in those patients without a repair involving a stabilizing annuloplasty ring (30,76).

IOE Assessment of MR Severity (Tables 30.12–30.14)

The intraoperative evaluation of patients presenting with known severe MR is focused on determining the mechanism of the dysfunction. However, there are circumstances where severity assessment is critical to the management of a patient.

| TABLE 30.12 | Intraoperative Assessment of MR Severity: Qualitative and Semiquantitative Assessment |

Parameter 2D Imaging	Utility/Advantages	Limitations	Mild	Moderate	Severe
LA size	LAE with chronic MR	Enlarged other conditions	Normal	Normal or dilated	LAE
	NI LA size excludes significant chronic MR	Severe acute MR may be normal			
LV size			Normal	Normal or dilated	Dilated enlarged
MV apparatus	Flail or ruptured PM; severe MR	Limited to flail and ruptured PM	Normal or abnormal	Normal or abnormal	Flail leaflet/ rupt PM
Doppler					
CF Doppler MJA	Efficient screen for mild or severe MR	Technical: wall filter, power, aliasing velocity, color gain, frequency	MJA < 4 cm²	Variable	MJA > 8 cm² PFC present Wall jet
Aliasing velocity 50–60 cm/s	Mechanism evaluation	Load dependent Wall impingement underestimates by 60%		Jet in LA	Circumferential
PW Doppler	A wave dominance excludes severe MR	Dependent on load, diastolic fx, MVA, a fib Indirect indication	Dominant A wave	Variable	Dominant E wave E > 1.2 m/s
PW Doppler PV flow	Systolic flow reversal indicates severe MR	Increased LAP, a fib, need R and L PV to call severe	Systolic dominance	Diastolic dominance	Systolic flow reversal
CW Doppler spectral density	Easy to perform	Qualitative	Faint envelope	Dense	"v" wave cut off sign
CW Doppler contour	Simple	Qualitative	Parabolic	Variable	Early peaking-triangular

In the assessment of patients undergoing MV surgery, the purpose is to confirm the presence of MV dysfunction and focus on better understanding of the underlying etiology and mechanism(s) of dysfunction. MR severity assessment becomes critical when previously undiagnosed MR is discovered or during the post-CPB exam when assessing the results of MV surgery. CF Doppler serves as a useful severity screening method capable of distinguishing mild from severe MR. However, intraoperative decisions based on the severity of MR (i.e., returning to CPB for further repair of the MV) should be founded on quantitative data such as ROA and VC diameter with PW Doppler of the MV inflow and pulmonary veins serving as supporting information. The data are weighted according to its quality and its ability to reliably quantify the severity of regurgitation. Zoghbi WA, Enriquez-Sarano M, Foster E, et al. Recommendations for evaluation of the severity of native valvular regurgitation with two-dimensional and Doppler echocardiography. J Am Soc Echocardiogr 2003;16(7):777–802.

TABLE 30.13	Proximal Isovelocity Surface Area		
Grade	PISA Radius (mm)	ROA r²/2 (Peak) (cm²)	Regurgitant Volume (Peak) (mL)
Mild	>18.9	0.02	<30
Mod	7.7–8.8	0.02–0.29	30–40
Mod–sev	6.3–7.6	0.3–0.39	45–59
Sev	<6.2	≥0.40	≥60

PFC radius and severity of MR—$V_{aliasing}$ = 40 cm/s or 1/12th (0.8) peak V_{MR}.

TABLE 30.14	Severity Assessment in MVRep

1. CF Doppler screening of entire MV coaptation plane
   - ME 4 Chr MV
   - ME 5 Chr MV (ant-lat comm)
   - ME lower 4 Chr MV (post-med comm) (aliasing velocity 50–60 cm/s)
2. If CF Doppler detects MR jet
   - Use 2D imaging to detect structural defect
   - Quantify amount
   - Use simplified PISA
     - Peak ROA > 0.3 cm² is moderately severe
   - VC diameter (VC > 0.3 cm is moderate)
     - CMM may clarify closing regurgitation jet
       - Short lived <40% systolic time interval
     - If moderate, integrate multiple methods
       - Weight toward quality of data obtained and quantitative reliability of parameter
   - Use other quantitative methods
     - PW Doppler PV: systolic reversal is severe
     - CW intensity of spectral envelope
     - MV inflow e > a more severe; e > 1.2 m/s
     - Other volumetric methods
3. When to return to CPB for further repair
   - Identified structural defect that will not
     - Improve though less than moderate
     - SAM with LVOTO and MR
     - Perforation, suture dehiscence identified mechanism
   - Greater than mild to moderate MR
     - ROA > 0.3 cm², regurgitant volume >40–45 mL/beat
     - VC > 0.3 cm
   - If additional CPB time would jeopardize patient modify indications for return to CPB

Assessing the severity of any valve disease integrates multiple parameters of severity with weighting of the parameter used, according to the quality of the data, the ability to more accurately quantify, and the limitations of the technique for particular types of regurgitant jets. The methods of severity assessment in MR are organized as 2D and Doppler-derived parameters of severity assessment (35,57).

Regurgitant jet timing is a factor that must be considered, especially if a short-lived regurgitant jet with a large spatial area is being used to determine if a patient should be returned to CPB for further repair of the MV (67). Other parameters will provide the integrated guidance in determining the significance of MR of short duration. The parameters used to assess regurgitant valves are either 2D or Doppler-derived parameters, demonstrating the direct and indirect cause and the effects of acute and chronic regurgitation. The post-CPB assessment of MR utilizes CF Doppler as an initial screen for significant MR and, if found, is relied upon in conjunction with 2D imaging to provide an understanding of mechanism(s) of unsuccessful MVRep and MVR.

Two-Dimensional IOE

2D imaging provides direct indications of the severity of MV dysfunction by evaluating the indirect effect of regurgitation on the receiving chamber and valve structure. Patients with significant chronic MR have enlarged left atria. Significant MR is rarely associated with normal MV structure. Patients with a flail segment usually have severe MR. This holds true even if the CF Doppler demonstrates a small regurgitant jet area (RJA), such as that seen with an eccentric wall hugging jet or one associated with acute MR that is directed into a noncompliant LA. TEE imaging does not lend itself to see the entire LA, but massively enlarged atria associated with chronic MR are apparent (57).

Doppler Assessment of MR

The regurgitant jet that is detected by CFD consists of a subvalvular zone of PFC, the narrowest portion of the jet (at or just distal to the valve orifice on the LA side), and the spatial jet area in the LA. All components may yield distinct information, which, when integrated together, provides a clearer understanding of the significance of the MV dysfunction. Doppler methods of severity assessment of MR have relied heavily on CF determination of the MJA.

Color Flow Doppler Maximal Jet Area (MJA)

MJA may be utilized as an effective means for screening patients with severe or trivial MR and to characterize the mechanism of MR. However, MJA is not able to distinguish subtle differences of severity grade (35,57). MJA may not reflect the severity of valve dysfunction in acute MR or with eccentric MR (57). In addition, there are a host of settings that impact the MJA. While the MJA (utilizing an aliasing velocity near 50–60 m/s) is generally predictive of the severity of MR, it may underestimate the severity if it is eccentric or acute in etiology (35,57). If the absolute jet area is greater than 8 cm², there is severe MR; if the absolute jet area is less than 4 cm², it is mild. All grades in between are not reliable as a stand-alone assessment of severity. The jet direction, however, is valuable in determining structural mechanisms of MR.

Vena Contracta Diameter (VCD)

Measuring the narrowest diameter of the regurgitant orifice at or distal to the anatomic orifice provides a more quantitative and accurate method of assessment. The VCD should be from an image plane that is perpendicular to the commissural line of MR. The VCD is not dependent on the flow rate, the LA-LV gradient, or the eccentricity of the MR jet. It does change throughout the cardiac cycle. Because of the small size of the VCD, focused zoom should be used to diminish the percentage of error. A VCD of less than 0.3 cm^2 is consistent with mild MR whereas greater than 0.6 to 0.8 cm^2 is severe (35,57). The presence of PFC and a width greater than 0.6 cm^2 confirm the severity of the MR. Multiple small jets are not additive by diameter.

Proximal Flow Convergence

PFC is based on the principle that blood increases in velocity as it approaches a regurgitant orifice, resulting in hemispheric velocity shells (66). The presence of PISAs with MR at an aliasing velocity of 50 to 60 cm/s is an indicator of clinically significant MR (35,57). When one does not see a flow convergence larger than 3 to 4 mm at an aliasing velocity of less than 30 cm/s, the MR would be trivial or at most mild. However, when the flow convergence is larger than 7 to 8 mm at the aliasing velocity

greater than 50 to 60 cm/s, the MR is severe (35). The size of the radius is strictly dependent on the aliasing velocity and alignment of the CFD parallel to the PISA. Not doing so will underestimate the severity of MR. The aliasing velocity must be adjusted down to obtain a hemispheric PFC. Assuming that the peak flow rate occurs simultaneously with the peak radius and peak regurgitant velocity, the (peak) ROA may be determined with the following formula:

$$(Peak)ROA = (6.28r^2 \times V_a)/peak\ V_{MR},$$

where r^2 is the aliasing radius between the orifice and interface, V_a represents the aliasing velocity, and V_{MR} is the peak regurgitant velocity measured with CWD. If there is wall impingement at the aliasing radius r, the wall constraint angle/180 degrees is multiplied by the ROA as a correction (Fig. 30.64) (65,66). An aliasing velocity must be hemispherical (decrease Nyquist limit or baseline shift in direction of jet) with the absence of wall impingement. Limitations apply to eccentric jets, nonhemispheric PFC, and variance of results using non-hemispheric aliasing velocities. Nonparallel alignment of the CW peak V_{MR} results in an underestimation of the velocity peak and an overestimation of the (peak) ROA. If the ROA is greater than 0.4 cm^2, there is severe MR; if the ROA is less than 0.2 cm^2, it is mild. By multiplying the ROA by the MR TVI, the regurgitant volume may be determined (35).

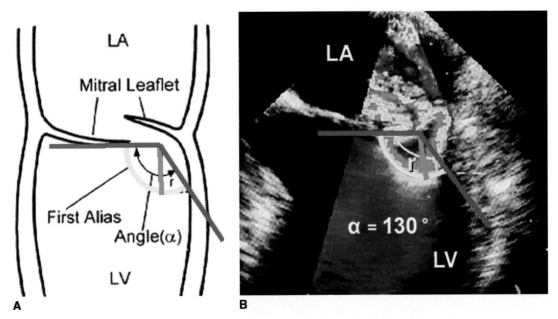

Figure 30.64. Peak ROA. Assuming that the peak flow rate is simultaneous with peak radius regurgitant velocity, the ROA (at peak flow rate) may be determined with the formula above (where r is the aliasing radius between the orifice and interface, V_a is the aliasing velocity, and V_{MR} is the peak regurgitant velocity). Using aliasing velocity for ROA is most reliable with a hemispheric PFC zone (adjust Nyquist limit down and/or baseline shift in direction of jet) and with absence of wall impingement. If there is wall impingement at the aliasing radius r, a reliable correction may be provided with the formula: ROA = (6.28r^2 × V$_a$)/peak V$_{MR}$ × angle/180° (66).

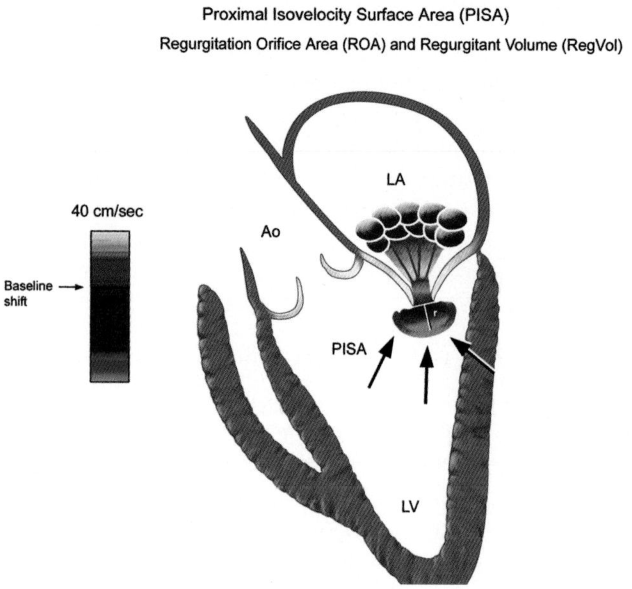

Proximal Isovelocity Surface Area (PISA)

Regurgitation Orifice Area (ROA) and Regurgitant Volume (RegVol)

A

PROXIMAL ISOVELOCITY SURFACE AREA

Regurgitant Orifice Area (ROA)
Regurgitant Volume (Reg Vol)

Flow rate = $2\pi\,r^2$ x $V_{aliasing}$

if $V_{aliasing}$ = 40 cm/sec
then Flow rate = 2(3.14) r^2 x 40 cm/sec
and Flow rate = 251.2 cc/sec

ROA = Flow rate / peak V_{MR}

if LA- LV systolic gradient = 100 mmHg
then peak V_{MR} = 5 m/sec = 500 cm/sec

∴ ROA = (r^2) 251.2 cc/sec / 500 cm/sec

or

ROA $\approx r^2/2$
Reg Vol = ROA x TVI_{MR}

B

Figure 30.65. This shorthand method for ROA is consistent with the intraoperative need for efficiency and reliability of quantitative measurement. Assuming that the systolic pressure gradient between the LV and LA is 100 mm Hg (120–20 mm Hg), via the Bernoulli equation the peak velocity is 5 m/s. (LV-LA gradient = 100 mm Hg = 4 peak V2 and therefore peak V = 5 m/s.) ROA = $(2\pi r^2 \times V_a)$/peak V_{MR} or ROA = r^2 (251/500) or $r^2/2$.

Simplified PISA Method (Fig. 30.65; Table 30.14)

This shorthand method for effective ROA is consistent with the intraoperative requirement for efficiency and simplicity of quantitative measurement in a multitasking environment. There are two simplified PISA methods (57,66).

If we assume that the systolic pressure gradient between the LV and LA is 100 mm Hg, then we understand from the Bernoulli equation that the gradient 100 mm Hg = 4 peak V^2 and therefore peak V = 5 m/s.
Method one:
Aliasing velocity set to 40 cm/s

$$(Peak)ROA = 2\pi r^2 \times V_a/V_P,$$

$$(Peak)ROA = \frac{6.28 \times 40\,cm/s\,r^2}{500\,cm/s} = \frac{251r^2}{500},$$

$$(Peak)ROA = \frac{1}{2}r^2.$$

Method two:
Aliasing velocity set to 32 cm/s. Because any ROA greater than 0.40 cm² is severe MR, if V_p is also assumed to be 500 cm/s, then the V_a must be 30 cm/s for the ROA to equal 0.4 cm²

$$V_a = \frac{0.4\,cm^2 \times 500\,cm/s}{6.28 \times r^2(1)},$$

$$V_a = \frac{200\,cm^3/s = 32\,cm/s}{6.28\,cm^2}.$$

Therefore, if the V_a is set at 30 cm/s and *r* is greater than 1 cm, the ROA is always greater than 0.4 cm².

The major advantages of the PISA method over the MJA method are that PISA is not influenced by color gain or affected by jet eccentricity.

Continuous Wave Doppler

The intensity of the spectral envelope signal is indicative of the severity of the MR. If the signal density is equivalent to the antegrade flow, the MR is significant. With more MR, the LA-LV gradient equilibrates quickly and there is a V wave cutoff (Fig. 30.62) (35,57,144).

Pulse Wave Doppler

Transmitral flow

PWD at the leaflet tips may be used as an indirect indication of the additional regurgitant flow resulting in increase flow across the MV in diastole. If the peak E wave velocity is greater than 1.2 m/s, it is consistent with severe MR (assuming no MS). PWD may also be used to calculate regurgitant fraction; however, in the cardiac operating room, it is rarely performed and only for guidance in borderline decisions. Borderline MR should not alter plans for MV surgery unless other complicating factors are present, placing the patient at extremely high risk for cannulation and CPB (35).

Pulmonary venous flow

PWD of the pulmonary vein inflow is an indirect method of assessing elevated LAP and is used to determine the presence of retrograde (reversal) of systolic pulmonary venous flow due to a severe MR jet. Systolic reversal in more than two pulmonary veins is indicative of severe MR. Placing the cursor parallel to left upper PV flow into the LA at a PW depth of at least 2 cm into the pulmonary vein results in optimal spectral tracings (57,60–62). Blunting of the systolic waves is indicative of increased LAP and not specific for MR.

Mitral Stenosis

Etiology and mechanisms of mitral stenosis

Etiology (Table 30.15A,B) MS most commonly results from long-standing rheumatic heart disease secondary to acute rheumatic fever. However, there are other potential causes of MS, including congenital, MAC (extending onto leaflets), parachute MV, obstructing masses (large atrial myxomas, thrombi), or endocarditis vegetations. Rarer causes of stenosis include valve abnormalities associated with inborn errors of metabolism, malignant carcinoid syndrome, systemic lupus, cardiac amyloid, and rheumatoid arthritis (41,42,44,46). The pathologic features of rheumatic valvular disease involving the MV include diffuse thickening, fibrosis, and calcification of the valve leaflets, commissures, and subvalvular chordae. This results in thickened rigid valves, commissural fusion, and shortened fused chordae producing a "fish-mouth"–shaped valve with both valvular and subvalvular stenosis. In addition, rheumatic nodules are deposited in the myocardium (Aschoff bodies), which may produce underlying myocarditis. The MS ultimately leads to elevated LA pressures, pulmonary artery hypertension, RV dysfunction, and TR (with or without rheumatic involvement). The chronic elevation of LA pressure may result in atrial enlargement, stagnant blood flow (detected as spontaneous contrast), and thrombus formation.

Mechanisms

Mechanisms of MS may be classified as those that are predominantly supravalvular (obstructing atrial myxoma, thrombus, or large obstructing vegetation), valvular (rheumatic, degenerative calcification), and subvalvular (rheumatic, parachute MV). Determining the mechanism of MS is essential for the purposes of MVRep. If there is significant subvalvular stenosis, repairing the valve apparatus may contribute to increased mobility, but the gradient will probably remain significantly elevated.

TABLE 30.15A	Acute and Chronic MR: Etiology and Pathology	
Etiology	**Pathologic Anatomy**	**IOE Assessment**
Rheumatic	1. Thickened fibrotic Ca²⁺ leaflets with basal commissural fusion, and retraction with "fish-mouth" deformity and reduced mobility	1. 2D imaging demonstrates decreased mobility, leaflet thickening, subvalvular chordal fusion, and stenosis
	2. Fibrotic Ca²⁺ of annulus with diminished mobility resulting in poor coaptation and MR	2. Planimetry of MV area in transgastric after TG 2 Chr CF Doppler confirms that subvalvular apparatus is not the most stenotic level; planimetry of the MV area TG SAX
	3. Subvalvular chordal fusion and obliteration of the effective interchordal orifice and subvalvular stenosis	3. Annulus is fibrotic and frequently calcified with reduced mobility
Mitral annular calcification	1. MAC²⁺ extends from posterior annulus into leaflet tips	1. 2D imaging shows Ca²⁺ in PMVL and annulus
	2. Subannular and valvular fibrosis with Ca²⁺ bars impeding LV inflow	2. Leaflet Ca²⁺ reduces mobility with incomplete coaptation
		3. Annular Ca²⁺ reduces mobility and contribution to coaptation
		4. Subannular Ca²⁺ for bars which impede LV inflow
LA thrombus	Associated with atrial fibrillation and associated with intermittent ball-valve occlusion of MV orifice	2D imaging demonstrates thrombus and spontaneous contrast with diminished LAA velocities under 0.5/s
LA myxoma	Attached to interatrial septum and, like thrombus, causes ball-valve type of abrupt obstruction of LV inflow	2D imaging demonstrates myxoma with stalk attachment to IAS

TABLE 30.15B	Etiology of MS and Pathologic Anatomy: Less Frequent Causes of MS

Etiology	Pathologic Changes Involving MV
Malignant carcinoid	Rare but may lead to thickening and immobility of valves
Systemic lupus	Inflammatory nodules (Libman-Sacks endocarditis resulting in inflammation and fusion of cusps)
Rheumatoid arthritis	Rheumatoid nodules and secondary inflammation
Hunter-Hurley	Mucopolysaccharide deposition in valve leaflets
Cortriatriatum	Membrane in LA
Amyloid deposits on rheumatoid valves	Rare presentation of amyloid, with amyloid deposition on rheumatic leaflets further decreasing mobility

Rheumatic MV disease most commonly results from long-standing rheumatic heart disease secondary to acute rheumatic fever. Rheumatic valvular disease involving the MV is characterized pathologically by diffuse thickening, fibrosis, calcification of the valve leaflets, commissures, and subvalvular apparatus, including the chordae and heads of the papillary muscle. Significant disease usually appears after a latent period of 20 to 25 years but may occur earlier with repeated exposures to rheumatic fever or active rheumatic myocarditis. The inflammatory process results in thickened and rigid valves, commissural fusion, and shortened fused chordae producing a "fish-mouth"–shaped valve with potential for valvular and subvalvular stenosis. If there is restricted leaflet motion of the leaflet edges, it may result in a classic "hockey stick" deformity of the AMVL. Chronic rheumatic inflammation produces stenosis or a combination of MS and MR. Isolated rheumatic MR is rare.

MAC is a degenerative disease associated with aging and is found in 54% of males over the age of 60 (56). It is associated with arteriosclerosis of the aorta and coronary arteries. It is usually seen at the base of the posterior PMVL and extends into the posterior LV wall. It may cause rigidity of the PMVL and calcific stenosis. The calcification and valve thickening progress from the annulus toward the edge of the leaflets. There is reduced mobility of the saddle-shaped annulus with MAC, and this may be associated with subvalvular calcific stenosis. The presence of annular calcification may require annular debridement and reconstruction for performance of either an annuloplasty or MV prosthesis, increasing the risk for pseudoaneurysms or annular disruption.

Pathophysiology

Rheumatic MS results in the development of an early diastolic gradient between the LA and LV. As the process continues, the gradient becomes elevated throughout late diastole. If there is coexisting MR, this may produce symptoms of pulmonary congestion earlier. The left atrium gradually dilates with MS, depending on the compliance changes in the atria. With enlarged LA, there is a propensity to develop atrial fibrillation, which, in the face of significant MS, may markedly reduce LV filling and overall forward cardiac output.

As the area of the MV decreases from 4.0 to 1.0 cm^2, the gradient between the LV and LA may increase to a peak gradient of 25 mm Hg with a mean greater than 10 mm Hg (56). This is manifest as a decreased E to A slope on CWD (55,56). Chronically, patients with greater than moderate MS have elevated LA pressures up to 30 mm Hg and associated pulmonary hypertension with RV dysfunction. The RV will chronically dilate, resulting in TV annular enlargement (>3.5 cm), a lack of coaptation, and significant tricuspid regurgitation and hepatic congestion (55,56).

Severity Assessment (Table 30.16)

As with MR, MS is best assessed using a weighted and integrated IOE approach of 2D assessment (splitability score and planimetry) and Doppler (CFD, PISA, MVA calculation, CW and PWD determination of MVA) using

TABLE 30.16	Echocardiographic Splitability Index Based on MV Morphology			
Grade	Mobility	Leaflet Thickening	Subvalvular	Calcification
1	Tips restricted	Normal 4–5 mm	<1/3 below leaflet	Area
2	Base to mid-normal	Mid normal	1/3 of chordae	Scattered areas on leaflet margins
3	Base normal	Throughout leaflet	2/3 of chordae	Bright to mid leaflet portion
4	No movement	Marked throughout >8–10 mm	No movement	Ca^{2+} throughout >8–10 mm

Wilkins GT, Weyman AE, Abascal VM, et al. Percutaneous balloon dilatation of the mitral valve: an analysis of echocardiographic variables related to outcome and the mechanism of dilatation. Br Heart J 1988;60:299–308.

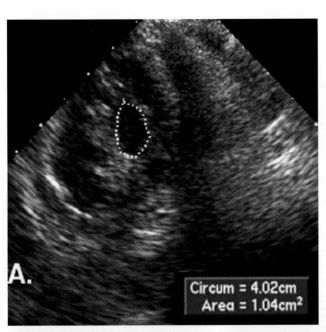

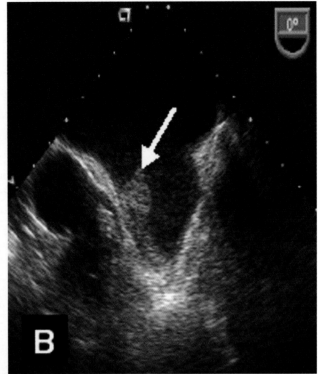

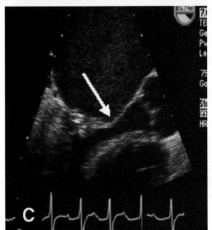

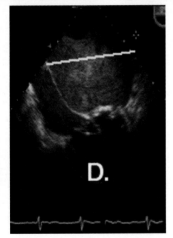

Figure 30.66. A: Rheumatic MV stenosis may be valvular or subvalvular. Using CF Doppler in the TF 2 Chr demonstrates PVC at the level of maximal stenosis. Using the TG basal SAX, the MV may be planimetered. Planimetry provides a reliable estimate of MVA if it is done at the level of the stenosis. **B–D:** Other findings in rheumatic valve disease include LAA thrombus (**B**), fusion of leaflet edges and a hockey stick deformity (**C**), and LA enlargement, which must be estimated using TEE (**D**).

the continuity equation and mean gradient, pressure half-time, and DT.

IOE Two-Dimensional Assessment of Severity of MS (Table 30.16)

Examination of the MVAp permits an identification of the underlying etiology. With more advanced rheumatic MS, features are pathognomonic. Unlike MS resulting from MAC, which extends from the base of the leaflets, rheumatic MS progresses from the leaflet tips toward the leaflet base. The TG basal SAX view aligned parallel to the annulus may demonstrate commissural fusion and restricted valve motion. However, the TG 2 Chr MV image plane with color determines the level of the most significant stenosis. From the TG basal SAX, at the level of the most significant narrowing, a digital image loop is captured and advanced to the frame demonstrating maximal opening. Planimetering the MVA electronically provides a reliable estimation of the true valve area (Fig. 30.66). Planimetry may underestimate the severity due to echogenic shielding from the presence of Ca^{2+} in the valve annulus and the subvalvular degree of flow obstruction.

In 1988, Wilkins et al. evaluated patients over a 6-month period, who had balloon valvuloplasty for rheumatic MS. As discussed previously, they developed an echo score correlating with a propensity to restenose (68). This score was subsequently applied to 100 consecutive patients who underwent a similar procedure—valvotomy—and discovered that only one patient with a score greater than 8 restenosed (Table 30.17). To validate the ability to utilize TEE imaging to reliably determine a patient's splitability score, Marwick et al. compared the TTE and TEE of 45 patients undergoing balloon valvuloplasty over 2 years. TEE was useful in MS, but there were significant differences between

TABLE 30.17	MV Stenosis Severity Assessment			
Left atrial size	LAE > 45 mm AP diameter			
	Exclude LAA thrombi			
PA pressure	$PASP = 4(V_{TR})^2 + CVP^a$			
	$PAM = (-0.45)AT + 79$			
Planimeter valve area	Difficult with heavy Ca^{2+}, previous commissurotomy			
Mean gradient	Integrated area of $MV_{diastolic}$ spectral envelope			
	With atrial fibrillation, average five consecutive diastoles gradient α flow across MV and MVA, therefore severe MR produces larger than expected gradient			
Continuity equation	$MVA = (D_{LVOT}^2 \times 0.785)(TVI_{LVOT})/TVI_{MV}$			
	No AR, LVOT obstruction, or MR			
Deceleration time	$MVA = 759/DT$			
	$PT_{1/2} = 0.29 \times DT$			
	Altered by diastolic dysfunction			
Pressure half time	$MVA = 220/PT_{1/2}$			
	Inaccurate with abnormal compliance (LA, LV), significant AR, or post valvuloplasty (AR reduces $PT_{1/2}$ and overestimates valve area)			
PISA (proximal isovelocity surface area)	$MVA = 2\pi R^2 \times V_{aliasing}/peak\ V_{MS} \times \alpha°/180°$			
	$V_{aliasing}$ = aliasing velocity of color Doppler			
	R = radius from orifice to PISA interface			
	Peak V_{MS} = peak CW diastolic Doppler velocity			
	Normal = 4–6 cm²	**Mild**	**Moderate**	**Severe**
	Planimetered area	1.5–2.0 cm²	1.0–1.5 cm²	≤0.9 cm²
	Mean gradient$_{diastolic}$	<6 mm Hg^a	6–12 mm Hg^a	>12 mm Hg^a
	Deceleration time	<517 m/s	517–690 m/s	>759 m/s
	Pressure half-time	<150 m/s	150–200 m/s	>220 m/s

Note: Symptoms = Gradient = MVA, if not, must explain (rest vs. exercise, other etiology).
^{a}Measured or estimated.

the TTE and TEE scores, with the TTE score 7.2 compared to TEE 5.9 ($p < 0.001$). The difference was thought to be subvalvular shielding by thickened and dense MV leaflets and a shielded transducer position on the LA side during esophageal imaging (145).

Doppler Methods of Severity Assessment

A semiquantitative method of estimating MVA is to measure the pressure gradient, using CWD interrogation across the MV inflow. A mean pressure gradient (from tracing the CW envelope) greater than 12 mm Hg signifies severe MS and less than 5 mm Hg gradient indicates less than moderate MS. Gradient is flow related, but if properly aligned, it has less probability of inducible human error (55,56). Quantitative methods of MS assessment are pressure half-time ($PT_{1/2}$), DT, continuity equation, or

PISA. The CW spectral envelope demonstrates increased flow velocity across the valve, which corresponds to the increased valve gradient demonstrating a flattened slope of a slower reduction in LA and LV gradient. $PT_{1/2}$ is the time it takes for the initial peak instantaneous pressure gradient ($4 \times$ peak V^2) to drop by 50% (Fig. 30.67). Using standard analysis programs available on most platforms, these calculations are automatically calculated based on relative diastolic properties of the LA and LV by dividing the constant 220 by the $PT_{1/2}$. Whenever $PT_{1/2}$ is ≥220 ms, there is severe MS with an estimated MVA less than 1.0 cm². There are circumstances that lead to miscalculation, including the fact that aortic regurgitation reduces $PT_{1/2}$ (more rapid equilibration of LA-LV gradient), which leads to overestimation of MVA. Aging, which reduces the compliance of the LV with the LA-LV gradient

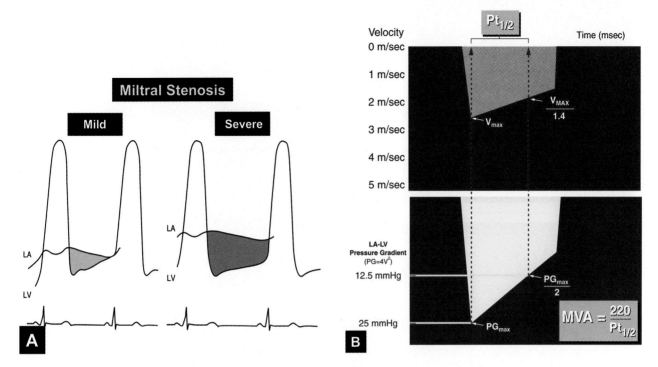

Figure 30.67A,B. The peak instantaneous gradient (using the simplified Bernoulli equation), where V is the initial peak instantaneous velocity. Determining the time it requires for the gradient to drop by 50%. The MVA is calculated by dividing 220 by $PT_{1/2}$. The constant 220 is based on the relative diastolic properties of the LA and LV. Since severe MS is classified as a MVA less than 1.0 cm², whenever $PT_{1/2}$ is greater than 220 ms, there is severe MS. There are circumstances that may lead to miscalculation including (a) the presence of AR leading to a reduced $PT_{1/2}$ and overestimation of MVA due to more rapid equilibration of LA and LV pressure gradient and (b) aging reduces the compliance of the LV, and the LA-LV gradient LV diastolic pressure rises faster than in normal complaint ventricles, hence a shorter $PT_{1/2}$ with and overestimation of MVA (55,56).

causing a shorter and faster $PT_{1/2}$ and overestimation of MVA (55,56).

The DT, or time it takes the peak velocity to reach 0 m/s along the interpolated slope, may be used to calculate the MVA. The relation is characterized by the formula MVA = 759/DT. $PT_{1/2}$ may be calculated from the DT ($PT_{1/2}$ = 0.29 × DT). Therefore, a DT greater than 760 is also suggestive of severe stenosis (55,56,71).

Another alternative for calculation of the MVA is utilizing the continuity equation based upon the principle that flow across one valve must equal flow across another (in the absence of regurgitation of either valve).

MV flow = LVOT flow and (MV_A × TVI_{MV} = $area_{LVOT}$ × TVI_{LVOT}).

Therefore:

$$MV_A = (area_{LVOT}) \times (TVI_{LVOT})/TVI_{MV}.$$

This technique involves obtaining the LVOT diameter at the aortic valve annulus in the ME LAX imaging plane, the PW Doppler VTI $_{LVOT}$, and the

CWD VTI across the MV. PISA can also be used to calculate MVA (Fig. 30.68A–F). Using the ME 4 Chr, CF Doppler interrogation of the MV is performed with a baseline shift to reduce the aliasing velocity away from the transducer. A digital loop is captured and the image is frozen in diastole to optimize the radius measurement of the first PISA interface zone. The atrial MV angle is then determined (Fig. 30.69). Rodriguez et al. validated a method for determining MV area, using the PFC method of calculating flow rate (hemispherical area × aliasing velocity) (146). With the convergence funnel not being hemispherical, an adjustment was made for the typical funnel angle by the formula:

MV flow rate = hemispherical area × velocity aliasing × (angle/180°),

$$\text{MV flow rate} = 2\pi r^2 (V_{aliasing}) \times (angle/180°),$$

MVA = hemishperical flow rate/peak(CW Doppler)V_{MS}.

Flow convergence method or PISA method (Fig. 30.74).

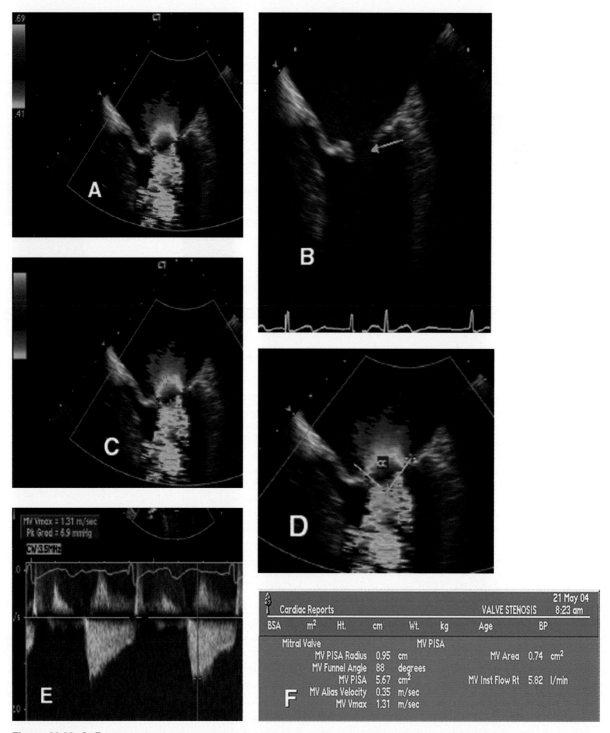

Figure 30.68. A–F: PISA PFC is also used to calculate MVA. Using the ME 4 Chr view, CF Doppler interrogation of the MV steno tic jet is performed with the zero baseline shifted upward to reduce the aliasing velocity away from the transducer. A digital loop is captured as the image is frozen in diastole to optimize the radius measurement of the first PISA interface zone. The atrial MV angle is then determined. Rodriguez et al. validated a method for determining MV area using the PVC velocity. Since the convergence funnel is not spherical, an adjustment is made for the funnel angle using the following:

$$\text{MV flow rate} = \text{spherical area} \times \text{velocity aliasing}(\text{angle}/180°)\text{MV flow rate}$$
$$= \text{spherical area} \times \text{velocity aliasing} \times (\text{angle}/180°),$$

$$\text{MV flow rate} = 2\pi r^2 (V_{\text{aliasing}}) \times (\text{angle}/180°)\text{MVA}$$
$$= \text{flow rate}/\text{peak}(\text{CW Doppler})\text{VMS}.$$

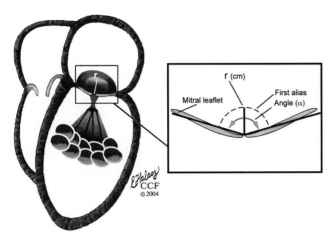

Figure 30.69. Rodriguez et al. validated a method for determining MV area using the PFC method of calculating flow rate (MV flow rate = spherical area × V_a). When the convergence funnel is not spherical, an adjustment was made based on the funnel angle by the formula:

$$\text{MV flow rate} = \text{spherical area} \times V_a(\text{angle } \alpha/180°)$$
$$= 2\pi r^2 V_a(\text{angle } \alpha/180°),$$

$$\text{MVA} = \text{flow rate/peak(CW Doppler)}.$$

IOE Findings Associated with MV Dysfunction

Secondary pathophysiology in mitral valve disease

In acute MR, blunting of the S wave is usually present in all pulmonary veins with a LAP greater than 15 mm Hg. Whereas in chronic MR, the left atrium may dilate to 70 mm (55,56). These patients may develop stagnant blood flow in the left atrial appendage, especially in patients with atrial fibrillation. Because of the regurgitant jet, left atrial appendage thrombi are extremely rare except in instances of atrial fibrillation with combined rheumatic MS-MR, or low flow states due to severe ventricular dysfunction. With chronic MS, associated stagnant left atrial blood flow secondary has an increased risk for the development of thrombi in the left atrium and appendage. Predictors include the presence of atrial fibrillation, left atrial enlargement, spontaneous contrast, and PW Doppler peak LAA velocities under 0.5 m/s (68). The presence of any of these risks is used as an indication for closure of the left atrial appendage. 2D imaging may demonstrate spontaneous contrast in the LA, and the PW Doppler of the LAA may demonstrate low velocity flows under 0.5 m/s, indicating that the patient is at an increased risk for developing LAA thrombi (73).

Up to 50% of patients undergoing MV surgery will have history of atrial fibrillation. Patients with transient paroxysmal atrial fibrillation often will have their inciting reentry focus at the junction of the pulmonary veins with the left atrium. In these patients, pulmonary vein isolation techniques achieve encouraging results when the LA is markedly enlarged. In patients who present to the OR in atrial fibrillation greater than 1 year duration, MV surgery is unlikely to remodel the LA enough to convert the patient back to normal sinus rhythm. The IOE exam in patients who have enlarged left atrium should document the LA dimensions in the two-chamber imaging plane and ME LAX imaging planes. The finding of an enlarged left atrium (>50 mm) indicates the potential for sustainable chronic atrial fibrillation (55,56). Patients who have undergone pulmonary vein isolation using percutaneous catheter ablation have demonstrated up to 23%–39% pulmonary vein stenosis within 3 days of their procedure. While this is not commonly reported with pulmonary vein isolation, documentation of pulmonary vein PW Doppler flows for future reference may prove useful.

Persisting elevations of left atrial pressure may eventually result in proliferation of the intramural musculature of the pulmonary resistance vessels. Estimations of the PA systolic, mean, and diastolic pressures are possible using CWD (Table 30.18) (33,56).

RV function is afterload dependent, and the presence of persistently increased RV afterload leads to RV failure with tricuspid annulus dilatation, with resulting tricuspid regurgitation and passive congestion of the liver. RV failure causes dilation, ischemia, and decreased RV contractility. The 2D IOE exam may demonstrate a septum that is flattened (D-shaped LV) and shifted toward the LV in systole with RV pressure overload, whereas, with RV volume overload associated with chronic TR, the septum is shifted in both systole and diastole.

Chronically, patients with significant MS or MR have elevated LA pressures (up to 30 mm Hg). These pressures are associated with pulmonary systolic pressures of 60 or greater. Eighty-nine percent of patients undergoing tricuspid valve repair do so as a result of secondary pathophysiologic changes associated with primary MV disease and surgery (56). Up to 67% of patients undergoing MV surgery for rheumatic MS and/or MR are discovered to have moderate or severe tricuspid regurgitation (73). In the presence of pulmonary hypertension with RV dilatation, the TV annulus dilates predominately at the bases of the anterior and posterior leaflets due to the basal septal leaflet incorporation into the central fibrous skeleton of the heart. Consequently, the regurgitant is frequently diffuse and directed septally and centrally. Klein et al. determined that tricuspid valve repair in MV surgery was associated with the most favorable outcome when both the mitral and tricuspid have greater than moderate TR (73). Other findings of severe TR are indicated by a TR jet area greater than 30% of the RA area or ≥6 cm, dense CW spectral envelope of the TR jet, hepatic plethora, VC greater than 0.7 cm, PISA greater than 0.6 to 0.9 cm with Nyquist at 28 cm/s, MJA greater than 7 to 10 cm², and hepatic vein systolic reversal (Table 30.19) (73). Duran et al. have also reported that tricuspid regurgitation, that is moderate or severe should be repaired (137,147).

With elevated RAP, the fossa ovalis may become distended, revealing a patent foramen ovale. In the presence of severe pulmonary hypertension, a right-to-left shunt may occur leading to hypoxemia.

Patients with chronically elevated RA pressures or significant TR may develop chronic congestion of the liver. Hepatic plethora is diagnosed by having a lack of

TABLE 30.18 Secondary Pathophysiology in MV Disease: Estimation of Hemodynamic Pressures

Pressure Estimated	Required Measurement	Formula	Normal Values (mm Hg)
Estimated CVP	Respiratory IVC collapse	$\geq$40% = 5 mm Hg	5–10 mm Hg
		<40%, (NI RV) = 10 mm Hg	
		0% and RV Dysfx = 15 mm Hg	
RV systolic (RVSP)	Peak velocity^{TR}	RVSP = $4(V_{TR})^2$ + CVP (no PS)	16–30 mm Hg
	CVP or measured		
RV systolic (with VSD)	Systemic systolic BP	RVSP = SBP − $4(V_{LV-RV})^2$ (no LVOT obstruction)	With VSD usually >50
	Peak V_{LV-RV}		
PA systolic (PASP)	Peak velocity^{TR}	PASP = $4(V_{TR})^2$ + CVP (no PS; use estimated or measured CVP)	16–30 mm Hg
	CVP estimated or measured		
PA diastolic (PAD)	End diastolic Velocity$_{PR}$	PAEDP = $4(V_{PR\,ED})^2$ + CVP	0–8 mm Hg
	CVP estimated or measured		
PA mean (PAM)	Acceleration time (AT) to peak V_{PA}	PAM = (−0.45)AT + 79	10–16 mm Hg
RV dP/dt	TR spectral envelope	RV dP = $4V_{TR(2\,m/s)}^2 - 4V_{TR(2\,m/s)}^2$	>150 mm Hg/ms
	$T_{TR(2\,m/s)} - T_{TR(1\,m/s)}$	RV dP/dt = $dP/T_{TR(2\,m/s)} - T_{TR(1\,m/s)}$	
LA systolic (LASP)	Peak V_{MR}	LASP = SBP − $4(V_{MR})^2$	100–140 mm Hg
	Systolic BP (SBP)	No LVOT gradient	
LA (PFO)	Velocity$_{PFO}$	LAP = $4(V_{PFO})^2$ + CVP	3–15 mm Hg
	CVP estimated or measured		
LV diastolic (LVEDP)	End diastolic Velocity$_{AR}$	LVEDP = DBP − $4(V_{AR})^2$	3–12 mm Hg
	Diastolic BP (DBP)		
LV dP/dt	MR spectral envelope	LV dP = $4V^2_{MR(2\,m/s)} - 4V^2_{TR(2\,m/s)}$	>800 mm Hg/ms
	$T_{MR(2\,m/s)} - T_{MR(1\,m/s)}$	LV dP/dt = $dP/T_{MR(2\,m/s)} - T_{MR(1\,m/s)}$	

respiratory change in the diameter of the hepatic veins by M-mode echocardiography. PW Doppler may indicate severe TR by demonstrating systolic flow reversal or a systolic directional change as demonstrated by CFD.

Associated Valvular or Coexisting Cardiac Pathology

Cleft MV leaflet abnormalities are commonly associated with specific congenital abnormalities: Endocardial cushion defects. Ostium primum atrial septal defect (ASD) have been reported to be associated with cleft MV leaflets in 87% of cases (Fig. 30.70) and secundum ASD in 13%.

In patients presenting with rheumatic MV disease, 47% have some combination of rheumatic disease in other valves. Based on autopsy studies, the most frequent is aortic valve disease (32%), followed by mitral-aortic-tricuspid combination (9%), and mitral-tricuspid (4%) (131). Consequently, the aortic and tricuspid valves should be carefully interrogated for evidence of leaflet thickening and restricted aortic valve opening with commissural fusion when patients present for rheumatic MV surgery. If the degree of aortic stenosis is greater than mild to moderate, consideration is often given for replacement at the time of MV surgery because of the potential for progression to moderate or severe stenosis over a 15-year period (148). Patients with recurrent episodes of rheumatic fever may develop an active rheumatic myocarditis, leading to LV dysfunction and eccentric dilatation, as demonstrated by 2D IOE.

Myxomatous MV disease is the etiology of MR in over 50% of cases (30). Similarly, myxomatous prolapse of the aortic valve is the most frequent cause of aortic regurgitation. While primary myxomatous degeneration of either of these valves is not associated with the other, prolapse of the mitral and aortic valves is seen in combination in patients with connective tissue disorders, such

TABLE 30.19	Intraoperative Assessment of TR Severity

Parameter 2D Imaging	Utility/ Advantages	Limitations	Mild	Moderate	Severe
RA/RV/IVC size					
RA diameter <4.6.cm	RAE and RVE indicate chronic TR	RAE not specific	Normal	Normal or dilated	Usually dilated
RV diameter <4.3.cm	Normal RA and RV exclude signs of chronic TR	RA normal in severe acute TR			
Tricuspid valve	Flail and poor coaptation with significant TR	Other findings not specific for significant TR	Normal	Normal or abnormal	Flail and poor coaptation
Doppler					
CF Doppler	Efficient screen for TR	Note: tech factors and load conditions	<5	5–10	>10
Max jet area (MJA) cm²		Underestimates eccentric jets			
Nyquist limit 50–60 cm/not valid eccentric jets					
PW Doppler	Simple	Blunting multiple causes	Systolic dominance	Systolic blunting	Systolic reversal
Hepatic vein flow					
CW Doppler	Simple	Qualitative	Soft	Dense	Dense
Jet density—contour	Readily available	Complementary data	Parabolic	Variable contour	Triangular with early peaking
Quantitative					
CF Doppler	Efficient	Intermediates direct need of other parameters confirmation	Not defined	<0.7	>0.7
Vena contracta diameter (VCD) (cm)	Quantitative				
	distinguishes mild from severe TR				
PISA radius (cm)	Quantitative	Validated in only a few studies	<0.5	0.6–0.9	>0.9
Baseline shift with Nyquist 28 cm/s					

In the assessment of patients undergoing MV surgery, the purpose of assessing the severity of tricuspid regurgitation is to determine the necessity of performing a TV repair. If the preoperative assessment of TR suggested the need for replacement, finding less TR should not be the determining factor in deciding not to proceed with TV repair.

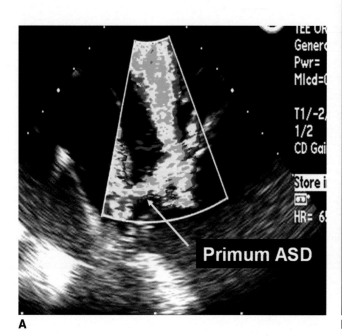

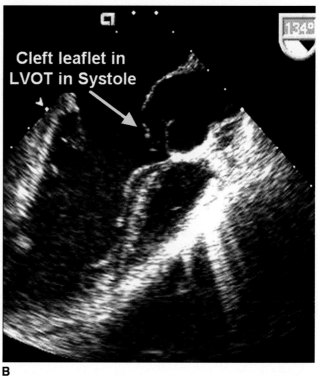

A   **B**

Figure 30.70. Cleft MV leaflet abnormalities are commonly associated with specific congenital abnormalities. Endocardial cushion defects (ostium primum ASD) have been reported to be associated with cleft MV leaflets in 87% of cases and secundum ASD in 13%.

as Ehlers Danlos, Marfans, and osteogenesis imperfecta. In these patients, if the severity of the AR is greater than moderate, consideration is given to repair of the aortic valve unless there is architectural dilatation or distortion of the aortic root. Myxomatous tricuspid prolapse with TR has been reported in more than half of patients with MV prolapse. Because of the ability to reliably repair significant TR, TV repair is frequently performed in these patients.

Calcific mitral and aortic valve disease is closely associated with aging. Calcific aortic stenosis is a frequent etiology of significant aortic stenosis in the elderly. Aronow et al. determined that calcific aortic stenosis may be present in 15% to 20% of elderly individuals over the age of 65 (25). In comparison, significant MR in the elderly is present in over 30% of the same population with MAC. In patients greater than 75 years old, more than one quarter of patients with calcific aortic stenosis may have coexisting MAC with varying degrees of stenosis. While there is no close association between MAC, both are encountered in the same population.

Aortic Stenosis or Regurgitation in Patient for MV Surgery

Coexistence of significant MR in the presence of AS or AR more frequently occurs in patients presenting for aortic valve surgery (see discussion below regarding moderate MR in patients with aortic valve stenosis). However, when significant AS or AR is found in the patient presenting for MVRep, it may be with an incorrect assumption that the

MR is secondary to coexisting ischemic heart disease. If there is greater than moderate aortic stenosis and dilatation of the LV, the replacement of the aortic valve is often considered in addition to MVRep. If, however, there is hypertrophy of the ventricle associated with the aortic valve disease, aortic valve replacement alone may correct the MR. If there is significant AR with ventricular dilatation, consideration is given to surgically correcting the aortic valve in addition to the MVRep. With the dilatation, it is probable that the MR is secondary to apical tethering of the MV leaflets with an associated central jet of MR.

Endocarditis of the Mitral and Aortic Valves

As previously discussed with MV endocarditis, it is unusual to have primary MV endocarditis without underlying MV disease or aortic valve endocarditis. Endocarditis involving multiple valves has been reported in more than 15% of cases, usually involving the aortic valve and MV (131).

MITRAL VALVE PROCEDURES

Introduction

When surgical intervention is indicated for the optimal long-term management of a patient's MV dysfunction, valve repair is always the procedure of choice (36,76,91,149,150). This is founded upon scientific evidence that, in comparison to MVR, MVRep offers lower operative mortality; improved long-term ventricular function; and greater freedom from thromboembolism, anticoagulant complications, endocarditis, and reoperation (76,91,149,150). While the repair of the MVAp is influenced by the underlying valve pathology and mechanism(s) of dysfunction, the precise application of repair techniques and the intraoperative assessment of the result of the surgical repair are guided by intraoperative echo. For patients undergoing MV surgery, there are issues related to the specific surgical intervention, which are addressed by the intraoperative examination. Those related to MVRep and MVR have been previously discussed.

Mitral Valve Repair Historical Perspective

Though MVRep was first suggested in 1902 by Sir Thomas Brunton for patients with rheumatic MS (151), it was not until the early 1920s when Allen, Cutler, and Souttar, working independently, first developed such techniques. Due to the nonexistence of antimicrobials and methods for dealing with blood loss, further progress was limited (151,152). The surgical treatment of MR was limited to a diversion of the regurgitant jet until the idea of circumferentially reshaping the mitral annulus was advanced by Glover and Davila in 1938. However, it was not until the Gibbons introduction of the heart-lung machine in 1953 that Lillehei first attempted the correction of pure MR by reconstruction of the annulus in 1957 (153). Further clinical development of this radical concept, however, was postponed by the enthusiasm surrounding the introduction of the mechanical valve by Starr and Edwards in 1961. It was not until 1971 that Carpentier et al. presented their revolutionary new concept of a physiologic classification of mechanisms of MR and resulting clinical success (126). Duran advanced the development of repair techniques for the patients with combined stenotic and regurgitant rheumatic MV disease (154). These developments revolutionized the world of cardiac surgery and the era of modern valve repair began. Surgeons in the United States envisioned potential benefits for older patient populations with degenerative and ischemic regurgitation (154). Over the ensuing 20 years, a number of contributions have been made by various surgeons and cardiac centers and have established MVRep as the procedure of choice for the management of all etiologies of MR.

MV Repair Compared to MV Replacement (Outcomes)

In 1987, Sand et al. first reported their remarkable results comparing MVRep with MVR (155). When they examined the outcome of 490 patients undergoing MVRep (101) and MVR (389) for MR, the 5-year survival was superior for MVRep (76% vs. 56%, $p = 0.005$) and superior for protection from endocarditis (0/101 vs. 11/389, $p = 0.08$). Because of this, a radical shift has occurred in

the management of patients with MV dysfunction caused by all etiologies (76).

MV Repair for Rheumatic Disease

The number of patients presenting for cardiac surgery with pure rheumatic MS has declined due to a decreased incidence of the disease and the number of patients receiving balloon valvuloplasty for its treatment (150,156). Rheumatic MV disease may produce a range of anatomic presentations, including MV prolapse associated with acute rheumatic valvulitis (rarely seen in United States) to the more chronic presentations of mixed MR and stenosis caused by the subvalvular thickening and fusion of the chordae, commissural fusion, and a fixed "fishmouth" deformity with the Type IIIa systolic and diastolic restriction. Current indications for surgical intervention in patients with MS and/or MR include onset of congestive symptoms and new onset atrial fibrillation. If patients have atrial fibrillation, they are frequently referred for surgery irrespective of their echocardiographic splitability score. Patients with rheumatic MV disease usually present with restricted leaflet motion, causing either pure MS or a combination of both. Patients with pure MS with high splitability scores (>8) or those with atrial fibrillation or those with mixed MS and MR are referred for surgery. David et al. demonstrated that even if patients have higher splitability scores (>8), repair may be possible if their anterior leaflets are pliable with a subvalvular structure that is not fused (138). In 2001, Carpenter et al. published their 20-year results of MVRep in degenerative MR (31). Between 1970 and 1994, they performed 951 reconstructive procedures (7% type I, 33% type II prolapse, 36% type III, and 24% combined type II AMVL and type III PMVL). Overall, they demonstrated a 10- and 20-year freedom of death (89% and 82%), freedom from reoperation (82% and 55%), and freedom from cardiac morbidity. Freedom from reoperation at 20 years was highest in type IIa/IIIp (65%), followed by type II (63%), and type III (46%). The main cause of reoperation was progression of MV fibrosis (31).

MV Repair for Endocarditis

Endocarditis involving the left-sided valve structures usually involves the aortic valve. If endocarditis involves the MV, it implies coexistence of degenerative or rheumatic valve disease or it is secondary to a jet lesion from a posteriorly directed regurgitant jet associated with aortic valve endocarditis. In MV endocarditis, the associated mechanism of regurgitation may be multiple mechanisms and includes the underlying valve abnormality, such as combined rheumatic MS-MR valve dysfunction or previously existing myxomatous degeneration of the MV. Endocarditis involving the MV produces a range of MVAp pathology, including isolated leaflet perforations (Type I) or secondary windsock defect from AR jet, vegetations attached to leaflets, ruptured chordae, and abscess cavities with erosion into the central intervalvular fibrosa (131). Repair of the MV in endocarditis involves patching of perforations, wide debridement and pericardial exclusion, and more aggressive reconstructive surgery where there is combined involvement of the aortic valve and intervalvular fibrosa. Muehrke et al. have reported an 80% success rate in repair of infected MVs (132).

MV Repair for Ischemic Heart Disease

Ischemic MR is classified as either transient or chronic. The chronic form involves an infarction and may result in a ruptured papillary muscle (type II), elongation of the papillary muscle head with leaflet prolapse (type II), or functional regurgitation associated with ventricular remodeling and apical tethering (type IIIb with or without type I annular dilatation) or a posterior and/or lateral infarct impacting the mitral apparatus in that region (IIIb). While all three are approachable by reconstructive technique, the decision to proceed with repair or replacement is patient dependent. Papillary muscle infarction, which results in chordal elongation, causes a focal prolapse of a segment of the AMVL or PMVL scallop. Often these patients are referred for surgical management of coexisting myxomatous and coronary disease. Recently, Reece et al. compared 110 CABG patients, with type IIIb with or without type I annular dilatation, which either had MVRep (54 undersized annuloplasty ring with or without a posterior patch) or MVR (subvalvular sparring technique) (141). Comparing the MVRep with the MVR group, they demonstrated a superior in-hospital mortality (1.9% vs. 10.7%), shorter length of stay (9.7 vs. 13.1 days), lower infection rate (9% vs. 13%), shorter CPB times (112 vs. 132 minutes), and shorter cross-clamp times (152 vs. 171 minutes) (137). They concluded that MVRep was superior to MVR with regard to perioperative mortality and morbidity. In 2001, Gillinov et al. reported on 482 patients with ischemic MR who underwent either MVRep or replacement and were propensity matched into a better-risk and poor-risk group (36). They found that MVRep compared to MVR in the better-risk group demonstrated superior survivals at 30 days, 1 year, and 5 years (94% vs. 81%, 82% vs. 56%, 58% vs. 36%; $p =0.08$) (36). There was no significant difference in the poor-risk group. Ischemic MR patients with papillary muscle rupture have a better long-term survival compared with those patients with chronic failure and apical tethering (36).

MV Repair for Myxomatous MV Disease

Myxomatous degeneration is the most common indication for MVRep, with 90% of such valves being repairable. In the general population, 4% to 5% of individuals may have MV prolapse potentially leading to surgical intervention in up to 5% (157). The surgical approaches that have been developed are directed at the underlying pathology of redundant myxomatous leaflets, thinned and elongated chordae—which are prone to rupture—and annular dilatation. Patients with significant MR secondary to structural abnormalities of the apparatus eventually require surgical intervention. If untreated, the

natural history indicates that patients will develop progressive heart failure and many will develop atrial fibrillation. Valve repair for myxomatous disease is accomplished in the majority of patients, using five surgical techniques, including a central or modified quadrilateral resection of the PMVL, chordal transfer, annuloplasty, commissural closure, and a sliding annuloplasty. Other surgical techniques include addition of gortex chords, chordal shortening, anterior leaf resection (Pomeroy procedure), and anterior leaflet plication.

Gillinov et al. reported on the long-term durability of MVRep at the Cleveland Clinic in 1,072 patients who underwent primary isolated MVRep for valvular regurgitation caused by degenerative disease between 1985 and 1997. In this study 1-, 5-, and 10-year freedom from reoperation were reported as 98.7%, 96.9%, and 92.9%, respectively. Freedom from reoperation was highest in those patients with PMVL prolapse or flail (98%, type II) and those who received an intraoperative assessment by transesophageal or epicardial echocardiography and annuloplasty with leaflet resection (76). Using multivariant analysis, they found that the risks of reoperation were decreased by use of IOE and use of an annuloplasty ring and were increased by use of chordal shortening and non-PMVL pathology. Of the 30 patients with late MV dysfunction, the repair failed in 16 (53%) as a result of progressive degenerative disease. Death before reoperation was increased in patients having isolated anterior leaflet prolapse, annular calcification, and by use of chordal shortening or annuloplasty alone.

Carpentier and Deloche reported their long-term, 20-year results in the first 162 consecutive patients who underwent nonrheumatic MVRep for degenerative MV regurgitation between 1970 and 1984 (31). The Carpentier mechanism was type II in 152 (PMVL 93, AMVL 28, bileaflet in 31). There were three postoperative deaths and three reoperations in the first month. The remaining patients with MVRep were followed for a median of 17 years. The survival was 48% for 20 years, which is similar to a normal population. The cardiac death and cardiac morbidity were 19% and 26%, respectively. For patients with PMVL involvement, the 10- and 20-year freedom from reoperation were 98.5% and 93%, whereas AMVL was 86.2% and bileaflet involvement was 88.1% and 82.6% (31).

Clinical Guidelines for MV Repair

In 1996, Ling et al. reported a study that evaluated the optimal timing of surgical intervention for 221 patients with severe MR caused by a myxomatous Carpentier type II flail or prolapse mechanism (28). These patients were separated into two groups that were designated as Group 1 (early surgery <1 month) and Group 2 (those patients who had surgery after 1 month or not at all). Both groups had similar comorbidities and no significant incidence of coronary disease by angiography in small subsets of either group. It was found that those patients who had earlier surgery (within 1 month of being diagnosed with clinically significant MR) had improved survival at 5 and

10 years ($p = 0.28$). In addition, the early surgery patients demonstrated decreased operative mortality ($p = 0.17$), a decreased likelihood of progressive congestive heart failure, and better long-term survival with diminished cardiovascular mortality ($p = 0.002$). The authors concluded by suggesting a strategy of earlier surgery in acceptable candidates, with severe MR, with a high probability of successful MVRep (28).

Because of this and similar studies, in 1998, the ACC and AHA Task Force on Guidelines in Valvular Heart Disease recommended the following as indications for MVRep surgery in patients with MR:

1. ≥ Functional Class II symptoms and severe MR
2. Asymptomatic patients with severe MR and LV dysfunction (LVESD > 45 mm) and MS
3. Functional Class III with MVA less than 1.5 cm²
4. With an echocardiography score less than 8, balloon valvuloplasty optional (33)

Moderate MR in Patients for Aortic Valve Surgery

When patients are discovered to have coexisting functional MR in the presence of significant aortic valve dysfunction, it is usually in the setting of primary aortic valve surgery. Christenson et al. evaluated 60 consecutive patients with aortic stenosis and MR to determine the effect of aortic valve replacement on the severity of MR. They found that unless there was irreversible eccentric remodeling, the repair or correction of the aortic valve dysfunction resulted in an improvement of the severity of MR (158). Conversely, if there is moderate MR and spherical remodeling, they found that it was unlikely that the MR would be diminished. Gillinov et al. reported a study evaluating 813 patients undergoing AVR in addition to either MVRep (295) or MVR (518) from 1975 to 1998. MVR was more common in patients with severe MS ($p = 0.0009$), atrial fibrillation ($p = 0.0006$), and in patients receiving a mechanical aortic prosthesis ($p = 0.0002$). Hospital mortality rate for MVR was 5.4% ($p = 0.4$). Survivals at 5, 10, and 15 years were 79%, 63%, and 46%, after MVRep, compared to 72%, 52%, and 34%, after replacement ($p = 0.01$). Late survival was increased by MVRep rather than replacement ($p = 0.03$) in all subsets of patients, including those with severe MS. In many patients with double valve disease, aortic valve replacement and MVRep may improve late survival rates and are the preferred strategy when MVRep is possible (159).

Mitral Valve Replacement

In MVR, the post-CPB echocardiographic evaluation focuses on the integrity of the valve, presence of perivalvular regurgitation, underlying LV function, and potential for valve strut interference with LVOT blood flow. Because of the left-sided systolic pressures, small spaces between the valvular sewing ring and mitral annulus may result in small, but high velocity, perivalvular regurgitation. Such high velocity has a propensity to cause hemolysis and requires further evaluation or repair of the sewing ring leak. It is imperative

that regurgitant jets associated with valve replacement be localized as either originating from within the sewing ring or as perivalvular. Localization and quantification of the regurgitant jet associated with prosthetic valves are one of the most difficult challenges in IOE due to the artifacts associated with an echo-dense valve ring or mechanical leaflets. Use of multiple imaging views and/or epicardial imaging is often necessary to achieve a confident conclusion. Helpful clues in this dilemma include the almost universal presence of small regurgitant jets with bioprosthetic valves and the characteristic regurgitant patterns of the various mechanical valves. In addition, the application of gentle manual pressure posteriorly on the sewing ring may obliterate some perivalvular leaks, confirming the diagnosis. In patients receiving a bileaflet (St. Jude, Carbomedics) or a tilting disc, it is important to visualize an appropriate range of motion of the individual leaflets or disc.

Nonchordal sparring MVR is associated with reduced ventricular function due to disruption of the mitral tensor apparatus. This is especially prevalent in those circumstances when the surgeon was not able to maintain the continuity of the mitral tensor apparatus. In addition, the propensity for disruption of the posterior LV or annulus is increased in such circumstances. Such disruption is preceded by identifiable intramyocardial areas of turbulence permitting the echocardiographer to alert the surgeon prior to a catastrophic myocardial rupture.

With the implantation of higher profile valves in the mitral position, the valve struts may protrude into the LVOT if not appropriately aligned. While some prosthetic valve models permit an in situ rotation of the valve, significant obstruction to LVOT flow may require reimplantation of the prosthetic valve.

Mitral Valve Homograft

Acar et al. reported on the use of MV homografts for patients who had MV dysfunction that was too extensive for successful repair (160). Forty-three patients underwent MVR with a cryopreserved mitral homograft in patients with acute endocarditis (14), rheumatic stenosis (26), systemic lupus endocarditis (2), and marasmic endocarditis (1). Partial homograft was performed in 21 and total in 22. Follow-up at 14 months demonstrated one reoperation for restenosis and one death (pulmonary neoplasm). Thirty-three patients were in sinus rhythm, no to minimal MR in 33, and mild MR in five with an average MVA of 2.4 cm². Since the initial experience, this procedure has been performed in selected institutions (160,161).

Pre-CPB IOE Exam

The IOE exam has unique requirements for confirming that the mechanism of dysfunction is irreparable. The homograft was matched to measurements provided by the pre-CPB or pre-OR TEE. Using the ME 4 Chr imaging plane, the diastolic "height" was measured from the hinge point to the distal edge. In systole, the anteroposterior diameter of the annulus was measured, as well as the distance between the annular planes in the image to the tip of the ALPM. These measured parameters (+3 mm) were matched with harvested mitral homographs.

Post-CPB IOE Exam

The post-CPB assessment of the homograft includes a determination of the presence of MR, MV area by planimetry, and the transvalvular gradient. MR was minimal in 15 patients and mild in six. The mean transvalvular gradient was 3 ± 2 mm Hg, and the valve area measured 2.5 cm^2 by planimetry (160).

Intraoperative Three-Dimensional Echocardiography of the Mitral Valve

One of the most exciting innovations in IOE is three-dimensional (3D) imaging. The concept was first developed in the early 1970s but only recently has it become practical in the intraoperative environment (162,163). This is primarily due to faster acquisition times and better methods to analyze the data obtained in the busy operating room environment. The 3D exam of the MV complements a complete 2D exam to develop a full understanding of mitral anatomy and mechanism of dysfunction, including the severity of disease (Fig. 30.71).

The MV is ideally suited for 3D echo imaging, given it is spatially close to the TEE probe tip and 90 degrees to the ultrasound beam. Since the TEE imaging plane can be centered on the MV, rational-gated reconstructed 3D data sets can be created that allow imaging of the MV anatomy to help determine mechanism of dysfunction and a large CF 3D Doppler area to analyze both regurgitant jets and mitral stenotic flow acceleration (Fig. 30.72). Recently, with the development of real-time 3D (RT3D) echocardiography, the incorporation of 3D analysis into the evaluation of the MV in a fast paced operating room environment is easily performed.

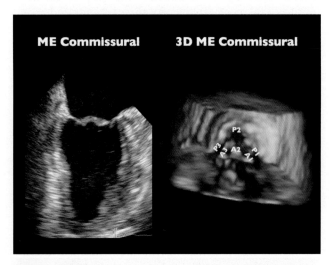

Figure 30.71. Complementary images showing the 2D midesophageal commissural view and a RT 3D midesophageal commissural view.

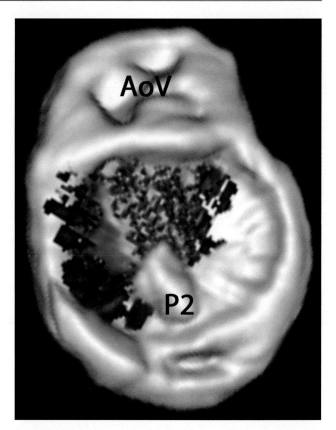

Figure 30.72. A 3D gated reconstruction of the MV with a flail P2 and jet directed anterior and laterally. AoV, aortic valve; P2, P2 segment (middle scallop) of the posterior mitral valve leaflet.

Intraoperative surgical planning depends on proper evaluation of the MVAp (164). The feasibility, accuracy, and value of intraoperative 3D echocardiography in valve surgery were studied by Abraham et al. (165). Intraoperative 2D and 3D reconstruction TEE examinations were performed on 60 patients undergoing valve surgery. 3D acquisitions were completed in 87% of the patients within a mean acquisition time of 2.8 ± 0.2 minutes and reconstruction time within 8.6 ± 0.7 minutes. 3D echocardiography detected all salient valve morphological pathology (leaflet perforations, fenestrations and masses), which was subsequently confirmed on pathological examination in 84% of the patients. In addition, intraoperative 3D TEE provided new additional information not obtained by 2D TEE in 15 patients (25%) and in one case influenced the surgeon's decision to perform a valve repair rather than a replacement. Furthermore, intraoperative 3DE provided worthwhile and complementary anatomic information that explained the mechanism of valve dysfunction demonstrated by 2D imaging and CFD.

The ability of 3DE to render new views not previously obtainable by 2DE, such as the "en face" and surgical views of the MV (Fig. 30.73), provides new insight and possible better communication with the surgeon. Ahmed et al. evaluated the potential utility of 3D TEE in identifying individual MV scallop prolapse in 36 adult patients undergoing surgical correction (166). Perfect correlation

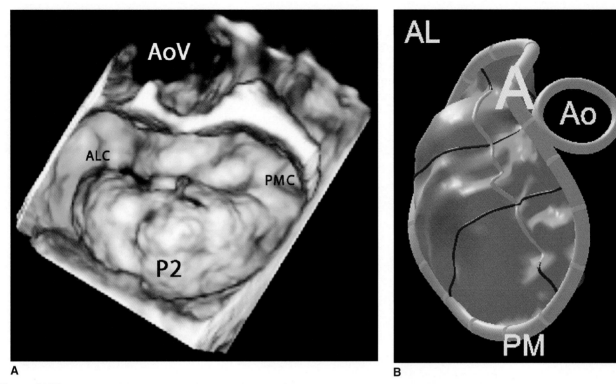

Figure 30.73. En face surgeon's view of the MV showing P2 prolapse (**A**) and digitally constructed model of the myxomatous valve (**B**). A, anterior annulus; AL, anterolatera annulus; PM, posteromedial annulus.

between 3D TEE and surgical findings was noted in 78% of the patients.

Being able to "cut" the MV in any plane from both atrial and ventricular views adds a new dimension to its evaluation. In studies comparing 2D versus 3D TEE for measuring MV area and volume in patients with stenosis undergoing percutaneous MV balloon valvuloplasty (PMTV), 3D TEE enabled a better description of valve anatomy including the identification of commissural splitting and leaflet tears post-PTMV (167–169). Two studies have shown that 3DE

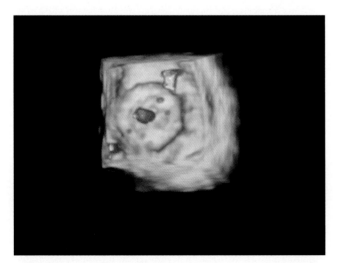

Figure 30.74. A gated color 3D reconstruction of a tilting-disc MVR showing the typical central jet inherent in the function of the valve and a perivalvular leak.

of the MV allows direct visualization and accurate planimetry of the ROA in patients with MR when compared to the PFC method (170,171). Sugeng et al. studied 3DE with CFD (172). The study looked at 46 patients with MR. 3D CFD was particularly helpful in patients with paravalvular leaks and eccentric jets (Fig. 30.74).

Several recent studies have highlighted the feasibility and utility of RT3D TEE for evaluating MV disease (173). In 211 patients, including patients with atrial fibrillation, there was excellent visualization of all MV leaflet scallops (anterior and posterior) in 85% to 91% of patients (174). In 47 patients, intraoperative diagnosis was used to confirm the RT3D TEE exam. Surgical findings correlated in 96% of the patients (175).

Although 3DE has shown promise, it still has drawbacks that need to be considered. 3D gated reconstruction requires additional time to acquire and reconstruct the images. Any type of motion artifact in the 2D images prior to reconstruction will make the 3D data set suboptimal. Patients with atrial fibrillation or an irregularity in their RR interval will prolong data acquisition and make the 3D reconstruction of poorer quality (stitching artifacts). RT3D TEE is a newer technology. Its ability to visualize near-field structures, such as the left atrium, atrial septum, MV and LV, appears superior to far-field structures, such as the tricuspid and pulmonic valves. RT 3D images have slower frame rates and decreased line density compared to traditional 2D imaging.

There is a learning curve to data acquisition and reconstruction. 3D echocardiography much more than 2D requires a complete understanding of the physics of ultrasound. The ultrasound frequency, line density, depth of the image, sector size, gain, and dynamic range (compression) settings must all be optimized based on the structure and pathology to be imaged. This will maximize both spatial and temporal resolution (frame rate) and minimize image dropout and other 3D artifacts.

KEY POINTS

■ The MVAp consists of the fibrous cardiac skeleton, saddle-shaped mitral annulus, MV leaflets, chordae, papillary muscles, and ventricular wall complex.

■ Pathologic processes may structurally alter the anatomic integrity of the components of the MVAp, resulting in MV dysfunction.

■ While the IOE exam confirms the presence of MV dysfunction and its (intraoperative) severity, its most significant role is refining the understanding of the structure and mechanism(s) of MV dysfunction.

■ MVRep is the treatment of choice for MV dysfunction resulting from all etiologies.

■ In MV surgery, the most significant surgical issues that the IOE exam resolves are the repairability of the MVAp, the necessity to perform other surgical interventions, and the post-CPB assessment of the surgical procedure and complications.

■ In addition to the expertise and experience of the surgical team, the probability of MVRep is dictated by etiology apparatus and mechanism of dysfunction. These are determined by the IOE exam in conjunction with the surgeon's direct inspection of the MVAp.

■ The IOE exam may be organized by priority to ensure that critical issues are addressed should the patient require the initiation of CPB.

■ The pre-CPB also determines the secondary or associated pathophysiology, cannulation-perfusion strategy, the potential for post-CPB complications, and provides an ongoing assessment of cardiac function.

■ The post-CPB exam provides a quality assurance safety net with the assessment of the surgical procedure and diagnosis of complications.

■ Consistent with the recommendations of the ASE Standards Committee and Task Force on Native Valve Regurgitation, the intraoperative exam relies on a weighted-integration method of severity assessment for all valve dysfunction. This may be efficiently performed in a multitasking environment.

■ CFD (MJA) is a useful screening method for determining the presence of ≥ severe or ≤ trivial MV regurgitation. More quantitative methods are recommended in addition to CFD (MJA).

■ The 3D echocardiographic exam of the MV complements a complete 2D exam.

REFERENCES

1. Johnson ML, Holmes JH, Spangler RD, et al. Usefulness of echocardiography in patients undergoing MV surgery. *J Thorac Cardiovasc Surg* 1972;64:922–928.
2. Frazin L, Talano JV, Stephanides L. Esophageal echocardiography. *Circulation* 1975;54:102–104.
3. Hisanga K, Hisanaga A, Nagata K, et al. A new trans-esophageal real-time two-dimensional echocardiographic system using a flexible tube and its clinical application. *Proc Jpn Soc Ultrason Med* 1977;32:43–45.
4. Hanrath P, Kremer P, Langenstein BA. Transosophageal echokardiographie: ein neues verfahren zur dynamischen ventrikelfunktionsanalyse. *Dtsch Med Wochenschr* 1981;106:533.
5. Kremer P, Roizen MT, Gutman J, et al. Cardiac monitoring by transesophageal 2-D echocardiography during abdominal aortic aneurysmectomy. *Circulation* 1982;66:II179 (abst).
6. Goldman ME, Mindich BP, Teichholz LE, et al. Intraoperative contrast echocardiography to evaluate MV operations. *J Am Coll Cardiol* 1984;4:1035–1040.
7. Takamoto S, Kyo S, Adachi H, et al. Intraoperative color flow mapping by real-time two-dimensional Doppler echocardiography for evaluation of valvular and congenital heart disease and vascular disease. *J Thorac Cardiovasc Surg* 1985;90:802–812.
8. Stewart WJ, Salcedo EE, Schiavone WA, et al. Intraoperative Doppler color flow mapping in valve conservation surgery. Proc Tenth World Congress Cardiology 1986:247 (abst).
9. Stewart WJ, Currie PJ, Agler DA, et al. Intraoperative epicardial echocardiography: technique, imaging planes, and use in valve repair for mitral regurgitation. *Dyn Cardiovasc Imaging* 1987;1:179–184.
10. Kyo S, Takamoto S, Matsumura M, et al. Immediate and early postoperative evaluation of results of cardiac surgery by transesophageal two-dimensional Doppler echocardiography. *Circulation* 1987;76:113–121.
11. Rankin JS, Livesey SA, Smith LR, et al. Trends in the surgical treatment of ischemic mitral regurgitation: effects of mitral valve repair on hospital mortality. *Semin Thorac Cardiovasc Surg* 1989;1:149–163.
12. Mishra M, Chauhan R, Sharma KK, et al. Real-time intraoperative transesophageal echocardiography—how useful? Experience of 5,016 cases. *J Cardiothorac Vasc Anesth* 1998;12:625–232.
13. Sutton DC, Kluger R. Intraoperative transesophageal echocardiography: impact on adult cardiac surgery. *Anesth Intensive Care* 1998;26:287–293.
14. Cheitlin MD, Armstrong WF, Aurigemma GP, et al. ACC/AHA/ASE 2003 guideline update for the clinical application of echocardiography—summary article: a report of the American College of Cardiology/American Heart Association Task Force on Practice guidelines (ACC/AHA/ASE Committee to Update the 1997 Guidelines for the Clinical Application of Echocardiography). *J Am Coll Cardiol* 2003;42(5):954–970.
15. Stewart WJ, Currie PJ, Salcedo EE, et al. Intraoperative Doppler color flow mapping for decision-making in valve repair for mitral regurgitation. Technique and results in 100 patients. *Circulation* 1990;81:556–566.
16. Kawano H, Mizoguchi T, Aoyagi S. Intraoperative transesophageal echocardiography for evaluation of mitral valve repair. *J Heart Valve Dis* 1999;8(3):287–293.
17. Abraham TP, Warner JG, Kon ND, et al. Feasibility, accuracy, and incremental value of intraoperative three-

dimensional echocardiography in valve surgery. *Am J Cardiol* 1997;80(12):1577–1582.

18. Aklog L, Filsoufi F, Flores KQ, et al. Does coronary artery bypass grafting alone correct moderate ischemic mitral regurgitation? *Circulation* 2001;104(12 Suppl. 1):I68–I75.

19. Savage RM, Lytle BW, Aronson S, et al. Intraoperative echocardiography is indicated in high-risk coronary artery bypass grafting. *Ann Thorac Surg* 1997;64:368–373.

20. Cohn LH, Rizzo RJ, Adams DH, et al. The effect of pathophysiology on the surgical treatment of ischemic mitral regurgitation: operative and late risks of repair versus replacement. *Eur J Cardiothorac Surg* 1995;9:568–574.

21. Bonow RO, Smith SC Jr. Cardiovascular manpower: the looming crisis. *Circulation* 2004;109(7):817–820.

22. National Center for Health Statistics, Owings MF, Lawrence L. *Detailed Diagnosis and Procedures: National Hospital Discharge Survey, 1997. Vital and Health Statistics. Series 13. No. 145.* Washington, DC: Government Printing Office, 1999.

23. 2003 United States Census Bureau Statistics.

24. Singh JP, Evans JC, Levy D, et al. Prevalence and clinical determinants of mitral, tricuspid, and aortic regurgitation (the Framingham Study). *Am J Cardiol* 1999;83:897–902.

25. Aronow WS, Ahn C, Kronzon I. Echocardiographic abnormalities in African-American, Hispanic, and white men and women aged >60 years. *Am J Cardiol* 2001;87(9):1131–1133.

26. Horstkotte D. Pathomorphological aspects, etiology and natural history of acquired mitral valve stenosis. *Eur Heart J* 1991;12(Suppl. B):55–60.

27. Supino PG, Borer JS, Yin A. The epidemiology of valvular heart disease: an emerging public health problem. *Adv Cardiol* 2002;39:1–6.

28. Ling LH, Sarano ME, Seward JB, et al. Clinical outcome of mitral regurgitation due to flail leaflet. *N Engl J Med* 1996;335:1417–1423.

29. Enriquez-Sarano M, Basmadjian AJ, Rossi A, et al. Progression of mitral regurgitation: a prospective Doppler echo-cardiographic study. *J Am Coll Cardiol* 1999;34(4):1137–1144.

30. Gillinov AM, Cosgrove DM. Mitral valve repair for degenerative disease. *J Heart Valve Dis* 2002;11(Suppl. 1):S15–S20.

31. Braunberger E, Deloche A, Berrebi A, et al. Very long-term results (more than 20 years) of valve repair with Carpentier's techniques in nonrheumatic mitral valve insufficiency. *Circulation* 2001;104(Suppl. I):I-8–I-11.

32. Enriquez-Sarano M. Timing of mitral valve surgery. *Heart* 2002;87(1):79–85.

33. Bonow R, Carabello B, Chatterjee K, et al. 2008 focused update incorporated into the ACC/AHA 2006 guidelines for the management of patients with valvular heart disease. A report of the American College of Cardiology/American Heart Association task force on practice guidelines (Writing committee to revise the 1998 guidelines for the management of patients with valvular heart disease). *J Am Coll Cardiol* 2008;52:1–142.

34. *The Society of Thoracic Surgeons National Cardiac Surgery Database: Executive Summary 2003.* Chicago: The Society of Thoracic Surgeons, 2003. STS National Database. Available at:ww.sts.org/sections/stsnationaldatabase/datamanagers/adultcardiacdb. Accessed Sep 6, 2006.

35. Zoghbi WA, Enriquez-Sarano M, Foster E, et al. Recommendations for evaluation of the severity of native valvular regurgitation with two-dimensional and Doppler echocardiography. *J Am Soc Echocardiogr* 2003;16(7):777–802.

36. Gillinov AM, Cosgrove DM, Lytle BW, et al. Surgery for acquired heart disease: reoperation for failure of mitral valve repair. *J Thorac Cardiovasc Surg* 1997;113:467–475.

37. Enriquez-Sarano M, Nkomo V, Mohty D, et al. Mitral regurgitation: predictors of outcome and natural history. *Adv Cardiol* 2002;39:133–143.

38. Chaliki HP, Click RL, Abel MD. Comparison of intraoperative transesophageal echocardiographic examinations with the operative findings: prospective review of 1918 cases. *J Am Soc Echocardiogr* 1999;12:237–240.

39. Sheikh KH, de Bruijn NP, Rankin JS, et al. The utility of transesophageal echocardiography and Doppler color flow imaging in patients undergoing cardiac valve surgery. *J Am Coll Cardiol* 1990;15:363–372.

40. Shah PM, Raney AA, Duran CM, et al. Multiplane transesophageal echocardiography: a roadmap for mitral valve repair. *J Heart Valve Dis* 1999;8:625–629.

41. Perloff JK, Roberts WC. The mitral apparatus: functional anatomy of mitral regurgitation. *Circulation* 1972;46:227.

42. Becker AE, de Wit APM. The mitral valve apparatus: a spectrum of normality relevant to mitral valve prolapse. *Br Heart J* 1980;42:680–689.

43. DePlessis LA, Marchand P. The anatomy of the mitral valve and its associated structures. *Thorax* 1964;19:221–227.

44. Rusted IE, Schiefley CH, Edwards JE. Studies of the mitral valve. I. Anatomic features of the normal mitral valve and associated structures. *Circulation* 1952;6:825–831.

45. Brock RC. The surgical and pathological anatomy of the mitral valve. *Br Heart J* 1952;14:489–513.

46. Zimmerman J, Bailey CP. The surgical significance of the fibrous skeleton of the heart. *J Thorac Cardiovasc Surg* 1962;44:701–712.

47. Kunzelman KS, Reimink MS, Cochran RP. Annular dilation increases stress in the mitral valve and delays coaptation: a finite element computer model. *Cardiovasc Surg* 1997;5(4):427–434.

48. Flashskampf FA, Chandra S, Gaddipatti A, et al. Analysis of shape and motion of the mitral annulus in subjects with and without cardiomyopathy by echocardiographic 3-dimensional reconstruction. *J Am Soc Echocardiogr* 2000;13(4):277–287.

49. Lam JHC, Ranganathan N, Wigle ED, et al. Morphology of the human mitral valve. I. Chordae tendineae: a new classification. *Circulation* 1970;41:449–458.

50. Stümper O, Fraser AG, Ho SY, et al. Transesophageal echocardiography in the longitudinal axis: correlation between anatomy and images and its clinical implications. *Br Heart J* 1990;64:282–288.

51. Voci P, Bilotta F, Caretta Q, et al. Papillary muscle perfusion pattern: a hypothesis for ischemic papillary muscle dysfunction. *Circulation* 1995;91:1714–1718.

52. Shanewise JS, Cheung AT, Aronson S, et al. ASE/SCA guidelines for performing a comprehensive intraoperative multiplane transesophageal echocardiography examination: recommendations of the American Society of Echocardiography Council for Intraoperative Echocardiography and the Society of Cardiovascular Anesthesiologists Task Force for Certification in Perioperative Transesophageal Echocardiography. *J Am Soc Echocardiogr* 1999;12(10):884–900.

53. Kumar N, Kumar M, Duran CMG. A revised terminology for recording surgical findings of the mitral valve. *J Heart Valve Dis* 1995;4:70–75.

54. Stewart WJ. Intraoperative echocardiography. In: Topol E, ed. *Textbook of Cardiovascular Medicine.* Baltimore, MA: Lippincott, 2003.

55. Otto C. Valvular stenosis: diagnosis, quantitation, and clinical approach. In: Otto C, ed. *Textbook of Clinical Echocardiography*. 2nd ed. Philadelphia, PA: WB Saunders, 2000: 229–264.

56. Carabello BA. Timing of surgery for mitral and aortic stenosis. *Cardiol Clin* 1991;9:229–38.

57. Thomas JD. Doppler echocardiographic assessment of valvar regurgitation. *Heart* 2002;88(6):651–657.

58. Grayburn P, Fehske W, Omran H, et al. Multiplane transesophageal echocardiographic assessment of mitral regurgitation by Doppler color flow mapping of the vena contracta. *Am J Cardiol* 1994;74:912–917.

59. Hall SA, Brickner ME, Willett DL, et al. Assessment of mitral regurgitant severity by Doppler color flow mapping of the vena contracta. *Circulation* 1997;95:636–642.

60. Klein AL, Stewart WJ, Bartlett J, et al. Effects of mitral regurgitation on pulmonary venous flow and left atrial pressure: an intraoperative transesophageal echocardiographic study. *J Am Coll Cardiol* 1992;20:1345–1352.

61. Pu M, Griffin BP, Vandervoort PM, et al. The value of assessing pulmonary venous flow velocity for predicting severity of mitral regurgitation: a quantitative assessment integrating left ventricular function. *J Am Soc Echocardiogr* 1999;12: 736–743.

62. Klein AL, Savage RM, Kahan F, et al. Experimental and numerically modeled effects of convergence altered loading conditions on pulmonary venous flow and left atrial pressure in patients with mitral regurgitation. *J Am Soc Echocardiogr* 1997;10(1):41–51.

63. Pu M, Vandervoort PM, Griffin BP, et al. Quantification of mitral regurgitation by the proximal convergence method using transesophageal echocardiography. Clinical validation of a geometric correction for proximal flow constraint. *Circulation* 1995;92:2169–2177.

64. Rivera JM, Vandervoort PM, Thoreau DH, et al. Quantification of mitral regurgitation using the proximal flow convergence method: a clinical study. *Am Heart J* 1992;124: 1289–1296.

65. Rodriguez L, Anconina J, Flachskampf FA, et al. Impact of finite orifice on proximal flow convergence: implications for Doppler quantification of valvular regurgitation. *Circ Res* 1992;70:923–930.

66. Pu M, Prior DL, Fan X, et al. Calculation of mitral regurgitant orifice area with use of a simplified proximal convergence method: initial clinical application. *J Am Soc Echocardiogr* 2001;14:180–185.

67. Schwammenthal E, Chen C, Giesler M, et al. New method for accurate calculation of regurgitant flow rate based on analysis of Doppler color flow maps of the proximal flow field. *J Am Coll Cardiol* 1996;27:161–172.

68. Wilkins GT, Weyman AE, Abascal VM, et al. Percutaneous balloon dilatation of the mitral valve: an analysis of echocardiographic variables related to outcome and the mechanism of dilatation. *Br Heart J* 1988;60:299–308.

69. Martin RP, Rakowski H, Kleiman JH, et al. Reliability and reproducibility of two dimensional echocardiograph measurement of the stenotic mitral valve orifice area. *Am J Cardiol* 1979;43:560–568.

70. Carabello BA, Crawford FA Jr. Valvular heart disease. *N Engl J Med* 1997;337(1):32–41 (erratum *N Engl J Med* 1997;337(7):507).

71. Hatle L, Brubakk A, Tromsdal A, et al. Noninvasive assessment of pressure drop in MS by Doppler ultrasound. *Br Heart J* 1978;40:131–140.

72. Enriquez-Sarano M, Freeman WK, Tribouilloy CM, et al. Functional anatomy of mitral regurgitation: accuracy and outcome implications of transesophageal echocardiography. *J Am Coll Cardiol* 1999;34:1129–1136.

73. Bajzer CT, Stewart WJ, Cosgrove DM, et al. Tricuspid valve surgery and intraoperative echocardiography: factors affecting survival, clinical outcome, and echocardiographic success. *J Am Coll Cardiol* 1998;32(4):1023–1031.

74. Newman MF, Wolman R, Kanchuger M, et al. Multicenter preoperative stroke risk index for patients undergoing coronary artery bypass graft surgery. Multicenter Study of Perioperative Ischemia (McSPI) Research Group. *Circulation* 1996;94(Suppl. 9):II-74–II-80.

75. Moisa RB, Zeldis SM, Alper SA, et al. Aortic regurgitation in coronary artery bypass grafting: implications for cardioplegia administration. *Ann Thorac Surg* 1995;60:665–668.

76. Gillinov AM, Cosgrove DM, Blackstone EH, et al. Durability of mitral valve repair for degenerative disease. *J Thorac Cardiovasc Surg* 1998;116:734–743.

77. Michel-Cherqui M, Ceddaha A, Liu N, et al. Assessment of systematic use of intraoperative transesophageal echocardiography during cardiac surgery in adults: a prospective study of 203 patients. *J Cardiothorac Vasc Anesth* 2000;14:45–50.

78. Stewart WJ, Currie PJ, Salcedo EE, et al. Evaluation of mitral leaflet motion by echocardiography and jet direction by Doppler color flow mapping to determine the mechanisms of mitral regurgitation. *J Am Coll Cardiol* 1992;20:1353–1361.

79. Foster GP, Isselbacher EM, Rose GA, et al. Accurate localization of mitral regurgitant defects using multiplane transesophageal echocardiography. *Ann Thorac Surg* 1998;65(4): 1025–1031.

80. Lambert AS, Miller JP, Merrick SH, et al. Improved evaluation of the location and mechanism of mitral valve regurgitation with a systematic transesophageal echocardiography examination. *Anesth Analg* 1999;88(6):1205–1212.

81. Omran AS, Woo A, David TE, et al. Intraoperative transesophageal echocardiography accurately predicts mitral valve anatomy and suitability for repair. *J Am Soc Echocardiogr* 2002;15(9):950–957.

82. Caldarera I, Van Herwerden LA, Taams MA, et al. Multiplane transesophageal echocardiography and morphology of regurgitant mitral valves in surgical repair. *Eur Heart J* 1995;16(7):999–1006.

83. Grewal KS, Malkowski MJ, Kramer CM, et al. Multiplane transesophageal echocardiographic identification of the involved scallop in patients with flail mitral valve leaflet: intraoperative correlation. *J Am Soc Echocardiogr* 1998;11:966–971.

84. Bach DS, Deeb GM, Bolling SF. Accuracy of intraoperative transesophageal echocardiography for estimating the severity of functional mitral regurgitation. *Am J Cardiol* 1995;76(7):508–512.

85. Marwick TH, Stewart WJ, Currie PJ, et al. Mechanisms of failure of mitral valve repair: an echocardiographic study. *Am Heart J* 1991;122(1 Pt 1):149–156.

86. Agricola E, Oppizzi M, Maisano F, et al. Detection of mechanisms of immediate failure by transesophageal echocardiography in quadrangular resection mitral valve repair technique for severe mitral regurgitation. *Am J Cardiol* 2003;91(2):175–179.

87. Schiavone WA, Cosgrove DM, Lever HM, et al. Follow-up of patients with left ventricular outflow tract obstruction after Carpentier ring mitral valvuloplasty. *Circulation* 1988;78(3 Pt 2):I60–I65.

88. Lee KS, Stewart WJ, Lever HM, et al. Mechanism of outflow tract obstruction causing failed mitral valve repair. Anterior displacement of leaflet coaptation. *Circulation* 1993;88:II24–II-29.

89. Carpentier A. The sliding leaflet technique. *Le Club Mitrale Newsletter* 1988;1:2–3.

90. Gillinov AM, Cosgrove DM III. Modified sliding leaflet technique for repair of the mitral valve. *Ann Thorac Surg* 1999;68(6):2356–2357.

91. Gillinov AM, Wierup PN, Blackstone EH, et al. Is repair preferable to replacement for ischemic mitral regurgitation. *J Thorac Cardiovasc Surg* 2001;122(6):1125–1141.

92. Maslow AD, Regan MM, Haering JM, et al. Echocardiographic predictors of left ventricular outflow tract obstruction and systolic anterior motion of the mitral valve after mitral valve reconstruction for myxomatous valve disease. *J Am Coll Cardiol* 1999;34(7):2096–2104.

93. Feindel CM, Tufail Z, David TE. Mitral valve surgery in patients with extensive calcification of the mitral annulus. *J Thorac Cardiovasc Surg* 2003;126(3):777–782.

94. David TE, Feindel CM, Armstrong S, et al. Reconstruction of the mitral annulus. A ten-year experience. *J Thorac Cardiovasc Surg* 1995;110(5):1323–1332.

95. David TE, Armstrong S, Sun Z. Left ventricular function after mitral valve surgery. *J Heart Valve Dis* 1995;4(Suppl. 2):S175–S180.

96. Fix J, Isada L, Cosgrove D, Savage RM, Blum J, Stewart WJ. Do patients with less than "echo perfect" results from mitral valve repair by intraoperative echocardiography have different outcome? *Circulation* 1993;88(2):38–48.

97. Davila-Roman VG, Barzilai B, Wareing TH, et al. Atherosclerosis of the ascending aorta. Prevalence and role as an independent predictor of cerebrovascular events in cardiac patients. *Stroke* 1994;25:2010.

98. Davila-Roman VG, Phillips KJ, Daily BB, et al. Intraoperative transesophageal echocardiography and epiaortic ultrasound for assessment of atherosclerosis of the thoracic aorta. *J Am Coll Cardiol* 1996;28:942–947.

99. Wareing TH, Davila-Roman VG, Barzilai B, et al. Management of the severely atherosclerotic ascending aorta during cardiac operations. A strategy for detection and treatment. *J Thorac Cardiovasc Surg* 1992;103:453–462.

100. Roach GW, Kacchuger M, Mangano C, et al. Adverse cerebral outcomes after coronary bypass surgery. *N Engl J Med* 1996;335:1857.

101. Konstadt SN, Reich DL, Quintana C, et al. The ascending aorta: how much does transesophageal echocardiography see? *Anesth Analg* 1994;78:240–244.

102. Morehead AJ, Firstenberg MS, Shiota T, et al. Intraoperative echocardiographic detection of regurgitant jets after valve replacement. *Ann Thorac Surg* 2000;69:135–139.

103. Thomas JD, Vandervoort PM, Pu M, et al. Doppler/echocardiographic assessment of native and prosthetic heart valves: recent advances. *J Heart Valve Dis* 1995;4(Suppl. 1):S59–S63.

104. Cohen GI, Davison MB, Klein AL, et al. A comparison of flow convergence with other transthoracic echocardiographic indexes of prosthetic mitral regurgitation. *J Am Soc Echocardiogr* 1992;5(6):620–627.

105. Nkomo VT, Gardin JM, Skelton TN, Gottdiener JS, Scott CG, Enriquez-Sarano M. Burden of valvular heart diseases: a population-based study. *Lancet* 2006;368:1005–1011.

105a. Enriquez-Sarano M, Schaff HV, Orszulak TA, et al. Valve repair improves the outcome of surgery for mitral regurgitation: a multivariate analysis. *Circulation* 1995;91:1022–1028.

106. David TE. Dynamic left ventricular outflow tract obstruction when the anterior leaflet is retained at prosthetic mitral valve replacement. *Ann Thorac Surg* 1988;45(2):229.

107. Grimm RA, Stewart WJ. The role of intraoperative echocardiography in valve surgery. *Cardiol Clin* 1998;16:477–489.

108. Fix J, Isada L, Cosgrove D, et al. Do patients with less than "echo-perfect" results from mitral valve repair by intraoperative echocardiography have a different outcome? *Circulation* 1993;88:II-39–II-48.

109. Freeman WK, Schaff HV, Khandheria BK, et al. Intraoperative evaluation of mitral valve regurgitation and repair by transesophageal echocardiography: incidence and significance of systolic anterior motion. *J Am Coll Cardiol* 1992;20:599–609.

110. Milas BL, Bavaria JE, Koch CG, et al. Case 8–2001. Resolution of systolic anterior motion after mitral valve repair with atrial pacing. *J Cardiothorac Vasc Anesth* 2001;15(5):641–648.

111. Gatti G, Cardu G, Trane R, et al. The edge-to-edge technique as a trick to rescue an imperfect mitral valve repair. *Eur J Cardiothorac Surg* 2002;22(5):817–820.

112. Saiki Y, Kasegawa H, Kawase M, et al. Intraoperative TEE during mitral valve repair: does it predict early and late postoperative mitral valve dysfunction? *Ann Thorac Surg* 1998;66(4):1277–1281.

113. Umana JP, Salehizadeh B, Oz M, et al. "Bow-tie" mitral valve repair: an adjuvant technique for ischemic mitral regurgitation. *Ann Thorac Surg* 1998;66(5):1640–1646.

114. Privitera S, Butany J, Cusimano RJ, et al. Images in cardiovascular medicine. Alfieri mitral valve repair: clinical outcome and pathology. *Circulation* 2002;106(21):173–174.

115. Ibrahim MF, David TE. Mitral stenosis after mitral valve repair for non-rheumatic mitral regurgitation. *Ann Thorac Surg* 2002;73(1):34–36.

116. Tingleff J, Joyce FS, Pettersson G. Intraoperative echocardiographic study of air embolism during cardiac operations. *Ann Thorac Surg* 1995;60:673–677.

117. Secknus MA, Asher CR, Scalia GM, et al. Intraoperative transesophageal echocardiography in minimally invasive cardiac valve surgery. *J Am Soc Echocardiogr* 1999;12(4):231–236.

118. Varghese D, Riedel BJ, Fletchker SN, et al. Successful repair of intraoperative aortic dissection detected by transesophageal echocardiography. *Ann Thorac Surg* 2002;73(3):953–955.

119. Tavilla G, Pacini D. Damage to the circumflex coronary artery during mitral valve repair with sliding leaflet technique. *Ann Thorac Surg* 1998;66(6):2091–2093.

120. Obarski TP, Loop FD, Cosgrove DM, et al. Frequency of acute myocardial infarction in valve repairs versus valve replacement for pure mitral regurgitation. *Am J Cardiol* 1990;65(13):887–890.

121. Genoni M, Jenni R, Schmid ER, et al. Treatment of left atrial dissection after mitral repair: internal drainage. *Ann Thorac Surg* 1999;68(4):1394–1396.

122. Ionescu AA, West RR, Proudman C, et al. Prospective study of routine perioperative transesophageal echocardiography for elective valve replacement: clinical impact and cost-saving implications. *J Am Soc Echocardiogr* 2001;14(7):659–667.

123. Mills WR, Barber JE, Skiles JA, et al. Clinical, echocardiographic, and biomechanical differences in mitral valve prolapse affecting one or both leaflets. *Am J Cardiol* 2002;89(12):1394–1399.

124. Robert WC. Morphologic aspects of cardiac valve dysfunction. *Am Heart J* 1992;123:1610.

125. Braunwald E. Mitral regurgitation: physiologic, clinical, and surgical considerations. *N Engl J Med* 1969;281(8):425–433.

126. Carpentier A, Deloche A, Dauptain J, et al. A new reconstructive operation for correction of mitral and tricuspid insufficiency. *J Thorac Cardiovasc Surg* 1971;61:1–13.

127. Waller BF, Morrow AG, Maron BJ, et al. Etiology of clinically isolated, severe, chronic, pure mitral regurgitation: analysis of 97 patients over 30 years of age having mitral valve replacement. *Am Heart J* 1982;104:276–288.

128. Fornes P, Heudes D, Fuzellier J, et al. Correlation between clinical and histologic patterns of degenerative mitral valve insufficiency: a histomorphometric study of 130 excised segments. *Cardiovasc Pathol* 1999;8(2):81–92.

129. Rosen SE, Borer JS, Hochreiter C, et al. Natural history of the asymptomatic/minimally symptomatic patient with severe mitral regurgitation secondary to mitral valve prolapse and normal right and left ventricular performance. *Am J Cardiol* 1994;74:374–380.

130. Kwan J, Shiota T, Agler DA, et al. Geometric differences of the mitral apparatus between ischemic and dilated cardiomyopathy with significant mitral regurgitation: real-time three-dimensional echocardiography study. *Circulation* 2003;107(8):1135–1140.

131. Karp RB. Role of surgery in infectious endocarditis. *Cardiovasc Clin* 1987;17:141.

132. Muehrcke DD, Cosgrove DM, Lytle BW, et al. Is there an advantage to sparing infected mitral valves? *Ann Thorac Surg* 1997;63:1718.

133. Marcus RH, Sareli P, Pocock WA, et al. The spectrum of severe rheumatic mitral valve disease in a developing country: correlations among clinical presentation, surgical pathologic findings, and hemodynamic sequelae. *Ann Intern Med* 1994;120:177–183.

134. Olson LJ, Subramanian R, Ackermann DM, et al. Surgical pathology of the mitral valve: a study of 712 cases spanning 21 years. *Mayo Clin Proc* 1987;62:22–34.

135. Carpentier A, Chauvaud S, Fabiani JN, et al. Reconstructive surgery of mitral valve incompetence, ten-year appraisal. *J Thorac Cardiovasc Surg* 1980;79:338–348.

136. Carpentier AF, Pellerin M, Fuzellier JF, et al. Extensive calcification of the mitral valve annulus: pathology and surgical management. *J Thorac Cardiovasc Surg* 1996;111(4):718–729; discussion 729–730.

137. Duran CM, Gometza B, Balasundaram S, et al. A feasibility study of valve repair in rheumatic mitral regurgitation. *Eur Heart J* 1991;12:34–38.

138. David TE. The appropriateness of mitral valve repair for rheumatic mitral valve disease. *J Heart Valve Dis* 1997;6(4):373–374.

139. Hanson TP, Edwards BC, Edwards JE. Pathology of surgically excised mitral valves: one hundred cases. *Arch Pathol Lab Med* 1985;109:823.

140. Carpentier A. Cardiac valve surgery: the "French Connection." *J Thorac Cardiovasc Surg* 1983;86:323.

141. Reece TB, Tribble CG, Ellman PI. Mitral repair is superior to replacement when associated with coronary artery disease. *Ann Surg* 2004;239(5):671–675; discussion 675–677.

142. Messas E, Pouzet B, Touchot B, et al. Efficacy of chordal cutting to relieve chronic persistent ischemic mitral regurgitation. *Circulation* 2003;108(Suppl. 1):II-111–II-115.

143. Levine RA, Hung J. Ischemic mitral regurgitation, the dynamic lesion: clues to the cure [comment]. *J Am Coll Cardiol* 2003;42(11):1929–1932.

144. Enriquez-Sarano M, Bailey KR, Seward JB, et al. Quantitative Doppler assessment of valvular regurgitation. *Circulation* 1993;87:841–848.

145. Marwick TH, Torelli J, Obarski T, et al. Assessment of the mitral valve splitability score by transthoracic and transesophageal echocardiography. *Am J Cardiol* 1991;68:1106–1107.

146. Rodriguez L, Thomas JD, Monterosso V, et al. Validation of the proximal flow convergence method. Calculation of orifice area in patients with mitral stenosis. *Circulation* 1993;88:1157–1165.

147. Duran CM. Tricuspid valve surgery revisited. *J Cardiac Surg* 1994;9:242–247.

148. Choudhary SK, Talwar S, Juneja R, et al. Fate of mild aortic valve disease after mitral intervention. *J Thorac Cardiovasc Surg* 2001;122:583.

149. McGoon DC. Repair of mitral insufficiency due to ruptured chordae tendineae. *J Thorac Cardiovasc Surg* 1960;39:357–362.

150. Gillinov AM, Cosgrove DM III, Shiota T, et al. Cosgrove-Edwards annuloplasty system: midterm results. *Ann Thorac Surg* 2000;69(3):717–721.

151. Brunton T. Preliminary note on the possibility of treating mitral stenosis by surgical methods. *Lancet* 1902;1:352.

152. Cutler EE, Levine SA, Beck CS. The surgical treatment of mitral stenosis: experimental and clinical studies. *Arch Surg* 1924;9:689–821, 104–105.

153. Lillehei CW, Gott VL, DeWall RA, et al. Surgical correction of pure mitral insufficiency by annuloplasty under direct vision. *Lancet* 1957;77:446–449.

154. Duran CG, Pomar JL, Revuelta JM, et al. Conservative operation for mitral insufficiency. Critical analysis supported by postoperative hemodynamic studies in 72 patients. *J Thorac Cardiovasc Surg* 1980;79:326.

155. Sand ME, Naftel DC, Blackstone EH, et al. A comparison of repair and replacement for mitral valve incompetence. *J Thorac Cardiovasc Surg* 1987;94(2):208–219.

156. Edwards JE. Pathology of mitral incompetence. In: Silver MD, ed. *Cardiovascular Pathology.* vol. 1. New York: Churchill Livingstone, 1983:575.

157. Gordis L. The virtual disappearance of rheumatic fever in the United States: lessons in the rise and fall of disease. T. Duckett Jones Memorial Lecture. *Circulation* 1985;72:1155.

158. Christenson JT, Jordan B, Bloch A, et al. Should a regurgitant mitral valve be replaced simultaneously with a stenotic valve? *Tex Heart Inst J* 2000;27:350–355.

159. Gillinov AM, Blackstone EH, White J, et al. Durability of combined aortic and mitral valve repair. *Ann Thorac Surg* 2001;72(1):20–27.

160. Acar C, Farge A, Ramsheyi A. Mitral valve replacement using a cryopreserved mitral homograft. *Ann Thorac Surg* 1994;57(3):746–748.

161. Chauvaud S, Waldmann T, d'Attellis N, et al. Homograft replacement of the mitral valve in young recipients: mid-term results. *Eur J Cardiothorac Surg* 2003;23(4):560–566.

162. Dekker DL, Piziaii RL, Dong E Jr. A system for ultrasonically imaging the human heart in three dimensions. *Comput Biomed Res* 1974;7:544–553.

163. Hung J, Lang R, Flachskampf F, et al. 3D echocardiography: a review of the current status and future directions. *J Am Soc Echocardiogr* 2007;20:213–233.

164. Mahmood F, Karthik S, Subramaniam B, et al. Intraoperative application of geometric three-dimensional mitral valve assessment package: a feasibility study. *J Cardiothorac Vasc Anesth* 2008;22:292–298.

165. Abraham T, Warner J, Kon N, et al. Feasibility, accuracy, and incremental value of intraoperative three-dimensional transesophageal echocardiography in valve surgery. *Am J Cardiol* 1997;80:1577–1582.

166. Ahmed S, Nanda N, Miller A, et al. Usefulness of transesophageal three-dimensional echocardiography in the identification of individual segment/scallop prolapse of the mitral valve. *Echocardiography* 2003;20:203–209.

167. Langerveld J, Valocik G, Plokker T, et al. Additional value of three-dimensional transesophageal echocardiography for patients with mitral valve stenosis undergoing balloon valvuloplasty. *J Am Soc Echo* 2003;16:841–849.

168. Applebaum RM, Kasliwal RR, Kanojia A, et al. Utility of three-dimensional echocardiography during balloon mitral valvuloplasty. *J Am Coll Cardiol* 1998;32:1405–1409.

169. Zomorano J, Cordeiro P, Sugeng L, et al. Real-time three-dimensional echocardiography for rheumatic mitral valve stenosis evaluation: an accurate and novel approach. *J Am Coll Cardiol* 2004;43:2091–2096.

170. Bredurda C, Griffin B, Rodriguez L, et al. Three-dimensional echocardiographic planimetry of maximal regurgitant orifice area in myxomatous mitral regurgitation: intraoperative comparison with proximal flow convergence. *J Am Coll Cardiol* 1998;32:432–437.

171. Lange A, Palka P, Donnelly E, et al. Quantification of mitral regurgitation orifice area by 3-dimensional echocardiography: comparison with effective regurgitant orifice area by PISA method and proximal regurgitant jet diameter. *Int J Cardiol* 2002;86:87–98.

172. Sugeng L, Spencer K, Mor-Avi V, et al. Dynamic three-dimensional color flow Doppler: an improved technique for the assessment of mitral regurgitation. *Echocardiography* 2003;20:265–273.

173. Shernan S, Shook D, Fox J. Feasibility of real time three-dimensional intraoperative transesophageal echocardiography using a matrix transducer. *JACC* 2007;49:119A.

174. Sugeng L, Shernan S, Salgo I, et al. Real-time three-dimension atransesophageal echocardiography using fully-sampled matrix array probe. *J Am Coll Cardiol* 2008;52(6):446–449.

175. Sugeng L, Shernan S, Weinert L, et al. Real-time 3D transesophageal echocardiography in valve disease: comparison with surgical findings and evaluation of prosthetic valves. *J Am Soc Echocardiogr* 2008;21:1347–1354.

QUESTIONS

1. Type IIIb leaflet motion is most associated with which of the following?
   A. Diastolic leaflet restriction
   B. Excessive systolic leaflet motion
   C. Ruptured chords
   D. Systolic leaflet restriction
   E. Leaflet perforation

2. Advancing the TEE probe from a midesophageal four-chamber view by 1 to 2 cm allows better imaging of this structure?
   A. LVOT
   B. A1
   C. P2
   D. A3
   E. Left atrial appendage

3. This is a predictor of periannular disruption during the pre-CPB exam?
   A. Bileaflet prolapse
   B. Severe mitral annular calcification
   C. Severely enlarged left atrium
   D. Dilated left ventricle
   E. Severe mitral stenosis

4. This term is given to mitral valve prolapse involving multiple segments of both the anterior and posterior leaflets?
   A. Barlow syndrome
   B. Myxomatous degeneration
   C. Bicommissural disease
   D. Fibroelastic deficiency
   E. Type IIIB leaflet motion

5. In a patient with restrictive diastolic dysfunction and low cardiac output syndrome which of the following is the best method to determine the severity of mitral stenosis in a patient with rheumatic valve disease?
   A. Peak mitral inflow velocity
   B. Pressure half time
   C. Mean pressure gradient
   D. Deceleration time
   E. Proximal isovelocity surface area

6. Which of the following patients is most likely to have post-repair mitral stenosis?
   A. Annuloplasty ring placement
   B. Quadrangular resection for P2 prolapse
   C. Type II leaflet motion on pre-CPB assessment
   D. Commissural prolapse with a commissuroplasty
   E. Mechanical mitral valve replacement

7. The simplified PISA method for determining the effective regurgitant orifice area in mitral regurgitation ($ROA = r^2/2$) should be modified in what way in patients with poor contractility?
   A. Need to use the angle correction alpha
   B. Need to change the Nyquist limit to 50 cm/s
   C. Should to use a different method to estimate ROA
   D. Need to change the Nyquist limit to 30 cm/s
   E. No change is needed

8. Real-time 3D echocardiography compared to 2D echocardiography typically has which of the following?
   A. Better temporal resolution
   B. Less artifacts
   C. Decreased line density
   D. Better visualization of far field structures
   E. Replaces the 2D exam

CHAPTER 31

Assessment in Aortic Valve Surgery

Ankur R. Gosalia ▪ Christopher A. Troianos

The prevalence of aortic valve disease among surgical patients is steadily increasing as our population ages. Aortic valve replacement (AVR) remains the most common valve replacement procedure in the United States and the second most common cardiac operation overall following coronary artery bypass grafting (CABG). The Society of Thoracic Surgeons' database reported that over 13,800 AVR procedures and nearly 4,000 combined AVR and CABG procedures were performed in the United States in 2005 (1). Operative mortality for AVR has remained constant over the past decade while perioperative complications have decreased significantly (2). A thorough and detailed understanding of the use of intraoperative transesophageal echocardiography (TEE) during aortic valve surgery has the potential to improve patient care by establishing new diagnoses, confirming the severity of known disease, and assisting with hemodynamic management, thus improving surgical decision making, and decreasing cost (3).

TEE provides high-resolution images of the aortic valve due to the close proximity of the valve to the esophagus. Evaluation of leaflet morphology and mobility, degree of calcification, aortic root disease, and etiology of valve dysfunction are important aspects of two-dimensional (2D) and 3D evaluation. Clinical information provided by TEE permits appropriate hemodynamic management for patients with aortic valve disease, which is particularly important in patients with manifestation of chronic aortic valve stenosis, regurgitation, or both. The application of Doppler echocardiography (pulsed wave, continuous wave, and color) with 2D and 3D imaging allows for the complete evaluation of stenotic and regurgitant lesions. A consensus statement from the American College of Cardiology, the American Heart Association, and the American Society of Echocardiography designated intraoperative TEE a Class I indication ("evidence and/or general agreement that a given procedure or treatment is useful and effective") in patients undergoing surgical repair of valvular lesions and many experts suggest the use of routine TEE during all AVRs (4,5). Numerous studies demonstrate modifications in therapy in 10% to 40% of cases when TEE is used intraoperatively (Table 31.1) (4). Accurate determination of aortic valve and root dimensions is important for guiding therapy and choosing the type and size of a prosthesis to implant, along with determining the likelihood of patient-prosthesis mismatch after replacement. Postoperative echocardiographic evaluation permits rapid assessment of complications associated with repair or replacement, and prompts surgical intervention to correct inadequate valve repair and reoperation for complications.

The transesophageal echocardiographic anatomy of the aortic valve and assessment of disease pathophysiology are presented in Chapter 14. This chapter will review the echocardiographic evaluation of the aortic valve with particular emphasis on critical issues that arise during aortic valve surgery including implications for surgical intervention, intraoperative hemodynamic management, and associated cardiovascular lesions.

TABLE 31.1	Usefulness of Intraoperative Echocardiography in Adult Cardiac Surgery			
Author	Year	N	New Information (%)	Change in Management (%)
Click	2000	3245	15	14
Couture	2000	851	—	14.6
Michel-Cherqui	2000	203	12.8	10.8
Mishra	1998	5016	22.9	—
Sutton	1998	238	38.6	9.7

From Cheitlin MD, et al. ACC/AHA/ASE 2003 Guideline update for the clinical application of echocardiography: summary article. JACC 2003;42:954–970.

CRITICAL ISSUES DURING AORTIC VALVE SURGERY

Echocardiography provides essential information in the evaluation of patients with aortic valve disease. Intraoperative echocardiography is used to confirm the preoperative diagnosis and etiology of valve dysfunction, determine the feasibility of repair versus replacement, measure the annulus and aortic root to estimate the valve size and type to be implanted, identify other associated cardiac pathology that may require surgical intervention, and evaluate the implanted or repaired valve function for complications. Preoperative valve sizing is important when valves of limited availability, such as homografts, are to be implanted (6). For patients undergoing AVR for aortic stenosis, intraoperative TEE alters the surgical plan in 13% of patients (Table 31.2) (7). During the intraoperative examination of the patient scheduled for AVR for aortic stenosis, it is imperative to rule out other causes of obstruction to left ventricle (LV) outflow such as subaortic and supravalvular stenosis. Subaortic stenosis (subaortic membrane or ridge, and asymmetric septal hypertrophy) and supravalvular stenosis (narrowed aortic root) mimic aortic stenosis but do not represent true valvular stenosis and are not normally treated by AVR, therefore requiring a change in the surgical plan. Many of the echocardiographic techniques used for hemodynamic assessment of the aortic valve, however, can also be used to evaluate the severity of subvalvular and supravalvular pathology.

The patient with mild to moderate aortic valve disease scheduled for non–aortic valve cardiac surgery, as well as the patient with previously unsuspected aortic valve disease, presents clinical dilemmas. Another clinical dilemma is the setting of low-gradient aortic stenosis, in which the valve appears restricted but does not have a high-pressure gradient across the aortic valve.

ROLE OF TEE IN SURGICAL DECISION MAKING

Intraoperative TEE among patients with known aortic valve disease undergoing valve replacement is used to confirm the preoperative diagnosis and determine the etiology of valve dysfunction. High-resolution images, owing to the close proximity of the valve and the esophagus, permit accurate diagnosis of the mechanism of valve dysfunction, a key aspect for determining the feasibility of repair versus replacement. The vast majority of aortic valves suitable for repair have regurgitant lesions rather than stenotic lesions. Valve repair for patients with aortic dissection involves resuspension of the cusps and is easily performed and highly successful in the absence of additional leaflet pathology.

Postoperatively, TEE is used to evaluate the success of repair or function of the prosthetic valve. The degree of residual aortic regurgitation (AR) is an important aspect of valve repair evaluation and determines the need for further surgery and possible valve replacement. The number and area of regurgitant jets present after AVR are less than after mitral valve replacement, but there is a similar percentage decrease of regurgitant jet area after protamine administration (8). Patients undergoing the Ross procedure for autograft replacement of their aortic valve also require evaluation of the prosthetic pulmonic valve.

Moderate Aortic Stenosis

Surgical decision making in patients with mild to moderate disease when discovered during CABG is important because of the higher mortality associated with reoperation in patients with aortic stenosis with previous CABG (9). The most recently published ACC/AHA Practice Guidelines emphasize the importance of describing aortic stenosis as a continuum, in that no single value defines severity. Instead, severity is graded on the basis of a variety of hemodynamic and natural history data,

---

TABLE 31.2	**Impact of Intraoperative TEE During AVR in 383 Patients**
New Findings	**Surgical Impact**
Before bypass	
7 PFO	2 closed
2 masses (TV fibroelastoma, LVOT accessory chordae)	2 removed
5 LAA thrombi	5 removed
10 homograft annular size measurements	10 sized
After bypass	
1 new wall motion abnormality	No change

PFO, patent foramen ovale; LAA, left atrial appendage; TV tricuspid valve: LVOT, left ventricular outflow obstruction.
From Nowrangi SK, Connolly HM, Freeman WK, et al. Impact of intraoperative transesophageal echocardiography among patients undergoing aortic valve replacement for aortic stenosis. J Am Soc Echocardiogr 2001;14:863–866.

TABLE 31.3	Grading Aortic Stenosis			
Indicator		Mild	Moderate	Severe
Jet velocity (m/s)		<3.0	3.0–4.0	>4.0
Mean gradient (mm Hg)		<25	25–40	>40
Valve area (cm²)		>1.5	1.0–1.5	<1.0
Valve area index (cm²/m²)				<0.6

Source: *Bonow RO, Carabello BA, Chatterjee K, et al. ACC/AHA 2006 guidelines for the management of patients with valvular heart disease. J Am Coll Cardiol 2006;48:e1–e148.*

specifically aortic jet velocity, mean pressure gradient, and valve area (Table 31.3) (10).

Patients with coronary artery disease and moderate aortic stenosis may be asymptomatic from their valve disease and would otherwise not be candidates for AVR. Consideration is made for concomitant AVR because they are undergoing CABG surgery. AVR is a class I indication for patients undergoing CABG with severe aortic stenosis (valve area < 1.0 cm², mean gradient > 40 mm Hg, jet velocity > 4.0 m/s) (10). AVR is a class IIb recommendation for patients with mild aortic stenosis (aortic valve area [AVA] > 1.5 cm², aortic valve gradient [AVG] < 25 mm Hg, jet velocity < 3.0 m/s), undergoing CABG. Most experts do not recommend performing combined CABG–AVR surgery in this setting due to the higher operative and 10-year mortality, 2% to 6% per year complication rate of prosthetic heart valves, and because only 12% of patients with mild aortic stenosis will progress to severe aortic stenosis within 10 years (11).

Patients with moderate aortic stenosis (AVA of 1.0–1.5 cm², AVG of 25–40 mm Hg, jet velocity 3.0–4.0 m/s) undergoing CABG present a clinical dilemma as to whether the patient should have CABG alone or combined AVR and CABG, but the most recent guidelines consider this to be a class IIa indication (10). Further considerations should be made in the setting of significant valve calcifications and rapid progression of aortic jet velocity in the setting of concomitant coronary artery disease because outcomes in this subset of patients with moderate aortic stenosis are worse than previously assumed (12). The presence of moderate tosevere calcification suggests that progression of aortic stenosis may be rapid (10).

The size of the annulus must also be considered when deciding whether a valve with mild tomoderate stenosis should be replaced. Patients with a small annular diameter may not derive as significant a benefit from AVR as patients in whom a larger valve could be implanted. The other point to consider is that AVR after previous CABG is associated with higher mortality than combined aortic valve and coronary bypass surgery (13). It is therefore important to identify moderate aortic stenosis during coronary bypass surgery so that the surgeon has the opportunity to perform combined coronary artery bypass with

valve replacement surgery in order to avoid the higher mortality associated with reoperation.

The degree of aortic stenosis is an important consideration for surgical management, as valves with a smaller valve area will progress more rapidly to severe aortic stenosis. The average annual rate of progression of aortic valvular stenosis is 0.1 cm² per year and factors including smoking, renal insufficiency, and hypercholesterolemia are associated with a more rapid rate of progression (14–16). A 1.5 cm² AVA will progress to a 1.0 cm² area within 5 years in the average patient, coupled with patient age and overall risk factors for a prolonged duration of cardiopulmonary bypass, are clinical issues to consider when making a decision regarding combined surgery for a moderately stenotic valve.

The planimetric method of area determination using the ME AV SAX view in two and three dimensions provides good correlation with other methods used for assessment of aortic stenosis (17) and is usually very accurate and easy to perform in patients with mild to moderate aortic stenosis (Figs. 31.1 and 31.2). This method of determining AVA is more difficult and less reliable if the valve is severely calcified. Calcium deposits, particularly

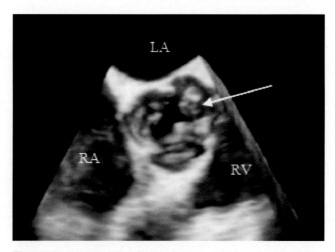

Figure 31.1. Three-dimensional transesophageal echocardiogram of the midesophageal aortic valve short-axis view during systole in a patient with moderate aortic stenosis. Arrow identifies calcification on the left coronary cusp. LA, left atrium; RA, right atrium; RV, right ventricle.

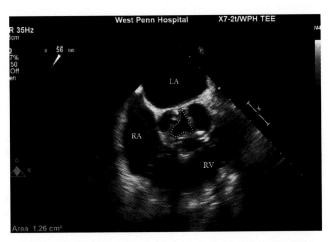

Figure 31.2. Two-dimensional transesophageal echocardiogram of the midesophageal aortic valve short-axis view during systole in a patient with moderate aortic stenosis (AVA = 1.26 cm²) determined with planimetry. LA, left atrium; RA, right atrium; RV, right ventricle.

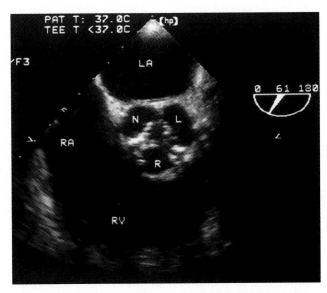

Figure 31.3. Transesophageal echocardiogram of the midesophageal aortic valve short-axis view during systole in a patient with severe calcific aortic stenosis. L, left coronary cusp; R, right coronary cusp; N, noncoronary cusp; LA, left atrium; RA, right atrium; RV, right ventricle.

if they are located along the posterior aspect of the valve, will shadow the anterior aspect of the valve and make it difficult to define the leaflet edges, making valve area determination with planimetry more challenging.

Low-Gradient Aortic Stenosis

A particularly challenging dilemma is the patient with aortic stenosis and low cardiac output, or "low-gradient aortic stenosis." The clinical question is whether the patient has a low gradient due to mild aortic stenosis or severe aortic stenosis and severe left ventricular dysfunction. A gradient across a stenotic orifice is dynamic because of its dependence on flow. As the flow (or cardiac output) through the valve decreases, the gradient also decreases. Systolic function is preserved until late in the progression of aortic stenosis when left ventricular dilation develops. Severe aortic stenosis (Fig. 31.3) has a dismal prognosis when associated with systolic dysfunction and congestive heart failure. Medical management in this setting only offers a 2-year survival, making AVR the most viable option (18). Systolic dysfunction due to aortic stenosis is usually reversible with valve replacement, but systolic dysfunction due to myocardial infarction, extensive coronary artery disease, or superimposed myocardial fibrosis may not improve after AVR and causes an underestimation of the severity of aortic stenosis by gradient determination (19). Patients with low-gradient aortic stenosis have a small valve area (<1.0 cm²), impaired systolic function, and a low mean transvalvular pressure gradient (<30 mm Hg). Although less than 5% of patients with aortic stenosis represent this subset, their management is the most controversial (20). Mortality for AVR in this setting is increased as high as 18% if the ejection fraction is less than 30% to 35%. Without surgical intervention, the 4-year survival is only 20% (18–22).

A recent study assessed the outcome of patient having AVR with low transvalvular pressure gradients and LV dysfunction. AVR combined with CABG despite poor contractile reserve, in the setting of low transvalvular gradient, was associated with improved functional status, albeit still with higher operative mortality. Surgical mortality was directly related to older age and smaller prosthesis size, suggesting that valve-prosthesis patient mismatch may play an important role in outcome in this subset of aortic stenosis patients with low gradients (18). There is increasing evidence that severe prosthesis-patient mismatch will lead to poor left ventricular mass regression. This may also be an independent risk factor of survival time after adjustment for age, ejection fraction, atrial fibrillation, serum creatinine level, hemoglobin level, and New York Heart Association heart failure class (23,24).

Intraoperative echocardiography when combined with the dobutamine stress test is useful in determining contractile reserve and perioperative risk. A 20% increase in stroke volume from baseline to peak dobutamine dose identifies contractile reserve (22,25). A large prospective, multicenter study revealed operative mortality of 5% and 32%, respectively, in patients with or without contractile reserve (26). Long-term survival was predicted by AVR and left ventricular contractile reserve. Six-year survival after AVR among patients with contractile reserve is greater than 75% (25) (Fig. 31.4). Dobutamine administration may also help to identify true severe anatomic aortic stenosis in the setting of low-gradient disease. Patients *without* true anatomically severe stenosis will exhibit an increase in valve area and little change in gradient with increased stroke volume. For example, a valve area increase of 0.2 cm² or greater with little change in gradient most likely does not represent true severe anatomic

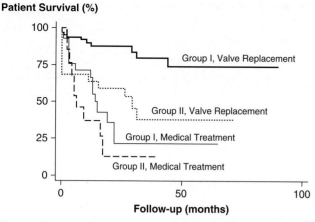

Figure 31.4. Kaplan-Meier survival estimates in patients with low-gradient aortic stenosis. Group I patients displayed positive contractile reserve with dobutamine administration. Group II patients did not display contractile reserve with dobutamine administration. (Monin JL, Quere JP, et al. Low-gradient aortic stenosis: operative risk stratification and predictors for long-term outcome: a multicenter study using dobutamine stress hemodynamics. *Circulation* 2003 Jul 22;108[3]:319–324.)

stenosis. In contrast, patients with an anatomically fixed stenotic valve will exhibit an increase in their gradient but no change in their valve area as stroke volume increases (10,26,27) (Fig. 31.5).

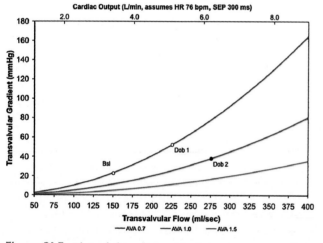

Figure 31.5. Plot of the relationship between mean gradient (y-axis) and transvalvular flow (x-axis), according to the Gorlin formula for three different AVA values (0.7, 1.0, and 1.5 cm²). Cardiac output is also shown (x-axis, top). At low transvalvular flows, mean gradient is low at all three values. Two different responses to dobutamine testing are shown. Baseline flow is 150 mL/s. Response *Dob 1* illustrates a significant increase in transvalvular gradient (area remains at AVA of 0.7 cm²) following dobutamine administration, signifying fixed severe aortic stenosis. Response *Dob 2* illustrates minimal change in transvalvular gradient (and an increase in functional AVA to 1.0 cm²) following dobutamine administration, signifying nonsevere nonfixed aortic stenosis. HR, heart rate; SEP, systolic ejection time. (Grayburn P. Assessment of low-gradient aortic stenosis with dobutamine. *Circulation* 2006;113:604–606.)

Hemodynamic Therapy with Altered Ventricular Compliance

TEE is important for guiding hemodynamic therapy during and after aortic valve surgery. An accurate evaluation of left ventricular function is important during the immediate postoperative period because of the inherently low ventricular compliance present among patients with left ventricular hypertrophy due to the adaptive mechanisms of long-standing aortic stenosis or chronic hypertension. Myocardial preservation during cardiopulmonary bypass in the setting of left ventricular hypertrophy with concomitant coronary artery disease is difficult secondary to the increased ventricular muscle mass, which may lead to significant postbypass ventricular dysfunction. Left ventricular volume and contractility are more accurately determined by 2D and 3D echocardiographic assessment of LV cavity size than by pulmonary artery catheter estimates of filling pressure (28). Characteristically, patients with low LV compliance often require volume infusion despite high filling pressures in the postbypass period. TEE also provides early indication of myocardial ischemia, even in the absence of coronary artery disease, by assessment of regional wall motion. An assessment of diastolic function using mitral valve inflow velocities, pulmonary venous pulse wave Doppler morphology, and tissue Doppler imaging of mitral annular excursion can also guide therapy aimed at improving ventricular filling time and adjusting the contractile state. TEE is utilized to diagnose and aid in the management of post-AVR mitral regurgitation (MR) following extensive decalcification of the aortic annulus and annular enlargement (29). Clinical information provided by TEE permits appropriate hemodynamic management for patients with aortic valve disease before, during, and after aortic valve surgery.

APPROACH

Focused Intraoperative Echocardiography Examination for Aortic Valve Surgery

A focused intraoperative echocardiography examination is a brief directed assessment of the anatomy and function most pertinent to the surgical approach. For patients in whom the preoperative diagnosis of aortic valve disease is confirmed and well established, this usually entails a verification of the preoperative findings including the elucidation of the etiology of valve dysfunction, an estimation of valve size, and an assessment of associated findings. A complete discussion of the echocardiographic evaluation of aortic stenosis and regurgitation is given in Chapter 14. The pertinent portions of that evaluation specific to the surgical decision-making process for aortic valve surgery are discussed in this section.

The diagnosis of severe aortic stenosis is confirmed simply by a 2D echocardiographic evaluation of the valve, utilizing the midesophageal aortic valve short-axis view (ME AV SAX) (Fig. 31.6). The valve appears severely restricted and heavily calcified. This view is important for tracing the aortic valve orifice area, using planimetry, and for identifying the site of AR, using color flow Doppler. Limitations to planimetry include the following:

1. Inability to obtain an adequate short-axis view where the valve appears circular in shape, all three cusps are viewed simultaneously, and they are equal in shape. A cross section that is oblique or inferior to the leaflet tips overestimates the orifice size (Fig. 14.19).
2. Heavy calcification (particularly posterior), which causes shadowing of the valve
3. The presence of "pinhole" aortic stenosis, in which the valve orifice cannot be identified

The presence of these elements suggests advanced disease or the likelihood of rapid progression of aortic stenosis, and favors a decision to replace the valve. The midesophageal aortic valve long-axis (ME AV LAX) (Fig. 31.7) view provides imaging of the left ventricular outflow tract (LVOT), aortic valve, and aortic root and allows differentiation of valvular from subvalvular and supravalvular pathology. An important sign of aortic stenosis is leaflet doming during systole (Fig. 31.8). The leaflets are curved toward the midline of the aorta instead of parallel to the aortic wall. Leaflet doming is such an important observation that this finding alone is sufficient for the qualitative diagnosis of aortic stenosis. Coincident with doming is reduced leaflet separation (<15 mm), which is appreciated in both the short- and long-axis views of the aortic valve.

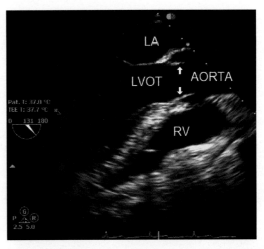

Figure 31.7. Two-dimensional transesophageal echocardiogram of the midesophageal aortic valve long-axis view during systole. A multiplane angle of 131 degrees provides a long-axis view of the left ventricular outflow tract, aortic valve, and aortic root. *Arrows* identify normal aortic valve leaflets that open parallel with the walls of the aorta. LA, left atrium; LVOT, left ventricular outflow tract; RV, right ventricle.

Quantifying the severity of stenosis by either gradient or area determination is usually not necessary during the focused examination of a patient whose diagnosis of aortic stenosis was firmly established preoperatively but is often included in a more comprehensive examination. Area determination by planimetry in patients with severe aortic stenosis may be difficult to perform due to shadowing of the valve from heavy calcification. A peak velocity measurement provides some indication of the severity

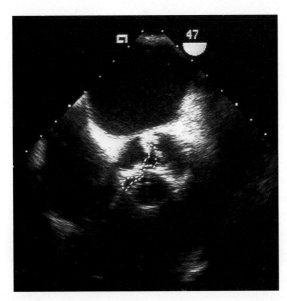

Figure 31.6. Transesophageal echocardiogram of the ME aortic valve short-axis view during systole in a patient with severe calcific aortic stenosis, using planimetry to measure AVA. Note the heavy calcifications and shadowing leading to difficult planimetry assessment.

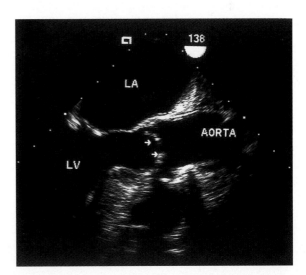

Figure 31.8. Two-dimensional transesophageal echocardiogram of the midesophageal aortic valve long-axis view during systole in a patient with severe aortic stenosis. A multiplane angle of 138 degrees provides this view of an aortic valve with doming leaflets (*arrows*). Leaflet doming is a qualitative sign of severe stenosis. LA, left atrium; LV, left ventricle.

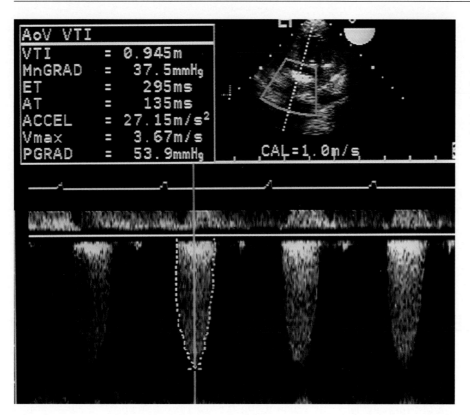

Figure 31.9. Continuous wave spectral Doppler velocities through a stenotic aortic valve. The fine, feathery appearance of the high (3.67 m/s) velocities with a midsystolic peak indicates flow through a stenotic aortic valve. The denser lower velocities near the baseline indicated flow through the LVOT.

of stenosis but must be taken in the context of the left ventricular function, as previously discussed (Fig. 31.9).

An accurate, comprehensive intraoperative examination must be performed for patients in whom the severity of disease is borderline or moderate because the data are important in the surgical decision-making process. The intraoperative echocardiography examination in these situations should utilize the full diagnostic potential of this tool and be performed by echocardiographers with advanced training (30). More than one method should be employed to assess the severity of disease, because the assessment will be used to guide the surgical decision. These include 2D echocardiography, 3D echocardiography, gradient determination by measurement of transaortic velocity, and area determination by planimetry and the continuity equation as described in Chapter 14.

The recent introduction of 3D echocardiography into clinical practice allows a more detailed evaluation of the LVOT and AVA, compared to 2D echocardiography (Fig. 31.10). Direct measurement of the aortic valve orifice and LVOT using off-line selection of specific planes allows the echocardiographer to precisely measure the desired orifice. Three-dimensional planimetry of aortic valve orifice area (Fig. 31.11) correlates better with invasive measurements and 2D planimetry than with the continuity equation (31). Real-time intraoperative 3D echocardiography is also useful for identifying aortic valve abnormalities such as quadricuspid aortic valve that are sometimes missed with 2D echocardiography (32).

A focused examination in patients with severe AR undergoing aortic valve surgery involves a 2D and 3D echocardiographic evaluation to determine the etiology of the regurgitation. Color flow Doppler interrogation of the LVOT and aortic valve allows for the evaluation of the severity (Table 31.4) (10) and etiology

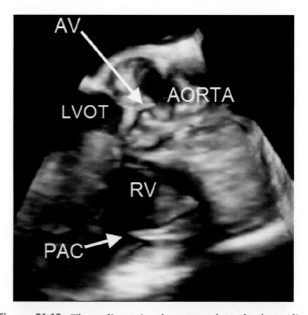

Figure 31.10. Three-dimensional transesophageal echocardiogram of the midesophageal aortic valve long-axis view during diastole with the arrow indicating the aortic valve. Using off-line selection of specific 3D planes, direct caliper measurements may be obtained of the valvular, subvalvular, and supravalvular apparatus. LVOT, left ventricular outflow tract; RV, right ventricle; PAC, pulmonary artery catheter; AV, aortic valve.

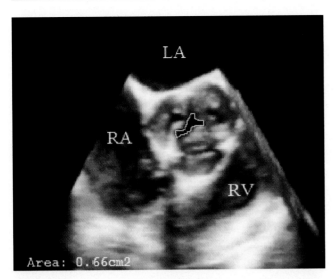

Figure 31.11. Three-dimensional transesophageal echocardiogram of the short-axis aortic valve view in the setting of severe aortic stenosis. Aortic valve orifice area is 0.66 cm², determined using planimetry.

of the regurgitation, respectively (Fig. 31.12). AR is caused by either intrinsic disease of the aortic cusps or secondarily from diseases affecting the ascending aorta. Intrinsic valvular problems include rheumatic, calcific, and myxomatous valvular disease; endocarditis; traumatic injury; and congenital abnormalities. Conditions affecting the ascending aorta that lead to AR include annular dilatation and aortic dissection (secondary to blunt trauma or hypertension), mycotic aneurysm, cystic medial necrosis, Marfan's syndrome, and chronic hypertension. The most common cause of pure AR is no longer postinflammatory due to the decreasing prevalence of rheumatic heart disease among cardiac surgical patients (33). Aortic root dilation (Fig. 31.13) is now the most common etiologic factor, due to the increased prevalence of degenerative disease, followed by postinflammatory disease and bicuspid valve disease.

It is important to note that in the setting of aortic stenosis, leaflets that dome during systole often do not completely coapt during diastole, causing AR. The etiology directs the surgeon as to the feasibility of repair versus replacement, and the techniques to be employed for repair. The postoperative assessment is important for ascertaining the success of the repair. The degree of residual AR is an essential aspect of valve repair evaluation and determines the need for further revisions or possible valve replacement.

For patients undergoing valve replacement, another aspect of the focused examination is determination of valve size and suitability of the implantation of specific valve types. The midesophageal aortic valve long-axis view in two and three dimensions is used to measure annular diameter and size of the aortic root. A size discrepancy greater than 10% between the diameters of the aortic annulus and sinotubular junction (STJ) makes implantation of a stentless aortic valve unfeasible. The points at which the measurements are made are indicated in Figure 31.14. The annular diameter measurement is the size used for implantation of mechanical and stented bioprosthetic valves, while the STJ diameter is the size used for implantation of stentless aortic valves.

Intraoperative echocardiography is not only critical in the evaluation of the aortic valve but in the evaluation of cardiac and vascular structures that are affected by the techniques employed during aortic valve surgery. Evaluation of left ventricular function is important, because patients with aortic stenosis develop left ventricular hypertrophy, decreased left ventricular compliance, and are prone to myocardial ischemia. TEE provides early indication of myocardial ischemia through monitoring of regional wall motion, and a global assessment of overall contractility and volume loading. Patients with aortic stenosis have decreased left ventricular compliance; therefore, assessment of preload using pulmonary artery catheter data is often misleading. TEE provides a more accurate assessment of preload by imaging intracavitary

TABLE 31.4	**Grading AR**		
Indicator	**Mild**	**Moderate**	**Severe**
Angiographic grade	1+	2+ and 3+	4+
Color Doppler jet width	<25% of LVOT	25%–64%	>64%
Doppler vena contracta width (cm)	<0.3	0.3–0.6	>0.6
Regurgitant volume (ml per beat)	<30	30–59	≥60
Regurgitant fraction (%)	<30	30–49	≥50
Regurgitant orifice area (cm²)	<0.10	0.10–0.29	≥0.30
Pressure half-time (*Supportive sign*)	>500 ms	200–500 ms	<200 ms

LVOT, left ventricular outflow tract; ms, milliseconds.
Source: *Bonow RO, Carabello BA, Chatterjee K, et al. ACC/AHA 2006 guidelines for the management of patients with valvular heart disease. J Am Coll Cardiol 2006;48:e1–e148.*

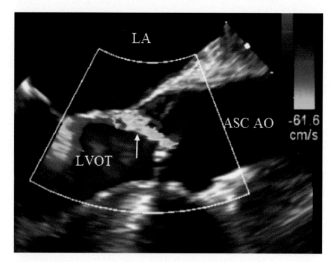

Figure 31.12. Transesophageal echocardiogram with color flow Doppler in a patient with eccentric AR. The AR (*arrow*) is identified by the color flow disturbance that originates from the aortic valve and directed toward the ante rior mitral valve leaflet. LVOT, left ventricular outflow tract; ASC AO, ascending aorta; LA, left atrium.

volume and global contractility. Patients with long-standing AR have chronic left ventricular volume overload. This leads to progressive left ventricular dilation over many years while systolic function remains preserved. Ejection fraction is initially normal with AR while end-diastolic dimensions are increased. In contrast to aortic stenosis, the ventricle remains relatively compliant until systolic dysfunction ensues late in the course of the disease process. Unlike aortic stenosis, the systolic dysfunction is not significantly reversible. Acute AR is not associated with left ventricular dilation because adaptive left ventricular dilation has not occurred. This lack of adaptation is associated with a decreased left ventricular compliance and

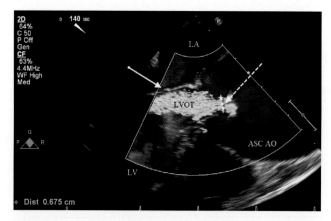

Figure 31.13. Two-dimensional transesophageal echocardiogram of the midesophageal aortic valve long-axis view with color flow Doppler in a patient with severe AR due to aortic root dilation. Vena contracta (*dashed arrow*) measures 0.675 cm. *Solid arrow* identifies anterior mitral valve leaflet. LA, left atrium; LV, left ventricle; LVOT, left ventricular outflow tract; ASC AO, ascending aorta.

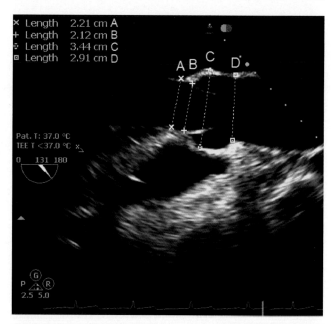

Figure 31.14. Two-dimensional transesophageal echocardiogram of the midesophageal aortic valve long-axis view, indicating measurements of the left ventricular outflow tract (*A*), AVA (*B*), sinuses of Valsalva (*C*), and the STJ (*D*) diameters.

a rapid onset of symptoms. It is imperative to ascertain changes in left ventricular filling and ejection patterns for both aortic stenosis and regurgitation during the intraoperative examination because the severity of the changes will alter the surgical plan and help guide the need for inotropic support during separation from cardiopulmonary bypass.

Patients with aortic valve disease develop diastolic dysfunction, which may also be evaluated and monitored with intraoperative echocardiography. Long-standing left ventricular dysfunction leads to MR, pulmonary hypertension, and ultimately right ventricular dysfunction. TEE is useful for managing these problems intraoperatively and for guiding surgical management decisions regarding the need for cardiac surgical intervention. MR as a consequence of aortic stenosis commonly improves after AVR with the resultant afterload reduction in the absence of mitral leaflet pathology. However, MR in patients with intrinsic mitral valve disease, left atrial dilation, or mitral calcifications may not improve after AVR (34). The surgical treatment of mitral valve regurgitation at the time of AVR still remains controversial. MR as a consequence of hypertrophic obstructive cardiomyopathy commonly worsens after AVR secondary to afterload reduction and hypovolemia. The presence of concomitant mitral stenosis causes an underestimation of the severity of aortic stenosis by gradient determination because of decreased trans-aortic blood flow. Christenson et al. (36) studied 60 consecutive patients with aortic stenosis and concluded that patient with concomitant MR may not benefit from mitral surgery in the absence of echocardiographic signs of chordal or papillary muscle rupture and absence of coronary artery disease (35). MR in this population either remained the same or improved. Moazami et al. (37) also studied patients undergoing isolated AVR among whom many had concomitant functional (1 to 4+) MR. Survival was directly related to the severity of preexisting MR prior to AVR. Patients with 1 to 2+ preoperative MR had a 3-year survival of 98% compared to patients with 3 to 4+ MR who had a 78% 3-year survival. The authors advocate repair of moderate-to-severe MR at the time of aortic valve surgery (36).

Dilation of the ascending aorta may be a consequence of long-standing aortic stenosis due to the body's adaptive mechanism in promoting left ventricular ejection, or may be secondary to intrinsic disease within the aortic walls. The latter is more likely to require surgical intervention, while the former does not require surgical correction unless the dilation is severe. Evaluation of the aorta is also important for determining the cannulation site and guiding perfusion strategies, and for identifying atheromatous disease in the proximal ascending aorta, which is implicated as a leading cause of neurologic injury. A high prevalence of aortic root dilation has been demonstrated in patients with bicuspid aortic valve (BAV), irrespective of valvular hemodynamics or age, suggesting a common developmental defect (37). BAV is also associated with increased ascending aortic diameter in patients greater than forty years of age (38). The progression of ascending aortic dilation has been shown to continue after BAV repair, suggesting that consideration should be made to concomitant replacement of the ascending aorta, if the diameter is greater than or equal to 4.5 cm (39).

Postoperatively, the echocardiographic examination is focused on the function of the prosthetic valve, postimplant or postrepair complications, and resolution of dynamic lesions not surgically addressed. Postbypass echocardiography is particularly important for patients undergoing valve repair to assess the success of repair. The presence of AR after aortic valve repair is a poor prognostic indicator, as these patients commonly require reoperation for definitive correction. Another major concern is the development of systolic anterior motion (SAM) of the anterior mitral valve leaflet after AVR for aortic stenosis. Although this condition is well recognized with asymmetric septal hypertrophy, SAM can also occur after AVR in patients with *symmetric* septal hypertrophy due to chronic aortic stenosis. This is usually a manifestation of the abrupt reduction in left ventricular afterload after AVR and hypovolemia in patients with septal or concentric hypertrophy. This left ventricular obstruction during systole leads to decreased cardiac output. There is associated MR because the anterior mitral leaflet is displaced into the LVOT during systole, rendering the mitral valve incompetent. The condition usually resolves with administration of volume, phenylephrine, and discontinuation of inotropic and chronotropic medications, and the condition must be excluded in all patients after AVR. Echocardiographic evaluation of the mitral valve and LVOT can predict the likelihood of SAM occurring based upon anatomic factors (40).

SPECIFIC AORTIC VALVE PROCEDURES

Aortic Valve Replacement

The role of intraoperative echocardiography for AVR is to confirm the diagnosis of aortic valve dysfunction and evaluate the LVOT, aortic annulus, and proximal ascending aorta for abnormalities that impact AVR, as well as evaluate secondary and associated abnormalities. An estimate of the valve size to be implanted allows the surgeon to consider prosthetic valve options and determine whether the annulus needs to be enlarged. The diameter of the annulus is measured trailing edge to leading edge at the point of leaflet attachment, using the midesophageal aortic valve long-axis view. The importance of correct sizing is magnified when the annulus is small (<21 mm) as complications related to aortic root enlargement and patient prosthetic mismatch become more common (41). The question is sometimes asked whether to make this measurement during systole or diastole. The annular size does not change significantly within the cardiac cycle, and certainly does not vary by an entire valve size. It is generally easier to make the measurement during systole because the point of leaflet attachment to the annulus is more easily identified (Fig. 31.15).

It is important to identify AR because of the impact on cardioplegia administration for myocardial protection. Severe AR necessitates an altered myocardial perfusion strategy, such as retrograde cardioplegia administration via a coronary sinus catheter, or selective antegrade cardioplegia via the coronary ostia. TEE is useful for guiding and confirming cannulation of the coronary sinus.

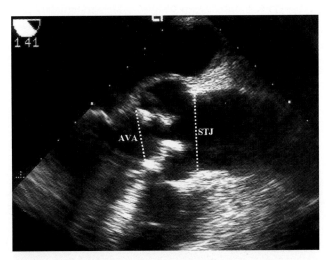

Figure 31.15. Two-dimensional transesophageal echocardiogram of the midesophageal aortic valve long-axis view with severe aortic stenosis, indicating where measurements are made of the AVA and STJ diameters.

Severe calcification within the aortic annulus may affect the ease of valve seating and the presence of paravalvular leaks after implantation. Atheromatous disease in the aortic root may necessitate debridement or aortic root replacement. Aneurysmal dilation and dissection involving the ascending aorta contribute to aortic valve dysfunction. These conditions require replacement of the ascending aorta concomitant with the aortic valve and are discussed later in this chapter. Issues of coronary reimplantation may arise depending on the procedure employed, hence the importance of evaluating regional and global left ventricular contractility before and after cardiopulmonary bypass.

Secondary abnormalities necessitate an intraoperative echocardiographic evaluation of mitral valve regurgitation, particularly for long-standing, end-stage aortic valve disease. Diastolic dysfunction, pulmonary hypertension, right ventricular dysfunction, and tricuspid regurgitation are frequently present and must be evaluated during the intraoperative examination of patients undergoing aortic valve surgery, as part of a complete examination.

Postoperatively, the TEE examination is focused on the function of the prosthetic valve, evaluation of post-implant complications, and resolution of dynamic lesions not surgically addressed. The prosthetic valve function is assessed after cardiopulmonary bypass by evaluating leaflet motion with 2D echocardiography. It is important to know the type of prosthetic valve implanted in order to make an accurate assessment of prosthetic valve function.

Some echocardiographers routinely measure the gradient across the prosthetic aortic valve during the postbypass period. Caution must be exercised to avoid unnecessary concern for valve dysfunction due to a higher than expected gradient determination immediately after cardiopulmonary bypass. The measured gradient is affected by flow through the prosthetic valve, the type of valve (bileaflet mechanical [Fig. 31.16] vs. trileaflet bioprosthetic [see Chapter 16, Fig. 16.18]), and the commonly seen hyperdynamic "high output" state immediately following bypass. The systemic vascular resistance is usually low, inotropes are being infused, and the patient may be hypovolemic and anemic. It is important to differentiate between prosthetic valve dysfunction, pressure recovery, and patient-prosthetic mismatch as explanations for a higher-than-expected gradient across an aortic valve after bypass. Pressure recovery is more likely to be observed when directing the Doppler beam through the smaller (higher velocity central) orifice of a bileaflet mechanical valve. The resultant higher peak velocity through this smaller orifice will yield a falsely elevated pressure gradient, which emphasizes the importance of evaluating leaflet mobility with 2D echocardiography, rather than relying solely on a Doppler derived estimate of the valve gradient. The phenomenon of patient-prosthetic mismatch is also associated with a higher-than-expected valve gradient. This should be considered in the clinical scenario when a smaller-than-desired valve is implanted in a relatively large patient, and when a high gradient persists beyond the hyperdynamic period shortly after bypass.

Large intravalvular leaks are not normal and require further investigation. Small intravalvular leaks immediately after bypass are not uncommon, depending on the type of prosthetic valve implanted. Bioprosthetic valves may have no intravalvular leaks or a small central leak. Mechanical valves may have one or several small intravalvular leaks and/or closure jets, depending on the type of valve implanted (Fig. 16.10). The presence of paravalvular leaks is usually a concern after AVR, but the degree of concern depends on the size of the leak and whether or not the leak persists after protamine administration. For a more comprehensive review of prosthetic valve evaluation, see Chapter 16, Assessment of Prosthetic Valves.

Stentless Aortic Valves

The ideal valve replacement for an aortic valve has a minimal transvalvular gradient, minimal risk of thromboembolism, and is durable for the life of the patient. Stentless valves and stented bioprosthetic valves do not require chronic anticoagulation therapy, but stentless valves offer a superior hemodynamic profile. The use of a stentless valve when compared to its stented equivalent has shown lower pressure gradients and earlier regression of left ventricular hypertrophy (42). The lack of a sewing ring and valve struts supporting the cusps makes implantation more time consuming and sometimes more difficult, but their absence results in a better hemodynamic profile. The pliability of stentless valves and the lack of struts allow for a more laminar flow pattern, lower pressure gradients, and a larger effective orifice size compared to a similar size stented bioprosthesis. There is also, theoretically, less stress on the leaflets of a stentless valve than a stented bioprosthesis, because the stress is distributed to the commissures and aortic wall, similar to a native aortic valve. Newer anticalcification treatments may reduce calcium deposit on these valves, prolonging their durability. The main disadvantage of these valves is the risk of distortion during implantation, leading to valve dysfunction.

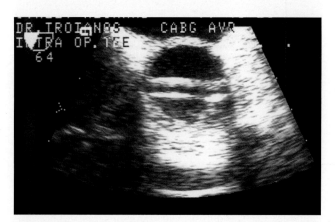

Figure 31.16. Two-dimensional TEE of the midesophageal short-axis aortic valve view during systole following AVR with a St. Jude bileaflet mechanical valve.

Proper valve sizing and implantation are crucial to the function of the stentless valve. Prebypass TEE provides a detailed assessment of native anatomic structures. Particular attention is directed to the annular and STJ diameters. Dilation of the aortic root at the STJ may result in significant valvular regurgitation. This condition must be communicated to the surgeon so that repair of the aortic root accompanies the use of a stentless valve (43). Measurements are made at the STJ and aortic valve annulus (AVA) to determine proper sizing because the valve is sewn both to the annulus (inflow sutures) and aortic wall (outflow suture line). The diameter of the annulus is measured trailing edge to leading edge at the point of leaflet attachment using the mid esophageal aortic valve long-axis view. The STJ diameter is measured trailing edge to leading edge at the top of the sinuses of Valsalva.

Stentless valves suitable for implantation in the aortic position include homografts, autografts, and manufactured or processed valves. Although there are several stentless manufactured or processed valves on the market and newer valves are being released and trialed across the globe, specific discussion in this chapter will be in reference to the most commonly used valves, the Toronto Stentless Porcine Valve (SPV) and the Medtronic Freestyle aortic root.

The Toronto SPV is an excised porcine aortic valve that has been trimmed, cross-linked, sterilized, preserved in glutaraldehyde, and wrapped in polyester fabric. The valve has the advantage of the more superior hemodynamic profile, similar to a homograft. This manufactured valve is available in sizes 21, 23, 25, 27, and 29 mm and is usually more readily available than homografts. Proper valve sizing and implantation are crucial to the function of the valve. Measurements are made at the STJ and AVA to determine proper sizing because the valve is sewn to both the annulus (inflow sutures) and aortic wall (outflow suture line) (Fig. 31.17). The diameter of the annulus is measured trailing edge to leading edge at the point of leaflet attachment using the midesophageal aortic valve long-axis view. The STJ diameter is measured trailing edge to leading edge at the top of the sinuses of Valsalva. The sizing of the Toronto SPV is based primarily on the STJ diameter rather than the annular diameter. The STJ diameter should not be more than 10% (or one valve size) greater

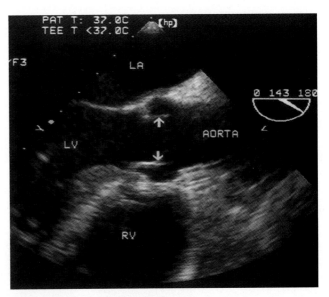

Figure 31.17 Illustration of the Toronto SPV valve indicating its position within the aortic root and two suture lines (inflow and outflow). (From St. Jude Medical, with permission.)

than the annular diameter (Table 31.5). Implantation of a valve that "fits" the annulus, but is too small for the STJ, will result in valve distortion and intravalvular regurgitation due to the leaflets being "pulled apart" by the aortic wall. Oversizing of the Toronto SPV may lead to leaflet buckling and asymmetric valve closure. A recent randomized prospective study by Chamber et al. (23) revealed no significant difference in echocardiographic hemodynamic profiles, regression of left ventricular hypertrophy, or clinical events between the Toronto SPV and the Perimount stented bovine pericardial valve; there is no significant difference in the early postoperative period (44).

Similar to the Toronto SPV, the Medtronic Freestyle aortic root is also obtained from the porcine aortic root and lacks rigid sewing and supporting struts. In contrast to the Toronto SPV, the ascending aorta is intact with ligated coronary arteries on the Freestyle valve and sculpted by the surgeon to one of three possible configurations (Fig. 31.18) (43). Two suture lines are used to implant this valve. The inflow sutures are placed into the annulus, similar to the Toronto SPV. The outflow sutures, however, vary according to the implantation technique

TABLE 31.5	Toronto SPV Valve Sizing (all values are in mm)	
Sinotubular Junction Diameter	**Annular Diameter**	**Toronto SPV Valve Size**
21	19–21	21
23	21–23	23
25	23–25	25
27	25–27	27
29	27–29	29

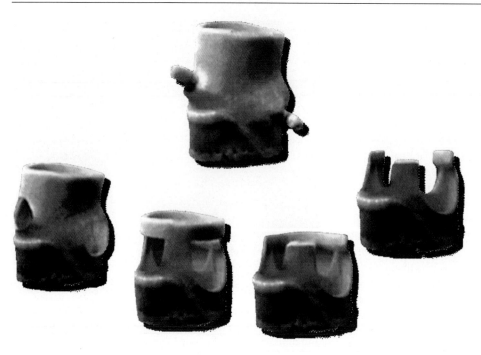

Figure 31.18. Illustration of the Medtronic Freestyle valve, indicating various configurations used for implantation. (From Medtronic Corporation, with permission.)

chosen: full root, root-inclusion, complete subcoronary, or modified subcoronary. The variety of implantation options provided by this valve is an advantage that reduces the problems associated with implanting the Toronto SPV in patients with greater than 10% annular-STJ diameter discrepancies. Disadvantages of the Freestyle aortic root bioprosthesis include the requisite expertise and sculpting necessary to implant the valve and the associated longer implantation time. Evaluation of regional wall motion and documentation of flow within the coronary arteries should be performed postbypass to exclude the possibility of native coronary artery occlusion.

When the annular diameter to sinotubular diameter difference is greater than 10%, either another valve option must be selected or the size of either the annulus or sinotubular ridge must be altered to accommodate the Toronto SPV. A recent study utilizing the Sorin Pericarbon stentless valve demonstrated better valve competence and a better hemodynamic profile when the valve size was 3 mm to 4 mm greater than the annular diameter. Patients with aortic root dilation underwent surgical revision of the noncoronary sinus to maintain the STJ diameter within 115% of the aortic annulus diameter (43).

Two- and three-dimensional echocardiography are used during the postbypass period to evaluate leaflet mobility, while color flow Doppler is used to detect abnormal flow patterns that may indicate valve malfunction. Leaflet prolapse or lack of leaflet coaptation may indicate problems with implantation, sizing, or malposition. Color flow Doppler provides confirmation that the valve malfunction is causing intravalvular or paravalvular leaks. Prolapse of a single leaflet would most likely result in an eccentric jet, while lack of leaflet coaptation would likely result in a central regurgitant jet. A small central jet of AR

is usually not cause for concern and most surgeons would not routinely reopen the aorta to evaluate a trace central jet of AR. Paravalvular leaks are generally uncommon with stentless valves because there are two suture lines. The outflow suture line is considered to be hemostatic. If the inflow suture line is not completely occlusive, *systolic* flow may be detected around the valve, but if the outflow suture line is incompetent, one should expect to see *diastolic* flow around the valve. Small paravalvular leaks often resolve with protamine administration. However, larger (moderate to severe) paravalvular or intravalvular leaks are not likely to resolve after protamine administration. Provided that leaflet mobility is normal, routine measurement of stentless valve gradients immediately after bypass is not required.

Stentless valves are easier to image with echocardiography than stented bioprosthetic valves and mechanical valves. The aortic wall appears thicker in the proximal ascending aorta due to the valve being sewn into the wall of the aorta, and an echolucent space may be observed between the porcine and native aortic walls (43). This paravalvular space should be interrogated with color flow Doppler, particularly if the space varies in size during the cardiac cycle. Expansion of the space with color entry during systole implies communication of the space with the LVOT, which may be expected if the inflow suture line is not hemostatic. Expansion of the space with color entry during diastole implies communication with the ascending aorta. The diagnosis of partial valve dehiscence is made in patients with significant paraprosthetic diastolic regurgitation visualized through an echolucent space (43). A paraprosthetic echolucent space that does not vary in size and lacks color flow Doppler disturbance does not require surgical exploration if valve function is not affected. A persistent or expanding paraprosthetic echolucent space that develops several weeks after implantation raises concerns for a paravalvular infection due to abscess formation (43).

Aortic Valve Homograft

Homograft valves have excellent durability, with a 92% 10-year freedom of reoperation rate from graft-related causes (45). These valves provide many desirable characteristics such as an excellent hemodynamic profile and resistance to infection, and do not require long-term anticoagulation therapy. These characteristics make homografts particularly suitable for younger patients and those with active endocarditis (46). Disadvantages have been a shortage of supply and tissue failure in the past. Recent advances have improved their durability and storage time, promoting a renewed interest in use of these valves (47).

Particular attention is directed to the annular and STJ diameters during the prebypass assessment of native anatomic structures. The annular diameter is measured in a manner similar to that described above for mechanical and stentless valves; however, for patients in whom a homograft is planned, internal annular diameter must accommodate the external diameter of the homograft. For this reason, a valve size 2 to 3 mm smaller than the measured native annulus (internal diameter) is selected as the homograft size. TEE is useful for measuring annular diameter and predicting the size of the homograft to be implanted (48). Accurate estimation of homograft size with intraoperative echocardiography reduces aortic cross-clamp and bypass times if the homograft is thawed before the surgeon directly measures the annular size after aortotomy. The difference between the aortic annular size measured with intraoperative echocardiography and the size measured by the surgeon is less than 1 mm in 94% of patients and less than 2 mm in all patients, with an average difference of 0.6 mm (49). It is also important to measure the STJ diameter so that the implanted homograft is proportional to the size of the supravalvular ridge (50).

Postbypass 2D echocardiography is used to evaluate leaflet mobility, while color Doppler is used to detect any abnormal flow disturbance that may indicate valve malfunction. The same issues previously discussed with stentless aortic valves, also applies to homografts. Homograft valves are prone to distortion and malposition during implantation due to the absence of a sewing ring. Leaflet prolapse or lack of leaflet coaptation may indicate problems with implantation, sizing, or malposition. Color flow Doppler is used to evaluate flow patterns across the valve and to detect intravalvular leaks. Prolapse of a single leaflet would most likely result in an eccentric jet, while lack of leaflet coaptation would result in a central regurgitant jet. The frequency of problems with homograft implantation requiring a return to cardiopulmonary bypass is higher (11.6%) (49), compared with implantation of a prosthetic valve. Intraoperative echocardiography is

valuable for identifying these problems (49), which are primarily AR and myocardial ischemia (with coronary reimplantation). Homografts implanted using an inclusion technique have the same issues regarding a thicker aortic wall and a potential space between the homograph and native aortic walls previously described for stentless aortic valves. Postbypass color flow Doppler interrogation and observing the size of the space throughout the cardiac cycle are important for identifying valve dehiscence.

Combined Aortic Valve–Aortic Root Replacement

Patients with aortic valve disease and aortic root disease (aneurysm, dissection) require a combined aortic valve–aortic root replacement. The role of intraoperative echocardiography is to evaluate the aortic valve for repair versus replacement and to identify the extent of disease in the aorta both proximally and distally. The pathophysiologic process affecting the aortic valve with both aneurysm and dissection is regurgitation. Otherwise normal leaflet anatomy allows for aortic valve repair by resuspension of the cusps in cases of dissection and annular placation in cases of aortic root dilation. Aortic valve repair is possible in 70% of patients with type A dissection (51,52). Patients with an abnormal aortic valve in the setting of dissection or aneurysm require a combined valve-conduit approach for replacement. Patients with significant aortic root pathology, due to cystic medial necrosis or a significantly dilated aortic root, require a valve conduit approach with coronary artery reimplantation into the graft. The graft is extended to replace the affected segment of diseased aorta.

It is important to identify coronary artery involvement with proximal extension of an aortic dissection, and involvement of the great vessels with extension of the dissection into the arch. Epiaortic ultrasound is a necessary adjunct to TEE for the intraoperative evaluation of the distal ascending aorta and proximal aortic arch because these areas cannot be imaged with TEE. The right main stem bronchus is interpositioned between these aortic segments and the esophagus, making these areas inaccessible for imaging by TEE. Aneurysmal involvement of these aortic segments can be appreciated by surgical inspection. The involvement of these aortic segments in the disease process has important implications in placement of the arterial perfusion and cardioplegia cannula, in addition to the surgical approach and the need for deep hypothermic circulatory arrest.

It is important to confirm cannulation of the true lumen when a femoral cannulation site is chosen for arterial perfusion during cardiopulmonary bypass. The true lumen is identified by systolic expansion, generally higher velocity flow, and absence of spontaneous echo contrast. True lumen cannulation is confirmed by observing a wire inserted into the femoral catheter threaded far enough to allow imaging of the wire in the thoracic aorta with TEE. The observation of fluid contrast with initiation of

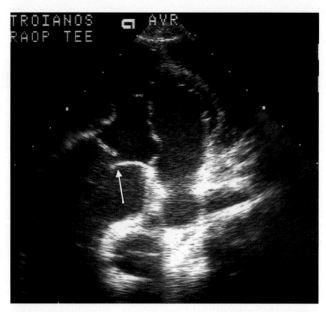

Figure 31.19. Two-dimensional deep transgastric view demonstrating single-leaflet prolapse (*arrow*) of the aortic valve suitable for repair.

cardiopulmonary bypass provides further confirmation of true lumen cannulation via the femoral artery. Intraoperative echocardiography is also used for identifying pericardial and pleural fluid, evaluating global and regional myocardial contractility, estimating the valve size (if not repairable), and measuring the diameter of the various aortic segments.

Postbypass echocardiography is used to evaluate the repaired native or prosthetic aortic valve, the aortic anastomoses, and left ventricular wall motion. Persistent regurgitation, paraprosthetic regurgitation, and new persistent wall motion abnormalities may indicate complications of

surgery that require a return to cardiopulmonary bypass for correction. The frequency of a return to cardiopulmonary bypass is 3.8% after aortic aneurysm surgery (52). The postbypass echocardiographic evaluation of patients undergoing surgery for aortic dissection should demonstrate reduced flow in the false lumen. Persistent flow and absence of thrombus in the false lumen are poor prognostic indicators and indicate a greater risk of the dissection extending within the aorta. These patients require more intensive observation, postoperatively. (53).

Aortic Valve Repair

Valve repair, when feasible, is usually preferred over replacement procedures, and the preoperative echocardiography examination plays a paramount role in identifying aortic valves suitable for repair. Stenotic valves and valves with regurgitation due to leaflet restriction (degenerative, calcific) or retraction (rheumatic) comprise the most common etiologies of AR, but unfortunately these valves are not amenable to repair. Repair is a suitable option among patients with AR due to single-leaflet prolapse of either a tricuspid or congenitally bicuspid valve (Fig. 31.19). Although leaflet prolapse is observed in tricuspid aortic valves, this lesion most commonly affects bicuspid valves (54). TEE provides a highly accurate anatomic assessment of all types of AR lesions, and the functional anatomy defined by TEE is an independent predictor of valve reparability and postoperative outcome. Agreement between TEE and surgical inspection has been shown to be as high as 93%, allowing for accurate prediction for the viability of repair versus replacement (55).

The prolapsing area of the leaflet is resected and reapproximated with suture (Figs. 31.20 and 31.21). Annuloplasty is often performed in association with the

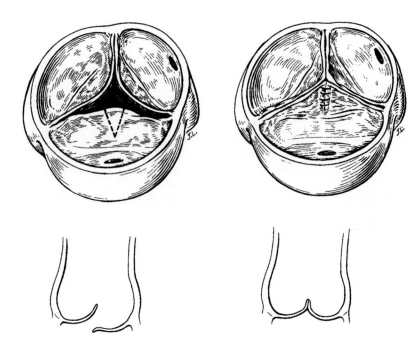

Figure 31.20. Aortic valve repair involving a tricuspid valve with a single-leaflet prolapse. Triangular resection of the free edge of the prolapsing cusp results in normal leaflet size and coaptation. (From Cosgrove DM, Rosenkranz ER, Hendren WG, et al. Valvuloplasty for aortic insufficiency. *J Thorac Cardiovasc Surg* 1991;102:571–577, with permission.)

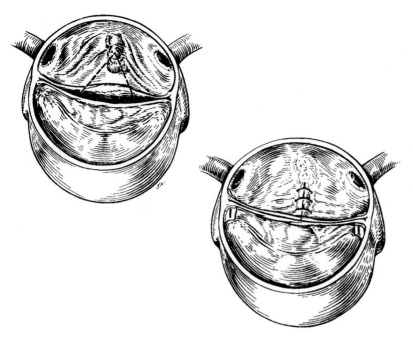

Figure 31.21. Aortic valve repair involving a bicuspid valve with leaflet prolapse involves resection of the raphe when present, triangular resection of the prolapsing cusp, and annuloplasty. (From Cosgrove DM, Rosenkranz ER, Hendren WG, et al. Valvuloplasty for aortic insufficiency. *J Thorac Cardiovasc Surg* 1991;102:571–577, with permission.)

triangular resection of the prolapsing leaflet. Results from the Cleveland Clinic suggest that repair of regurgitant BAVs is superior (0% immediate postrepair replacement rate) when compared with attempted repair of regurgitant tricuspid aortic valves (15% immediate postrepair replacement rate) (56). Calcification limits the potential for valve reconstruction and is usually included in the resected portion of the leaflet. Due to the technical difficulty of the procedure, the failure rate for valve repair is higher for aortic valves (14%) as compared with mitral valve repair (6.6%) (53).

Regurgitant lesions with anatomically normal leaflets and mobility are commonly caused by aortic root dilation and have a characteristic central jet of regurgitation. Annular dilation secondary to aortic root dilation can be repaired, if annular dilation is limited and the leaflets are otherwise anatomically normal. The size and morphology of the aortic root are determined with TEE. A normal aortic root consists of three sinuses of Valsalva that are symmetrical in shape and at most 2 mm to 3 mm larger than the

valve annulus (52). Carpentier's technique of correcting annular dilation employs continuous circumferential horizontal mattress sutures placed through the annulus (54,57). Cosgrove's technique places sutures at the commissures to advance the sinotubular ridge inward and allow central coaptation (Fig. 31.22) (54,57). This method provides selected plication to the most affected areas of the valve (usually the commissures).

The valve sparing procedure for patients with AR due to aortic dissection involves resuspension of the cusps, and is easily performed and highly successful in the absence of additional leaflet pathology. Leaflet perforation caused by endocarditis can be repaired by patch or primary closure if destruction is limited to a small perforation of a single leaflet.

Intraoperative echocardiography after aortic valve repair identifies residual AR and the mechanism of valve dysfunction. Even with a perfect result in the course of repairing a prolapsing leaflet of a congenitally bicuspid valve, the leaflets appear thickened, bicuspid, and mildly

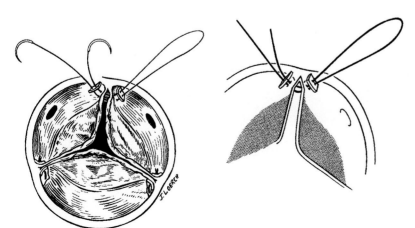

Figure 31.22. Aortic valve annuloplasty is performed by placing horizontal mattress sutures buttressed with Teflon felt at each commissure. Care is taken to avoid leaflet contact as the suture passes through the annulus, into the outflow tract, and back through the annulus. (From Cosgrove DM, Rosenkranz ER, Hendren WG, et al. Valvuloplasty for aortic insufficiency. *J Thorac Cardiovasc Surg* 1991;102:571–577, with permission.)

stenotic (with leaflet doming) (54). The mechanism of valve dysfunction aids the surgeon to decide whether to attempt additional repair or to replace the valve. The presence of AR after aortic valve repair is a poor prognostic indicator as these patients commonly require reoperation for more definitive correction.

Ross Procedure

The Ross procedure involves excision of the patient's own pulmonic valve, implantation of the autograft into the aortic position, and implantation of a homograft or bioprosthetic valve into the pulmonic position (Fig. 31.23). The pulmonary-aortic switch results in an excellent hemodynamic profile, durability, and resistance to infection, and obviates the need for long-term anticoagulant therapy. There is also the potential for growth of this living tissue, making this an attractive option for younger patients (58). Disadvantages to this procedure are the required technical expertise of the surgeon and suitability of the patient. The tissue is difficult to work with given the absence of a sewing ring, and the coronary arteries must be reimplanted.

The presence of significant aortic valve disease is confirmed and the etiology of the valve disease is identified. Identification of etiology is important because progressive

valvulitis is a cause of early postoperative valve dysfunction in patients with rheumatic valve disease (59). An important aspect of the intraoperative evaluation, besides confirming the presence of aortic valve disease, is the suitability of the pulmonic valve for transplantation into the aortic position. First and foremost, the pulmonic valve itself must be a functionally normal tricuspid valve without significant stenosis or regurgitation. The size of the pulmonic valve must also be suitable for transplantation into the aortic position. Epicardial echocardiography is an important adjunct for the intraoperative evaluation of the pulmonic valve due to its anterior location and difficult imaging with TEE. Patients with a difference in the aortic and pulmonic valve diameters of less than 3 mm have less postbypass and postoperative autograft regurgitation (60). Dilation of the aortic annulus or proximal ascending aorta may indicate unrecognized connective tissue disease that progresses after autograft implantation, leading to annular dilation.

The postbypass TEE examination focuses on the function of the autograft, the pulmonary allograft, and regional left ventricular contractility. Particular attention should be devoted to evaluation of leaflet coaptation, leaflet prolapse, and restriction of leaflet mobility. Color flow Doppler is used to detect AR. The degree of regurgitation is best determined with the long-axis view, while the location of

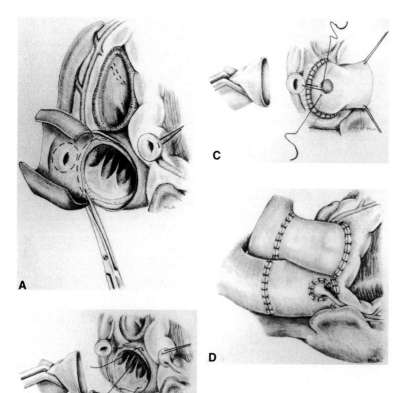

Figure 31.23. Ross Procedure root replacement technique. **A:** Generous cuffs of aorta are left attached to the right and left coronary ostia. Minimal mobilization of these arteries is performed. The remaining proximal aorta is excised, transecting the aorta below the aortic annulus in the interleaflet triangle. **B:** The pulmonary autograft is in an anatomic position with the posterior sinus of the autograft becoming the new left coronary sinus (stay sutures omitted from drawing). The remaining sutures for orientation are placed to position the new right coronary sinus and to trifurcate the aortic annulus. **C:** Completion of the pulmonary autograft root implantation with selection of the site of implantation of the right coronary artery with the autograft distended. **D:** The pulmonary homograft reconstruction of the right ventricle outflow tract is done with two continuous suture lines. (From Elkins RC. Aortic valve: Ross procedure. In: Kaiser LR, Kron IL, Spray TL, eds. *Mastery of Cardiothoracic Surgery*. Philadelphia, PA: Lippincott-Raven, 1998.)

the coaptation defect is identified using the short-axis view. More than a minimal amount of regurgitation indicates possible valve distortion during implantation and a need for return to cardiopulmonary bypass for correction (61). The pulmonary allograft is similarly evaluated using 2D and color flow Doppler for both leaflet mobility and regurgitation, respectively. Epicardial imaging may be required to adequately evaluate valve function. The aortic root and proximal pulmonary artery are evaluated for narrowing at the anastomotic site and for dilation of the proximal ascending aorta. Baseline measurements are important for long-term follow-up given the propensity for disease progression. Sievers et al. (64) discussed their experience over fifteen years and 228 patients who underwent the Ross procedure. The midterm results demonstrated a preservation of the aortic root and excellent hemodynamic profiles with a subcoronary or inclusion technique (62).

The septal perforator branch of the left anterior descending coronary artery lies in close proximity to the pulmonic valve; hence, compromise of septal perforator artery flow is a potential complication during pulmonic valve harvesting. TEE is used to evaluate left ventricular contractility, particularly myocardial thickening and radial shortening in the basal anteroseptal segment to assess patency of the septal perforator. Regional contractility is assessed in other areas of the left and right ventricles for coronary malperfusion due to problems that may arise from coronary reimplantation or bleeding.

Percutaneous Aortic Valve Surgery

Percutaneous aortic valve surgery is a new procedure in development that involves the placement of a prosthesis across the aortic valve, using an intravascular approach. The general principle utilizes a collapsible bioprosthetic valve mounted within an expandable stent. Lutter et al. (65) described their experience with a porcine aortic valve mounted into a self-expandable nitinol stent by means of a suture technique (63). They implanted six valves in the descending aorta and eight valves in a subcoronary position in the ascending aorta of 14 anesthetized pigs, via the left iliac artery or infrarenal aorta. One animal died of ventricular fibrillation, and technical failure (stent twisting) occurred in two animals. The remaining 11 valve stents demonstrated low transvalvular gradients, physiologic regurgitation in only eight animals, and mild regurgitation in three animals (63). Color Doppler indicated no regurgitation in 5 of 5 cases and minor paravalvular leakage in one.

The first human implantation of a percutaneous aortic valve was reported by Cribier et al. (66) in a 57-year-old man with calcific aortic stenosis, cardiogenic shock, subacute leg ischemia, and other associated noncardiac medical problems (64). Valve replacement was declined for this patient. Although balloon valvuloplasty had been performed, the results were nonsustained. The investigators used an antegrade transseptal approach to successfully implant the percutaneous heart valve within the diseased

aortic valve. Their valve was composed of three bovine pericardial leaflets mounted within a balloon-expandable stent (Fig. 31.24) (65). The placement was accurate and stable with no impingement of coronary artery blood flow or interference with mitral valve function. A mild degree of paravalvular regurgitation was present after implantation. Valvular function remained satisfactory for 4 months after the procedure, assessed with sequential transesophageal echocardiograms without the recurrence of heart failure. The patient died 17 weeks after implantation due to noncardiac complications from worsening leg ischemia, amputation, and infection (64). Cribier et al. (66) followed up their original case study with a case series of six additional patients in whom percutaneous AVR was performed. The patients had severe calcific aortic stenosis with New York Heart Association functional class IV congestive heart failure and ranged in age from 57 to 91 years. All patients were not surgical candidates due to multiple comorbidities. Their outcomes are described in Table 31.6.

Grube et al. (69) reported results on 86 patients with aortic stenosis who underwent percutaneous aortic valve implantation via a 21-French and 18-French CoreValve aortic valve prosthesis (CoreValve Inc., Irvine, California) (65,66) (Fig. 31.25). Successful device implantation resulted in a marked reduction of aortic transvalvular gradients with AR grade remaining unchanged. Acute procedural success rate was 74% with procedural mortality of 6%. Overall 30-day mortality rate was 12%, while the combined rate of death, stroke, and myocardial infarction was 22% (67). The smaller 18-French device allowed

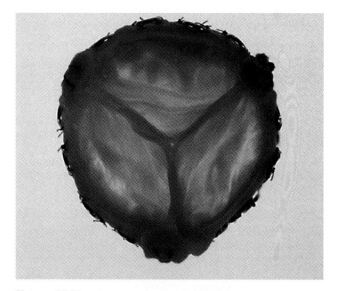

Figure 31.24. The percutaneously implanted heart valve is composed of three bovine pericardial leaflets mounted within a balloon-expandable steel stent structure that is crimped onto a percutaneous delivery balloon. (From Davidson M, Baim D. Percutaneous aortic valve interventions. In: Cohn L, ed. *Cardiac Surgery in the Adult.* New York: McGraw-Hill, 2008:963–971.)

TABLE 31.6 Patient Outcomes in Cribier Study

Patient	Age(y)	Sex	Comorbidities	Mean Gradient mm Hg)[a] Pre/Postimplant	Aortic Regurgitation[b] Pre/Postimplant	Ejection Fraction (%)[a] Preimplant/Follow-up	Outcome
1	57	M	Severe PAD, lung cancer s/p left lobectomy, silicosis, chronic pancreatitis	35/8	0/1	10/22	Died at 18 weeks, after leg amputation
2	80	M	Severe AR, recent stroke, CRI, asbestosis, prostate cancer	—	—	—	Died during procedure
3	91	M	Pacemaker, decubitus ulcers	56/6	2/3	29/40	Died at 4 weeks of acute abdominal syndrome
4	63	M	Rectal adenocarcinoma, severe COPD, CRF	30/4	0/1	28/42	Died at 2 weeks of rectal hemorrhage
5	80	F	HTN, breast cancer with lung and bone metastases, COPD, kyphoscoliosis	38/6	1/1	34/53	Alive
6	77	M	IMI, stroke, CRF	31/13	2/3	19/48	Alive

[a]Follow-up measurement of mean gradient and ejection fraction performed at 2 weeks in patient 3 and at 4 weeks in patients 1, 4, 5, and 6.
[b]Postimplant assessment of AR performed immediately after implantation.
AR, aortic regurgitation; PAD, peripheral arterial disease; CRI, chronic renal insufficiency; COPD, chronic obstructive pulmonary disease; CRF, chronic renal failure; HTN, hypertension; IMI, inferior myocardial infarction.
Table data from Cribier A, Eltchaninoff H, Tron C, et al. Early experience with percutaneous transcatheter implantation of heart valve prosthesis for the treatment of end-stage inoperable patients with calcific aortic stenosis. J Am Coll Cardiol 2004;43:698–703.

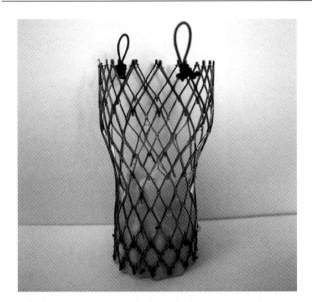

Figure 31.25. The Core valve system consists of pericardial leaflets attached to a self-expanding nitinol frame shown in the deployed state. The flared distal end anchors the device in the ascending aorta. The stent covers the coronary ostia, but cell size is designed to allow later coronary catheterization. (From Davidson M, Baim D. Percutaneous aortic valve interventions. In: Cohn L, ed. *Cardiac Surgery in the Adult.* New York: McGraw-Hill, 2008:963–971.)

implantation using only local anesthesia and without hemodynamic support.

Berry et al. (70) evaluated the role of TEE during percutaneous AVR. Eleven patients who underwent percutaneous surgery and TEE had excellent visual agreement between fluoroscopic and TEE images of prosthetic positioning and deployment. Perioperative TEE provided immediate information on prosthetic position and function, LV function, and associated mitral pathology (68).

A trial of transcatheter implantation of a balloon-expandable stent valve using the femoral arterial approach

reported similar results. Webb et al. (71) described the learning curve as procedural success increased from 76% to 96%, malposition decreased from 8% to zero, and procedural mortality decreased from 4% to zero in a comparison of the first 25 patients to the latter 25 patients (69).

Zierer et al. (72) has described their success with 26 consecutive patients treated with transapical AVR performed via a limited anterolateral incision at the fifth intercostal space to access the LV apex (70). A 23-mm or 26-mm stent mounted valve was introduced into the LV through purse string sutures, while TEE and fluoroscopy were used to guide the prosthesis into proper position in the annulus (Fig. 31.26). Temporary rapid ventricular pacing may be required to reduce left ventricular ejection and unwanted movement during deployment. The valve is placed in coaxial alignment with the long axis of the ascending aorta and perpendicular to the AVA. All valves in the study were successfully deployed (Fig. 31.27) with good hemodynamic function and transvalvular gradients of 6 ± 2 mm Hg. Thirty day mortality was 15%, and two patients required stent angioplasty due to partial left main stem coronary artery obstruction by the prosthesis. Although surgical complications requiring conversion to an open procedure are higher, the transapical approach to AVR may provide a viable option in the setting of severe peripheral vascular disease that prohibits a femoral approach (70,71).

TEE will continue to play a critical role in the evaluation of patients suitable for percutaneous aortic valve implantation, sizing, placement, stabilization of the device, and postimplantation evaluation for complications. These complications include movement of the device, obstruction of coronary artery blood flow, and damage to the mitral valve. Patients with calcific disease face complications similar to balloon valvuloplasty, such as embolic events associated with the procedure. The use of 3D echocardiography in the setting of percutaneous mitral balloon valvotomy enables a better description of

Figure 31.26. Schematic view (**left**) of valve positioning of Edwards Sapien prosthesis (Edwards Lifesciences, Irving, California) on a balloon catheter within the AVA via transapical approach using stay sutures. Fluoroscopic (**right**) and echocardiographic guidance are used to confirm proper placement. (From Walther T, Dewey T, Borger M, et al. Transapical aortic valve implantation: step-by-step. *Ann Thorac Surg* 2009;87:276–283.)

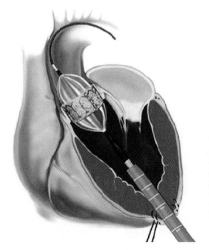
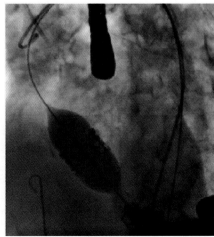

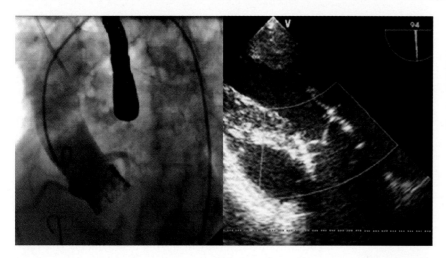

Figure 31.27. Continuous fluoroscopic (**left**) and echocardiographic (**right**) imaging are performed to confirm proper deployment of the Edwards Sapien prosthesis after removal of the balloon catheter. (From Walther T, Dewey T, Borger M, et al. Transapical aortic valve implantation: step-by-step. *Ann Thorac Surg* 2009;87:276–283.)

valve anatomy before and after surgery (72). Continued improvements in the device, implantation techniques, and the ability to three-dimensionally assess function after surgical therapy may provide similar benefits in the treatment of patients with aortic valve disease.

CONCLUSIONS

Intraoperative echocardiography plays an important role during aortic valve surgery by providing critical information for surgical decision making and hemodynamic management. TEE helps to confirm the preoperative diagnosis, evaluate the severity of aortic valve disease, determine the feasibility of aortic valve repair versus replacement, and evaluate the success of surgical correction. In addition, a careful and systematic transesophageal echocardiographic evaluation in the operating room can lead to new diagnoses, altered surgical management, and improved patient care. Clinical information provided by TEE guides appropriate hemodynamic management for patients with aortic valve disease, which is particularly important in patients with manifestation of chronic disease, whether it be stenosis, regurgitation, or both.

Intraoperative TEE evaluation is particularly important in the patient who presents for non–aortic valve surgery who is discovered to have previously unsuspected but significant aortic valve disease. The issue of whether or not to intervene in patients with mild to moderate disease is more important for patients with stenosis rather than regurgitation, because of the higher mortality associated with reoperation in patients with aortic stenosis who have had previous CABG (45). The particularly challenging dilemma of evaluating the patient with low-gradient aortic stenosis requires the echocardiographer to make a determination as to whether the low gradient is due to mild aortic stenosis or due to severe aortic stenosis with severe left ventricular dysfunction. Two- and three-dimensional imaging combined with pulsed wave, continuous wave, and color Doppler echocardiography allow

quantitative evaluation of stenotic and regurgitant lesions to identify the etiology of valve dysfunction and to aid in the management of this and other challenging intraoperative dilemmas. As percutaneous aortic valve surgery develops, TEE will play a critical role in the evaluation of patients suitable for percutaneous aortic valve implantation, sizing, placement, stabilization of the device, and postimplantation evaluation for complications.

The recent introduction of real-time 3D TEE will undoubtedly enhance the ability of the echocardiographer to better define and quantify aortic valve pathology, communicate a more accurate description of the valve dysfunction to the surgeon, and direct percutaneous interventions with safer deployment of these devices. The prospect of new applications for this technology is exciting as the medical community awaits clinical trials and more experience for validation of its usefulness for evaluating the aortic valve.

KEY POINTS

- Epiaortic, epicardial, and TEE are valuable intraoperative tools for the complete evaluation of the aortic valve and ascending aorta. Two- and three-dimensional imaging combined with pulsed wave, continuous wave, and color Doppler allow quantitative evaluation of stenotic and regurgitant lesions.
- Focused and comprehensive echocardiographic examinations are performed during aortic valve surgery to confirm the preoperative diagnosis, evaluate the severity of aortic valve disease, determine the feasibility of aortic valve repair versus replacement, and evaluate the success of surgical correction.
- Intraoperative echocardiography during AVR is used to estimate the size of the valve to be implanted, assess the function of the prosthetic valve, assess de-airing maneuvers, evaluate ventricular function, and evaluate the thoracic aorta.

- Implantation of a stentless aortic valve requires measurements of both the aortic annulus and STJ.
- Preoperative TEE for patients undergoing homograft implantation is useful for determining homograft size before aortotomy, reducing cross-clamp time, and ensuring availability of this valve.
- Combined aortic root and aortic valve procedures are long, technically demanding, and associated with serious complications that can be diagnosed with intraoperative echocardiography.
- Aortic valve repair is a suitable option for patients with AR due to single-leaflet prolapse of either a tricuspid or congenitally bicuspid valve. Moderate-to-severe regurgitation is a cause for concern after repair, and often necessitates return to cardiopulmonary bypass for further correction.
- The Ross procedure involves the use of the patient's own pulmonic valve as an autograft replacement of the aortic valve and an allograft replacement of the pulmonic valve. Echocardiography plays an important role in determining the suitability of the patient for this procedure and identifying complications that may arise. These complications include valve dysfunction, aortic root dilation due to disease progression, proximal pulmonary artery stricture, and inadequate coronary perfusion.
- Percutaneous aortic valve surgery involves the placement of a bioprosthetic, collapsible aortic valve mounted on an expandable stent through a percutaneous approach. As this technology develops, TEE will play a critical role in the evaluation of patients suitable for percutaneous aortic valve implantation, sizing, placement, stabilization of the device, and postimplantation evaluation for complications.

REFERENCES

1. The Society of Thoracic Surgeons Adult CV Surgery National Database – STS Spring 2006 Executive Summary Report; http://www.sts.org/documents/pdf/STS-ExecutiveSummarySpring2006.pdf.
2. Hanayama N, Fazel S, Goldman B, et al. Contemporary trends in aortic valve surgery: a single centre 1-year clinical experience. *J Cardiac Surg* 2004;19:552–558.
3. Ionescu A, West R, Proudman C, et al. Prospective study of routine perioperative transesophageal echocardiography for elective valve replacement: clinical impact and cost-saving implications. *J Am Soc Echocardiogr* 2001;14:659–667.
4. Cheitlin MD, Armstrong WF, Aurigemma GP, et al. ACC/AHA/ASE 2003 Guideline update for the clinical application of echocardiography: summary article. *JACC* 2003;42:954–970.
5. Qizilbash B, Couture P, Denault A, et al. Impact of perioperative transesophageal echocardiography in aortic valve replacement. *Semin Cardiothor Vasc Anesth* 2007;11:288–300.
6. Oh CC, Click RL, Orszulak TA, et al. Role of intraoperative transesophageal echocardiography in determining aortic annulus diameter in homograft insertion. *J Am Soc Echocardiogr* 1998;11:638–642.
7. Nowrangi SK, Connolly HM, Freeman WK, et al. Impact of intraoperative transesophageal echocardiography among patients undergoing aortic valve replacement for aortic stenosis. *J Am Soc Echocardiogr* 2001;14:863–866.
8. Morehead AJ, Firstenberg MS, Shiota T, et al. Intraoperative echocardiographic detection of regurgitant jets after valve replacement. *Ann Thorac Surg* 2000;69:135–139.
9. Filsoufi F, Aklog L, Adams DH, et al. Management of mild to moderate aortic stenosis at the time of coronary artery bypass grafting. *J Heart Valve Dis* 2002;11(Suppl. 1):S45–S49.
10. Bonow RO, Carabello BA, Chatterjee K, et al. ACC/AHA 2006 guidelines for the management of patients with valvular heart disease. *J Am Coll Cardiol* 2006;48:e1–e148.
11. Eslami M, Rahimtoola S. Prophylactic aortic valve replacement in older patients for mild aortic stenosis during coronary bypass surgery. *Am J Geriatric Cardiol* 2003;12:197–200.
12. Rosenhek R, Klaar U, Schemper M, et al. Mild and moderate aortic stenosis: natural history and risk stratification by echocardiography. *Eur Heart J* 2004;25:199–205.
13. Odell JA, Mullany CJ, Schaff HV, et al. Aortic valve replacement after previous coronary artery bypass grafting. *Ann Thorac Surg* 1996;62:1424–1430.
14. Bahler RC, Desser DR, Finkelhor RS, et al. Factors leading to progression of valvular aortic stenosis. *Am J Cardiol* 1999;84:1044–1048.
15. Palta S, Pai AM, Gill KS, et al. New insights into the progressions of aortic stenosis: implications for secondary prevention. *Circulation* 2000;101:2497–2502.
16. Kume T, Kawamoto T, Akasaka T, et al. Rate of progression of valvular aortic stenosis in patients undergoing dialysis. *J Am Soc Echocardiogr* 2006;19(7):914–918.
17. Hoffmann R, Flachskampf FA, Hanrath P. Planimetry of orifice area in aortic stenosis using multiplane transesophageal echocardiography. *J Am Coll Cardiol* 1993;22:529–534.
18. Connolly H, Oh J, Schaff H, et al. Severe aortic stenosis with low transvalvular gradient and severe left ventricular dysfunction: result of aortic valve replacement in 52 patients. *Circulation* 2000;101:1940–1947.
19. Vaquette B, Corbineau H, Laurent M, et al. Valve replacement in patients with critical aortic stenosis and depressed left ventricular function: predictors of operative risk, left ventricular function recovery, and long term outcome. *Heart* 2005;91(10):1324–1329.
20. Tarantini G, Buja P, Scognamiglio R, et al. Aortic valve replacement in severe aortic stenosis with left ventricular dysfunction: determinants of cardiac mortality and ventricular function recovery. *Eur J Cardiothorac Surg* 2003;24(6):879–885.
21. Pereira JJ, Lauer MS, Bashir M, et al. Survival after aortic valve replacement for severe aortic stenosis with low transvalvular gradients and severe left ventricular dysfunction. *J Am Coll Cardiol* 2002;39(8):1356–1363.
22. Chambers J. Low "gradient", low flow aortic stenosis. *Heart* 2006;92:554–558.
23. Florath I, Albert A, Rosendahl U, et al. Impact of valve prosthesis-patient mismatch estimated by echocardiographic-determined effective orifice area on long-term outcome after aortic valve replacement. *Am Heart J* 2008;155:1135–1142.
24. Kato Y, Suehiro S, Shibata T, et al. Impact of valve prosthesis-patient mismatch on long-term survival and left ventricular mass regression after aortic valve replacement for aortic stenosis. *J Cardiac Surg* 2007;22:314–319.

25. Bermejo J, Yotti R. Low-gradient aortic valve stenosis. Value and limitations of dobutamine stress testing. *Heart* 2006;93(3):298–302.

26. Monin JL, Quere JP, Monchi M, et al. Low-gradient aortic stenosis: operative risk stratification and predictors for long-term outcome: a multicenter study using dobutamine stress hemodynamics. *Circulation* 2003;108(3):319–324.

27. Grayburn P. Assessment of low-gradient aortic stenosis with dobutamine. *Circulation* 2006;113:604–606.

28. Kumar A, Anel R, Bunnell E. Pulmonary artery occlusion pressure and central venous pressure fail to predict ventricular filling volume, cardiac performance, or the response to volume infusion in normal subjects. *Crit Care Med* 2004;32(3):691–699.

29. Islamoglu F, Apaydin A, Degirmenciler K, et al. Detachment of the mitral valve anterior leaflet as a complication of aortic valve replacement. *Tex Heart Inst J* 2006;33(1):54–56.

30. Cahalan MK, Abel M, Goldman M, et al. American Society of Echocardiography; Society of Cardiovascular Anesthesiologists. American Society of Echocardiography and Society of Cardiovascular Anesthesiologists task force guidelines for training in perioperative echocardiography. *Anesth Analg* 2002;94:1384–1388.

31. Khaw AV, von Bardeleben RS, Strasser C, et al. Direct measurement of left ventricular outflow tract by transthoracic real-time 3D-echocardiography increases accuracy in assessment of aortic valve stenosis. *Int J Cardiol* 2008, doi:10.1016/j. ijcard.2008. 04.070.

32. Armen TA, Vandse R, Bickle K, et al. Three-dimensional echocardiographic evaluation of an incidental quadricuspid aortic valve. *Eur J Echocardiogr* 2008;9:318–320.

33. Cosgrove DM, Rosenkranz ER, Hendren WG, et al. Valvuloplasty for aortic insufficiency. *J Thorac Cardiovasc Surg* 1991;102:571–577.

34. Tassan-Mangina S, Metz D, Nazeyllas P, et al. Factors determining early improvement in mitral regurgitation after aortic valve replacement for aortic valve stenosis: a transthoracic and transesophageal prospective study. *Clin Cardiol* 2003;26(3):127–131.

35. Christenson J, Jordan B, Bloch A, et al. Should a regurgitant mitral valve be replaced simultaneously with a stenotic aortic valve? *Tex Heart Inst J* 2000;27(4):350–355.

36. Moazami N, Diodato M, Moon M, et al. Does functional mitral regurgitation improve with isolated aortic valve replacement? *J Cardiac Surg* 2004;19(5):444–448.

37. Hahn RT, Roman MJ, Mogtader AH, et al. Association of aortic dilation with regurgitant, stenotic and functionally normal bicuspid aortic valves. *J Am Coll Cardiol* 1992;19:283–288.

38. Cecconi M, Manfrin M, Moraca A, et al. Aortic dimensions in patients with bicuspid aortic valve without significant valve dysfunction. *Am J Cardiol* 2005;95:292–294.

39. Borger MA, Preston M, Ivanov J, et al. Should the ascending aorta be replaced more frequently in patients with bicuspid aortic valve disease? *J Thorac Cardiovasc Surg* 2004;128:677–683.

40. Maslow AD, Regan MM, Haering JM, et al. Echocardiographic predictors of left ventricular outflow tract obstruction and systolic anterior motion of the mitral valve after mitral valve reconstruction for myxomatous valve disease. *J Am Coll Cardiol* 1999;34(7):2096–2104.

41. Pibarot P, Dumesnil JG. Hemodynamic and clinical impact of prosthesis-patient mismatch in the aortic valve position and its prevention. *J Am Coll Cardiol* 2000;36(4):1131–1141.

42. Dunning J, Graham R, Thambyrajah J, et al. Stentless vs. stented aortic valve bioprostheses: a prospective randomized controlled trial. *Eur Heart J* 2007;28(19):2369–2374.

43. Bach DS. Echocardiographic assessment of stentless aortic bioprosthetic valves. *J Am Soc Echocardiogr* 2000;13(10):941–948.

44. Chambers J, Rimington H, Hodson F, et al. The subcoronary Toronto stentless versus supra-annular Perimount stented replacement aortic valve: early clinical and hemodynamic results of a randomized comparison in 160 patients. *J Thorac Cardiovasc Surg* 2006;131(4):878–882.

45. Doty JR, Salazar JD, Liddicoat JR, et al. Aortic valve replacement with cryopreserved aortic allograft: ten-year experience. *J Thorac Cardiovasc Surg* 1998;115:371–379.

46. Petrou M, Wong K, Albertucci M, et al. Evaluation of unstented aortic homografts for the treatment of prosthetic aortic valve endocarditis. *Circulation* 1994;90:II-198–II-204.

47. Oh CC, Click RL, Orszulak TA, et al. Role of intraoperative transesophageal echocardiography in determining aortic annulus diameter in homograft insertion. *J Am Soc Echocardiogr* 1998;11:638–642.

48. Fan CM, Liu X, Panidis JP, et al. Prediction of homograft aortic valve size by transthoracic and transesophageal two-dimensional echocardiography. *Echocardiography* 1997;14:345–348.

49. Stewart WJ, Gillam L, Morehead AJ, et al. Impact of intraoperative echocardiography on homograft aortic valve surgery. *J Am Coll Cardiol* 1993;21:17A.

50. Kunzelman KS, Grande KJ, David TE, et al. Aortic root and valve relationships. Impact on surgical repair. *J Thorac Cardiovasc Surg* 1994;107:162–170.

51. Jex RK, Schaff HV, Piehler JM, et al. Repair of ascending aortic dissection: influence of associated aortic valve insufficiency on early and late results. *J Thorac Cardiovasc Surg* 1987;93:375–384.

52. Mazzucotelli JP, Deleuze PH, Baufreton C, et al. Preservation of the aortic valve in acute aortic dissection: long-term echocardiographic assessment and clinical outcome. *Ann Thorac Surg* 1993;55(6):1513–1517.

53. Grimm RA, Stewart WJ. The role of intraoperative echocardiography in valve surgery. *Cardiol Clin* 1998;16:477–489.

54. Cosgrove DM, Rosenkranz ER, Hendren WG, et al. Valvuloplasty for aortic insufficiency. *J Thorac Cardiovasc Surg* 1991;102:571–577.

55. le Polain de Waroux J, Pouleur A, Goffinet C, et al. Functional anatomy of aortic regurgitation: accuracy, prediction of surgical repairability, and outcome implications of transesophageal echocardiography. *Circulation* 2007;116(11):I-264–I-269.

56. Faber CN, Smedira NG. Surgical considerations in aortic valve surgery. In: Savage RM, Aronson S, eds. *Comprehensive Textbook of Intraoperative Transesophageal Echocardiography*. 1st ed. Philadelphia, PA: Lippincott Williams & Wilkins, 2005:537.

57. Erbel R, Oelert H, Meyer J, et al. Effect of medical and surgical therapy on aortic dissection evaluated by transesophageal echocardiography. Implications for prognosis and therapy. The European Cooperative Study Group on Echocardiography. *Circulation* 1993;87:1604–1615.

58. Carpentier A. Cardiac valve surgery—"the French correction." *J Thorac Cardiovasc Surg* 1983;86:323–337.

59. Walls JT, McDaniel WC, Pope ER, et al. Documented growth of autogenous pulmonary valve translocated to the aortic valve position. *J Thorac Cardiovasc Surg* 1994;107:1530–1531.

60. al-Halees Z, Kumar N, Gallo R, et al. Pulmonary autograft for aortic valve replacement in rheumatic disease: a caveat. *Ann Thorac Surg* 1995;60(2 Suppl):S172–S175.

61. Stewart WJ, Secknus MA, Thomas JD, et al. Intraoperative echocardiography in the Ross procedure. *J Am Coll Cardiol* 1996;27:190A.

62. Sievers H, Dahmen G, Graf B, et al. Midterm results of the Ross procedure preserving the patient's aortic root. *Circulation* 2003;108(10):II-55–II-60.

63. Lutter G, Kuklinski D, Berg G, et al. Percutaneous aortic valve replacement: an experimental study. I. Studies on implantation. *J Thorac Cardiovasc Surg* 2002;123:768–776.

64. Cribier A, Eltchaninoff H, Bash A, et al. Percutaneous transcatheter implantation of an aortic valve prosthesis for calcific aortic stenosis: first human case description. *Circulation* 2002;106:3006–3008.

65. Davidson M, Baim D. Percutaneous aortic valve interventions. In: Cohn L, ed. *Cardiac Surgery in the Adult*. New York: McGraw-Hill, 2008:963–971.

66. Cribier A, Eltchaninoff H, Tron C, et al. Early experience with percutaneous transcatheter implantation of heart valve prosthesis for the treatment of end-stage inoperable patients with calcific aortic stenosis. *J Am Coll Cardiol* 2004;43:698–703.

67. Grube E, Schuler G, Buellesfeld L, et al. Percutaneous aortic valve replacement for severe aortic stenosis in high-risk patients using the second- and current third-generation self-expanding CoreValve prosthesis: device success and 30-day clinical outcome. *J Am Coll Cardiol* 2007;50:69–76.

68. Berry C, Oukerraj L, Asgar A, et al. Role of transesophageal echocardiography in percutaneous aortic valve replacement with the Core Valve Revalving system. *Echocardiography* 2008;25(8):840–848.

69. Webb JG, Pasupati S, Humphries K, et al. Percutaneous transarterial aortic valve replacement in selected high-risk patients with aortic stenosis. *Circulation* 2007;116:755–763.

70. Zierer A, Wimmer-Greinecker G, Martens S, et al. The transapical approach for aortic valve implantation. *J Thorac Cardiovasc Surg* 2008;136(4):948–953.

71. Walther T, Dewey T, Borger M, et al. Transapical aortic valve implantation: step-by-step. *Ann Thorac Surg* 2009;87:276–283.

72. Langerveld J, Valocik G, Plokker H, et al. Additional value of three-dimensional transesophageal echocardiography for patients with mitral valve stenosis undergoing balloon valvuloplasty. *JASE* 2003;16(8):841–849.

QUESTIONS

1. The planimetry method of determining AVA is
   A. more reliable using 2D echocardiography than using 3D echocardiography
   B. more difficult and less reliable if the valve is severely calcified
   C. performed using the midesophageal aortic valve long-axis view between 110 and 150 degrees
   D. difficult to perform when calcifications are located along the anterior aspect of the valve

2. Which of the following statements regarding low-gradient aortic stenosis is TRUE?
   A. Patients with true anatomically severe stenosis will exhibit an increase in valve area and little change in pressure gradient during dobutamine infusion.
   B. Survival after AVR among patients with low-gradient aortic stenosis with and without preoperative contractile reserve is the same.
   C. Systolic dysfunction due to aortic stenosis is usually reversible with valve replacement, but systolic dysfunction due to myocardial infarction, extensive coronary artery disease, or superimposed myocardial fibrosis may not improve after AVR.
   D. The presence of concomitant mitral stenosis causes an overestimation of the severity of aortic stenosis by gradient determination because of increased trans-aortic blood flow.

3. Which of the following valve pathologies would be most suitable for repair?
   A. Aortic regurgitation with calcific aortic stenosis
   B. Aortic stenosis with rheumatic valve disease
   C. Aortic regurgitation with single-leaflet prolapse
   D. Aortic regurgitation with annular dilatation from an ascending aortic aneurysm

4. Which of the following methods are considered viable approaches to percutaneous aortic valve surgery?
   A. Antegrade venous-to-arterial transseptal approach via the femoral vein
   B. Retrograde approach via the femoral artery
   C. Antegrade transapical approach via a limited anterolateral incision
   D. All of the above

Surgical Considerations and Assessment in Aortic Surgery

Edward G. Soltesz ■ Lars G. Svensson

INTRODUCTION

Surgery of the thoracic aortic has evolved considerably over the past decades and now can be performed with relative safety in most elective situations. In sharp contrast to current methods of aortic surgery, the early operative treatment of thoracic aortic disease was mainly palliative, including wrapping of an aneurysm sac with cellophane to induce periarterial fibrosis. Before the use of cardiopulmonary bypass, thoracic aneurysm surgery was limited to the resection of discrete saccular aneurysms. Soon after the development of cardiopulmonary bypass, Cooley and DeBakey reported the resection of an ascending aortic aneurysm and replacement with a graft in 1956. In 1957, DeBakey et al. replaced the ascending aorta and arch with a homograft using separate innominate and left carotid artery perfusion. It was not until 1975 that Griepp described the technique of circulatory arrest for the complete replacement of the aortic arch and ushered in the technique of the "open distal anastomosis." Finally, in the 1980s, Borst and Svensson developed and refined the technique of the "elephant trunk" to treat extensive disease of the aortic arch and descending thoracic aorta (1). Over the past decade, endovascular treatment of the aorta has begun to replace traditional surgical approaches. This exciting new technology avoids the large incisions, need for circulatory support, and surgical hemorrhage associated with open repair techniques. Although present endovascular techniques only allow for repair of descending aortic, thoracoabdominal, and abdominal aneurysms, new graft designs are in the pipeline to treat ascending aortic and arch disease as well.

This chapter will review the anatomy of the thoracic aorta and guide the reader through a synopsis of surgical diseases of the aorta with a focus on their echocardiographic appearance. Emphasis will be placed on obtaining necessary transesophageal echocardiographic (TEE) information to assist in surgical decision making in the operating room.

ANATOMY OF THE THORACIC AORTA

The thoracic aorta begins at the ventriculo-aortic junction and continues to the diaphragmatic hiatus where it then becomes the abdominal aorta. The aortic annulus is the fibrous structure that attaches the aortic root to the left ventricle (LV) and is, thus, the transition into the thoracic aorta. Surgically, the thoracic aorta is divided into four segments: the aortic root, the ascending aorta, the aortic arch, and the descending thoracic aorta.

The *aortic root* consists of the aortic annulus, the aortic cusps, the aortic sinuses of Valsalva, and the sinotubular junction. All these structures function together as a unit. The normal aortic valve has three cusps, each of which has a semilunar shape. The base of each cusp is attached to the aortic annulus in a crescent fashion. The point where the free margin of each cusp joins its base is the commissure, and the ridge in the aortic wall that lies immediately above the commissures is the sinotubular junction, the point that marks the transition to the ascending aorta. The spaces contained between the aortic annulus and the sinotubular junction are the aortic sinuses of Valsalva. There are three cusps and three sinuses: left cusp and sinus, right cusp and sinus, and noncoronary cusp and sinus. The left main coronary artery arises from the left aortic sinus and the right coronary artery from the right aortic sinus. The normal aortic annulus measures 27 mm in diameter or less.

The *ascending aorta* refers to the portion of the thoracic aorta that lies between the sinotubular junction and the origin of the innominate artery.

The *aortic arch*, or sometimes called the transverse aorta, refers to the segment of the aorta that forms a leftward and backward curve and contains the origins of the epiaortic vessels. The innominate artery, left common carotid artery, and left subclavian artery arise from the aortic arch and typically have separate orifices. A "bovine" arch configuration refers to the anatomic variant in which the innominate and left common carotid arteries arise from a single trunk off the aortic arch.

The *descending thoracic aorta* begins distal to the left subclavian artery and terminates at the diaphragm where the aorta becomes the abdominal aorta. The aortic isthmus is a region just distal to the left subclavian artery, which can have a slight narrowing due to previous ductal tissue.

OVERVIEW OF THORACIC AORTIC DISEASES

Aneurysms

An *aneurysm* is defined as an enlargement of more than 50% of normal aortic diameter, while *ectasia* is the term applied to an enlargement that falls short of a true aneurysm. Aortic aneurysms can be broadly classified according to their morphology (saccular, fusiform, or diffuse) as well as their location within the thoracic aorta. Most thoracic aortic authorities would consider an aortic segment that is more than 4 cm in maximal diameter to be aneurysmal. Aneurysms may be congenital or acquired and generally result from weakening of the aortic wall. Congenital aneurysms are caused by connective tissue disorders such as Marfan syndrome and Ehlers Danlos syndrome, while acquired aneurysms are more common and result from various destructive processes affecting the aortic wall. Degenerate aortic aneurysms are the most common form of aneurysm and reflect the pathologic effects of advanced age, smoking, hypertension, and hypercholesterolemia on the aortic wall. Sixty-five percent of aneurysms only involve the abdominal aorta, while 11% involve the thoracoabdominal aorta, and 6% affect the distal thoracic aorta and arch (2).

The incidence of newly diagnosed thoracic aneurysms in the United States approximates 5.9 per 100,000 person-years with a lifetime probability of rupture of 75% to 80% (3). If left untreated, 5-year survival rates range from 10% to 20%. In nondissecting thoracic aortic aneurysms, absolute size is a major predictor of median time to rupture. Aneurysms which are larger than 6 cm have a 43% risk of rupture within 1 year, while those larger than 8 cm have an 80% risk (4). Other factors which independently predict risk of rupture include advanced age, pain, and chronic obstructive pulmonary disease.

Thoracoabdominal aortic aneurysms are categorized according to the Crawford classification (Fig. 32.1). Type I aneurysms originate in the proximal descending thoracic aorta and end above the renal arteries; Type II begin in the proximal descending thoracic aorta and terminate below the renal arteries; Type III originate in the mid-descending thoracic aorta, while Type IV originate at the diaphragm.

Dissections

Aortic dissections are a true surgical emergency and result from an intimal tear that allows blood to escape from the true lumen and create a false lumen within layers of aortic media. Blood within this false channel then can extend proximally or distally and compromise branch vessels, freely rupture into the pericardium or thoracic cavity, or detach the aortic valve leaflets to cause acute aortic insufficiency. The incidence of aortic dissection is approximately five per million population per year. Independent risk factors for dissection include hypertension, advanced age, connective tissue disorders (Marfan and Erlos-Danlos syndromes), and thoracic trauma.

Two classifications systems are used to describe the extent of aortic dissections: the DeBakey system and the Stanford system (5,6). DeBakey classifies dissections into three types: Type I—intimal tear in the ascending aorta with extension of the dissection to the descending aorta; Type II—tear in the ascending aorta with dissection confined to the ascending aorta; and Type III—tear beginning in the descending aorta. The Stanford classification system is simpler and uses two groups: Type A dissections involve the ascending aorta, and Type B dissections do not involve the ascending aorta (Fig. 32.2). The Stanford classification not only simplifies the topographic description of the dissection but also identifies the preferred line of therapy based on risk. Type A dissections carry a mortality of 90% to 95% without surgical intervention

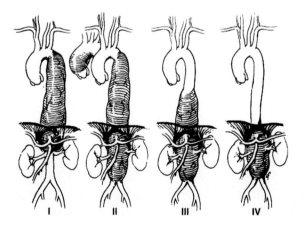

Figure 32.1. Crawford classification of thoracoabdominal aneurysms according to the extent of involvement (From Crawford ES, Svensson LG, Hess HE, et al. A prospective randomized study of cerebrospinal fluid drainage to prevent paraplegia after high-risk surgery on the thoracoabdominal aorta. *J Vasc Surg* 1991;13:37, with permission).

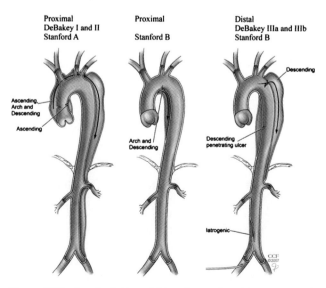

Figure 32.2. Stanford (A and B) and DeBakey (Types I, II, III) classification of aortic dissection.

and account for approximately 65% to 70% of all aortic dissections. Due to a 1% per hour mortality, they require urgent repair (7). Type B dissections carry a 40% mortality, and medical management is the preferred type of therapy except for Type B dissections, which involve the aortic arch.

Intramural hematomas constitute a particular variant of aortic dissections. In about 13% of aortic dissections, there is no evidence of an intimal tear. It is believed that in these cases the inciting event is an intramural hematoma (caused by hemorrhage into the media from a penetrating ulcer). An intramural hematoma should be treated the same as an aortic dissection (8).

Traumatic Injuries

Traumatic injuries to the thoracic aorta can result from blunt or penetrating trauma. Blunt trauma, usually the result of motor vehicle accidents, results in a decelerating force exerting sheer stress on transition points of the aorta. Damage typically occurs at the aortic isthmus, the region just beyond the fixed aortic arch and the mobile descending thoracic aorta. Of the 100,000 blunt chest trauma hospital admissions per year, 3,000 have aortic injuries requiring surgery (9). Survival in these situations is poor, party due to the severity of other organ injury in these patients.

Atherosclerotic Disease

Atherosclerotic disease of the thoracic aorta is pathologically similar to the disease process that affects other arterial systems and results in the formation of various amounts of arterial wall plaque. A penetrating atherosclerotic ulcer (PAU) can result from erosion of an atherosclerotic plaque into the aortic media. A PAU can eventually expand and result in an aneurysm, dissection, or frank rupture. Atherosclerotic plaque in the ascending aorta and arch has been linked to an increased risk of stroke, peripheral embolization, perioperative stroke, as well as neuropsychological dysfunction after open heart surgery. Atheroemboli, thromboemboli, and plaque thickness greater than 4 mm correlate with embolic risk. In patients undergoing cardiopulmonary bypass with identifiable aortic atheroma, the risk of stroke is as high as 12%, far above the usual 1% to 2% stroke rate (10,11).

Coarctation and Other Congenital Anomalies

The most common congenital anomalies of the thoracic aorta include coarctation, aortic arch anomalies, and patent ductus arteriosus. Coarctation is the most common and can present in early adulthood with upper extremity hypertension and weak pulses in the lower body. If left untreated, chronic increased afterload can result in heart failure.

TRANSESOPHAGEAL ECHOCARDIOGRAPHY IN THE EXAMINATION OF THE AORTA

Multiplane TEE in the operating room can visualize nearly the entire course of the thoracic aorta except for the most distal ascending aorta and proximal portion of the aortic arch (12). Here, the trachea and left main stem bronchus obscure imaging. The examination begins with evaluation of the ascending aorta. The midesophageal aortic valve long-axis view at 120 degrees is obtained first to clearly visualize the sinus segment of the ascending aorta, the sinotubular junction, and the proximal ascending aorta (Fig. 32.3). Slight withdrawal of the probe and rotation of the angle back to 45 degrees allows further visualization of the ascending aorta. Complete examination of the ascending aorta is not complete until a short-axis view is completed by rotating the probe between 0 and 45 degrees (Figs. 32.4 and 32.5). In this and the long-axis views, the diameter of the ascending aorta, sinus segment,

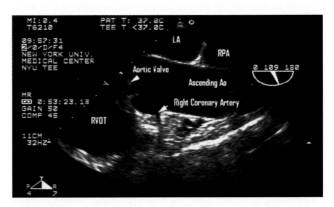

Figure 32.3. Longitudinal (109 degrees) view of the ascending aorta showing the aortic valve and right coronary ostium. (Reprinted from Konstadt SN, Shernan SK, Oka Y. *Clinical Transesophageal Echocardiography*. Philadelphia: Lippincott Williams & Wilkins, 2003, with permission.)

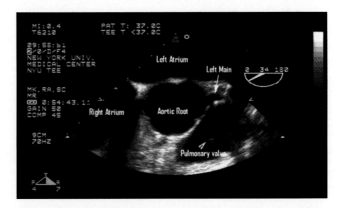

Figure 32.4. Slightly oblique transverse (34 degrees) view of the base of the heart through the aortic root showing the ostium of the left main coronary artery. (Reprinted from Konstadt SN, Shernan SK, Oka Y. *Clinical Transesophageal Echocardiography*. Philadelphia: Lippincott Williams & Wilkins, 2003, with permission.)

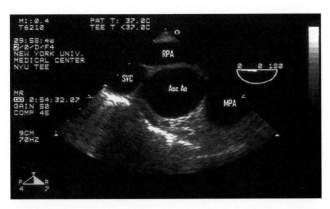

Figure 32.5. Transverse (0 degree) view of the ascending aorta at the base of the heart just superior to the sinotubular junction. (Reprinted from Konstadt SN, Shernan SK, Oka Y. *Clinical Transesophageal Echocardiography*. Philadelphia: Lippincott Williams & Wilkins, 2003, with permission.)

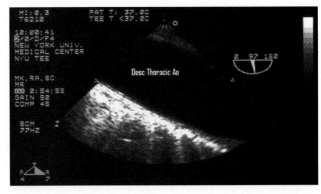

Figure 32.7. Longitudinal (97 degrees) view of the descending thoracic aorta. (Reprinted from Konstadt SN, Shernan SK, Oka Y. *Clinical Transesophageal Echocardiography*. Philadelphia: Lippincott Williams & Wilkins, 2003, with permission.)

and annulus can be measured. Care must be taken during this examination to identify the Swan Ganz catheter so as to not mistake this for an aortic pathology (e.g., intimal flap).

The descending aortic transesophageal examination begins by turning the probe to the left from the midesophageal four-chamber view until a circular structure appears in the upper center of the echo image (Fig. 32.6). Called the descending aorta short-axis view, the image should be enlarged to a depth of 6 to 8 cm to optimize visualization. The long-axis view of the descending thoracic aorta can be obtained simply by rotating the probe to 90 degrees (Fig. 32.7). The operator should withdraw the probe until the left subclavian artery origin is visualized, then re-advance the probe caudally to visualize the entire descending thoracic and upper abdominal aorta. Descriptions of descending aortic pathologies should include a distance from the left subclavian artery for localization.

The aortic arch is brought into view by withdrawing the probe at an angle of 0 degrees during which the circular structure of the descending thoracic aorta becomes an elliptical structure, the aortic arch (Fig. 32.8). This view is called the upper-esophageal aortic arch long-axis view, with the distal arch to the right of the image and the proximal arch to the left (Fig. 32.9). Turning the probe to the right and the left will allow complete visualization of the aortic arch, with the posterior wall at the top and the anterior wall at the bottom of the image. Visualization of the aortic arch vessels can be more challenging. Starting with the upper esophageal aortic arch long-axis view, withdrawing the probe cranially and rotating the probe from 20 to 40 degrees brings the proximal left subclavian and carotid arteries into view. The innominate artery is obscured by the trachea.

Results of the thoracic aortic transesophageal survey should be reported in a systematic fashion by using at least two planes and color Doppler. Maximal diameters at the level of the aortic annulus, midsinus segment, sinotubular junction, midascending aorta, proximal descending thoracic aorta, middescending aorta, and diaphragmatic

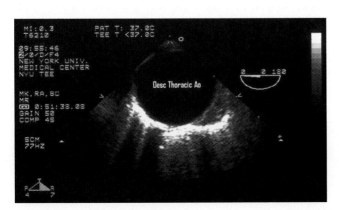

Figure 32.6. Transverse (0 degree) view of the descending thoracic aorta. (Reprinted from Konstadt SN, Shernan SK, Oka Y. *Clinical Transesophageal Echocardiography*. Philadelphia: Lippincott Williams & Wilkins, 2003, with permission.)

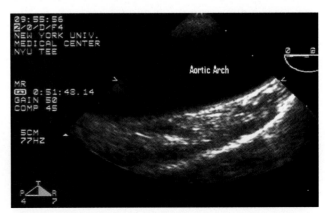

Figure 32.8. Transverse (0 degree) view of the distal aortic arch. (Reprinted from Konstadt SN, Shernan SK, Oka Y. *Clinical Transesophageal Echocardiography*. Philadelphia: Lippincott Williams & Wilkins, 2003, with permission.)

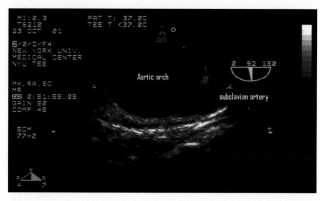

Figure 32.9. Longitudinal (92 degrees) view of the midaortic arch showing the origin on the left subclavian artery. (Reprinted from Konstadt SN, Shernan SK, Oka Y. *Clinical Transesophageal Echocardiography*. Philadelphia: Lippincott Williams & Wilkins, 2003, with permission.)

aorta should be recorded along with corresponding degree of atheroma (13).

Grade	Description
1	Normal aorta
2	Extensive intimal thickening
3	Protrudes <5mm into aortic lumen
4	Protrudes >5mm into aortic lumen
5	Mobile atheroma

INTRAOPERATIVE ROLE OF TEE IN AORTIC DISEASE

Type A Aortic Dissections

Type A aortic dissections carry an extremely high mortality, and urgent surgical repair is indicated at the time of diagnosis. TEE is an important diagnostic tool and should be utilized both preoperatively and intraoperatively. Historically, aortography was the gold standard for diagnosing an aortic dissection, yet more recently, computerized tomography (CT scan), TEE, and magnetic resonance imaging (MRI scan) have been shown to be useful (14). CT scans can be performed quickly and safely in almost all patients suspected of having an aortic dissection. Unfortunately, CT scans cannot provide information about aortic regurgitation, coronary artery involvement, or the site of intimal tear. MRI scans, on the other hand, are very sensitive and specific for diagnosing an aortic dissection and can identify the location of the intimal tear quite well. Many patients with acute aortic syndromes, however, are not hemodynamically stable enough to undergo a complete MRI scan; additionally, MRI examination is contraindicated in some patients owing to pacemakers, certain types of aneurysm clips, and orthopedic hardware.

TEE has recently emerged as a singularly sufficient study for the diagnosis of a Type A aortic dissection. Multiple studies over the past decade have substantiated TEE's role in the diagnosis of an aortic dissection (15). Sensitivity was consistently high, ranging from 97% to 100%, while specificity was anywhere from 77% to 100%. The more recent use of multiplanar technology has further increased the accuracy of TEE in aortic dissection diagnosis with sensitivities reported between 98% and 100% and specificity between 94% and 100% (16,17).

Intraoperative TEE evaluation of an aortic dissection is crucial for successful operative management (18). Specific findings on TEE will direct the surgical approach and lead to surgeon to consider different cannulation sites, root or valve replacement, bypass grafting, and arch replacement in addition to the usual repair techniques. At the Cleveland Clinic, our minimum standard approach to a Type A aortic dissection involves right axillary artery cannulation, reconstruction of the dissected layers (without the use of glue), placement of a supracoronary graft after aortic valve resuspension, and creation of an open distal anastomosis under deep hypothermic circulatory arrest. Intraoperative TEE by an experienced operator is quintessential to the success of the surgical endeavor. The goals of intraoperative TEE during a Type A dissection repair include

1. Confirmation of the diagnosis;
2. Assessment of the aortic root, including the size of the sinus segment, the degree of aortic insufficiency, and patency of the coronary ostia;
3. Assessment of global LV and right ventricular (RV) function and localization of any regional wall-motion abnormalities;
4. Monitoring for LV distension during cooling in the setting of aortic insufficiency;
5. Postrepair assessment of LV and RV functions, aortic valve competence, and coronary ostial patency.

Confirmation of the Diagnosis

The pathognomonic echocardiographic appearance of an aortic dissection is an undulating linear density (intimal flap) within the aortic lumen which separates the true from the false lumen (Figs. 32.10 and 32.11). Each of these lumens will have different Doppler flow patterns. Importantly, a clear linear flap may not be completely visualized owing to either ineffective probe positioning or to the topographic nature of the dissection flap itself. Nonetheless, whenever a single aortic wall appearance is replaced by two separate echo densities, an aortic dissection should be suspected. Other clues to the presence of an aortic dissection include central displacement of intimal calcification and separation of the intimal layers from wall thrombus. Often, the location of the intimal tear can be identified by TEE as a turbulent jet of color flowing from true to false lumen. Most studies report that 70% of primary initial tears occur in the ascending aorta, 20% in the arch, and the remainder in the descending thoracic aorta (14).

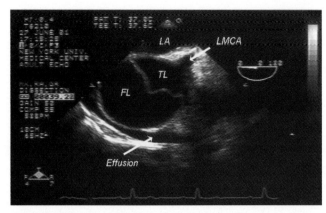

Figure 32.10. Transverse view of a Type A aortic dissection at the level of the left main coronary artery. A small pericardial effusion is also present.

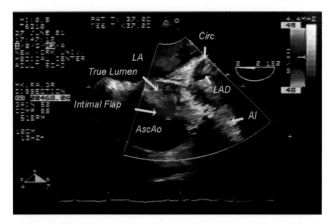

Figure 32.12. Longitudinal view of a Type A aortic dissection with aortic insufficiency.

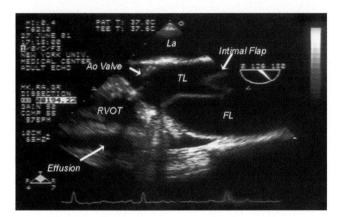

Figure 32.11. Longitudinal view of a Type A aortic dissection.

Assessment of the Aortic Root, Aortic Valve, and Coronary Ostia

TEE evaluation of the aortic valve is crucial in aortic dissection surgical decision making. Aortic insufficiency is present in nearly 70% of Type A aortic dissections and can result from a number of mechanisms including (a) aortic root dilatation alone without commissural detachment, (b) destruction of commissural support, and (c) dissection flap prolapse into LV outflow tract (19).

TEE must evaluate the size of the sinus segment (i.e., the aortic root) as well, since aortic root dilatation with aortic insufficiency may require a root replacement (Fig. 32.12). Patients with Marfan syndrome who have significant aortic root enlargement with aortic insufficiency usually require full root replacement to obviate the poor long-term durability of valve repair techniques.

Finally, evaluation of the integrity of the coronary ostia is critical in planning surgical repair. The coronary ostia are involved in the dissection process in approximately 20% of patients and alert the surgical team for the possible need of coronary bypass grafting (19). Often, coronary malperfusion usually affects the right coronary artery and can be seen clearly upon visual inspection of the aortic

root. Earlier detection of coronary artery involvement, especially in the setting of accompanying regional wall motion abnormality, can alert the surgical team and allow earlier harvest of saphenous vein conduit.

Assessment of Global and Regional Myocardial Function

Intraoperative TEE should provide a clear assessment of global ventricular function. Global dysfunction can result from coronary artery involvement, severe aortic insufficiency, pericardial tamponade, or a preexisting cardiomyopathy. Regional wall motion abnormalities usually signal coronary malperfusion or preexisting coronary artery disease. Most patients undergoing repair of a Type A dissection do not undergo preoperative coronary angiography, and discovery of a regional wall motion abnormality should alert the surgical team to the likely need for coronary artery bypass to the affected territory. At the Cleveland Clinic, we will routinely harvest saphenous vein and bypass the territory that has evidence of regional ischemia.

Monitoring for LV distention cooling

Repair of a Type A dissection almost always requires a period of active cooling to a core temperature of 18°C during which time ventricular fibrillation will occur. Depending on the degree of aortic insufficiency, the LV may begin to distend and result in poor myocardial perfusion and protection. Intraoperative TEE can be useful here to monitor LV distension and alert the surgical team to the need for either aortic cross-clamping with cardioplegic arrest or placement of a LV vent catheter.

Postrepair Assessment

Following completion of the repair, TEE should focus on the degree of residual aortic insufficiency, the overall ventricular function, and assessment of intracardiac air. Residual aortic insufficiency of 2+ or more will usually prompt the surgical team to re-arrest the heart and replace the aortic valve. Additionally, a regional wall motion abnormality may prompt the need for an additional coronary bypass to the affected territory. Close communication between the TEE operator and the surgeon is essential to a successful and durable repair of a Type A dissection.

Type B Aortic Dissections

The role of intraoperative TEE during open surgery for a complicated Type B aortic dissection involves identification of the primary intimal tear, which is usually near the left subclavian artery. In most instances, circulatory arrest will be necessary since there will not be a safe place to place a cross-clamp on the fragile aortic arch. During the cooling phase, intraoperative TEE must carefully monitor for LV distension, especially in situations where there is more than 1+ aortic insufficiency. Since the surgeon cannot reliably identify LV distension from a left thoracotomy, the TEE operator must remain vigilant for this situation until the circulation is stopped.

Thoracic Aortic Plaque

The presence of thoracic aortic atheroma has been correlated with perioperative strokes in multiple studies (13). The ability to detect significant atheromatous or calcific burden within the portions of the ascending aorta can direct the surgical team to alternate methods of cannulation and even overall surgical strategy in order to prevent untoward events of brain embolization. From an echocardiographic perspective, the ascending aorta has been divided into six zones corresponding to sites of surgical manipulation (20). Zones 1 through 3 correspond to the proximal, mid, and distal ascending aorta and represent sites for aortotomies, proximal anastomoses/vent catheters, and cross-clamping, respectively. Zone 4 is the proximal aortic arch and typically the site of aortic cannulation. Zones 5 and 6, which are the distal arch and proximal descending thoracic aorta, are rarely manipulated during standard open heart surgeries. Royse demonstrated that adequate intraoperative TEE imaging of zone 3 occurred in only 58% of cases and zone 4 in only 42% of cases. Additionally, manual surgical palpation detects only 50% of important aortic disease identified by epiaortic ultrasonography. As such, TEE has an important role as a screening tool for disease of the ascending aorta and proximal aortic arch. If significant atheroma or calcification is identified in zones 1, 2, 5, or 6, then epiaortic scanning should be performed by the surgeon (Figs. 32.13 and 32.14). Finally, identification of mobile thrombi in zone 6 should alert the surgeon to the possibility of disrupting this plaque if an intraaortic balloon should need to be placed.

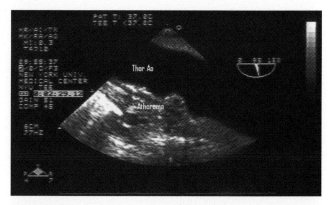

Figure 32.13. Transverse view of the distal aortic arch showing a mobile atheroma.

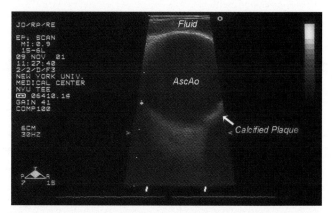

Figure 32.14. Epiaortic scan of the ascending aorta using a 7.5-MHz probe; there is a small plaque posteromedially.

Endovascular Stent Grafting

The increased use of thoracic endovascular stents for the management of complicated Type B aortic dissections and descending thoracic aortic aneurysms has led to a new use for intraoperative TEE. The success of a thoracic endograft depends on correct anchoring within a portion of normal-sized aorta at its proximal and distal ends (i.e., proximal and distal landing zones). Intraoperative TEE can be useful to confirm stiff-guidewire position within the aorta (usually "parked" just above the aortic valve), aid in device placement, and finally confirm the absence of endoleak. Intraoperative TEE currently serves as an adjunct to angiography.

Percutaneous Aortic Valves

Transapical or transfemoral placement of percutaneous aortic valves relies on expert intraoperative TEE to confirm the diameter of the aortic root (long-axis view) and evaluate the amount and pattern of calcification of the native aortic valve cusps (short-axis view). Intraoperative TEE is an essential adjunct to angiography during valve deployment. After guidewire advancement, TEE is used to confirm valve placement (typically one third of the stent placed above the annulus) as well as assess valve function postdeployment. After the valve has been expanded into position, the amount of aortic insufficiency must be identified to determine the need for repeat balloon dilatation. Additionally, wall motion abnormalities must be quickly identified since these signal either coronary embolization or cusp impingement. The detection of a wall motion abnormality or global ventricular dysfunction signals the immediate need for emergency coronary catheterization.

CONCLUSIONS

Intraoperative TEE has an important role in the assessment of the aorta as it relates to open heart surgery. Careful dialogue between the TEE operator and the surgeon is essential in order to derive all the benefits this imaging technology has to offer. Newer, less invasive techniques such as endovascular stenting and percutaneous aortic valves have an important place for the use of intraoperative TEE.

KEY POINTS

■ The thoracic aorta is divided into four segments: the aortic root (aortic annulus, the aortic cusps, the aortic sinuses of Valsalva, and the sinotubular junction), the ascending aorta (sinotubular junction to innominate artery), aortic arch (origins of epiaortic vessels), and descending thoracic aorta (left subclavian artery to diaphragm).

■ An *aneurysm* is an enlargement of more than 50% of normal aortic diameter classified according to their morphology (saccular, fusiform, or diffuse) as well as their location within the thoracic aorta.

■ Thoracoabdominal aortic aneurysms are categorized according to the Crawford classification. Type I originate in the proximal descending thoracic aorta and end above the renal arteries; Type II begin in the proximal descending thoracic aorta and terminate below the renal arteries; Type III originate in the mid-descending thoracic aorta, while Type IV originate at the diaphragm.

■ Aortic dissections result from an intimal tear with creation of a false lumen within layers of aortic media. That may extend proximally or distally and compromise branch vessels, freely rupture into the pericardium or thoracic cavity, or detach the aortic valve leaflets to cause acute aortic insufficiency.

■ Two classifications systems of aortic dissections are used, describing the extent of dissection: (a) DeBakey classifies dissections into three types: Type I—dissection confined to ascending aorta and Type III. (b) Stanford system classifies into two groups:

Type A dissections involve the ascending aorta and Type B dissections.

■ Traumatic injuries to the thoracic aorta can result from blunt or penetrating trauma with damage at the aortic isthmus, the region just beyond the fixed aortic arch and the mobile descending thoracic aorta.

■ Atherosclerotic disease of the thoracic aorta includes atherosclerotic plaque atherosclerotic ulcer (PAU), aneurysm, dissection, or frank rupture.

■ Multiplane TEE visualizes the entire course of the thoracic aorta except for the most distal ascending aorta and proximal portion of the aortic arch.

■ In Type A aortic dissections, TEE is an important diagnostic tool utilized both preoperatively and intraoperatively. The goals of intraoperative TEE during a Type A dissection repair include confirmation of diagnosis, aortic root assessment, degree of aortic insufficiency, and patency of coronary ostia.

■ Goals of intraoperative TEE during a Type A dissection repair include confirmation of the diagnosis, aortic root assessment, and patency of the coronary ostia.

■ TEE for complicated Type B aortic dissection includes identification of intimal tear identification of place to cross clamp the aorta. During cooling phase, TEE monitors LV distension.

■ TEE during thoracic endovascular stents for complicated Type B aortic dissections and descending thoracic aortic aneurysms to identify correct anchoring, confirm stiff-guidewire position within the aorta, aid in device placement, and confirm absence of endoleak.

■ Transapical or transfemoral placement of percutaneous aortic valves relies on expert intraoperative TEE to (a) confirm diameter of the aortic root (long-axis view); (b) evaluate calcification of native aortic valve cusps. TEE is used to confirm valve placement and assess valve function postdeployment. Detection of a wall motion abnormality or global ventricular dysfunction signals the immediate need for emergency coronary catheterization.

REFERENCES

1. Svensson LG. Rationale and technique for replacement of the ascending aorta, arch, and distal aorta using a modified elephant trunk procedure. *J Card Surg* 1992;7:301–312.
2. Crawford ES, Svensson LG, Hess KR, et al. A prospective randomized study of cerebrospinal fluid drainage to prevent paraplegia after high-risk surgery on the thoracoabdominal aorta. *J Vasc Surg* 1991;13:36–45; discussion 45–46.
3. Bickerstaff LK, Pairolero PC, Hollier LH, et al. Thoracic aortic aneurysms: a population-based study. *Surgery* 1982;92:1103–1108.

4. Szilagyi DE, Elliott JP, Smith RF. Clinical fate of the patient with asymptomatic abdominal aortic aneurysm and unfit for surgical treatment. *Arch Surg* 1972;104:600–606.

5. DeBakey ME, McCollum CH, Crawford ES, et al. Dissection and dissecting aneurysms of the aorta: twenty-year follow-up of five hundred twenty-seven patients treated surgically. *Surgery* 1982;92:1118–1134.

6. Daily PO, Trueblood HW, Stinson EB, et al. Management of acute aortic dissections. *Ann Thorac Surg* 1970;10:237–247.

7. Scholl FG, Coady MA, Davies R, et al. Interval or permanent nonoperative management of acute type A aortic dissection. *Arch Surg* 1999;134:402–405;discussion 405–406.

8. Sundt TM. Intramural hematoma and penetrating atherosclerotic ulcer of the aorta. *Ann Thorac Surg* 2007;83:S835–S841; discussion S846–S850.

9. von Segesser LK, Fischer A, Vogt P, et al. Diagnosis and management of blunt great vessel trauma. *J Card Surg* 1997;12:181–186; discussion 186–192.

10. Roach GW, Kanchuger M, Mangano CM, et al. Adverse cerebral outcomes after coronary bypass surgery. Multicenter Study of Perioperative Ischemia Research Group and the Ischemia Research and Education Foundation Investigators. *N Engl J Med* 1996;335:1857–1863.

11. Marschall K, Kanchuger M, Kessler K, et al. Superiority of transesophageal echocardiography in detecting aortic arch atheromatous disease: identification of patients at increased risk of stroke during cardiac surgery. *J Cardiothorac Vasc Anesth* 1994;8:5–13.

12. Kanchuger M, Delphin E. Assessment of surgery of the aorta. In: Savage RW, Aronson S, Thomas JD, et al, eds. *Comprehensive Textbook of Intraoperative Transesophageal Echocardiography*, 1st ed. Philadelphia: Lippincott Williams & Wilkins, 2004:569.

13. Katz ES, Tunick PA, Rusinek H, et al. Protruding aortic atheromas predict stroke in elderly patients undergoing cardiopulmonary bypass: experience with intraoperative transesophageal echocardiography. *J Am Coll Cardiol* 1992;20:70–77.

14. Cigarroa JE, Isselbacher EM, DeSanctis RW, et al. Diagnostic imaging in the evaluation of suspected aortic dissection. Old standards and new directions. *N Engl J Med* 1993;328:35–43.

15. Willens HJ, Kessler KM. Transesophageal echocardiography in the diagnosis of diseases of the thoracic aorta: part 1. Aortic dissection, aortic intramural hematoma, and penetrating atherosclerotic ulcer of the aorta. *Chest* 1999;116:1772–1779.

16. Sommer T, Fehske W, Holzknecht N, et al. Aortic dissection: a comparative study of diagnosis with spiral CT, multiplanar transesophageal echocardiography, and MR imaging. *Radiology* 1996;199:347–352.

17. Keren A, Kim CB, Hu BS, et al. Accuracy of biplane and multiplane transesophageal echocardiography in diagnosis of typical acute aortic dissection and intramural hematoma. *J Am Coll Cardiol* 1996;28:627–636.

18. Payne KJ, Ikonomidis JS, Reeves ST. Transesophageal echocardiography of the thoracic aorta. In: Perrino AC, Reeves ST, eds. *A Practical Approach to Transesophageal Echocardiography*, 2nd ed. Philadelphia: Lippincott Williams & Wilkens, 2007:321–343.

19. Ballal RS, Nanda NC, Gatewood R, et al. Usefulness of transesophageal echocardiography in assessment of aortic dissection. *Circulation* 1991;84:1903–1914.

20. Royse C, Royse A, Blake D, et al. Screening the thoracic aorta for atheroma: a comparison of manual palpation, transesophageal and epiaortic ultrasonography. *Ann Thorac Cardiovasc Surg* 1998;4:347–350.

QUESTIONS

1. Median time to rupture in nondissecting thoracic aortic aneurysms is most closely correlated with
   A. degree of hypertension
   B. presence of a congenital aortic wall abnormality
   C. absolute size of the aorta
   D. rate of increase of the size of the aorta

2. Type B aortic dissections which involve the aortic arch should be treated with
   A. medical management alone with antihypertensives
   B. urgent surgical repair
   C. delayed surgical repair
   D. stent graft repair

3. During aortic dissection repair, intraoperative TEE is needed for monitoring during the cooling phase of cardiopulmonary bypass in order to assess for

A. LV distension due to aortic insufficiency in the setting of ventricular fibrillation
B. mitral insufficiency during ventricular fibrillation
C. change in the dissection flap dynamics
D. aortic leakage

4. Aortic plaque identified in zone 5 or 6 prior to routine CABG would necessitate
   A. no definite change in distal aortic annulation
   B. always a need for axillary cannulation
   C. always a need for aortic arch replacement
   D. cancellation of the case

5. Mortality in Type A aortic dissections approach
   A. 1%/day
   B. 1%/hour
   C. 40%
   D. 5%/hour

Surgical Considerations and Assessment of Endovascular Management of Thoracic Vascular Disease

Teng C. Lee ■ Madhav Swaminathan ■ G. Chad Hughes

INTRODUCTION

Diseases of the thoracic aorta are serious and can be life threatening. Conventional surgical therapy is associated with relatively high morbidity and mortality. Since the first successful use of stent grafts to treat thoracic aortic pathology by Volodos et al. (1), there has been considerable worldwide enthusiasm for adoption of this technique. Initial results by Dake et al. (2) at Stanford using early generation stent grafts were promising. Since that time, there have been significant advances in the technology, which has been used to treat a variety of thoracic aortic pathologies. However, the treatment of aneurysmal disease is the only indication currently approved by the U.S. Food and Drug Administration (FDA). The early results of thoracic stent-grafting have been excellent, with 30-day morbidity and mortality rates lower than those observed following conventional open repair (3–8). However, long-term durability remains less clear, with mid-term results just starting to appear in the literature (9–16).

The majority of thoracic endovascular aortic repairs (TEVAR) are performed in the operating room with fluoroscopic capabilities under general anesthesia. The use of fluoroscopy in the deployment of thoracic endografts is currently the gold standard. Transesophageal echocardiography (TEE) has become a useful adjunct in some institutions to confirm the accuracy of deployment and to detect endoleaks (17–20). Studies involving a limited number of cases have suggested that TEE is more sensitive and specific than angiography in detecting endoleaks (21–23). TEE is also an extremely sensitive tool to detect aortic dissections (24). Although the majority of patients presenting for endovascular repair of the thoracic aorta have undergone a variety of imaging studies to determine the extent and severity of their aortic disease, TEE may detect coexisting aortic pathology not seen on other imaging modalities (25). The technique is also very sensitive for detecting atheromatous plaque in the aorta, which may be useful in guiding safe placement of stent grafts

and wires so as to minimize the potential for embolic complications.

In the following text, thoracic aortic anatomy, pathology, endovascular approaches, and the utility of TEE will be discussed.

ANATOMY OF THE THORACIC AORTA

The aorta shares a close relationship with the esophagus throughout its length in the thorax. Echocardiographic views must keep this relationship in perspective at all times. The thoracic aorta can be divided into three anatomic segments: the ascending, arch, and descending aorta. In adults, the ascending aorta is approximately 5 cm in length; the initial segment of the ascending aorta, the aortic root (sinus of Valsalva segment), originates at the aortic valve annulus and becomes the tubular ascending aorta at the level of the sinotubular junction. The tubular ascending aorta then extends rightward around the main pulmonary artery trunk, crosses the right pulmonary artery anteriorly, and ascends rightward and anteriorly until it meets the aortic arch at the origin of the brachiocephalic (innominate) artery at the level of the second intercostal space. The diameter of the ascending aorta increases with age; the diameter is smallest at the aortic annulus and largest at the sinuses of Valsalva, varying from 2 to 3.7 cm in an average adult.

The aortic arch curves in a posterior and leftward direction with a cephalad convexity. The proximal portion of the arch is poorly visualized by TEE due to the anatomical interposition of the air-filled trachea between the esophagus and the aorta at this level. Three major vessels, the brachiocephalic (innominate), left common carotid, and left subclavian arteries, typically arise from the arch, although multiple variants exist including the so-called bovine arch, whereby the innominate and left common carotid arise from a common trunk, as well as a four-vessel arch in which the left vertebral artery arises directly from the arch, rather than its usual origin from the left subclavian artery (LSCA). These anatomic variants may have surgical significance in both open and endovascular thoracic aortic repairs.

The descending thoracic aorta begins just distal to the origin of the LSCA, at the level of the 4th thoracic vertebral body. The descending aorta then courses slightly anteriorly and rightward toward the diaphragm. It is anterior and to the left of the esophagus at the level of the 4th thoracic vertebral body, becoming directly posterior at the level of the diaphragm. Therefore, at the lower esophageal position, the heart and aorta are on opposite sides of the esophagus or TEE probe.

Branches of the intercostal arteries may variably be seen using TEE, and blood flow may be imaged using color flow Doppler (CFD). In some cases, the celiac artery may be seen arising off the anterior aortic wall with the probe in the transgastric position. Imaging the aortic branches assumes importance in assessment of branch vessel involvement in aneurysms and dissections, potential coverage by stent grafts, and as a source of type 2 endoleaks. Endoleaks are further described later in this text.

The aortic wall is composed of an intima, media, and adventitia. The intima is a thin layer of endothelium, while the media consists of a thick layer of elastic tissue and smooth muscle. The adventitia is a loose layer of tissue containing collagen, lymphatics, and the vasa vasorum. The media accounts for up to 80% of the aortic wall thickness and is responsible for both its strength and elasticity. Using TEE, the aortic wall may be assessed for intimal tears, aneurysmal dilatation, and atheroma quantification.

THORACIC AORTIC ANEURYSMS

An aneurysm is defined as a dilatation of the aorta to twice the diameter of the contiguous normal aortic caliber. Therefore, in an average-height person with an average distal arch diameter of 2.8 cm, a diameter of 5.6 cm or greater is defined as aneurysmal (26). The estimated annual incidence is 6 cases per 100,000 persons, with 40% of these involving the descending thoracic aorta. Thoracic aortic aneurysms (TAA) are most commonly due to medial degeneration and luminal atherosclerosis. Other causes include connective tissue disorders such as the Marfan syndrome, Ehlers-Danlos syndrome, or Loeys-Dietz syndrome, trauma, infection, and pseudoaneurysms after previous aortic surgery. Chronic dissections can also lead to aneurysmal dilatation. TEVAR is generally utilized in the treatment of descending thoracic aneurysms located between the level of the left common carotid artery and celiac axis, although aneurysms of the arch and thoracoabdominal aorta may be treated as well using currently available devices if proximal and/or distal seal zone ("landing zone") is created via a combination of open surgery and endovascular repair (27). These so-called "hybrid" procedures create landing zone via translocation or debranching of great vessels arising from

the aorta, allowing them to be subsequently covered by the endografts. Although beyond the scope of this chapter, a complete discussion of "hybrid" thoracic aortic repair has recently been presented (28).

The timing of intervention for thoracic aneurysms is based upon calculating the risk of the procedure versus the expected risk of death, rupture, or dissection in the absence of treatment. Recommendations regarding the size criteria for intervention have been suggested based upon population studies by Coady et al. (29). Due to the exponential increase in event rates observed when an aneurysm reaches a diameter of 7 cm in the descending aorta, the authors suggested that intervention at 6.5 cm in asymptomatic patients would preempt most ruptures and dissections. However, a recent consensus statement from the Society of Thoracic Surgeons recommends intervention for descending aneurysms at a diameter of 5.5 cm for fusiform aneurysms and 2 cm for saccular aneurysms in asymptomatic patients (26). Further, in patients with the Marfan syndrome, Loeys-Dietz syndrome, or other connective tissue disease, repair is generally performed sooner because of the higher risk of rupture or dissection in these patients at smaller aortic diameters. However, the presence of a connective tissue disorder is considered a contraindication to TEVAR, with the exception being the patient in whom both proximal and distal landing zones are within previously placed Dacron grafts, rather than genetically abnormal aorta. Likewise, a significant family history of adverse aortic events may prompt intervention at smaller diameters. Finally, patients who are symptomatic should be treated regardless of aortic size, assuming there are no contraindications to surgery. Typical symptoms include chest or back pain, hoarseness (from left recurrent laryngeal nerve involvement), and dysphagia (esophageal displacement).

THORACIC AORTIC DISSECTIONS

Thoracic aortic dissections result in significant morbidity and mortality, even with optimal surgical and/or medical management. The incidence is about 5 to 30 cases per million, with a male predominance. Thoracic aortic dissections are generally due to tears in the aortic intima. In nontraumatic situations, these occur due to degeneration of the aortic media or cystic medial necrosis. Tears in the intima lead to the creation of a false lumen, which allows blood to course within the wall of the aorta ("double-barrel aorta"). This false lumen generally occurs in the outer one third of the media, and thus the outer wall of the aorta constraining the false lumen consists only of the adventitia and outer media. As such, the false lumen may rupture resulting in exsanguination. Alternatively, the blood flow in the pressurized false lumen may compress the true lumen, potentially causing organ ischemia due to branch vessel compromise (so-called dynamic malperfusion). Finally, the dissection process may extend out into aortic branch vessels themselves, causing distal occlusion (static malperfusion). Either type of malperfusion syndrome increases the risk of death from dissection significantly.

Risk factors for dissection include chronic hypertension, connective tissue disorders (Marfan, Ehlers-Danlos, Loeys-Dietz syndromes), aortic coarctation, bicuspid aortic valve, and iatrogenic trauma. Thoracic aortic dissections are classified as Stanford type A when the ascending aorta is involved and Stanford type B when only the descending aorta is involved. Although not the focus of this chapter, acute Type A dissection is a surgical emergency and mandates immediate open repair in most cases. With regard to acute Type B dissection, medical management remains the standard of care for uncomplicated cases. However, for acute Type B dissection complicated by impending or frank rupture or malperfusion syndromes, endovascular management has become increasingly popular given the significant improvement in outcomes compared with open repair in this scenario (26). The use of TEVAR for this indication is not currently approved by the FDA, although clinical trials to gain approval for this application are ongoing. The use of TEVAR for aneurysmal degeneration secondary to chronic Type B dissection remains controversial at the current time (26), and additional data regarding this application are needed.

THORACIC AORTIC TRANSECTIONS

Traumatic aortic transections are usually due to blunt trauma and have been associated with significant morbidity and mortality rates when managed by open repair in the acute setting. As such, endovascular repair has gained widespread popularity in recent years in this area, although like dissection, this remains an off-label application. One major advantage of TEVAR for transection is that endovascular repair may be performed using low-dose or even no heparin administration, which is especially beneficial in patients with significant head or solid organ injury. Further, unlike open repair, operative delay is generally not necessary given that TEVAR imposes minimal additional physiologic insult to patients already critically ill as a result of their associated traumatic injuries. A recent review of current data by Hoffer et al. (30) supports the use of stent-grafting for blunt thoracic trauma, with mortality and paraplegia rates being reduced by half as compared to open surgery. TEE may play an important role here as well for both diagnosis and stent graft positioning and deployment, especially if preoperative imaging has been limited due to patient condition.

OTHER AORTIC PATHOLOGIES

Intramural hematoma (IMH) is a variant of aortic dissection falling into the category of acute aortic syndrome. It is believed to be caused by spontaneous bleeding into the media from the vasa vasorum or resulting from a penetrating aortic ulcer (PAU). It can progress to aortic dissection and even rupture. The incidence of this disorder appears to be increasing with the more liberal use of CT scanning for the diagnosis of acute aortic syndromes. On TEE, IMH is seen as a layered thickening of the aortic wall without an intimal flap. IMH of the descending thoracic aorta is typically managed medically, similar to uncomplicated acute Type B dissection, unless impending or frank rupture is present, in which case TEVAR may be utilized. TEVAR should include coverage of the associated PAU if present.

PAU are due to a disruption of atherosclerotic plaque in the media, exposing the media to pulsatile blood flow, frequently resulting in IMH or formation of a focal saccular aneurysm. Indications for surgical or endovascular repair include symptoms (typically back pain) or, in the asymptomatic patient, a diameter ≥ 20 mm for the saccular component, as this pathology is felt to carry a higher risk for rupture than fusiform aneurysm (26). Fortunately, the majority of PAU occur in the descending thoracic aorta and are usually amenable to endovascular repair if indicated.

CURRENT PRACTICE OF ENDOVASCULAR REPAIR OF THE THORACIC AORTA

The basic concept of a stent has not changed since the development of coronary stents. Most stent grafts are made of thin woven dacron (polyethylene terephthalate) or polytetrafluoroethylene (PTFE) supported by a fine metal skeleton, usually made of nitinol or stainless steel, that is radio-opaque. Endografts may be self-expanding after deployment from a surrounding sheath or require expansion (molding) with a balloon after deployment. Several stent grafts are available on the market, and a number of them have been used for thoracic aortic pathology. Currently, in the United States, there are three FDA-approved endografts for the thoracic aorta. The first to be approved (March, 2005) was the TAG thoracic stent graft (W.L. Gore and Associates, Flagstaff, Arizona). The Medtronic Talent (Medtronic Inc., Minneapolis, Minnesota) and Zenith TX-2 (Cook Medical Inc., Bloomington, Indiana) devices received approval in the summer of 2008. Each has its own advantages and disadvantages and none is ideal.

The Talent device has been the most widely used worldwide, with over 20,000 implants to date. This device consists of a polyester graft with nitinol stents and comes in diameters ranging from 22 to 46 mm. This broad range of available sizes represents the main advantage of the Talent graft. However, the device comes only in lengths of approximately 11 cm, which is a major disadvantage when long lengths of aorta need to be covered.

The Zenith TX2 device consists of stainless steel Z-stents attached to a polyester fabric. This device is designed with proximal and distal components and comes in diameters from 28 to 42 mm. A unique feature of this device is the presence of "barbs" on the proximal and distal ends to prevent migration. Unlike the other devices, which require a 2-cm proximal and distal landing zone, the TX2 device requires 2.5 cm for the larger diameter endografts, which represents a potential disadvantage. Advantages of this device include the availability of tapered devices, as well as the fact that the stainless steel frame is more easily visualized under fluoroscopy than nitinol.

The Gore TAG device is a flexible, nitinol-supported PTFE graft available in diameters ranging from 26 to 40 mm, allowing treatment of a range of aortic sizes similar to the TX2 device. Advantages of this device include ease of deployment, as well as the fact that the device is passed via a separate sheath and thus does not require each device to be passed up individually through the iliofemoral access vessels, an issue which may be important if these vessels are diseased.

To ensure maximal patient safety, the FDA has mandated that physicians using these devices receive appropriate supervised training as well as proctoring by company clinical specialists, for their early cases prior to gaining full unlimited access to the devices. The number of proctored cases varies depending on the physicians' previous endovascular experience.

Endovascular Procedure

The goal of an endovascular aortic stent-graft procedure is to deploy a stent graft that seals in normal diameter aorta above and below an aneurysm, thus excluding the aneurysm sac from systemic blood flow, distending arterial pressure, and eliminating the risk of aneurysm rupture.

Endovascular procedures are accomplished either in a specialized radiology suite or in an operating room outfitted with appropriate fluoroscopic equipment. The choice of anesthetic is variable; the majority of procedures for the thoracic aorta are performed under general anesthesia, although regional techniques have also been used successfully. However, with the increasing use of TEE for TEVAR, general anesthesia is an obvious choice.

Patients with long-segment coverage of the thoracic aorta may be at an increased risk of spinal cord ischemia. In these patients, intraoperative neurological monitoring may include transcranial motor evoked potentials (tc-MEP) and/or somatosensory evoked potentials (SSEP) for online assessment of spinal cord function (31). Cerebrospinal fluid (CSF) drains may be inserted to allow monitoring of CSF pressure as well as therapeutic CSF drainage to increase spinal cord perfusion pressure (Spinal cord perfusion pressure = MAP – CSF pressure). These drains are inserted in the lumbar position either in the awake patient or after induction of general anesthesia. The CSF catheter is connected to a pressure transducer and drainage system. The CSF pressure is usually maintained at 10 to 12 mm Hg and fluid is drained in 10- to 20-mL increments, if this pressure is exceeded. Patients are usually prepared for evoked potential monitoring

prior to general anesthesia. A total intravenous anesthetic technique may be chosen for tc-MEP monitoring since the use of muscle relaxants and volatile agents may interfere with interpretation of evoked potentials (31,32).

Patients are positioned supine for the procedure, and the abdomen is prepared for either groin or lower abdominal aortic access. The stent grafts come mounted onto insertion devices or "delivery systems," which are large bore (20–24 French) and somewhat inflexible catheters. Patients with small, tortuous, or heavily calcified femoral or iliac vessels may require a lower abdominal transplant-type incision for retroperitoneal delivery via the iliac artery or distal aorta, rather than the femoral route. The femoral arteries are cannulated via a small transverse incision for device delivery on one side and percutaneously on the other, although, as mentioned, more proximal access to the iliac arteries or aorta is occasionally necessary. Once the aorta has been accessed, aortography is performed to clearly establish the aortic pathology and location of "landing zones" for stent-graft deployment, including the location of important branch vessels in the aortic arch or visceral segment.

Devices that must be placed more proximally in the thoracic aorta may necessitate coverage of the left subclavian or left common carotid artery (Fig. 33.1). This may require a concomitant bypass procedure to maintain branch vessel flow once the origin of the vessel(s) has been covered by the endograft. In general, left common carotid coverage mandates adjunctive bypass, whereas left subclavian coverage requires revascularization only in selected circumstances as discussed in more detail below.

Careful positioning of the devices over guidewires is essential to allow for accurate deployment and to

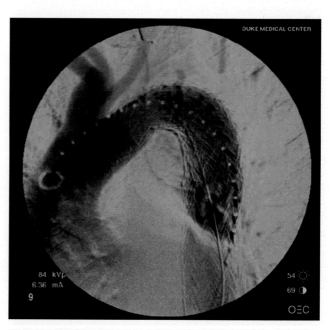

Figure 33.1. Intraoperative angiogram of the thoracic aorta, demonstrating an endovascular stent graft after deployment. The LSCA has been covered by the endograft.

minimize graft migration with deployment. During digital subtraction angiography with the device in the aortic lumen, the surgeon will usually request that respiration be held during contrast injection. The TEE probe may have to be pulled out into the proximal esophagus to allow for unimpeded angiographic imaging of the aorta (Fig. 33.2). Care must be taken to ensure that tachycardia and hypertension are avoided. In early cases of TEVAR, extreme measures were taken to ensure a "still" field, including ventricular asystole with adenosine (33), or ventricular fibrillation (34). However, with newer, self-deploying stents, such extreme maneuvers are not required. Once the stent graft has been deployed, its position is confirmed by various imaging modalities, including TEE, and if required, the proximal and distal ends of the stent graft are "sealed" to the aortic wall by endoluminal balloon inflation. During this transient balloon occlusion of the aorta, the patient may experience significant hemodynamic stress, especially if baseline cardiac function is poor. Vasopressors and inotropes must be available at hand to manage hemodynamic emergencies. Some newer balloons incorporate a multilobed structure that allows the stent graft to be sealed without total occlusion of the aorta (Fig. 33.3).

Blood loss is often difficult to quantify, since it is lost around the sheaths and catheters, under drapes, and can even be retroperitoneal in the case of injury to femoral or iliac vessels if they have been used for access to the aorta. Hemoglobin should be checked during the procedure, especially if the patient becomes unstable. Endovascular procedures also involve the use of radiographic contrast to assist in appropriate deployment of the graft, ensure exclusion of the aneurysmal sac, and determine branch

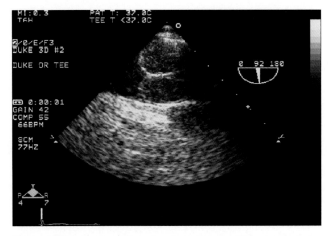

Figure 33.3. Midesophageal echocardiographic view of the descending thoracic aorta with an endovascular balloon shown filled with saline. The multilobed nature of the balloon can be appreciated as a feature that prevents total occlusion of the aorta during balloon inflation.

vessel patency. It is important to ensure that patients are adequately hydrated during the procedure and in the postoperative period, to minimize the possibility of contrast-induced nephropathy.

An important anatomic consideration during TEVAR with which the anesthesiologist should be familiar is coverage of the LSCA. By covering the LSCA, an adequate proximal landing zone can often be achieved for endovascular treatment of proximal descending thoracic aortic pathology in which 2 cm may not be available between the aneurysm and the LSCA origin. In general, LSCA coverage is well tolerated with early studies suggesting that 10% or fewer patients develop subsequent arm or posterior circulation symptoms (35). This study also demonstrates that the proximal portion of the LSCA that comes off the aorta thromboses following stent-graft coverage. This proximal thrombosis may prevent the development of type II endoleak via backflow through the LSCA. Similarly, the arm generally remains asymptomatic due to numerous collateral sources, most notably the left vertebral artery. These patients will have a pressure differential of approximately 50 mm Hg between the right and left arms, and should therefore have blood pressure monitoring done in the right arm to obtain an accurate reflection of central aortic pressure.

However, a more recent analysis of subclavian coverage showed that up to 41% of patients in whom the LSCA was covered required preoperative or postoperative subclavian revascularization (36). There are several definite contraindications to left subclavian coverage without preceding or concomitant revascularization including a patent pedicled left internal mammary artery bypass graft arising from the LSCA, an arteriovenous fistula/graft for renal dialysis, a dominant left vertebral artery that contributes the majority of flow to the posterior circulation, and a left vertebral artery that arises directly off the aortic arch, as these latter patients will develop arm symptoms

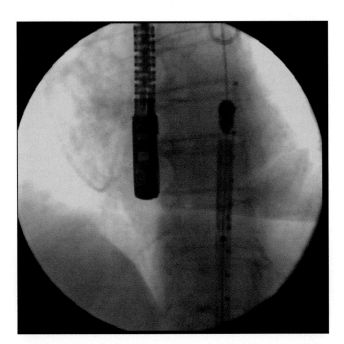

Figure 33.2. Angiogram demonstrating the proximity of the TEE probe to the descending thoracic aorta. There is a stent delivery system in the aorta ready for deployment.

from a lack of collateral flow to the arm via the vertebral. In general, the posterior circulation and circle of Willis should be investigated electively with CT angiography or magnetic resonance angiography (MRA) preoperatively whenever LSCA coverage is planned. Another relative contraindication to LSCA coverage without prior revascularization is planned endografting of the entire thoracic aorta in a patient with prior repair of an abdominal or TAA. Prior aortic surgery and extensive aortic coverage are major risk factors for paraplegia with TEVAR, and coverage of the LSCA further diminishes collateral flow via the vertebral arteries to the upper spinal cord (37). Our standard protocol in cases where LSCA coverage is planned is to place bilateral radial arterial lines preoperatively. After LSCA coverage, one typically sees dampening in the left-sided trace with a decrease in arterial blood pressure relative to the right arm of between 20 and 50 mm Hg. However, pulsatility in the waveform is generally maintained; a loss of pulsatility or greater decreases in blood pressure beyond that expected should prompt consideration of adjunctive LSCA revascularization to prevent left arm ischemia.

Surgical complications of TEVAR can include damage to iliofemoral access vessels (dissection, rupture), distal embolization of atheromatous debris, adverse reactions from radiographic contrast, retrograde Type A dissection, postimplantation syndrome, and neurologic deficits from occlusion of intercostal arteries. Exclusion of the aneurysm sac by the device is critical to prevent future rupture of the aneurysm. A great deal of discussion exists in the surgical literature about the appropriate management of endoleaks (classified below). Type I endoleak, due to incomplete seal of the device at proximal or distal attachment sites, is considered unacceptable and requires further intervention. Intraoperative TEE is a sensitive imaging modality for detecting endoleaks.

Endoleaks and Their Classification (38)

Endoleak is defined as the persistence of blood flow outside the lumen of the stent graft but within the aneurysm sac or adjacent vascular segment being treated by the graft (39,40). Endoleaks may occur due to misplacement or poor sizing of a stent graft (technical error), material fatigue, displacement or distortion of the stent-graft material (device failure), or by reactions to the stent graft within the aneurysmal sac environment (patient factors). Endoleaks are classified based on location and/or mechanism, and by timing of occurrence.

Persistent flow around the attachment site (proximal or distal) of the stent graft due to ineffective seal at the graft ends is classified as a Type I endoleak. This type of leak, if seen early, is most often due to a technical error, whereas late Type I endoleaks may be due to loss of endograft seal from device migration or seal zone dilation. An endoleak may also occur due to retrograde flow into the aneurysmal sac from a patent collateral branch vessel. This is known as a

Type II endoleak, and, following TEVAR, is most commonly due to retrograde flow from the LSCA or intercostal arteries. Flow into the aneurysmal sac due to a tear or defect in the stent-graft fabric or due to leakage between modular segments of a stent graft is classified as a Type III endoleak. This may be more common in the thoracic region due to greater hemodynamic stress causing early or late graft material fatigue. Flow detected in the aneurysmal sac after completion angiography may also occur due to highly porous graft material and is essentially due to the nature of the stent-graft fabric itself rather than device failure. This is termed a Type IV endoleak and may be difficult to distinguish from other types of graft leakage. Fortunately, with newer generation devices, this is almost never seen. In cases where the source of leakage cannot be identified, the endoleak is classified as "endoleak of undefined origin." Type I endoleaks are also subclassified as I-A or I-B depending on whether only an inflow channel can be imaged as opposed to an inflow and outflow channel, respectively.

Endoleaks are also classified on the basis of timing of occurrence. Endoleaks detected within the first 30 days of deployment are considered "Primary," while those detected later in the postoperative period are termed "Secondary." Secondary endoleaks may be Types I or III and require reintervention to prevent aneurysm rupture. Type II endoleaks are rarely serious and can be left alone to thrombose or may be occluded by embolization techniques. Endoleaks may either be monitored for effect on aneurysm size or treated by percutaneous embolization, secondary stent-graft placement, or open surgical repair. In general, all Type I or III endoleaks, which transmit systemic pressure to the aneurysm sac, should be treated, and the presence of persistent Type I or III endoleak following TEVAR is considered a treatment failure (38).

ASSESSMENT OF THORACIC AORTIC PATHOLOGIES

Angiography had traditionally been the gold standard for the diagnosis of thoracic aortic pathologies. However, in recent years, multidetector computed tomography (MDCT) scans have become the *de facto* gold standard worldwide. The sensitivity of CT for the diagnosis of aortic dissection ranges from 83% to 100%, with a specificity of 100% (41,42). This is in contrast to the sensitivity of 88% and specificity of 94% for conventional angiography. The advantages of MDCT include easy access at most hospitals and the ability to perform scans in a short period of time. Other pathologies in the chest can also be determined. CT is also extremely helpful in multitrauma patients when injuries elsewhere in the body can be seen.

Magnetic resonance imaging, specifically contrast-enhanced three-dimensional (3D) MRA, has also recently become a useful adjunct in the diagnosis of aortic pathologies. Sensitivity is in the range of 92% to 96% with a specificity of 100% for both acute and chronic dissection.

TABLE 33.1	Transesophageal Echocardiographic Imaging Views that Provide Adequate Visualization of the Thoracic Aorta		
Window (Depth from Incisors)	Imaging View	Multiplane Angle	Structures Visualized
Upper esophageal (20–25 cm)	Aortic arch long axis	0	Aortic arch
	Aortic arch short axis	90	Aortic arch, PA
Midesophageal (30–45 cm)	Ascending aortic short axis	0–60	Ascending aorta, SVC, PA
	Ascending aortic long axis	100–150	Ascending aorta, right PA
	Descending aorta short axis	0	Descending aorta, left pleural space
	Descending aorta long axis	90–110	Descending aorta, left pleural space

PA, pulmonary artery; SVC, superior vena cava.

The advantages of MRA include the lack of radiation and avoidance of potentially nephrotoxic iodinated-contrast agents. The main disadvantage is the limited availability and long scan times, which limit usefulness of the modality in an emergency situation.

TEE has been increasingly used to provide an accurate diagnosis of aortic dissection since Erbel et al. (43) published his series in 1989. The sensitivity for the diagnosis of aortic dissection ranges from 97% to 99%, although the specificity has been as low as 77% to 85%. However, with the advent of multiplanar TEE, the ascending aorta can be viewed in multiple imaging planes, which has increased the sensitivity and specificity to 98% and 95%, respectively (44).

ROLE OF TRANSESOPHAGEAL ECHOCARDIOGRAPHY

Introduction

The success of endovascular repair of thoracic aortic pathologies is critically dependent upon the demonstration of satisfactory stent-graft deployment by various imaging modalities. Conventional angiography has been the gold standard, but TEE can add significant information regarding sizing and positioning of stent grafts, the presence or absence of endoleaks, valvular competency, and cardiac function. It is an extremely important adjunct in guiding the placement of stent grafts in the true lumen during repair of dissection.

Views

Care must be exercised while inserting a TEE probe in a patient with known aneurysmal dilatation of the thoracic aorta. This is especially true in cases where a preoperative history of dysphagia, hoarseness (recurrent nerve palsy), or stridor is present. Since the thoracic aorta is in close

proximity with the esophagus, views are usually obtained at an imaging depth of 5 to 7 cm. Excellent resolution is obtained with higher frequency transducers. According to the SCA/ASE guidelines, the six standardized views of the thoracic aorta provide a comprehensive assessment of most aortic pathology (Table 33.1) (45).

Patients with aortic aneurysms require a thorough assessment of aneurysm size and extent, as well as involvement of branch vessels. In the descending aorta, TEE assessment of branch vessel involvement and distal extent of the aneurysm are important. In endovascular repair, an assessment of the stent-graft "landing zone" can be made.

In aortic dissection, a search for the site of intimal tear is extremely useful, although it may not always be easily recognized. Care must be taken to avoid false positives with TEE, since mirror images ("double barrel aorta") are common in this region (Fig. 33.4). CFD is more useful for aortic dissections than aneurysms. The differential flow

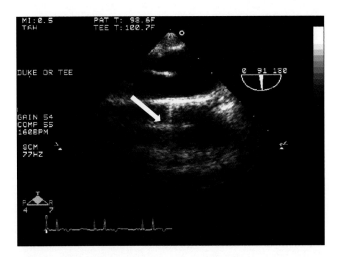

Figure 33.4. Midesophageal echocardiographic image of descending thoracic aorta in long axis, demonstrating a mirror image of an intraaortic balloon pump outside the wall of the aorta (*arrow*). This may create an erroneous impression of a dissection flap.

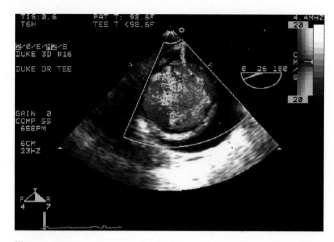

Figure 33.5. Midesophageal echocardiographic image of the descending aorta in short axis, demonstrating higher velocity flow by CFD in the true lumen following dissection.

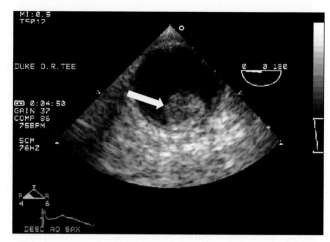

Figure 33.6. Midesophageal echocardiographic image of the descending thoracic aorta in short axis, demonstrating a large intraluminal atheromatous plaque (*arrow*).

between the true and false lumens can be appreciated with the CFD modality (Fig. 33.5). Postoperative echocardiographic assessment includes evaluation of residual dissection, adequacy of repair, and restoration of distal aortic or branch vessel flow.

Confirming Pathology

TEE is a sensitive tool for diagnosing aortic dissections and aneurysms. However, patients presenting for endovascular repair in the operating room usually have already been subjected to a variety of imaging tests to determine the extent and severity of their aortic disease. The anesthesiologist, therefore, has a small role to play in contributing to the principal diagnosis. However, coexisting aortic pathology may be diagnosed by careful observation of the descending thoracic and upper abdominal aorta. Patients with TAAs are prone to develop aneurysms at multiple sites. Coexisting aneurysms may be detected by TEE and may potentially alter the course of the procedure. Since most TAAs result from degenerative changes caused by atherosclerosis, it is common to find atheromatous plaques and calcified deposits throughout the thoracic aorta (Fig. 33.6). These findings are also important since they may indicate where positioning of the endograft is hazardous or result in detachment of atheromatous lesions. Aortic atheromatous disease is commonly implicated in patients with stroke. Identification of the extent and severity of aortic atherosclerosis by TEE can alert the surgical team to the increased risk of an adverse neurological event. TEE can be also helpful in distinguishing type B from type A dissection before an endovascular procedure.

Guiding Stent-Graft Placement

Precise placement of the stent graft is essential to ensure exclusion of the aneurysmal sac from aortic flow. Fluoroscopy is performed to confirm size and length of the aneurysm and select optimal landing zones. In aortic

dissections, TEE can be invaluable in determining the placement of the guidewire in the true lumen. The stent-graft system can be clearly visualized in the aorta, from guidewire insertion to balloon inflation and stent expansion. The guidewire is visible as a bright echo-dense structure in both short- and long-axis views of the descending aorta on the TEE image (Fig. 33.7). The TEE probe also serves as a useful marker of aortic level on fluoroscopy without contrast injection (Fig. 33.2).

Monitoring Cardiac Performance

Myocardial responses to aortic cross-clamping are well-known. The higher the level of the clamp, the greater is the hemodynamic disturbance. Unlike open aortic aneurysm repair, endovascular techniques do not involve extended periods of aortic occlusion. There is usually a brief period of aortic occlusion due to inflation of the endovascular balloon that enables fixation of the stent graft to the aortic

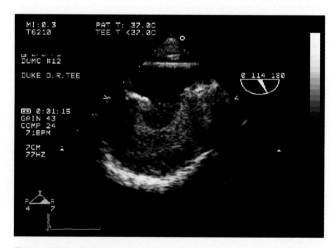

Figure 33.7. Midesophageal echocardiographic long-axis view of the descending thoracic aorta, demonstrating a guidewire inside the aortic lumen. A large saccular aneurysm can also be seen in the lower half of the image.

wall; the balloon is usually deflated within 15 to 20 seconds. As mentioned earlier, induction of pharmacologic bradycardia and hypotension may be required for accurate endograft deployment, and are achieved by various means that place significant stresses on the heart. Patients with coronary artery disease or left ventricular dysfunction may respond poorly to these stresses and run a high risk of myocardial ischemia. Cardiac performance should be monitored by TEE during the acute hemodynamic disturbances of stent-graft deployment and ballooning and appropriate remedial action taken. Most echocardiography machines are capable of performing complex calculations, which enable rapid assessment of systolic and diastolic function of the left ventricle. Diastolic dysfunction may be the only manifestation of a perioperative myocardial injury that remains undetected by any other monitoring modality.

Detecting Endoleaks

The timely detection of endoleaks may be one of the most important benefits of TEE during endovascular repair of TAAs. Type 1 endoleaks may occur in up to 24% of endovascular repairs of the thoracic aorta. CFD is a sensitive technique for assessment of blood flow in any area. Even small endoleaks may be identified by CFD. In many instances, TEE may detect an endoleak that angiography cannot confirm. The disadvantage of angiography in this setting is that it relies on a fixed volume of contrast to circulate within the endoleak. Small leaks may be missed because the volume of contrast within the leak may not be detectable by fluoroscopy or the imaging angle may not be accurate enough to detect the leak. TEE has been shown to be more sensitive than angiography in detecting endoleaks after endovascular TAA repair. Endoleak may also be indicated by the development of spontaneous echo contrast, or echocardiographic "smoke" within the aneurysmal sac after stent-graft deployment (46) (Fig. 33.8). The sudden development of "smoke" in a previously quiescent aneurysmal sac should alert the anesthesiologist to the possibility of an endoleak. A distinction should be made between swirling echo contrast in an aneurysmal sac and static contrast. Contrast that swirls around the sac suggests continued flow within the sac, which may indicate an endoleak, while static contrast implies no movement or flow within the sac, signifying the absence of any endoleak. Gradually, blood within the sac will form a coagulum and organize, leading to an echocardiographic appearance similar to surrounding tissue, rather than blood. Type 2 endoleaks are less common than Type 1 leaks but may also be detected by intraoperative TEE.

Limitations of TEE

Most of the distal abdominal aorta is inaccessible for imaging by standard TEE probes. That makes assessment of infrarenal AAAs, as well as the distal extent of many aortic dissections and thoracoabdominal aortic aneurysms

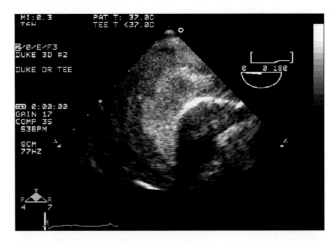

Figure 33.8. Echocardiographic view of the proximal descending aorta after deployment of an endovascular stent, demonstrating the bright echo-dense shadow of echocardiographic "smoke" indicating absence of endoleak.

(TAAA), extremely difficult, if not impossible. As such, intravascular ultrasound (IVUS) plays an important role in these latter scenarios, as outlined in more detail below. If the aorta is tortuous along its length, imaging may become difficult and interpretation inaccurate because the aorta may disappear from view at crucial locations. The introduction of stent-graft hardware into the aorta may make imaging of the aneurysm difficult due to the high echodensity of the equipment. The "fallout" due to the echodensity does not permit Doppler color evaluation, and detection of endoleak may be difficult.

ROLE OF INTRAVASCULAR ULTRASOUND

IVUS has become increasingly utilized as an adjunct in endovascular procedures. It was first developed in the 1970s and since then has been used in a variety of settings in both the coronary and peripheral vasculature. The IVUS catheters operate in high-resolution B mode and allow one to visualize the entire aortic circumference (Fig. 33.9). They are introduced either percutaneously or through an arteriotomy during an open procedure. They track over 0.025 or 0.035-in guidewires and can be maneuvered within the lumen of the blood vessel. The best images are obtained when the catheter is parallel to the vessel wall and the ultrasound beam is directed at 90 degrees to the luminal surface, which can be challenging in tortuous vessels. Images are typically obtained as the catheter is withdrawn through the lumen rather than during advancement.

IVUS is very helpful during endovascular interventions for aortic dissection as the technique allows determination of whether or not the guidewire is in the desired location in the true lumen; this is critical for endograft deployment in the true lumen. IVUS also allows one to determine the entry and reentry sites of the dissection. Branch vessels are also easily identified to allow precise deployment of stent grafts.

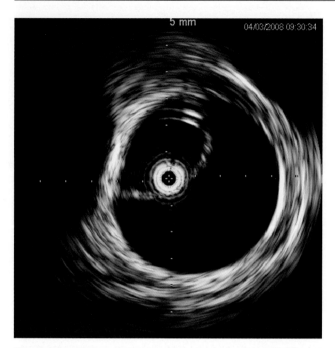

Figure 33.9. IVUS image of a dissected thoracic aorta demonstrating location of IVUS probe in the true aortic lumen.

IVUS can also be used to determine the diameter of the aortic lumen for stent-graft sizing. Studies in abdominal aortic aneurysms have validated the correlation of neck diameters, as measured by computer tomography and IVUS, with a coefficient of variation of 9% (47). IVUS results tended to underestimate aneurysm neck diameters in the infrarenal aorta, although the reverse is true in the thoracic aorta two thirds of the time (48). This is due to increasing tortuosity in the thoracic aorta.

IVUS has also been used for performance of endografting without angiography (49). The potential advantages of this approach are a reduction in radiation exposure and the lack of contrast use in patients with renal insufficiency.

SUMMARY AND FUTURE DIRECTIONS

Endovascular management of aortic disease has evolved since its introduction in the early 1990s. It is now rapidly replacing open repair as the preferred technique for treatment of a majority of descending aortic pathologies (50). Imaging is crucial not only for the diagnosis of aortic disease, but also for performance of TEVAR procedures and postoperative follow-up. As experience with the current generation of stent grafts grows, we will begin to tackle pathology of the aortic arch and ascending thoracic aorta with endovascular techniques. There are currently a number of centers around the world, including our own, that have placed stent grafts in the aortic arch in combination with ascending aorta-based arch debranching, carotid-carotid bypass, or carotid-subclavian bypass in a "hybrid" fashion (28).

Similar "hybrid" approaches to TAAA have been utilized as well (27). We are beginning to see fenestrated stent grafts being used in the aortic arch in Europe for a totally endovascular approach. These have been used in limited centers and the experience has been positive so far. Future stent grafts will include multiple fenestrations and side branches to handle the supra-aortic and visceral vessels to enable a totally endovascular approach to arch and thoracoabdominal pathology (51). Devices for the ascending aorta have already been deployed in San Francisco, Cleveland, and Malmo, Sweden (52).

As we move proximally along the aortic arch, precision deployment of stent grafts becomes even more crucial, especially with deployment utilizing more than one branch or fenestration. As such, TEE will play an ever-increasing role in the future.

KEY POINTS

- Thoracic aortic pathologies are common, are complex, and can be life threatening.
- Management has evolved to include endovascular stent grafting as a viable and durable treatment modality.
- Hybrid approaches involve a combination of open and endovascular techniques to achieve optimal results.
- Endovascular procedures that are accompanied by a high risk of spinal cord ischemia usually require prophylactic insertion of lumbar spinal fluid drainage catheters.
- Transesophageal echocardiography (TEE) is an excellent imaging technique for the thoracic aorta but is limited by poor imaging of the distal ascending aorta and proximal aortic arch due to the interposition of the air-filled trachea.
- Endovascular repair may involve coverage of the left subclavian artery.
- Timely detection of endoleaks may be an important advantage of TEE versus other imaging modalities.

REFERENCES

1. Volodos NL, Karpovich IP, Troyan VI, et al. Clinical experience of the use of self-fixing synthetic prostheses for remote endo-prosthetics of the thoracic and the abdominal aorta and iliac arteries through the femoral artery and as intraoperative endoprosthesis for aorta reconstruction. *Vasa Suppl* 1991;33:93–95.
2. Dake MD, Miller DC, Semba CP, et al. Transluminal placement of endovascular stent-grafts for the treatment of descending thoracic aortic aneurysms. *N Engl J Med* 1994;331(26): 1729–1734.
3. Dake MD, Miller DC, Mitchell RS, et al. The "first generation" of endovascular stent-grafts for patients with aneurysms of the descending thoracic aorta. *J Thorac Cardiovasc Surg* 1998;116(5):689–703; discussion 703–704.

4. Ehrlich M, Grabenwoeger M, Cartes-Zumelzu F, et al. Endovascular stent graft repair for aneurysms on the descending thoracic aorta. *Ann Thorac Surg* 1998;66(1):19–24; discussion 24–25.

5. Mitchell RS, Miller DC, Dake MD, et al. Thoracic aortic aneurysm repair with an endovascular stent graft: the "first generation". *Ann Thorac Surg* 1999;67(6):1971–1974; discussion 1979–1980.

6. Greenberg R, Resch T, Nyman U, et al. Endovascular repair of descending thoracic aortic aneurysms: an early experience with intermediate-term follow-up. *J Vasc Surg* 2000;31(1 Pt 1): 147–156.

7. Buffolo E, da Fonseca JH, de Souza JA, et al. Revolutionary treatment of aneurysms and dissections of descending aorta: the endovascular approach. *Ann Thorac Surg* 2002;74(5):S1815–S1817; discussion S1825–S1832.

8. Criado FJ, Clark NS, Barnatan MF. Stent graft repair in the aortic arch and descending thoracic aorta: a 4-year experience. *J Vasc Surg* 2002;36(6):1121–1128.

9. Greenberg RK, O'Neill S, Walker E, et al. Endovascular repair of thoracic aortic lesions with the Zenith TX1 and TX2 thoracic grafts: intermediate-term results. *J Vasc Surg* 2005;41(4): 589–596.

10. Makaroun MS, Dillavou ED, Kee ST, et al. Endovascular treatment of thoracic aortic aneurysms: results of the phase II multicenter trial of the GORE TAG thoracic endoprosthesis. *J Vasc Surg* 2005;41(1):1–9.

11. Appoo JJ, Moser WG, Fairman RM, et al. Thoracic aortic stent grafting: improving results with newer generation investigational devices. *J Thorac Cardiovasc Surg* 2006;131(5):1087–1094.

12. Dias NV, Sonesson B, Koul B, et al. Complicated acute type B dissections—an 8-years experience of endovascular stent-graft repair in a single centre. *Eur J Vasc Endovasc Surg* 2006;31(5):481–486.

13. Fattori R, Nienaber CA, Rousseau H, et al. Results of endovascular repair of the thoracic aorta with the Talent Thoracic stent graft: the Talent Thoracic Retrospective Registry. *J Thorac Cardiovasc Surg* 2006;132(2):332–339.

14. Patel HJ, Williams DM, Upchurch GR Jr, et al. Long-term results from a 12-year experience with endovascular therapy for thoracic aortic disease. *Ann Thorac Surg* 2006;82(6):2147–2153.

15. Wheatley GH III, Gurbuz AT, Rodriguez-Lopez JA, et al. Midterm outcome in 158 consecutive Gore TAG thoracic endoprostheses: single center experience. *Ann Thorac Surg* 2006;81(5):1570–1577; discussion 1577.

16. Xu SD, Huang FJ, Yang JF, et al. Endovascular repair of acute type B aortic dissection: early and mid-term results. *J Vasc Surg* 2006;43(6):1090–1095.

17. Koschyk DH, Nienaber CA, Knap M, et al. How to guide stent-graft implantation in type B aortic dissection? Comparison of angiography, transesophageal echocardiography, and intravascular ultrasound. *Circulation* 2005;112(9 Suppl.):I260–I264.

18. Rocchi G, Lofiego C, Biagini E, et al. Transesophageal echocardiography-guided algorithm for stent-graft implantation in aortic dissection. *J Vasc Surg* 2004;40(5):880–885.

19. Schutz W, Gauss A, Meierhenrich R, et al. Transesophageal echocardiographic guidance of thoracic aortic stent-graft implantation. *J Endovasc Ther* 2002;9(Suppl. 2):II14–II19.

20. Rapezzi C, Rocchi G, Fattori R, et al. Usefulness of transesophageal echocardiographic monitoring to improve the outcome of stent-graft treatment of thoracic aortic aneurysms. *Am J Cardiol* 2001;87(3):315–319.

21. Fattori R, Caldarera I, Rapezzi C, et al. Primary endoleakage in endovascular treatment of the thoracic aorta: importance of intraoperative transesophageal echocardiography. *J Thorac Cardiovasc Surg* 2000;120(3):490–495.

22. Gonzalez-Fajardo JA, Gutierrez V, San Roman JA, et al. Utility of intraoperative transesophageal echocardiography during endovascular stent-graft repair of acute thoracic aortic dissection. *Ann Vasc Surg* 2002;16(3):297–303.

23. Swaminathan M, Lineberger CK, McCann RL, et al. The importance of intraoperative transesophageal echocardiography in endovascular repair of thoracic aortic aneurysms. *Anesth Analg* 2003;97(6):1566–1572.

24. Penco M, Paparoni S, Dagianti A, et al. Usefulness of transesophageal echocardiography in the assessment of aortic dissection. *Am J Cardiol* 2000;86(4A):53G-56G.

25. Evangelista A, Avegliano G, Elorz C, et al. Transesophageal echocardiography in the diagnosis of acute aortic syndrome. *J Card Surg* 2002;17(2):95–106.

26. Svensson LG, Kouchoukos NT, Miller DC, et al. Expert consensus document on the treatment of descending thoracic aortic disease using endovascular stent-grafts. *Ann Thorac Surg* 2008;85(1 Suppl.):S1–S41.

27. Hughes GC, Nienaber JJ, Bush EL, et al. Use of custom dacron branch grafts for "hybrid" aortic debranching during endovascular repair of thoracic and thoracoabdominal aortic aneurysms. *J Thorac Cardiovasc Surg* 2008; 136:21–28.

28. Hughes GC, McCann RL, Sulzer CF, et al. Endovascular approaches to complex thoracic aortic disease. *Semin Cardiothorac Vasc Anesth* 2008;12:298–319.

29. Coady MA, Rizzo JA, Hammond GL, et al. Surgical intervention criteria for thoracic aortic aneurysms: a study of growth rates and complications. *Ann Thorac Surg* 1999;67(6):1922–1926; discussion 1953–1958.

30. Hoffer EK, Forauer AR, Silas AM, et al. Endovascular stent-graft or open surgical repair for blunt thoracic aortic trauma: systematic review. *J Vasc Interv Radiol* 2008;19(8):1153–1164.

31. Husain AM, Swaminathan M, McCann RL, et al. Neurophysiologic intraoperative monitoring during endovascular stent graft repair of the descending thoracic aorta. *J Clin Neurophysiol* 2007; 24:328–335.

32. Scheufler KM, Zentner J. Total intravenous anesthesia for intraoperative monitoring of the motor pathways: an integral view combining clinical and experimental data. *J Neurosurg* 2002;96(3):571–579.

33. Dorros G, Cohn JM. Adenosine-induced transient cardiac asystole enhances precise deployment of stent-grafts in the thoracic or abdominal aorta. *J Endovasc Surg* 1996;3(3):270–272.

34. Kahn RA, Marin ML, Hollier L, et al. Induction of ventricular fibrillation to facilitate endovascular stent graft repair of thoracic aortic aneurysms. *Anesthesiology* 1998;88(2):534–536.

35. Gorich J, Asquan Y, Seifarth H, et al. Initial experience with intentional stent-graft coverage of the subclavian artery during endovascular thoracic aortic repairs. *J Endovasc Ther* 2002;9(Suppl. 2):II39–II43.

36. Reece TB, Gazoni LM, Cherry KJ, et al. Reevaluating the need for left subclavian artery revascularization with thoracic endovascular aortic repair. *Ann Thorac Surg* 2007;84(4):1201–1205; discussion 1205.

37. Buth J, Harris PL, Hobo R, et al. Neurologic complications associated with endovascular repair of thoracic aortic pathology: Incidence and risk factors. a study from the European Collaborators on Stent/Graft Techniques for Aortic Aneurysm Repair

(EUROSTAR) registry. *J Vasc Surg* 2007;46(6):1103–1110; discussion 1110–1111.

38. Chaikof EL, Blankensteijn JD, Harris PL, et al. Reporting standards for endovascular aortic aneurysm repair. *J Vasc Surg* 2002;35(5):1048–1060.

39. White GH, Yu W, May J, et al. Endoleak as a complication of endoluminal grafting of abdominal aortic aneurysms: classification, incidence, diagnosis, and management. *J Endovasc Surg* 1997;4(2):152–168.

40. White GH, Yu W, May J. Endoleak—a proposed new terminology to describe incomplete aneurysm exclusion by an endoluminal graft. *J Endovasc Surg* 1996;3(1):124–125.

41. Nienaber CA, von Kodolitsch Y, Nicolas V, et al. The diagnosis of thoracic aortic dissection by noninvasive imaging procedures. *N Engl J Med* 1993;328(1):1–9.

42. Hayter RG, Rhea JT, Small A, et al. Suspected aortic dissection and other aortic disorders: multi-detector row CT in 373 cases in the emergency setting. *Radiology* 2006;238(3):841–852.

43. Erbel R, Engberding R, Daniel W, et al. Echocardiography in diagnosis of aortic dissection. *Lancet* 1989;1(8636):457–461.

44. Keren A, Kim CB, Hu BS, et al. Accuracy of biplane and multiplane transesophageal echocardiography in diagnosis of typical acute aortic dissection and intramural hematoma. *J Am Coll Cardiol* 1996;28(3):627–636.

45. Shanewise JS, Cheung AT, Aronson S, et al. ASE/SCA guidelines for performing a comprehensive intraoperative multiplane transesophageal echocardiography examination: recommendations of the American Society of Echocardiography Council

for Intraoperative Echocardiography and the Society of Cardiovascular Anesthesiologists Task Force for Certification in Perioperative Transesophageal Echocardiography. *Anesth Analg* 1999;89(4):870–884.

46. Swaminathan M, Mackensen GB, Podgoreanu MV, et al. Spontaneous echocardiographic contrast indicating successful endoleak management. *Anesth Analg* 2007;104(5):1037–1039.

47. van Essen JA, Gussenhoven EJ, van der Lugt A, et al. Accurate assessment of abdominal aortic aneurysm with intravascular ultrasound scanning: validation with computed tomographic angiography. *J Vasc Surg* 1999;29(4):631–638.

48. Fernandez JD, Donovan S, Garrett HE Jr, et al. Endovascular thoracic aortic aneurysm repair: evaluating the utility of intravascular ultrasound measurements. *J Endovasc Ther* 2008;15(1):68–72.

49. von Segesser LK, Marty B, Ruchat P, et al. Routine use of intravascular ultrasound for endovascular aneurysm repair: angiography is not necessary. *Eur J Vasc Endovasc Surg* 2002;23(6):537–542.

50. Hughes GC, Daneshmand MA, Swaminathan M, et al. "Real world" thoracic endografting: results with the Gore TAG endoprosthesis 2 years following U.S. FDA approval. *Ann Thorac Surg* 2008;86:1530–1538.

51. Chuter TA. Branched and fenestrated stent grafts for endovascular repair of thoracic aortic aneurysms. *J Vasc Surg* 2006;43(Suppl. A):111A–115A.

52. Ohrlander T, Sonesson B, Ivancev K, et al. The chimney graft: a technique for preserving or rescuing aortic branch vessels in stent-graft sealing zones. *J Endovasc Ther* 2008;15(4):427–432.

QUESTIONS

1. A 45-year old man is scheduled to undergo endovascular stent repair of a 5.5 cm aortic aneurysm that originates at the distal arch and extends to the diaphragmatic level of the descending aorta. Monitoring includes a left radial arterial line, a central venous catheter, and a five-lead EKG. Immediately following stent graft deployment, the mean arterial pressure decreases to 30 mm Hg with an unchanged heart rate and central venous pressure. Which of the following best explains this hemodynamic change?
   A. Inadvertent aortic rupture
   B. Sudden vasodilation
   C. Coverage of the left subclavian artery
   D. Acute type A aortic dissection
   E. Acute myocardial ischemia

2. Which of the following is most useful for distinguishing between the true and false lumens of an aortic dissection by transesophageal echocardiography?
   A. Identification of an intimal flap
   B. Echo contrast ("smoke") in both lumens
   C. Holodiastolic flow reversal in either lumen
   D. M-mode pattern of flap motion
   E. Harmonic imaging of the intimal flap

3. A "double barrel" aorta refers a phenomenon in which there is an appearance of a parallel aortic image

in transesophageal echocardiography. Which of the following is most likely responsible for this phenomenon?
   A. Ghosting artifact
   B. Mirror image
   C. Type B dissection
   D. Pleural effusion
   E. Intraaortic balloon pump

4. Which of the following is most likely to be mistaken for a Type A dissection on intraoperative TEE imaging?
   A. Pulmonary artery catheter
   B. Pleural effusion
   C. Pericardial effusion
   D. Pulmonary thrombus
   E. Intraaortic balloon pump

5. In a patient with a Type A dissection and gradually deteriorating mental status in the setting of stable hemodynamics, which of the following is the most likely finding?
   A. Ascending aortic atheroma
   B. Carotid dissection
   C. Pericardial effusion
   D. Pleural effusion
   E. Intramural hematoma

CHAPTER 34

Echocardiographic Assessment of Cardiomyopathies

Jordan K.C. Hudson ■ Christopher C. C. Hudson ■ G. Burkhard Mackensen

INTRODUCTION

Cardiomyopathies represent a spectrum of diseases of the myocardium causing cardiac dysfunction; nonischemic cardiomyopathies are the underlying etiology of 15% of heart failure cases in adults (1,2). In 1850, chronic myocarditis was the earliest known cause of heart muscle disease, and the term "cardiomyopathy" was first used a mere half-century ago in 1957 (3). The World Health Organization (WHO) identifies five classifications of cardiomyopathies: dilated, hypertrophic, restrictive, arrhythmogenic right ventricular (RV), and unclassified (Table 34.1) (2).

Traditional methods of defining cardiomyopathies may not be sufficient to classify an individual patient's disease due to the wide spectrum of possible pathophysiologic derangements. Our increasing understanding of the anatomic and functional manifestations, as well as genetic factors responsible for the development of cardiomyopathies prompted the American Heart Association (AHA) to release an updated definition and classification system in 2006 (4). The AHA proposed a revised definition of cardiomyopathies as "a heterogeneous group of diseases of the myocardium associated with mechanical and/or electrical dysfunction that usually (but not invariably) exhibit inappropriate ventricular hypertrophy or dilation, and are due to a variety of causes that frequently are genetic" (4). The AHA suggests cardiomyopathies be classified as primary or secondary, with primary cardiomyopathies further subdivided as genetic, acquired, or mixed. However, for the purposes of this chapter, the widely cited WHO classification system was chosen to discuss cardiomyopathies.

Initial assessment of the patient with cardiomyopathy serves to classify the type and underlying etiology. In patients with heart failure, echocardiography is used to assess right and left heart function, screen for associated pulmonary hypertension, determine the underlying etiology, aid prognostication, and guide treatment (1). While more invasive testing may be required for definitive diagnosis, echocardiography is the first imaging test of choice in patients with suspected cardiomyopathy (5). This chapter will review the various classes of cardiomyopathy, the echocardiographic findings specific to each, and discuss the role of echocardiography in estimating prognosis and guiding treatment. A summary of common echocardiographic findings for the cardiomyopathies may be found in Table 34.2.

DILATED CARDIOMYOPATHY

Dilated cardiomyopathy (DCM) manifests as dilation and impairment of systolic function of one or both ventricles (2). Ischemic heart disease is the most common cause of DCM, due to remodeling following an acute myocardial infarction or chronic systolic heart failure (6).

TABLE 34.1	WHO Classification of Cardiomyopathies
Cardiomyopathy	**Definition**
Dilated	Dilatation and impaired contraction of the LV or both ventricles
Hypertrophic	Left and/or RV hypertrophy, usually asymmetric and involves the interventricular septum
Restricted	Restrictive filling and reduced diastolic volume of either or both ventricles with normal or near-normal systolic function and wall thickness
Arrhythmogenic RV	Progressive fibrofatty replacement of RV myocardium
Unclassified	Cases that do not fit readily into any group defined above

Source: *Richardson P, McKenna W, Bristow M, et al. Report of the 1995 World Health Organization/International Society and Federation of Cardiology Task Force on the Definition and Classification of cardiomyopathies. Circulation 1996;93:841–842.*

TABLE 34.2	Echocardiographic Features of Cardiomyopathies
Dilated	Dilated left (± right) ventricle
	Global hypokinesis
	Atrial enlargement
	Dilated mitral annulus with MR
	Spontaneous echo contrast in left atrium
	Diastolic dysfunction
Hypertrophic	Septal hypertrophy
	LV hypertrophy (global or focal)
	SAM of anterior mitral leaflet
	LVOT obstruction
	Dynamic pressure gradient across LVOT
	Diastolic dysfunction
Restrictive	Impaired ventricular filling
	Biatrial enlargement
	Diastolic dysfunction
	Normal ventricular size and wall thickness
	Normal systolic function
Arrhythmogenic RV	RV regional or global enlargement or dysfunction
	Diastolic outpouchings and systolic aneurysms

TABLE 34.3	Causes of DCM
Ischemic cardiomyopathy
Idiopathic DCM
Hypertensive heart disease
Valvular heart disease
Tachycardia-induced cardiomyopathy
PPCM
Familial DCM
Infectious/inflammatory cardiomyopathy
Coxsackie B, HIV, Hepatitis C, Tryposoma, Toxoplasma
Toxic cardiomyopathy
Alcohol, cocaine, amphetamines, chemotherapeutic agents
Metabolic cardiomyopathy
Carnitine deficiency

Other forms of DCM are familial, idiopathic, or viral and/or immune while mechanical, neurohormonal, and genetic factors may all contribute to the development of DCM (Table 34.3). The common final pathway of all of etiologies associated with DCM is progressive decline in myocardial function with fibrosis and necrosis, leading to ventricular dilation and further worsening of myocardial function.

The presentation of DCM may vary significantly depending on the underlying cause, but the end-pathway is one of left ventricular (LV) or biventricular dilation and failure leading to a low cardiac output state. In addition to symptoms of congestive heart failure, patients may develop mitral regurgitation (MR) because of annular dilation and disruptions of the conducting system resulting in ventricular and supraventricular arrhythmias enhancing the risk for thromboembolism. The clinical course is often unpredictable, with 2-year mortality as high as 60% in highly symptomatic patients (7). Predictors of poorer prognosis include male gender, increased LV dilation, RV involvement, and increased severity of heart failure symptoms (8).

Echocardiographic Features

DCM is often diagnosed in the presence of decreased LV ejection fraction (<30%) and marked LV dilation. End-systolic and end-diastolic volumes are typically increased (Fig. 34.1). RV dilation and dysfunction may also be present. Common findings in DCM include atrial enlargement, mitral annular dilation resulting in MR (Carpentier Type 1), decreased stroke volume and cardiac output, diastolic dysfunction, and presence of spontaneous echo contrast with or without presence of atrial and/or apical ventricular thrombi due to a low-flow state. Advanced stages of DCM require surgical intervention with either placement of a LV assist device or heart transplantation (Fig. 34.2). Global LV hypokinesis is typically seen, and regional wall motion abnormalities may also be present, particularly in cases of ischemic DCM. While LV mass is uniformly increased, wall thickness varies among patients. Doppler assessments of patients with advanced stage of DCM are consistent with diastolic dysfunction of the LV, usually with a restrictive pattern (increased E/A ratio and decreased E wave deceleration time, blunting of the S wave in the pulmonary venous flow pattern) (9). Elevated left ventricular end-diastolic pressure (LVEDP) is indicated by a shorter transmitral A-wave compared to the pulmonary venous inflow A-wave. Signs of pulmonary hypertension are also common with high-velocity tricuspid regurgitation (TR) jets assessed with continuous wave Doppler (CWD) and pulmonary acceleration times less than 90 millisecond. Patients exhibiting high-velocity TR (>2.5 m/s) appear to have a higher mortality and more symptoms of congestive heart failure compared to patients with lower-velocity TR (≤2.5 m/s) (10). It is not possible to distinguish the underlying etiology of DCM by echocardiographic features.

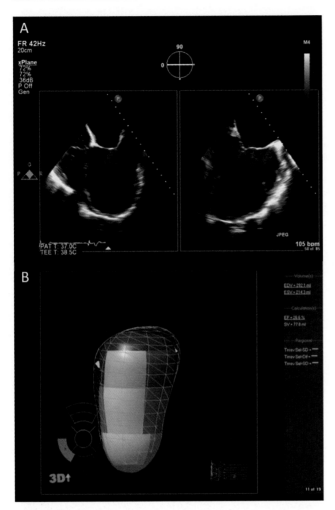

Figure 34.1. A. TEE, midesophageal biplane view of DCM, with left image showing a four-chamber view at 0 degree and right image showing a two-chamber view at 90 degrees, demonstrating increased ventricular dimensions. **B.** 3D model of LV (QLAB, Philips Healthcare, Inc, Andover, MA version 6.0) in same patient demonstrating increased end-systolic and end-diastolic volumes (indicated by mesh), and reduced ejection fraction of 26.6%.

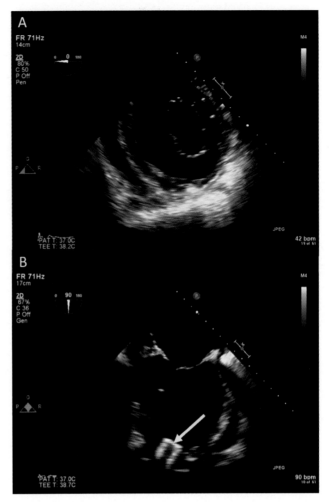

Figure 34.2 TEE transgastric basal view of the LV (**A**), demonstrating increased ventricular dimensions. The lower half of this panel (**B**) shows a TEE midesophageal two-chamber view at 90 degrees in the same patient with a LV assist device cannula placed in the apex (*arrow*).

HYPERTROPHIC CARDIOMYOPATHY

Hypertrophic cardiomyopathy (HCM) is the most common genetic cardiac disease, with an incidence of 0.2% among adults (11,12). HCM is an autosomal dominant disorder caused by mutations in any of ten genes encoding sarcomeric proteins, leading to LV hypertrophy in the absence of other cardiac or systemic disease. While it has received much notoriety as the most common cause of sudden death in young persons, hypertrophic obstructive cardiomyopathy (HOCM) with obstruction of the left ventricular outflow tract (LVOT) at rest occurs in only 30% of patients with HCM (13). However, up to 70% of patients with HCM will show evidence of obstructive disease if tested with exercise echocardiography (13). Although isolated asymmetric hypertrophy of the anterior

septum is classically described, there is no consistent pattern of LV hypertrophy, with many patients experiencing diffuse ventricular hypertrophy and one third experiencing hypertrophy of a single segment (11).

While classically described as a disease of young adults, improvements in screening and diagnosis have broadened our understanding of HCM. It may be diagnosed at any age and present with a wide variety of phenotypes. While the overall mortality rate is approximately 1% annually, patients with more severe disease (LVOT obstruction, congestive heart failure, and ventricular dysrhythmias) have a mortality rate greater than 5% annually (11).

Echocardiographic Features

Echocardiography is the preferred noninvasive method to diagnose HCM and HOCM and to differentiate them from left ventricular hypertrophy (LVH). The addition of three-dimensional (3D) echocardiography to standard

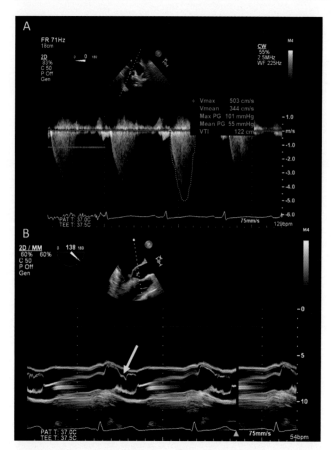

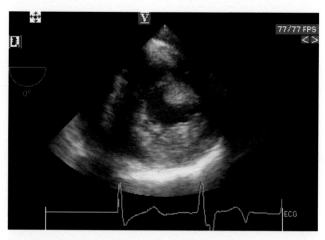

Figure 34.4 TEE transgastric mid short-axis view in a patient with HCM, demonstrating concentric hypertrophy of the LV.

Figure 34.3 A: CWD obtained from a TEE deep transgastric long-axis view in a patient with HCM, demonstrating increased flow velocity (>5 m/s; >100 mm Hg gradient) across the LVOT, resulting in a Doppler spectrum with a characteristic late-peaking (middle to late systole) dagger-shaped appearance. **B:** Mid-systolic partial closure and flutter of the AV (*arrow*) in the same patient with HOCM as demonstrated by M-mode imaging.

two-dimensional (2D) echocardiography has improved the diagnostic sensitivity and specificity to 93.3% and 100%, respectively (14). During systole, the hallmarks of HOCM include systolic anterior motion (SAM) of the mitral valve (MV), LVOT obstruction due to septal hypertrophy, turbulent flow in the LVOT with a late peaking gradient (dagger-shaped appearance of the CWD spectrum), early closure of one or more aortic valve (AV) cusps, and diminished systolic LV cavity size (Fig. 34.3). Echocardiographic assessment of the patient with HCM should focus on assessment of global LV function, distribution of LV hypertrophy (Fig. 34.4), presence of regional wall motion abnormalities, presence of LVOT obstruction, and SAM of the MV (Fig. 34.5). Obstruction of the LVOT is an important pathophysiological component of HCM. When present under resting conditions, LVOT obstruction is an independent predictor of adverse clinical events such as progressive heart failure and cardiovascular death (15). Although asymmetric septal hypertrophy is the most common type of morphologic pattern, HCM can present with concentric, apical, or free wall LV hypertrophy (16).

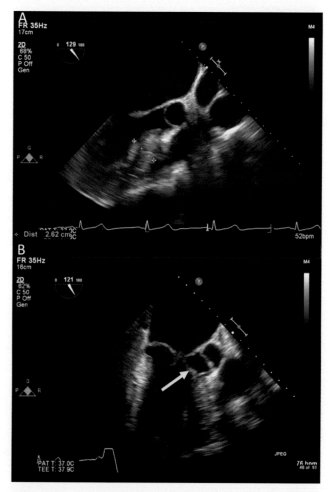

Figure 34.5 TEE midesophageal AV long-axis view in a patient with HCM (**A**), demonstrating a hypertrophied basal septum (2.62 cm), which narrows the LVOT and provides conditions for dynamic obstruction. TEE midesophageal AV long-axis view of HCM (**B**), demonstrating SAM of the MV (*arrow*), resulting in anterior leaflet-septal contact and subaortic obstruction to outflow.

LV systolic function is usually normal to supranormal, with high ejection fraction. The dynamic obstruction in HOCM results in a narrowed LVOT with increased systolic velocity of blood flow. In patients scheduled for intervention, exact measurements should be taken of the outflow gradient and septal thickness. The MV should also be carefully examined to assess the need for concomitant MV repair or replacement (17). The distance from the AV to the point of septal contact should be measured to ensure that the myectomy will extend beyond that point.

MR associated with SAM is thought to be due to the Venturi effect and drag forces within the LVOT. The subsequent anterior displacement of the MV causes mitral leaflet-septal contact and subaortic obstruction, as well as the development of a funnel-shaped interleaflet gap as the posterior MV leaflet is unable to follow the displacement of the anterior MV leaflet anteriorly toward the ventricular septum. MR is common with a posteriorly directed jet that usually peaks in mid or late systole (Fig. 34.6). LVOT obstruction may also cause the AV to close prematurely, recognized best by M mode echocardiography as AV fluttering (see Fig. 34.3). In patients with HCM, the MV is often enlarged, with an elongated anterior mitral leaf-

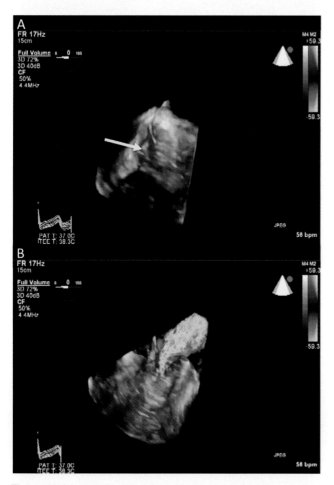

Figure 34.6 **A:** TEE midesophageal 3D image illustrating near-complete occlusion of the LVOT during SAM of the MV (*yellow arrow*). **B:** 3D TEE color flow Doppler image of the same patient, demonstrating MR directed posteriorly into the left atrium.

let (12). Measurements of the mitral annular diameters and leaflet lengths should be made, and features such as MV prolapse and leaflet restriction should also be communicated to the surgeon. This is important because for patients with HOCM and MR not due to independent MV disease, myomectomy significantly reduces the degree of regurgitation, without requirement for additional MV surgery (17).

Patients with HCM typically have diastolic dysfunction (abnormal relaxation; decreased E/A ratio) secondary to the hypertrophic myocardium (18). Findings may include prolongation of isovolumic relaxation time and early diastolic peak flow velocity, as well as slower deceleration and reduced maximal flow velocity in early diastole (18). As an apparent compensation for impaired relaxation and early diastolic filling, the atrial contribution to LV filling increases. At this time, LV filling may be substantially dependent on atrial contraction. Over time, the LV becomes less compliant, and left atrial pressure increases, causing early filling to increase and deceleration time to decrease. Late in the evolution of diastolic dysfunction, a restrictive type of diastolic filling defect may become evident, in which a high atrial pressure results in an increased rate and volume of filling during the rapid filling period with reduced filling during atrial systole (16). Because the deceleration time is markedly prolonged at baseline in patients with HCM, the same degree of left atrial pressure increase does not produce similar deceleration time shortening as it does in patients with DCM. Thus, no correlation exists between deceleration time and LV filling pressures in patients with HCM (19). Patients with HCM typically demonstrate redistribution of intracavitary flow during isovolumic relaxation due to asynchronous myocardial relaxation, which may lead to erroneous interpretation of mitral inflow velocities and the mitral inflow velocity profile.

Not all cases of dynamic LVOT obstruction are due to HCM. Patients with basal septal hypertrophy who develop hyperdynamic systolic ventricular function may also exhibit dynamic LVOT obstruction (20). Following AV replacement for aortic stenosis, patients may develop acute LVOT obstruction as well. Other less common causes of dynamic LVOT obstruction include cardiac amyloidosis, myocardial infarction, and subaortic stenosis, among others.

Interventions that reduce LV contractility, increase peripheral vascular resistance, or both are considered beneficial (21). Interventions that lower peripheral vascular resistance and increase myocardial contractility are thought to be detrimental (21). The occurrence of atrial fibrillation in HCM is also associated with clinical deterioration. Beta-blockers are considered the basic treatment for patients with HCM.

Surgical repair of HOCM is generally reserved for those individuals who remain refractory to medical therapy. Criteria include an intraventricular gradient at rest of ≥30 or ≥60 mm Hg with provocation and a septum measuring more than 18 mm in thickness (21). Patients should also exhibit typical SAM of the MV. Surgical repair is via myomectomy, which consists of removing ventricular septal tissue through a transaortic approach (thus, widening the LVOT). Isolated septal myomectomy has been demonstrated to be effective in eliminating LVOT obstruction and sudden death, as well as improving functional status, with low perioperative morbidity and mortality (22). Intraoperative Transesophageal echocardiography (TEE) is very useful in determining the site of septal contact by the anterior MV leaflet during SAM and determining the thickness of the interventricular septum, helping the surgeon decide the extent and depth of the myomectomy. The presence of asymmetric septal hypertrophy and severe SAM of the MV apparatus predicts a good outcome after septal myectomy (23). 3D-TEE may allow for spatial assessment of the extent of maximal septal thickness, the degree of LVOT obstruction, and the intimate relationship between MV and LVOT (e.g., the extent of systolic mitral leaflet-to-septal contact)—important information that may assist the surgeon to optimize the site and size of the septal myomectomy.

Following septal myomectomy, TEE is indispensable to assess the adequacy of the procedure and to rule out any potential complications. Insufficient septal resection can result in persistent LVOT obstruction, detectable in 20% of patients by postbypass TEE (Fig. 34.7) (24). 3D TEE may be superior to 2D TEE in assessing the extent and location of the myomectomy. Excessive septal resection produces a ventricular septal defect in 0% to 2% of cases, with increased incidence in the elderly and in patients undergoing concomitant coronary artery bypass grafting (12). Other potential complications of myomectomy include complete heart block and creation of a coronary artery LV fistula. Postoperatively, it is also important to determine the severity of residual MR. SAM of the MV apparatus may persist following myomectomy even though the LVOT gradient is reduced.

The beneficial effects of myomectomy led to the concept of nonsurgical myocardial reduction, which involves infusion of desiccated alcohol distal to an angioplasty balloon into the first major septal perforator of the left anterior descending coronary artery (producing septal infarction) (21).

RESTRICTIVE CARDIOMYOPATHY

Restrictive cardiomyopathy (RCM) is the rarest of the cardiomyopathies and may be idiopathic or secondary to other diseases such as amyloidosis or endomyocardial disease. In contrast to DCM, in which systolic ventricular dysfunction is the predominant defect, RCM is characterized by restrictive filling patterns and impaired ventricular relaxation (diastolic dysfunction), usually in the presence of normal systolic function (25). The clinical

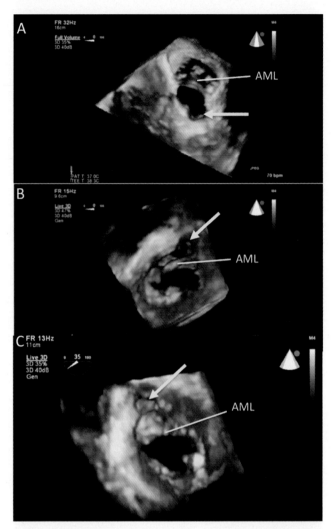

Figure 34.7 3D TEE assessment of two patients who underwent septal myomectomy. **A:** The first image shows a good surgical result with myomectomy (*arrow*) in the mid-portion of the ventricular septum as seen en face from the AV side. **B:** The second image demonstrates partial septal myomectomy (*arrow*) lateral from the midportion of the hypertrophied septum associated with continued (partial) dynamic obstruction as seen from the LV perspective. **C:** The third image was taken in the same patient as in 33.7.A, and it shows a large myomectomy (*arrow*) of the midportion of the hypertrophied septum from the LV side. AML, anterior mitral valve leaflet.

presentation is typically one of worsening diastolic dysfunction and heart failure. Disease progression and prognosis vary depending on the underlying etiology, with poor long-term survival overall. Advanced stages of RCM result in congestive heart failure with pulmonary and venous vascular congestion due to high filling pressures required to maintain an adequate cardiac output. A summary of causes of RCM can be found in Table 34.4. Echocardiography is often performed to distinguish between RCM and constrictive pericarditis: while few management options exist for RCM (with the exception of hemochromatosis), constrictive pericarditis can be surgically treated. However, distinguishing RCM from

TABLE **34.4** **Causes of RCM**
Primary RCM
Idiopathic RCM
Endomyocardial fibrosis
Loeffler eosinophilic endomyocardial disease
Secondary RCM
Hemochromatosis
Amyloidosis
Sarcoidosis
Scleroderma
Carcinoid
Radiation
Metastatic disease
Fabry disease
Glycogen storage diseases
Anthracycline toxicity

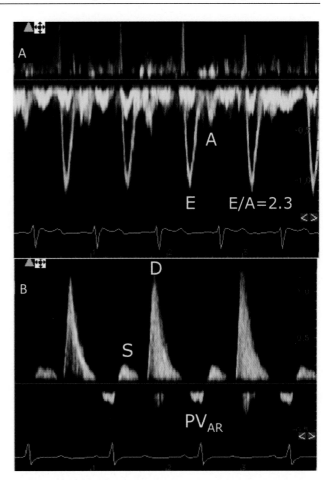

Figure 34.8. Mitral inflow pattern (**A**) and pulmonary venous flow pattern (**B**) in a patient with RCM. The mitral inflow demonstrates an increased E/A ratio (restrictive physiology). The pulmonary venous flow pattern confirms the diagnosis of restrictive physiology with a blunted systolic component (S).

constrictive pericarditis is not trivial as both entities may present with similar features (e.g., both have preserved LV function and evidence of impaired LV filling). Some patients may even present with a combination of the two disease states. Pericardial thickening and relatively preserved diastolic function (i.e., a mitral annular tissue Doppler E´ ≥ 8 cm/s) are more consistent with constrictive pericarditis (26).

Echocardiographic Features

A combination of 2D, M-mode, and Doppler echocardiography is used to differentiate RCM from constrictive pericarditis, although endomyocardial biopsy is required for definitive diagnosis. Impaired diastolic function of one or both ventricles is the hallmark finding in RCM. Diastolic dysfunction may manifest with impaired ventricular filling, elevated filling pressures, shortened isovolumic relaxation time, increased transmitral E/A ratio, and systolic blunting of the pulmonary vein waveform. In the early stages of the disease, impaired relaxation is seen with decreased peak transmitral E velocities, E/A ratios less than 1, and prolonged deceleration of the E wave. As the disease progresses, a "pseudonormal" flow pattern can be distinguished from a normal transmitral flow pattern by the presence of the S wave attenuation in the pulmonary venous inflow pattern, or "unmasking" the pseudonormalization during a Valsalva maneuver. Furthermore, the pulmonary venous A velocity is increased with pseudonormalization. A truly restrictive pattern is seen in the final stages of the disease. The E/A ratio is increased (>2), E wave deceleration time is shortened (<150 ms), the isovolumetric relaxation

time is decreased (<60 ms), the systolic component of the pulmonary venous flow pattern is attenuated, and the pulmonary venous A wave is increased due to high LVEDP (Fig. 34.8). Decreased color M-mode Doppler propagation velocity consistent with diastolic dysfunction can also be demonstrated in patients with RCM (Fig. 34.9). Other changes consistent with pulmonary hypertension include increased peak TR velocities measured with CWD and shortened pulmonary acceleration time measured with pulse wave Doppler. Right-sided heart failure may be present when there is RV involvement. In contrast to constrictive pericarditis, patients with RCM frequently have biatrial enlargement.

TEE typically shows nondilated ventricles that may be somewhat thickened with normal systolic function and no regional wall motion abnormalities. Thickened ventricular walls are especially seen if the underlying etiology is infiltrative as in cases of amyloidosis, which may mimic HCM when visualized with echocardiographic imaging. A granular or speckled myocardium may be seen in infiltrative disorders.

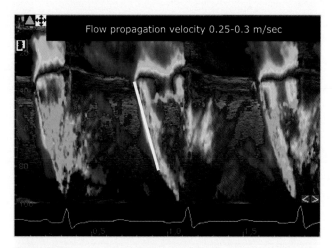

Figure 34.9. Decreased color M-mode Doppler propagation velocity (*white line*) consistent with diastolic dysfunction in a patient with RCM shown as the slope of the first aliasing velocity during early filling of the LV. A propagation velocity of more than 55 cm/s is associated with normal diastolic function in healthy young adults.(From Garcia MJ, Thomas JD, Klein AL. New Doppler echocardiographic applications for the study of diastolic function. *J Am Coll Cardiol* 1998;32:865–875.)

ARRHYTHMOGENIC RIGHT VENTRICULAR CARDIOMYOPATHY

Arrhythmogenic right ventricular cardiomyopathy (ARVC) is characterized by three features: progressive fibrofatty replacement of RV myocardium, strong familial association, and presentation with symptomatic arrhythmias or sudden death (27). It is a well-known cause of sudden cardiac death in previously healthy young adults. Early changes typically involve regions of the RV, followed by global RV and some LV changes. Sparing of the ventricular septum is frequently seen (2). End-stage ARVC is clinically similar to DCM, with fibrofatty degeneration detectable only on biopsy or autopsy. ARVC is familial in 50% of cases, typically autosomal dominant although rare recessive forms have been described (27).

ARVC typically presents in young adulthood, with symptomatic arrhythmias, left or right heart failure, or sudden cardiac death. This diagnosis should be suspected in a young adult presenting with cardiac symptoms, or in those with a family history of ARVC or sudden death. Noninvasive testing for ARVC includes EKG, Holter monitoring, and echocardiography, with cardiac MRI being helpful if other noninvasive tests are inconclusive (28,29).

Echocardiographic Features

Fibrofatty dysplasia of the RV can occur regionally or globally and leads to RV enlargement and failure. The three most common areas for dysplasia which occur in early ARVC are the RV outflow tract, inflow, and apex, otherwise know as the "triangle of dysplasia" (27).

Manifestations of regional dysplasia may include RV aneurysms and outpouchings of the ventricle during diastole. These findings in the presence of clinical suspicion are strongly suggestive of ARVC.

On echocardiographic evaluation of a patient with possible ARVC, it is important to assess for other causes of RV dysfunction: congenital anomalies, valvular dysfunction, and shunts. A patient in the early stages of ARVC may present with a normal echocardiogram.

UNCLASSIFIED CARDIOMYOPATHIES

The category of unclassified cardiomyopathies is reserved for cases that do not fit into any of the aforementioned classes: this includes systolic dysfunction without dilation, fibroelastosis, noncompacted myocardium, and mitochondrial disease (2). In addition, certain cases may meet criteria for multiple cardiomyopathies, such as amyloidosis with hypertrophic and restrictive features. A standard comprehensive echocardiographic evaluation should be performed in such cases. Peripartum cardiomyopathy (PPCM) is a rare and poorly understood condition. The etiology of PPCM is unknown, but viral, autoimmune, and idiopathic causes may contribute. Clinically, PPCM is defined as the onset of cardiac failure with no identifiable cause in the last month of pregnancy or within 5 months after delivery, in the absence of heart disease before the last month of pregnancy (30). Echocardiographic criteria for the diagnosis include an ejection fraction of less than 45%, fractional shortening less than 30% (or both), and a LV end-diastolic volume of more than 2.7 cm/m²/BSA (31). Echocardiography is not only essential in the diagnosis of PPCM but also in determining the severity of disease.

ROLE OF ECHOCARDIOGRAPHY: PROGNOSTICATION AND TREATMENT

As described in the preceding sections, echocardiography is useful to diagnose cardiomyopathies and may provide clues to their underlying etiology. Increasingly, echocardiography may also be used in prognostication and to predict response to treatment. Echocardiographic assessment, when combined with clinical variables, may be useful for risk stratification of patients with HCM (32). Among all patients with heart failure, echocardiographic predictors of mortality include mitral E-point to septal separation, increased LV end-systolic dimension, and end-systolic radius to wall thickness ratio (1).

Valvular disease is common in patients with cardiomyopathy, either as a result of ventricular remodeling or as a preexisting contributor to cardiac dysfunction. Echocardiographic assessment is useful to identify patients who may benefit from valvular repair or replacement (1).

In patients with heart failure, a combination of M-mode echocardiography and tissue Doppler imaging allows assessment of LV dyssynchrony in 96% of patients, thus identifying patients who could benefit from LV resynchronization therapy (33). Sensitivity and specificity for tissue Doppler imaging are 90% and 82%, respectively. In patients who receive LV assist devices or other forms of ventricular support, the addition of strain and strain rate imaging to standard echocardiographic techniques may provide additional information on ventricular remodeling and recovery (34).

SUMMARY

Echocardiography is a useful clinical tool in the assessment of patients with known or suspected cardiomyopathy. While heterogeneity exists within the cardiomyopathies (both clinical and echocardiographic), each class has a subset of commonly found echocardiographic features. Echocardiography can be used to assess right and left heart function, screen for associated pulmonary hypertension, determine the underlying etiology and uncover treatable etiologies, and is increasingly being used to aid prognostication and guide treatment.

KEY POINTS

■ Cardiomyopathies are defined as diseases of the myocardium associated with cardiac dysfunction, and are classified by the WHO as DCM, HCM, RCM, ARVC, and unclassified cardiomyopathies.

■ 2D echocardiographic findings characteristic of DCM include increased end-diastolic and end-systolic ventricular dimensions and volumes, and decreased ventricular systolic function.

■ Doppler and color-flow echocardiographic findings characteristic of DCM include either an abnormal relaxation (decreased E/A ratio) or restrictive physiology (increased E/A ratio) mitral inflow velocity profile, and varying degrees of mitral and/or tricuspid insufficiency.

■ 2D echocardiographic findings characteristic of HCM include LV and/or RV hypertrophy (usually asymmetric) predominantly involving the interventricular septum and SAM of the MV apparatus, resulting in mitral insufficiency.

■ Doppler and color-flow echocardiographic findings characteristic of HCM include increased flow velocity (and pressure gradient) across the LVOT (dagger-shaped appearance of spectral wave form analysis), varying degrees of mitral insufficiency, and an abnormal relaxation (decreased E/A ratio) mitral inflow velocity profile.

■ Intraoperative TEE plays a pivotal role in guiding surgical management of HCM (e.g., extent and depth of myectomy, evaluation of MV, assessing postmyectomy LVOT velocity, and pressure gradient) and in assessing potential complications (residual mitral insufficiency, ventricular septal defect, coronary artery-LV fistula, etc.).

■ Characteristic echocardiographic findings of RCM include normal ventricular cavity size and wall thickness, relatively preserved global systolic function, biatrial enlargement, a restrictive physiology (increased E/A ratio) mitral inflow velocity profile, and alterations in pulmonary venous flow velocities (decreased systolic, increased diastolic).

■ Characteristic echocardiographic findings of ARVC include increased end-diastolic and end-systolic RV dimensions and volumes, decreased RV systolic function, and varying degrees of tricuspid insufficiency.

REFERENCES

1. Vitarelli A, Tiukinhoy S, Di Luzio S, et al. The role of echocardiography in the diagnosis and management of heart failure. *Heart Fail Rev* 2003;8:181–189.

2. Richardson P, McKenna W, Bristow M, et al. Report of the 1995 World Health Organization/International Society and Federation of Cardiology Task Force on the Definition and Classification of cardiomyopathies. *Circulation* 1996;93:841–842.

3. Brigden W. Uncommon myocardial diseases: the noncoronary cardiomyopathies. *Lancet* 1957;273:1243–1249.

4. Maron BJ, Towbin JA, Thiene G, et al. Contemporary definitions and classification of the cardiomyopathies: an American Heart Association Scientific Statement from the Council on Clinical Cardiology, Heart Failure and Transplantation Committee; Quality of Care and Outcomes Research and Functional Genomics and Translational Biology Interdisciplinary Working Groups; and Council on Epidemiology and Prevention. *Circulation* 2006;113:1807–1816.

5. Rosendorff C. *Essential Cardiology: Principles and Practice.* 2nd Ed. Totowa, NJ: Humana Press, 2005;34:641–647.

6. Jessup M, Brozena S. Heart failure. *N Engl J Med* 2003;348:2007–2018.

7. Stewart RA, McKenna WJ, Oakley CM. Good prognosis for dilated cardiomyopathy without severe heart failure or arrhythmia. *Q J Med* 1990;74:309–318.

8. Dec GW, Fuster V. Idiopathic dilated cardiomyopathy. *N Engl J Med* 1994;331:1564–1575.

9. Rihal CS, Nishimura RA, Hatle LK, et al. Systolic and diastolic dysfunction in patients with clinical diagnosis of dilated cardiomyopathy. Relation to symptoms and prognosis. *Circulation* 1994;90:2772–2779.

10. Abramson SV, Burke JF, Kelly JJ Jr, et al. Pulmonary hypertension predicts mortality and morbidity in patients with dilated cardiomyopathy. *Ann Intern Med* 1992;116:888–895.

11. Maron BJ. Hypertrophic cardiomyopathy: a systematic review. *JAMA* 2002;287:1308–1320.

12. Sherrid MV, Chaudhry FA, Swistel DG. Obstructive hypertrophic cardiomyopathy: echocardiography, pathophysiology, and the continuing evolution of surgery for obstruction. *Ann Thorac Surg* 2003;75:620–632.

13. Maron MS, Olivotto I, Zenovich AG, et al. Hypertrophic cardiomyopathy is predominantly a disease of left ventricular outflow tract obstruction. *Circulation* 2006;114:2232–2239.

14. Caselli S, Pelliccia A, Maron M, et al. Differentiation of hypertrophic cardiomyopathy from other forms of left ventricular hypertrophy by means of three-dimensional echocardiography. *Am J Cardiol* 2008;102:616–620.

15. Maron MS, Olivotto I, Betocchi S, et al. Effect of left ventricular outflow tract obstruction on clinical outcome in hypertrophic cardiomyopathy. *N Engl J Med* 2003;348:295–303.

16. Wigle ED, Rakowski H, Kimball BP, Williams WG. Hypertrophic cardiomyopathy. Clinical spectrum and treatment. *Circulation* 1995;92:1680–1692.

17. Yu EH, Omran AS, Wigle ED, et al. Mitral regurgitation in hypertrophic obstructive cardiomyopathy: relationship to obstruction and relief with myectomy. *J Am Coll Cardiol* 2000;36:2219–2225.

18. Maron BJ, Spirito P, Green KJ, et al. Noninvasive assessment of left ventricular diastolic function by pulsed Doppler echocardiography in patients with hypertrophic cardiomyopathy. *J Am Coll Cardiol* 1987;10:733–742.

19. Nishimura RA, Appleton CP, Redfield MM, et al. Noninvasive doppler echocardiographic evaluation of left ventricular filling pressures in patients with cardiomyopathies: a simultaneous Doppler echocardiographic and cardiac catheterization study. *J Am Coll Cardiol* 1996;28:1226–1233.

20. Topol EJ, Traill TA, Fortuin NJ. Hypertensive hypertrophic cardiomyopathy of the elderly. *N Engl J Med* 1985;312:277–283.

21. Roberts R, Sigwart U. New concepts in hypertrophic cardiomyopathies, part II. *Circulation* 2001;104:2249–2252.

22. Smedira NG, Lytle BW, Lever HM, et al. Current effectiveness and risks of isolated septal myectomy for hypertrophic obstructive cardiomyopathy. *Ann Thorac Surg* 2008;85:127–133.

23. McCully RB, Nishimura RA, Bailey KR, et al. Hypertrophic obstructive cardiomyopathy: preoperative echocardiographic predictors of outcome after septal myectomy. *J Am Coll Cardiol* 1996;27:1491–1496.

24. Marwick TH, Stewart WJ, Lever HM, et al. Benefits of intraoperative echocardiography in the surgical management of hypertrophic cardiomyopathy. *J Am Coll Cardiol* 1992;20:1066–1072.

25. Wilmshurst PT, Katritsis D. Restrictive cardiomyopathy. *Br Heart J* 1990;63:323–324.

26. Ha JW, Ommen SR, Tajik AJ, et al. Differentiation of constrictive pericarditis from restrictive cardiomyopathy using mitral annular velocity by tissue Doppler echocardiography. *Am J Cardiol* 2004;94:316–319.

27. McRae AT III, Chung MK, Asher CR. Arrhythmogenic right ventricular cardiomyopathy: a cause of sudden death in young people. *Cleve Clin J Med* 2001;68:459–467.

28. Gear K, Marcus F. Arrhythmogenic right ventricular dysplasia/cardiomyopathy. *Circulation* 2003;107:e31–e33.

29. Marcus FI, Zareba W, Calkins H, et al. Arrhythmogenic right ventricular cardiomyopathy/dysplasia clinical presentation and diagnostic evaluation: results from the North American Multidisciplinary Study. *Heart Rhythm* 2009;6:984–992.

30. Pearson GD, Veille JC, Rahimtoola S, et al. Peripartum cardiomyopathy: National Heart, Lung, and Blood Institute and Office of Rare Diseases (National Institutes of Health) workshop recommendations and review. *JAMA* 2000;283:1183–1188.

31. Hibbard JU, Lindheimer M, Lang RM. A modified definition for peripartum cardiomyopathy and prognosis based on echocardiography. *Obstet Gynecol* 1999;94:311–316.

32. Sorajja P, Nishimura RA, Ommen SR, et al. Use of echocardiography in patients with hypertrophic cardiomyopathy: clinical implications of massive hypertrophy. *J Am Soc Echocardiogr* 2006;19:788–795.

33. Bleeker GB, Schalij MJ, Boersma E, et al. Relative merits of M-mode echocardiography and tissue Doppler imaging for prediction of response to cardiac resynchronization therapy in patients with heart failure secondary to ischemic or idiopathic dilated cardiomyopathy. *Am J Cardiol* 2007;99:68–74.

34. Havemann L, McMahon CJ, Ganame J, et al. Rapid ventricular remodeling with left ventricular unloading postventricular assist device placement: new insights with strain imaging. *J Am Soc Echocardiogr* 2006;19:355 e359–355 e311.

1. Which of the following echocardiographic signs is most consistent with a diagnosis of late stage, DCM ?
   A. Decreased E/A ratio
   B. Increased E wave deceleration time
   C. Increased pulmonary venous S/D ratio
   D. Pulmonary acceleration times greater than 90 millisecond
   E. Shorter transmitral A-wave compared to the pulmonary venous A-wave

2. Which of the following echocardiographic signs is least commonly seen in patients with HOCM?
   A. Delayed closure of the AV
   B. Diminished systolic LV cavity size
   C. Late peaking LVOT CWD profile
   D. LV septal hypertrophy
   E. SAM of the MV

3. SAM of the MV is least likely to occur in which of the following clinical conditions?
   A. DCM
   B. Following MV ring annuloplasty
   C. Following AV replacement for aortic stenosis
   D. HCM
   E. Infiltrative cardiomyopathy

4. Which of the following echocardiographic findings is most consistent with diastolic dysfunction associated with early HCM?

A. Increased atrial contribution to LV filling
B. Increased transmitral E-wave peak flow velocity
C. Reduced isovolumic relaxation time
D. Reduced transmitral E-wave deceleration time

5. Surgical repair of HOCM is generally reserved for individuals with which one of the following echocardiographically determined criteria?
   A. Apical tethering of the MV leaflets
   B. Intraventricular gradient ≥ 40 mm Hg with provocation
   C. Intraventricular gradient at rest of ≥ 20 mm Hg
   D. Interventricular septum measuring more than 18 mm in thickness

6. Which of the following echocardiographically diagnosed complications is most common following septal myomectomy for HOCM?
   A. MV prolapse
   B. Creation of a coronary artery-to-LV fistula
   C. Persistent LVOT obstruction
   D. Ventricular septal defect

7. Which of the following locations is least likely to manifest with fibrofatty dysplasia of the RV?
   A. Apex
   B. Free wall
   C. Inflow tract
   D. Outflow tract

CHAPTER 35

Surgical Considerations and Assessment in Heart Failure Surgery

Alina M. Grigore ■ Christopher A. Thunberg ■ Robert M. Savage ■ Nicholas J. Smedira

IMPACT OF CONGESTIVE HEART FAILURE ON THE POPULATION

Congestive heart failure (CHF) has been defined as a complex clinical syndrome caused by any structural or functional cardiac disorder that impairs the ability of the ventricles to maintain adequate cardiac output (CO) (Table 35.1). In the United States, more than 5.7 million people have CHF, and its incidence is estimated at 7 per 1,000 in people over the age of 65. The incidence of heart failure has not decreased in over 20 years, but the survival after diagnosis is improving (1). It is likely that the number of patients with end-stage CHF will grow as the average age of our population rises (see Fig. 28.1). The number of hospital discharges for heart failure is greater than 1 million annually. The estimated cost of heart failure care in 2009 will be 37.2 billion dollars (2).

TABLE 35.1	Pathophysiology of Heart Failure—From Injury to Clinical Syndrome

1. Causes
   a. Myocardial injury
      i. ischemia
      ii. toxins
      iii. volume overload
      iv. pressure overload
   b. Genetic perturbation
2. Cardiac remodeling
   a. Myocyte growth
      i. concentric hypertrophy
      ii. eccentric hypertrophy
   b. Interstitial fibrosis
   c. Apoptosis
   d. Sarcomere slippage
   e. Chamber enlargement
3. Clinical heart failure milieu
   a. Pump performance
   b. Circulatory dynamics
   c. Metabolic abnormalities
   d. Symptoms
   e. Physical findings

TRENDS IN MANAGEMENT OF PATIENTS WITH CONGESTIVE HEART FAILURE

CHF is a complex syndrome in which myocardial injury and the resulting hemodynamic changes perturb many neuroendocrine, humoral, and inflammatory feedback loops (Fig 35.1). Early in the course of the disease, ventricular contractility is maintained by adrenergic stimulation, activation of renin-angiotensin-aldosterone, and other neurohormonal and cytokine systems (3,4). However, these compensatory mechanisms become less effective over time, so that ventricular dilation and fibrosis occur and cardiac function deteriorates. This produces a chronic state of low perfusion that ends in multisystem failure and death unless adequate circulation is restored.

Strategies for treating end-stage CHF aim to improve quality of life, limit disease progression, and prolong life. Medical therapies, such as angiotensin-converting enzyme inhibitors (ACEI), β-blockers, diuretics, inotropic agents, and antiarrhythmics, represent the usual standard of care for CHF management. However, even multidrug regimens may not prevent progression toward end-stage CHF; when this occurs, surgery is the only effective intervention.

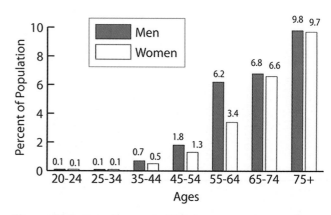

Figure 35.1. Prevalence of CHF by age and sex. (From Zoghbi WA, Enriquez-Sarano M, Foster E. et al. Recommendations for evaluation of the severity of native valvular regurgitation with two-dimensional and Doppler echocardiography. *J Am Soc Echocardiogr* 2003;16[7]:777–802.)

Cardiac transplantation is the "gold-standard" surgical treatment for end-stage CHF. It is associated with excellent 1-year survival (>80%), 5-year survival (60%), and functional capacity (5). While the 1-year survival rate after transplantation is 85%, patients in New York Heart Association (NYHA) class IV have a 1-year mortality rate of 40% to 50% (6). Additionally, the small number of donors limits the number of CHF patients who can benefit from cardiac transplantation. Over the past decade, the number of transplant recipients older than 65 years has quadrupled, but the number of donors has remained the same and transplantation waiting times have increased steadily. As a result, even though more than 10,000 people per year could benefit from cardiac transplantation, only 2,200 heart transplantations are available each year (7). The mismatch between the growing number of cardiac transplant candidates and the limited number of donors has led to increasing use of alternative advanced surgical therapies intended to unload the heart and allow myocardial reverse remodeling and recovery. Included among these advanced procedures are mechanical ventricular assist device (VAD) implantation, ventricular remodeling procedures in conjunction with revascularization and mitral valvuloplasty (i.e., endoventricular circular patch plasty [EVCPP], partial ventriculectomy), newer procedures intended to reduce ventricular dilatation (i.e., external or internal splinting), and total artificial heart (TAH) implantation.

CRITICAL ISSUES ADDRESSED BY INTRAOPERATIVE ECHOCARDIOGRAPHY: PATIENTS UNDERGOING PROCEDURES FOR CHF

Intraoperative echocardiography (IOE) (consisting of both transesophageal echocardiography [TEE] and epicardial echocardiography) can be used to identify the important aspects of a particular case of end-stage CHF and promote successful surgical intervention (Table 35.2).

Determine the Etiology and Mechanism of CHF

Advanced CHF is caused by a variety of diseases that affect the myocardium. Based on their functional and morphologic features, cardiomyopathies (CMP) can be classified as dilated, hypertrophic, or restrictive. Dilated CMP is the result of viral, bacterial, or parasitic disease of toxic insult. It can also occur in association with pregnancy. Long-term severe myocardial ischemia and chronic regurgitant valvular disease, such as mitral or aortic insufficiency, could also lead to dilated CMP (Figs. 35.2 and 35.3). Hypertrophic CMP is either genetically inherited or is the result of long-standing hypertension or valvular disease, such as aortic stenosis. Infiltrative processes (amyloidosis, hemochromatosis) and inflammatory disease (sarcoidosis) are

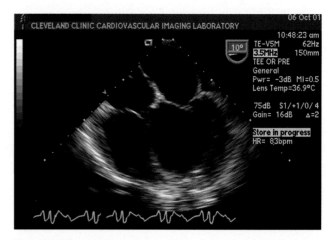

Figure 35.2. Dilated cardiomyopathy: ME 4-chamber view.

the most common causes of restrictive CMP. IOE is an important diagnostic tool due to its unique ability to evaluate cardiac morphology and function and to differentiate among various types of CMP (Tables 35.3 and 35.4) (8).

Assessment of Left and Right Ventricular Function

Assessment of left ventricular (LV) and right ventricular (RV) function is critical to the proper evaluation and perioperative management of patients with end-stage CHF. Using IOE can provide excellent qualitative and quantitative information on RV and LV function.

Dilated CMP is characterized by dilation of both ventricular and atrial chambers associated with systolic heart failure (9). Both motion mode (M-mode) and two-dimensional (2D) echocardiography can be used for the evaluation of LV systolic function. The high time resolution of M-mode echocardiography enables it to accurately measure ventricular internal dimension and wall thickness. Additionally, placing the M-mode beam at the mitral chordal level to obtain a transgastric (TG) short-axis view

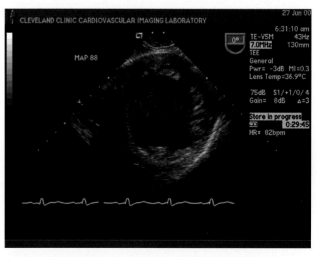

Figure 35.3. Dilated cardiomyopathy: TG midpapillary SAX view.

TABLE 35.2	Application of IOE During Surgical Procedures for CHF		
Surgical Procedure	**Critical IOE Issues**	**Pre-CPB**	**Post-CPB**

LVAD implantation	RV function
	Sequelae of CHF
	  MR, pulmonary HTN
	  Diastolic dysfunction
	  Mural thrombi (LA, LV)
	Potential R → L shunt
	Potential Ao → LV circuit
	Cannulation-perfusion
	LVAD cannula inflow/outflow
	  Position and function
	LVAD function
	  LV volume
	  Valve competence
	Complications of CPB
		Global RV Fx, RV FAC
		MR (grade, mechanism)
		LAA or LV mural thrombi
		PW of MV inflow pulmonary vein
		CFD, contrast with valsalva
		CFD of AV
			Global RV Fx, RV FAC
			
			PW of MV and pulmonary vein
			
			CFD of AV
			TEE and EPE
			Apical inflow position
			  CW, CFD
			Aortic outflow
			  Air embolism
			Hypovolemia, flow <1.5 m/s
			Regurgitant LVAD flow
			2D ascending and descending aorta

BI-VAD, ECMO	RV function
	Sequelae of CHF
	
	  MR, pulmonary HTN
	  Diastolic dysfunction
	  Mural thrombi (LA, LV)
	Potential R → L shunt
	Potential Ao → LV circuit
	Cannulation-perfusion
	LVAD cannula inflow/outflow
	  Position and function
	LVAD function
	  LV volume
	  Valve competence
	Complications of CPB
	cannula positioning
	  LA, PA, LV, Ao
	LA thrombus formation
			Global RV Fx, RV FAC
			PW of MV and pulmonary vein
			CFD of AV
			TEE and EPE
			Apical inflow position
			  CW, CFD
			Aortic outflow
			  Air embolism
			Hypovolemia, flow <1.5 m/s
			Regurgitant LVAD flow
			2D ascending and descending aorta

Dor procedure
Ventricular reconstruction
  Remodeling LV
  Coronary artery bypass grafting (CABG)
  MV repair
	RV function
	LV function and scar
	Sequelae of CHF
	  MR, pulmonary HTN
	
	  Diastolic dysfunction
	
	  Mural thrombi
	Potential R → L shunt
	Embolic source (LA, LV)
	Cannulation-perfusion strategy
	Myocardial viability
	MR severity and mechanism
		Global RV Fx, RV FAC, TR
		RWMA, scar
		
		MR (severity and mechanism)
		PWD MW and pulmonary vein
		Contrast
		CFD, contrast and valsalva
		
		EPE
		
		Resting RWMA
		Low-dose dobutamine stress
			Global RV Fx, RV FAC
			PW of MV and pulmonary vein
			CFD of AV
			TEE and EPE
			Apical inflow position
			
			  CW, CFD
			Aortic outflow
			  Air embolism
			Hypovolemia, flow <1.5 m/s
			
			Regurgitant LVAD flow
			2D ascending and descending aorta

(continued)

Surgical Procedure	Critical IOE Issues	Pre-CPB	Post-CPB
Revascularization	Myocardial viability	Resting RWM Low-dose dobutamine stress Mitral valve function	Assess for new RWMA Comprehensive IOE focusing on complications of cannulation, perfusion, myocardial protection, and valve function
MV repair	Mitral regurgitation	MR severity and mechanism Pathoanatomy, annulus size	Success of repair Complications
External and internal splinting	Size LV, Systolic LV/RV Fx, MR, diastolic Fx Position of mechanical splints	As above, LV dimensions, LV and RV dimensions, Ej Fx MR mechanism/severity, mitral inflow, pulmonary vein CW	Diastolic function Filling RV function
Total artificial heart	Atrial shunts Pulmonary vein flow Inferior vena cava flow Superior vena cava flow PVR	Atrial shunts PVR Intracardiac thrombus	Gradients and flows through right and left inflow valves Gradients and flows through right and left outflow valves Patency of the aortic and pulmonary anastomosis PVR

RWM, regional wall motion.

of the LV (Fig. 35.4) makes it possible to compute LV fractional shortening, a rough measurement of LV systolic function with a normal range of 25% to 45%, using the following formula:

$$\text{Fractional shortening (\%)} = (LVID_d - LVID_s) / LVID_d \times 100\%$$

$LVID_d$ = left ventricular internal diameter at end-diastole; $LVID_s$ = left ventricular internal diameter at end-systole.

The 2D echocardiography provides both qualitative and quantitative evaluation of systolic ventricular function. Midesophageal four-chamber (ME 4-chamber) and two-chamber (ME 2-chamber) views and the ME long-axis

---

TABLE 35.3	**Typical Features of the Three Physiologic Types of Cardiomyopathy**

	Dilated	Hypertrophic	Restrictive
LV systolic function	Moderately to severely ↓	Normal	Normal
LV diastolic function	May be abnormal	Abnormal	Abnormal
LV hypertrophy	↑ LV mass due to LV dilation with normal wall thickness	Asymmetric LV hypertrophy	Concentric LV hypertrophy
Chamber dilation	All four chambers	LA and RA dilation if MR is present	LA and RA dilation
Outflow tract obstruction	Absent	Dynamic LV outflow tract obstruction may be present	Absent
Left ventricular end-diastolic pressure	Elevated	Elevated	Elevated
Pulmonary artery pressures	Elevated	Elevated	Elevated

LV, Left ventricular; ↓, decreased; ↑, increased.
From Otto CM. The cardiomyopathies, hypertensive heart disease, post-cardiac-transplant patient and pulmonary heart disease. In: Textbook of Clinical Echocardiography. Philadelphia: W.B. Saunders, 2000:183–212, with permission.

TABLE 35.4	Echocardiographic Approach to the Patient with a Suspected Cardiomyopathy	
	Qualitative	**Quantitative**
2D/M-mode imaging	Chamber dimensions	LV-EDV, LV-ESV
	Degree and pattern of LV hypertrophy	LV mass
	Evidence for dynamic outflow tract obstruction	
	SAM of mitral valve	
	AV midsystolic closure	
LV systolic function	Visual estimate of EF	Apical biplane EF
Doppler echo	Associated valvular regurgitation	Maximum and mean ΔP
	Pattern of LV diastolic filling	PA pressures
	Pattern of LA filling (pulmonary venous inflow)	
	Velocity curve of dynamic outflow tract obstruction	
	Localization of the level of obstruction	

2D, Two-dimensional; LA, left atrial; LV, left ventricular; EDV, end-diastolic volume; ESV, end-systolic volume; SAM, systolic anterior motion; P, pressure gradient; PA, pulmonary artery; EF, ejection fraction.
From Otto CM. The cardiomyopathies, hypertensive heart disease, post-cardiac-transplant patient and pulmonary heart disease. In: Textbook of Clinical Echocardiography. Philadelphia: W.B. Saunders, 2000:183–212, with permission.

(ME LAX) view, TG short-axis (TG SAX) views (basal, midpapillary, and apical), and the TG LAX view allow assessment of both global and regional ventricular function. The 2D quantitative measures of LV systolic function include ventricular dimensions, volume, stroke volume (SV), CO, ejection fraction (EF), and regional wall motion abnormalities (Figs. 35.5 and 35.6). Left ventricular ejection fraction (LVEF) can be calculated from LV end-systolic volume (LVESV) and end-diastolic volume (LVEDV) as the ratio (LVEDV – LVESV)/LVEDV (Fig 35.5). CO can be calculated using the area-length formula across a cardiac valve (most commonly the aortic valve [AV]):

$$CO = 0.785 \times LVOT\ D^2 \times LVOT_{VTI} \times HR$$

[LVOT, left ventricular outflow tract; D, LVOT diameter; $LVOT_{VTI}$, velocity time integral (VTI), measured with Doppler spectrum across the LVOT; HR, heart rate]. IOE determination of CO is helpful, even when a pulmonary artery (PA) catheter is used, because some patients with dilated CMP present with some degree of tricuspid valve (TV) regurgitation, which renders the thermodilution technique inaccurate.

In addition, patients with end-stage CHF often present with coexisting pathology such as acquired left ventricle aneurysm (LVA). LVA is the final expression of transmural infarct expansion and is often accompanied by anterior

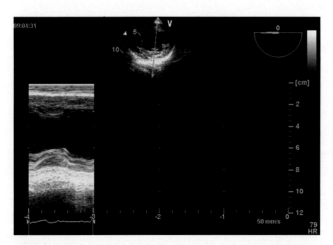

Figure 35.4. Dilated cardiomyopathy: LV M-mode TG midpapillary SAX view.

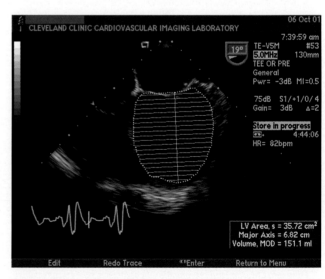

Figure 35.5. Dilated cardiomyopathy, LV dimensions, and volume: ME 4-chamber view.

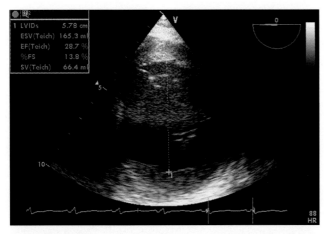

Figure 35.6. Dilated cardiomyopathy, LV dimension, and volume: TG SAX midpapillary view.

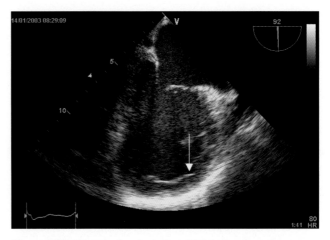

Figure 35.8. Ventricular thrombus: ME 2-chamber view.

infarction in the area of the distribution of the left anterior descending coronary artery (Fig. 35.7). Thrombi are frequently detected within aneurysms and are often associated with systemic embolization (Fig. 35.8). Therefore, careful echocardiographic assessment is mandatory if cardiopulmonary bypass (CPB) is to be successful.

Evaluation of RV systolic function is a critical part of the intraoperative management of patients with end-stage CHF. Preexisting pathologic conditions in the RV, such as ischemia, infarction, CMP, and pulmonary hypertension (PHTN), are major risk factors for RV failure. Sometimes, the extent of RV dysfunction becomes apparent only when a sudden increase in venous return challenges an already impaired RV. With dilated CMP, there is an increase in systolic ventricular interaction, making RV systolic performance more dependent on the LV to generate pressure (10). Under these circumstances, sudden LV unloading may depress RV function further.

The standard 2D TEE views used to evaluate RV function are the ME 4-chamber view, the ME RV inflow-outflow view, the TG mid-SAX view, and the TG RV inflow view. Signs of RV dysfunction include hypokinesis or akinesis of the RV free wall and RV dilation caused by volume or pressure overload. Normally, the RV end-diastolic cross-sectional area is less than 60% of the LV end-diastolic cross-sectional area. With dilatation, however, the RV changes its shape from triangular to round, with concomitant enlargement of the right ventricular outflow tract (RVOT), and flattening of the bulge in the interventricular septum from right to left can be seen in the ME 4-chamber view and the ME RV inflow-outflow view (Figs. 35.9 and 35.10). With RV pressure overload, a maximal leftward septal shift is noted at end-systole, whereas RV volume overload is associated with a maximum reversed septal curvature in mid-diastole. As RV dilation becomes moderate or severe, the RV replaces the LV in forming the cardiac apex in the ME 4-chamber view, and the end-diastolic cross-sectional area of the RV may equal or exceed that of the LV (Fig 35.11). Wall thickness greater than 5 mm as measured by M-mode is considered abnormal and suggests elevated PA pressure, pulmonary valve (PV) stenosis, or infiltrative CMP. In severe cases of RV dysfunction, pulsed-wave Doppler examination of blood flow in the hepatic veins may show attenuation of the systolic inflow wave.

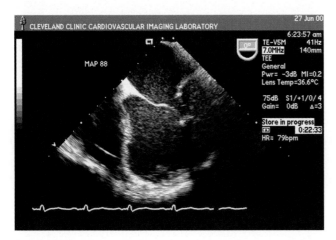

Figure 35.7. LV aneurysm: ME 4-chamber view.

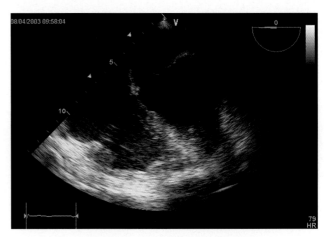

Figure 35.9. Biventricular failure: ME 4-chamber view.

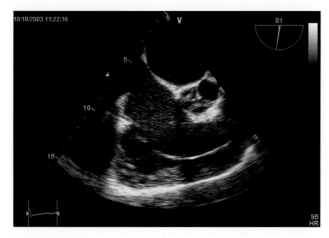

Figure 35.10. RV failure: ME RV inflow-outflow view.

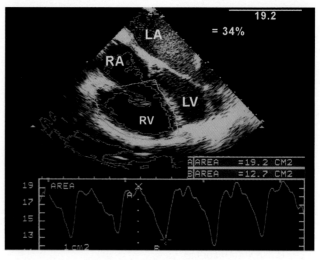

Figure 35.12. RV function: ME 4-chamber view.

Quantitative echocardiographic assessment of RV systolic function is difficult due to the complex geometry of the chamber. An estimate of RV systolic function can be obtained in the ME 4-chamber view by using RV fractional area change (RVFAC) (11) (Fig. 35.12).

$$RVFAC = [(\text{end-diastolic area} - \text{end-systolic area})/\text{end-diastolic area}] \times 100\%$$

A value greater than 35% is considered normal. The calculation of RVFAC can be tedious and time-consuming when the endocardial border is poorly visualized, but automated border detection software may speed the calculation.

An alternative method of assessing RV systolic function is tricuspid annular plane systolic excursion (TAPSE), in which the M-mode cursor is placed across the lateral tricuspid annulus in the ME 4-chamber view. During systole, the tricuspid plane is displaced toward the RV apex due to lengthwise shortening of the RV free wall and interventricular septum. In normal individuals, TAPSE is at least

25 mm, while individuals with RV dysfunction may have a TAPSE of less then 20 mm (12) (Fig. 35.13). TAPSE correlates well radionuclide-based determinations of RVEF and data obtained from right heart catheterization, and it is much simpler to obtain (13).

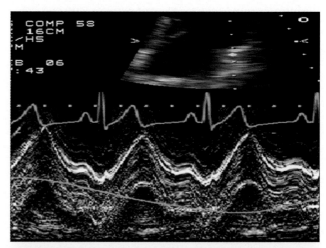

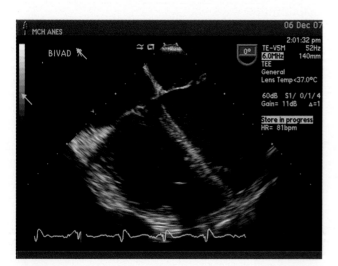

Figure 35.11. RV failure: ME 4-chamber view.

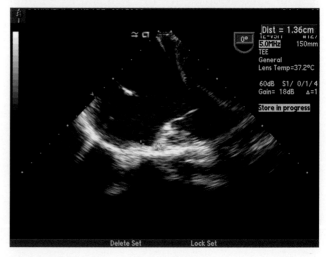

Figure 35.13. **A, B:** RV function: TAPSE.

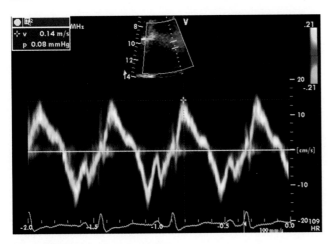

Figure 35.14. RV function: TDI.

Techniques employing tissue Doppler imaging (TDI) have also been used to assess RV function. Pulsed-wave TDI of the lateral tricuspid annulus is analogous to TAPSE, except that velocity, not displacement, of the tricuspid annulus is measured. Peak tricuspid annular systolic velocity (S_a) less than 10 cm/s is predictive of reduced RVEF, severe PHTN, and elevated transpulmonary gradient (14) (Fig. 35.14). Strain analysis, another tissue Doppler technique, measures myocardial deformation (shortening) of the RV free wall during the cardiac cycle. Systolic shortening is impaired in individuals with impaired RV function due to PHTN and improves with vasodilator therapy, as shown in Fig. 35.15A and B (15).

PA pressure estimates remain one of the most important quantitative measures of RV systolic function. As RV dysfunction progresses, dilation of TV annulus occurs, causing varying degrees of tricuspid regurgitation (TR) (Fig. 35.16). Measuring the velocity and pressure gradient of the tricuspid regurgitant jet (Fig. 35.17) reveals the gradient between RV and right atrial (RA) pressure and, when added to an estimate of RA pressure (transduced from the central venous line), allows calculation of RV systolic pressure (Table 35.5). RV SV and CO can be measured directly by imaging the RVOT tract and PA in the upper esophageal aortic arch SAX (UE aortic arch SAX) view (Fig. 35.18). By measuring the diameter (D) of PA annulus and using PWD mode to determine VTI across pulmonic valve, RV SV and CO can be calculated using the formulas $SV = PA\ D^2 \times 0.785 \times PA_{VTI}$ and $CO = SV \times HR$.

Growing evidence suggests that both systolic and diastolic dysfunction play important roles in the clinical presentation and prognosis of patients with end-stage CHF. Patients with hypertrophic, infiltrative, or primary restrictive CMP may report symptoms of heart failure despite normal EF, a condition known as diastolic heart failure (16,17). In addition, in patients with preexisting systolic dysfunction, abnormalities in diastolic dysfunction may be significantly related to the severity of cardiac symptoms and prognosis in patients with CHF (18). Diastole is

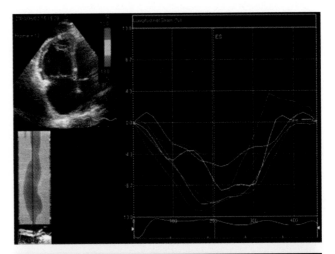

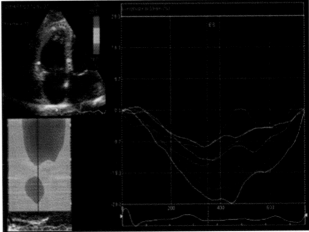

Figure 35.15. A,B: RV strain curves, effect of vasodilator therapy.

the interval between AV closure and mitral valve closure and can be divided into four phases:

1. Isovolumic relaxation
2. Early rapid diastolic filling
3. Diastasis
4. Late diastolic filling caused by atrial contraction (Fig. 35.19).

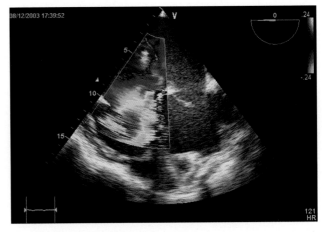

Figure 35.16. Severe TR: ME 4-chamber view.

TABLE 35.5	Estimation of Intracardiac Pressures		
Pressure Estimated	**Required Measurement**	**Formula**	**Normal Valves (mm Hg)**
Estimated CVP	Respiratory IVC collapse	>40% = 5 mm Hg	5–10
		<40%, (nl RV) = 10 mm Hg	
		0% and RV Dysfx = 15 mm Hg	
RV systolic pressure (RVSP)	Peak velocity$_{TR}$	RVSP = $4(V_{TR})^2$ + CVP	16–30
	CVP or measured	(No PS)	
RV systolic (with VSD)	Systemic systolic BP	RVSP = SBP – $4(V_{LV-RV})^2$	With VSD usually >50
	Peak V_{LV-RV}	(No LVOT obstruction)	
PA systolic	Peak velocity$_{TR}$	PASP = $4(V_{TR})^2$ + CVP	16–30
PASP	CVP* or measured	(No PS)	
PA diastolic (PAD)	End diastolic	PAEDP = $4(V_{PR\ ED})^2$ + CVP	0–8
	Velocity$_{PR}$		
	CVP* or measured		
PA mean (PAM)	Acceleration time (AT) to peak V_{PA}	PAM = (–0.45) AT + 79	10–16
RV dP/dt	TR spectral envelope	RV dP = $4V^2_{TR(2m/s)}$ – $4V^2_{TR(2m/s)}$	>150 mm Hg/ms
	$T_{TR(2\ m/s)}$ – $T_{TR(1\ m/s)}$	RV dP/dt = dP/$T_{TR(2\ m/s)}$ – $T_{TR(1\ m/s)}$	
LA systolic (LASP)	Peak V_{MR}	LASP = SBP – $4(V_{MR})^2$	100–140
	Systolic BP (SBP)	(No LVOT gradient)	
LA (PFO)	Velocity$_{PFO}$	LAP = $4(V_{PFO})^2$ + CVP	3–15
	CVP* or measured		
LV diastolic (LVEDP)	End diastolic	LVEDP = DBP – $4(V_{AR})^2$	3–12
	Velocity$_{AR}$		
	Diastolic BP (DBP)		
LV dP/dt	MR spectral envelope	LV dP = $4V^2_{TR(2m/s)}$ – $4V^2_{TR(2m/s)}$	>800 mm Hg/ms
	$T_{MR(2\ m/s)}$ – $T_{MR\ (1\ m/s)}$	LV dP/dt = dP/$T_{MR\ (2\ m/s)}$ – $T_{MR\ (1\ m/s)}$	

RVSP, right ventricular systolic pressure.

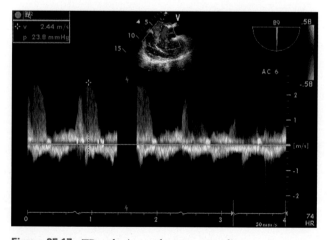

Figure 35.17. TR, velocity, and pressure gradient.

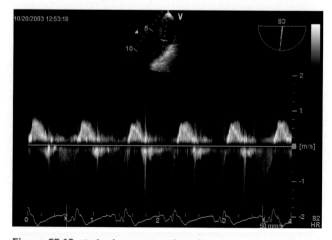

Figure 35.18. Pulsed wave Doppler of PA.

DIASTOLE

Figure 35.19. The relationship among LV, LA, and aortic pressures.

Parameters of diastolic function include ventricular relaxation, myocardial compliance, and chamber compliance. Ventricular relaxation is measured by isovolumic relaxation time (IVRT), the rate of pressure decline (dP/dT), and time constant of relaxation (τ). Myocardial compliance is estimated by the ratio of change in volume to change in pressure

(dV/dP). Chamber compliance is assessed by measuring early diastolic LV filling (E wave), deceleration time (DT), late diastolic LV filling (A_M wave), the A_p wave (reversed) of LA contraction, the s wave of the systolic LA filling phase, and the d wave of the LA diastolic filling phase.

The earliest stage of abnormal diastolic filling is *impaired relaxation* with inverse E/A ratio as the major Doppler abnormality (Table 35.6). With progression of the disease to moderate diastolic dysfunction, *pseudonormalization of diastolic filling flow* occurs because of impaired myocardial relaxation balanced by elevation of mean LA pressures (Table 35.6). The diagnosis is confirmed by abnormal PV flow or response to Valsalva maneuver. The *restrictive filling pattern* is the most advanced form of diastolic dysfunction that can be associated with either normal or abnormal systolic function. It may accompany advanced infiltrative CMP, such as amyloidosis, advanced hypertensive disease, or dilated CMP. The hallmark of the disease is elevated LA pressures with increased LV stiffness that cause a large E wave, short DT, a small A_M wave, and a very small s/d ratio on PV PWD trace (Figs. 35.20 and 35.21; Table 35.7) (19).

Assessment of Coexisting or Secondary Pathology

Mitral regurgitation (MR) is commonly encountered in CHF as a consequence of dilated cardiomyopathy (20–22). Mitral annular dilation caused by LV dilation and papillary muscle dysfunction are the most common mechanisms behind the development of regurgitation in dilated cardiomyopathy. Abnormal papillary muscle alignment and abnormal leaflet apposition during systole are caused by changes in the shape of the LV chamber during both

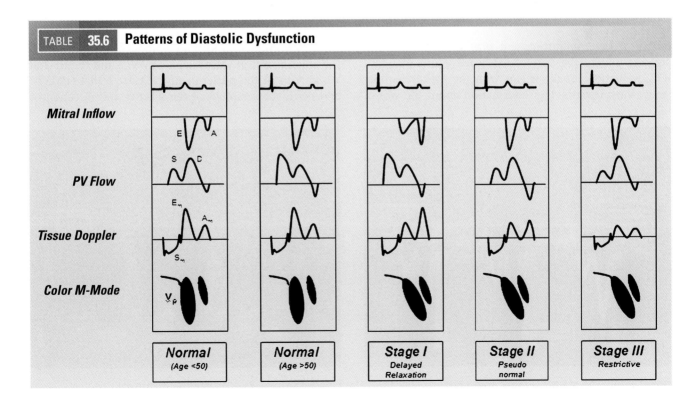

| TABLE | 35.6 | Patterns of Diastolic Dysfunction |

TABLE 35.7	Distinguishing the Patterns of Diastolic Dysfunction			
Parameter	Normal Filling	Impaired Filling Stage 1	Pseudonormal Filling Stage 2	Restrictive Filling Stages 3 and 4
E wave				
DT	160–240 ms	>240 ms	160–200 ms	<160 ms
IVRT	70–90 ms	>90 ms	<90 ms	<70 ms
E:A	1–2	<1	1–1.5	>1.5
A_M:A_P duration	AM ≥ AP	AM > AP	AM < AP	AM << AP
PVS:PVD	PVS > PVD	PVS >> PVD	PVS < PVD	PVS << PVD
VE' MA:VA' MA	VE' MA > VA' MA	VE' MA < VA' MA	VE' MA < VA' MA	VE' MA < VA' MA
Valsalva	Decreased	Decreased	Reversal	Decreased
E:A		<1		
Volume loading	—	AM < AP	AM << AP	AM <<< AP
A_M:A_P duration				

the systolic and the diastolic periods (23). Color flow Doppler (CFD) imaging has been used to quantify the severity of MR, whereas PWD is used to measure regurgitant SV and regurgitant fraction (24,25). TR can be encountered either in isolation or in conjunction with MR. The regurgitant tricuspid jet is usually directed toward the interatrial septum in patients with dilated CMP. RV dysfunction, PHTN, patent foramen ovale (PFO), and aortic regurgitation AR) are other pathophysiologies that may accompany end-stage CHF.

Standard Intraoperative Echocardiographic Examination

IOE is a key monitoring and diagnostic modality in patients undergoing surgery for heart failure. Standard IOE evaluation usually begins with the ME 4-chamber view. This view provides information about the size of the left and right cardiac chambers; the thickness of ventricular walls and the basal, mid, and apical segments of LV lateral and septal walls; the apical and basal portion of RV free wall; and MV and TV function. PWD assessment of the left upper pulmonary vein (LUPV) and left lower pulmonary veins (LLPV), the right upper pulmonary vein (RUPV), and MV diastolic flow can be used to estimate the severity of MR and the extent of diastolic impairment. Next, the multiplane angle is rotated 30 degrees into the ME AV SAX view, which allows examination of morphology and function of the AV cusps. The ME RV inflow-outflow view is obtained at 60 degrees and provides information about RV diaphragmatic free wall motion, RVOT size, and PV and TV function. The ME mitral commissural view provides information about the A2 scallop of the anterior mitral valve leaflet (AMVL) and the P1 and P2 scallops of the posterior mitral valve leaflet (PMVL) and permits assessment of the severity and direction of

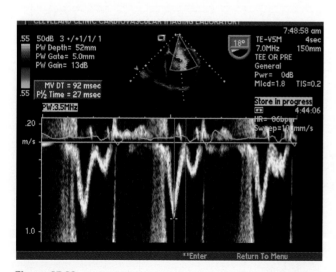

Figure 35.20. Pulsed wave Doppler: transmitral diastolic flow.

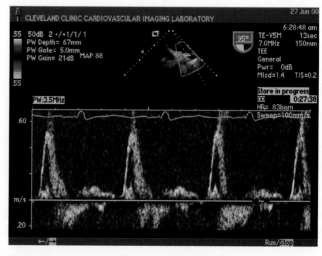

Figure 35.21. LUPV PWD: restrictive pattern.

the MV regurgitant jet, if present. The ME 2-chamber view at 90 degrees allows evaluation of the basal, mid, and apical segments of the anterior and inferior LV walls as well as examination of the left atrial appendage (LAA) for mural thrombi. The ME LAX view at 120 degrees shows both basal and midanteroseptal segments, basal and mid-posterior segments, the LVOT, and the AV. The ME bicaval view is the image of choice for evaluating PFO by CFD and contrast study. This view provides information about the size of and blood flow through the RA, the left atrium (LA), and the right lower pulmonary vein (RLPV) using PW Doppler. TG views are obtained by advancing the probe into the stomach and flexing the tip anteriorly. TG basal and mid-SAX views are the views of choice for the examination of LV regional wall motion abnormalities. In addition, the TG basal SAX view provides a SAX view of the MV that allows further location of the regurgitant jets using CFD. Rotating the multiplane angle 90 degrees to the TG two-chamber view allows further assessment of the LV anterior and posterior walls, the MV, and the LAA. The TG LAX view at 120 degrees provides a longitudinal view of the AV and allows measurement of pressure gradients across the AV using continuous wave Doppler (CWD) and pulse wave Doppler (PWD). Turning the probe to the right and to 120 degrees to the TG RV inflow view allows evaluation of the RV diaphragmatic and free walls, TV function, and RA dimensions. The deep TG LAX view provides a longitudinal view of the LV and AV and allows measurement of AV gradients and calculation of the AV area using CWD and PWD. Atherosclerotic disease in the descending aorta can be detected with the probe in a gastric position and the tip rotated posteriorly into the left descending aortic SAX (descending aortic SAX) view. A longitudinal view of the descending aorta can be obtained at 90 degrees in the descending aortic long-axis (descending aortic LAX) view. The ME ascending aortic SAX/LAX views and UE aortic arch LAX/SAX views are used to examine the ascending aorta and should be used to guide cannulation and cross-clamping of the aorta. Doppler examination of the PV is best achieved using the UE aortic arch SAX view (26).

Surgical Procedure–Related Issues

Surgical approaches to end-stage CHF are rapidly becoming more numerous and sophisticated. Substantial advances have been made in myocardial revascularization, mitral valvuloplasty, ventricular remodeling (i.e., EVCPP and LV partial resection), ventricular constraint techniques (i.e., Acorn CorCap external splinting, Myosplint internal splinting), mechanical ventricular support, TAH, and heart transplantation. During the period before CBP is initiated, IOE focuses on the evaluation of

1. RV function, severity of TR, and the potential need for RV mechanical support
2. Baseline LV function

3. Potential sequelae of end-stage-dilated cardiomyopathy, such as LVA, LA mural thrombi, MR, and diastolic dysfunction
4. Potential right-to-left shunting through PFO, which may contribute to hypoxemia
5. The presence of AR or mitral stenosis (MS)
6. The presence of ascending aortic atheroma, which necessitates changing the cannulation strategy and myocardial protection

This information guides the development of CPB strategy. At the time of separation from CPB, IOE is useful for evaluating the adequacy of deairing of the cardiac chambers. It is also important at that time to establish a comprehensive baseline study for future comparison and to assess LV and RV filling patterns, native valve function, the quality of the valve repair, and the presence of any intracardiac shunts. Given the importance of RV function in the outcome of the procedure, an objective qualitative assessment of RV systolic and diastolic function by RVFAC, RVEDV, RV dP/dT, TV annulus diameter, and severity of TR is important. These parameters will allow comparison between baseline and postoperative RV performance and dictate postoperative management in the event of acute deterioration of RV function, which is often seen when respiratory insufficiency occurs.

Transplantation

Please see Chapter 36, "Assessment of Cardiac Transplantation."

Complications of Surgical Procedures for CHF

Right Ventricular Dysfunction

The success of surgical procedures for end-stage CHF depends on postoperative RV performance. Unfortunately, right-sided circulatory failure is a common postoperative complication in patients undergoing surgical procedures for CHF. Patients with end-stage CHF often develop substantial passive PHTN secondary to elevated LA and pulmonary venous pressures, a condition that is reversible with LV unloading. When pulmonary disease is also present, irreversible elevated pulmonary vascular resistance (PVR) complicates the clinical picture. RV function is significantly afterload dependent, and the presence of pulmonary congestion in association with high PVR can have a tremendous impact on RV systolic and diastolic performance. RV failure causes dilation, ischemia, and decreased RV contractility. It is associated with decreased pulmonary blood flow and a leftward septal shift that subsequently lowers LV filling pressure and reduces systemic CO. Treatment of RV is difficult (Table 35.8).

IOE plays an important role in the diagnosis and treatment of RV failure. It allows estimation of intracardiac pressures, such as central venous pressure (CVP); RV systolic pressure; and PA systolic, diastolic, and mean

TABLE 35.8	Perioperative Management of Right-Sided Heart Failure Goals

1. Preserving coronary perfusion through maintenance of systemic blood pressure
2. Optimizing RV preload
3. Reducing RV afterload by decreasing PVR
4. Limiting pulmonary vasoconstriction through optimal ventilation
    a. High inspired oxygen concentration (100% FiO_2)
    b. Hyperventilation to $PaCO_2$ of 25–30 mm Hg
    c. Optimal tidal volumes
    d. Correction of acid-base abnormalities
5. Supporting RV function
    a. Pharmacological agents
    b. Intra-aortic balloon pump
    c. RV assist devices

pressures (Table 35.2). In addition, RV afterload can be computed by dividing the mean PA pressure by the CO. RV dP/dT calculation is helpful in assessing the extent of diastolic dysfunction. Optimal mechanical ventilatory settings and mode can be guided by serial measurement of the above-mentioned parameters. Echocardiographic monitoring of the effect of different pharmacological interventions (Tables 35.9 and 35.10) on PVR and RV performance can also be used during the post-CPB and early postoperative periods.

Right-to-Left Shunt

Right-to-left shunt is a condition that may be encountered during the post-CPB period when the RV is dilated, and there is TR and increased RA pressure. Distension of RA and elevation of RA pressure increase the pressure gradient across the interatrial septum that can cause the opening of a previously sealed PFO or the unmasking of a previously partially closed PFO. Moreover, when right-to-left shunt is accompanied by severe TR, the regurgitant jet is directed along the interatrial septum, which can amplify the hemodynamic effects of elevated right-side pressure. The bicaval view allows PWD interrogation, measurement of the PFO orifice, and calculation of the shunt volume. Significant right-to-left shunting may be caused by right-side distension and can lead to severe hypoxia, acidosis, and hemodynamic decompensation.

Hemodynamic Instability

Hemodynamic instability is frequently present during the early post-CPB period and can be caused by LV dysfunction, low systemic vascular resistance (SVR), and hypovolemia. IOE is a helpful tool in differentiating among cardiogenic, vasodilatory, and hypovolemic shock and in assessing the effects of various interventions. The 2D

TABLE 35.9	Pulmonary Vasodilator Agents

1. **Phosphodiesterase-III inhibitors**
    Inhibition of myocardial type III phosphodiesterase → increase in myocardial cAMP → increase in intracellular Ca^{2+} influx → positive inotropic effect
    Unique mechanism of inotropic effects independent of β-receptor stimulation
    Bypass β-adrenergic receptors in patients with preexisting heart failure
    Additive effect with catecholamines
    Pulmonary vasodilation
    Coronary vasodilation

2. **B-type natriuretic peptide**
    Recombinant human B-type natriuretic peptide
    Site of action: guanylate cyclase receptor of vascular smooth muscle and endothelial cells
    Effect: increased intracellular cGMP and smooth muscle cell relaxation, dose-dependent reduction in PCWP, and systemic arterial pressure in patients with heart failure
    Increased permeability of vascular endothelium
    Inhibition of renin-angiotensin-aldosterone axis
    Dose: 2 g/kg bolus followed by 0.01–0.03 µg/kg/min infusion
    Plasma half-life 18 minutes

3. **Prostaglandin I_2 (PGI_2)**
    Endogenous prostaglandin
    Synthesized by cyclooxygenase arm of arachidonic acid metabolic pathway
    Potent vasodilator
    Inhibits neutrophil activation
    Stabilized cell membranes
    Enhances myocardial inotropy by activating adenylate cyclase and increasing intracellular cAMP

4. **Nitric oxide**
    Selective pulmonary dilator less potent than inhaled prostacyclin
    Activation of guanylate cyclase
    Improves ventilation-perfusion distribution
    No effect on cardiac index and stroke index
    Complex and expensive technology implied for safe and effective use
    Could cause rebound pulmonary vasoconstriction with prolonged use
    Toxic metabolites nitrogen dioxide and methemoglobin

5. **Prostaglandin E_1 (PGE_1)**
    Endogenous prostaglandin
    Synthesized by cyclooxygenase arm of arachidonic acid metabolic pathway
    Potent pulmonary and systemic vasodilator
    Cleared from the circulation during its first pass through the lung

TABLE **35.10** **Pharmacological Agents**

TABLE **35.10**	**Pharmacological Agents**

1. Isoproterenol
   Nonselective beta-adrenergic agonist
   Positive chronotropic and inotropic agent
   Pulmonary and systemic vasodilator

2. Dobutamine
   Beta-adrenergic receptor agonist with minimal
   alpha-adrenergic receptor agonist activity
   Positive chronotropic and inotropic agent
   Pulmonary and systemic vasodilator

3. Epinephrine
   Alpha- and beta-adrenergic receptor agonist
   Beta-adrenergic receptor predominance at lower
   doses
   Potent RV inotrope
   Significant arrhythmogenic potential

4. Levosimendan
   Calcium sensitizer, stabilizes calcium-troponin C
   interaction, increases contractility
   Open ATP-dependent potassium channels in vascular smooth muscle, vasodilation
   Does not increase O_2 consumption or increase
   intracellular calcium levels

echocardiography and Doppler modalities provide useful information about overall LV contractility, regional wall motion abnormalities, valve function, and adequacy of preload. TG views are extremely helpful in assessing LV loading and contractility as well as calculating CO (SV × HR). Measurements of LV end-diastolic pressure, LVEDV, and LVESV allow calculation of LVEF and may indicate the use of vasoactive therapy. CWD and PWD modes can be used to detect different degrees of diastolic dysfunction that may occur either in isolation or in conjunction with systolic dysfunction (Tables 35.5–35.7). Vasomotor collapse frequently occurs during the post-CPB period,

TABLE **35.11**	**Arginine Vasopressin**

Endogenous peptide with osmoregulatory and
vasomotor properties end-organ effect mediated by

V_1 receptor present in vascular smooth muscle

    Promotes vasoconstriction by activation of G pro-
tein and phospholipase C with release of calcium
from sarcoplasmic reticulum

V_2 receptor present in the distal and collecting
tubules

    Promotes water resorption by increase in intra-
cellular levels of cAMP and activation of protein
kinase A

possibly resulting from a CPB-induced systemic inflammatory response, sepsis, anaphylaxis, arginine vasopressin deficiency, or preoperative administration of ACE inhibitors or amiodarone, or intraoperative administration of milrinone or dobutamine. Vasopressin is a useful vasoactive drug for the treatment of vasomotor collapse (Table 35.11). The TG SAX view reveals a hyperdynamic LV, decreased LVEDV and LVEDP, elevated CO, and decreased SVR. Hypovolemic shock is characterized by a hyperdynamic LV with adequate contractility, decreased CO, and normal-to-elevated SVR.

INTRAOPERATIVE ECHOCARDIOGRAPHY IN SURGICAL PROCEDURES FOR CHF

Mitral Valve Repair or Replacement

Mitral valve competence depends on the integrity of all components of the MV apparatus, including the MV annulus, leaflets, chordae tendinae, and papillary muscle, as well as the function of the underlying ventricular myocardium. End-stage CHF is often associated with moderate or severe MR (20–22). The presence of MR in patients with dilated CMP is associated with deterioration of clinical status, diminished response to medical therapy, and reduced survival rate (23,27,28). Thus, MR detection, qualitative and quantitative assessment, and surgical correction (when indicated) are desirable to improve survival and quality of life in patients with end-stage CHF. Annular dilation and change in LV morphology with papillary muscle dysfunction are the most common mechanisms of MR (23).

IOE is extremely helpful in the assessment of the cause and severity of MR. The 2D echocardiography provides information about MV morphology, such as leaflet motion, prolapse or restriction, and leaflet coaptation. Baseline measurements of MV annulus diameter, AMVL A3 scallop, and PMVL P1 scallop are taken in the ME 4-chamber view. As the multiplane angle is rotated forward to about 60 degrees into the ME mitral commissural view, the A2 scallop of the AMVL is seen in the middle, with the PMVL P1 scallop on the left and the P3 scallop on the right. The ME 2-chamber view at 90 degrees provides information about the A1 and P3 MV scallops, and the ME LAX view shows the A2 and P2 scallops. The ME views should be repeated with CFD, with the color flow sector extended over the LA and over the ventricular portion of MV. Transmitral flow velocity is examined with PWD, with the sample volume placed between the tips of the open MV leaflets, to evaluate the presence and extent of diastolic dysfunction (Fig. 35.20). The TG SAX view visualizes the posteromedial and anterolateral commissures and provides an overall view of the entire MV in the short axis, which allows the detection of leaflet abnormalities and sites where abnormal flows originate. A baseline area of MV can be measured by planimetry in this view. Abnormal motion or fibrosis of papillary muscles can be seen in the TG mid-SAX view. The TG two-chamber view is extremely useful for assessing the entire MV apparatus (26). Apical tethering, posterior restriction (secondary to posterolateral infarction), papillary muscle fibrosis, and chordal ribboning are the most common pathologic findings associated with MR in end-stage CHF patients. In addition, 2D echocardiography allows the measurement of the Lana diameter of greater than 5 mm that is considered dilated. The ratio of CFD maximum jet area to LA area has been used to quantify the severity of MR. MR greater than 40% or maximum jet area higher than 8 to 10 cm² is classified as severe, 20% to 40% MR is moderate, and MR <20% is considered mild (29,30).

CFD has certain limitations. In the presence of eccentric jets, maximum jet area is poorly correlated with regurgitant grade because jet impingement on the LA wall produces a smaller color flow area that does not correlate with regurgitant jet size (i.e., the Cowanda effect). In addition, CFD imaging is dependent on the pressure difference between LV and LA, LV systolic function, compliance of LA, gain setting, pulsed repetition frequency, and field depth. Therefore, even though CFD is extremely sensitive in detecting MR, quantitation of the severity of MR is difficult and limited by the significant overlap in jet sizes among patients with mild, moderate, and severe regurgitation (24).

Evaluating pulmonary vein flow with PWD helps to quantify the severity of MR. The systolic component is blunted (s < d) as LA pressure increases, and severe MR causes a systolic flow reversal (31). All four PVs should be carefully examined when there are eccentric jets that may produce flow reversal in only the pulmonary vein at which they are directed. With severe MR, antegrade mitral flow velocity is increased (E wave peak velocity >1.5 m/s) and regurgitant jet velocity decreases below 4 m/s because of an increase in LA pressure that reduces the transmitral systolic gradient.

Doppler echocardiographic quantitation of regurgitant SV (MV RV) and regurgitant fraction (MV RF)

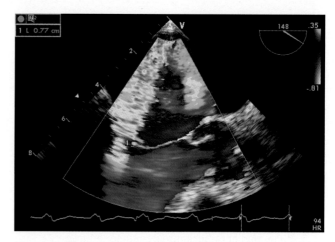

Figure 35.23. Calculation of PISA: ME LAX view.

can also be used to quantify the severity of MR by using continuity equations after measurement of MV annulus diameter (MV D), MV VTI, LVOT diameter (LVOT D), LVOT VTI, and calculation of mitral valve SV (MV SV) and LVOT SV

$$MV\ RV = MV\ SV - LVOT\ SV$$

$$MV\ SV = 0.785 \times MV\ D^2 \times MV\ VTI$$

$$LVOT\ SV = 0.785 \times LVOT\ D^2 \times LVOT\ VTI$$

$$MV\ RF = MV\ RV\ /\ MV\ SV \times 100\%$$

Effective regurgitant orifice (ERO) can be calculated as

$$MV\ ERO = MV\ RV\ /\ MV\ TVI$$

Proximal isovelocity surface area (PISA) is another quantitative method of measuring the severity of MR (Figs. 35.22–35.24). Its advantages are that it is independent of color gain settings and it is not influenced by the eccentricity of

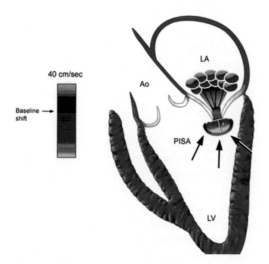

Figure 35.22. Proximal isovelocity surface area.

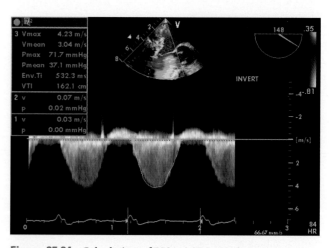

Figure 35.24. Calculation of PISA: ME LAX view.

the MR jet (32). It is used to calculate MV regurgitant flow rate, volume, and ERO, and is achieved by

1. Optimizing color-flow imaging of MR jet
2. Expanding the image of the regurgitant MV by using zoom
3. Shifting color flow baseline to 10 to 30 cm/s to set the negative aliasing velocity (Vr)
4. Measuring the radius (r) of the proximal isovelocity hemisphere
5. Measuring the angle of the isovelocity hemisphere to the leaflets and dividing it by 180 degrees
6. Obtaining peak velocity (V) (in cm/s) and TVI of the MR jet (in cm)
7. Calculating the MR flow rate: flow rate (mL/s) = $2\pi r^2 \times$ Vr = $6.28 \times r^2 \times$ Vr, in which $2\pi r^2$ is the proximal isovelocity hemispheric surface area at radial distance r from the surface
8. Calculating ERO = flow rate/V(MR)
9. Calculating MV regurgitant volume (mL): MV RV = ERO × MR VTI

A relationship between the severity of MR and PISA radius has been established. A PISA radius of less than 2 mm correlates to mild MR, 4 to 7 mm to mild-to-moderate MR, 7 to 10 mm to moderate-to-severe MR, and greater than 10 mm to severe MR (32).

Usually, severe MR is diagnosed if one or more of the following conditions are present: CFD area >8 cm² or >40% of LA area, RV >60 mL, RV >55%, ERO >0.35 cm², pulmonary vein systolic flow reversal, dense continuous-wave Doppler signal, decreased maximum velocity of the regurgitant jet (<3 m/s), increased E velocity (>1.5 m/s), LV diastolic size >7 cm, and LA size ≥5.5 cm.

Functional MR creates a vicious cycle of increasing volume load, increasing MR, and further LV dilatation. Elevated right-side pressure often occurs in association with severe MV as the result of high pressures in the LA and pulmonary vein. As a result, PHTN, RV dysfunction, TR, and hepatic congestion often accompany severe MR. When MR is associated with severely distorted LV or LVA, alternative surgical procedures for ventricular reconstruction should be considered. Early pre-CPB detection of such conditions can improve postoperative management and surgical outcome.

Intraoperative diagnosis of the cause and severity with MR is crucial for the surgical management of patients with end-stage heart failure. IOE findings, in conjunc-

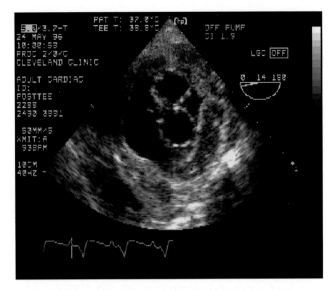
Figure 35.26. LV remodeling–Alfieri repair of mitral valve.

tion with direct examination of the valve, help the surgical team decide among annuloplasty, reconstruction, or replacement of the MV (Fig. 35.25) (33–36). With dilated CMP, the MR jet is typically central because of the symmetrical restriction of the tensor apparatus to the AMVL and PMVL, and the MV annulus is usually greater than 35 mm, a condition requiring an annuloplasty ring. One may also use an Aliferi repair technique, which involves suturing the A2 and P2 segments of the AMVL and PMVL, resulting in a double-barreled MV orifice with an increased MV leaflet coaptation area (Fig. 35.26). During the post-CPB period and early postoperative care, IOE examination should be focused on the assessment of the quality of valve repair or replacement, RV and LV performance, PHTN, and guiding medical management and the use of vasoactive medication when indicated.

In a cohort of patients with severe MR and LVEF < 25%, Bolling et al. performed successful MV reconstruction with undersized flexible annuloplasty rings (Fig. 35.27). In addition, they also performed concomitant coronary artery bypass grafting and TV repair on several patients (34,35). Actuarial survival rates were 82% at 12 months,

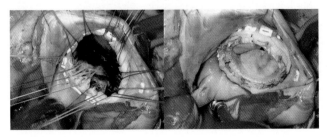
Figure 35.25. Chordal sparing mitral valve replacement.

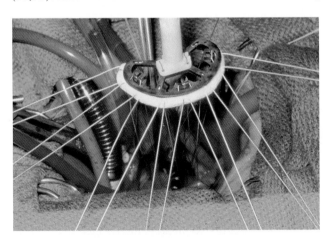
Figure 35.27. Undersized flexible annuloplasty ring.

71% at 24 months, and 56% at 5 years. Moreover, the authors reported postoperative improvements in NYHA status and LVEF (34,35).

Ventricular Reconstruction Surgery

Partial Left Ventriculectomy (Batista Procedure)

Partial left ventriculectomy is intended to reverse LV dilatation by removing a portion of viable myocardium from the LV lateral free wall. This reduces LV diameter and LV wall stress. Some authors have reported performing concomitant MV repair in 85% of patients who underwent the Batista procedure (36,37).

Endoventricular Circular Patch Plasty (Dor Left Ventricular Aneurysm Repair)

The Dor procedure, or infarction excision surgery, reduces LV size by surgical reconstruction of ischemic ventricles distorted by dyskinetic or akinetic infarcted myocardium. After coronary revascularization and MV repair (if indicated), EVCPP is used to reconstruct the LV. Endocardectomy and cryotherapy are used to prevent ventricular arrhythmia (38).

Patients with severe LV dysfunction, LVEF <30%, frequent ventricular arrhythmias, and distended LV benefit the most from EVCPP procedures (39). EVCPP (in conjunction with MV repair when indicated) has been shown to improve myocardial ischemia by myocardial revascularization, to diminish ventricular volume, to restore the LV to a more physiologic shape, and to further diminish LVEPD (36). Several studies have reported a significant increase in LVEF, a significant reduction in LV volume, an improvement of NYHA status, a reduction in the rate of ventricular arrhythmias, and an overall 18-month survival rate of 89% in patients who received EVCPP (39–43). Yamaguchi et al. (44), in a small retrospective study, reported a superior 5-year survival rate in patients who received surgical ventricular restoration (SVR) in addition to bypass surgery versus patients who received bypass surgery alone. However, recently, Jones et al. (45), in a large prospective randomized trial, found that even though adding SVR to bypass surgery was associated with a decrease in end-systolic LV volume, this was not associated with an improvement in primary outcomes, death, acute myocardial infarction, and stroke.

IOE examination of patients undergoing EVCPP should focus on evaluating LV volume and function, assessing the severity of MR, examining myocardial viability issues, and checking for comorbid TR, PHTN, RV dysfunction, and apical thrombus. Myocardial viability can be assessed with IOE stress testing with low-dose dobutamine. Because reducing LV volume is the central aim of this procedure, accurate calculation of LV volume is desirable. LVEF is calculated as (LVEDV – LVESV)/LVEDV. In the presence of LVA, LV is distorted from its symmetrical shape; this limits the usefulness of TEE because the 2D method assumes that the geometry of the LV is symmetrical. Recent studies found three-dimensional (3D) echocardiography to be more accurate in estimating LV volume (46). At the present time, 3D echocardiography has major limitations, mostly related to the system's size, complexity, and low image resolution. However, as the technology advances, 3D echocardiography might become the method of choice for determining absolute LV volume and EF.

VENTRICULAR CONSTRAINT TECHNIQUES

Recently, new approaches to treating dilated CMP have evolved. These are designed to unload the heart and promote reverse ventricular remodeling (Fig. 35.28). Some authors have hypothesized that merely limiting remodeling can improve long-term outcomes and quality of life in patients with end-stage CHF.

The Acorn CorCap (for external splinting) is a mesh-like implantable cardiac support device that is positioned around the heart (47). Its purpose is to stop the myocardial remodeling process by reducing LV wall stress and myocyte overstretching—the chief components of postinfarction progressive LV dilation and contractile dysfunction. The mesh-like material of the CorCap has a unique bidirectional compliance that allows the device to conform to the ellipsoidal surface of the heart. When the device is fit snugly, it produces an immediate reduction in the circumference of the heart (47). Candidates for Acorn CorCap implantation are adults with dilated CMP (either ischemic or idiopathic) and LVEF < 35%. MV surgery and myocardial revascularization have been performed concomitantly with the implantation of this device. A large, randomized, multicenter trial is presently underway in Europe and the United States. Patients in this trial have NYHA class III or IV (with or without MR and TR) and dilated cardiomyopathy (ischemic or nonischemic with LVEF < 35% or < 45% in the presence of mild MR); are stable; are on optimal medical management;

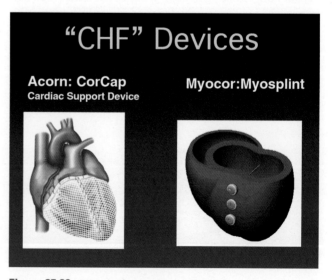

Figure 35.28. Ventricular constraint devices.

CorCap Global Implant Trials

Figure 35.29. CorCap global implant trials.

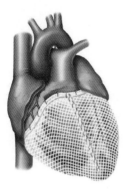
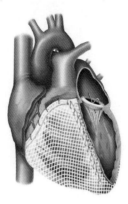
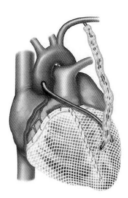

CorCap only
27 pts

Mitral valve repair/
replacement
59 pts

CABG
(Europe and Asia only)
25 pts

and have acceptable renal, hepatic, and pulmonary function. Two clinical studies evaluated the initial safety of the device and reported similar results (Fig. 35.29). The Acorn CorCap was shown to improve NYHA functional status, LVEDV, and LVEF at 12 months after surgery (48,49). The authors found no evidence of constrictive physiology. The actuarial survival rate after device implantation was 73% at 12 months and 68% at 24 months (49).

The Myosplint (for internal splinting) is another myocardial restraint device that uses transventricular splints and epicardial pads to constrain the ventricle at the upper, mid, and low ventricular levels (Figs. 35.30 and 35.31). This device can be implanted in isolation or in conjunction with MV repair. It is designed to reduce LV wall stress and improve cardiac function by changing LV geometry and reducing LV radius (50). Safety and feasibility studies of the device in patients are currently in progress in Europe and United States.

Both the Acorn CorCap and the Myosplint implantation procedures require IOE evaluation similar to that used to guide other surgical approaches for end-stage CHF. In addition, it is necessary to assess the impact of ventricular constraint procedures on systolic and diastolic function. This may be accomplished by determining global EF using volumetric calculations, global estimation of function, and PWD interrogation of the mitral inflow and pulmonary veins. The appropriate device size is determined by the basal, midpapillary, and apical diameters of LV as measured by IOE. ME SAX views are used to guide the positioning of the device and to confirm its proper placement after surgery (Fig. 35.32). The presence of device-induced constrictive physiology can be evaluated using pressure-volume loop analysis, right and left end-diastolic pressures, RA pressure, and RV pressure ratios. The 3D IOE has also been used to demonstrate the impact of ventricular constraint procedures

Myosplint® Concept

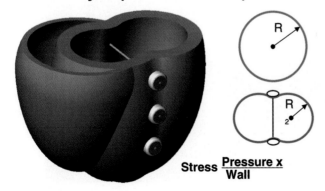

Stress $\dfrac{\text{Pressure x}}{\text{Wall}}$

Figure 35.30. Myosplint concept.

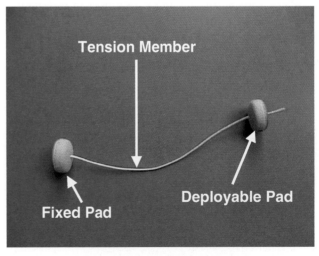

Tension Member

Fixed Pad

Deployable Pad

Figure 35.31. Myosplint epicardial pad and tension member.

Short Axis TM Positioning

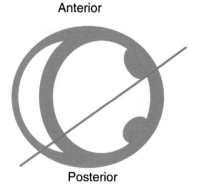

Figure 35.32. SAX tension member positioning.

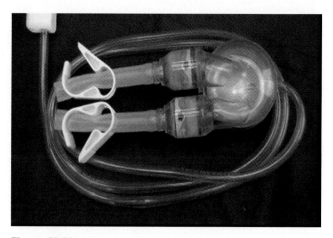

Figure 35.33. The ABIOMED BVS 5000.

on wall stress and overall LV performance. Given the increasing number of patients who are candidates for ventricular constraint procedures, the outcomes of these surgical interventions will become an expanding area of research and clinical responsibility for the cardiovascular anesthesiologist.

MECHANICAL CIRCULATORY SUPPORT

Mechanical circulatory support (MCS) includes a wide variety of devices designed to connect to the heart or to be placed within the heart to assume some of the workload and to allow the ventricle to rest, undergo reverse remodeling, and recover some of its contractile function. It has been demonstrated previously that the myocardium is able to repair itself during a period of unloading, after which some patients experience an improvement in quality of life (51,52). Therefore, VADs have many clinical applications, ranging from temporary support of the ventricle to long-term support, including bridging to heart transplantation. The mismatch between the growing number of cardiac transplant candidates and the limited number of donors has led to a significant increase in the use of mechanical assist devices as bridges to cardiac transplantation (53) or as destination therapy (54).

The indications for mechanical assistance include

1. Reversible ventricular dysfunction after cardiac surgery
2. Bridging to heart transplantation
3. Destination therapy for patients who are not transplant candidates

Compared to medical therapy, left ventricular assist devices (LVADs) for destination therapy result in a significantly better survival rate and quality of life at 1 year and 2 years of support (54). Improvements in patient selection, postoperative medical management, and enhanced durability of the LVAD devices have led to an overall

improvement in mortality, quality of life, and at reduced costs (55,56).

Currently, various cardiac assist devices are available for short- and long-term support. VADs may be classified as either continuous flow or pulsatile (Table 35.12) depending on the type of blood flow they produce. Alternatively, when the site of the pump is taken into account, VADs may be categorized as extracorporeal or intracorporeal. Most extracorporeal devices, whether pulsatile or nonpulsatile, are used for short- or medium-term support. Continuous flow devices are designed with either centrifugal, axial, or mixed flow patterns.

Pulsatile assist devices provide an intermittent flow and can generate a CO of 6 to 10 L/min, depending on the filling pressure. Currently, FDA-approved pulsatile VADs in the United States include the AbioMed BVS and AB 5000 (Fig. 35.33) (57,58), the Thoratec iVAD/pVAD Systems (59) (Fig. 35.34), and the Heartmate XVE

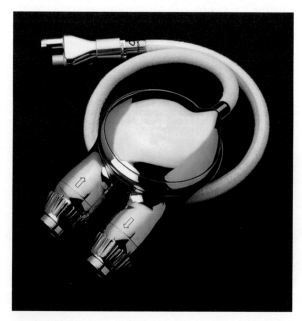

Figure 35.34. Thoratec iVAD.

| TABLE 35.12 | Types of VADs | | | | |

Type	Device	Length of Support	Position	Ventricular Support	Drive Mechanism
Pulsatile	Abiomed BVS/AB 5000	Short-term support	Extracorporeal	LV, RV, BV	Atrial and ventricular chambers (BVS) pneumatically driven
	Thoratec iVAD/ pVAD	Short- to medium-term support	Extracorporeal	LV, RV, BV	Pneumatically driven sac
	HeartMate XVE	Long-term as a bridge to transplantation, recovery, or destination therapy (HeartMate VE)	Intracorporeal, abdominal (pre- or intraperitoneal)	LV	Flexible textured polyurethane diaphragm electrically driven
	AbioCor TAH	Long-term support	Intracorporeal	BV	Electric
Continuous flow	CentriMag (centrifugal flow)	Short-term	Extracorporeal	LV, RV, BV	Electric
	Tandem Heart (centrifugal-flow)	Short-term	Extracorporeal	LV	Electric
	Impella (axial-flow pump)	Short term	Extracorporeal	LV	Electric
	Jarvik Flowmaker (axial-flow)	Long-term support	Intracorporeal	LV	Electric
	DeBakey LVAD (axial-flow)	Long-term support	Intracorporeal	LV	Electric
	HeartMate II (axial flow pump)	Short-term	Intracorporeal	LV	Electric
	HeartWare HVAD (centrifugal flow)	Long-term	Intracorporeal (Pericardial)	LV	Electric (MagLev)
	Duraheart (centrifugal flow)	Long-term	Intracorporeal	LV	Electric
	Synergy (mixed flow)	Long-term	Intracorporeal (Subcutaneous)	LV	Electric

IP, implantable pneumatic; VE, vented electric; LV, left ventricle; VAD, ventricular assist device; TAH, total artificial heart.

(vented electric) (Figs. 35.35) (60). The Heartmate XVE is the only mechanical device approved by the FDA for both bridge to transplantation and long-term destination therapy.

Continuous flow pumps have the advantage of being small, silent, valveless, and fully implantable. Additionally, these devices have a single moving component, the impeller, which results in a high degree of reliability when compared to the pulsatile pumps. Continuous flow pumps have flow patterns that are either axial, centrifugal, or a mixed flow. During support, blood flow is continuous throughout the cardiac cycle from either the right or left heart to the PA or aorta, depending on whether there is RV support (right ventricular assist device [RVAD]), left ventricular sup-

port (LVAD), or biventricular assist device (BiVAD) support. The HeartMate II (Thoratec Corp., Pleasanton, CA) (Fig. 35.36) (61), Jarvik 2000 (Jarvik Heart Inc., New York, NY) (Fig. 35.37) (62), and Debakey-Micromed VAD (Micromed Cardiovascular Inc., Houston, TX) (Fig. 35.38) (63) are implantable axial flow LVADs that are intended for long-term support. The HeartMate II has been commercially approved for bridge to heart transplant (64), and approval for destination therapy is pending as of September 2009. The Jarvik 2000 and Debakey-Micromed VAD are in clinical trials in the United States for bridge to heart transplant. All three axial flow devices have CE Mark approval in Europe and are available throughout Asia.

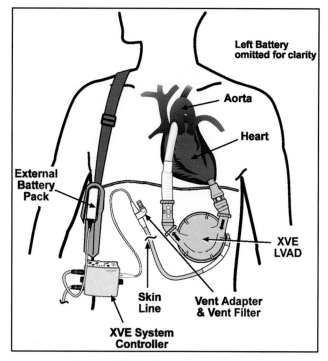

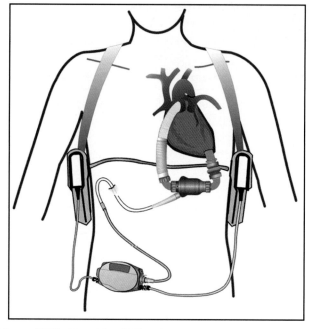

Figure 35.36. HeartMate II Electric.

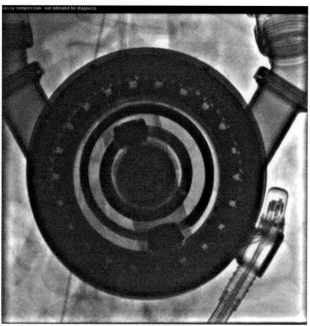

Figure 35.35. HeartMate XVE LVAS Electric.

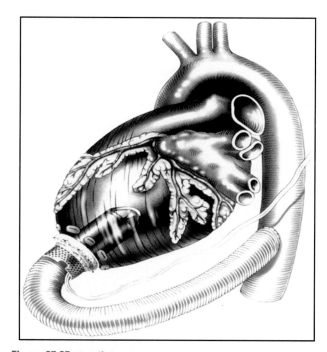

Figure 35.37. Jarvik 2000.

Recently, a new generation of blood pump has entered clinical trials and offers the hope for long-term support with a very high degree of reliability by using magnetically levitated impellers, which are frictionless and warless. This new generation of blood pump may improve long-term outcomes for patients being supported for destination therapy. The HVAD (HeartWare International, Miami Lake, FL) (Fig. 35.39) (65), Duraheart (Terumo, Ann Arbor, MI) (Fig. 35.40) (66), and Levacor (Worldheart Inc, Oakland, CA) (Fig. 35.41) (67) are third generation, fully magnetically levitated LVADs that have recently

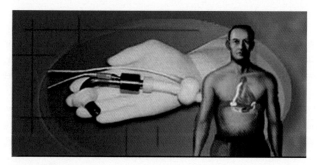

Figure 35.38. DeBakey-Micromed.

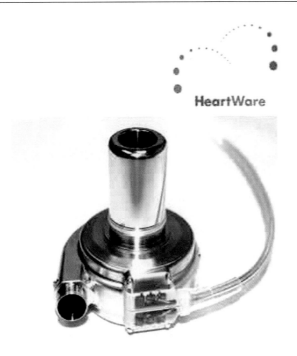

HeartWare Ventricular Assist Device

Figure 35.39. HeartWare (HVAD).

begun clinical trials. In addition to the frictionless movement of the impeller without component wear in these devices, that absence of heat generation may prove to offer reduced thrombogenicity. These devices are also considerably smaller than the first generation of pulsatile LVAD.

The Synergy VAD (Circulite, Saddle Brook, NJ) utilizes a small blood pump that is about the size of an AA battery and is placed subcutaneously in the anterior chest wall (Fig 35.42) (68). Inflow to the Synergy pump is from a cannula that is placed transseptally into the LA. Outflow from the pump is from a graft anastomosed to the subclavian artery. The Synergy system can provide up to 3 L/min and can be used in adults and children for chronic partial circulatory support.

The use of temporary devices, to stabilize patients as a bridge to decision, allows for better patient selection for the implantable devices. Improved patient selection will

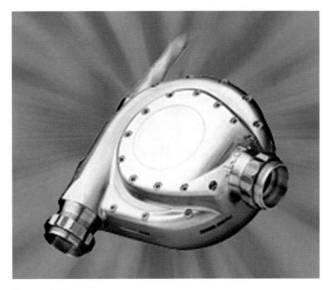

Figure 35.41. Levacor.

continue to enhance survival rates and help to minimize cost. The TandemHeart pVAD (Cardiac Assist, Pittsburgh, PA) (Fig. 35.43) (69) and the Impella 2.5/5.0 devices (Fig. 35.44) (70) can be inserted percutaneously for LVAD support and allow for rapid support and stabilization of patients with cardiogenic shock. The CentiMag (Levitronix LLC, Waltham, MA) is another temporary support device that is commonly used for postcardiotomy shock (Fig. 35.45A, B) (71). Centers using these short-term devices as bridges to decision, transplant, or implantable LVAD have shown good survival rates for patients who have a very high expected mortality (72–75).

The use of mechanical assist devices as bridges to cardiac transplantation or destination therapy has been found to improve the survival rates and outcomes of patients with decompensated heart failure and cardiogenic shock. The newer VAD technology is more reliable, biocompatible, smaller, and easier to implant. Thus, mechanical assistance has become an important tool in the surgical management of patients with failing hearts.

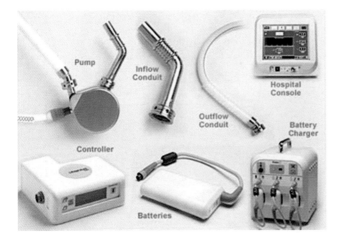

Figure 35.40. Duraheart.

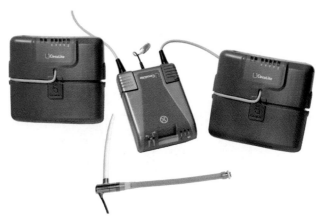

Figure 35.42. CircuLite.

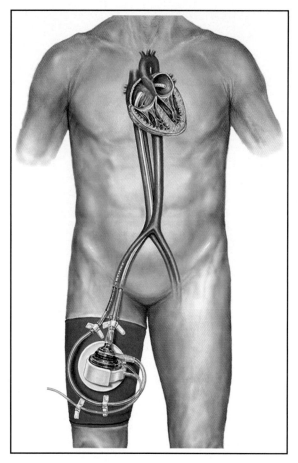

Figure 35.43. TandemHeart.

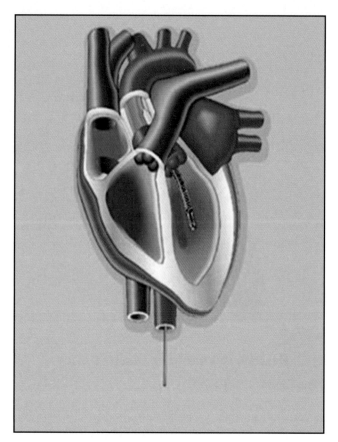

Figure 35.44. Impella.

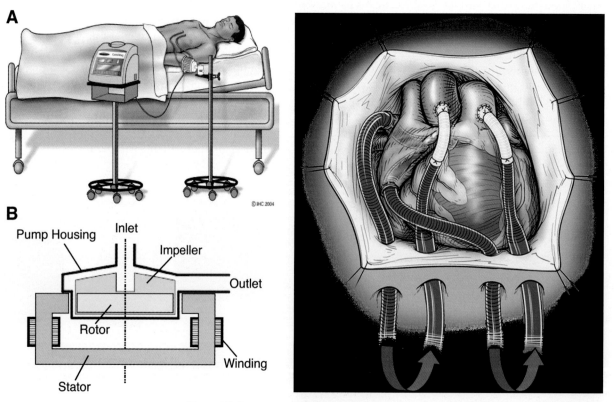

Figure 35.45. **A–C:** Lexitronix Centimag.

The HeartMate XVE was approved for bridge to transplantation in 1998 and then was approved for destination therapy at the completion of the REMATCH trial in 2002. Support with the XVE was shown to be superior to medical therapy for both applications (54); however, the long-term durability of this device and persistent complications related to implantation limited the effectiveness of this therapy. In the REMATCH trial, the 1-year survival rate for patients supported by the XVE was 52%, compared to the only 25% for the medical therapy group. In a post-REMATCH study after device improvements had been made, the survival rate had increased to 56% in one study (55) and 61% in another (76). In addition to the improved durability of the XVE, refinements in selection of the patients and care protocols have contributed to the better outcomes.

Other important advances in survival for LVAD-supported patients have been reported with the use of the HeartMate II continuous flow device. In the bridge to transplant trial with the HeartMate II that led to commercial approval, the 1-year survival rate was 68%, which showed a further progression in survival (64). In a follow-up study including 281 patients supported by the HeartMate II, the survival rate at 18 months after implant had increased to 72% (77). The continued improvement in survival rate is attributed not only to the experience gained in patient care but also to better VAD technology which is now associated with fewer adverse events. The new smaller VAD devices allow for less invasive implantation leading to less postoperative bleeding, and there is less infection because of the fewer bleeding events and the smaller surface area of the device. Echocardiography, intraoperatively and serially throughout VAD support, is essential for successful outcomes for VAD recipients (78). Ideally, echocardiographic assessments should be performed before, during, and after VAD implantation (Table 35.2).

Assessment Before Cardiopulmonary Bypass Is Initiated for VAD Implantation

During the pre-CPB period, a careful examination for intracardiac shunts is mandatory. Right-to-left shunting of unoxygenated blood through a PFO, atrial septal defect (ASD), or ventricular septal defect (VSD) may lead to systemic desaturation and paradoxical embolization when the LVAD is activated (79,80). With a RVAD, left-to-right shunting will produce excessive pulmonary blood flow, decreased systemic blood flow leading to hypotension, pulmonary edema, and cardiogenic shock. The bicaval view allows detection of ASD when color-flow mapping and rapidly agitated saline contrast injection are used (Figs. 35.46 and 35.47).

RV function is the most important factor in the postoperative management and outcome of patients with VADs. RV dysfunction can occur in 20% of patients with isolated LVAD support (81). LVAD inflow is dependent on LA fill-

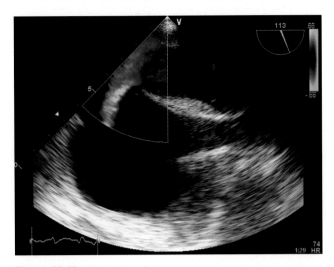

Figure 35.46. PFO: bicaval view.

ing pressures and subsequently, on RV performance. With passive, reversible PHTN and normal transpulmonary pressure gradients, LVAD support will reduce PA pressure and RV afterload, leading to an improvement in RV performance. In the presence of fixed, irreversible PHTN, LVAD support will cause an acute increase in the preload and no change in the afterload of an already impaired RV. Therefore, RV function, severity of TR, and the potential need for biventricular VAD (BiVAD) support should be carefully assessed during the pre-CPB period. The ME 4-chamber view, the RV inflow-outflow view, and TG SAX/LAX RV inflow views can be used to assess RV function (Figs. 35.9, 35.10, and 35.16–35.18). RVFAC, TAPSE, tricuspid annulus plane velocity, and strain analysis can be measured as described previously (Figs. 35.13–35.15).

Valvular abnormalities need to be diagnosed and corrected before VAD support is initiated. With regard to the AV, AR has been found in 22% of patients undergoing LVAD placement. Activation of the pump can increase the pressure gradient across the incompetent AV and cause regurgitant flow from the aorta to the LV, leading to continuous shunting of blood through the device. This con-

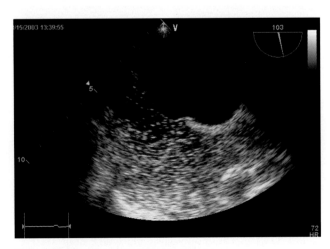

Figure 35.47. Contrast study: bicaval view.

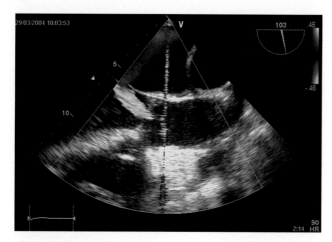

Figure 35.48. Aortic insufficiency: ME LAX view.

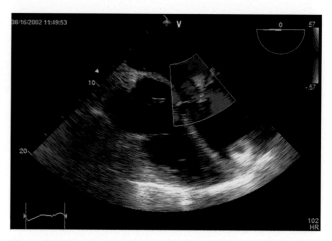

Figure 35.50. LVAD, MR: ME 4-chamber view.

dition prevents LV decompression and decreases the total device output, systemic perfusion, and CO (Figs. 35.48 and 35.49) (11). Moderate to severe AR mandates valve replacement with a bioprosthetic valve or closure of the aortic outlet.

MS should be identified during the pre-CPB period because it can severely impair LVAD inflow and cause hemodynamic instability when LVAD support begins. Additionally, MR is frequently encountered in the LVAD patient population. MR usually improves with LVAD decompression and has only a minor impact on LVAD output (Fig. 35.50).

TR is often encountered in conjunction with RV dysfunction. Twenty-five percent of patients undergoing LVAD implantation have preexisting TR, and another 19% develop it when the pump is activated. TR can affect thermodilution CO measurements (11). In patients with passive PHTN, the severity of TR decreases with LVAD support. Color-flow mode and Doppler measurements are used to assess the severity of TR (Fig. 35.17). RA dilation, dilation of superior and inferior vena cava, and hepatic vein systolic flow reversal are also associated with severe TR (Fig. 35.51).

LV or LAA thrombi are potential sequelae of end-stage dilated CMP. Their presence should be ruled out before CBP begins to reduce the risk of serious thromboembolic events during or after surgery (Fig. 35.8).

The aortic cannulation site should be evaluated for the presence of atheroma using the ME ascending aortic LAX view or epiaortic scanning. Cannulating a severely diseased aorta, particularly in the presence of mobile plaques, increases the risk of thromboembolic events and poor outcome. The descending aorta should also be scanned for atherosclerotic plaques with mobile components because intra-aortic balloon pumps (IABP) are frequently used during the postoperative period, which could dislodge plaques and cause organ embolization.

Weaning from CPB and Assessment after CPB

Adequate deairing of the VAD and the cardiac chambers is the most critical step in weaning patients from CPB. The ME LAX view is used to assess the efflux of microair emboli from the LVAD into the ascending aorta. When a significant amount of air is noted in the ascending aorta, the graft can be reclamped and the aorta vented.

LVAD inlet and outlet cannulas must be assessed for their position and patency. The inflow cannula is evaluated in the ME 4-chamber view, the ME 2-chamber view, and the ME LAX views (Figs. 35.52 and 35.53). CFD mode and Doppler examination are used to assess flow through the LVAD and measure the LV-LVAD inflow gradient (Figs. 35.54–35.56). Alignment of the inflow cannula with mitral valve needs to be established. Misaligned LVAD inflow cannula could lead to inflow obstruction (Fig. 35.57). If the inlet is partially obstructed, high-velocity aliased flow at the cannula orifice will be noted in association with LV distension and an elevated LV-LVAD gradient (Fig. 35.58). The outlet cannula can be visualized in the ME LAX views (Fig. 35.59). Inlet and outlet flow velocities of 3 m/s or less are considered indicative of laminar flow pattern and are adequate. Velocities CFD mode and Doppler analysis can also be used to assess

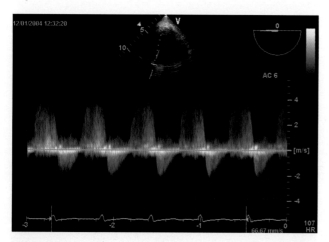

Figure 35.49. Aortic insufficiency and CWD: deep TG LAX view.

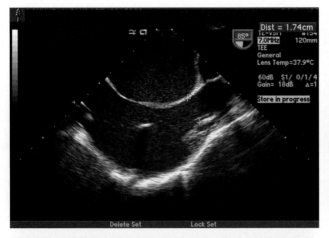

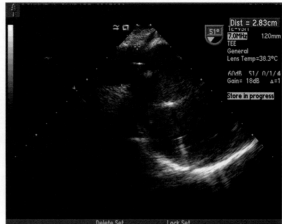

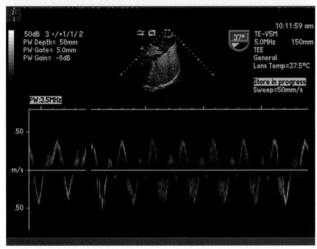

Figure 35.51. Dilation of superior and inferior vena cava, hepatic vein flow reversal.

LVAD output. Different flow patterns are seen with pulsatile and continuous flow devices (Fig. 35.60A,B). With chest closure, LVAD inlet and outlet obstruction can occur; reassessment of flow pattern is advisable at that point.

Adequacy of LV decompression should be also assessed in the ME 4-chamber, ME 2-chamber, TG SAX/LAX,

and deep TG views (Fig. 35.61A,B). The supported ventricle should be relatively empty, with no deviation of the interventricular septum toward the decompressed chamber (Fig. 35.61B). Mitral valve and LVAD inlet flow patterns can be used to adjust the pump flow rates to achieve the desired loading conditions.

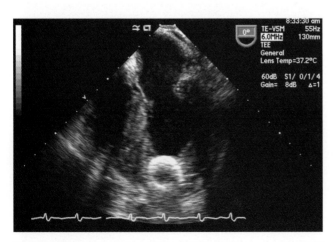

Figure 35.52. HeartMate XVE LVAD inflow cannula: ME 4-chamber view.

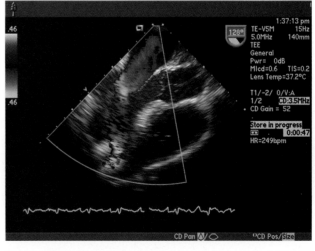

Figure 35.53. HeartMate XVE LVAD inflow cannula: ME LAX view.

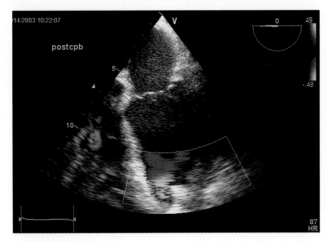

Figure 35.54. HeartMate XVE LVAD inflow cannula: ME 4-chamber view.

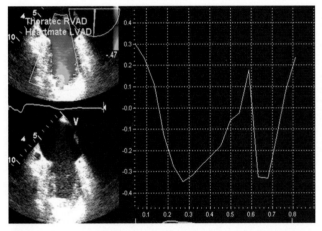

Figure 35.55. HeartMate XVE LVAD inflow cannula biphasic flow: ME 2-chamber view.

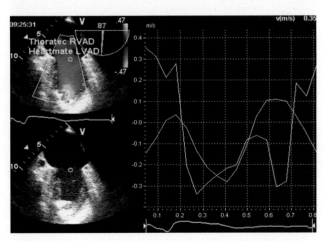

Figure 35.56. LVAD mitral valve and inflow cannula flow: ME 2-chamber view.

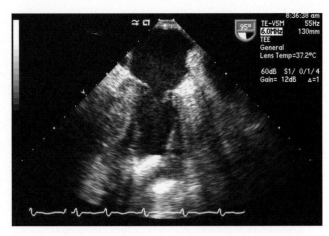

Figure 35.57. HeartMate II LVAD inflow cannula-malposition: ME 2-chamber view.

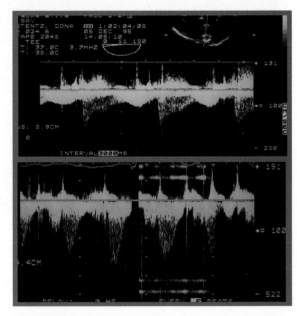

Figure 35.58. HeartMate XVE LVAD inflow cannula—obstructed flow.

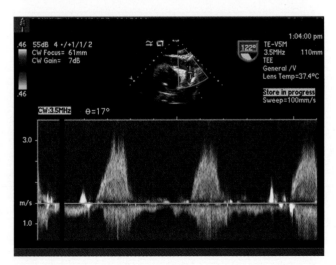

Figure 35.59. HeartMate XVE LVAD inflow cannula: ME LAX view.

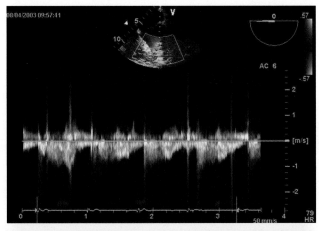

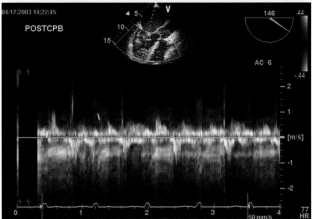

Figure 35.60. LVAD flow patterns pulsatile (**A**), continuous (**B**).

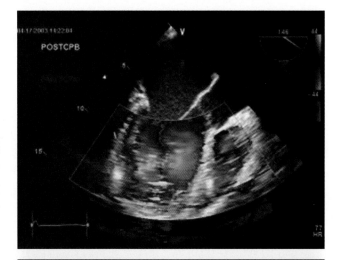

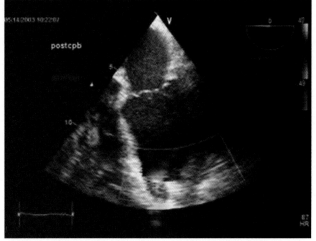

Figure 35.61. A: LV overloaded. **B:** LV decompressed Heart-Mate XVE LVAD.

For the continuous flow VADs, once CPB is discontinued, the proper speed setting of the VAD is assessed by determining changes in ventricular size and the frequency of AV opening. After the patient's intravascular volume is stabilized, the VAD speed should be adjusted so that the ventricular chamber size is in normal range, there is little or no septal shift, and the AV is opening intermittently. There is an inverse correlation of pulse pressure with pump speed (Fig. 35.62A,B) (82). The pulse pressure becomes smaller as pump speed is increased, as the result of decreased output across the AV. Pump speed should be adjusted to a pulse pressure of approximately 15 to 20 mm Hg in order to provide adequate AV opening with each systole and to prevent blood stagnation and thrombosis of the aortic root (Fig. 35.63) (83,84).

Ruling out the presence of PFO during the post-CPB period is also important. Activating the pump when the RV is distended can increase the pressure gradient across the interatrial septum, which may cause iatrogenic PFO. Reinstitution of CBP for PFO closure is recommended because PFO can cause significant shunting and systemic desaturation that can complicate the clinical picture and postoperative management (Fig. 35.64A,B).

For short-term devices, such as Levitonix Centrimag, in addition to LV approach, inlet cannula can also be placed either through the left upper and lower pulmonary veins

(Fig. 35.65). Proper placement and assessment of patency of inflow cannulas are important, as with short-term devices the cannula can be displaced (Fig. 35.66). When LV support is temporarily achieved with Tandem Heart, frequent assessment of the inflow cannula is recommended since it could migrate and it could be associated with significant hemodynamic instability (Fig. 35.67A,B).

Successful weaning from bypass depends on adequate RV function. Once the deairing process is complete, the pump is started at a low rate of output and RV function is assessed. In patients with fixed PHTN, the RV distends, causing acute severe TR, decreased LV preload, and the collapse of the LV (Fig. 35.68). Additionally, air can be trapped in the cardiac chambers as the result of increased negative pressure generated by the empty device, leading to air embolism of the coronary and systemic circulation. Additionally, the inflow cannula can become obstructed when LVAD preload decreases. Under these circumstances, pharmacological and mechanical RV support is indicated (Tables 35.9 and 35.10).

The AbioMed BVS 5000 and the Thoratec VAD System have been approved by the FDA for short- and

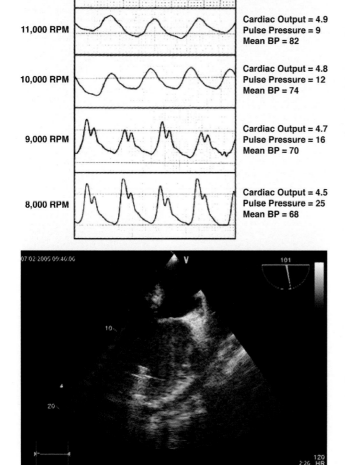

12,000 RPM	Cardiac Output = 5.1	Pulse Pressure = 6
	Mean BP = 87	
11,000 RPM	Cardiac Output = 4.9	Pulse Pressure = 9
	Mean BP = 82	
10,000 RPM	Cardiac Output = 4.8	Pulse Pressure = 12
	Mean BP = 74	
9,000 RPM	Cardiac Output = 4.7	Pulse Pressure = 16
	Mean BP = 70	
8,000 RPM	Cardiac Output = 4.5	Pulse Pressure = 25
	Mean BP = 68	

Figure 35.62. **A:** LV supported by Jarvik. **B:** Pulse pressures and pump speeds: Jarvik.

medium-term RV support, respectively (Table 35.12; Fig. 35.35). Levitronix CentiMag, is approved for 6 hours of support as an LVAD and may be used for up to 30 days as an RVAD (Fig. 35.69). These devices can be used for either

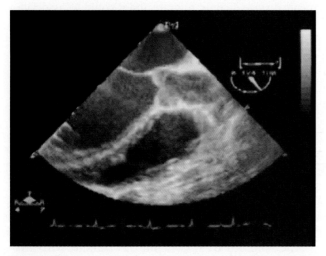

Figure 35.63. Thrombosis of the aortic root: Jarvik.

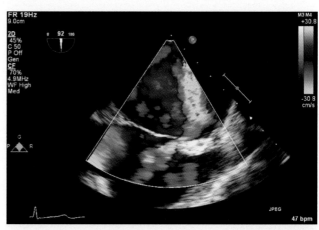

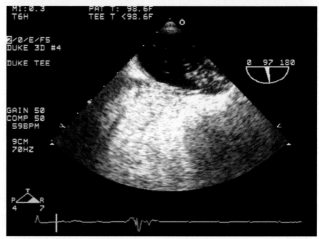

Figure 35.64. **A,B:** PFO-CFD and contrast.

isolated RV support or biventricular support, according to the patient's needs. Traditionally, RVAD inflow cannula is placed in RV (Fig. 35.70). More recently, inflow cannula has been placed in RA, in order to preserve RV function and help with RV recovery. Redundant Eustachian valve could inadvertently obstruct RV inflow cannula, a condition readily diagnosed with IOE (Fig. 35.71). Additionally, these devices can be used in conjunction with

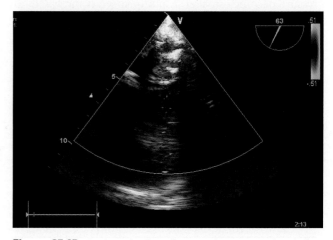

Figure 35.65. Levitronix Centrimag pulmonary veins inflow cannulas.

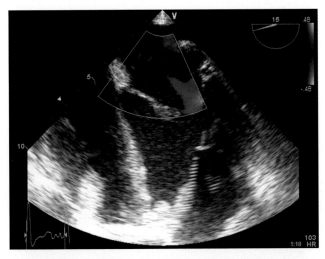

Figure 35.66. Levitronix Centrimag LVAD inflow cannula impinging on anterolateral papillary muscle of mitral valve.

any LVAD designed for long-term support (Table 35.12). ME 4-chamber and ME bicaval views are used to assess the position and patency of RVAD inflow cannulas and to examine blood flow in the superior vena cava. Inadequate RA decompression with leftward deviation of interatrial septum may occur if the RVAD inflow cannula is posi-

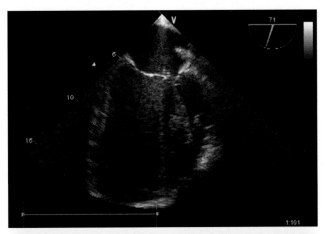

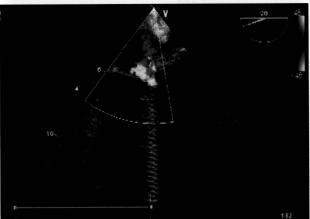

Figure 35.67. A,B: Malposition of Tandem Heart inflow cannula.

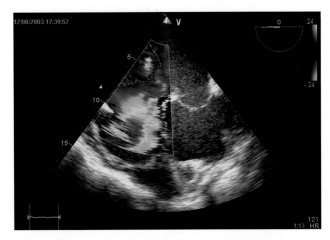

Figure 35.68. LVAD, severe TR: ME 4-chamber view.

tioned incorrectly (Fig. 35.72A,B). Proper repositioning of the cannula restores adequate right-side decompression. In patients undergoing BiVAD support, IOE is valuable for confirming the adequate loading of both right and left chambers. The goal of volume management and adjustment of the pump flow rates is to keep the interatrial and interventricular septa close to the midline (Fig 35.72B).

Biventricular mechanical support is important for the management of acute or chronic severe biventricular heart failure (Table 35.13). IOE issues are similar to those previously described for LVAD and RVAD implantation. Echocardiography can ensure that the loading conditions of both right and left chambers are adequate. Optimal preload and pump flow rates are achieved when both interatrial and interventricular septa are in the midline position. Doppler analysis of blood flow in the pulmonary veins as well as hepatic vein, inferior vena cava, and SVC provides additional information for assessing the volume status of the patient. As clinicians have gained experience over the years with the management of patients with BiVADs, the medical management of these patients has improved. This has led to better outcomes for patients

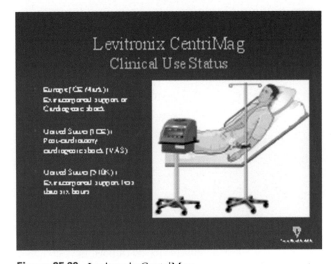

Figure 35.69. Levitronix CentriMag.

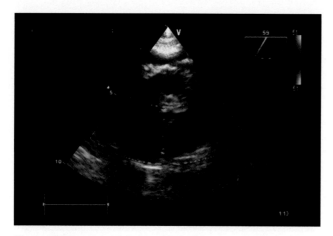

Figure 35.70. Levitronix CentriMag RV inflow cannula.

with biventricular failure who require biventricular support as a bridge to heart transplantation. In a recent study, Magliato et al. (85) reported a 59% rate of survival to transplantation of patients on biventricular support and a 90% posttransplant survival rate. Nonetheless, with the advent of new technologies, TAH may become a better alternative for the treatment of biventricular failure.

The Total Artificial Heart

Unfortunately, VAD support is not feasible for patients with certain conditions such as irreversible ventricular failure requiring high pump outputs, LV thrombus, arrhythmias, severe AR, aortic prosthesis, acquired VSD, and severe PHTN. Currently, there are two TAH systems available for clinical use, CardioWest and AbioCor. The SynCardia CardioWest TAH is a biventricular orthotopic pulsatile dual pump that is pneumatically driven from an external power source (86). Each pump has a smooth blood-contacting diaphragm, two intermediate diaphragms separated by thin coatings of graphite. The inflow (27 mm) and outflow (25 mm) Medtronic-Hall

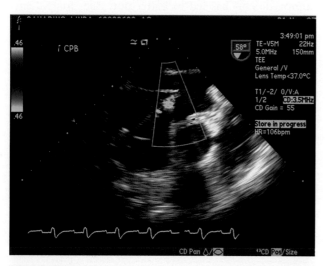

Figure 35.71. Obstruction of RVAD inflow by Eustachian valve.

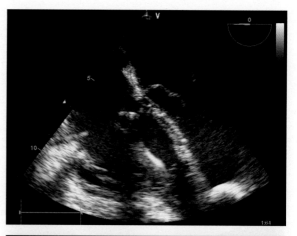

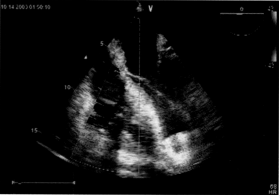

Figure 35.72. A: Malposition of RVAD inflow cannula with overdistension of RV. **B:** Reposition of RVAD inflow cannula with adequate RV decompression.

TABLE 35.13	Biventricular Support

Precardiotomy shock
    Acute myocardial infarction
    Viral myocarditis
    Rheumatic pancarditis
    Intractable arrhythmia
    Spontaneous coronary dissection
    Failed coronary angioplasty

Postcardiotomy shock
    Coronary artery bypass grafting
    Postinfarction ventral septal defect
    Postinfarction MR
    Aortic or mitral valve procedures
    LV remodeling procedures
    RV failure
    Acutely failed transplant

Chronic conditions
    Cardiomyopathies
    Chronic rejection
    Infiltrative disorders
    Nontransplant candidates

From Samuels L. Biventricualar mechanical replacement. Surg Clin N Am 2004;84;309–321, with permission.

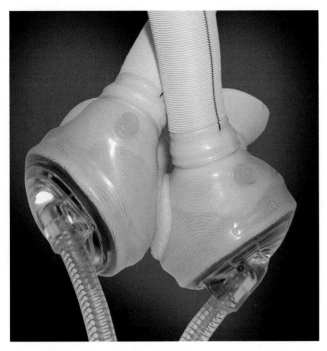

Figure 35.73. CardioWest TAH.

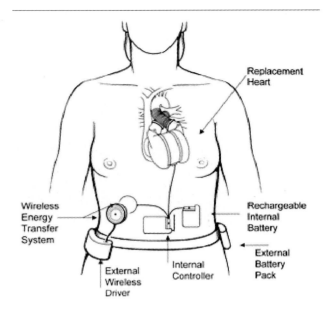

Figure 35.74. The AbioCor TAH system.

valves provide the proper direction of blood flow. The ventricles can fill and eject up to 70 mL/beat and provide 9 L/min CO (Fig. 35.73). Currently, the CardioWest is the only TAH in use for bridging to heart transplantation and is commercially approved for this indication (87). When used as a bridge to transplant, the reported survival rate is as high as 90% a year after support and transplant (88).

The AbioCor replacement heart is the first completely implantable TAH (89–93). The first phase of a multi-center trial of this device has been completed and is now commercially available as a humanitarian use device. Recipients are patients with severe, irreversible, inotrope-dependent biventricular failure. These patients have no potential for myocardial recovery and are not candidates for other therapies, including transplantation or VAD support. TAH candidates are already receiving pharmacologic or MCS and may have overt changes in the hepatic, renal, and coagulation systems. As a group, their predicted 30-day mortality is higher than 70%. Although the AbioCor TAH is used in patients who are not eligible for heart transplantation, supported patients may eventually become heart transplant candidates if their conditions improve sufficiently.

The AbioCor is made primarily of titanium and a proprietary polyurethane. The device is designed to fit inside the body and operate without penetrating the skin so that the recipient can remain mobile (Figs. 35.74 and 35.75). The internal components of the AbioCor system consist of a thoracic unit, an internal transcutaneous energy transfer (TET) coil, a controller, and a battery (91). The thoracic unit (blood pump) weighs approximately 2 lb and comprises two artificial ventricles, four valves, and a motor-driven hydraulic pumping system. The hydraulic pumping system uses pressure to move blood between the

chambers, from the artificial RV to the lungs, and from the artificial LV to the systemic circulation. The pump's motor rotates at 6,000 to 8,000 rpm, producing sufficient hydraulic fluid pressure to compress the diaphragm around the blood chamber and eject the blood. A miniaturized electronics package, which is implanted in the patient's abdomen, monitors and controls the pump rate, the right-left hydraulic fluid balance, and the speed of the hydraulic motor. A unique feature of the AbioCor is the right-left flow balancing mechanism that compensates for the natural right-left flow imbalance and eliminates the need for an external vent or internal compliance chamber.

The AbioCor TAH uses the TET system to provide external power and radiofrequency communication to control the implanted device. An internal rechargeable battery, also positioned within the abdomen, functions as a backup power source. The internal battery is continually recharged with power received through the TET, and

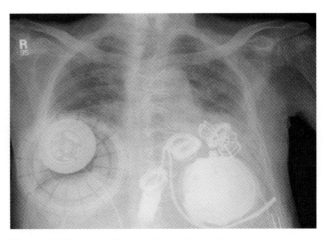

Figure 35.75. Chest X-ray of the AbioCor in situ.

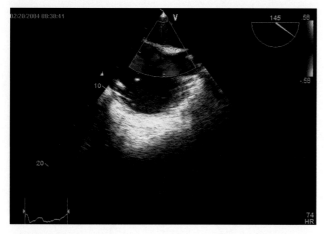

Figure 35.76. CFD of interatrial septum: bicaval view pre-CPB.

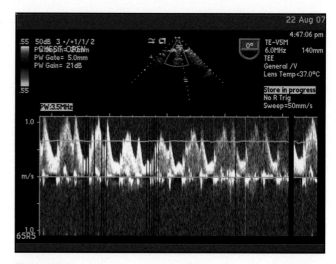

Figure 35.78. LLPV obstruction PWD.

it can provide up to 30 minutes of tether-free operation while disconnected from the main power source. Therefore, unlike many LVAD systems, this system does not require any percutaneous connections, either electrical or mechanical. The external components include a computer console, the external TET coil, and battery packs. The computer receives information about pump performance through the radiofrequency communication system.

IOE has an important role in the perioperative management of TAH recipients. Failure to recognize and correct a PFO can result in postimplantation systemic desaturation because the negative pressures generated in the device may shunt venous blood into the systemic circulation. Both CFD and contrast techniques are helpful in ruling out the presence of PFO (Figs. 35.76 and 35.77). Evaluation of baseline pulmonary flow velocities from all four PVs is important for the detection of pulmonary flow obstruction during the post-CPB period, at the time of chest closure, and during early postoperative care (Fig. 35.78); this obstruction may require repositioning of the device. PWD of hepatic vein blood flow is helpful to establish adequate preload conditions and to rule out any possible flow obstruction that might occur with

chest closure (Fig. 35.79). IOE is also helpful in assessing the adequacy of deairing of the native atria when CPB is discontinued. If further deairing becomes necessary, the aorta is reclamped and CPB is reestablished with the TAH turned off. During the post-CPB period, IOE provides useful information about blood flow across the right and left polyurethane valves into the device and through the outflow conduit and inferior vena cava (Figs. 35.80 and 35.81). Because TAH recipients do not need inotropic support, vasoactive therapy can be directed at the peripheral (both systemic and pulmonary) circulation. However, adequate volume must be maintained because the negative pressures generated in the TAH make it possible for air to enter through the new suture line if preload is very low.

Frequent assessment of pulmonary artery pressures (PAP) and PVR during postoperative period is important and challenging for transplant candidates on TAH support, because invasive monitoring and PA catheters cannot be used. Thus, noninvasive Doppler measurement of PAP and PVR makes TEE and IOE a crucial tool for the man-

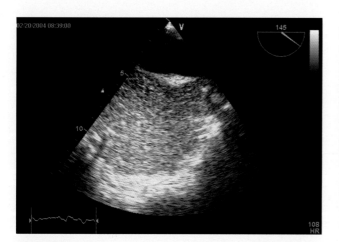

Figure 35.77. Contrast study: bicaval view pre-CPB.

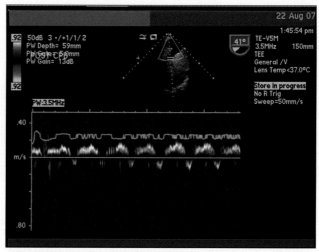

Figure 35.79. Hepatic vein flow PWD.

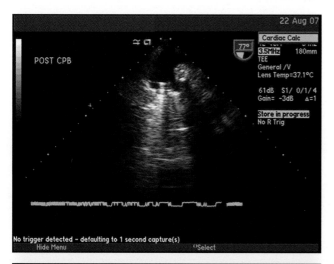

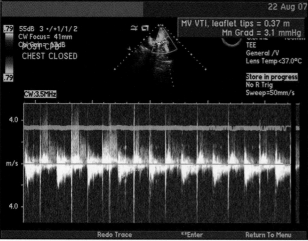

Figure 35.80. Left inflow valve: 2D (**A**), CWD (**B**).

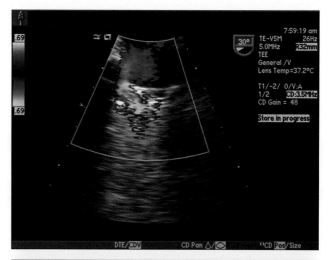

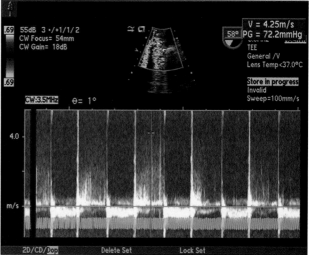

Figure 35.81. Right inflow valve: CFD (**A**), CWD (**B**).

agement of the TAH patients and establishment of their eligibility for transplantation. Some authors reported that the ratio between the PA acceleration time (AT) and right ventricular ejection time (RVET) of less than 0.3 ± 0.06 (Fig. 35.82) was found to indicate PHTN (94). Others found that PVR can be calculated as (Fig 35.83A, B)

$$PVR = 10 \times TRV\,(m/s)\,/\,VTI_{RVOT}\,(cm) + 0.16$$

A ratio of TRV (m/s)/VTI_{RVOT} (cm) greater than 0.175 is highly suggestive of PHTN (95) (Fig 35.83A, B). TRV (m/s)/VTI_{RVOT} (m) ratio of 38 indicates PVR of 8 Wood unit with 100% specificity (96). Mean PA can also be calculated as Mean PA= 90 − (0.62 × AT) (Fig. 35.84) (97).

For patients supported by TAH, PVR can also be calculated as

$$PVR = (Mean\ PA - PCWP)/CO$$

$$Mean\ PA = 90 - (0.62 \times AT)$$

$$CO = Pump\ output$$

$$PCWP = LAP$$

$$LAP = LEP - PG_{LRJ}$$

where LEP is left ejection pressure generated by the device and PG_{LRJ} is regurgitant pressure gradient of left inflow valve (Fig. 35.85).

Future Directions

The number of people with advanced heart failure continues to grow worldwide and there are no definitive therapies currently available. Heart transplantation is limited by the number of heart donors and medical therapy remains suboptimal. Therefore, the demand is for MCS to be widely available to a broad population of heart failure patients. VAD technology has advanced in recent years and its use is increasing. Clinical experience over the past two decades has led to important advances in patient selection and postoperative care, which has resulted in improved survival rates for patients with severe heart failure (55,64,77). Continued improvement in the design

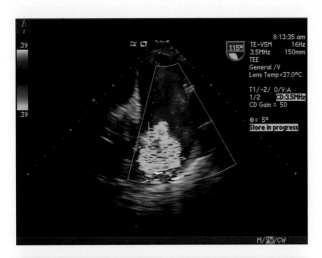

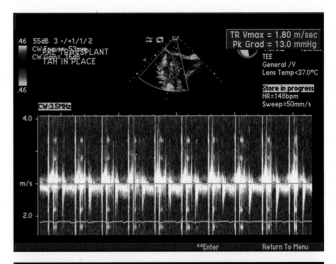

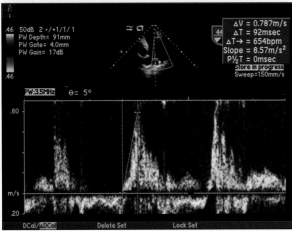

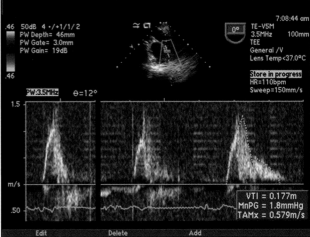

Figure 35.82. Pulmonary flow: CFD (**A**), PWD (**B**).

Figure 35.83. A, B: Calculation of pulmonary vascular resistance: $PVR = 10 \times TRV\ (m)/VTI_{RVOT}(cm) + 0.16$; PVR= 1,17WU (94).

of VAD technology along with refinements in care should help to more effectively treat heart failure.

The temporary use of a percutaneous VAD can help stabilize patients with cardiogenic shock until there is recovery of myocardial function, or in the absence of recovery, a long-term VAD can be implanted electively and more safely.

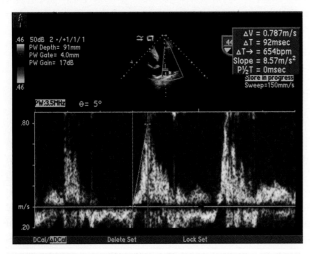

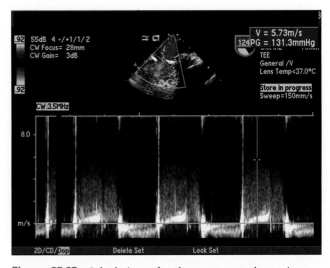

Figure 35.84. Calculation of mean PA pressure; mean PA = $90 - (0.62 \times AT)$, mean PA = 33 mm Hg (96).

Figure 35.85. Calculation of pulmonary vascular resistance; PVR= (Mean PA – pulmonary capillary wedge pressure [PCWP])/CO; Mean PA = $90 - (0.62 \times AT)$; CO = Pump output; PCWP = LAP; LAP = LEP – PG_{LRJ}. LEP, left ejection pressure; PG_{LRJ}, regurgitant pressure gradient of left inflow valve.

This bridging to decision with a temporary VAD has the potential to save the lives of many patients who have a very high expected mortality. Also, the use of long-term LVADs in combination with drug or gene therapy that improves myocardial function adequately to allow pump removal has great potential to further enhance survival (98).

Most heart failure patients are not given the option to be treated with VAD support due to the significant cost associated with the placement of the device or due to the lack of availability of advanced heart failure care services (99). Increasing the use of VAD technology to treat more patients will require a greater acceptance by the public, the medical community, government agencies, and insurance providers. Greater acceptance is dependent on improving outcomes and reducing the frequency of adverse events. The smaller and more reliable VAD technology, along with improvements in patient selection and care, has improved outcomes, but implanting VADs in less sick patients is an important next step. Once primary care physicians and cardiologists refer heart failure patients earlier for VAD support, the survival rate of VAD-supported patients could equal heart transplantation.

CONCLUSION

CHF has proven to be one of the greatest challenges in medicine, and it will continue to be in the next century. At present, the treatment of heart failure is a specialty in itself. The best treatment currently available is a combination of medical and surgical therapy. Patients with end-stage CHF have complex, highly individual diseases, and establishing specific and uniform criteria for treatment selection is impractical. As a result, IOE has become an invaluable tool for the diagnosis of heart failure, the selection of appropriate surgical procedures, and the overall perioperative management of heart failure patients. Surgical therapies for end-stage CHF are constantly evolving and will continue to improve as existing treatments are refined and new ones are developed.

KEY POINTS

■ In the United States, more than 4.5 million people have CHF, and its prevalence is estimated at 6.8% in people over the age of 65. It is likely that the number of patients with end-stage CHF will grow as the average age of our population increases.

■ CHF is a complex syndrome in which myocardial injury and the resulting hemodynamic changes alter many neuroendocrine, humoral, and inflammatory feedback loops.

■ Strategies for treating end-stage CHF include medical therapies such as ACEI, beta-blockers, diuretics, inotropic agents, and antiarrhythmics. Multifaceted pharmacologic regimens may not prevent progression toward end-stage CHF, and surgical intervention is required.

■ Cardiac transplantation is the "gold-standard" surgical treatment for end-stage CHF, while the 1-year survival rate after transplantation is 85%. Unfortunately, only 2,400 heart transplants are performed annually. Class IV patients awaiting transplant have a 1-year mortality rate of 40% to 50% with an ever expanding mismatch between the number of cardiac transplant candidates and the limited number of donors.

■ This mismatch has led to increasing use of alternative surgical therapies, including mechanical VAD, ventricular remodeling procedures in conjunction with revascularization and mitral valvuloplasty (i.e., EVCPP, partial ventriculectomy), newer procedures intended to reduce ventricular dilatation (i.e., external or internal splinting), and TAH implantation.

■ Critical issues addressed by IOE in patients undergoing procedures for CHF include determining the etiology and mechanism of CHF, assessment of ventricular function and coexisting or secondary pathology, surgical procedure–related issue, and the diagnosis of post-CPB bypass complications.

ACKNOWLEDGMENT

The authors would like to thank Mr. Tim Myers and Dr. O.H. Frazier for their help with the preparation of this chapter.

REFERENCES

1. Roger VL, Weston SA, Redfield MM. Trends in heart failure incidence and survival in a community-based population. *JAMA* 2004;292:344–350.

2. American Heart Association. Heart Disease & Stroke Statistics AHA – 2009 Update At A-Glance. 2009; http://www.american-heart.org/downloadable/heart/1240250946756LS-1982%20 Heart%20and%20Stroke%20Update.042009.pdf.

3. Francis GS, Goldsmith SR, Levine TB, et al. The neurohumoral axis in congestive heart failure. *Ann Intern Med* 1984;101:370–377.

4. Levine B, Kalman J, Mayer L, et al. Elevated circulating levels of tumor necrosis factor in severe chronic heart failure. *N Engl J Med* 1990;323:236–241.

5. Taylor DO, Edwards LB, Boucek MM, et al. The registry of the international society for heart and lung transplantation: twenty-first official adult heart transplant report—2004. *J Heart Lung Transplant* 2004;23:796–803.

6. The SOLVD Investigators. Effect of enalapril on survival in patients with reduced left ventricular ejection fractions and congestive heart failure. *N Engl J Med* 1991;325:293–302.

7. Miller LW, Lietz K. Candidate selection for long-term left ventricular assist device therapy for refractory heart failure. *J Heart Lung Transplant* 2006;25:756–764.

8. Otto CM. The cardiomyopathies, hypertensive heart disease, post-cardiac-transplant patient and pulmonary heart disease. In: Otto CM. *Textbook of Clinical Echocardiography*. Philadelphia: W.B. Saunders, 2000:183–212.

9. Jessup M, Brozena S. Heart failure. *N Engl J Med* 2003;348:2007–2018.

10. Farrar DJ, Chow E, Brown CD. Isolated systolic and diastolic ventricular interactions in pacing-induced dilated cardiomyopathy and effects of volume loading and pericardium. *Circulation* 1995;92:1284–1290.

11. Scalia GM, McCarthy PM, Savage RM, et al. Clinical utility of echocardiography in the management of implantable ventricular assist devices. *J Am Soc Echocardiogr* 2000;13:754–763.

12. Hammarstrom E, Wrannc B, Pinto FJ, et al. Tricuspid annular motion. *J Am Soc Echocardiogr*1991;4:131–139.

13. Kaul S, Tei C, Hopkins J. Assessment of right ventricular function using two-dimensional echocardiography. *Am Heart J* 1984;107:526–531.

14. Rajagopalan N, Saxena N, Simon M, et al. Correlation of tricuspid annular velocities with invasive hemodynamics in pulmonary hypertension. *Congest Heart Fail* 2007;13:200–204.

15. Borges A, Knebel F, Eddicks S, et al. Right ventricular function assessed by two-dimensional strain and tissue Doppler echocardiography in patients with pulmonary arterial hypertension and effects of vasodilator therapy. *Am J Cardiol* 2006;98:530–534.

16. Zile MR, Brutsaert DL. New concepts in diastolic dysfunction and diastolic heart failure: Part I: diagnosis, prognosis, and measurements of diastolic function. *Circulation* 2002;105:1387–1393.

17. Gaasch WH, Zile MR. Left ventricular diastolic dysfunction and diastolic heart failure. *Ann Rev Med* 2004;55:373–394.

18. Werner GS, Schaefer C, Dirks R, et al. Prognostic value of Doppler echocardiographic assessment of left ventricular filling in idiopathic dilated cardiomyopathy. *Am J Cardiol* 1994;73:792–798.

19. Rakowski H, Appleton C, Chan KL, et al. Canadian consensus recommendations for the measurement and reporting of diastolic dysfunction by echocardiography: from the Investigators of Consensus on Diastolic Dysfunction by Echocardiography. *J Am Soc Echocardiogr* 1996;9:736–760.

20. Johnson RA, Palacios I. Dilated cardiomyopathies of the adult (first of two parts). *N Engl J Med* 1982;307:1051–1058.

21. Lewis JF, Webber JD, Sutton LL, et al. Discordance in degree of right and left ventricular dilation in patients with dilated cardiomyopathy: recognition and clinical implications. *J Am Coll Cardiol* 1993;21:649–654.

22. Shah PM. Echocardiography in congestive or dilated cardiomyopathy. *J Am Soc Echocardiogr* 1988;1:20–30.

23. Kono T, Sabbah HN, Stein PD, et al. Left ventricular shape as a determinant of functional mitral regurgitation in patients with severe heart failure secondary to either coronary artery disease or idiopathic dilated cardiomyopathy. *Am J Cardiol* 1991;68:355–359.

24. Castello R, Lenzen P, Aguirre F, et al. Variability in the quantitation of mitral regurgitation by Doppler color flow mapping: comparison of transthoracic and transesophageal studies. *J Am Coll Cardiol* 1992;20:433–438.

25. Enriquez-Sarano M, Bailey KR, Seward JB, et al. Quantitative Doppler assessment of valvular regurgitation. *Circulation* 1993;87:841–848.

26. Shanewise JS, Cheung AT, Aronson S, et al. ASE/SCA guidelines for performing a comprehensive intraoperative multiplane transesophageal echocardiography examination: recommendations of the American Society of Echocardiography Council for Intraoperative Echocardiography and the Society of Cardiovascular Anesthesiologists Task Force for Certification in Perioperative Transesophageal Echocardiography. *J Am Soc Echocardiogr* 1999;12:884–900.

27. Junker A, Thayssen P, Nielsen B, et al. The hemodynamic and prognostic significance of echo-Doppler-proven mitral regurgitation in patients with dilated cardiomyopathy. *Cardiology* 1993;83:14–20.

28. Blondheim DS, Jacobs LE, Kotler MN, et al. Dilated cardiomyopathy with mitral regurgitation: decreased survival despite a low frequency of left ventricular thrombus. *Am Heart J* 1991;122:763–771.

29. Helmcke F, Nanda NC, Hsiung MC, et al. Color Doppler assessment of mitral regurgitation with orthogonal planes. *Circulation* 1987;75:175–183.

30. Spain MG, Smith MD, Grayburn PA, et al. Quantitative assessment of mitral regurgitation by Doppler color flow imaging: angiographic and hemodynamic correlations. *J Am Coll Cardiol* 1989;13:585–590.

31. Klein AL, Obarski TP, Stewart WJ, et al. Transesophageal Doppler echocardiography of pulmonary venous flow: a new marker of mitral regurgitation severity. *J Am Coll Cardiol* 1991;18: 518–526.

32. Enriquez-Sarano M, Tajik AJ, Bailey KR, et al. Color flow imaging compared with quantitative Doppler assessment of severity of mitral regurgitation: influence of eccentricity of jet and mechanism of regurgitation. *J Am Coll Cardiol* 1993;21:1211–1219.

33. Carpentier AF, Lessana A, Relland JY, et al. The "physio-ring": an advanced concept in mitral valve annuloplasty. *Ann Thorac Surg* 1995;60:1177–1185.

34. Bolling SF, Pagani FD, Deeb GM, et al. Intermediate-term outcome of mitral reconstruction in cardiomyopathy. *J Thorac Cardiovasc Surg* 1998;115:381–386.

35. Bolling SF, Smolens IA, Pagani FD. Surgical alternatives for heart failure. *J.Heart Lung Transplant* 2001;20:729–733.

36. Batista RJ, Verde J, Nery P, et al. Partial left ventriculectomy to treat end-stage heart disease. *Ann Thorac Surg* 1997;64:634–638.

37. Kass DA. Surgical approaches to arresting or reversing chronic remodeling of the failing heart. *J Card Fail* 1998;4:57–66.

38. Dor V, Sabatier M, Di Donato M, et al. Efficacy of endoventricular patch plasty in large postinfarction akinetic scar and severe left ventricular dysfunction: comparison with a series of large dyskinetic scars. *J Thorac Cardiovasc Surg* 1998;116:50–59.

39. Dor V, Sabatier M, Di Donato M, et al. Late hemodynamic results after left ventricular patch repair associated with coronary grafting in patients with postinfarction akinetic or dyskinetic aneurysm of the left ventricle. *J Thorac Cardiovasc Surg* 1995;110:1291–1299.

40. Menicanti L, Di Donato M. The Dor procedure: what has changed after fifteen years of clinical practice? *J Thorac Cardiovasc Surg* 2002;124:886–890.

41. Di Donato M, Sabatier M, Dor V, et al. Akinetic versus dyskinetic postinfarction scar: relation to surgical outcome in patients

undergoing endoventricular circular patch plasty repair. *J Am Coll Cardiol* 1997;29:1569–1575.

42. Athanasuleas CL, Stanley AW Jr, Buckberg GD, et al. Surgical anterior ventricular endocardial restoration (SAVER) in the dilated remodeled ventricle after anterior myocardial infarction. RESTORE group. Reconstructive Endoventricular Surgery, returning Torsion Original Radius Elliptical Shape to the LV. *J Am Coll Cardiol* 2001;37:1199–1209.

43. Shiota T, McCarthy PM. Volume reduction surgery for end-stage ischemic heart disease. *Echocardiography* 2002;19: 605–612.

44. Yamaguchi A, Adachi H, Kawahito K, et al. Left ventricular reconstruction benefits patient with dilated ischemic cardiomyopathy. *Ann Thorac Surg* 2005;79:456–461.

45. Jones RH, Velazquez EJ, Michler RE, et al. Coronary bypass surgery with or without surgical ventricular reconstruction. *N Engl J Med* 2009;360:1705–1717.

46. Qin JX, Jones M, Shiota T, et al. Validation of real-time three-dimensional echocardiography for quantifying left ventricular volumes in the presence of a left ventricular aneurysm: in vitro and in vivo studies. *J Am Coll Cardiol* 2000;36: 900–907.

47. Oz MC. Passive ventricular constraint for the treatment of congestive heart failure. *Ann Thorac Surg* 2001;71:S185–S187.

48. Konertz, WF, Kleber, FX, Dushe S, et al. Efficacy trends with the Acorn cardiac support device in patients with advanced heart failure. *J Heart Fail* 2001;7:39.

49. Oz MC, Konertz WF, Kleber FX, et al. Global surgical experience with the Acorn cardiac support device. *J Thorac Cardiovasc Surg* 2003;126:983–991.

50. Fukamachi K, Inoue M, Doi K, et al. Device-based left ventricular geometry change for heart failure treatment: developmental work and current status. *J Card Surg* 2003;18(Suppl. 2): S43–S47.

51. Frazier OH, Benedict CR, Radovancevic B, et al. Improved left ventricular function after chronic left ventricular unloading. *Ann Thorac Surg* 1996;62:675–681.

52. Bick RJ, Poindexter BJ, Buja LM, et al. Improved sarcoplasmic reticulum function after mechanical left ventricular unloading. *Cardiovasc Pathobiol* 1998;2:159–166.

53. Hunt SA, Frazier OH. Mechanical circulatory support and cardiac transplantation. *Circulation* 1998;97:2079–2090.

54. Rose EA, Gelijns AC, Moskowitz AJ, et al. Long-term mechanical left ventricular assistance for end-stage heart failure. *N Engl J Med* 2001;345:1435–1443.

55. Lietz K, Long JW, Kfoury AG, et al. Outcomes of left ventricular assist device implantation as destination therapy in the post-REMATCH era: implications for patient selection. *Circulation* 2007;116(5):497–505.

56. Miller LW, Nelson KE, Bostic RR, et al. Hospital costs for left ventricular assist devices for destination therapy: lower costs for implantation in the post-REMATCH era. *J Heart Lung Transplant* 2006;25(7):778–784.

57. Zhang L, Kapetanakis EI, Cooke RH, et al. Bi-ventricular circulatory support with the Abiomed AB5000 system in a patient with idiopathic refractory ventricular fibrillation. *Ann Thorac Surg* 2007;83(1):298–300.

58. Taoka M. Acute experimental study of Abiomed BVS5000 as a V-A bypass to cardiogenic shock models. *Ann Thorac Cardiovasc Surg* 2007;13(5):308–315.

59. Reichenbach SH, Farrar DJ, Hill JD. A versatile intracorporeal ventricular assist device based on the thoratec VAD system. *Ann*
Thorac Surg 2001;71(3 Suppl.):S171–S175; discussion S183–S174.

60. Pagani FD, Long JW, Dembitsky WP, et al. Improved mechanical reliability of the HeartMate XVE left ventricular assist system. *Ann Thorac Surg* 2006;82(4):1413–1418.

61. Frazier OH, Gemmato C, Myers TJ, et al. Initial clinical experience with the HeartMate II axial-flow left ventricular assist device. *Tex Heart Inst J* 2007;34(3):275–281.

62. Frazier OH, Myers TJ, Gregoric ID, et al. Initial clinical experience with the Jarvik 2000 implantable axial-flow left ventricular assist system. *Circulation* 2002;105(24):2855–2860.

63. Noon GP, Morley D, Irwin S, et al. Development and clinical application of the MicroMed DeBakey VAD. *Curr Opin Cardiol* 2000;15(3):166–171.

64. Miller LW, Pagani FD, Russell SD, et al. Use of a continuous-flow device in patients awaiting heart transplantation. *N Engl J Med* 2007;357(9):885–896.

65. Tuzun E, Roberts K, Cohn WE, et al. In vivo evaluation of the HeartWare centrifugal ventricular assist device. *Tex Heart Inst J* 2007;34(4):406–411.

66. Morshuis M, El-Banayosy A, Arusoglu L, et al. European experience of DuraHeart magnetically levitated centrifugal left ventricular assist system. *Eur J Cardiothorac Surg* 2009;35: 1020–1027.

67. Pitsis AA, Visouli AN, Vassilikos V, et al. First human implantation of a new rotary blood pump: design of the clinical feasibility study. *Hellenic J Cardiol* 2006;47(6):368–376.

68. Meyns B, Ector J, Rega F, et al. First human use of partial left ventricular heart support with the Circulite synergy micropump as a bridge to cardiac transplantation. *Eur Heart J* 2008;29(20):2582.

69. Kar B, Adkins LE, Civitello AB, et al. Clinical experience with the TandemHeart percutaneous ventricular assist device. *Tex Heart Inst J* 2006;33(2):111–115.

70. Lee MS, Makkar RR. Percutaneous left ventricular support devices. *Cardiol Clin* 2006;24(2):265–275, vii.

71. Mueller JP, Kuenzli A, Reuthebuch O, et al. The CentriMag: a new optimized centrifugal blood pump with levitating impeller. *Heart Surg Forum* 2004;7(5):E477–E480.

72. Cheng JM, den Uil CA, Hoeks SE, et al. Percutaneous left ventricular assist devices vs. intra-aortic balloon pump counterpulsation for treatment of cardiogenic shock: a meta-analysis of controlled trials. *Eur Heart J* 2009;30(17):2102–2108.

73. Bhama JK, Kormos RL, Toyoda Y, et al. Clinical experience using the Levitronix CentriMag system for temporary right ventricular mechanical circulatory support. *J Heart Lung Transplant* 2009;28(9):971–976.

74. Vecchio S, Chechi T, Giuliani G, et al. Use of Impella Recover 2.5 left ventricular assist device in patients with cardiogenic shock or undergoing high-risk percutaneous coronary intervention procedures: experience of a high-volume center. *Minerva Cardioangiol* 2008;56(4):391–399.

75. Seyfarth M, Sibbing D, Bauer I, et al. A randomized clinical trial to evaluate the safety and efficacy of a percutaneous left ventricular assist device versus intra-aortic balloon pumping for treatment of cardiogenic shock caused by myocardial infarction. *J Am Coll Cardiol* 2008 (19):1584–1588.

76. Long JW, Kfoury AG, Slaughter MS, et al. Long-term destination therapy with the HeartMate XVE left ventricular assist device: improved outcomes since the REMATCH study. *Congest Heart Fail.* 2005;11(3):133–138.

77. Pagani FD, Miller LW, Russell SD, et al. Extended mechanical circulatory support with a continuous-flow rotary left ventricular assist device. *J Am Coll Cardiol* 2009;54(4):312–321.

78. Catena E, Milazzo F. Echocardiography and cardiac assist devices. *Minerva Cardioangiol* 2007;55(2):247–265.

79. Baldwin RT, Duncan JM, Frazier OH, et al. Patent foramen ovale: a cause of hypoxemia in patients on left ventricular support. *Ann Thorac Surg* 1991;52:865–867.

80. Shapiro GC, Leibowitz DW, Oz MC, et al. Diagnosis of patent foramen ovale with transesophageal echocardiography in a patient supported with a left ventricular assist device. *J Heart Lung Transplant* 1995;14:594–597.

81. Santamore WP, Gray LA Jr. Left ventricular contributions to right ventricular systolic function during LVAD support. *Ann Thorac Surg* 1996;61:350–356.

82. Nussmeier NA, Probert CB, Hirsch D, et al. Anesthetic management for implantation of the Jarvik 2000 left ventricular assist system. *Anesth Analg* 2003;97:964–971.

83. Siegenthaler MP, Martin J, van de Loo A, et al. Implantation of the permanent Jarvik 2000 left ventricular assist device: a single-center experience. *J Am Coll Cardiol* 2002;39:1764–1772.

84. Myers TJ, Bolmers M, Gregoric ID, et al. Assessment of arterial blood pressure during support with an axial flow left ventricular assist device. *J Heart Lung Transplant* 2009;28:423–427.

85. Magliato KE, Kleisli T, Soukiasian HJ, et al. Biventricular support in patients with profound cardiogenic shock: a single center experience. *ASAIO J* 2003;49:475–479.

86. El-Banayosy A, Arusoglu L, Morshuis M, et al. CardioWest total artificial heart: Bad Oeynhausen experience. *Ann Thorac Surg* 2005;80(2):548–552.

87. Copeland JG, Smith RG, Arabia FA, et al. The CardioWest total artificial heart as a bridge to transplantation. *Semin Thorac Cardiovasc Surg* 2000;12(3):238–242.

88. Roussel JC, Senage T, Baron O, et al. CardioWest (Jarvik) total artificial heart: a single-center experience with 42 patients. *Ann Thorac Surg* 2009;87(1):124–129; discussion 130–179.

89. Dowling RD, Gray L, Etoch SW, et al. Initial experience with the AbioCor implantable replacement heart system. *J Thorac Cardiovasc Surg* 2004;127:131–141.

90. Myers TJ, Robertson K, Pool T, et al. Continuous flow pumps and total artificial hearts: management issues. *Ann Thorac Surg* 2003;75:S79–S85.

91. Dowling RD, Gray LA, Etoch SW, et al. The AbioCor implantable replacement heart. *Ann Thorac Surg* 2003;75:S93–S99.

92. Frazier OH. Prologue: ventricular assist devices and total artificial hearts: a historical perspective. *Cardiol Clin* 2003;21:1–13.

93. Thielmeier KA, Pank JR, Dowling RD, et al. Anesthetic and perioperative considerations in patients undergoing placement of totally implantable replacement hearts. *Sem Cardiothorac Vasc Anesth* 2001;5:335–344.

94. Kitabake A, Inoue M, Asao M, et al. Noninvasive evaluation of pulmonary hypertension by a pulsed Doppler technique. *Circulation* 1983;68:302–309.

95. Abbas AE, Fortuin D, Schiller NB, et al. A simple method for noninvasive estimation of pulmonary vascular resistance. *J Am Coll Cardiol* 2003;41:1021–1027.

96. Vlahos AP, Feinstein JA, Schiller NB, et al. Extension of Doppler-derived echocardiographic measures of pulmonary vascular resistance to patients with or severe pulmonary vascular disease. *J Am Soc Echocardiogr* 2008;21:711–714.

97. Dabestani A, Mahan G, Gardin JM, et al. Evaluation of pulmonary artery pressure and resistance by pulsed Doppler echocardiography. *Am J Cardiol* 1987;59:662–668.

98. Birks EJ, Tansley PD, Hardy J, et al. Left ventricular assist device and drug therapy for the reversal of heart failure. *NEJM* 2006;355(18):1873–1884.

99. Joyce DL, Conte JV, Russell SD, et al. Disparities in access to left ventricular assist devic therapy 2008. *J Surg Res* 2009;152:111–117.

QUESTIONS

1. What percent of patients over the age of 65 have congestive heart failure (CHF)?
   A. 7%
   B. 14%
   C. 21%
   D. 28%
   E. 35%

2. The overall postorthotopic heart transplant 1-year survival rate is
   A. 95%
   B. 90%
   C. 85%
   D. 80%
   E. 75%

3. Hypertrophic cardiomyopathy may be associated with which of the following patterns of diastolic dysfunction?
   A. Normal
   B. Abnormal relaxation
   C. Reversible restrictive physiology
   D. Irreversible restrictive physiology
   E. All of the above

4. The most important determinant of success of surgical procedures for end-stage CHF is
   A. LV ejection fraction (EF)
   B. left atrial (LA) pressure
   C. etiology of LV dysfunction
   D. RV function
   E. hematocrit

5. Which of the following is a contraindication to LVAD implantation?
   A. Moderate aortic regurgitation (AR)
   B. Atrial septal defect (ASD)
   C. Severe mitral regurgitation (MR)
   D. Patent foramen ovale (PFO)
   E. Active systemic infection

CHAPTER 36

Assessment of Cardiac Transplantation

Mihai V. Podgoreanu ■ Joseph P. Mathew

Although Barnard performed the first human cardiac transplant in 1967, it was only by the early 1980s that it gained widespread acceptance as a realistic therapeutic option for patients with end-stage heart disease. The consistent advancements in donor management, surgical techniques, immunosuppressive therapy, and antibiotic therapy resulted in a dramatic growth of cardiac transplantation in the 1980s and have led to successful heart-lung and lung transplantation. In 2001, the Registry of the International Society for Heart and Lung Transplantation listed a cumulative total of 57,818 heart transplants and 2,861 heart-lung transplants performed in 211 centers worldwide (1). The annual number of heart transplants reached a plateau in the mid-1990s at approximately 4,500 per year, and has been declining in recent years (1). The limiting factor has been a shortage of suitable donors, further compounded by a tendency to relax the recipient selection criteria in an effort to extend the benefits of transplantation. As of January 2002, the United Network for Organ Sharing national cardiac transplant waiting list (www.unos.org) included 4,119 patients, whereas only 2,197 heart transplants were performed in the United States in the year 2000 (2). Although the majority of heart transplant recipients cluster between the ages of 35 and 64 years, 12.4% of all cardiac transplants in the year 2000 were performed in pediatric patients (<18 years old) and 9.8% in patients 65 years and older, with the recipients being predominantly male (73.3%) and white (83.2%) (2). The most common indications for adult cardiac transplantation are coronary artery disease (46.1%) and cardiomyopathy (45.3%), with valvular heart disease and congenital heart disease contributing only 3.6% and 1.6%, respectively (1). The retransplantation rate in the year 2000 was 3.1% (1,2).

The overall 1-year survival for cardiac transplantation is 80%, with a subsequent mortality rate of 4% per year (1). Risk factors for 1- and 5-year mortality in adult heart transplantation have been associated with recipient factors (repeat transplant, ventilator dependence, pulmonary vascular resistance [PVR], ischemic or congenital heart disease, ventricular assistance, older age, female gender, risk for primary cytomegalovirus infection, panel reactive antibody, body length, body mass index), medical center factors (volume of heart transplants performed, ischemic time), and donor factors (advanced age, female). Early

mortality is most frequently due to primary nonspecific graft failure, intermediate-term deaths are caused by acute rejection or infection, whereas late deaths after cardiac transplantation are most frequently due to allograft vasculopathy, lymphoproliferative or other malignancies, and chronic rejection (1).

The expanding role of transesophageal echocardiography (TEE) in adult cardiac surgery has included its use as a perioperative diagnostic and monitoring technique during cardiac transplantation. There are currently five categories of applications of TEE in the assessment of cardiac transplantation:

1. Cardiac donor screening
2. Intraoperative monitoring in the pretransplantation period
3. Intraoperative evaluation of cardiac allograft function and surgical anastomoses in the immediate posttransplantation period
4. Management of early postoperative hemodynamic abnormalities in the intensive care unit
5. Postoperative follow-up studies of cardiac allograft function

THE ROLE OF TEE IN CARDIAC DONOR SCREENING

The chronic shortage of ideal donor hearts has led some cardiac transplant centers to liberalize the originally established donor selection criteria (3,4) to include older donors and marginally acceptable hearts, such that, of all the hearts transplanted in the year 2000, 11.5% were harvested from donors greater than 50 years old (1).

Echocardiography has become an integral component in the evaluation of potential cardiac transplant donors (5). This evaluation should be performed at a time when dosages of intravenous inotropic agents have been lowered to a minimum compatible with adequate blood pressure and cardiac output (CO), and after adequate fluid resuscitation. The echocardiographic assessment allows for the inclusion of donor hearts demonstrating normal function in patients otherwise considered at risk for cardiac injury by clinical criteria (known chest trauma, prolonged hypotension, hemodynamic instability requiring high doses of catecholamines). Additionally, it can circumvent the need for costly and time-consuming direct surgical inspection or cardiac catheterization in potential donors with severely depressed cardiac function (5). However, transthoracic echocardiography (TTE) is technically inadequate in up to 29% of mechanically ventilated brain-dead potential donors (6). In these patients, TEE consistently allows for unobstructed tomographic imaging of the heart, becoming a safe and useful adjunct in the assessment of ventricular function, chamber sizes, valvular structure and function, and septal wall motion and integrity (6).

Brain death is associated with hemodynamic deterioration and biventricular dysfunction, which is usually reversible shortly after transplantation. Studies in potential clinical donors and in experimental animals have suggested that brain death can have major histopathological and functional effects on the myocardium, with very typical focal lesions consisting of petechial subendocardial hemorrhage, contraction bands, and coagulative myocytolysis. Although the mechanism of myocardial injury and contractile dysfunction after brain death remains incompletely understood, it is believed to be caused by a catecholamine excess that occurs during the process of brain death, resulting in cytosolic calcium overload (7–9). Previous studies have shown that segmental wall motion abnormalities and global left ventricular (LV) systolic dysfunction (fractional area change [FAC] < 50%) are frequent in brain-dead donors (67.5% and 36%, respectively), improve shortly after heart transplantation, and remain improved 15 months later (4,10), thus suggesting that potential cardiac donors should not be excluded on the basis of segmental wall motion abnormalities. A recent multiinstitutional study, however, identified wall motion abnormalities on the donor echocardiogram as an independent powerful predictor of fatal early graft failure (relative risk of 1.7), especially with increasing donor age and prolonged ischemic time (11). As of yet, the lowest FAC enabling the heart to be transplanted without risk is not known, but one study recommends harvesting and heart transplantation when the FAC is above 35% if there are no other severe cardiac abnormalities (right ventricular [RV] failure or valvular dysfunction) (5). One retrospective study suggests that the presence of left ventricular hypertrophy (LVH) in the donor heart increases the incidence of early graft dysfunction (12). Such marginal donor hearts should not be used in high-risk recipients (those on ventilator support, with prior sternotomies, or in renal failure, for example), and should be carefully monitored postoperatively for allograft dysfunction (13).

INTRAOPERATIVE MONITORING IN THE PRETRANSPLANTATION PERIOD

The vast majority of patients referred for cardiac transplantation suffer from ischemic or idiopathic cardiomyopathy with a dilated LV and depressed ejection fraction. The currently accepted indications for transplantation,

however, include impaired functional status (peak VO_2 < 14 mL/kg/min) and/or refractory hemodynamic decompensation, manifested as severe ischemia not amenable to revascularization, or recurrent symptomatic ventricular arrhythmias despite optimal medical management (14). As such, these patients have a relatively fixed low stroke volume (SV) and depend on appropriate preload and heart rate to maintain a marginal CO. Due to the characteristics of the end-systolic pressure volume relationship in the myopathic heart, even mild increases in afterload can markedly decrease the SV (15). Sympathetic tone is increased in patients with heart failure, leading to generalized vasoconstriction as well as salt and water retention. The combination of vasoconstriction and ventricular dilation results in a substantial increase in myocardial wall tension. Moreover, in patients with long-standing left-sided cardiac failure, RV impairment may result by a process of ventricular interdependence, independent of neurohumoral or circulatory effects, and can be further compromised by elevations in PVR (16). Almost all cardiac transplant candidates will be maintained on a combination of vasodilators for afterload reduction (usually angiotensin-converting enzyme inhibitors [ACE-I]), diuretics to minimize volume overload, and antiarrhythmics (usually amiodarone). This combination therapy was associated with a decrease in the overall 1-year mortality, as well as a decrease in the incidence of sudden death in end-stage heart failure (17). The average waiting time for patients at home is currently more than 18 months and continues to lengthen, but patients who develop refractory hemodynamic decompensation will require continued hospitalization for hemodynamic monitoring, prolonged inotropic therapy, or various degrees of mechanical assistance as a bridge to transplantation (intraaortic balloon counterpulsation [IABP], univentricular or biventricular assist devices). In the United States, priority (Status I) is accorded to hospitalized patients requiring assist devices or intravenous inotropic therapy in intensive care units; all other patients are Status II. In the year 2000, 56.6% of heart transplant recipients were reported to be on life support at the time of transplantation, of which 32.3% were in the intensive care unit (2).

The main goal during the prebypass period is to maintain adequate end-organ perfusion. However, in these patients with end-stage heart failure, cardiovascular decompensation during induction or maintenance of anesthesia can result from multiple mechanisms. Decreases in sympathetic outflow (especially when the renin-angiotensin system is blocked by ACE-I) with resultant hypotension and impaired coronary perfusion, alterations in preload (hypovolemia from exaggerated diuresis), decreases in heart rate (with absent compensatory preload reserve), or increases in PVR can be extremely deleterious (15).

In these patients with precarious hemodynamic status, TEE is ideally suited to evaluate and guide intraoperative management decisions in the pretransplantation period. A complete TEE examination will often reveal information not readily available from other sources. Some examples follow.

Left Ventricular Volume

Due to a right shift in the LV pressure-volume relationship, the failing heart requires a larger preload to maintain marginal performance. Moreover, superimposed diastolic dysfunction results in a poor correlation between LV filling pressures and volumes, further compounded by the effects of positive-pressure ventilation. Thus, optimization of LV filling is best achieved by monitoring LV volumes under TEE guidance.

Left Ventricular Contractility

Performed in conjunction with the assessment of LV preload, monitoring global LV systolic function in the pretransplantation period may help achieve hemodynamic stability in the face of reductions in sympathetic outflow associated with induction of anesthesia, by guiding the adjustments in inotropic infusions.

Intracavitary Thrombus

Particular attention should be paid to the LV apex, the most common site for ventricular thrombus associated with cardiomyopathy or apical infarcts. The left atrial (LA) appendage should be inspected for possible thrombi, especially in atrial fibrillation. If intracavitary thrombi are identified, manipulation of the heart should be limited and dissection should proceed with great caution prior to cardiopulmonary bypass (CPB) to avoid systemic embolization (Fig. 36.1).

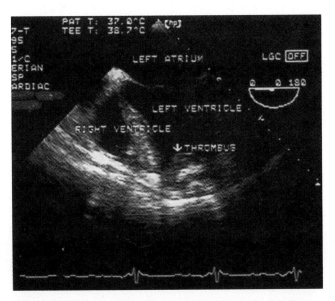

Figure 36.1. TEE image of laminated intraventricular thrombus in the native LV apex. (From Quinlan JJ, et al. Anesthesia for heart, lung, and heart-lung transplantation. In: Kaplan JA, ed. *Cardiac Anesthesia*, 4th ed. Philadelphia: WB Saunders, 1999:461, with permission.)

Atherosclerosis of the Ascending Aorta and Aortic Arch

Aortic atheroma burden is assessed well by TEE, and should guide aortic cannulation site and cross-clamp placement. The ascending aorta and aortic arch can be assessed in the midesophageal aortic valve long-axis, ascending aortic short-axis, and long-axis views and in the upperesophageal aortic arch long-axis and short-axis views (18). The descending aorta is also assessed for the presence of mobile atheroma, in case an intraaortic balloon pump is required posttransplant. This can be achieved in the descending aortic short-axis and long-axis views (18).

Right Ventricular Dilation or Hypertrophy

Their presence would be suggestive of long-standing pulmonary hypertension and should heighten the awareness for possible acute RV dysfunction in the transplanted heart.

Assessment of Left Ventricular Assist Device Explant

In patients who required mechanical circulatory assistance as a bridge to transplant, microperforations can occur at the time of left ventricular assist device (LVAD) explant, during the lengthy dissection onto the inlet cannula and its connections. This can result in air entrainment and subsequent ejection into the aorta (19). TEE monitoring for such an event can be performed in the midesophageal aortic valve long-axis view (18) (see Chapter 36).

Hemodynamic Calculations

Most cardiac anesthesiologists agree that a pulmonary artery catheter (PAC) is useful in the hemodynamic evaluation of patients undergoing cardiac transplantation. However, floating the PAC into correct position may be difficult due to cardiac chamber dilation and severe tricuspid regurgitation (TR). Furthermore, PAC placement may be more prone to induce dysrhythmias, resulting in rapid hemodynamic decompensation in these patients with marginal cardiovascular reserve. Consequently, the PAC may be placed in a sterile sheath with the tip advanced to the end of the cordis introducer, during the prebypass period, and subsequently advanced by the surgeon under direct vision before the completion of the right atrial anastomosis. This minimizes the risk of blindly passing the PAC across fresh surgical suture lines. When a PAC cannot be placed, TEE can be used to determine the CO and pulmonary artery (PA) pressures in the prebypass period.

The area-length formula can be used to calculate the SV across a cardiac valve:

$$SV = \text{cross-sectional area (CSA)} \times \text{velocity time integral (VTI)}$$

The SV across a valve can be subsequently used to calculate the CO, if there is no stenosis and/or regurgitation across that valve. Because most of these patients with dilated cardiomyopathies present with various degrees of mitral regurgitation (MR), the aortic valve is usually used for CO measurements. The left ventricular outflow tract (LVOT) diameter is measured from the midesophageal aortic valve long-axis view; the $LVOT_{VTI}$ is measured from the LVOT Doppler spectrum in the transgastric long-axis or deep transgastric long-axis views, which provide windows for continuous wave Doppler interrogation, which is nearly parallel to aortic flow (18). The final formula for CO (in L/min) becomes

$$CO = 0.785 \ (LVOT \ diameter)^2 \\ \times LVOT_{VTI} \times heart \ rate \ / \ 1,000$$

This TEE determination of CO in the prebypass period should be performed even if the PAC has been successfully advanced into the PA because most of these patients present with various degrees of TR, which renders thermodilution CO measurements inaccurate (20).

Doppler echocardiography is an ideal tool for determining PA pressures. In the presence of TR, the systolic pulmonary artery pressure (PAS) can be calculated using the simplified Bernoulli equation from the peak velocity of the TR jet (V_{TR}, measured by continuous wave Doppler in the midesophageal RV inflow-outflow view) (18) and the central venous pressure (CVP) as

$$PAS = 4 \ (V_{TR})^2 + CVP$$

In the presence of pulmonic regurgitation (PR), the diastolic pulmonary artery pressure (PAD) can be calculated in a similar fashion, using the end-diastolic velocity of the PR jet (V_{PR}, measured by continuous wave Doppler in the upperesophageal aortic arch short-axis view) and the CVP as

$$PAD = 4 \ (V_{TR})^2 + CVP$$

As with all Doppler measurements, the ultrasound beam must be parallel to the regurgitant flows or the velocities (hence the PA pressures) will be underestimated.

Intraoperative Monitoring in the Posttransplantation Period

The pathophysiology of the transplanted heart is dependent upon several factors, including the amount of donor inotropic support, the degree of subclinical myocardial damage, the ischemic time, the myocardial protection during the ischemic interval, cardiac denervation, and the degree of pulmonary hypertension in the recipient.

Assisting with Venting and De-Airing Maneuvers

Prior to weaning from CPB, TEE is used to detect retained intracardiac air and to assist the de-airing maneuvers. The most common sites of air retention are the right and left

upper pulmonary veins, the LV apex, the LA, and the right coronary sinus of Valsalva (21). Reports of acute RV dysfunction caused by air embolization to the right coronary artery exist in the literature (22). Detection of echogenic material by TEE in the LA or LV after the heart is allowed to fully eject, followed by RV dilatation, loss of contraction, and ST segment changes in inferior leads, should raise the suspicion of right coronary air embolus. Full CPB should be reinstituted and the coronary perfusion elevated to allow the dissolution of the coronary embolus. Without the aid of TEE, the real cause of RV dysfunction in this scenario may be missed (see also "Assessment of the Right Ventricle," below).

In the majority of cardiac transplantations, separation from CPB is readily achieved. After separation from CPB, TEE allows for the online assessment of biventricular function and flow dynamics across the surgical anastomoses, with important diagnostic and prognostic implications.

Assessment of the Left Ventricle

The global and segmental LV systolic function should be assessed in the midesophageal four-chamber, two-chamber, and long-axis views, as well as in the transgastric mid short-axis, basal short-axis, and long-axis views (18). To minimize intraobserver and interobserver variability, the LV FAC should always be measured in the transgastric midpapillary muscle short-axis tomographic plane, by manually tracing the endocardial border, or defined with an automated border detection system. Intraoperative TEE assessment of allograft LV systolic function early after separation from CPB, in contrast to routinely measured hemodynamic variables, has been shown to better predict early requirements for inotropic and mechanical support, particularly in patients with longer ischemic times (23).

The following 2D-echocardiographic findings of the LV, which would be considered abnormal in the general population, are characteristic of transplant recipients:

1. An increase in LV wall thickness (especially the posterior and septal walls), LV mass, and LV mass index may be observed. It has been hypothesized to represent myocardial edema, resulting from the manipulation and transport of the heart (24–26).
2. Paradoxical or flat interventricular septal motion, and decreased interventricular septal systolic thickening compared to normals (31% vs. 44%) (24).
3. Because the donor heart is normal in size, it is typically smaller than the original dilated failing heart and, therefore, it is positioned more medially in the mediastinum and tends to be rotated clockwise. This usually necessitates nonstandard transducer locations and angles for echocardiography. Residual fluid accumulations in the posterior pericardial space contribute to the common small postoperative pericardial effusions (27).

Assessment of LV Diastolic Function

The postischemic condition of the allograft decreases diastolic compliance of both ventricles, necessitating greater than normal filling pressures to adequately preload the heart. The echocardiographic assessment of LV diastolic function in the transplanted heart is complicated by the variability of the Doppler velocity profiles from the atrioventricular valves, which may be observed when the remnant recipient atria retain mechanical activity. This results in asynchronous atrial contractions, modifying the filling patterns of both ventricles (24–26,28,29). The beat-to-beat variations in transmitral (and tricuspid) diastolic velocities, assessed by pulsed wave Doppler, relate to the timing of contraction of the recipient atria within the cardiac cycle. Therefore, it is important to locate the recipient P waves within the donor cardiac cycle before making the required Doppler measurements. When the recipient P waves occur between late systole and mitral valve opening, the flow signals should not be used to measure diastolic indices. Recipient P waves occurring during this time frame decrease isovolumic relaxation time and pressure half-time, and increase the mitral inflow peak E-wave velocity. If the recipient P waves occur anywhere from late diastole through midsystole, the flow signals may be used (24,25,28) (Table 36.1).

Several studies have demonstrated an abnormal transmitral flow pattern compatible with restrictive diastolic LV dysfunction in orthotopic heart transplant recipients (reduced late maximum flow velocity, increased early-to-late diastolic maximum flow velocity ratio) (26,30). Similarly, an abnormal pulmonary venous flow pattern characterized by reduced peak flow velocity and reduced time velocity integral in the systolic phase with relatively enhanced flow during the diastolic phase has been observed (23,30). This decreased systolic to diastolic maximum pulmonary venous flow velocity ratio, found despite normal pulmonary capillary wedge pressures and associated with a reduced LA area change and a reduced

mitral annulus motion is suggestive of LA dysfunction (26) secondary to altered atrial anatomy and dynamics (31). Beat-to-beat variability of all pulmonary venous flow parameters was found to be higher in transplant recipients than in controls, especially in the systolic phase parameters (26).

Therefore, mitral Doppler inflow analysis alone appears to be inadequate for the assessment of diastolic LV function in heart transplant recipients, as LV diastolic dysfunction cannot be differentiated from atrial dysfunction, and should be therefore corroborated with the analysis of pulmonary venous flow patterns. The assessment is further complicated by the various pacing modalities used in the perioperative period.

Assessment of the Right Ventricle

Etiology, Pathophysiology, and Diagnosis of Acute RV Dysfunction

Despite advances in perioperative management, ISHLT registry data show that RV dysfunction accounts for 50% of all cardiac complications and 19% of all early deaths in patients after heart transplantation (1). Acute RV dysfunction in heart transplant recipients is of multifactorial etiology, resulting either from an increase in PVR in the recipient, or from a loss of contractility in the donor heart (9,32).

Recipient pulmonary hypertension represents an important risk factor for acute RV failure and for other postoperative morbidity (posttransplant infections, arrhythmias) (32) and is attributed to the inability of the donor RV myocardium to acutely compensate for the recipient's elevated PVR (9). Pulmonary hemodynamic indices represent a spectrum of values associated with postoperative mortality, but this relationship is by no means linear. The literature confirms the absence of threshold hemodynamic values beyond which RV failure is certain to occur and heart transplantation is contraindicated; there are no values below which

TABLE 36.1	**Mitral Inflow Doppler Velocities**			
Timing of recipient atrial contraction	Peak E-wave	Peak A-wave	Isovolumic relaxation time	Deceleration time
Early diastole	Normal	Decreased	Normal	Normal
Late diastole	Normal	Increased	Normal	Normal
Early systole	Decreased	Normal	Normal	Increased
Late systole	Increased	Normal	Decreased	Decreased
Overall E/A variability (%)	28 ± 15			

Modified from Suriani RJ. Transesophageal echocardiography during organ transplantation. J Cardiothorac Vasc Anesth 1998;12(6):686–698; Bouchart F, Derumeaux G, Mouton-Schleifer D, et al. Conventional and total orthotopic cardiac transplantation: a comparative clinical and echocardiographical study. Eur J Cardiothorac Surg 1997;12:555–559, with permission.

RV failure is always avoidable (32). Although patients with preoperative fixed pulmonary hypertension are excluded from cardiac transplantation, unfortunately normal preoperative PVR does not rule out the potential for pulmonary hypertension and acute RV failure after heart transplantation, resulting from the effects of CPB on the pulmonary circulation, the administration of protamine, or from the simple act of awakening from anesthesia (25,32).

A loss of contractility in the donor heart may be related to the myocardial changes occurring after brain death, which is known to be associated with donor organ dysfunction, cardiovascular deterioration, and metabolic and hormonal changes (7–9). Additionally, adaptation by the donor heart may be impaired by ischemia, reperfusion injury associated with organ preservation, and the deleterious effects that CPB has upon ventricular function. As mentioned above, acute RV dysfunction can occasionally be caused by air embolization to the right coronary artery (22). This is usually a transient event, and the recovery is uneventful with reinstitution of full CPB.

Irrespective of its etiology, acute RV failure after heart transplantation results in further dilation, ischemia, and decreased contractility. Decreased pulmonary blood flow and leftward shift of the interventricular septum subsequently lead to reduced LV filling and decreased systemic CO.

The complex geometry of the RV, further compounded by the inadequate definition of the RV free wall, makes direct echocardiographic assessment of RV function difficult. Numerous methods of assessing the RV have been developed, including geometry-dependent (i.e., relying on models that assume a specific geometric shape, planimetry), geometry-independent (tricuspid annular plane systolic excursion [TAPSE], Doppler echocardiography, myocardial performance index), quantitative (RV ejection fraction [RVEF]), or qualitative methods (septal curvature, real-time visual assessment) (25,33) (see Chapter 11).

Planimetry of the RV is performed in the midesophageal four-chamber view or in the transgastric mid short-axis view, with the endocardial border manually traced or defined by an automated border detection system (acoustic quantification; Fig. 36.2). Comparison of serial measurements is difficult because of the irregularity of RV anatomy and difficulty in ensuring that the same tomographic plane is obtained during each measurement (25).

The use of TAPSE to estimate RV function is based on the concept that, during RV systole, lengthwise shortening of both the interventricular septum and the RV free wall occurs. The technique was found to closely correlate with RVEF as measured by radionuclide angiography (RVEF = 3.2 × TAPSE), and attempts to avoid the geometric assumptions involved in extrapolating two-dimensional (2D) measurements (i.e., planimetry) to RV

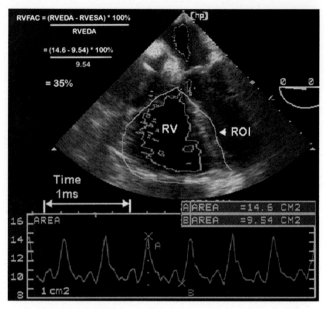

Figure 36.2. Midesophageal four-chamber view with automatic border detection and region of interest (ROI) around the RV. The area-versus-time curve is used to generate end-diastolic (**A**) and end-systolic (**B**) right ventricular areas (RVEDA, RVESA). The equation is then used to calculate right ventricular fractional area change as a percentage (RVFAC). (From Scalia GM, et al. Clinical utility of echocardiography in the management of implantable ventricular assist devices. *J Am Soc Echocardiogr* 2000;13:757, with permission.)

volumes (33). TAPSE is measured in the midesophageal four-chamber view as the excursion (in mm) of the junction point of the tricuspid valve with the RV free wall between end-diastole and end-systole.

The maximum acceleration of blood in the PA can be used as an index of RV ejection. This can be obtained in the midesophageal ascending aortic short-axis view, where the main PA is nearly parallel to the spectral Doppler beam. The maximum acceleration of pulmonary blood flow is defined as the tangent to the upstroke of the velocity profile and is easily measured using the internal calculation software in most echocardiographic machines. Changes in the maximum acceleration of blood in the PA have been shown to correlate with changes in the thermodilution RVEF (34).

The RV function can be qualitatively assessed by visually estimating the RV size, the systolic motion of RV free wall, and RVEF, and by examining the interventricular septum for systolic thickening and paradoxical curvature in the midesophageal four-chamber view and in the transgastric mid short-axis view. Normally, the septum bulges from left to right due to the higher left-sided interventricular pressure, but this situation can be reversed during acute RV dysfunction, when the right-sided interventricular pressure exceeds the LV pressure (35). Paradoxical septal shift occurs in late diastole with RV volume overload and at end-systole and early diastole with RV pressure overload (25,36).

Management of Acute RV Dysfunction

Goals in the treatment of acute RV failure include

1. Preserving coronary perfusion through maintenance of aortic pressure
2. Optimizing RV preload
3. Reducing RV afterload by decreasing PVR
4. Limiting pulmonary vasoconstriction through ventilation with high-inspired oxygen concentrations, increased tidal volume, and optimal PEEP ventilation

Optimizing RV preload should be performed under echocardiographic guidance to avoid overdistending an ischemic RV, and in conjunction with CVP and serial CO measurements. Inotropes and inodilators are often used to increase RV contractility and decrease PVR. Isoproterenol and phosphodiesterase III inhibitors (milrinone) are the mainstays of therapy, often in combination with alpha-adrenergic agonists (norepinephrine) to maintain systemic vascular resistance and coronary perfusion. Inhaled nitric oxide can be used immediately after heart transplantation to prevent or to treat RV failure due to its potent, rapidly acting, and selective pulmonary vasodilator properties. Additionally, inhaled nitric oxide can improve hypoxemia by optimizing the ventilation-perfusion relationship.

IABP can be employed in patients with LV dysfunction, and may be of benefit in patients with acute RV dysfunction resulting from ischemia, preservation injury, or reperfusion injury. In acute RV failure, RV hypertension and distension may cause reduced coronary blood flow to the RV and impair LV function by reduced filling and altered septal dynamics. In the setting of early postoperative low CO syndrome characterized predominantly by RV failure, IABP placement has been shown to improve hemodynamics and peripheral tissue perfusion (37). The mechanisms involved include improved myocardial perfusion through enhanced coronary filling and improved LV mechanics through afterload reduction. Optimal LV function ultimately indirectly relieves RV dysfunction through reduced RV afterload and PVR (32) and improved ventricular interdependence (37).

The decision regarding RV assist device implantation is dependent upon a stepwise review of overall hemodynamics after the institution of maximal inotropic and vasodilator support. The assessment includes an evaluation of the size and function of both ventricles by TEE, the status of mediastinal bleeding, oxygenation, presence of arrhythmias, and urine output. This assessment usually takes place after several unsuccessful attempts to separate the patient from CPB and approximately 1 hour after removal of the aortic cross-clamp. The observation of a small hyperdynamic LV and a dilated RV by TEE, marginal urine output, arrhythmias, or coagulopathy should prompt the insertion of a RV assist device. The presence of coagulopathy will require ongoing volume resuscitation with blood products, likely resulting in a worsening of pulmonary hypertension, pulmonary edema, and RV failure with its secondary effects on CO and end-organ perfusion. Reduction of elevated right-sided pressures following RV assist device implantation is a positive predictor for survival (32). Still, the need for RV mechanical assistance after heart transplantation increases the early mortality to over 50% (38).

Assessment of the Atria and Atrial Anastomoses

The vast majority of heart transplantation procedures are orthotopic, with heterotopic transplants representing only 0.3% of the procedures performed in the year 2000 (2). Three different orthotopic heart transplantation techniques have been described: standard biatrial, bicaval, and total orthotopic heart transplantation (39). The resultant atrial size and geometry, and the donor-recipient atrial anastomoses are entirely dependent upon the transplantation technique employed. TEE is ideally suited to assess the interatrial septum, atrial free walls, and atrial appendages in the transplanted heart, providing unique information on the sites of atrial anastomoses. This should be performed in the midesophageal four-chamber, two-chamber, and midesophageal bicaval views (18).

In the standard biatrial orthotopic heart transplant technique, originally described by Lower and Shumway, the posterior and lateral portions of the recipient atria and the posterior part of the interatrial septum are left in situ and serve to anchor the corresponding parts of the donor atria. Thus, the size and geometry of both atria are remodeled during the operation (31), and several anatomic and functional abnormalities occur in the recipients. These include biatrial enlargement, asynchronous contraction of the donor and recipient atria, and intraluminal protrusion of the atrial anastomoses, creating distorted "hour-glass" or "snowman" configurations of the new atria (31,39). The atrial suture lines appear prominently as echodense ridges, which give mass-like effects in the atria (25,40,41), are nonmobile and nonpedunculated, and should not be confused with thrombi (Fig. 36.3). These anastomotic protrusions are particularly prominent at the LA free wall and, occasionally, systolic contact between the protruding suture and the posterior mitral leaflet has been reported to occur (31). Stenotic LA suture lines, causing hemodynamically significant obstruction to blood flow with systemic hypotension and elevated PA pressures, have been described in the literature (42–46), and are due to a mismatch of the donor and recipient LA cuff circumferences, worsened by a purse-string effect of the anastomotic suture line. The deformity has been coined *acquired cor triatriatum* (44–46) due to the similarity to the congenital cardiac anomaly in which the LA is subdivided into two chambers by a perforated fibromuscular septum (Fig. 36.4). Occasionally, acquired cor triatriatum can result from an infolding of redundant donor (45) or recipient (46) LA tissue and not the atrial suture line. Intraoperative TEE is clinically crucial in identifying such stenotic suture lines or tissue infoldings, prompting early surgical revision. In the midesophageal four-chamber or two-chamber views, TEE reveals a

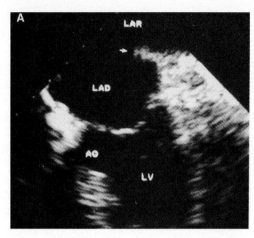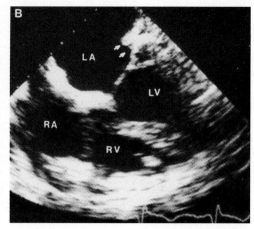

Figure 36.3. A: Prominent suture (*arrow*) between the donor (LAD) and recipient (LAR) components of LA. **B:** Systolic contact (*arrows*) between posterior mitral valve leaflet and suture. AO, aortic root; LV, left ventricle; RV, right ventricle; RA, right atrium. (From Angermann CE, et al. Anatomic characteristics and valvular function of the transplanted heart: transthoracic versus transesophageal echocardiographic findings. *J Heart Transplant* 1990;9:333, with permission.)

markedly enlarged atrial remnant with a reduced LV volume, and the suture line protrusion can be measured. Additionally, detection of turbulent flow by color flow Doppler, "fluttering" of the mitral valve leaflets, and elevated transstenotic blood-flow velocities by pulsed wave Doppler confirm the presence of a LA pressure gradient and LV inflow obstruction (44). Failure to identify such LV inflow obstruction may result in unexplained pulmonary hypertension and RV failure in the early postoperative period.

Most heart transplant recipients show some phasic excursion of the interatrial septum during the cardiac cycle. This cyclic septal motion is called "pseudoaneurysm" if a portion of the atrial septum bulges at least 10 mm beyond the atrial septal plane and if the base of the bulging part is at least 15 mm in diameter (47). By these criteria, the incidence of posttransplant atrial septal pseudoaneurysms

in one study was 35% (31). The integrity of the interatrial septum should be assessed intraoperatively by using both color flow Doppler and contrast echocardiography (saline microcavitation). Shunts can occur either at the atrial anastomotic site or through a patent foramen ovale (PFO) in the recipient atrial septum. Although uncommon, right-to-left shunting through a PFO that is not apparent preoperatively may become hemodynamically significant postoperatively as the relative pressure difference between the atria changes because of RV dysfunction or TR, and can present as refractory postoperative hypoxemia (48). Identification of a left-to-right shunt across the interatrial anastomosis should also prompt surgical repair, as it can contribute to progressive RV volume overload and TR (40).

Dissociation of the mechanical performance of recipient and donor atria, a consequence of the persisting independent electrical activity in both atrial components,

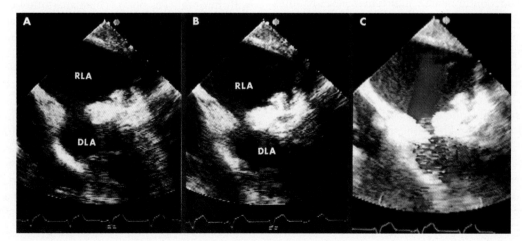

Figure 36.4. Acquired cor triatriatum. **A:** Intraoperative TEE image of recipient left atrium (RLA) and donor left atrium (DLA) during systole. **B:** Intraoperative TEE image during diastole shows the dynamic narrowing of the intra-atrial channel. **C:** TEE image during diastole with color flow Doppler imaging of the intra-arterial channel. (From Bjerke RJ, et al. Early diagnosis and follow-up by echocardiography of acquired cor triatriatum after orthotopic heart transplantation. *J Heart Lung Transplant* 1992;11:1073–1077.)

can be visualized by TEE and has important implications for both left and right heart function. Several studies have reported LA spontaneous echo contrast (SEC) in heart transplant recipients (29,31,40,41,49). The combination of disturbed atrial hemodynamics caused by asynchronous contraction of the atria and atrial enlargement might contribute to slow blood flow within the atrial cavities and explain the relatively high incidence of SEC (25%–55%) despite normal ventricular function in these patients (29,31,40,41). This is usually confined to the donor atrial component and is characterized by multiple microechoes slowly swirling within the enlarged atrial cavity and disappearing after passage through the mitral valve. SEC is visible at normal gain settings, and the characteristic motion pattern allows clear discrimination from noise echoes or reverberations (31). The importance of diagnosing LA SEC in heart transplant recipients stems from its association with LA thrombi and systemic embolic events on postoperative follow-up studies (31,41,49). In most cases, the thrombi are attached to the atrial free wall underneath the protruding suture in a niche formed after partial removal of the LA appendage during transplantation (31,41) but can also be localized on the posterior LA wall or on the suture line (29). Occasionally, protruding suture ends, endocardial tags, or other tissue remnants may have an echocardiographic appearance of thrombus-like structures (Fig. 36.5). Therefore, the presence of LA SEC on intraoperative TEE should prompt postoperative follow-up studies to assess for the presence of atrial thrombi and the need for antiplatelet or anticoagulation therapy.

Previous studies have demonstrated that synchronous atrial contraction is an important compensatory response to RV dysfunction (50). Intact right atrial function may be important in preventing the development of RV failure after orthotopic heart transplantation or in limiting its severity, particularly in patients with elevated PVR (39).

In 1990, Reitz (51) introduced the bicaval anastomotic technique at Stanford University, as a modification of the standard biatrial technique. Using this technique, the donor and recipient superior and inferior venae cavae are anastomosed in an end-to-end fashion, completely avoiding a right atrial suture line. Several reports confirm that the bicaval technique improves atrial function, decreases atrial conduction abnormalities, and decreases the incidence of TR (52,53). When combined with an everting suture for the LA anastomosis, the incidence of LA SEC and subsequent LA thrombi and systemic embolic events on postoperative follow-up is decreased (49).

In an attempt to further minimize left and right atrial dysfunction and electrophysiologic abnormalities, Dreyfus (54) and Yacoub (55) devised a technique of total orthotopic heart transplantation. This technique incorporates the bicaval anastomosis for the implantation of the right atrium and a direct anastomosis between the donor and recipient pulmonary veins to implant the LA. Thus, an anatomic replacement of the heart is achieved (39), with normal atrial morphology and normal atrioventricular interactions. When compared to the standard technique, total heart transplantation significantly reduces the incidence of postoperative rhythm disturbances and pacemaker dependence, atrioventricular valve regurgitation (39), and LA SEC and thrombi (29).

Assessment of the Pulmonary Artery Anastomosis

The main PA anastomosis should be evaluated for stenosis or possible kinking or torsion by 2D-echocardiography, color flow Doppler to detect turbulent flow, and by continuous wave Doppler to measure the pressure gradient across the anastomosis. The main PA can be imaged in the midesophageal RV inflow-outflow or in the midesophageal ascending aortic short-axis views, with the latter

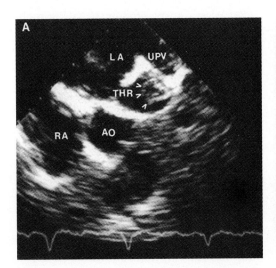 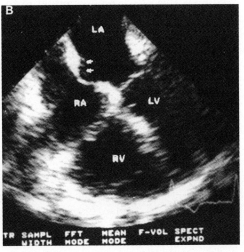

Figure 36.5. A: Atrial thrombus (THR) attached to the LA free wall. **B:** Small thrombus-like structures (*arrows*) attached to atrial septum. UPV, upper pulmonary vein; RA, right atrium; RV, right ventricle; LV, left ventricle; AO, aortic root. (From Angermann CE, et al. Anatomic characteristics and valvular function of the transplanted heart: transthoracic versus transesophageal echocardiographic findings. *J Heart Transplant* 1990;9:335, with permission.)

offering the best beam alignment for Doppler interrogation (18). Several reports describe PA anastomotic kinking (56) or torsion (57), recognized intraoperatively or early postoperatively, and manifested as elevated RV pressures and high-pressure gradients across the PA anastomoses. The kinking was the result of the excess length of the combined donor and recipient PA segments, whereas PA torsion was related to marked size mismatch between donor and recipient hearts and consequent malalignment of the PA stumps. Occasionally, recipient valve remnants, surface raggedness, or protruding suture lines can be identified (42).

Assessment of the Pulmonary Venous Anastomoses

When the total orthotopic heart transplantation technique is employed, intraoperative TEE assessment of individual pulmonary venous anastomoses should be performed, including pulmonary vein diameter, color flow pattern, and pulsed wave Doppler profile. Identification of hemodynamically significant suture line stenosis or torsion should prompt early surgical revision.

Assessment of the Atrioventricular Valves

Mild to moderate degrees of mitral and TR are commonly found on color flow Doppler imaging after cardiac transplantation. MR occurs with an incidence ranging from 48% to 87% depending on the study quoted (31,41,58,59), and is usually mild in severity, with an eccentric jet pointing toward the LA free wall. TR found in 85% of transplant recipients, occurs immediately after heart transplantation, and is usually moderate, with an eccentric jet direction pointing toward the interatrial septum (31,59). We found no association between the incidence and severity of TR immediately after cardiac transplantation and the presence of RV dysfunction (60). Quantification of the severity of TR by color flow Doppler is best achieved using the ratio of the maximum area of the regurgitant jet to the right atrial area (61). This method has been validated in heart transplant recipients and was found to correlate better with the thermodilution-derived tricuspid regurgitant fraction than the maximum jet area or the maximum jet length (Table 36.2) (62). Still, the area of the color Doppler regurgitant jet may be underestimated because of jet eccentricity.

The etiology of atrioventricular valve regurgitation in the transplanted heart is still controversial, but because no structural valvular abnormalities could be found, it is thought to be caused by the distorted atrial geometry and the tension generated on the muscular parts of the annuli by the enlarged atria (31,59). With the standard biatrial technique, donor-recipient size mismatch is more evident on the right atrial side because the LA anastomosis is performed first, allowing a better degree of adaptation of the LA walls, and might explain the higher incidence of TR in the transplanted heart (59). The severity of posttransplant TR correlates with echocardiographic indices of atrial distortion (recipient to

TABLE 36.2	Ratio of Jet Area to Right Atrial Area
Trivial TR	
Mild TR 10% to 24%	
Moderate TR 25% to 49%	
Severe TR ≥ 50%	

From Chan MCY, Giannetti N, Kato T, et al. Severe tricuspid regurgitation after heart transplantation. J Heart Lung Transplant 2001;20: 709–717, with permission.

donor atrial area ratio) and the systolic shortening of the tricuspid annulus (59). The significantly reduced incidence of moderate and severe TR with the bicaval anastomotic technique (52,53,63,64), and both TR and MR after total orthotopic heart transplantation (39), further supports this hypothesis. Distortion of the tricuspid annulus may also be caused by a size mismatch of the donor heart and recipient pericardial cavity. In one study, if greater than mild TR was detected by intraoperative echocardiography after discontinuation of CPB, pericardial reduction plasty was performed that successfully prevented TR up to 8 weeks of follow-up (65). Yet other investigators suggested that multivalvular regurgitation observed after heart transplantation might be a result of mild edema of the cardiac structures, as they found a significant LV mass reduction within the first postoperative weeks with a progressive resolution of valvular regurgitation (66). The natural history of these regurgitant lesions varies, but the incidence of severe TR appears to increase with time, and some patients may require tricuspid valve replacement for refractory symptoms (61).

Rarely, MR secondary to systolic anterior motion (SAM) of the anterior mitral valve leaflet has been reported after heart transplantation (67). This might be caused or aggravated by the common use of the β-adrenergic agonist isoproterenol, with resultant vasodilation, tachycardia, and increased myocardial contractility, along with iatrogenic hypovolemia to prevent graft distension, and increased LV wall thickness observed in the transplanted heart. Intraoperative TEE diagnosis of SAM of the anterior mitral valve leaflet with associated MR is facilitated by the systematic assessment of the mitral valve and LVOT in the midesophageal five-chamber, midesophageal aortic valve long-axis, and transgastric long-axis views (18). Characteristic features include SAM of the anterior mitral valve leaflet, mid-systolic notching of the aortic valve, posteriorly directed MR jet, flow turbulence at the site of LVOT obstruction with a dagger-shaped continuous wave Doppler tracing and significant LVOT pressure gradient (>50 mm Hg). These findings should be managed by optimizing the LV volume, changing the inotrope to one with more α-adrenergic effects (e.g., isoproterenol to dopamine) to decrease the heart rate and increase the afterload, and follow-up echocardiographic assessments of SAM and MR.

MANAGEMENT OF EARLY POSTOPERATIVE HEMODYNAMIC ABNORMALITIES IN THE INTENSIVE CARE UNIT

TEE has become an invaluable tool in the management of seriously ill intensive care unit patients in whom transthoracic acoustic images may be particularly poor. Particular uses in these circumstances include assessment of biventricular function, anastomotic problems (kinks, torsions, stenoses), valvular abnormalities, sources of systemic emboli, and the exclusion of pericardial fluid (see Chapters 21 and 29).

POSTOPERATIVE FOLLOW-UP STUDIES OF CARDIAC ALLOGRAFT FUNCTION

Echocardiography plays an increasingly important role in the follow-up of recipients after cardiac transplantation as one of the most important potential noninvasive means of diagnosing transplant rejection. Proposed echocardiographic indicators of rejection in cardiac transplantation include

1. Increasing LV mass/LV wall thickness
2. Increased myocardial echogenicity
3. New or increasing pericardial effusion
4. A greater than 10% decrease in LV ejection fraction
5. Restrictive LV filling pattern (>20% decrease in MV pressure half-time, 20% decrease in isovolumic relaxation time)
6. New onset MR

Additionally, 2D echocardiography may be utilized to guide transvenous endomyocardial biopsies and prevent inadvertent damage to the tricuspid valve and its supporting apparatus. Dobutamine stress echocardiography has been used in the detection of allograft vasculopathy and has a high negative predictive value for determining future cardiac events and death in heart transplant recipients (68).

KEY POINTS

■ Cardiac transplantation has become the gold standard treatment of advanced heart failure in selected patients during the last 20 years, but the numerical disparity between donors and recipients continues to increase.

■ In an effort to expand the donor criteria, TEE is a useful adjunct to TTE in the screening of brain-dead potential cardiac donors when the latter is technically inadequate.

■ In the pretransplantation period, intraoperative TEE is useful in maintaining cardiovascular stability, performing hemodynamic calculations, and monitoring ventricular assist explantation.

■ In the posttransplantation period, intraoperative TEE assists with the de-airing maneuvers, the assessment of global and regional LV systolic and diastolic function, the diagnosis and management of acute RV dysfunction, and should be used in the decision to institute mechanical support for the failing allograft; moreover, intraoperative TEE can be used in diagnosing mechanical complications in the transplanted heart by assessing the atrial and PA anastomoses.

■ It is important to recognize the 2D echocardiographic and Doppler changes characteristic of transplant recipients, to avoid diagnostic errors.

■ TEE can be used to manage the hemodynamically unstable heart transplant recipient in the intensive care unit.

■ Echocardiography aids in the follow-up assessment of cardiac allograft function as one of the most important noninvasive methods of diagnosing transplant rejection.

REFERENCES

1. Hosenpud JD, Bennett LE, Keck BM, et al. The registry of the international society for heart and lung transplantation: eighteenth official report-2001. *J Heart Lung Transplant* 2001;20:805–815.
2. 2001 Annual Report of the U.S. Organ Procurement and Transplantation Network and the Scientific Registry for Transplant Recipients: Transplant Data 1991–2000. Department of Health and Human Services, Health Resources and Services Administration, Office of Special Programs, Division of Transplantation, Rockville, MD; United Network for Organ Sharing, Richmond, VA; University Renal Research and Education Association, Ann Arbor, MI. The data and analyses reported in the 2001 Annual Report of the U.S. Organ Procurement and Transplantation Network and the Scientific Registry of Transplant Recipients have been supplied by UNOS and URREA under contract with HHS.
3. Livi U, Bortolotti U, Luciani GB, et al. Donor shortage in heart transplantation. Is extension of donor age limits justified? *J Thorac Cardiovasc Surg* 1994;107:1346–1355.
4. Kron IL, Tribble CG, Kern JA, et al. Successful transplantation of marginally acceptable thoracic organs. *Ann Surg* 1993;217:518–524.
5. Vedrinne JM, Vedrinne C, Coronel B, et al. Transesophageal echocardiographic assessment of left ventricular function in brain-dead patients: are marginally acceptable hearts suitable for transplantation? *J Cardiothorac Vasc Anesth* 1996;10(6):708–712.
6. Stoddard MF, Longaker RA. The role of transesophageal echocardiography in cardiac donor screening. *Am Heart J* 1993;125:1676–1681.

7. Powner DJ, Hendrich A, Nyhuis A, et al. Changes in serum catecholamine levels in patients who are brain dead. *J Heart Lung Transplant* 1992;11:1046–1053.

8. Shivalkar B, Van Loon J, Wieland W, et al. Variable effects of explosive or gradual increase of intracranial pressure on myocardial structure and function. *Circulation* 1993;87(1):230–239.

9. Bittner HB, Chen EP, Biswas SS, et al. Right ventricular dysfunction after cardiac transplantation: primarily related to status of donor heart. *Ann Thorac Surg* 1999;68:1605–1611.

10. Seiler C, Laske A, Gallino A, et al. Echographic evaluation of left ventricular wall motion before and after transplantation. *J Heart Lung Transplant* 1992;11:867–874.

11. Young JB, Hauptman PJ, Naftel DC, et al. Determinants of early graft failure following cardiac transplantation, a 10 year multi-institutional, multi-variable analysis. *J Heart Lung Transplant* 2001;20:212.

12. Aziz S, Soine LA, Lewis SL, et al. Donor left ventricular hypertrophy increases risk for early graft failure. *Transpl Int* 1997;10:446–450.

13. Mudge GH, Goldstein S, Addonizio LJ, et al. 24th Bethesda conference: Cardiac transplantation. Task Force 3: Recipient guidelines/prioritization. *J Am Coll Cardiol* 1993;22(1):21–31.

14. Dinardo J. Anesthesia for heart, heart-lung and lung transplantation. In: *Anesthesia for Cardiac Surgery*, 2nd ed. New York: Appleton & Lange, 1998:201–239.

15. Bove A, Santamore W. Ventricular interdependence. *Prog Cardiovasc Dis* 1981;23:363–388.

16. Stevenson W, Stevenson L, Middlekauff H, et al. Improving survival for patients with advanced heart failure: a study of 737 consecutive patients. *J Am Coll Cardiol* 1995;26:1417–1423.

17. Dickstein M. Anesthesia for heart transplant. *Semin Cardiothorac Vasc Anesth* 1998;2:131–139.

18. Shanewise JS, Cheung AT, Aronson S, et al. ASE/SCA guidelines for performing a comprehensive intraoperative multiplane transesophageal echocardiography examination: recommendations of the American Society of Echocardiography Council for Intraoperative Echocardiography and the Society of Cardiovascular Anesthesiologists Task Force for certification in perioperative transesophageal echocardiography. *Anesth Analg* 1999;89:870–884.

19. Scalia GM, McCarthy PM, Savage RM, et al. Clinical utility of echocardiography in the management of implantable ventricular assist devices. *J Am Soc Echocardiogr* 2000;13:754–763.

20. Heerdt P, Pond C, Blessios G, et al. Inaccuracy of cardiac output determination by thermodilution during acute tricuspid regurgitation. *Ann Thorac Surg* 1992;53:706–708.

21. Orihashi K, Matsuura Y, Hamanaka Y, et al. Retained intracardiac air in open heart operations examined by transesophageal echocardiography. *Ann Thorac Surg* 1993;55(6):1467–1471.

22. Donica SK, Saunders CT, Ramsay MA. Right ventricular dysfunction during cardiac transplantation: an essential role for transesophageal echocardiography. *J Cardiothorac Vasc Anesth* 1992;6(6):775–776.

23. Kaye DM, Bergin P, Buckland M, et al. Value of postoperative assessment of cardiac allograft function by transesophageal echocardiography. *J Heart Lung Transplant* 1994;13:165–172.

24. Homans D, Ulstad V. Echocardiography in heart transplantation. In: Letourneau JG, Day DL, Ascher NL, eds. *Radiology of Organ Transplantation*. St. Louis: Mosby Year Book, 1991:308–321.

25. Suriani RJ. Transesophageal echocardiography during organ transplantation. *J Cardiothorac Vasc Anesth* 1998;12(6):686–694.

26. Spes CH, Tammen AR, Fraser AG, et al. Doppler analysis of pulmonary venous flow profiles in orthotopic heart transplant recipients: a comparison with mitral flow profiles and atrial function. *Z Kardiol* 1996;85:753–760.

27. Weitzman LB, Tinker WP, Krozon I, et al. The incidence and natural history of pericardial effusion after cardiac surgery; an echocardiographic study. *Circulation* 1984;69:506–511.

28. Valantine HA, Appleton CP, Hatle LK, et al. Influence of recipient atrial contraction on left ventricular filling dynamics of the transplanted heart assessed by Doppler echocardiography. *Am J Cardiol* 1987;59:1159–1163.

29. Bouchart F, Derumeaux G, Mouton-Schleifer D, et al. Conventional and total orthotopic cardiac transplantation: a comparative clinical and echocardiographical study. *Eur J Cardiothorac Surg* 1997;12:555–559.

30. St. Goar FG, Gibbons R, Schnittger I, et al. Left ventricular diastolic function—Doppler echocardiographic changes soon after cardiac transplantation. *Circulation* 1990;82:872–878.

31. Angermann CE, Spes CH, Tammen A, et al. Anatomic characteristics and valvular function of the transplanted heart: transthoracic versus transesophageal findings. *J Heart Lung Transplant* 1990;9:331–338.

32. Stobierska-Dzierzek B, Awad H, Michler RE. The evolving management of acute right-sided heart failure in cardiac transplant recipients. *J Am Coll Cardiol* 2001;38:923–931.

33. Kaul S, Tei C, Hopkins JM, et al. Assessment of right ventricular function using two-dimensional echocardiography. *Am Heart J* 1984;107:526–531.

34. Dickstein ML, Jackson DT, Dephia E, et al. Validation of maximum acceleration of pulmonary blood flow as an index of right ventricular function in the dog. In: *Proceedings of the Fourteenth Annual Meeting of the Society of Cardiovascular Anesthesiologists*. Boston, May 3–6, 1992:191.

35. Ellis J, Lichtor J, Feinstein S, et al. Right heart dysfunction, pulmonary embolism, and paradoxical embolization during liver transplantation. *Anesth Analg* 1989;68:777–782.

36. Louis EK, Rich S, Levitsky S, et al. Doppler echocardiographic demonstration of the differential effects of right ventricular pressure and volume overload on left ventricular geometry and filling. *J Am Coll Cardiol* 1992;19:84–90.

37. Arafa OE, Geiran OR, Andersen K, et al. Intraaortic balloon pumping for predominantly right ventricular failure after heart transplantation. *Ann Thorac Surg* 2000;70:1587–1593.

38. Barnard SP, Hasan A, Forty J, et al. Mechanical ventricular assistance for the failing right ventricle after cardiac transplantation. *Eur J Cardiothorac Surg* 1995;9:297–299.

39. Magliato KE, Trento A. Heart transplantation—surgical results. *Heart Failure Rev* 2001;6:213–219.

40. Polanco G, Jafri SM, Alam M, et al. Transesophageal echocardiographic findings in patients with orthotopic heart transplantation. *Chest* 1992;101:599–602.

41. Derumeaux G, Mouton-Schleifer D, Soyer R, et al. High incidence of left atrial thrombus detected by transesophageal echocardiography in heart transplant recipients. *Eur Heart J* 1995;16:120–125.

42. Wolfsohn AL, Walley VM, Masters RG, et al. The surgical anastomoses after orthotopic heart transplantation: clinical

complications and morphologic observations. *J Heart Lung Transplant* 1994;13:455–465.

43. Ulstad V, Braunlin E, Bass J, et al. Hemodynamically significant suture line obstruction immediately after heart transplantation. *J Heart Lung Transplant* 1992;11:834–836.

44. Bjerke RJ, Ziady GM, Matesic C, et al. Early diagnosis of acquired cor triatriatum after orthotopic heart transplantation. *J Heart Lung Transplant* 1992;11:1073–1077.

45. Oaks TE, Rayburn BK, Brown ME, et al. Acquired cor triatriatum after orthotopic cardiac transplantation. *Ann Thorac Surg* 1995;59:751–753.

46. Law Y, Belassario A, West L, et al. Hypertrophied native atrial tissue as a complication of orthotopic heart transplantation. *J Heart Lung Transplant* 1997;16:922–925.

47. Hanley PC, Tajik AJ, Hynes JK, et al. Diagnosis and classification of atrial septal aneurysm by two-dimensional echocardiography: report of 80 consecutive cases. *J Am Coll Cardiol* 1985;6:1370–1382.

48. Ouseph R, Stoddard MF, Lederer ED. Patent foramen ovale presenting as refractory hypoxemia after heart transplantation. *J Am Soc Echocardiogr* 1997;10:973–976.

49. Riberi A, Ambrosi P, Habib G, et al. Systemic embolism: a serious complication after cardiac transplantation avoidable by bicaval technique. *Eur J Cardiothorac Surg* 2001;19:307–312.

50. Goldstein JA, Harada A, Yagi Y. Hemodynamic importance of systolic ventricular interaction, augmented right atrial contractility and atrioventricular synchrony in acute right ventricular dysfunction. *J Am Coll Cardiol* 1990;16:181–189.

51. Reitz BA. Heart and lung transplantation. In: Baumgartner WA, Reitz BA, Achuff SC, eds. *Heart and Heart-Lung Transplantation.* Philadelphia: Saunders, 1990.

52. Deleuze PH, Benvenuti C, Mazucotelli JP, et al. Orthotopic cardiac transplantation with direct caval anastomosis: is it the optimal procedure? *J Thorac Cardiovasc Surg* 1995;109:731–737.

53. Leyh R, Jahnke AW, Kraatz EG, et al. Cardiovascular dynamics and dimensions after bicaval and standard cardiac transplantation. *Ann Thorac Surg* 1995;59:1495–1500.

54. Dreyfus G, Jebara V, Mihaileanu S, et al. Total orthotopic heart transplantation: an alternative to the standard technique. *Ann Thorac Surg* 1991;52(5):1181–1184.

55. Yacoub M, Mankad P, Ledingham S. Donor procurement and surgical techniques for cardiac transplantation. *Semin Thorac Cardiovasc Surg* 1990;2:153–161.

56. Dreyfus G, Jebara VA, Couetil JP, et al. Kinking of the pulmonary artery: a treatable cause of acute right ventricular failure after heart transplantation. *J Heart Lung Transplant* 1990;9:575–576.

57. De Marchena E, Futterman L, Wozniak P, et al. Pulmonary artery torsion: a potentially lethal complication after orthotopic heart transplantation. *J Heart Lung Transplant* 1989;8:499–502.

58. Stevenson LW, Dadourian BJ, Kobashigawa J. Mitral regurgitation after cardiac transplantation. *Am J Cardiol* 1987;60:119–122.

59. De Simone R, Lange R, Sack FU, et al. Atrioventricular valve insufficiency and atrial geometry after orthotopic heart transplantation. *Ann Thorac Surg* 1995;60:1686–1693.

60. Lombard FW, Swaminathan M, Podgoreanu MV, et al. The association of tricuspid regurgitation with right ventricular dysfunction after cardiac transplant surgery. *Anesth Analg* 2002;93:SCA66.

61. Chan MCY, Giannetti N, Kato T, et al. Severe tricuspid regurgitation after heart transplantation. *J Heart Lung Transplant* 2001;20:709–717.

62. Mugge A, Daniel WG, Herrmann G, et al. Quantification of tricuspid regurgitation by Doppler color flow mapping after cardiac transplantation. *Am J Cardiol* 1990;66(10):884–887.

63. Blanche C, Valenza M, Czer LSC, et al. Orthotopic heart transplantation with bicaval and pulmonary venous anastomoses. *Ann Thorac Surg* 1994;58:1505–1509.

64. Aziz TM, Burgess MI, Rahman AN, et al. Risk factors for tricuspid valve regurgitation after orthotopic heart transplantation. *Ann Thorac Surg* 1999;68(4):1247–1251.

65. Haverich A, Albes JM, Fahrenkamp G, et al. Intraoperative echocardiography to detect and prevent tricuspid valve regurgitation after heart transplantation. *Eur J Cardiothorac Surg* 1991;5(1):41–45.

66. Cladellas M, Abadal ML, Pons-Llado G, et al. Early transient multivalvular regurgitation detected by pulsed Doppler in cardiac transplantation. *Am J Cardiol* 1986;58(11):1122–1124.

67. Chatel D, Paquin S, Oroudji M, et al. Systolic anterior motion of the anterior mitral leaflet after heart transplantation. *Anesthesiology* 1999;91:1535–1537.

68. Akosah KO, Olsovsky M, Kirchberg D, et al. Dobutamine stress echocardiography predicts cardiac events in heart transplant recipients. *Circulation* 1996;94(Suppl. 9):283–288.

QUESTIONS

1. All of the following are characteristic two-dimensional (2D) echocardiographic changes in the left ventricle (LV) of transplant recipients *except*
   A. Septal wall motion abnormalities
   B. Residual posterior pericardial effusion
   C. Altered mediastinal anatomy requiring nonstandard TEE transducer locations and angles
   D. Decreased LV wall thickness, LV mass, and LV mass index

2. Which of the following statements regarding the assessment of LV diastolic function in the transplanted heart is true?
   A. Transmitral Doppler velocity profiles should be interpreted as usual in the transplanted heart.
   B. Diastolic indices should be measured in transmitral flow signals generated by recipient P waves occurring in late systole.
   C. Recipient P waves occurring from late diastole through midsystole result in decreased isovolumic relaxation time and pressure half-time.
   D. Transmitral Doppler inflow analysis should be corroborated with pulmonary vein flow analysis to differentiate LV diastolic dysfunction from left atrial (LA) dysfunction.

3. Which of the following echocardiographic findings supports an indication for right ventricular assist device (RVAD) implantation in a transplanted heart?
   A. An underfilled, hypocontractile right ventricle (RV)
   B. A dilated, hypocontractile RV after administration of protamine in a patient with no preexisting pulmonary hypertension
   C. A small hyperdynamic LV, dilated RV, and paradoxical interventricular septal shift, associated with marginal urine output, arrhythmias, or coagulopathy
   D. An acutely dilated, hypocontractile RV associated with electrocardiographic ST segment changes following TEE detection of echogenic material in the left heart

4. Which of the following statements regarding intraoperative TEE detection of LA spontaneous echo contrast (SEC) in the transplanted heart is false?
   A. It represents slow blood flow within the atria, caused by a combination of asynchronous contraction and atrial enlargement.
   B. Because it is not associated with systemic embolic events, further postoperative follow-up or therapy is not indicated.
   C. It is characterized by multiple swirling microechoes visible at normal gain settings, confined to the donor atrial component, and disappearing after passage through the mitral valve.
   D. The incidence of SEC is highest with the standard biatrial orthotopic heart transplant technique.

5. Characteristics of tricuspid regurgitation (TR) in transplant recipients include all of the following, *except*
   A. A ratio of the maximum area of the regurgitant jet to the right atrial area greater than 30% constitutes severe TR.
   B. Regurgitation is not associated with the incidence and severity of RV dysfunction.
   C. Occurs with high frequency immediately after heart transplantation, is usually moderate, with an eccentric jet pointing toward the interatrial septum.
   D. The incidence and severity of TR are reduced with bicaval anastomotic technique.

CHAPTER 37 Assessment in Cardiac Intervention

Domnik Wiktor ■ E. Murat Tuzcu ■ Patrick L. Whitlow ■ Robert M. Savage

Although many challenges remain in the field of percutaneous coronary intervention (PCI), the lessons learned over the last three decades have generally made these procedures very safe. More than 1 million PCIs are performed annually in the United States. During this time, noncoronary cardiac intervention in adult patients was restricted largely to the treatment of aortic, mitral, and pulmonic stenosis, using balloon valvuloplasty techniques. However, over the last 10 years, the field of noncoronary cardiac intervention has rapidly evolved and its scope has extended well beyond the treatment of stenotic valves.

There is no doubt that the dominant force behind these new developments is the proliferation of new technologies. In concert with these developments has come the realization that surgical therapies can be replaced by effective endovascular alternatives. In fact, a number of the newer endovascular technologies have been initiated by cardiothoracic surgeons, seeking to replicate their surgical techniques, using endovascular devices. This burgeoning field presents a tremendous opportunity to offer novel and alternative therapies, but significant challenges, too. Compared with coronary artery disease, the disease states being treated during noncoronary cardiac intervention vary significantly, which necessitates a multidisciplinary approach to patient management. Another challenge is the requirement for high-quality echocardiographic imaging during preprocedural evaluation, the procedure itself (Table 37.1), and the postprocedural management of these patients. Although the development of intracardiac echocardiography (ICE) has provided some autonomy for the interventionalist during some procedures, a successful noncoronary cardiac intervention program cannot be built without the support and expertise offered by our echocardiographer colleagues.

TABLE 37.1	Utility of Various Echocardiographic Imaging Modalities During Noncoronary Cardiac Intervention		
Procedure	**Echocardiographic Technique**		
	TTE	TEE	ICE
Alcohol septal ablation	++++	–	–
ASD closure	–	++++	++++
PFO closure	–	++	++
Aortic valve replacement	–	++	++
MV repair	–	++++	–
Annuloplasty	–	++++	+++
Edge-to-edge repair	–	++++	++
LAA exclusion	–	++++	+++
Pericardiocentesis	++++	++	
Myocardial biopsy	++++	–	+++
Mitral balloon valvuloplasty	++++	++++	–
Radiofrequency ablation	–	++	++

TTE, transthoracic echo; TEE, transesophageal echo; LAA, left atrial appendage; ++++, vital for the procedure; ++, helpful for the procedure; –, not helpful/not required for the procedure.

In this chapter, the principal noncoronary cardiac interventions that are currently performed by cardiac interventionalists requiring echocardiographic guidance are described. Some of these are well-established techniques with good clinical data supporting their efficacy. Others are at an early stage of development and, while holding great promise, further study is required before they can gain widespread acceptance.

PERCUTANEOUS AORTIC VALVE REPLACEMENT

For patients with acquired calcific aortic stenosis, aortic valve replacement is the treatment of choice, providing effective symptomatic relief and a survival benefit (1). However, some patients are not deemed operative candidates due to the presence of serious comorbid conditions that predict high operative mortality. The introduction of percutaneous balloon aortic valvuloplasty (PBAV) in the mid-1980s offered a new therapeutic option for these patients. While the short-term outcomes of PBAV were encouraging, long-term follow-up demonstrated near 100% restenosis rates at 2 years (2). PBAV is currently used only to provide palliation or to serve as a bridge toward aortic valve replacement. The limitation of PBAV has provided the impetus to develop percutaneous aortic valve replacement techniques for the treatment of patients with severe aortic stenosis not amenable to surgical valve replacement.

Following ex vivo and animal testing of a variety of valve bioprostheses and techniques, Cribier et al. (3,4) performed the first percutaneous transcatheter implantation of an aortic valve prosthesis (Percutaneous Valve Technologies, Inc., Fort Lee, NJ) in April 2002. The valve consists of three bovine (subsequently changed to equine) pericardial leaflets that are sutured to a stainless

steel stent frame (14 mm long, 21–23 mm diameter) (Fig. 37.1A), which in turn is mounted on a commercially available Z-MED II (NuMED, Inc., Hopkinton NY, USA; 30 mm long, 23 mm diameter) balloon valvuloplasty catheter (Fig. 37.1B). In brief, the prosthesis is introduced over a continuous wire loop (360 cm stiff guidewire) extending from the femoral vein to the right atrium (RA), across the septum into the left atrium (LA), mitral valve (MV), left ventricle (LV), aorta, and femoral artery. To prepare for valve placement, ballon aortic valvuloplasty (BAV) is performed (23 mm balloon). Currently, a 24 Fr sheath in the femoral vein is required to allow delivery of the aortic valve prosthesis, which is positioned at the midsection of the native aortic valve, using the valvular calcifications as a marker. Rapid and full inflation of the balloon followed by rapid deflation results in delivery of the valve prosthesis (Fig. 37.2). To date, a total of 14 such procedures have been performed in 12 patients with functional class IV symptoms and two patients with cardiogenic shock (unpublished data). Successful implantation of the prosthesis was achieved in 12 patients (86%). Successful implantation is associated with an impressive reduction of the mean aortic gradient (44 ± 13 to 5 ± 0.5 mm Hg) and increase in aortic valve area (0.5 ± 0.1 to 1.7 ± 0.1 cm²). There was one procedural death, and four late noncardiac deaths. The latter finding is not surprising, given the clinical context in which device implantation is performed in these patients.

All of these procedures are performed under transesophageal echocardiography (TEE) guidance, and both transthoracic echocardiography (TTE) and TEE are essential in the accurate follow-up of these patients. During the procedure, TEE is most helpful in assessing outcome following implantation of the prosthesis. TEE allows measurement of the stent diameter, which should be between 21 and 23 mm, and assessment of

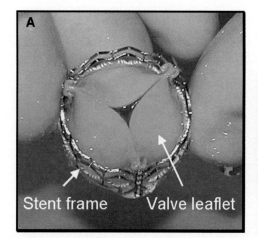
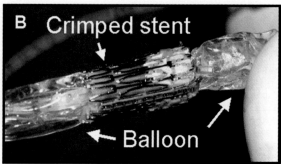

Figure 37.1. **A:** Appearance of prosthetic aortic heart valve when expanded. Valve consists of three leaflets attached to a metal stent. **B:** Appearance of valve when crimped onto balloon for delivery into patient via femoral sheath. (Reproduced from Eltchaninoff H, et al. *J Interv Cardiol* 2003;16(6):515–521, with permission.)

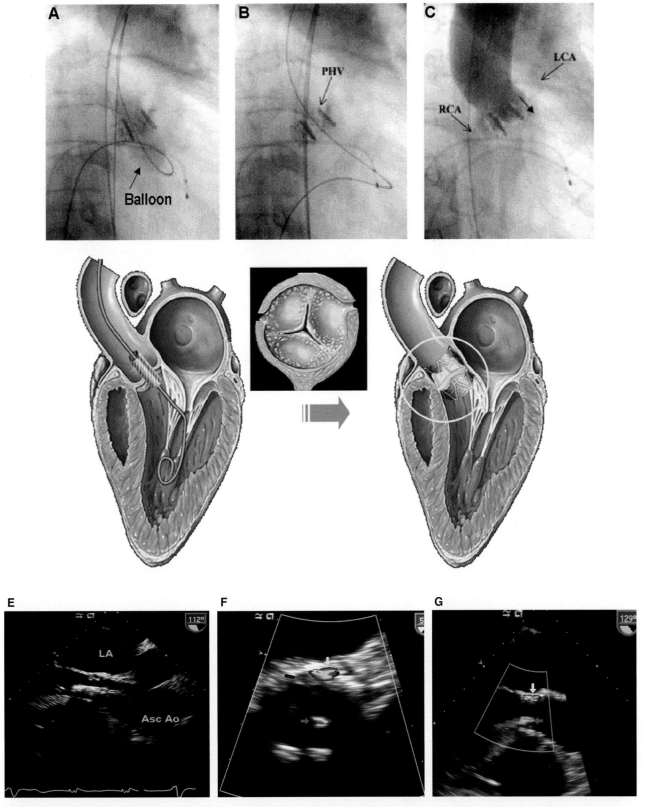

Figure 37.2. **A:** The prosthetic aortic valve is deployed by inflation of the 23 mm balloon on which the stent valve is delivered. **B:** Radiographic appearance of prosthetic valve following deployment. **C:** Aortography following placement of prosthetic aortic valve demonstrating patent right and left coronary arteries above the prosthesis. (Reproduced from Cribier A, et al. *Circulation* 2002;106:3006–3008, with permission.) **D:** Illustration depicting positioning of undeployed device across native aortic valve and subsequent appearance after deployment. **E:** TEE guidance images of undeployed device positioned for deployment. **F:** TEE assessment of valvular (*pink arrow*) and perivalvular aortic regurgitation (*yellow arrow*) in short-and long-axis views (**G**).

stent geometry, which should ideally be circular. TEE is also helpful in assessing paravalvular regurgitation, which reflects failure of apposition of the prosthesis with the native calcific valve. Severe paravalvular regurgitation (∼ +3) was present in one third of patients immediately following placement of the aortic prosthesis. Along with this, the increasing use of three-dimensional (3D) TEE enables more precise placement of stents as well as affording an "en face" or surgical view of the aortic valve after deployment. Follow-up TEE and TTE allow assessment of the prosthetic leaflets, valvular and paravalvular regurgitation, planimetry of the aortic valve area, aortic valve gradients, and LV function.

MITRAL VALVE REPAIR

Percutaneous catheter-based approaches to the management of functional and structural mitral regurgitation (MR) in human subjects are at an early stage of development but represent a potentially dramatic advance (5). Functional MR has a complicated pathogenesis but is felt to result from mitral annular dilatation and altered ventricular geometry, which causes incomplete leaflet coaptation. The resultant MR begets further LV dysfunction and mitral annular dilatation, setting up a vicious perpetuating spiral of progressive MR and LV failure. Surgical repair generally involves a ring- or suture-based mitral annuloplasty, which reshapes the annulus and promotes leaflet coaptation. Several groups have attempted to mimic this strategy, using percutaneous methods by exploiting the relationship of the coronary sinus and great cardiac vein with the posterior aspect of the mitral annulus (Fig. 37.3). Although different types of device are in development

(C-Cure, ev3/Mitralife, Santa Rosa, CA, USA; Viacor, Inc., Wilmington, MA), in essence, they each consist of a metal constraint device that is inserted into the coronary sinus, using the internal jugular venous access site. The goal is to apply tension on the underlying annulus, resulting in an approximately 25% reduction in annular diameter. TEE guidance during the procedure is essential to monitoring the annular diameter and the associated change in MR. Published data have been limited to small animal studies, where insertion of the device was associated with an impressive reduction in mitral annular diameter (4.17 ± 0.14 to 3.24 ± 0.11 cm), severity of MR, and a consistent improvement in hemodynamic assessments (cardiac output, pulmonary capillary wedge pressure) (6). While this therapy is promising, both short- and long-term clinical data are required. The complexity of functional MR mandates a clear demonstration of efficacy in human subjects before acceptance of the technique. Additionally, a number of safety concerns exist including coronary sinus perforation and thrombosis, coronary ischemia secondary to impingement on the circumflex artery, and arrhythmias. These complications were not seen in the early human experience of a group in Venezuela, but given the small sample size, caution is still warranted (unpublished data).

Structural MR is caused by pathology of the valve leaflets or supporting structures (i.e., chordae, papillary muscles). Since the early 1990s, Alfieri (7) has championed the double-orifice technique of surgical mitral repair for more complicated cases of structural MR with excellent clinical outcomes. Most commonly, the technique involves suturing the middle scallops of the anterior and posterior mitral leaflets, and it is used to treat bileaflet or anterior leaflet prolapse (7). Building on this technique, a percutaneous catheter-based edge-to-edge technique using a V-shaped, polyester-covered metal clip for repair of structural MR has been developed and undergone Phase I safety and feasibility and long-term durability testing.(Evalve, Inc., Redwood City, CA) (Fig. 37.4) (8,9). The procedure is outlined in Figures 37.5 and 37.6. In summary, using the femoral venous access site, and transseptal puncture, a steerable guiding catheter is placed in the LA above the MV. The V clip is attached to the delivery catheter and then advanced through the guide and opened in the LA. The opened clip crosses the MV perpendicular to the line of leaflet coaptation and in the same vertical plane as the middle scallops of the anterior and posterior leaflets. Once in the LV and below the free edges of the leaflets, the clip is retracted and the leaflets grasped. A thorough two-dimensional (2D) and color Doppler echocardiographic assessment is performed to confirm adequate placement with complete or near-complete elimination of MR. In all cases, complex spatial orientation and optimal clip placement are best facilitated by simultaneous bi-plane imaging of the MV afforded by 3D TEE.

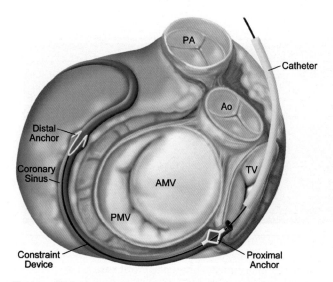

Figure 37.3. Schematic of percutaneous mitral annular reduction technique for treatment of functional MR. A metal constraint device is positioned in coronary sinus opposite the posterior aspect of the MV.

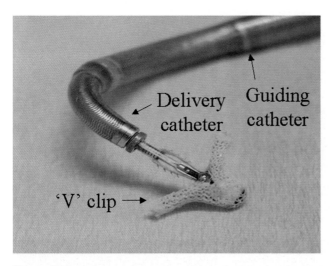

Figure 37.4. Polyester covered metal V-shaped clip used to perform percutaneous edge-to-edge repair of MV.

If device placement is unsatisfactory, the device may be released and redeployed until successful placement is achieved. The importance of TEE guidance during each step of this procedure cannot be overemphasized

(Fig. 37.6). (9,10). Of 107 patients with 3 to 4+ MR in the EVEREST cohort treated with the MitraClip system, 79 achieved acute postprocedural success with 64% of these patients eventually being discharged from the hospital with MR < or = 1+ (9). The technical expertise required by both the interventionalist and echocardiographer for this procedure is significantly greater than that for the mitral annular reduction technique. Clearly, this technique is in its infancy, and despite encouraging safety, efficacy, and durability data, extensive clinical testing will be required before the technique can be applied in routine clinical practice. It is likely that the ultimate success of percutaneous treatments for structural MR will be determined by the ability to use endovascular techniques to treat both the structural defect *and* mitral annular dilatation, as currently practiced by cardiothoracic surgeons during most surgical repairs. While current technologies offer some promise toward that end, their niche will initially be restricted to nonsurgical candidates. Beyond this patient group, the burden of proof will rest heavily on percutaneous techniques to prove their equivalency or superiority to established surgical techniques.

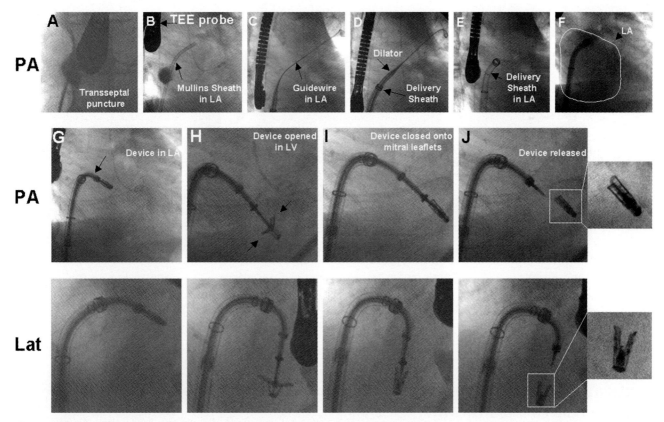

Figure 37.5. Fluoroscopic procedural images from patient undergoing endovascular edge-to-edge repair of MV using E-valve system. **A–F:** Following transseptal puncture (**A**), a Mullins sheath is placed in the LA (**B**). A stiff guidewire is placed in the LA and the Mullins sheath is exchanged for a 24 Fr guide (**C–E**). The device is advanced through the guide into the LA (**G**), opened (**H**), advanced across the MV, retracted against the MV, and then closed, grasping the leaflets (**G–I**). Once adequate device placement is determined by echocardiography, the device is released (**J**).

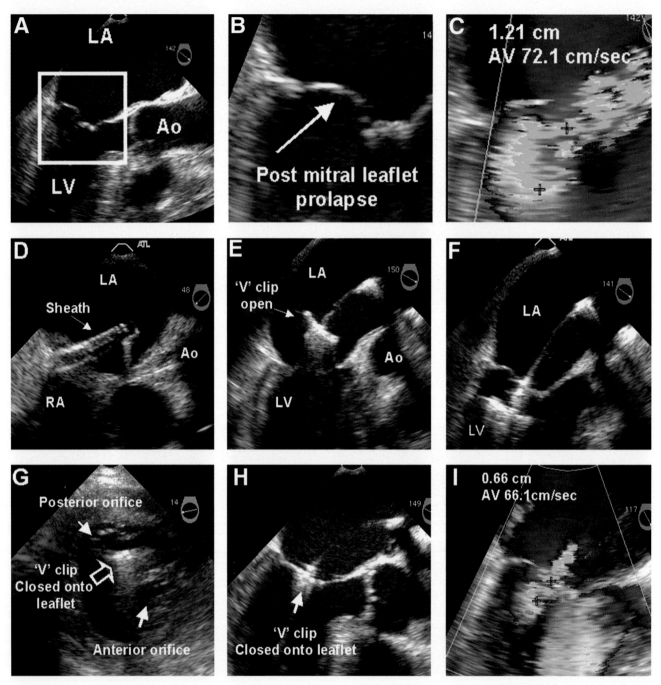

Figure 37.6. TEE images from same patient described in Figure 37.5. **A–C:** Images demonstrating prolapse of the posterior mitral leaflet and associated anteriorly directed MR at baseline. **D:** Guide catheter in LA. **E,F:** Device opened in LA and advanced into LV. **G,H:** Transgastric (**G**) and esophageal (**H**) views demonstrating appearance of MV, following capture of the middle scallops of the anterior and posterior mitral leaflets by the V clip. **I:** Color Doppler of mitral flow following device placement.

NONSURGICAL SEPTAL REDUCTION FOR HYPERTROPHIC CARDIOMYOPATHY

Significant left ventricular outflow tract (LVOT) obstruction is present in 10% of patients with hypertrophic cardiomyopathy (HCM), and is believed to contribute significantly to symptoms of angina, dyspnea on exertion, and syncope (11). Until the early 1990s, surgical myectomy was the only therapeutic option for patients who were refractory to medical therapy. At this time, observational data regarding implantation of DDD pacemakers in these patients showed some promise, but subsequent randomized studies failed to demonstrate any objective improvement in functional status, and this therapy has largely been abandoned (12,13). In 1995, Sigwart (14) reported a novel therapeutic approach that involved the injection of absolute alcohol into the first septal perforator branch, producing a circumscribed myocardial infarction involving the portion of septum in contact with the anterior mitral leaflet during the typical systolic anterior motion (SAM) of the leaflet observed in HCM (Fig. 37.7). Clinical outcomes were impressive, and subsequent larger series, involving hundreds of patients, demonstrated an early and sustained reduction in LVOT gradient (90%), and resolution or effective relief of symptoms in greater than 90% of patients during long-term follow-up (15,16).

The majority of operators use TTE guidance for alcohol septal ablation procedures. The critical function of TTE guidance is to help select the target septal perforator, supplying the area of septum in contact with the anterior mitral leaflet during SAM. This is sometimes challenging because of the tremendous interindividual variation in the number, distribution, and overlap in distribution of the septal perforator branches. Following inflation of a balloon in the selected perforator branch, an echo contrast agent is injected through the balloon lumen

(diluted 1:8 with saline). Imaging from the apical and parasternal views allows a determination of the myocardium perfused by the septal perforator branch (Fig. 37.7D). In some patients, this procedure may have to be repeated with the balloon in various branches or sub-branches to confirm the optimal location for injection of alcohol. By more effective localization of the targeted myocardium, the use of myocardial contrast echocardiography (MCE) during alcohol ablation has been associated with improved hemodynamic results, despite a reduction in the total infarct size (15). The safety of the procedure is improved by identifying perforator branches whose perfusion distribution involves the posterior free wall and papillary muscles, making them unsuitable targets. Additionally, the incidence of complete heart block, which occurred in 20% to 40% of patients in an early series, has been reduced to 5% to 10% in a series using MCE guidance (17). TTE may also be used to monitor the effects of the procedure on the LVOT gradient at rest and during provocation (e.g., amyl nitrate, post-PVC), and to document the resolution or improvement in SAM and the associated posteriorly directed MR (Fig. 37.8). In summary, TTE

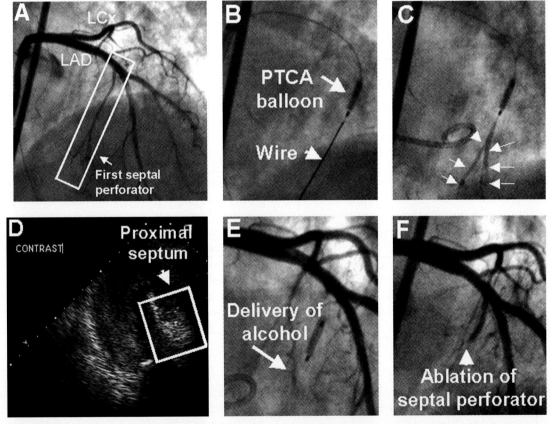

Figure 37.7. A: Angiogram of left coronary artery demonstrating location of the first septal perforator branch of the left anterior descending artery (LAD). **B:** The septal perforator branch is wired and a balloon positioned in the proximal portion of the vessel. **C:** Injection of contrast through the balloon demonstrates anatomy of first septal perforator branch. **D:** Echo contrast injection through the balloon confirms that the selected septal perforator branch perfused the proximal septum and is an appropriate target for alcohol ablation. **E:** Absolute alcohol is injected through the balloon. **F:** Final appearance of the perforator branch following alcohol ablation. LAD, left anterior descending artery; LCx, left circumflex artery; PTCA, percutaneous transluminal coronary angioplasty.

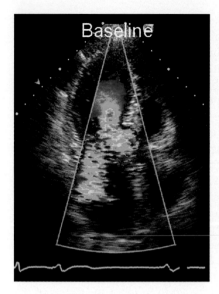
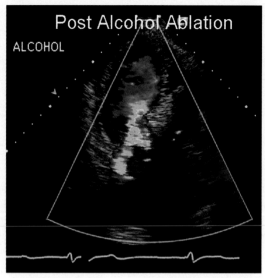

Figure 37.8. A: Apical five-chamber view demonstrating severe posteriorly directed jet of MR at baseline in patients undergoing alcohol ablation. **B:** Marked reduction in MR immediately following alcohol ablation due to resolution of SAM of the anterior mitral leaflet.

and MCE make alcohol septal ablation a safer and more effective procedure. They should be regarded as mandatory components of the technique.

Patent Foramen Ovale/Atrial Septal Defect Closure

Mills and King (18) performed the first nonoperative atrial septal defect (ASD) closure in 1976, using a double-umbrella device. Although further attempts to develop more user-friendly devices were made by individual investigators, the procedure did not gain acceptance until the development of the Clamshell device in the late 1980s. Despite the initial technical limitations of this device (metal arm fractures and high rates of residual shunting), it formed the basis for further generations of similar devices and other novel devices that have been successfully employed in 40,000 percutaneous ASD closures (secundum-type). The late 1980s also saw an appreciation of the role of patent foramen ovale (PFO) in cryptogenic stroke due to paradoxical embolism (19). Many of these same ASD closure devices were applied in PFO closure, and other specific devices for PFO closure were developed.

The ASD/PFO closure devices currently in use are double-disc devices, with right and LA disc components that oppose the atrial septum, and a central connecting waist element that rests in the PFO or ASD joining the discs (Fig. 37.9). The discs are composed of a metal frame (most commonly nitinol) that supports a fabric. Both components are important in promoting the formation of a thrombotic layer on the surface of the device with subsequent endothelialization of the device surfaces, which results in closure of the defect. In the United States, the CardioSEAL/STARFlex and Amplatzer PFO/ASD occluder devices represent the majority of the devices used. The basic technique for ASD/PFO closure utilizing the former devices is illustrated in Figure 37.10. Essentially, the defect is crossed with a diagnostic catheter, which facilitates the placement of a supportive wire in the pulmonary

vein. Over this wire, a delivery sheath is placed in the LA. Through this sheath, the device attached to a delivery catheter is passed and the LA disc is deployed in the LA. Withdrawal of the sheath and delivery catheter together results in the LA disc abutting the atrial septum. At this point, the sheath is withdrawn, which results in deployment of the RA disc. Detachment of the delivery catheter from the device results in final release of the device. The use of adjunctive imaging modalities during percutaneous PFO/ASD closure is variable, both with respect to usage and the type of adjunctive imaging utilized. TEE and ICE are the best imaging modalities to guide these procedures. ICE is a relatively new imaging modality that is performed by the interventionalist. Potential advantages over TEE include elimination of the need for sedation or general anesthesia required with TEE, improved visualization of the inferoposterior portion of the interatrial septum, and greater autonomy for the interventionalist. The system consists of a 10 Fr ultrasound catheter (AcunavTM) transducer that is interfaced with the SequioaTM, AspenTM, or CypressTM ultrasound imaging platforms. Within the catheter tip, there is a multifrequency 5.0 to 10 MHz, 64-element vector, phased array transducer that provides high-resolution 2D and Doppler imaging (including color Doppler). The catheter is introduced through an 11 Fr sheath in the femoral vein and positioned in the RA to visualize the RA and LA and atrial septum.

For ASD closure, adjunctive TEE or ICE during percutaneous closure is essential (Fig. 37.11). Prior to closure, the stretch balloon diameter of the defect is determined by both fluoroscopy and echo (Fig. 37.11E). This is a critical measurement because it determines the device size to use. With the balloon inflated across the defect, it is also imperative to examine the remainder of the septum using 2D imaging and color Doppler to ensure the absence of additional defects, which may be present in up to 15% of cases (Fig. 37.11F). Although fluoroscopy and tactile sensation are usually adequate to determine the appropriate

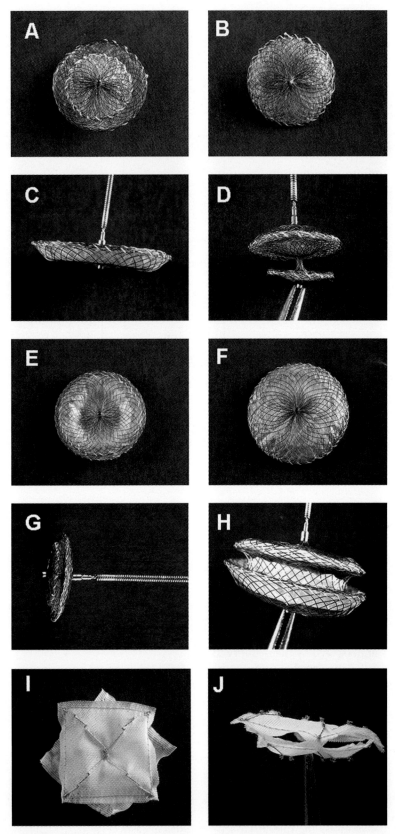

Figure 37.9. Sample of PFO/ASD devices most commonly used in the United States. **A–D:** Amplatzer PFO occluder device as viewed from LA side (**A**), RA side (**B**), in side profile (**C**), and in side profile with both atrial components pulled apart to demonstrate the waist portion of the device (**D**). **E,F:** Amplatzer ASD occluder device as viewed from LA side (**E**), RA side (**F**), in side profile (**G**), and in side profile with both atrial components pulled apart to demonstrate the waist portion of the device (**H**). **I,J:** CardioSEAL device in en-face view (**I**) and in side profile (**J**).

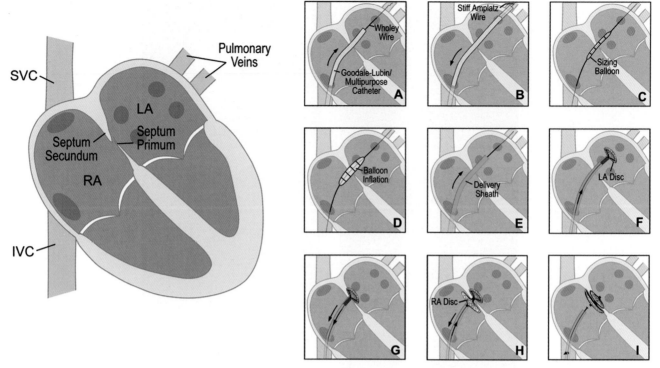

Figure 37.10. Schematic illustration of the technique used to perform percutaneous PFO/ASD closure (device illustrated is Amplatzer PFO device). **A,B:** A catheter is used to cross the defect, and a supportive wire is positioned in the pulmonary vein. **C,D:** The size of the defect is determined using a sizing balloon inflated across the defect. **E:** The delivery sheath is positioned in the LA. **F–H:** The LA and RA components of the device are deployed across the defect. **I:** The device is released by detaching the device from the delivery catheter. (Reproduced from Casserly I, et al. Percutaneous patent foramen ovale and atrial septal defects. In: *Manual of Peripheral Vascular Intervention.* Lippincott Williams & Wilkins, with permission.)

location for deployment of the right and LA components of the device, echo guidance provides additional confirmation. Following deployment of the device and prior to release, TEE or ICE provides invaluable information regarding the appropriate positioning of the device. To be confident of device stability, it is imperative to visualize the atrial septum between both the right and LA components superoanterior and inferoposterior to the defect. The importance of this step is underscored by the inability to reliably retrieve the device following detachment from the delivery catheter. Additionally, echo guidance allows the operator to determine if adjacent vital structures (e.g., right upper pulmonary vein, MV, coronary sinus, and superior/inferior vena cava) are impinged by the device. This is particularly relevant in the closure of large ASDs where the LA disc diameter approaches the diameter of the atrial septum.

For PFO closure, adjunctive imaging is very helpful but probably not essential, provided the patient has had a preprocedural TEE to adequately assess the interatrial septum and that the operator has an adequate procedural experience. The presence of a long interatrial tunnel and an associated atrial septal aneurysm is generally an indication to use a larger device for PFO closure. Adjunctive imaging certainly provides reassurance of appropriate

device placement prior to release of the device, and is always useful where untoward events occur during the procedure. For example, occasionally, the RA component of the device becomes entangled in a prominent eustachian valve or Chiari network. A steerable catheter can be used to displace these structures under echo guidance.

Left Atrial Appendage Occlusion

Atrial fibrillation (AF) is associated with a threefold to fivefold increase in stroke risk in patients aged 50 to 90 years (20). Due to the increased prevalence of AF with age (reaching ~10% in octogenarians), the percentage of strokes attributable to AF also increases with age, reaching 23.5% in persons aged 80 to 89 years (20). With the decline in rheumatic valvular disease in developed countries, the majority of AF is now related to nonvalvular etiologies. In patients with nonvalvular AF, the left atrial appendage (LAA) is the location of LA thrombus in approximately 90% of cases (Fig. 37.12) (21). While oral anticoagulation with warfarin (achieving an INR 2-3) has demonstrated efficacy in reducing the risk of stroke in this population (22), issues related to maintenance of a therapeutic INR and bleeding complications limit the efficacy and application of this therapy. This is underscored by a 1996 survey

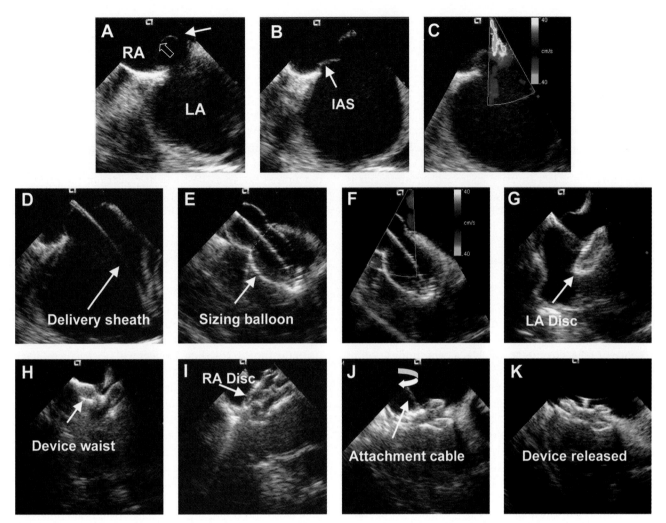

Figure 37.11. Series of images obtained using ICE during closure of a secundum type ASD with an Amplatzer ASD occluder. **A–C:** Baseline images demonstrating mobile interatrial septum (*open arrow*) with secundum type ASD. **D:** Delivery sheath is positioned in the LA. **E:** Sizing balloon positioned across defect with measurement of waist diameter. **F:** Color flow of septum during balloon inflation to examine for additional defects. **G–I:** Deployment of right and LA components of the device across the defect. **J–K:** Device is detached from delivery cable by counterclockwise rotation of cable. (Reproduced from Casserly I, et al. Percutaneous patent foramen ovale and atrial septal defects. In: *Manual of Peripheral Vascular Intervention*. Lippincott Williams & Wilkins, with permission.)

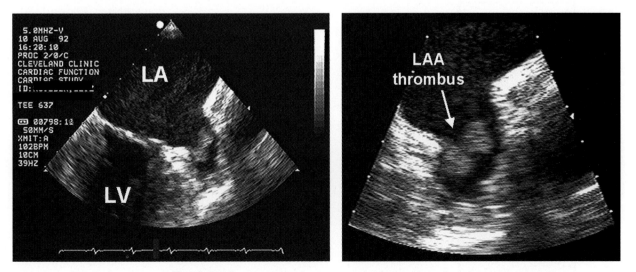

Figure 37.12. TTE image from patient with LAA thrombus.

in which the utilization rate for warfarin in patients with AF who met criteria for anticoagulation was only 33% (23). This highlights the need for alternative therapies to prevent stroke from embolization of LAA thrombus in the group of patients who are currently inadequately treated.

Since the late 1940s, surgeons have performed exclusion of the LAA during MV surgery in patients with mitral stenosis (MS) in an effort to reduce the risk of subsequent stroke (24). More recently, thoracoscopic closure techniques have been reported for isolated LAA exclusion (25). However, a less invasive endovascular approach is required if the strategy of LAA exclusion is to be applied to a broader population of AF patients. To this end, two endovascular LAA exclusion devices have been developed that are at different stages of clinical testing (Percutaneous Left Atrial Appendage Transcatheter Occlusion device, PLAATOTM, Appriva Medical; WATCHMAN left atrial appendage filter system [26,27]) (Fig. 37.13). The basic technique is similar for both devices, and current protocols mandate TEE guidance during the procedure. Prior to the procedure, TEE is also required to document the absence of LAA thrombus, which is a contraindication to device implantation. Following a transseptal puncture, a specially designed 12 Fr delivery sheath is positioned in the LAA appendage. An angiogram of the appendage in orthogonal views, together with TEE measurements of the diameter of the LAA ostium, allows a determination of the device size to be used (Fig. 37.14). Generally, the device size chosen is 20% to 40% larger than the LAA orifice diameter. The diameter of the LAA orifice can vary markedly and enlarges significantly in patients with AF. In a postmortem study of 220 patients, the maximal and minimal diameters of the ostium varied from 5 to 27 mm and 10 to 40 mm, respectively (28). Although the device shapes and designs differ, they both consist of a self-expandable nitinol metal frame and a covering membrane material (ePTFE in the PLATTO device, and PET in the WATCHMAN device). The device is delivered through the sheath and released into the appendage. Following angiographic and TEE confirmation of appropriate device position and adequate sealing of the appendage, the device is detached from its delivery catheter. At a small number of centers in the United States and Europe, operators have used the Amplatzer ASD occluder device in a small group of patients for LAA exclusion (n = 16) with adequate outcomes (29). In a 103- patient registry of the PLAATO device, successful implantation was achieved in 98% of cases (unpublished data). In follow-up, there were two strokes at 6 months, and three nonprocedure/nondevice-related deaths within the first year (30–32). Clinical experience with the WATCHMAN device is limited to a registry of 38 patients from Germany. Successful implantation was achieved in 30 patients (79%), which likely reflects a learning curve with the technique, and the need to refine the device and associated equipment (33). Clinical follow-up with this device is forthcoming.

In the short term, these devices will be strictly reserved for patients who have contraindications to long-term anticoagulant therapy and are deemed at high risk for stroke from AF (presence of one or more of the following risk factors: hypertension, heart failure, history of transient ischemic attack [TIA]/stroke, diabetes mellitus, and clinical coronary artery disease)(32). Broader application will require that these devices be tested in a head-to-head fashion against warfarin for patients who are warfarin eligible. Such studies are necessary to determine if percutaneous LAA exclusion offers any advantages over oral anticoagulation, or if any subgroups (e.g., high-risk groups) benefit from this more invasive approach to stroke prevention in AF patients (33).

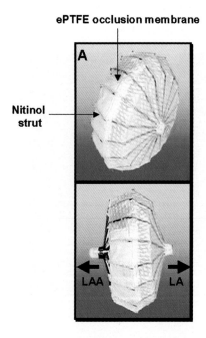

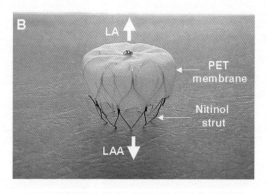

Figure 37.13. Illustration of the PLAATO (percutaneous LAA transcatheter occlusion) (**A**) and WATCHMAN devices (**B**) under investigation for percutaneous LA appendage occlusion. (Reproduced with modification from Sievert H, et al. *Circulation* 2002;105(16): 1887–1889.)

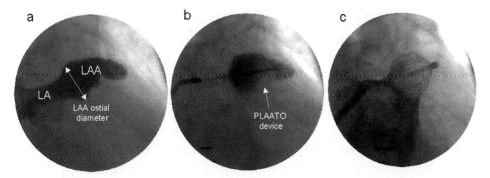

Figure 37.14. Angiography of LAA and LA during implantation of LAA occlusion device. **A:** Baseline LAA angiogram allows determination of the diameter of LAA ostium. **B:** Injection of contrast through a lumen in the device documents stagnation of contrast distal to the sealing surface of the device. **C:** Angiography in LA following release of device documents sealing of the appendage. (Reproduced from Sievert H, et al. *Circulation* 2002;105:1887–1889, with permission.)

PERICARDIOCENTESIS FOR CARDIAC TAMPONADE

The echocardiographic diagnosis of cardiac tamponade in the presence of a large pericardial effusion is established by specific criteria (Fig. 37.15A). These include LA or RA wall inversion, right ventricular (RV) diastolic inversion, hepatic plethora (Fig. 37.15B), and respiratory variation in the flow and volume of the hepatic vein (Fig. 37.15C) and cardiac chambers. The use of echocardiography to guide pericardiocentesis has been previously reported and validated by Armstrong et al. (34). The procedure is performed with the patient in the supine position with the effusion localized by TEE or TTE. The puncture site is chosen based on direct distance to the pericardial effusion and vicinity of vital structures (RV, RA, coronary arteries,

and internal mammary artery). The most frequent approach is subcostal; however, it may also be parasternal or apical. The advance of the aspiration needle is guided and monitored echocardiographically. Between 1996 and 2002, 450 echo-guided pericardiocenteses were performed at the Cleveland Clinic. Complications included pneumothorax (1), vasovagal reaction (2), RV puncture (3), and pneumopericardium (1). There were no iatrogenic procedure-related deaths. The success of the procedure was monitored echocardiographically (Fig. 37.15D).

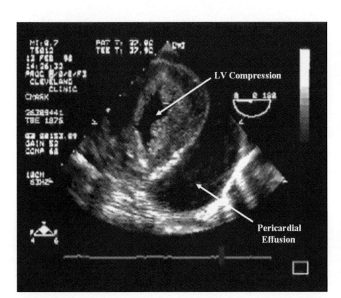

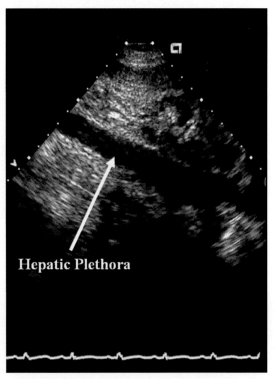

Figure 37.15. TTE and TEE are utilized in the diagnosis of cardiac tamponade and the guidance of percutaneous pericardiocentesis. **A:** The pericardial effusion and ventricular compression associated with cardiac tamponade are noted. **B:** Hepatic vein engorgement is consistent with the diagnosis of tamponade.

(Continued)

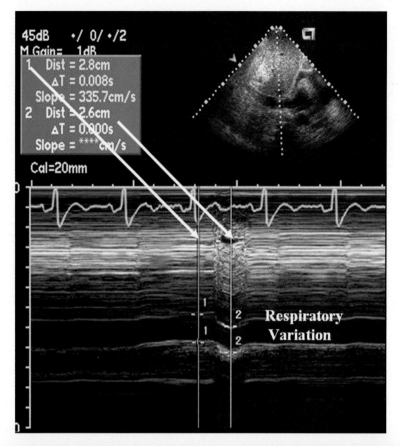

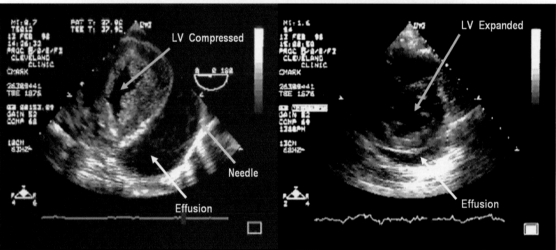

Figure 37.15. (*Continued*). **C:** M-mode echo demonstrates the respirator dependence on mediastinal blood flow. **D:** Comparison of effusion during the pericardiocentesis and postpericardiocentesis.

MYOCARDIAL BIOPSY

Endocardial biopsy is a diagnostic intervention, which is used most commonly to establish the clinical course of rejection following orthotopic heart transplantation. However, as illustrated in Figure 37.16, it is also used diagnostically in patients with cardiac masses, infiltrative cardiac disease, restrictive cardiomyopathy, chemotherapy-induced cardiomyopathy, and other diagnostic dilemmas

involving the heart (cardiac sarcoid and amyloid) (35–38). Endomyocardial biopsy has been associated with perforation of the RA and ventricle, and trauma to the tricuspid valve. Tricuspid regurgitation following myocardial biopsy has been reported in up to 85% of heart transplant recipients and is associated with traumatic flail (8%–15%), perforated leaflets, and RV dysfunction secondary to pulmonary hypertension (39–41). To reduce the incidence of complications associated with this necessary diagnostic,

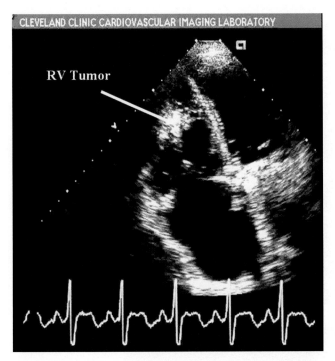

Figure 37.16. RV tumor demonstrated using apical four-chamber TTE.

the first reported use of echo-guided endomyocardial biopsy was reported in 1988 (41). Pandian et al. (38) have utilized ICE to guide endomyocardial biopsy.

MITRAL BALLOON VALVULOTOMY

The value of TEE in patients with MS undergoing percutaneous valvuloplasty has long been established in the diagnosis of LAA thrombi, grading the severity of MS

and regurgitation, and assessing the results of balloon valvuloplasty (42). Wilkins et al. (43) first reported the ability of an echocardiographic score to predict the long-term course of patients undergoing percutaneous valvuloplasty. While it is understood that the scoring parameters are influenced by instrument settings (gain, wall filter, intensity, and resolution) and transducer frequency, TEE has proven a useful adjunct in the evaluation of the qualitative assessment of rheumatic mitral disease. For anesthetized patients undergoing balloon dilatation of stenotic MVs, TEE has provided diagnostic guidance in the baseline assessment of the severity of stenosis and regurgitation, positioning of the balloon, and the serial evaluation of the results of the intervention (Fig. 37.17). Frequently repeated inflations are required as determined by persistence of a significant gradient in the presence of insignificant regurgitation. Ramondo compared the success of performing TEE-guided balloon valvuloplasty with the traditional fluoroscopy-guided procedure. As determined by the absence of significant complications (cardiac tamponade, large residual atrial shunting, and severe MR) and a satisfactory MV area, 96% of the echo-monitored procedures were successful, whereas only 40% of the procedures conducted without echocardiographic control achieved a satisfactory final result (44).

RADIOFREQUENCY ABLATION

ICE has become more relied upon for ablation of anatomically dependent arrhythmias. Since the establishment of the cavotricuspid isthmus as an important structure in the reentrant circuit of typical atrial flutter, ICE has been used to identify the cavotricuspid isthmus and also to directly observe the ablating catheter tip during the ablation procedure (45). This ability to visualize the direct interaction

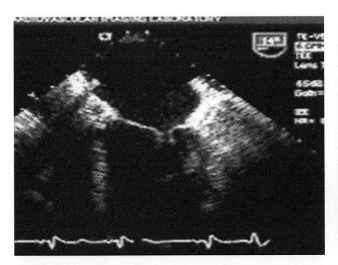 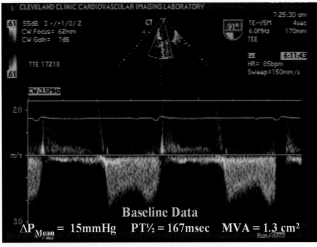

Figure 37.17. TEE is utilized to successfully guide the Inoue balloon valvuloplasty procedure **A:** Midesophageal (ME) four-chamber TEE image plane, demonstrating rheumatic MS with a splitability score of 7. **B:** Baseline transvalvular gradient and pressure half-time. **C:** Inoue balloon positioned across MV.

(Continued)

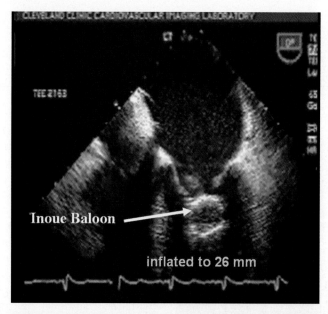

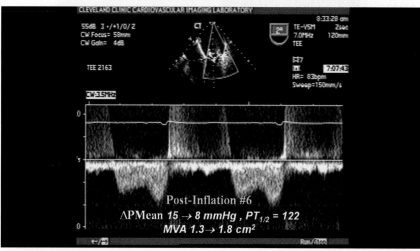

Figure 37.17. (*Continued*). **D:** Reduced pressure gradient and pressure half-time. Postballoon valvuloplasty. Initial pressure half-time may not be as accurate due to LA and LV compliance changes associated acutely with the procedure.

between the catheter tip and underlying tissue is important when considering that typical atrial flutter ablation is 95% to 98% successful after complete interruption of the atrial accessory pathway in the cavotricuspid isthmus. In addition to cavotricuspid isthmus ablation, ICE has most commonly been utilized during both linear atrial ablation and pulmonary vein isolation (PVI) for the treatment of AF. The ability to identify the number and location of the pulmonary veins, as well as directly visualize the guiding catheter positioning at the pulmonary vein ostia has vastly increased the precision, safety, and success of these procedures (46,47).

Along with facilitating more precise and predictable ablation, ICE has afforded electrophysiologists the benefit of being able to directly visualize potential complications before they become otherwise apparent. LA and catheter-tip thrombosis are easily visualized on ICE and in turn may decrease the risk of thromboembolic complications

associated with AF ablations (48). ICE also plays an important role in enabling operators to visualize developing pericardial effusions much earlier than tamponade physiology manifests itself clinically. Additionally, the observation of microbubble formation on ICE is possibly more accurate than catheter-tip temperature monitoring when assessing heat generation and tissue overheating during ablation procedures (49).

CONCLUSION

The current definition of noncoronary cardiac intervention extends well beyond the traditional realm of treating stenotic cardiac valves. This is an exciting field that is expanding and is likely to continue to do so in the coming decades in the same way that PCI has over the last three decades. The use of echocardiographic support at all stages of patient management cannot be overemphasized and is clearly essential for appropriate patient selection, successful procedural outcome, and adequate surveillance following the procedure.

> ### KEY POINTS
>
> ■ Percutaneous cardiac intervention has traditionally involved myocardial revascularization.
>
> ■ Experience with percutaneous balloon valvuloplasty, electrophysiologic procedures, and PFO closure demonstrated the potential for other noncoronary applications.
>
> ■ With the cumulative experience of more than one million percutaneous cardiac interventions annually, other noninvasive approaches to cardiac disease include the management of shunt closure (ASD, PDA, VSD), LAA closure, valvular disease (pulmonic and aortic valve replacement, MV repair), septal reduction in hypertrophic obstructive cardiomyopathy (HOCM), and major vascular intervention (carotid and aortic stenting).
>
> ■ Echocardiography has been utilized to successfully facilitate the safe implementation of new interventional procedures. TTE and TEE hasten the learning curve for the inventional specialist and enable the immediate diagnosis of complications related to the procedure.
>
> ■ The use of echocardiographic guidance in the newer interventional procedures is essential for appropriate patient selection, successful procedure outcome, and patient safety. Incorporating echocardiography with the collaborative and interdisciplinary management of patients undergoing cutting-edge approaches to cardiovascular disease will enable a realistic determination of the full capabilities of these new and exciting developments.

REFERENCES

1. Schwarz F, Baumann P, Manthey J, et al. The effect of aortic valve replacement on survival. *Circulation* 1982;66(5):1105–1110.
2. Cribier A, Eltchaninoff H, Letac B. Advances in percutaneous techniques for treatment of aortic and mitral stenosis. In: Topol EJ, ed. *Textbook of Interventional Cardiology*, 4th ed. Philadelphia: Elsevier Science, 2003:941–953.
3. Cribier A, Eltchaninoff H, Bash A, et al. Percutaneous transcatheter implantation of an aortic valve prosthesis for calcific aortic stenosis: first human case description. *Circulation* 2002;106(24):3006–3008.
4. Eltchaninoff H, Tron C, Cribier A. Percutaneous implantation of aortic valve prosthesis in patients with calcific aortic stenosis: technical aspects. *J Interv Cardiol* 2003;16(6):515–521.
5. Condado JA, Velez-Gimon M. Catheter-based approach to mitral regurgitation. *J Interv Cardiol* 2003;16(6):523–534.
6. Kaye DM, Byrne M, Alferness C, et al. Feasibility and short-term efficacy of percutaneous mitral annular reduction for the therapy of heart failure-induced mitral regurgitation. *Circulation* 2003;108(15):1795–1797.
7. Alfieri O, Maisano F, De Bonis M, et al. The double-orifice technique in mitral valve repair: a simple solution for complex problems. *J Thorac Cardiovasc Surg* 2001;122(4):674–681.
8. Feldman T, Wasserman HS, Herrmann HC, et al. Percutaneous mitral valve repair using edge-to-edge techniques: six-month results of the EVEREST Phase I Clinical Trial. *J Am Coll Cardiol* 2005;46(11):2134–2140.
9. Feldman T, Kar S, Rinaldi M, et al. Percutaneous mitral repair with the MitraClip system: safety and midterm durability in the initial EVEREST (Endovascular Valve Edge-to-Edge Repair Study) cohort. *J Am Coll Cardiol* 2009;54(8):686–694.
10. Silvestry FE, Rodriguez LL, Herrmann HC, et al. Echocardiographic guidance and assessment of percutaneous repair for mitral regurgitation with the Evalve MitraClip: Lessons learned from EVEREST I. *J Am Soc Echocardiogr* 2007;20:1131–1140.
11. Kimmelstiel CD, Maron BJ. Role of percutaneous septal ablation in hypertrophic obstructive cardiomyopathy. *Circulation* 2004;109(4):452–456.
12. Maron BJ, Nishimura RA, McKenna WJ, et al. Assessment of permanent dual-chamber pacing as a treatment for drug-refractory symptomatic patients with obstructive hypertrophic cardiomyopathy. A randomized, double-blind, crossover study (M-PATHY). *Circulation* 1999;99(22):2927–2933.
13. Nishimura RA, Trusty JM, Hayes DL, et al. Dual-chamber pacing for hypertrophic cardiomyopathy: a randomized, double-blind, crossover trial. *J Am Coll Cardiol* 1997;29(2):435–441.
14. Sigwart U. Non-surgical myocardial reduction for hypertrophic obstructive cardiomyopathy. *Lancet* 1995;346(8969):211–214.
15. Ruzyllo W, Chojnowska L, Demkow M, et al. Left ventricular outflow tract gradient decrease with non-surgical myocardial reduction improves exercise capacity in patients with hypertrophic obstructive cardiomyopathy. *Eur Heart J* 2000;21(9):770–777.
16. Lakkis NM, Nagueh SF, Dunn JK, et al. Nonsurgical septal reduction therapy for hypertrophic obstructive cardiomyopathy: one-year follow-up. *J Am Coll Cardiol* 2000;36(3):852–855.
17. Seggewiss H, Faber L. Percutaneous septal ablation for hypertrophic cardiomyopathy and mid-ventricular obstruction. *Eur J Echocardiogr* 2000;1(4):277–280.
18. Mills NL, King TD. Nonoperative closure of left-to-right shunts. *J Thorac Cardiovasc Surg* 1976;72(3):371–378.
19. Lechat P, Mas JL, Lascault G, et al. Prevalence of patent foramen ovale in patients with stroke. *N Engl J Med* 1988;318(18):1148–1152.
20. Kannel WB, Wolf PA, Benjamin EJ, et al. Prevalence, incidence, prognosis, and predisposing conditions for atrial fibrillation: population-based estimates. *Am J Cardiol* 1998;82(8A):2N–9N.
21. Blackshear JL, Odell JA. Appendage obliteration to reduce stroke in cardiac surgical patients with atrial fibrillation. *Ann Thorac Surg* 1996;61(2):755–759.
22. Hart RG, Halperin JL, Pearce LA, et al. Lessons from the stroke prevention in atrial fibrillation trials. *Ann Intern Med* 2003;138(10):831–838.

23. Stafford RS, Singer DE. Recent national patterns of warfarin use in atrial fibrillation. *Circulation* 1998;97(13):1231–1233.

24. Madden J. Resection of the left auricular appendix. *JAMA* 1948;140:769–772.

25. Odell JA, Blackshear JL, Davies E, et al. Thoracoscopic obliteration of the left atrial appendage: potential for stroke reduction? *Ann Thorac Surg* 1996;61(2):565–569.

26. Nakai T, Lesh MD, Gerstenfeld EP, et al. Percutaneous left atrial appendage occlusion (PLAATO) for preventing cardioembolism: first experience in canine model. *Circulation* 2002;105(18):2217–2222.

27. Sievert H, Lesh MD, Trepels T, et al. Percutaneous left atrial appendage transcatheter occlusion to prevent stroke in high-risk patients with atrial fibrillation: early clinical experience. *Circulation* 2002;105(16):1887–1889.

28. Al-Saady NM, Obel OA, Camm AJ. Left atrial appendage: structure, function, and role in thromboembolism. *Heart* 1999;82(5):547–554.

29. Meier B, Palacios I, Windecker S, et al. Transcatheter left atrial appendage occlusion with Amplatzer devices to obviate anticoagulation in patients with atrial fibrillation. *Catheter Cardiovasc Interv* 2003;60(3):417–422.

30. Blackshear JL, Johnson WD, Odell JA, et al. Thoracoscopic extracardiac obliteration of the left atrial appendage for stroke risk reduction in atrial fibrillation. *J Am Coll Cardiol* 2003;42(7):1249–1252.

31. Crystal E, Lamy A, Connolly SJ, et al. Left Atrial Appendage Occlusion Study (LAAOS): a randomized clinical trial of left atrial appendage occlusion during routine coronary artery bypass graft surgery for long-term stroke prevention. *Am Heart J* 2003;145(1):174–178.

32. Pennec PY, Jobic Y, Blanc JJ, et al. Assessment of different procedures for surgical left atrial appendage exclusion. *Ann Thorac Surg* 2003;76(6):2168–2169.

33. Bartel T, Konorza T, Arjumand J, et al. Intracardiac echocardiography is superior to conventional monitoring for guiding device closure of interatrial communications. *Circulation* 2003;107(6):795–797.

34. Armstrong G, Cardon L, Vilkomerson D, et al. Localization of needle tip with color Doppler during pericardiocentesis: in vitro validation and initial clinical application. *J Am Soc Echocardiogr* 2001;14(1):29–37.

35. Lynch M, Clements SD, Shanewise JS, et al. Right-sided cardiac tumors detected by transesophageal echocardiography and its usefulness in differentiating the benign from the malignant ones. *Am J Cardiol* 1997;79(6):781–784.

36. Keefe DL. Anthracycline-induced cardiomyopathy. *Semin Oncol* 2001;28(4 Suppl. 12):2–7.

37. Shammas RL, Movahed A. Sarcoidosis of the heart. *Clin Cardiol* 1993;16(6):462–472.

38. Pandian NG, Hsu TL. Intravascular ultrasound and intracardiac echocardiography: concepts for the future. *Am J Cardiol* 1992;69(20):6H–17H.

39. Reddy SCB, Rath GA, Ziady GM, et al. Tricuspid flail leaflets after orthotopic heart transplant: a new complication of endomyocardial biopsy. *J Am Soc Echocardiogr* 1993;6:223–226.

40. Williams MJA, Lee MY, DiSalvo TG, et al. Biopsy-induced flail tricuspid leaflet and tricuspid regurgitation following orthotopic cardiac transplantation. *Am J Cardiol* 1996;77:1339–1344.

41. Miller LW, Labovitz AJ, McBride LA, et al. Echocardiography-guided endomyocardial biopsy. *Circulation* 1988;78(Suppl. III):III-99–III-102.

42. Miche E, Bogunovic N, Fassbender D, et al. Predictors of unsuccessful outcome after percutaneous mitral valvotomy including a new echocardiographic scoring system. *J Heart Valve Dis* 1996;5:430–435.

43. Wilkins GT, Weyman AE, Abascal VM, et al. Percutaneous balloon dilatation of the mitral valve: an analysis of echocardiographic variables related to outcome and the mechanism of dilatation. *Br Heart J* 1988;60:299–308.

44. Ramondo A, Chirillo F, Dan M, et al. Value and limitations of transesophageal echocardiographic monitoring during percutaneous balloon mitral valvotomy. *Int J Cardiol* 1991;31(2):223–233.

45. Morton JB, Sanders P, Davidson NC, et al. Phased-array intracardiac echocardiography for defining cavotricuspid isthmus anatomy during radiofrequency ablation of typical atrial flutter. *J Cardiovasc Electrophysiol* 2003;14:591–597.

46. Martin RE, Ellenbogen KA, Lau YR, et al. Phased-array intracardiac echocardiography during pulmonary vein isolation and linear ablation for atrial fibrillation. *J Cardiovasc Electrophysiol* 2002;13:873–879.

47. Arruda M, Wang ZT, Patel A, et al. Intracardiac echocardiography identifies pulmonary vein ostea more accurately than conventional angiography. *J Am Coll Cardiol* 2000;35:110A.

48. Ren JF, Marchlinski FE, Callans SJ. Left atrial thrombus associated with ablation for atrial fibrillation: identification with intracardiac echocardiography. *J Am Coll Cardiol* 2004;43:1861–1867.

49. Asirvatham S, Packer DL, Johnson SB. Ultrasound vs. temperature feedback monitoring microcatheter ablation in the canine atrium [abstract]. *Pacing Clin Electrophysiol* 1999;22:822A.

1. The role of TEE in deployment of the percutaneous aortic valve stent includes which of the following except?
   A. Assessment of AS severity
   B. Assessment of AR mechanism
   C. Determining proper deployment of balloon inflation pressure
   D. Positioning of the device prior to deployment
   E. Verifying coronary ostia patency after deployment

2. Which of the following are determinants of a successful mitral balloon valvuloplasty?
   A. Degree of calcification of leaflets
   B. Valve leaflet thickness and mobility restriction
   C. Degree of subvalvular apparatus involvement
   D. Commissural calcification
   E. All of the above

3. The E-Valve MitraClip is based on which previous experience?

   A. Balloon valvuloplasty
   B. Coronary sinus stenting
   C. Mitral valve (MV) annuloplasty
   D. Alfieri repair

4. TEE is used in percutaneous MV procedures for which of the following?
   A. Baseline MR severity and mechanism
   B. Measurement of coaptation gap
   C. Determine location of transseptal puncture
   D. Alignment of device before MV leaflet capture
   E. All of the above

5. All of the following criteria are used to diagnose cardiac tamponade in the presence of large pericardial effusion except?
   A. Right ventricular (RV) diastolic inversion
   B. Respiratory variation in the flow and volume of the hepatic vein
   C. Left ventricular (LV) wall motion abnormalities
   D. Left- or right-atrial wall inversion

CHAPTER 38

Perioperative Applications of New Modalities: Strain Echocardiography and Three-Dimensional Echocardiography

Nikolaos J. Skubas ■ Feroze Mahmood ■ Douglas C. Shook ■ Stanton K. Shernan

INTRODUCTION

Transesophageal echocardiography (TEE) has advanced the role of cardiovascular anesthesiologists and increased their participation in perioperative decision making during cardiac surgical procedures and intensive care (1–4). TEE is considered safe with a very low rate of complications (5).

The echocardiographic assessment of global and regional left ventricular (LV) function consists of two-dimensional (2D) or Doppler evaluation of cardiac structures and their interaction with blood flow. The techniques used are mostly visual and subjective (6,7), thus not always accurate or error free. Adequate visualization and accurate tracing of the endocardial-blood pool interface during the cardiac cycle (8), precise measurement of an orifice diameter, and parallel orientation between the Doppler beam and direction of blood flow (9) are paramount in producing unidimensional (fractional shortening) or 2D estimates (fractional area change, stroke volume, and ejection fraction [EF]) (10) as suggested by published guidelines (8). The evaluation of regional LV function based on the degree of systolic myocardial thickening is highly subjective (7) and inaccurate if imaging is suboptimal, when myocardial segments lay parallel to the propagation of ultrasound or when the epicardium is not even seen. Furthermore, impairment of regional function does not cause reduction in LVEF unless several segments are involved.

Conventional TEE methods cannot discriminate the effects of load on contractility (i.e., impaired contractility and falsely high EF in severe mitral regurgitation or intact contractility and falsely low EF in severe aortic stenosis). Calculation of the rate of LV systolic pressure rise (LV+dp/dt) requires the presence of a mitral regurgitation jet (11), while contractility indices such as end-systolic elastance, preload recruitable stroke work, or myocardial performance index are too complicated for clinical application (12). Additionally, all conventional echocardiographic methods examine only a single LV diameter or tomographic plane at a time. Taking into consideration the frequent LV foreshortening that occurs in the midesophageal (ME) tomographic planes or the presence of segmental abnormalities particularly in patients with coronary artery disease, it is easy to realize why true representation of global LV function is not always feasible with these methods.

The recent technological advances in signal processing in Doppler (Doppler tissue imaging [DTI] and Doppler strain echocardiography [DSE]) and ultrasound (2D speckle tracking imaging [STI]) enable measurement of tissue velocity and deformation in one or two dimensions; provide high quality, precise, and objective information regarding regional and/or global myocardial function in real time, decrease the subjectivity of the interpretation, and increase the diagnostic accuracy. This section will present the physiological principles and modalities (DTI, DSE, and STI) of tissue echocardiography, offer a guide on how to acquire data, and explore their clinical benefits.

MYOCARDIAL STRUCTURE AND MOTION

Newer insights into myocardial structure have shown that myocardial fibers are organized in layers and form a leftward helix in epicardium, a rightward helix in endocardium, and are circumferentially orientated in mid myocardium (Fig. 38.1). Myocardial tissue is incompressible and LV muscle volume remains constant during the cardiac cycle. Consequently, the aforementioned myocardial fiber arrangement results in longitudinal shortening and circumferential thinning and radial thickening during systole, while opposite direction changes occur in diastole (13).

This global cardiac motion cannot be appreciated during conventional TEE imaging, where only radial motion (inward endocardial excursion and myocardial thickening in ME or transgastric [TG] views), related to mid myocardium function, is evaluated. Longitudinal (ME views) and circumferential motion (TG views), both related to epicardial and endocardial fibers, are also difficult to appreciate. However, both radial and longitudinal motions are important since (a) it has been shown that during systole, a 40% radial thickening is accompanied by 14%

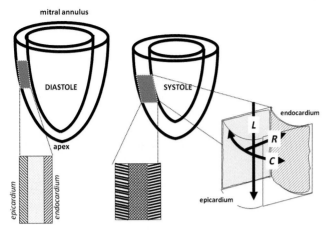

Figure 38.1. Myocardial architecture consists of helical (left-handed in epicardium and right-handed in endocardium) and circumferential (in mid-myocardium) layers of myocardial fibers. This fiber arrangement results in longitudinal (L) (mitral annulus to apex), radial (R) (epicardium to endocardium), and circumferential (C) (tangentially to epicardium) motions during systole and diastole.

longitudinal shortening (12), and (b) the first myocardial layer affected by ischemia is the subendocardium (14), which contributes to longitudinal motion. The subjective evaluation of regional LV motion (segmental function) is also limited since the passive motion of a noncontracting segment, due to tethering to adjacent segments, cannot be reliably excluded using conventional TEE visual analysis. Many of these limitations can be overcome by assessing myocardial deformation.

DEFORMATION

Strain means deformation (15). Myocardial strain (S or ε) is the deformation of a myocardial fiber, normalized to its original length:

$$S = L_1 - L_0 / L_0 (\%)$$

where L_0 is the baseline (end-diastolic) length and L_1 is the end-systolic length of the myocardial fiber. By definition, strain is positive when two locations are moving apart (the systolic dimension increases, i.e., the myocardial fiber is lengthening or the LV segment thickens, i.e., the segment expands). Alternatively, strain is negative when two locations move near (the systolic dimension decreases, i.e., the myocardial fiber shortens or is compressed). Therefore, radial thickening is associated with positive strain ($L_1 > L_0$) while longitudinal shortening and circumferential thinning are associated with negative strain ($L_1 < L_0$).

Natural strain is the deformation when the reference value (L_0) is continuously changing. *Lagrangian* strain is the instantaneous strain, in relation to time (t): ε(t) = [L(t) − L(t_0)]/L(t_0), where baseline strain is measured

at time (t_0). In the echocardiographic evaluation of myocardial function, we measure Lagrangian strain, where L(t_0) is the end-diastolic shape. For a 2D object, deformation occurs along both the x-axis and the y-axis (*normal* strain: the motion is normal to the borders of the object) and parallel to the borders of the object (*shear* strain). For a three-dimensional (3D) object, such as a myocardial segment, there are three *normal* strains (along the x-, y-, and z-axes), and six shear strains (along the combinations of the different axes) (16).

Because myocardial deformation is caused by fiber contraction, strain is a measure of myocardial contractile function. Myocardial deformation can be measured echocardiographically with Doppler velocity gradients (DSE) (17) or non-Doppler speckle tracking (STI) (18).

Strain rate (SR) reflects how fast regional myocardial deformation (strain) occurs (SR = the speed of deformation):

$$SR = S/t (\%/s)$$

where t is the time duration of this deformation (Fig. 38.2).

Strain measurements with either technique have been validated against sonomicrometry (18,19) and magnetic resonance (20,21) (r = 0.94 for SR; and r = 0.96 for strain) (22). For normal myocardium, SR reflects regional contractile function because it is relatively independent of heart rate, whereas systolic strain reflects changes in stroke volume (23,24). Evaluated with DTI or tagged cardiac MRI, LV regional strains increase slightly from base to apex and from endocardium to epicardium (16,25,26). Longitudinal right ventricular (RV) strain and SR values are inhomogeneous and higher than those of LV (27). Radial strain relates to motion from the endocardium to the epicardium. Circumferential strain relates to motion

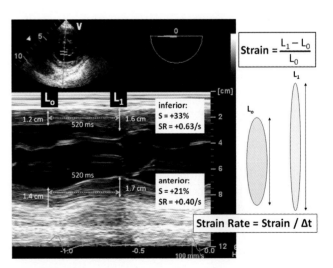

Figure 38.2. Illustrative example of estimation of strain and SR of mid inferior and mid anterior LV segments using M-mode. L_0, end-diastolic length; L_1, end-systolic length; Δt, systolic time interval.

along the circumference (curvature) of the LV. Normal values are −16% to −24% (longitudinal strain), +48% (radial strain) and −20% (circumferential strain) (27–29). Some have found significantly higher strain values in women than in men (30). Strain and SR offer complementary information and both should be calculated. Prolonged contraction may yield normal strain despite low SR. Consequently, SR is considered more sensitive than strain in revealing disease.

SR during isovolumic contraction showed good correlation with +dP/dt (r = 0.74) and with −dP/dt during isovolumic relaxation (r = 0.67) (31). Strain is load dependent (19,30) and does not appear to be less load-insensitive than EF, fractional shortening, and other traditional measures of systolic function. For example, withdrawal of 500 mL of blood from healthy subjects leads to decreased longitudinal DTI strain (−28 ± 8% to −21 ± 4%) while SR remained unchanged (−1.5 ± 0.35 to −1.4 ± 0.4/s) (32). Similarly, STI is preload and afterload dependent: longitudinal strain decreased after hemodialysis in end-stage renal disease patients (−18.4 ± 2.9% to −16.9 ± 3.2%) (33) and radial strain increased immediately postoperatively after aortic valve (AV) replacement for aortic stenosis (from 22.7 ± 2% to 23.7 ± 1.8%) and decreased (23.1 ± 3.5% to 21 ± 3.8%) after valve replacement for aortic regurgitation (34). However, others have shown that longitudinal strain values (recorded with DTI in healthy subjects) remain unchanged during preload manipulation (baseline −18 ± 3%, increased preload with Trendelenburg −18 ± 3%, reduced preload with venodilator −17 ± 3%), while myocardial velocities are affected (35). Discrepancies in the previous findings are explained by study design, techniques used for strain measurement, and degrees of preload manipulation. Therefore, it would be "safer" not to consider strain as a load-independent parameter of systolic function.

PRINCIPLES OF DOPPLER TISSUE IMAGING AND DOPPLER STRAIN ECHOCARDIOGRAPHY

A shift in frequency is caused when transmitted ultrasound is reflected off a moving target (Doppler phenomenon). In conventional echocardiography, the Doppler algorithms have been set up to interrogate only returning signals from the blood pool using high-gain settings (to amplify the low-amplitude signal) and a high-pass filter (to reject the "noise" generated by the slow-moving myocardium). Modification of these filter settings (reduction of gain amplification and bypass of the high-pass wall filter) will reject data from moving blood and permit recording of the stronger (approximately 40 dB higher amplitude) and slower (<25 cm/s) myocardial motion signal, respectively, thus enabling DTI and DSE (36). The principles of DTI along with applications and limitations have been reviewed recently (37).

For DSE, color DTI is obtained in the same manner as conventional color flow Doppler; that is, a color DTI sector is positioned over the myocardial wall of interest while mean myocardial velocities are computed using autocorrelation analysis and displayed in blue color if directed away from and in red color if directed toward the transducer. The color myocardial velocities are superimposed on a gray scale, 2D tomographic views (Fig. 38.3A) (38). DSE is performed by placing a sample volume (see step-by-step explanation below) over the myocardial area of interest while utilizing color DTI (Fig. 38.3B). The velocity gradient within this sample volume is used to calculate the deformation parameters SR (Fig. 38.3C) and strain (Fig. 38.3D):

$$SR = (V_2 - V_1)/\Delta x \sim (L_2 - L_1)/(1/\Delta t)/(1/\Delta x)$$
$$\sim \Delta L/(1/\Delta x)/(1/\Delta t) \sim S/(1/\Delta t)$$

Strain is derived by temporal integration of SR.

Strain can overcome limitations associated with myocardial velocity. Tethering to a functioning neighboring segment will cause displacement and recording of myocardial velocity giving the false impression of a moving segment. This can be graphically simulated by the example of a towed car: although the engine of the towed car is not functioning, the car has velocity. However, if no velocity gradient exists within the segment, there will be no deformation, and SR (and strain) will be 0.

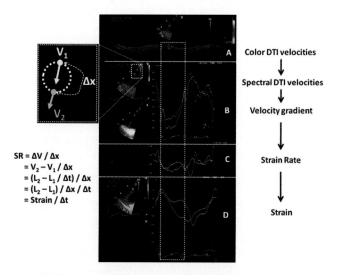

Figure 38.3. Doppler Strain and SR. **A:** Activation of DTI function allows imaging of myocardial velocities in color, here with M-mode (from the inferior wall in a midesophageal two-chamber view). The velocities are directed away from the transducer in systole (and colored *blue*) and toward the transducer in diastole (and colored *red*). **B:** Spectral display of myocardial velocities from within sample volumes (insert panel at **left**) demonstrates a velocity gradient (ΔV). Basal (V₁) velocity is greater than apical (V₂) velocity as the inferior wall shortens along its long axis. **C:** The velocity gradient (ΔV) of these points is used to calculate SR. **D:** Integration of SR over time (Δt) derives strain.

Strain (and SR) calculated from myocardial velocity gradients has been validated over a wide range of strain values using sonomicrometry in animal (19,39) and 3D tagged-magnetic resonance imaging in humans (20,40). However, systolic strain correlates with MRI better in healthy than diseased individuals (41). DTI-derived strain and SR are strong noninvasive indices of LV contractility (24). DTI strain and SR increased with dobutamine, decreased with esmolol, and correlated well with peak LV elastance in experimental settings.

While not limited by tethering or translation effects, thus being superior to DTI velocities in the evaluation of regional myocardial function, DSE is time-consuming and technically demanding and does have important limitations. Reverberation or dropout artifacts from neighboring structures can affect the measured velocity gradient and interfere with calculation of strain and SR. The most important limitation of DSE arises from the fact that it is a Doppler technique, which displays deformation along a single dimension only, that of the ultrasound plane. Therefore, the displayed value (SR and strain) may not relate to the true longitudinal, radial, or circumferential deformation. As a result, when using TEE, longitudinal strain (and SR) should be recorded only from ME views and radial strain (and SR) from TG views. Furthermore, the angle between the Doppler and motion planes will underestimate the true myocardial velocity gradient (and the calculated strain and SR) if greater than 20 degrees (39). At an angle of 45 degrees, the measured DTI strain is 0 (19). In ME views, when ultrasound beam is parallel to the myocardial wall, the actual (longitudinal) velocity can be accurately measured, but the velocity of radial (transverse) deformation will be 0 since radial motion will be perpendicular to the ultrasound beam. With any angle deviation from 0 degree, the contribution of radial deformation to the measured velocity increases (42). This becomes more problematic in the presence of regional wall motion abnormalities (43). Because of this angle dependency, DTI is used primarily to assess longitudinal deformation parameters.

STEP-BY-STEP GUIDE ON HOW TO OBTAIN DOPPLER STRAIN

To obtain Doppler strain parameters, the echocardiographic system must have a preset function to image tissue velocity. Of outmost importance is 2D imaging of optimal quality with clear definition between the blood pool and myocardium. This may be facilitated by using second harmonic imaging. In order to show the subtle changes in myocardial velocity, high acquisition frames are required (usually >100 frames/s). This is accomplished by narrowing the sector width over the myocardial wall of interest. Optimal ECG tracing with clear definition of QRS and P is essential, as well as pulse wave (PW) or continuous wave (CW) Doppler of transmitral and aortic flows for

timing purposes. These temporal recordings should be concurrent with strain data acquisition.

The first important elements of a successful DTI examination involves manipulation of the TEE probe in such a way that myocardial motion and ultrasound plane are parallel to each other (or with an angle of −20 degrees) (37). This may require turning the probe, to align the myocardium with the ultrasound beam. The examination sequence should be standardized or the views labeled because the narrow sector removes neighboring structures used for reference. Next, DTI is applied and a low Nyquist limit is chosen, usually in the range of <20 to +20 cm/s, to avoid aliasing. A lower velocity range will increase spatial and temporal resolution. The sector width and depth are then optimized. The operator has two options: either a conventional sector width, which enables side-by-side comparison of diametrically opposite segments and walls, or a narrow sector with the option of shallow depth, which maximizes the frame rate (DSE is optimal at >180 frames/s). The ventilator may be switched off during acquisition of images, which are then reviewed and digitally stored. At least 3 beats (in sinus rhythm) or up to 8 beats (in arrhythmia) should be captured and digitally stored (44). TEE images used for Doppler strain include the three standard ME views (for long-axis myocardial deformation) and the basal and mid TG mid-short-axis (SAX) views. Selection of these tomographic planes is dictated by the requirement for parallel orientation between the motion plane under examination and ultrasound direction as described above. Addition of an M-mode line to the color DTI velocities will display a velocity pattern along the M-mode beam with good temporal resolution (Fig. 38.3A) (45).

Further analysis is performed either on the primary echocardiographic system, or on a dedicated workstation. Currently, DSE techniques use proprietary software and are only able to analyze digitally stored images from the same system. An appropriately sized sample volume (6 × 10 mm) is placed on the desired LV region, keeping in mind that larger sample volumes result in "smoothing" of the strain signals while at the same time temporal and spatial resolution decreases. The size of the sample volume determines the length (L_0) over which the velocity gradient is calculated. In order to keep the region of interest within the myocardial borders, L_0 is typically 10 mm for longitudinal data sets and 5 mm for radial data sets (46). "Drift compensation," a default setting that corrects for drift (i.e., when myocardium does not return to its original length at end-diastole) in the strain curves, can introduce error in the evaluations and should be taken into account as well. Since strain is the temporal integral of SR, it is a "smoother" curve than SR. The SR curve should be inspected, because a noisy SR curve indicates suboptimal tracking of the region of interest and drift and may require repositioning of the sample volume.

The sample volumes are placed along the length of the myocardial wall (basal, mid and apical segments) toward

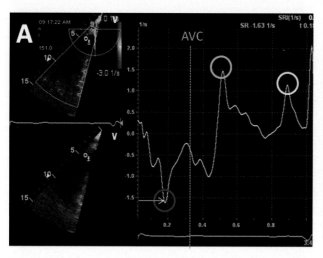
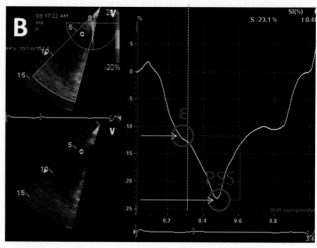

Figure 38.4. Measurements in DSE include **A**: peak systolic (SR_S), early diastolic (SR_D), and late diastolic (SR_A) SR and **B**: end-systolic strain (ε). Strain recorded after aortic valve closure (AVC) is called postsystolic strain (PSS).

the endocardial surface (ME views) or in the middle of myocardium (TG views) and should "track" (travel with) the segment throughout the cardiac cycle. The operator should verify that this happens by scrolling frame by frame and observing the concurrent motion of the sample volume with the myocardial segment. From each sample volume, SR, strain, and timing of peak values with respect to QRS are calculated (Fig. 38.4). The reproducibility of strain measurements is reported to be less than 15% (44). The suggested measurements and calculations are shown in Table 38.1.

PRINCIPLES OF SPECKLE TRACKING IMAGING AND 2D STRAIN

The 2D strain is recorded with STI and is based on scattering, reflection, and interference of ultrasound with myocardium. These interactions result in generation of a finely gray-shaded, speckled pattern. This speckled pattern is unique for each myocardial region and relatively stable throughout the cardiac cycle. The speckles function as acoustic markers, are equally distributed within the myocardium, and change their position from frame-to-frame

TABLE 38.1	Strain Echocardiography Measurements and Calculations
End-diastole	R wave of ECG
End-systole	Aortic Valve Closure (AVC)
End-systolic strain (S_{SYS})	Magnitude of systolic deformation between end-diastole and end-systole (AVC)
Peak strain (S_{PEAK})	Maximum systolic deformation over a mean RR interval
	• Lowest value for longitudinal or circumferential strain
	• Highest value for radial strain
Postsystolic strain (S_{PS} or PSS)	The difference between S_{PEAK} and S_{SYS}
	$S_{PS} = S_{PEAK} - S_{SYS}$
Postsystolic strain index (PSI)	Represents the relative amount of ischemia-related segment thickening or shortening, found to occur after AVC
	$PSI = S_{PS}/S_{PEAK} = (S_{PEAK} - S_{SYS})/S_{PEAK}$
Systolic SR (SR_{peak})	Maximum SR prior to end-systole
Peak systolic SR (SR_{peak})	Maximum SR
Rotation	Base rotates clockwise (initial, early systolic rotation is counterclockwise): (+)ve ° values
	Apex rotates counterclockwise (initial, early systolic rotation is clockwise): (−)ve ° values
Torsion	Basal rotation − apical rotation

in accordance with the surrounding myocardial deformation/tissue motion. The acoustic markers within a predefined region of interest are followed automatically frame by frame, and the change in their geometric position (which corresponds to local tissue movement) is used to extract strain, SR, velocity and displacement. Because these acoustic markers can be followed in any direction, STI is a non-Doppler, angle-independent technique for calculation of cardiac deformation along two dimensions. Therefore, radial and longitudinal deformation can be measured in the ME views and radial and circumferential deformation in the SAX views (42). Although considered as the only scientifically sound methodology for measuring cardiac deformation (43), this non-Doppler technique has limitations including (a) decreased sensitivity due to applied smoothing; (b) incorrect calculation of deformation, which is produced by erroneous tracking of stationary reverberations (when tissue moves, the speckle interference pattern may not move in exact accordance with tissue motion) (45); (c) necessity of clear visualization of the endocardial border for reliable radial and transverse tracking; and (d) undersampling during tachycardia since the optimal frame rate should be less than 100 frames/s (42). Equally important, STI algorithms require that the entire myocardium is visualized throughout the cardiac cycle. Echo dropout and mitral annulus calcification attenuate myocardial appearance in the TG or ME views, respectively, and do not allow adequate tracking of echocardiographic speckles.

SHEAR STRAIN AND TORSION

The myocardial architecture is such that epicardial fibers are left-handed oriented, while endocardial fibers are oriented in right-handed direction (Fig. 38.1). This will produce shear strain during the cardiac cycle (deformation parallel to the reference plane) and will result in the base and the apex of the heart rotating in opposite directions. From a TEE perspective, the base rotates clockwise (preceded by an early systolic counterclockwise rotation) and the apex counterclockwise (preceded by an early systolic clockwise rotation), producing torsion of the ventricle (the difference in apical and basal rotation), similar to wringing out a towel dry (12). The early systolic rotations are due to earlier activation of subendocardial fibers. As a result, during the cardiac cycle there is a systolic twist and an early diastolic untwist of the LV along its long axis because of opposite directed apical and basal rotations. Rotation angles and torsion can be measured with STI (47,48), and correlate well with sonomicrometry and tagged MRI. Since basal and apical rotations are in opposite directions, somewhere between them there exists a level (the "equator") where rotation changes from one direction to the other (48).

LV torsion occurs mainly by the counterclockwise apical rotation. Torsion is considered the mechanical link

between systolic and diastolic function: systolic twisting stores elastic energy, which, released during the isovolumic phase of diastole, produces untwisting and generates intraventricular pressure gradients and allows LV filling to proceed at low filling pressure (12). In healthy subjects during systole, the torsion increases and the LV volume decreases, but during diastole, the relation between rapid untwisting (uncoiling) and increasing volume is nonlinear. Initiation of untwisting is an early and key mechanism that promotes early diastolic relaxation and early diastolic filling, possibly more important than recoil of systolic basal descent (49).

LV twist is preload dependent and is increased with inotropy (50). Approximately 40% of LV untwisting occurs during the isovolumic relaxation period, reaching a maximum just after mitral valve (MV) opening, when approximately 20% of the stroke volume had entered the LV. By the peak of transmitral early filling (E wave, [TMF-E]), approximately 80% to 90% of untwisting is completed and essentially finished by the end of TMF-E wave, with the subsequent LV volume increase due to expansion in the short and long axes. LV systolic torsion and rapid untwisting increase significantly with exercise storing additional potential energy, which is released as increased diastolic suction. That is why the heart can increase the diastolic filling rate despite the shortened diastolic period during tachycardia. Patients with hypertrophic cardiomyopathy showed delayed untwisting that was not significantly augmented with exercise (51). That explains the inability of patients to increase filling during exercise without a significant increase in left atrial pressure.

The magnitude of torsion depends critically on the measurement level relative to LV base or other reference point. A limitation of STE in recording torsion is the in-out motion of the image plane as the LV moves along its longitudinal axis. Selection of reproducible anatomic landmarks is important for measuring and reporting reproducible values. At the basal level, reproducible image planes are easier to obtain, since the fibrous mitral ring is used for orientation. For apical recordings, the image plane should be just basal to the level with luminal closure at end-systole (there should be a recognizable apical cavity at end-systole).

STEP-BY-STEP GUIDE ON HOW TO PERFORM STI

The technique of non-Doppler strain analysis has been described for the ambulatory cardiac patient (42,52). As compared to DSE, STI is less demanding and is closer to standard imaging with a normal frame rate and without a Doppler requirement. The steps to perform STI in the anesthetized cardiac surgical patient are similar and are described in detail below. For the time being, analysis and measurements of 2D speckle strain parameters are only possible offline, using a dedicated workstation (EchoPAC,

GE Vingmed, Norway; Q-labs, Philips Healthcare, Inc., Andover, MA). As of this time, analysis is possible only on digitally acquired and stored images of the same vendor since there is no "cross-talk" from systems between different vendors.

The operator starts by acquiring 2D echocardiographic images of the LV, which are digitally stored. Three ME views (4C, 2C, and LAX) and three TG views (basal, mid, and apical) are acquired with a frame rate between 40 and 80/s, with adequate sector width and depth in order to image both endocardium and epicardium. In the anesthetized patient, it is better to temporarily stop ventilating to avoid image translation. Equally important is to acquire optimal quality 2D images and eliminate any myocardial areas with echo "dropout"—no speckles, no analysis!

Onset of systole is based on the ECG-R wave, and end of systole is defined using M-mode tracings of the AV or pulsed wave Doppler of the transaortic valve flow. This interval is then used by the software to define the systolic time. Therefore, it is practical to initiate postprocessing in a ME LAX view, where the AV is seen before moving to the other ME and TG views. Additionally, it is important to acquire images rapidly and ensure that heart rate (and rhythm) as well as hemodynamics remains stable. Otherwise, the systolic interval needs to be redefined prior to each strain analysis.

In each LV view stored, the operator manually traces the LV endocardium in a systolic frame where it is best defined/imaged. Based upon this initial endocardial tracing, the software generates a region of interest, which encompasses the entire thickness of the cardiac wall between the LV epicardium and endocardium. This region of interest can be adjusted manually by the operator, so that the inner border is tracing the endocardium and the region of interest "covers" the entire myocardium throughout the cardiac cycle. After approval of the software-generated myocardial wall delineation, speckle tracking analysis is done from within this region for one cardiac cycle at a time. In each view, the LV myocardium is automatically divided in six segments, and the tracking quality is scored as either acceptable or nonacceptable. If more than two segments have nonacceptable quality, the region of interest should be redefined or a different beat chosen. The more important reasons for poor quality (i.e., nonacceptable segments) are myocardial dropout and poor 2D image resolution. Neither can be corrected with postprocessing.

If tracking quality is acceptable, the operator approves the sampled segments and the software provides for each segment various deformation parameters: strain, SR, velocity, displacement, and rotation (torsion) (42,53). Examples of non-Doppler strain measurements are seen in Figure 38.5. Since acquisition of 2D images (in the ME and TG views) is standard procedure during a comprehensive TEE examination, appropriately stored 2D images with good quality can be analyzed offline provided that the analysis system is of the same manufacturer and is capable of providing STI parameters.

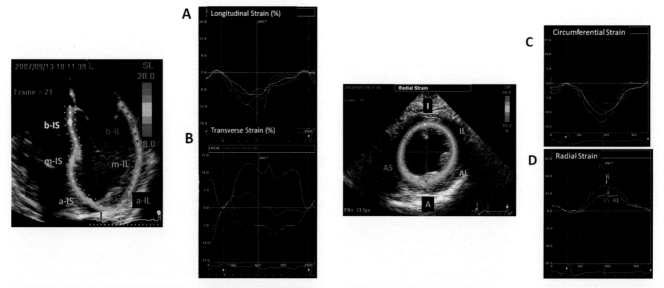

Figure 38.5. Speckle Tissue Imaging (STI). Longitudinal strain (**A**) and transverse strain (**B**) from a midesophageal four-chamber LV view. The white dotted line represents the global (average) longitudinal strain. Each myocardial segment is color coded. Longitudinal strain is abnormal in basal inferolateral (b-IL) segment (longitudinal expansion). Transverse strain is normal in only basal and mid inferoseptal (IS) segments (transverse thickening). Circumferential (**C**) and radial (**D**) strain from a TG mid papillary short-axis view of the LV. The white dotted line represents the global (average) circumferential strain. Deformation is uniform (as compared with panels **A** and **B**). a, apical; b, basal.

A three-click method (automated function imaging [AFI]), whereby the operator "anchors" three points, at each side of the mitral annulus and at the apex of the LV in the ME views, further simplifies the process of tracking and analyzing peak systolic strain based on 2D strain. The computerized assessment is able to present the data in parametric (color), anatomic M-mode, strain curves, and "bull's eye" displays. The usefulness of AFI is that deformation data are produced in an effortless manner and are comprehended easier by an inexperienced operator.

The differences between Doppler and non-Doppler strain measurements are summarized in Table 38.2 (42). Deformation values are shown in Table 38.3.

CORRELATION OF STRAIN BETWEEN DTI AND STI

If either DTI or STI measure deformation accurately, the respective strain values should correlate and give identical values. In 30 patients none of whom had acute myocardial infarction (MI), longitudinal strain values differed only by $0.6 \pm 6.0\%$ (r = 0.53, P < 0.001) and radial strain values differed by $1.8 \pm 13.4\%$ (r = 0.46, P < 0.001) (40). Using receiver-operating characteristic curve, STI showed greater area under the curve to discriminate among dysfunctional segments than DTI strain. Similarly, DTI and STI values were identical in normal subjects as well as patients with cardiomyopathy (25–28).

TABLE 38.2	**Strain Echocardiography: Imaging Modalities**	
	Doppler Tissue Imaging (DTI)	**Speckle Tracking Imaging (STI)**
Technique	Manipulation of Doppler signal	Tracking of acoustic markers
	• Elimination of wall filter	Gray speckles within myocardium are tracked frame by frame
	• Low-gain amplification	
	Strain is calculated from velocity gradients, measured against a fixed reference (transducer)	Strain is directly measured from tracking of acoustic markers (speckles)
Display	Color map (±M-mode)	Color map
	PW at a specific space (regional values only)	Spectral display (regional and global values)
Measurements	From color map (off-line):	• SR
	• SR	• Strain (Lagrangian)
	• Strain (Lagrangian)	• Velocity
	• Velocity (mean)	• Displacement
	• Displacement	• Torsion
	From PW (real-time):	
	• Velocity (peak)	
	• Displacement	
Limitations	Only deformation parallel to ultrasound beam is measured	Requires lower frame rate (time between collection of consecutive image frames ≥10 ms)—interpretation may be more reliable if tissue contains some stronger scattering structures
	Affected by translation and tethering	
	Requires high frame rate	
		Off-line implementation (not real-time)
		Different image resolution in axial and lateral beam directions (longitudinal vs. radial in ME and radial vs. circumferential in TG views)
		Dependent on optimal imaging
		Basal motion may result in poor spatial resolution

PW, pulsed wave.

TABLE 38.3	Deformation Values			
Reference	**Strain Mode**	**Normal**	**Impaired Myocardial Function**	**Comment**
Reisner (29)	STI	n = 12 GLS = −24.1 ± 2.9% GL SR = −1.02 ± 0.09/s	n = 27 post-MI GL S = −14.7 ± 5.1% GL SR = −0.57 ± 0.23/s	Good correlation with WMS Cutoff: GLS <−21% GL SR <−0.9/s for detection of post-MI patients
Jamal (62)	DTI	n = 14 L S: Basal: −18 ± 5% Mid: 21 ± 8% Apex: −20 ± 9% L SR: Basal: −1.1 ± 0.4/s Mid: −1.3 ± 0.5/s Apex: −1.3 ± 0.3/s	n = 40 post-MI (WMS = 2): L S: Basal: −10 ± 6% Mid: −12 ± 6% Apex: −11 ± 9% L SR: Basal: −0.7 ± 0.3/s Mid: −0.8 ± 0.4/s Apex: −0.8 ± 0.5/s (WMS = 3): L S: Basal: −4 ± 4% Mid: −7 ± 6% Apex: −6 ± 6% L SR: Basal: −0.4 ± 0.2/s Mid: −0.6 ± 0.3/s Apex: −0.6 ± 0.4/s	Cutoff: S <−13% SR <−0.8/s for infarcted segments
Serri (25)	DTI	n = 45 LS −19.12 ± 3.39%		
	STI	n = 45 LS −18.92 ± 2.19%		
Bogaert (16)	MRI tagged	n = 87 healthy LS −17% R S 38% C S −40%		
Kowalski (27)	DTI	n = 40		
		L S −20%		Higher L S and SR for RV wall
		L SR −1.5–2.0/s		Inhomogeneous values for RV
		R S 46%		
		R SR 3/s		
Hurlburt (30)	STI	n = 60 L S = −18.4 ± 4% (male); and −20.8 ± 4.3% (female) C S = −20.9 ± 4.3% (male); and −25.4 ± 6.3% (female) RS = 35 ± 10.2% (male); and 40 ± 15.6% (female)		
Andersen (35)	DTI	n = 32 LS = −17.93 ± 2.65%		

(continued)

Reference	Strain Mode	Normal	Impaired Myocardial Function	Comment
Abali (32)	DTI	n = 101 L S = –28 ± 8% L SR = –1.5 ± 0.35/s		
Zhang (68)	DTI	n = 720 segments L SR = –1.58 ± 0.38/s		
Kukulski (59)	DTI	n = 20 L S = –18.9 ± 3.7% R S = 25 ± 14%		
Andersen (26)	DTI	n = 55 L SR = –1.5 ± 0.3/s	Basal L SR = –1.8 ± 0.6/s Mid L SR = –1.4 ± 0.3/s Apical L SR = –1.4 ± 0.3/s	
Simmons (75)	DTI	n = 13 (septum) LS = –0.17 ± 0.04% n = 11 (inferior) LS = –0.13 ± 0.04%		
Mizuguchi (70)	STI	n = 30 L S = –22 ± 2.1% R S = 73.2 ± 10.5% C S = 22.1 ± 3.4% Tor = 19.3 ± 7.2°		
Helle-Valle (48)	STI	n = 29 Basal rotation: 4.6 ± 1.3 degrees Apical rotation: –10.9 ± 3.3 degrees Tor: –14.5 ± 3.2 degrees		
Opdahl (50)	STI	n = 18 Basal rotation: –5.9 ± 1.3 degrees Apical rotation: 12.2 ± 3.8 degrees Tor: 17.8 ± 3.7 degrees	n = 9 (EF > 50%) Basal rotation: –6 ± 3 degrees Apical rotation: 13.6 ± 2.1 degrees Tor: 19.1 ± 4.1 degrees	n = 18 (EF < 50%) Basal rotation: –4.8 ± 2.9 degrees Apical rotation: 7.6 ± 3 degrees Tor: 11.6 ± 3.9 degrees
Takeuchi (79)	STI	n = 15 R basal S = 52.8 ± 11.5% R apical S = 26.5 ± 13.5% C basal S = –16.2 ± 3.4% C apical S = –20.6 ± 3.3% Tor = 9.3 ± 3.6 degrees	WMI = 16 (EF > 45%) R basal S = 35.8 ± 10.7% R apical S = 16.5 ± 9% C basal S = –13.7 ± 4% C apical S = –13.5 ± 4.1% Tor = 9.8 ± 4 degrees	WMI = 14 (EF < 45%) R basal S = 27.4 ± 10.3% R apical S = 12.8 ± 5.4% C basal S = –10.7 ± 5.1% C apical S = –7.3 ± 2.6% Tor = 5.6 ± 2.6 degrees
Teske (74)	DTI STI	n = 22 RV L S = –30 ± 7.6% RV L SR = –1.77 ± 0.55/s RV L S = –29.4 ± 5.6 RV L SR = –1.75 ± 0.55		
Chow (80)	STI	n= 27 RV L S = 26.3 ± 2.9% RV L SR = 1.33 ± 0.23/s		

DTI, Doppler Tissue imaging; MI, myocardial infarction; RV, right ventricle; S, strain; SR, strain rate; STI, speckle tracking imaging; WMS, wall motion score; L, longitudinal; R, radial; C, circumferential; GL, global; Tor, torsion.

The diagnostic ability of STI (performed with TTE) in patients undergoing dobutamine stress test was less in the right and left circumflex territories than in the anterior circulation (54). Contrary to DTI, STI depends on image quality. Poor imaging will result in decreased speckled appearance and poor tracking of the myocardium.

APPLICATIONS OF DTI- AND STI-DERIVED STRAIN

DTI-derived strain accurately measures cardiac deformation (20), is sensitive to early ischemia (55), and is useful in assessing myocardial viability after MI better than DTI velocities or wall motion scoring (56). DTI strain in regions remote from ischemia will remain normal, contrary to spectral DTI velocities, which are affected by tethering (19,39).

Ischemia Detection

Acute regional ischemia causes a rapid decrease in segmental contraction during ejection, with the magnitude of regional shortening/thickening reduced proportionally to the reduction in myocardial blood flow. Following systole, myocardial relaxation is delayed as post-systolic shortening (PSS)/thickening occurs.

DTI strain may be an important supplement to the visual assessment of regional LV dysfunction. DTI strain and SR are more direct measures of regional function than tissue velocities, which are also influenced by contractile function of other myocardial regions due to tethering (19). In 17 patients with left anterior descending (LAD) disease (>75% obstruction) and normal baseline EF and wall motion score, DTI strain detected systolic longitudinal expansion in apical segments (baseline −17.7 ± 7.2% vs. 7.5 ± 6.5%) or reduced compression in mid septal segment (baseline −21.8 ± 8.2% vs. −13.1 ± 4.1%) in nearly all patients during balloon occlusion of LAD. Segments not supplied by LAD did not exhibit any strain changes. DTI strain is more sensitive than DTI velocities in detecting regional ischemia. The latter revealed longitudinal expansion in only two thirds of the involved segments (57).

Post-systolic deformation (PSS) is an important feature of ischemic myocardium. When associated with systolic hypokinesis or akinesis, PSS indicates actively contracting, therefore, potentially viable myocardium. In view of the findings from experimental and clinical studies, PSS should be considered an expression of myocardial asynchrony. A segment that does not deform during contraction when LV pressure increases, but does so when LV pressure decreases markedly during isovolumic relaxation, is not likely to be moving passively. DTI can quantify PSS. In an experimental setting, PSS was recorded during moderate (hypokinetic or akinetic myocardium) as well as, severe ischemia (dyskinetic myocardium) (58). During a 50% reduction of LAD flow, hypokinesis was accompa-

nied by decreased longitudinal DTI systolic strain (from 12.3 ± 1.1% to 6.6 ± 1.3%) and substantial PSS (from 0.9 ± 0.2% to 5.1 ± 0.9%). Concurrent LV pressure-segment length and LV stress-segment length loop analysis indicated that PSS was active. If afterload is increased, dyskinesis, for example, may be accompanied by even more marked PSS (58).

DTI strain indexes differentiate acutely ischemic myocardium from normal and dysfunctional myocardium, even in segments that appear visually normal. An acute reduction in regional myocardial blood flow induces, within seconds, a local contractile dysfunction which alters the regional deformation pattern. Consequently, during systole, the radial thickening and circumferential/longitudinal shortening of the ischemic segment are decreased. In addition, the segmental relaxation is considerably impaired during the ischemic insult, and the physiologic early diastolic radial thinning and circumferential/longitudinal lengthening are replaced by ongoing post-systolic thickening and shortening, respectively. Such consistent changes in early diastolic deformation have been proposed as an early marker of regional ischemia. In a population of 90 consecutive coronary artery patients who underwent balloon percutaneous coronary angioplasty (PTCA) of a coronary artery with greater than 90% obstruction, the baseline strain values in the at-risk segments (which had normal wall motion scores [WMS]) were similar to those observed in control patients (radial: 49 ± 6.9% vs. 56.3 ± 11.7%, longitudinal: −21.2 ± 4.5% vs. −23.3 ± 4.7%). At-risk segments with abnormal WMS had decreased strain values (radial: 21.9 ± 11%, longitudinal: −5.2 ± 4.5%) and increased post-systolic deformation (radial: 0.18 ± 0.14%, longitudinal: 0.32 ± 0.26%) as compared to normal and at-risk segments with normal WMS. Coronary occlusion resulted in a 50% reduction of radial and longitudinal strain, which peaked early in diastole and increased post-systolic deformation in all at-risk segments (irrespective of WMS). These changes were reversible, and after 2 minutes of coronary reperfusion, segmental deformation parameters returned to the preocclusion state. Neighboring segments did not exhibit any changes, and presence of collaterals diminished the occlusion-associated changes (less post-systolic strain) (59). DTI myocardial velocities changed during coronary occlusion only in segments with abnormal baseline function and had lower diagnostic accuracy when compared with strain (60).

In clinical settings, patients with regional wall motion abnormalities may have normal DTI myocardial velocities, due to tethering and translational effects. Only strain and SR offer quantitative and objective parameters indicating ischemia. As observed during dobutamine-exercise testing, DTI strain decreased and markedly increased during ischemia, while DTI myocardial velocities did not reveal any changes (61).

Using STI, global longitudinal strain less than −21% (normal: −24.1 ± 2.9%) and SR less than −0.9/s (normal: −1.02 ± 0.09/s) had good sensitivity and specificity

(92% and 89%, and 92% and 96%, respectively) for detection of post-MI with a good linear correlation with WMS index (29). STI-derived circumferential and radial strain is sensitive to acute reduction of myocardial perfusion. During balloon occlusion, there was a significant decrease in circumferential strain (baseline $-18.5 \pm 7.2\%$ to $-10.5 \pm 3.8\%$) and radial strain (baseline $46.5 \pm 19.4\%$ to $35.7 \pm 20.8\%$) and prolongation of the time to peak circumferential and radial strain (53).

Regional Function, Normal Versus Abnormal

Longitudinal deformation parameters are potentially superior to visual WMS in identification and quantification of subtle ischemia-induced changes in regional contractility. When DTI strain parameters were correlated with coronary angiogram, systolic strain and SR were significantly reduced in normokinetic segments supplied by a stenosed coronary artery (>70%) but not in normokinetic segments supplied by a coronary artery without significant lumen narrowing (62). When compared to myocardial velocities, systolic strain and SR differentiated abnormal from normal contracting segments. Infarct-involved segments were differentiated from normal myocardium using cutoff values of less than -13% for strain and less than $-0.8/s$ for SR (62).

DTI radial SR agrees well with wall motion and is significantly reduced in hypokinetic and akinetic segments ($-0.6 \pm 0.5/s$ and $-0.008 \pm 0.3/s$, respectively) than in normokinetic segments ($-2 \pm 0.6/s$). SR reflects changes in WMS induced by dobutamine challenge—it increased in those segments, which revealed augmented wall motion (from $-2 \pm 0.7/s$ to $-4.7 \pm 1.7/s$) and decreased in those segments, which showed deteriorating or unchanged wall motion (from -2.1 ± 1 to $-1.7 \pm 0.8/s$) (63).

Radial and circumferential STI strain enable distinction between normokinetic, hypokinetic, and akinetic segments at rest (defined by cMRI), in a highly reproducible manner and with small intraobserver and interobserver variability ($5.3 \pm 2.6\%$ and $8.4 \pm 3.7\%$, respectively) (64). A cutoff value of radial strain less than 29% differentiated hypokinetic from normokinetic segments with sensitivity and specificity of 83% and a cutoff value of radial strain less than 21% akinetic from hypokinetic segments with sensitivity of 83% and specificity of 94%.

Similar discriminatory ability of STI radial strain was found when transmurality of MI was analyzed using contrast-enhanced cardiac MRI. Radial strain decreased significantly with increased relative hyper-enhancement: $27.7 \pm 8\%$ (normal segments) versus $20.5 \pm 9.7\%$ (nontransmural infarction segments) versus $11.6 \pm 8.5\%$ (transmural infarction segments). Nontransmural infarction was distinguished from transmural infarction segments by radial strain cutoff value of greater than 16.5% (65).

In an experimental model of acute LAD ischemia-reperfusion, extent of infarct correlated well with radial and circumferential STI strain. Myocardial segments with greater than 50% area of infarct (verified by post-mortem

histology) had lower end-systolic radial and circumferential strain and longer time to peak strain versus areas with less than or equal to 50% or no infarct. End-systolic radial strain less than 2% had 88% sensitivity and 95% specificity for detecting infarcted area greater than 50% (66).

The use of STI strain for combined assessment of LAX and SAX cardiac function may allow differentiation of transmurality of chronic infarction and therefore overcome limitations of DTI strain, which is angle limited and can evaluate only longitudinal function reliably. In subendocardial infarction, STI radial strain ($32.4 \pm 20\%$) and circumferential strain ($-15.4 \pm 6.9\%$) are preserved, while longitudinal strain is reduced ($-13.2 \pm 5.6\%$). In contrast, in transmural infarcts both SAX and LAX STI strain are significantly reduced (cutoff value for circumferential strain $<-13.6\%$, sensitivity 73%, specificity 72%) (67).

Recovery

Accurate identification of infarcted, nonviable myocardium from viable, hypokinetic segments has important clinical implications: revascularization benefits only patients with a sufficient amount of viable myocardium while it is unlikely to benefit those with transmural MI. In post-MI patients, in contrast to DTI myocardial velocities, longitudinal DTI SRs of transmurally infarcted segments ($-0.51 \pm 0.17/s$) were significantly decreased when compared with nontransmural ($-1.06 \pm 0.29/s$), subendocardial ($-1.21 \pm 0.41/2$), and normal segments ($-1.58 \pm 0.38/s$). SRs were also significantly reduced in subendocardial infarction compared with normal segments. A cutoff value of SR greater than $-0.59/s$ identified transmural from nontransmural and subendocardial MI and a cutoff value of $-0.98/s > SR > -1.26/s$ identified a subendocardial infarction from normal segments (68).

STI radial strain is able to identify myocardial dysfunction and predict recovery of function using a cutoff value of peak radial strain greater than 17.2%. Segments that failed to recover had lower peak radial strain ($15.2 \pm 7.5\%$) than those which showed functional improvement following surgical or percutaneous revascularization ($22.6 \pm 6.3\%$). This predictive value (sensitivity of 70.2% and specificity of 85.1%) was similar to that of hyper-enhancement by contrast-enhanced MRI (69).

Among patients with cardiovascular risk factors but no overt cardiac disease, longitudinal strain and SR are decreased and circumferential strain is increased in those with apparently normal mitral inflow velocities (E/A > 1). This may imply that LV systolic function and filling are compensated by circumferential shortening at ventricular systole (70).

Right Ventricular Function

Assessment of RV function is important. However, the complex geometric shape and thin wall structure of RV do not allow accurate quantification with conventional 2D and M-mode techniques. In the experimental setting, systolic strain values obtained by DTI, in either inflow or outflow tract, were found to be comparable to those obtained by sonomicrometry (a method, where the actual myocardial length change is measured), independent of the RV loading conditions (71). RV longitudinal function is dominant over short-axis function, and RV inflow tract, represented by the basal RV free wall, is the major contributor in global RV systolic and diastolic function. Therefore, measurement of longitudinal RV inflow deformation, which has better reproducibility of measurements than radial (27), offers valuable insights into global RV function. DTI longitudinal strain measurements showed an insignificant decline with age (average value of 31%, in 54 healthy adults) (72). In laboratory experiments with opened pericardium, increased afterload after pulmonary artery constriction resulted in a shift of myocardial shortening from early-mid to end-systole or even diastole (PSS), whereas a reduction in preload caused by inferior vena cava occlusion induced earlier systolic shortening (71). However, in healthy ambulatory subjects, DTI strain of RV inflow (recorded from the basal segment, lateral to tricuspid annulus) did not change with preload or afterload increase (73). DTI and STI RV peak systolic strain values correlate well (r = 0.73), with DTI values being always higher, slightly overestimating peak systolic strain (74). The correlation for SR was superior (r= 0.90) (74).

Deformation in the Operating Room

Doppler strain is a sensitive means for detecting and localizing myocardial ischemia, as opposed to myocardial velocities. Intraoperative TEE measurements of DTI strain are comparable with transthoracic assessment, and pericardiotomy does not affect them (75). As is expected, Doppler strain measurements are not easily obtained in the radial direction due to Doppler angle and translation cardiac motion (76). DTI-based strain is better suited for the study of longitudinal cardiac deformation. DTI strain was found to be superior to myocardial velocity measurements in detecting and assessing regional myocardial ischemia during off-pump LAD revascularization. DTI strain demonstrated systolic lengthening of the apical septum and reduced longitudinal shortening of the mid septum during interrupted LAD flow. These changes occurred with concomitant deterioration of wall motion and were confined in the LAD territory, while there were no changes in the basal septum, supplied by the right coronary artery (77). At the same time, DTI velocities remained unchanged in the apical septum during interrupted LAD flow, probably explained by traction from the basal segments.

Rotation and Twist

Apical rotation (12.2 ± 3.8 degrees) represents the dominant contribution to LV twist (73 ± 15%) and reflects LV twist over a wide range of hemodynamic conditions, making it a noninvasive, feasible clinical index of LV twist (50). Estimation of LV twist from apical rotation eliminates the requirement of two separate recordings, one for

the base and one for the apex, and a possible calculation problem because of beat-to-beat variation in rotation, as well as the move-through of the LV image plane. In patients with chronic ischemia but preserved LV ejection fraction (LVEF), rotation and twist were similar to healthy subjects, but in those with depressed LVEF, apical rotation and twist were reduced (50). In patients with diastolic dysfunction (DTI E′ < 8 cm/s), peak LV twist is increased in early-stage diastolic dysfunction, mainly because of more vigorous and increased LV apical rotation (78). It is currently unknown if the mechanism of LV twisting and untwisting is independent of the underlying myocardial relaxation in patients with diastolic heart failure, or if is dependent of filling pressure (decreased twist with increased filling pressure) (78).

Systolic twist was depressed and diastolic untwisting prolonged in patients with anterior wall MI and abnormal LV systolic function. These abnormalities were related to reduced apical rotation and associated with the reduction of apical circumferential strain (79). In contrast, systolic twist was maintained in patients with anterior wall MI and LVEF greater than 45%. This is a result of the mild reduction of circumferential strain in the apex that may affect LV twist behavior in mild manner.

Imaging of cardiac deformation offers a new insight into regional and global myocardial function. However, like any ultrasound modality, both DSE and STI depend on image quality and are time-consuming and technically demanding for the novice operator. Although not currently part of the mainstream echocardiographic examination, introduction of DSE and STI in the everyday clinical practice can provide significant objective quantification of LV and RV function.

THREE-DIMENSIONAL ECHOCARDIOGRAPHY

There are numerous commercially available 3D echocardiography systems available which range from traditional ECG-gated reconstruction and real-time 3D (RT3D) transthoracic echocardiography (TTE) to RT3D TEE. The size of the TEE transducer and the computational processing power have historically been considered the main impediments to the development of a practical and clinically useful 3D TEE system. The development of a computer capable of rotational TEE image acquisition/immediate volume rendering and the more recent introduction of a matrix TEE transducer, which permits live RT3D imaging, have been landmark developments in the field of 3D echocardiography.

Real-Time Three-Dimensional Transesophageal Echocardiography

In 2007, Philips Healthcare, Inc. (Andover MA) introduced the first live RT3D TEE imaging system for clinical use. A TTE transducer based on the same matrix array

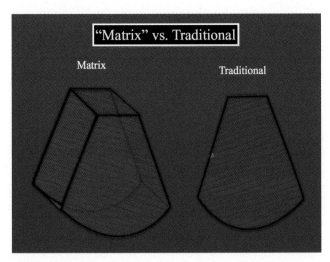

Figure 38.6. Traditional 2D versus volumetric three-dimensional echocardiography with a matrix array.

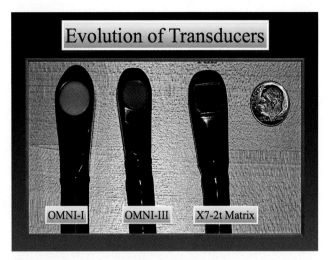

Figure 38.8. Comparison of TEE transducer probe tip relative size (Philips Healthcare, Inc., Andover, MA).

design has been available for several years. Instead of a linear phased array transducer with 128 piezoelectric crystals in a single row, which is the basis of the conventional 2D imaging, this latest development in TEE transducers incorporates 50 rows and 50 columns of crystals (2,500 elements), thus creating a "matrix." Hence, the ultrasound scan generated by a matrix transducer has true 3D characteristics in both elevational and azimuthal planes (Figs. 38.6 and 38.7). RT3D transducers have evolved over the years from bulky and awkward transthoracic devices to the newer matrix arrays, which are similar in size to conventional 2D TEE probes (Fig. 38.8). Significant advancements in transducer technology and data transfer have overcome the major impediment of the transducer size, which had kept this technology from being available for routine clinical use.

The RT3D matrix TEE transducer (X7-2t; Philips Healthcare, Inc; Andover, MA) is capable of conventional multi-planar 2D and Doppler imaging (except DTI) in addition to the RT3D imaging. The TEE probe length is about 10 cm longer than a conventional probe, while the diameter and width of the transducer head are similar to the conventional 2D transducer. Matrix array RT3D image acquisition is obtained via the following modes:

1. "Live 3D" (Fig. 38.9): Generates a pyramidal-shaped ultrasound beam with elevational and azimuthal characteristics. The displayed image is "live" and changes dynamically with probe manipulation. However, only the structures spanned by the width of the beam are displayed on the monitor (Fig. 38.10).
2. "Live Zoom 3D": In this mode of "live" viewing, a "region of interest" is identified within the 3D beam to display a smaller volume of tissue, which is magnified (i.e., "zoom") for better viewing (Fig. 38.11). Although the image is magnified and the structure of

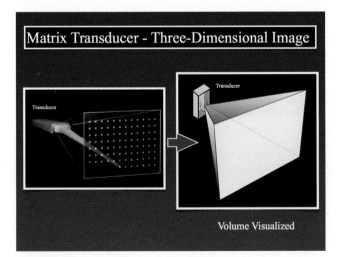

Figure 38.7. Generation of a three-dimensional echocardiographic beam with a matrix transducer.

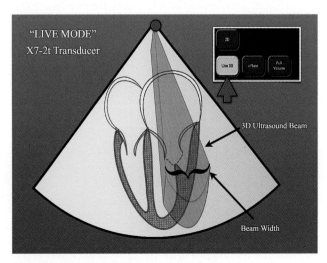

Figure 38.9. A pyramid shape ultrasound beam generated during "Live" 3D imaging with a matrix array.

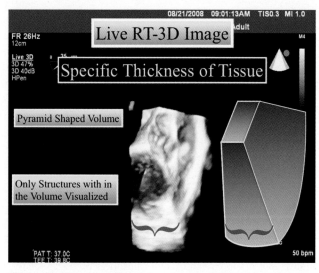

Figure 38.10. Pyramidal shape ultrasound beam and the cardiac structures visualized during the "live" imaging with a matrix array. Note that only the structures within the span of the ultrasound beam can be seen.

interest (e.g., MV) is visualized more closely, there is a certain degree of compromise on the frame rate and some deterioration of spatial orientation as compared to the "Live 3D" image. Live images can be rotated and cropped in multiple orientations in three dimensions, thus permitting the MV, for example, to be visualized from the left atrial as well as LV perspectives.

3. "Volumetric Imaging" (Fig. 38.12): The volumetric imaging is an EKG R-wave gated sequential acquisition of data that requires hybrid reconstruction. In this mode, multiple (4–7) pyramidal-shaped R-wave gated ultrasound beams are generated to visualize a "volume" of tissue. The main advantages of volumetric imaging are that cardiac structures can be interrogated in three dimensions that are larger than the width of a

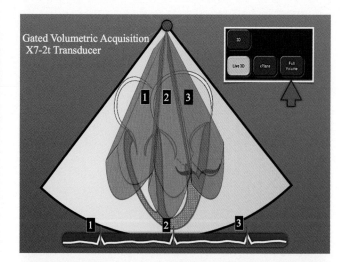

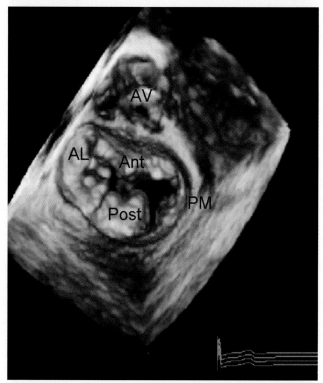

Figure 38.12. A: Volumetric imaging with the X7-2t matrix transesophageal echocardiographic transducer (Philips Healthcare, Inc.). Four to seven individual pyramidal-shaped volumes gated to the "R" wave of the EKG (*red lines*) are generated to create a "full" volume. **B:** Example of a "full volume" image of the MV. AL, antero-lateral commissure; PM, postero-medial commissure; Ant, anterior leaflet; Post, posterior leaflet; AV, aortic valve.

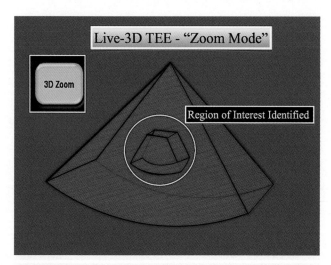

Figure 38.11. Principle of "Live 3D" imaging in "Zoom" mode with a matrix array, which enables the system to focus and zoom on an identified image of interest.

single matrix beam and with significant improvement in spatial resolution and frame rate to improve image quality. For optimal volumetric imaging, the gated volumes have to be "spatially aligned" without motion of the probe or patient and "temporally aligned," which requires acquisition at regularly spaced "R" waves to accurately align multiple volumes in time and space. Volumetric imaging is subject to motion artifacts (respiration and patient movement) and is difficult or sometimes impossible to perform in patients with arrhythmias. Patient and probe movements as well as electrical interference with cautery can significantly compromise the quality of the acquired image.

4. Volumetric imaging with "Color-Flow Doppler": Incorporation of color-flow Doppler (CFD) into the 3D image can currently only be performed in the gated volume acquisition, hybrid reconstruction mode. The acquisition steps are similar to volumetric imaging and are therefore equally subject to motion artifact and dependence on a regular rhythm for optimal acquisition. There is also a significant reduction in the frame rate with simultaneous display of the CFD information and gray scale image during gated volumetric acquisition. However, the image can be manipulated and cropped in multiple dimensions to precisely localize and pinpoint the location of regurgitation jets. Linear and area measurements cannot be made directly from the 2D volumetric or the CFD data sets, and hence the diameter, width of the vena-contracta, or the area estimation of the regurgitant jet cannot be calculated.

The IE-33 ultrasound machine comes equipped with a robust 3D software analysis program (Q-Labs; Philips Healthcare, Inc) for volumetric assessment of LV, as well as geometric reconstruction of MV. The geometric analysis can be performed on a MV image acquired either in the "live mode" or through gated volumetric acquisition.

Mitral Valve Q-Lab (MVQ)

MVQ is based on a "work-flow" arrangement, which enables analysis of the MV in series of sequential steps. Each step has to be completed before advancing to the next step. At the completion of the analysis, a static graphic model of MV is generated, which is color rendered with leaflet contour analysis (Fig. 38.13). In addition, valve

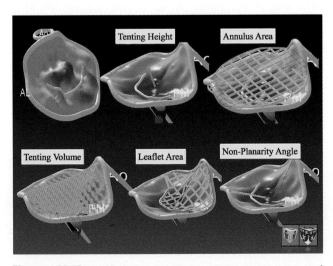

Figure 38.13. Different geometric parameters generated with Q-Lab analysis (3DQ: Philips Healthcare, Inc.) of the MV volumetric data. Ao, aortic valve; AL, antero-lateral; PM, postero-medial.

diameters, leaflet lengths and areas, a nonplanarity angle, and the aorto-mitral angle are automatically calculated (Fig. 38.13).

Left Ventricular Volume (3DQ)

Q-labs is also equipped with the ability to perform volume analysis of the LV (3DQ) based upon a gated volume acquisition with the TEE probe in the ME position. During LV volume analysis, reference points are first identified in the end-systolic and end-diastolic frames. An automated sequence analysis then generates a dynamic stroke volume assessment for the number of beats acquired during triggered acquisition. Global measures of LV function including calculated stroke volume and EF are provided, along with a graphic geometric model of the LV with identification of the individual segments and regional wall motion assessment based on standardized terminology. The accuracy of stroke volume and cardiac output determination is dependent upon a well-defined endocardial border and identification of LV apex.

Classic Reconstruction Three-Dimensional Echocardiography

Three-Dimensional TEE imaging based on ECG R-wave gated reconstruction (Siemens Medical Systems; Mountainview, CA) currently uses a proprietary "On-line Perspective Box" and "Four-Sight TEE" software manufactured by TomTec© (GmBH Germany). The system otherwise only requires a single universal multiplane 2D transducer V5M (Siemens Medical Systems; Mountainview, CA) and rotational acquisition of images. The TomTec© software is also available as stand-alone software for off-line reconstruction of R-wave gated volumetric data sets from any manufacturer systems, provided that system is compatible and equipped with the TomTec© software.

Synchronization of image acquisition with the EKG R-wave is essential for 3D reconstruction. The absolute dependence of image acquisition and reconstruction on R-wave gating makes 3D reconstruction echocardiography very difficult or nearly impossible in patients with arrhythmias or when there is electrocautery interference. The R-wave gated acquisition is performed by progressive automatic rotation of the scan plane from 0 to 180 degrees in three to five degree increments (Fig. 38.14). Immediately after acquisition, multiple 2D slices (i.e., 36 slices for five-degree acquisition, and 60 slices for three-degree acquisition) are volumetrically rendered automatically to generate a 3D image (Fig. 38.15). Depending upon the heart rate, the total time from acquisition to generation of a volumetrically rendered image is generally less than a minute.

Manipulation and reconstruction of images can be performed within the software environment, and multiple orthogonal 2D views can be displayed for orientation, cropping, and rotation. Of particular significance is the "Dart Tool" in the controls, which allows a particular

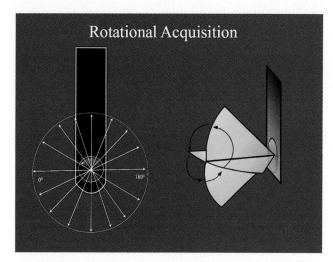

Figure 38.14. An image of V5M transducer (Siemens Medical Systems) showing the principles of rotational acquisition.

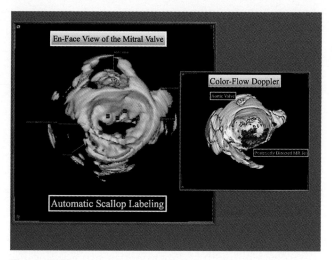

Figure 38.16. En face view of the MV generated with the "MV Assessment Package Software" (TomTec Corp. GmBH Germany) from geometric, rotational acquisition, 3D reconstruction. Note labeled leaflet scallops (**left**) and an en face view of MV with CFD data (**right**).

view of the MV to be selected, and automatically renders the image volumetrically in all dimensions, thus simplifying a very complex and time-consuming reconstruction process. The image is displayed as an en face view of the MV, which can be rotated to view the MV from the LV perspective (Fig. 38.16). Another advantage of the system is the ability to incorporate the CFD information during image acquisition, and display it at the same time as the gray scale image (Fig. 38.16). The 3D controls allow for stop-motion and individual frame advancement for making caliper measurements on the 3D image. The ability to make linear measurements with this software is a very useful and practical tool for routine clinical use. The quality of 3D image depends upon avoidance of motion artifact by keeping the TEE probe still, and acquiring the images during a brief period of apnea and stable EKG rhythm without electrical interference.

In addition to the "Four-Sight TEE" 3D reconstruction software, the On-line Perspective box can be equipped with the "MV Assessment Package Software" (TomTec© Corp. GmBH Germany) for geometric reconstruction of MV. Geometric reconstruction of MN can also be performed on a "work-flow" arrangement of identifying landmarks on selected images in a sequential manner. At the end of the analysis, dynamic en face views of the MV are generated with automatic labeling of the scallops/commissures and the adjoining structures (e.g., AV). In addition, the mitral annulus and the coaptation line between the two leaflets can be superimposed on the en face view of the MV for visualization of the 3D geometry of the mitral annulus from multiple perspectives. Furthermore, CFD imaging can also be incorporated during volumetric acquisition.

Geometric reconstruction generates MV diameters in different orientations in 3D (Fig. 38.17). The geometric analysis can be performed within a few minutes of volumetric data acquisition. If the initial image acquisition was performed with CFD information, the software permits "digitally subtraction" to specifically locate the origin of regurgitation jets.

Traditional "Live" RT3D imaging (TTE or TEE) is limited by the size of the ultrasound beam; thus, intracardiac structures with sizes larger than the dimensions of the 3D ultrasound beam have to be viewed by gated volumetric, hybrid reconstruction imaging. Recently a "Single-Beat Full-Volume Acquisition" (Siemens Medical Systems; Mountainview, CA) of a large volume of tissue has been introduced, in which the transducer generates a 3D beam, which is wide enough to include the whole heart. This technology allows for instantaneous real-time full volumes to be acquired with incorporation of CFD

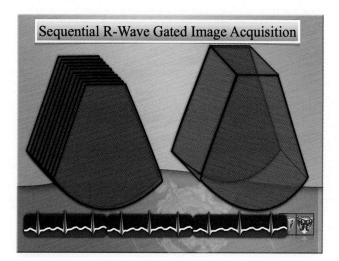

Figure 38.15. Generation of volumetric data based on rotational acquisition of 2D ultrasound slices, gated to "R" wave of EKG (*red lines*).

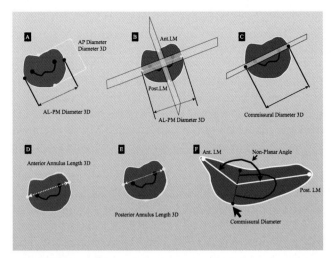

Figure 38.17. Geometric reconstruction with off-line analysis generates MV diameters in different orientations. AP diameter, antero-posterior diameter; AL-PM diameter, anterolateral-posteromedial diameter; Ant.LM, anterior landmark; Post. LM, posterior landmark.

information and therefore has potential applications for real-time quantification of regurgitation and ventricular volume as well as synchrony analysis. However, this technology is currently only with a TTE transducer.

Single-beat full-volume acquisition has been achieved by a special design of a transducer which generates a 900 by 900 volume at 16 cm depth of 2D imaging and a 400 by 400 volume during color-flow imaging (Fig. 38.18). Single-beat full-volume imaging has the potential to eliminate motion-generated "stitch artifacts" and electrical interference. Also, this technology allows the incorporation of CFD information during "live" acquisition, thereby permitting visualization of all ventricular walls, synchrony analysis, and segmental LV systolic function.

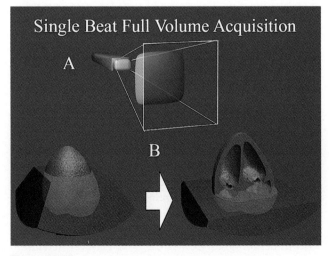

Figure 38.18. Single-beat full-volume acquisition.

Perioperative Applications of Three-Dimensional Echocardiography

Although the concept of 3D echocardiography was first introduced in the early 1970s, its utility in the perioperative environment has only recently acquired appropriate recognition (80). Advantages of both conventional 3D reconstruction and RT3D techniques for enhancing the diagnostic value of conventional echocardiography in the perioperative period have begun to emerge in the literature (81). Primary areas of interest have included the utility of various 3D echocardiography imaging techniques (i.e., TTE; TEE; epicardial) in preoperative surgical planning, intraoperative assessment of the surgical procedure, and postoperative early and long-term follow-up to determine the need for further intervention (82).

The utility of 3D echocardiographic techniques in providing preoperative, noninvasive imaging of intracardiac lesions from the surgeon's visual perspective has been demonstrated in patients with congenital heart and valvular lesions. Lange et al. (83) compared preoperative 2D and 3D reconstruction TTE evaluations with intraoperative findings in 15 patients with atrioventricular septal defect (VSD) morphology. In comparison with preoperative 2D echocardiography, 3D reconstruction TTE provided superior imaging of the MV and tricuspid valve (TV) function. In addition, in this study, 3D reconstruction TTE provided a more precise description of primum atrial septal defect (ASD) size, secundum ASD fenestrations, and VSD size. Acar et al. (84) also performed preprocedural 3D reconstruction TTE in 62 consecutive patients aged 2 to 18 years with ASDs scheduled for either transcatheter (n = 42) or surgical (n = 20) closure. Preprocedural 3D reconstruction TTE measurement of ASD size correlated well with findings obtained intraoperatively and during transcatheter closure. A similar degree of accuracy for 3D reconstruction TTE evaluation of VSD size prior to closure has also been demonstrated (85). Additional reported applications for preoperative 3D echocardiography have included a complementary role to conventional echocardiographic techniques in facilitating surgical planning for defining the shape, dimensions, location, origin, mobility, and valve involvement of cardiac tumors (86). Preoperative 3D reconstruction echocardiography has also been shown to enhance accurate imaging of the spatial relationship between mobile LV thrombi, the myocardial wall, and the valvular apparatus, which subsequently influenced the selection of the most appropriate surgical approach for urgent thrombectomy (87). Finally, several studies have demonstrated the utility of preoperative 3D reconstruction for defining complex MV pathology to facilitate surgical planning. Macnab et al. (88) sought to compare 3D reconstruction with 2D multiplane TEE in the assessment of regurgitant MV morphology in 75 patients prior to valve repair. Using surgical findings as the gold standard in this study, 2D and 3D reconstruction TEE were compared for image quality and accurate detection of functional MV morphology. Adequate recognition of individual leaflet scallops was more frequently obtained with 3D reconstruction imaging (97% of leaflet segments by 3D reconstruction vs. 90% by 2D TEE), especially for commissural pathology. 3D reconstruction TEE was more accurate in defining MV pathology using surgical findings as the gold standard, achieving exact functional description in 92% of segments versus 79% segments with 2D TEE. Specifically, 3D reconstruction TEE was more accurate for identifying commissural and anterior leaflet pathology but not posterior leaflet lesions. Pepi et al. (89) compared the accuracy of 2D and RT3D preoperative TTE with intraoperative 2D and 3D reconstruction TEE for identifying the mechanism of MV prolapse in 112 consecutive patients, using surgical inspection during MV repair as a gold standard (Fig. 38.19). The 3D techniques were performed in a relatively short time (RT3D TTE: 7 ± 4 minutes; 3D reconstruction TEE: 8 ± 3 minutes), with good (RT3D TTE 55%; 3D reconstruction TEE 35%) and optimal (RT3D TTE 21%; 3D reconstruction TEE 45%) imaging quality in the majority of cases. RT3D TTE allowed more accurate identification (95.6% accuracy) of all MV lesions in comparison with other techniques. RT3D TTE and 2D TEE had similar accuracies (90% and 87%, respectively), whereas the accuracy of 2D TTE (77%) was significantly lower. The authors concluded that RT3D TTE and 3D reconstruction TEE are feasible and useful methods in identifying the location of MV prolapse, were superior in the description of pathology in comparison with the corresponding 2D techniques,

and should be regarded as an important adjunct to standard 2D examinations in decisions regarding MV repair. Fabricius et al. (90) evaluated the feasibility, accuracy, and limitations of preoperative 3D reconstruction TEE in 51 patients with MV disease. The width of the anterior leaflet was measured with both 2D and 3D reconstruction TEE, and compared with operative findings. The 3D dynamic sequences of the reconstructed MV were shown preoperatively to the surgeon and later compared with the intraoperative finding. The quality of the 3D reconstruction TEE was graded as good in 25 patients (49.0%), fair in 16 patients (31.4%), and poor in 10 patients (19.6%) where atrial fibrillation did not allow ECG gating. Based on intraoperative findings, sensitivity for the diagnosis of MV prolapse using 2D TEE and 3D reconstruction TEE was 97.7% and 92.9% (P = ns), respectively, and specificity was 100% by both methods. Sensitivity for the diagnosis of rupture of chordae tendinae using 2D TEE and 3D reconstruction TEE was 92.3% and 30.8%, respectively (P < 0.05), and specificity was 100% by both methods. The authors concluded that dynamic 3D reconstruction echocardiography allows adequate preoperative planning when reconstruction is being considered. However, dynamic 3D reconstruction may be limited by the quality of the original 2D echo cross-sectional images, which can be adversely affected by minimal patient movements, respiration, or cardiac arrhythmia. Thus, preoperative 3D echocardiography may facilitate surgical planning by providing superior imaging of intracardiac structures, although ECG and respiratory gating requirements may be more limiting for reconstructive techniques, compared to RT3D echocardiography.

The accuracy, feasibility, and value of 3D echocardiography have also been demonstrated in the intraoperative environment. Abraham et al. (91) performed intraoperative 2D and 3D reconstruction TEE examinations on 60 patients undergoing valve surgery. In this study, 3D reconstruction acquisitions were completed in 87% of the patients within a mean acquisition time of 2.8 ± 0.2 minutes and reconstruction time within 8.6 ± 0.7 minutes. 3D reconstruction TEE detected all salient valve morphological pathology (leaflet perforations, fenestrations, and masses), which was subsequently confirmed on pathological examination in 84% of the patients (Fig. 38.20). In addition, intraoperative 3D reconstruction TEE provided new additional information not obtained by 2D TEE in 15 patients (25%) and in one case influenced the surgeon's decision to perform a valve repair rather than a replacement. Furthermore, intraoperative 3D reconstruction TEE provided worthwhile and complementary anatomic information that explained the mechanism of valve dysfunction demonstrated by 2D imaging and color flow Doppler (Fig. 38.21). Ahmed et al. (92) evaluated the potential utility of 3D reconstruction TEE in identifying individual MV scallop prolapse in 36 adult patients with undergoing surgical correction. Perfect correlation between 3D reconstruction TEE and surgical findings was

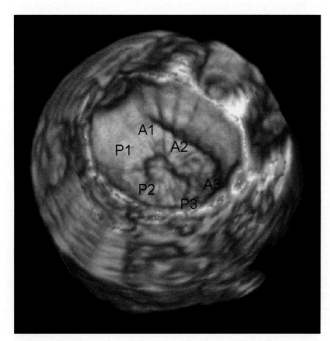

Figure 38.19. Transesophageal 3D echocardiographic reconstructed en face view of a MV with prolapse of the P2 (middle) scallop of the posterior leaflet. A1, anterior-lateral; A2, anterior-middle; A3, anterior-medial; P1, posterior-lateral; P3, posterior-medial.

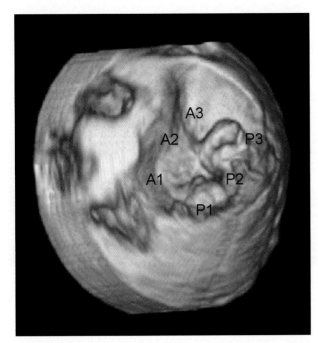

Figure 38.20. Transesophageal 3D echocardiographic reconstructed en face view of a MV with prolapse of the P2 (middle) and P1 (lateral) scallops, and an endocarditis vegetation on the P3 (medial) scallop of the posterior leaflet. A1, anterior-lateral; A2, anterior-middle; A3, anterior-medial.

42 consecutive patients, undergoing MV repair for mitral regurgitation, that intraoperative RT3D TEE is a feasible and efficient method for identifying specific MV pathology in the setting of complex disease, and is superior to 2D TEE imaging specifically in the diagnosis of P1, A2, A3, and bileaflet disease (P < 0.05) (Figs. 38.22–38.26). Intraoperative 3D TEE may be particularly useful in the evaluation of prosthetic valves in the mitral position. Sugeng et al. evaluated the quality of intraoperative RT3D TEE images of prosthetic valves in 47 patients undergoing MV surgery (94) (Figs. 38.27 and 38.28). The quality was considered superior and in addition, RT3D TEE imaging had 96% agreement with surgical findings.

Intraoperative 3D echo may also provide unique perspectives into dynamic valve lesions (Fig. 38.29). For example, in a case report by Jungwirth et al., intraoperative RT3D TEE datasets revealed additional information about the abnormalities of the MV apparatus in a patient with hypertrophic obstructive cardiomyopathy (HOCM) and MV systolic anterior motion (SAM) with persistent left ventricular outflow tract (LVOT) obstruction and MR following an initial LV septal myectomy (95). Specifically intraoperative RT3D TEE enabled the spatial assessment of the extent of maximal septal thickness, the degree of LVOT obstruction, and the intimate relationship between MV and LVOT including specific leaflet scallops involved and the extent of systolic mitral leaflet-to-septal contact. In addition, intraoperative 3D TEE has been used to identify distortion and folding of the mitral annulus as a cause of functional mitral stenosis or worsening mitral regurgitation during beating heart surgery while positioning to access the back of the heart (96). Thus, intraoperative

noted in 78% of the patients. Similarly, De Castro et al. demonstrated superior concordance between intraoperative 3D reconstruction TEE and surgical identification of prolapsing anterior and posterior MV scallops compared to 2D TEE (14,93). Grewal et al. also demonstrated in

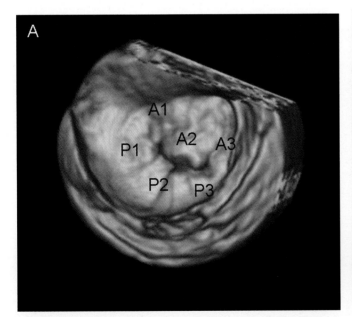

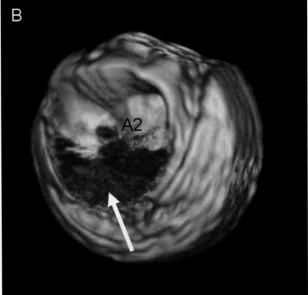

Figure 38.21. A: Transesophageal 3D echocardiographic reconstructed en face view of a MV with prolapse of the A2 (middle) scallop of the anterior leaflet. **B:** Superimposed color flow Doppler demonstrates significant jet of mitral regurgitation (*arrow*). A1, anterior-lateral; A3, anterior-medial; P1, posterior-lateral; P2, posterior-middle; P3, posterior-medial.

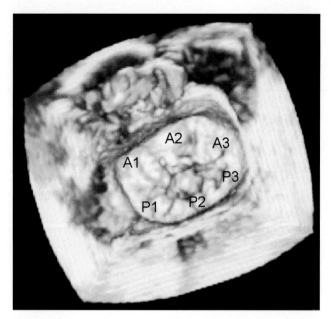

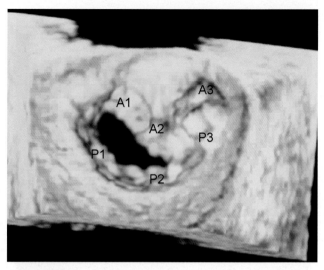

Figure 38.24. Transesophageal 3D echocardiographic full volume en face view of a MV obtained with a matrix array, which demonstrates fusion of the P3 (medial) and A3 (medial) scallops of the respective leaflets, in a patient with rheumatic valve disease. A1, anterior-lateral; A2, anterior-middle; P1, posterior-lateral; P2: posterior-middle.

Figure 38.22. Transesophageal 3D echocardiographic full volume en face view of a MV obtained with a matrix array, which demonstrates a flail P2 (middle) scallop of the posterior leaflet. A1, anterior-lateral; A2, anterior-middle; A3, anterior-medial; P1, posterior-lateral; P3, posterior-medial.

3D echocardiography may not only be useful for delineating MV pathology but may also be used to guide surgical decision making by providing unique insight into the dynamic mechanism of complex valve dysfunction (Fig. 38.30).

Native AV, TV, and pulmonic valve (PV) pathologies may be less easy to define with 3D TEE techniques compared to MV disease due to thinner leaflet tissue and often their oblique orientation to the probe. In 211 patients studied by Sugeng et al. (97) using RT3D TEE, AV cusps were optimally visualized in only 18% to 21% of patients (Fig. 38.31), while TV cusps (Fig. 38.32) were optimally

visualized only 11% of the time. The PV may be the most difficult to image. Despite the poorer image quality of the AV, 3D reconstruction TEE with color flow Doppler may be helpful in identifying the location and extent of AV dehiscence (98);the location of vegetations and extent of damage caused by endocarditis (99); and measurement of hemodynamic, anatomic, and functional changes after transcatheter-based transapical AV implantation (100). Finally, intraoperative 3D echocardiography has also been reported to be useful in facilitating surgical decision making pertaining to congenital lesions including VSDs (101), mitral leaflet clefts (102) (Fig. 38.33), intracardiac tumors (103), and left atrial appendage pathology (104,105).

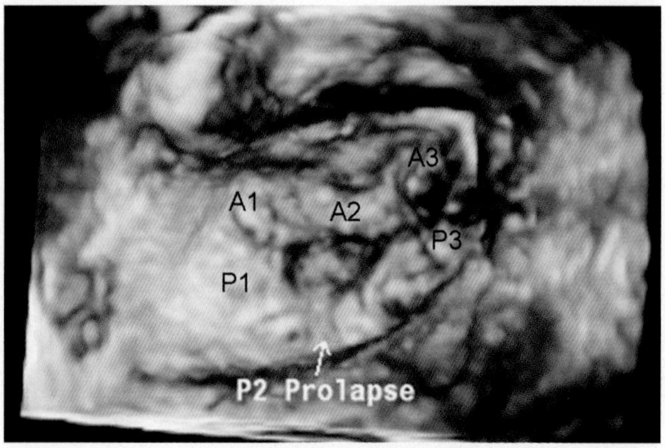

While 3D reconstruction (106) and the recent introduction of a sophisticated miniaturized transducers with matrix arrays capable of RT3D volume rendering (107) have facilitated the acceptance and endorsement of 3D TTE and TEE into perioperative clinical practice, it is also important to remember the potential value of intraoperative epicardial echocardiography, especially in patients in whom TEE probe placement may be difficult or contraindicated (108). Comprehensive RT3D epicardial examinations can be efficiently performed, and permit rapid acquisition of immediately available data to assist intraoperative surgical decision making. De Castro et al. (109) evaluated the feasibility, effectiveness, and incremental value of intraoperative RT3D epicardial echocardiography performed before and after CPB in 30 consecutive cardiac surgical patients with AV (N = 18) and MV (N = 12) disease (Fig. 38.34). The authors reported that RT3D epicardial echocardiography was feasible in all patients and

Figure 38.23. Transesophageal 3D echocardiographic full volume en face view of a MV obtained with a matrix array, which demonstrates prolapse of the P2 (middle), P3 (medial), and A3 (medial) scallops of the respective leaflets. A1, anterior-lateral; A2, anterior-middle; P1, posterior-lateral.

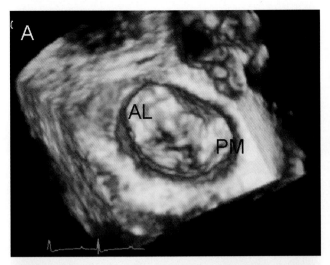

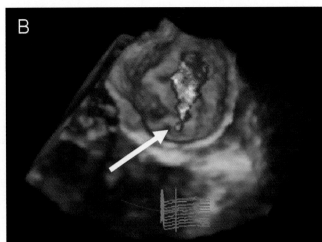

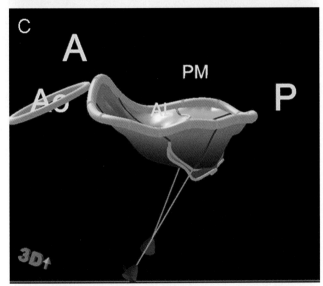

Figure 38.25. **A:** Transesophageal 3D echocardiographic en face view of a MV obtained with a matrix array, which demonstrates apical tethering of the P2 (middle) and A2 (middle) scallops of the respective leaflets in a patient with functional mitral regurgitation. **B:** Superimposed color flow Doppler demonstrates significant jet of mitral regurgitation (*arrow*). **C:** Computer-generated model of the MV (Q-Labs; MVQ; Philips Healthcare, Inc.) demonstrating apical tethering of the anterior and posterior leaflets. A, anterior; P, posterior; AL, anterolateral commissure; PM, postero-medial commissure; Ao, aortic valve.

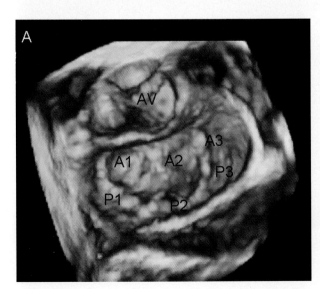

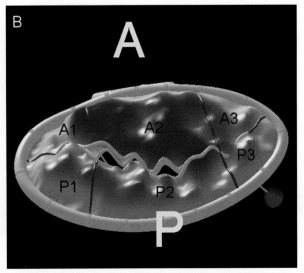

Figure 38.26. **A:** Transesophageal 3D echocardiographic full volume en face view of a MV obtained with a matrix array, which demonstrates diffuse prolapse of both leaflets, in a patient with myxomatous degeneration. **B:** Computer-generated model of the MV (Q-Labs; MVQ; Philips Healthcare, Inc.) demonstrating diffuse prolapse of both anterior (A) and posterior (P) leaflets. A1, anterior-lateral; A2, anterior-middle; A3, anterior-medial; P1, posterior-lateral; P2, posterior-middle; P3, posterior-medial.

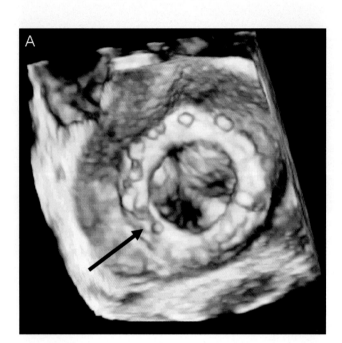

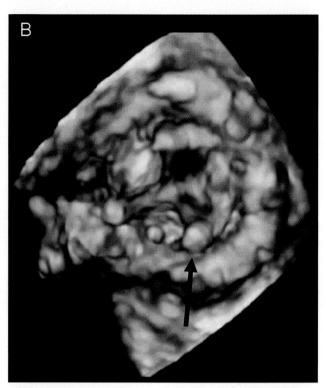

Figure 38.27. **A:** Transesophageal 3D echocardiographic full volume en face view from the left atrial perspective, of a bioprosthetic MV replacement. *White arrow*: bioprosthetic valve ring. **B:** Same bioprosthetic MV replacement rotated to view from the LV perspective. *Black arrow*: bioprosthetic valve strut.

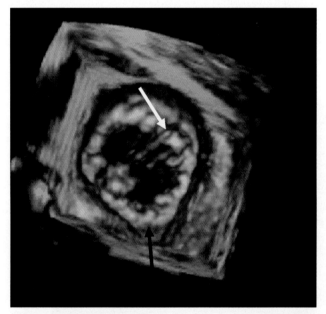

Figure 38.28. Bileaflet mechanical MV transesophageal 3D echocardiographic full volume en face view from the left atrial perspective, of a bi-leaflet mechanical MV replacement. *White arrow*: mechanical valve strut; *black arrow*: mechanical valve ring.

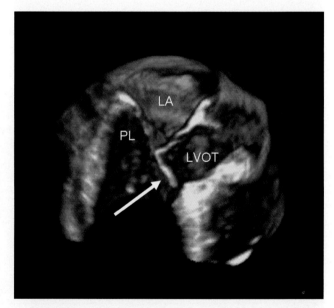

Figure 38.29. Transesophageal 3D echocardiographic reconstructed view, demonstrating SAM of the anterior leaflet (*arrow*) of the MV. LA, left atrium; PL, posterior leaflet; LVOT, left ventricular outflow tract.

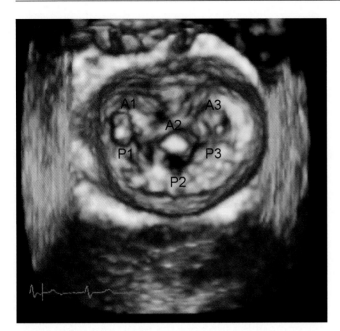

Figure 38.30. Transesophageal 3D echocardiographic full volume en face view of a MV obtained with a matrix array, which demonstrates A2 (middle) prolapse and a flail P1 (lateral) scallop of the respective leaflets. A1, anterior-lateral; A3, anterior-medial; P2, posterior-middle; P3, posterior-medial.

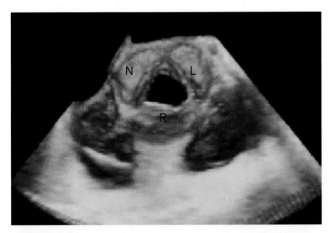

Figure 38.31. Transesophageal 3D echocardiographic full volume en face view of a normal AV obtained with a matrix array. N, noncoronary cusp; L, left coronary cusp; R, right coronary cusp.

superior in depicting aortic cusp morphologic lesions; LVOT spatial relationships with mitral apparatus and aortic root; and both anterior and posterior mitral leaflet scallops, particularly at the posterior commissure. The utility of intraoperative RT3D epicardial echocardiography has been reported in a patient with HOCM undergoing septal myomectomy, for enhancing the spatial assessment, extent of septal thickening, MV SAM, and postsurgical LVOT patency (110). Qin et al. also performed intraoperative epicardial and postoperative RT3D TTE to evaluate changes in LV volume and function in cardiac surgical

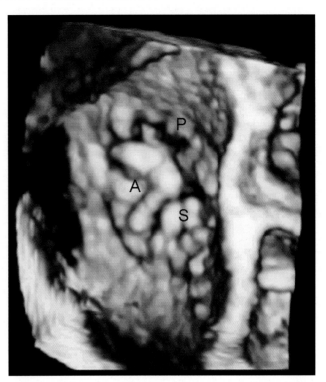

Figure 38.32. Transesophageal 3D echocardiographic full volume en face view of a TV from the right atrial perspective obtained with a matrix array, demonstrating prolapse of the anterior (A) and septal (S) leaflets. P, posterior leaflet.

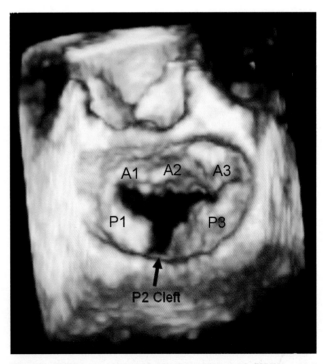

Figure 38.33. Transesophageal 3D echocardiographic full volume en face view of a MV obtained with a matrix array, demonstrating a cleft in P2 (middle) scallop (*arrow*). A1, anterior-lateral; A2, anterior-middle; A3, anterior-medial; P1, posterior-lateral; P3, posterior-medial.

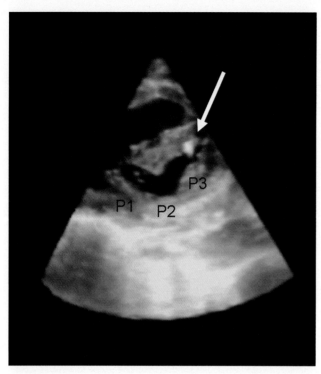

Figure 38.34. Epicardial 3D echocardiographic en face view of a MV obtained with a matrix array, demonstrating an endocarditis vegetation (*arrow*) on the A3 (medial) scallop of the anterior leaflet. P1, posterior-lateral; P2, posterior-middle; P3, posterior-medial.

patients undergoing infarct exclusion surgery for ischemic cardiomyopathy (111). In contrast to 3D echocardiographic imaging, conventional 2D methods may not accurately quantify LV volumes in patients with severe ischemic cardiomyopathy, especially in the presence of significant geometric changes due to an LV aneurysm.

While not necessarily considered a classic intraoperative environment, the electrophysiology and cardiac catheterization laboratories also provide opportunities for demonstrating the unique utility of cutting-edge 3D echocardiographic periprocedural imaging techniques (112). The main potential benefit of 3D echocardiography in the electrophysiology laboratory lies in real-time guidance of complex ablation procedures and precise assessment of cardiac dyssynchrony (113). For example, Mackensen et al. (114) reported the successful application of RT3D TEE to confirm stable catheter position along the entire length of the ligament of Marshall during left atrial catheter ablation for atrial fibrillation. In addition, RT3D TEE has been shown to be beneficial in guiding percutaneous closure of paravalvular leaks following valve surgery (115–117); percutaneous ASD (118) and post-MI VSD closure (119), as well as less invasive percutaneous valve repair and replacement techniques. Furthermore, in studies comparing 2D versus 3D TEE for measuring MV area and volume in patients with stenosis undergoing percutaneous MV balloon valvuloplasty, 3D TEE enabled a better description of valve anatomy including

the identification of commissural splitting and leaflet tears post valvuloplasty (120–122).

Finally, the accuracy, feasibility, and value of 3D echocardiography have also been demonstrated in the postoperative period following cardiac surgery. Kronzon et al. (123) sought to assess the use of RT3D TEE in the evaluation of postoperative MV dehiscence in 18 consecutive patients who previously underwent surgery, and were found postoperatively to have annuloplasty or prosthetic valve ring dehiscence (Fig. 38.35). The authors hypothesized that the unique diagnostic images obtained using RT3D TEE would allow (a) evaluation of the MV and ring anatomy; (b) diagnosis of the presence of dehiscence and delineation of its characteristics; and (c) evaluation of whether the mitral regurgitation could be treated without the need for reoperation with identification of potential candidates for percutaneous occlusion of the paravalvular orifice (Fig. 38.36). RT3D TEE allowed accurate evaluation of the pathology, including definition of the type of ring or prosthesis used; description of the site, size, shape, and area of the dehisced segment; and clear definition of the mitral regurgitation origin that could be used to help in planning the most appropriate corrective intervention. Qin et al. (124) also used RT3D TTE to accurately quantify LV volumes following ventricular reconstruction for dyskinetic or akinetic segments in 30 patients with ischemic cardiomyopathy to determine the impact of surgery due to complicated geometric changes. RT3D epicardial echocardiography studies were initially performed before and after infarct exclusion surgery, followed by RT3D TTE 42 ± 67 days after surgery in 22 of the patients. Significant decreases in LV end-diastolic volume indices (EDVI)

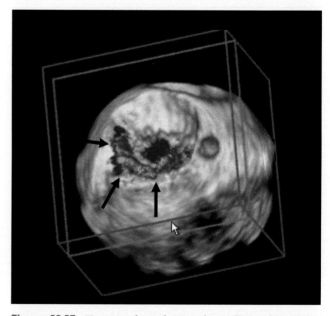

Figure 38.35. Transesophageal 3D echocardiographic reconstructed en face view of a dehisced bioprosthetic MV with a significant mitral regurgitation jet along the posterior annulus (*black arrows*).

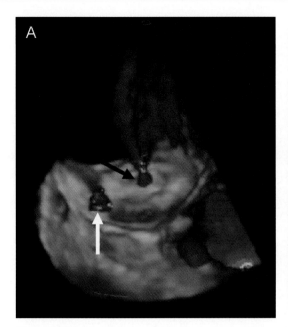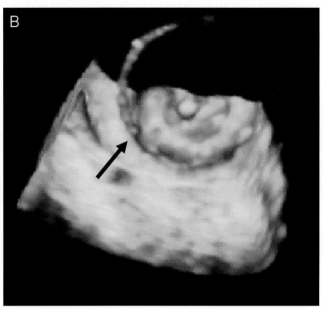

Figure 38.36. **A:** Transesophageal 3D echocardiographic en face view with color flow Doppler obtained with a matrix array, demonstrating a single-tilting-disc mechanical MV with a normal central washing jet (*black arrow*), and large perivalvular leak (*white arrow*). **B:** Real-time "live" transesophageal 3D echocardiography with a matrix array used to guide an occluder device wire (*black arrow*) across the perivalvular leak.

and end-systolic volume indices (ESVI) were apparent immediately after infarct exclusion surgery and in follow-up (EDVI 99 ± 40, 67 ± 26, and 71 ± 31 mL/m², respectively; ESVI 72 ± 37, 40 ± 21, and 42 ± 22 mL/m², respectively; P < 0.05). LV EF increased significantly and remained higher (0.29 ± 0.11, 0.43 ± 0.13, and 0.42 ± 0.09, respectively, P < 0.05). Smaller end-diastolic and end-systolic volumes, measured with RT3DE immediately after infarct exclusion surgery, were closely related to improvement in New York Heart Association functional class at clinical follow-up. The authors concluded that RT3DE can be used to quantitatively assess changes in LV volume and function after complicated LV reconstruction, and that decreased LV volume and increased EF imply a reduction in LV wall stress after infarct exclusion surgery and are predictive of symptomatic improvement.

Perioperative 3D TEE may offer some primary advantages over 2D echocardiography. Three-dimensional echocardiography can provide a potentially more efficient process for acquiring a comprehensive echocardiographic examination, which may be particularly important in the volatile intraoperative environment where timely and effective clinically relevant decision-making may be critical. By enabling the inclusion of depth and volume, more data are available for interpretation in a given imaging window for evaluating global and regional ventricular function. 3D echocardiography may also be superior to 2D techniques for defining important geometric relationships between components of complex intracardiac structures such as the mitral apparatus (125). Furthermore, the ability to rotate and crop whole volume data sets without any directional restriction enables an infinite

number viewing perspectives of cardiac and great vessel infrastructure. In addition to enabling potentially greater efficiency in performing a comprehensive intraoperative TEE examination, 3D TEE may also permit more accurate diagnoses and more effective communication with interventionalists. Unique imaging windows of the MV and TV as well as the left atrial appendage, which are not readily obtainable with 2D, can be presented in en face views to better appreciate anatomy and functional geometry and help communicate relevant diagnostic information to those less familiar with echocardiographic displays. These unique views may be more familiar to cardiac surgeons and cardiology interventionalists, and may therefore facilitate a better understanding of abnormal anatomy and associated pathology. Finally, 3D echocardiography can also assist in determining mechanisms and severity of dynamic pathophysiological states which often require surgical intervention including functional mitral regurgitation, HOCM, and SAM of the MV.

While the direct impact of 3D TEE on surgical outcomes has yet to be determined, perioperative 3D echocardiography will undoubtedly continue to improve upon the efficiency, accuracy, and communication of important diagnoses related to cardiovascular disease, thereby facilitating perioperative clinical decision making. Thus, assuming inevitable growth in the technological development of more sophisticated ultrasound transducers in the near future, the introduction of improvements in image acquisition, processing speed, real-time volume rendering, and transducer miniaturization may promote RT3DE into becoming the technique of choice for noninvasive intraoperative cardiac imaging.

KEY POINTS

- Myocardial *strain* (S or ε) is the deformation of a myocardial fiber, normalized to its original length: $S = L_1 - L_0/L_0$ (%) where L_0 is the baseline (end-diastolic) length and L_1 is the end-systolic length of the myocardial fiber. *Strain* is positive when two points are moving apart and negative when two points move near. Therefore, radial thickening is associated with positive strain ($L_1 > L_0$), while longitudinal shortening and circumferential thinning are associated with negative strain ($L_1 < L_0$).

- SR reflects the speed of myocardial deformation (strain): $SR = S/t$ (s − 1), where t is the time duration of this deformation. For normal myocardium, SR reflects regional contractile function because it is relatively independent of heart rate, whereas systolic strain reflects changes in stroke volume.

- DTI-derived strain accurately measures cardiac deformation, is sensitive to early ischemia, and is better than DTI velocities or wall motion scoring in assessing myocardial viability after MI. DTI strain in regions remote from ischemia will remain normal, contrary to spectral DTI velocities, which are affected by tethering.

- A conventional linear phased array transducer has 128 piezoelectric crystals aligned in a single row. Alternatively, RT3D transesophageal imaging uses a matrix array that incorporates 50 rows and 50 columns of crystals (2,500 element "matrix") to permit the simultaneous display of both elevational and azimuthal planes in live and hybrid reconstructed, full-volume modes

- The 3D reconstruction using 2D, multiplane phased array transesophageal probes requires synchronization (i.e., "gating") of image acquisition with the EKG R-wave and respiration. The absolute dependence of image acquisition and reconstruction on R-wave gating makes 3D reconstruction echocardiography very difficult or nearly impossible in patients with arrhythmias or when there is electrocautery interference. The R-wave gated acquisition is performed by progressive automatic rotation of the scan plane from 0 to 180 degrees in 3 to 5 degree increments to acquire multiple 2D slices which subsequently are volumetrically rendered automatically to generate a 3D image.

- Single-beat full-volume imaging has the potential to eliminate motion-generated "stitch artifacts" and electrical interference, and allows the incorporation of "live" color flow Doppler, thereby permitting visualization of all ventricular walls, synchrony analysis, and segmental LV systolic function.

REFERENCES

1. Click RL, Abel MD, Schaff HV. Intraoperative transesophageal echocardiography: 5-year prospective review of impact on surgical management. *Mayo Clin Proc* 2000;75:241–247.
2. Couture P, Denault AY, McKenty S, et al. Impact of routine use of intraoperative transesophageal echocardiography during cardiac surgery. *Can J Anesth* 2000;47:20–26.
3. Kolev N, Brase R, Swanevelder J, et al. The influence of transoesophageal echocardiography on intra-operative decision making. A European multicentre study. *Anaesthesia* 1998;53:767–773.
4. Denault AY, Couture P, McKenty S, et al. Perioperative use of transesophageal echocoardiography by anesthesiologists: impact in noncardiac surgery and in the intensive care unit. *Can J Anesth* 2001;49:287–293.
5. Kallmeyer IJ, Collard CD, Fox JA, et al. The safety of intraoperative transesophageal echocardiography: a case series of 7200 cardiac surgical patients. *Anesth Analg* 2001;92:1126–1130.
6. London MJ. Assessment of left ventricular global systolic function by transesophageal echocardiography. *Ann Card Anaesth* 2006;9:157–163.
7. Bergquist BD, Leung JM, Bellows WH. Transesophageal echocardiography in myocardial revascularization: I. Accuracy of intraoperative real-time interpretation. *Anesth Analg* 1996;82:1132–1138.
8. Lang RM, Bierig M, Devereux R, et al. Recommendations for chamber quantification: a report from the American Society of Echocardiography's Guidelines and Standards Committee and the Chamber Quantification Group, developed in conjunction with the European Association of Echocardiography, a branch of the European Society of Cardiology. *J Am Soc Echocardiogr* 2005;18:1440–1463.
9. Quinones MA, Otto CM, Stoddard M, et al. Recommendations for quantification of Doppler echocardiography: a report from the Doppler quantification task force of the nomenclature and standards committee of the American Society of Echocardiography. *J Am Soc Echocardiogr* 2002;15:167–184.
10. Marwick TH. Techniques for comprehensive two dimensional echocardiographic assessment of left ventricular systolic function. *Heart* 2003;89(Suppl. III):iii2–iii8.
11. Chen C, Rodriguez L, Guerrero JL, et al. Noninvasive estimation of the instantaneous first derivative of left ventricular pressure using continuous-wave pressure echocardiography. *Circulation* 1991;83:2101–2110.
12. Thomas JD, Popovic ZB. Assessment of left ventricular function by cardiac ultrasound. *J Am Coll Cardiol* 2006;48:2012–2025.
13. Sengupta PP, Korinek J, Belohlavek M, et al. Left ventricular structure and function. Basic science for cardiac imaging. *J Am Coll Cardiol* 2006;48:1988–2001.
14. Gallagher KP, Matsuzaki M, Koziol JA, et al. Regional myocardial perfusion and wall thickening during ischemia in conscious dogs. *Am J Physiol* 1984;247:H727–H738.
15. Marwick TH. Measurements of strain and strain rate by echocardiography. Ready for prime time? *J Am Coll Cardiol* 2006;47:1313–1327.
16. Bogaert J, Rademakers F. Regional nonuniformity of normal adult human left ventricle. *Am J Physiol Heart Circ Physiol* 2001;280:H610–H620.
17. Marwick TH. Clinical applications of tissue Doppler imaging: a promise fulfilled. *Heart* 2003;89:1377–1378.

18. Korinek J, Wang J, Sengupta PP, et al. Two-dimensional strain—a Doppler-independent ultrasound method for quantification or regional deformation: validation in vitro and in vivo. *J Am Soc Echocardiogr* 2005;18:1247–1253.
19. Urheim S, Edvardsen T, Torp H, et al. Myocardial strain by Doppler echocardiography. Validation of a new method to quantify regional myocardial function. *Circulation* 2000;102:1158–1164.
20. Edvardsen T, Gerber BL, Garot J, et al. Quantitative assessment of intrinsic regional myocardial deformation by Doppler strain rate echocardiography in humans: validation against three-dimensional tagged magnetic resonance imaging. *Circulation* 2002;106:50–56.
21. Amundsen BH, Helle-Valle T, Edvardsen T, et al. Noninvasive myocardial strain measurement by speckle tracking echocardiography. Validation against sonomicrometry and tagged magnetic resonance imaging. *J Am Coll Cardiol* 2006;47:789–793.
22. Modesto KM, Cauduro S, Dispenzieri A, et al. Two-dimensional acoustic pattern derived strain parameters closely correlate with one-dimensional tissue Doppler derived strain measurements. *Eur J Echocardiogr* 2006;7:315–321.
23. Weidemann F, Jamal F, Sutherland GR, et al. Myocardial function defined by strain rate and strain during alterations in inotropic states and heart rate. *Am J Physiol Heart Circ Physiol* 2002;283:H792–H799.
24. Greenberg NL, Firstenberg MS, Castro PL, et al. Doppler-derived myocardial systolic strain is a strong index of left ventricular contractility. *Circulation* 2002;105:99–105.
25. Serri K, Reant P, Lafitte M, et al. Global and regional myocardial function quantification by two-dimensional strain. Application in hypertrophic cardiomyopathy. *J Am Coll Cardiol* 2006;47:1175–1181.
26. Andersen NH, Poulsen SH. Evaluation of the longitudinal contraction of the left ventricle in normal subjects by Doppler tissue tracking and strain rate. *J Am Soc Echocardiogr* 2003;16:716–723.
27. Kowalski M, Kukulski T, Jamal F, et al. Can natural strain and strain rate quantify regional myocardial deformation? A study in healthy subjects. *Ultrasound Med Biol* 2001;27:1087–1097.
28. Leitman M, Lysyanski P, Sidenko S, et al. Two-dimensional strain—a novel software for real-time quantitative echocardiographic assessment of myocardial function. *J Am Soc Echocardiogr* 2004;17:1021–1029.
29. Reisner SA, Lysyanski P, Agmon Y, et al. Global longitudinal strain: a novel index of left ventricular systolic function. *J Am Soc Echocardiogr* 2004;17:630–633.
30. Hurlburt HM, Aurigemma GP, Hill JC, et al. Direct ultrasound measurement of longitudinal, circumferential, and radial strain using 2-dimensional strain imaging in normal adults. *Echocardiography* 2007;24:723–731.
31. Hashimoto I, Li X, Hejmadi Bhat A, et al. Myocardial strain rate is a superior method for evaluation of left ventricular subendocardial function compared with tissue Doppler imaging. *J Am Coll Cardiol* 2003;42:1574–1583.
32. Abali G, Tokgozoglu L, Ozcebe OI, et al. Which Doppler parameters are load independent? A study in normal volunteers after blood donation. *J Am Soc Echocardiogr* 2005;18:1260–1265.
33. Choi J-O, Shin D-H, Cho SW, et al. Effect of preload on left ventricular longitudinal strain by 2D speckle tracking. *Echocardiography* 2008;25:873–879.
34. Becker M, Kramann R, Dohmen G, et al. Impact of left ventricular loading conditions on myocardial deformation parameters: analysis of early and late changes of myocardial deformation parameters after aortic valve replacement. *J Am Soc Echocardiogr* 2007;20:681–689.
35. Andersen NH, Terkelsen CJ, Sloth E, et al. Influence of preload alterations on parameters of systolic left ventricular long-axis function: a Doppler tissue study. *J Am Soc Echocardiogr* 2004;17:941–947.
36. Waggoner AD, Bierig SM. Tissue Doppler imaging: a useful echocardiographic method for the cardiac sonographer to assess systolic and diastolic ventricular function. *J Am Soc Echocardiogr* 2001;14:1143–1152.
37. Skubas NJ. Intraoperative Doppler tissue imaging is a valuable addition to cardiac anesthesiologists' armamentarium: a core review. *Anesth Analg* 2009;108:48–66.
38. Wilkenshoff UM, Sovany A, Wigström L, et al. Regional mean systolic myocardial velocity estimation by real-time color Doppler myocardial imaging: a new technique for quantifying regional systolic function. *J Am Soc Echocardiogr* 1998;11:684–692.
39. Skulstad H, Urheim S, Edvardsen T, et al. Grading of myocardial dysfunction by tissue Doppler echocardiography. A comparison between velocity, displacement, and strain imaging in acute ischemia. *J Am Coll Cardiol* 2006;47:1672–1682.
40. Cho G-Y, Chan J, Leano R, et al. Comparison of two-dimensional speckle and tissue velocity based strain and validation with harmonic phase magnetic resonance imaging. *Am J Cardiol* 2006;97:1661–1666.
41. Herbots L, Maes F, D'hooge J, et al. Quantifying myocardial deformation throughout the cardiac cycle: a comparison of ultrasound strain rate, grey-scale M-mode and magnetic resonance imaging. *Ultrasound Med Biol* 2004;30:591–598.
42. Teske AJ, De Boeck BWL, Melman PG, et al. Echocardiographic quantification of myocardial function using tissue deformation imaging, a guide to image acquisition and analysis using tissue Doppler and speckle tracking. *Cardiovasc Ultrasound* 2007;5:27–46.
43. Thomas G. Tissue Doppler echocardiography—a case of right tool, wrong use. *Cardiovasc Ultrasound* 2004;2:12–18.
44. Gilman G, Khanderia BK, Hagen ME, et al. Strain and strain rate: a step-by-step approach to image and data acquisition. *J Am Soc Echocardiogr* 2004;17:1001–1020.
45. Sutherland GR, Bijnens B, McDicken WN. Tissue Doppler echocardiography. Historical perspectives and technological considerations. *Echocardiography* 1999;16:445–453.
46. D'hooge J, Bijnens B, Thoen J, et al. Echocardiographic strain and strain-rate imaging: a new tool to study regional myocardial function. *IEEE Trans Med Imag* 2002;9:1030.
47. Notomi Y, Lysyanski P, Setser RM, et al. Measurement of ventricular torsion by two-dimensional ultrasound speckle tracking imaging. *J Am Coll Cardiol* 2005;45:2034–2041.
48. Helle-Valle T, Crosby J, Edvardsen T, et al. New noninvasive method for assessment of left ventricular rotation: speckle tracking echocardiography. *Circulation* 2005;112:3149–3156.
49. Foster E, Lease KE. New untwist on diastole. What goes around comes back. *J Am Coll Cardiol* 2006;113:2477–2479.
50. Opdahl A, Helle-Valle T, Remme EW, et al. Apical rotation by speckle tracking echocardiography: a simplified bedside index of left ventricular twist. *J Am Soc Echocardiogr* 2008;21:1121–1128.
51. Notomi Y, Martin-Miklovic MG, Oryszak SJ, et al. Enhanced ventricular untwisting during exercise. A mechanistic manifestation of elastic recoil described by Doppler tissue imaging. *J Am Coll Cardiol* 2006;113:2524–2533.

52. Perk G, Tunick PA, Kronzon I. Non-Doppler two-dimensional strain imaging by echocardiography-from technical considerations to clinical applications. *J Am Soc Echocardiogr* 2007;20:234–243.

53. Winter R, Jussila R, Nowak J, Brodin L-Å. Speckle tracking echocardiography is a sensitive tool for the detection of myocardial ischemia: a pilot study from the catheterization laboratory during percutaneous coronary intervention. *J Am Soc Echocardiogr* 2007;20:974–981.

54. Hanekom L, Cho G-Y, Leano R, et al. Comparison of two-dimensional speckle and tissue Doppler strain measurement during dobutamine stress echocardiogarphy: an angiographic correlation. *Eur Heart J* 2007;28:1765–1772.

55. Voigt J-U, Exner B, Schmiedehausen K, et al. Strain-rate imaging during dobutamine stress echocardiography provides objective evidence of inducible ischemia. *Circulation* 2003;107:2120–2126.

56. Hoffmann R, Altiok E, Nowak B, et al. Strain rate measurement by Doppler echocardiography allows improved assessment of myocardial viability in patients with depressed left ventricular function. *J Am Coll Cardiol* 2002;39:443–449.

57. Edvardsen T, Skulstad H, Aakhus S, et al. Regional myocardial systolic function during acute myocardial ischemia assessed by strain Doppler echocardiography. *J Am Coll Cardiol* 2001;37:726–730.

58. Skulstad H, Edvardsen T, Urheim S, et al. Postsystolic shortening in ischemic myocardium. Active contraction or passive recoil? *Circulation* 2002;106:718–724.

59. Kukulski T, Jamal F, Herbots L, et al. Identification of acutely ischemic myocardium using ultrasonic strain measurements. A clinical study in patients undergoing coronary angioplasty. *J Am Coll Cardiol* 2003;41:810–819.

60. Kukulski T, Jamal F, D'hooge J, et al. Acute changes in systolic and diastolic events during clinical coronary angioplasty: a comparison of regional velocity, strain rate, and strain measurement. *J Am Soc Echocardiogr* 2002;15:1–12.

61. Voigt J-U, Nixdorff U, Bogdan R, et al. Comparison of deformation imaging and velocity imaging for detecting regional inducible ischaemia during dobutamine stress echocardiography. *Eur Heart J* 2004;25:1517–1525.

62. Jamal F, Kukulski T, Sutherland GR, et al. Can changes in systolic longitudinal deformation quantify regional myocardial function after an acute infarction? An ultrasonic strain rate and strain study. *J Am Soc Echocardiogr* 2002;15:723–730.

63. Nakatani S, Stugaard M, Hanatani A, et al. Quantitative assessment of short axis wall motion using myocardial strain rate imaging. *Echocardiography* 2003;20:145–149.

64. Becker M, Bilke E, Kuehl H, et al. Analysis of myocardial deformation based on pixel tracking in two dimensional echocardiographic images enables quantitative assessment of regional left ventricular function. *Heart* 2006;92:1102–1108.

65. Becker M, Hoffmann R, Kuehl H, et al. Analysis of myocardial deformation based on ultrasonic pixel tracking to determine transmurality in chronic myocardial infarction. *Eur Heart J* 2006;27:2560–2566.

66. Migrino RQ, Zhu X, Pajewski N, et al. Assessment of segmental myocardial viability using regional 2-dimensional strain echocardiography. *J Am Soc Echocardiogr* 2007;20:342–351.

67. Chan J, Hanekom L, Wong C, et al. Differentiation of subendocardial and transmural infarction using two-dimensional strain rate imaging to assess short-axis and long-axis myocardial function. *J Am Coll Cardiol* 2006;48:2026–2033.

68. Zhang Y, Chan AKY, Yu C-M, et al. Strain rate imaging differentiates transmural from non-transmural myocardial infarction. *J Am Coll Cardiol* 2005;46:864–871.

69. Becker M, Lenzen A, Ocklenburg C, et al. Myocardial deformation imaging based on ultrasonic pixel tracking to identify reversible myocardial dysfunction. *J Am Coll Cardiol* 2008;51:1473–1481.

70. Mizuguchi Y, Oishi Y, Miyoshi H, et al. The functional role of longitudinal, circumferential, and radial myocardial deformation for regulating the early impairment of left ventricular contraction and relaxation in patients with cardiovascular risk factors: a study with two-dimensional strain imaging. *J Am Soc Echocardiogr* 2008;21:1138–1144.

71. Jamal F, Bergerot C, Argaud L, et al. Longitudinal strain quantitates regional right ventricular contractile function. *Am J Physiol Heart Circ Physiol* 2003;285:2842–2847.

72. Kjaergaard J, Sogaard P, Hassager C. Quantitative echocardiographic analysis of the right ventricle in healthy individuals. *J Am Soc Echocardiogr* 2006;19:1365–1372.

73. Kjaergaard J, Snyder EM, Hassager C, et al. Impact of preload and afterload on global and regional right ventricular function and pressure: a quantitative echocardiography study. *J Am Soc Echocardiogr* 2006;19:515–521.

74. Teske AJ, De Boeck BWL, Olimulder M, et al. Echocardiographic assessment of regional right ventricular function: a head-to-head comparison between 2-dimensional and tissue Doppler-derived strain analysis. *J Am Soc Echocardiogr* 2008;21:275–283.

75. Simmons LA, Weidemann F, Sutherland GR, et al. Doppler tissue velocity, strain, and strain rate imaging with transesophageal echocardiography in the operating room: a feasibility study. *J Am Soc Echocardiogr* 2002;15:768–776.

76. Norrild K, Pedersen TF, Sloth E. Transesophageal tissue Doppler echocardiography for evaluation of myocardial function during aortic valve replacement. *J Cardiothorac Vasc Anesth* 2007;21:367–370.

77. Skulstad H, Andersen K, Edvardsen T, et al. Detection of ischemia and new insight into left ventricular physiology by strain Doppler and tissue velocity imaging: assessment during coronary bypass operation of the beating heart. *J Am Soc Echocardiogr* 2004;17:1225–1233.

78. Park SJ, Miyazaki C, Bruce CJ, et al. Left ventricular torsion by two-dimensional speckle tracking echocardiography in patients with diastolic dysfunction and normal ejection fraction. *J Am Soc Echocardiogr* 2008;21:1129–1137.

79. Takeuchi M, Nishikage T, Nakai H, et al. The assessment of left ventricular twist in anterior wall myocardial infarction using two-dimensional speckle tracking imaging. *J Am Soc Echocardiogr* 2007;20:36–44.

80. Matsumoto M, Matsuo H, Kitabatake A, et al. Three-dimensional echocardiograms and two-dimensional echocardiographic images at desired planes by a computerized system. *Ultrasound Med Biol* 1977;3:163–178.

81. Hung J, Lang R, Flaschkampf F, et al. 3D echocardiography: a review of the current status and future directions. *J Am Soc Echocardiogr* 2007;20:213–33.

82. Gunasegaran K, Yao J, De Castro S, et al. Three-dimensional transesophageal echocardiography (TEE) and other future directions. *Cardiol Clin* 2000;18:893–910.

83. Lange A, Mankad P, Walayat M, et al. Transthoracic 3-D echocardiography in the preoperative assessment of atrioventricular defect morphology. *Am J Cardiol* 2000;85:630–635.

84. Acar P, Roux D, Dulac Y, et al. Transthoracic 3-D echocardiography prior to closure of atrial septal defects in children. *Cardiol Young* 2003;13:58–63.

85. Acar P, Abdel-Massih T, Douste-Blazy M, et al. Assessment of muscular VSD closure by transcatheter or surgical approach: a 3-D echocardiographic study. *Eur J Echocardiogr* 2002;3:185–191.

86. Borges AC, Witt C, Bartel T, et al. Preoperative two-dimensional and three-dimensional echocardiographic assessment of heart tumors. *Ann Thorac Surg* 1996;61:1163–1167.

87. Muller S, Bartel T, Laube H. Left ventricular thrombus after pregnancy: choice of surgical access using dynamic three-dimensional echocardiography. *Echocardiography* 1996;13:293–296.

88. Macnab A, Jenkins NP, Bridgewater BJ, et al. Three dimensional echocardiography is superior to multiplane transoesophageal echo in the assessment of regurgitant mitral valve morphology. *Eur J Echocardiogr* 2004;5:212–222.

89. Pepi M, Tamborini G, Maltagliati A, et al. Head-to-head comparison of two- and three-dimensional transthoracic and transesophageal echocardiography in the localization of mitral valve prolapse. *J Am Coll Cardiol* 2006;48:2524–2530.

90. Fabricius AM, Walther T, Falk V, et al. Three-dimensional echocardiography for planning of mitral valve surgery: current applicability? *Ann Thorac Surg* 2004;78:575–578.

91. Abraham T, Warner J, Kon N, et al. Feasibility, accuracy, and incremental value of intraoperative three-dimensional transesophageal echocardiography in valve surgery. *Am J Cardiol* 1997;80:1577–1582.

92. Ahmed S, Nanda N, Miller A, et al. Usefulness of transesophageal three-dimensional echocardiography in the identification of individual segment/scallop prolapse of the mitral valve. *Echocardiography* 2003;20:203–209.

93. De Castro S, Salandin V, Cartoni D, et al. Qualitative and quantitative evaluation of mitral valve morphology by intraoperative volume-rendered three-dimensional echocardiography. *J Heart Valve Dis* 2002;11:173–180.

94. Sugeng L, Shernan S, Weinert L, et al. Real-Time 3D transesophageal echocardiography in valve disease: comparison with surgical findings and evaluation of prosthetic valves. *J Am Soc Echocardiogr* 2008;21:1347–1354.

95. Jungwirth B, Adams DB, Mathew JP, et al. Mitral valve prolapse and systolic anterior motion illustrated by real time three-dimensional transesophageal echocardiography. *Anesth Analg* 2008;107:1822–1824.

96. George S, Al-Russeh S, Amrani M. Mitral annulus distortion during beating heart surgery: a potential cause for hemodynamic disturbance—a three-dimensional echocardiographic reconstruction study. *Ann Thorac Surg* 2002;73:1424–1430.

97. Sugeng L, Shernan S, Salgo I, et al. Real-time three-dimensional transesophageal echocardiography using fully-sampled matrix array probe. *J Am Coll Cardiol* 2008;52:446–449.

98. Mukhtari O, Horton C, Nanda N, et al. Transesophageal color doppler three-dimensional echocardiographic detection of prosthetic aortic valve dehiscence: correlation of surgical findings. *Echocardiography* 2001;18:393–397.

99. Nemes A, Lagrand W, McGhie J, et al. Three-dimensional transesophageal echocardiography in the evaluation of aortic valve destruction by endocarditis. *J Am Soc Echocardiogr* 2006;19:355.e13–355.e14.

100. Scohy TV, Soliman OI, Lecomte PV, et al. Intraoperative real time three-dimensional transesophageal echocardiographic measurement of hemodynamic, anatomic and functional changes after aortic valve replacement. *Echocardiography* 2009;26:96–99.

101. Chen FL, Hsiung MC, Nanda N, et al. Real time three-dimensional echocardiography in assessing ventricular septal defects: an echocardiographic-surgical correlative study. *Echocardiography* 2006;23:562–568.

102. Nomoto K, Hollinger I, DiLuozzo G, et al. Recognition of a cleft mitral valve utilizing real-time three-dimensional transoesophageal echocardiography. *Eur J Echocardiogr* 2009;10:367–369.

103. Scohy TV, Lecomte PV, McGhie J, et al. Intraoperative real time three-dimensional transesophageal echocardiographic evaluation of right atrial tumor. *Echocardiography* 2008;25:646–649.

104. Mizuguchi KA, Burch TM, Bulwer BE, et al. Thrombus or bilobar left atrial appendage? Diagnosis by real-time three-dimensional transesophageal echocardiography. *Anesth Analg* 2009;108:70–72.

105. Matyal R, Karthik S, Subramaniam B, et al. Real-time three-dimensional echocardiography for left atrial appendage ligation. *Anesth Analg* 2009;108(5):1467–1469.

106. Mahmood F, Karthik S, Subramaniam B, et al. Intraoperative application of geometric three-dimensional mitral valve assessment package: a feasibility study. *J Cardiothorac Vasc Anesth* 2008;22:292–229.

107. Fischer G, Salgo I, Adams D. Real-time three-dimensional transesophageal echocardiography: the matrix revolution. *J Cardiothorac Vasc Anesth* 2008;22:904–912.

108. Reeves ST, Glas KE, Eltzschig H, et al. Guidelines for performing a comprehensive epicardial echocardiography examination: recommendations of the American Society of Echocardiography and the Society of Cardiovascular Anesthesiologists. *Anesth Analg* 2007;105:22–28.

109. De Castro S, Salandin V, Cavarretta E, et al. Epicardial real-time three-dimensional echocardiography in cardiac surgery: a preliminary experience. *Ann Thorac Surg* 2006;82:2254–2259.

110. Nash P, Agler D, Shin J, et al. Epicardial real-time 3-dimensional echocardiography during septal myectomy for obstructive hypertrophic cardiomyopathy. *Circulation* 2003;108:e54–e55.

111. Qin J, Shiota T, Asher C, et al. Usefulness of real-time three-dimensional echocardiography for evaluation of myectomy in patients with hypertrophic cardiomyopathy. *Am J Cardiol* 2004;94:964–966.

112. Silvestry F, Kerber R, Brook M, et al. Echocardiography-guided interventions. *J Am Soc Echocardiogr* 2009; 22:213–231.

113. Kautzner J, Peichl P. 3D and 4D echo-applications in EP laboratory procedures. *J Interv Card Electrophysiol* 2008;22:139–144.

114. Mackensen B, Hegland D, Rivera D, et al. Real-time 3-dimensional transesophageal echocardiography during left atrial radiofrequency catheter ablation for atrial fibrillation. *Circ Cardiovasc Imaging* 2008;1;85–86.

115. Little SH, Kleiman N, Guthikonda S. Percutaneous paravalvular repair: guidance using live 3-dimensional transesophageal echocardiography. *J Am Coll Cardiol* 2009;53:1467.

116. Hammerstingl C, Lickfett L, Nickenig G. Real-time three-dimensional transoesophageal echocardiography for guidance of interventional closure of paravalvular leakage. *Eur Heart J* 2009;30:915.

117. Biner S, Rafique AM, Kar S, Siegel RJ. Live three-dimensional transesophageal echocardiography-guided transcatheter closure of a mitral paraprosthetic leak by Amplatzer occluder. *J Am Soc Echocardiogr* 2008;21:1282.e7–1282.e9.

118. Roman KS, Nii M, Golding F, et al. Images in cardiovascular medicine. Real-time subcostal 3-dimensional echocardiography for guided percutaneous atrial septal defect closure. *Circulation* 2004;109:e320–e321.

119. Halpern DG, Perk G, Ruiz C, et al. Percutaneous closure of a post-myocardial infarction ventricular septal defect guided by real-time three-dimensional echocardiography. *Eur J Echocardiogr* 2009;10:569–571.

120. Langerveld J, Valocik G, Plokker T, et al. Additional value of three-dimensional transesophageal echocardiography for patients with mitral valve stenosis undergoing balloon valvuloplasty. *J Am Soc Echocardiogr* 2003;16:841–849.

121. Applebaum RM, Kasliwal RR, Kanojia A, et al. Utility of three-dimensional echocardiography during balloon mitral valvuloplasty. *J Am Coll Cardiol* 1998;32:1405–1409.

122. Zamorano J, Cordeiro P, Sugeng L, et al. Real-time three-dimensional echocardiography for rheumatic mitral valve stenosis evaluation: an accurate and novel approach. *J Am Coll Cardiol* 2004;43:2091–2096.

123. Kronzon I, Sugeng L, Perk G, et al. Real-time 3-dimensional transesophageal echocardiography in the evaluation of postoperative mitral annuloplasty ring and prosthetic valve dehiscence. *J Am Coll Cardiol* 2009;53:1543–1547.

124. Qin J, Shiota T, McCarthy P, et al. Real-time three-dimensional echocardiographic study of left ventricular function after infarct exclusion surgery for ischemic cardiomyopathy. *Circulation* 2000;102:III-101–III-106.

125. Salcedo E, Quaife R, Seres T, et al. A framework for systematic characterization of the mitral valve by real-time three-dimensional transesophageal echocardiography. *J Am Soc Echocardiogr* 2009;22:1087–1099.

QUESTIONS

1. Which of the following statements pertaining to strain is incorrect?
   A. Longitudinal shortening and circumferential thinning are associated with negative strain ($L_1 < L_0$)
   B. Myocardial strain is the deformation of a myocardial fiber, normalized to its original length
   C. Radial thickening is associated with positive strain ($L_1 > L_0$)
   D. Strain is load independent
   E. Strain is positive when two locations are moving apart

2. Which of the following characteristics of DTI-derived strain is not correct?
   A. DTI longitudinal strain can be measured in TEE midesophageal (ME) views
   B. DTI strain is angle dependent
   C. DTI strain measures deformation along multiple dimensions
   D. DTI strain is limited by dropout artifact
   E. DTI strain is limited by reverberation artifact

3. Which of the following characteristics of 2D strain recorded with speckle tracking imaging (STI) is not correct?
   A. It is a non-Doppler technique
   B. It is angle dependent

C. Radial and circumferential deformation can be measured in TEE short-axis views
D. Radial and longitudinal deformation can be measured in TEE ME views

4. Which of the following characteristic of speckle track imaging is not correct?
   A. Tracking algorithms require the entire myocardium to be visualized throughout the cardiac cycle
   B. Sensitivity is decreased due to applied smoothing
   C. Visualization of the endocardial border is necessary for clear and reliable radial and transverse tracking
   D. Incorrect calculation of deformation is possible by erroneous tracking of stationary reverberations
   E. Requires imaging at a high frame rate

5. Which of the following statements pertaining to three-dimensional (3D) transesophageal echocardiographic imaging using a matrix array is correct?
   A. Highest spatial and temporal resolution in the ZOOM mode
   B. Image display in only the azimuthal plane
   C. Requirement for ECG gating in the LIVE mode
   D. More accurate imaging of mitral valve (MV) commissural pathology compared to conventional 2D imaging

CHAPTER 39

Echocardiographic Evaluation of Pericardial Disease

Edwin G. Avery ■ Stanton K. Shernan

PERICARDIAL ANATOMY

The pericardium is most simply described as a two-layered sac measuring approximately 2 mm in overall thickness that encloses the myocardium along with its appendages and proximal portions of its vascular connections to the circulatory system. The two layers of the pericardium are separated by a potential space that variably contains between 5 and 50 mL of pericardial fluid under normal physiologic conditions. The inner layer of the pericardium is directly adherent and continuous with the epicardium; this thin layer of tissue is termed the visceral pericardium. The outer layer of the pericardium is thicker and is termed the parietal pericardium. The pericardial layers join together at various points to form reflections that create sinuses within the pericardium. Figure 39.1 demonstrates the relationships between the pericardial layers and the myocardium. The pericardial reflections around the vena cavae and pulmonary veins create the oblique pericardial sinus. The reflections around the proximal aorta and pulmonary artery create the transverse sinus, as depicted in Figure 39.2A and B.

Each pericardial layer is composed of an interdigitated monolayer of serosal mesothelial cells along with its loose underlying connective tissue. The underlying loose connective tissue contains nerves, arteries, lymph nodes, and lymphatics that supply the pericardium.

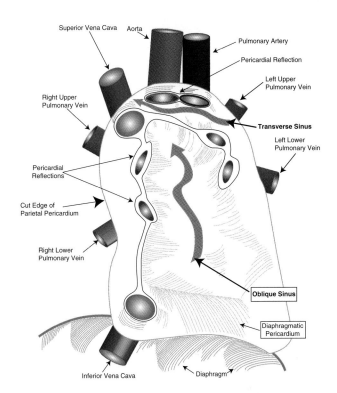

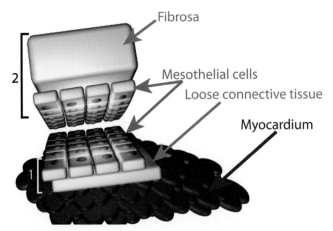

Figure 39.1. Pericardial layers and their relationship to the myocardium. 1: Visceral pericardium or epicardium; 2: Parietal pericardium.

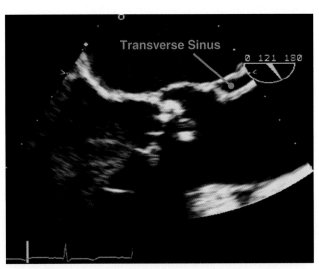

Figure 39.2. A: Pericardial space and sinuses with myocardium and visceral pericardium removed. **B:** TEE midesophageal long-axis view of the transverse sinus. Transverse sinus is indicated by the orange marker.

The mesothelial cells have microvillous projections. The grossly transparent visceral pericardium is continuous with the epicardium at its basal lamina. The grossly translucent parietal pericardium is a continuation of the same mesothelial layer that makes up the visceral pericardium but is distinct in that its outer covering contains the fibrosa. The addition of the fibrosa, a collection of fibrocollagenous tissue, imparts thickness, increased density, and strength to the pericardium. The pericardial fluid is a plasma ultrafiltrate that is secreted by the microvilli-lined mesothelial cells (1).

PERICARDIAL PHYSIOLOGY

Macrophysiology

The definitive function of the pericardium is not completely understood although it does appear to maintain the characteristic "heart-shaped" appearance of the organ. Myocardium that is not bound by intact pericardium assumes a more globular shape, although this does not appear to have a significant effect on cardiac function. The pericardium provides restraint to the heart in that if the heart is overloaded with volume acutely it will limit the amount of volume that the heart can accept in diastole and thus may also prevent acute atrioventricular valvular incompetence. The fibrosal layer of the parietal pericardium has ligamentous attachments at the central tendon of the diaphragm and throughout the mediastinum; these attachments are thought to anchor the heart and prevent excessive motion of the myocardium within the mediastinum. The microvilli and the unevenly distributed pericardial fluid are thought to help reduce friction between the pericardial layers during the cardiac cycle.

Microphysiology

In general, the microphysiologic function of the pericardium is not well understood but appears to be complex. The mesothelial microvilli secrete biochemical mediators into the pericardial fluid (e.g., prostacyclin) and may therefore play an undefined role in regulating epicardial coronary vascular tone and possibly myocardial contractility. Other biochemicals secreted into the pericardial space serve a fibrinolytic function in that smaller amounts of blood that enter the pericardial space remain fluid, rather than clotting. Additional fluid that accumulates in the pericardial space will initially find its way into the various recesses and sinuses. Once the pericardial sinuses and recesses are full with accumulating fluid, the mesothelial cells of the pericardium will begin to reorganize in order to accommodate the additional fluid, provided that it occurs slowly (1). Rapidly accumulating fluid (i.e., over hours to days) will not allow adequate time for mesothelial reorganization and hypertrophy to occur and tamponade physiology will ensue. The pressure volume relationships

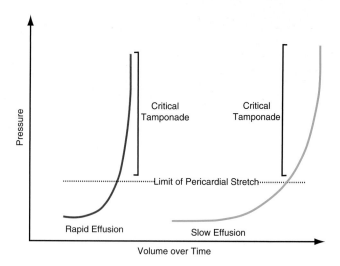

Figure 39.3. Pressure to volume relationships in slowly versus rapidly accumulating pericardial fluid collections in an animal model.

that characterize both acute and chronic accumulation of pericardial fluid are presented in Figure 39.3 (2).

Respirophasic Variation

In order to more completely understand how ultrasound assessment of pericardial physiology is conducted, the concept of respirophasic variation must be introduced. Respirophasic variation describes changes in flow into, out of, and within the heart coincident with pressure dynamics in the intrapleural cavity. Normally during spontaneous respiration changes in intrathoracic or intrapleural pressures are nearly equally transmitted to the pericardial space and intracardiac chambers. The pericardial pressure commonly approximates pleural pressure and will vary with the respiratory cycle demonstrating pressures of approximately −6 mm Hg at end inspiration and −3 mm Hg at end expiration (i.e., as measured by a fluid-filled, non–balloon-tipped catheter). It is the lowering of intrathoracic and pericardial pressure during inspiration that permits increased filling of the right-sided chambers in that venous return is augmented. The true filling pressure of the heart is determined by transmural pressure, which is calculated by subtracting the pericardial pressure from the intracardiac pressure. Figure 39.4A presents a sample calculation of the true right heart filling pressure during inspiration. The same inspiratory negative intrapleural pressures create a pooling of the increased right ventricular (RV) output in the pulmonary circulation, which reduces left atrial (LA) pulmonary venous return. The decrease in LA return results in a decrease in left ventricular (LV) stroke volume and output. Additionally, the decrease in intrathoracic pressure during spontaneous inspiration relative to higher extrathoracic systemic arterial pressures may contribute to a decrease in left heart output related to a relatively higher afterload

True RA Filling Pressure = RAP - Pericardial Pressure
(at end inspiration)

RAP = 6 mm Hg (directly measured)
Pericardial Pressure ≅ Intrapleural Pressure = -8 cm H_2O
X cm H_2O / 1.36 = mm Hg (allows conversion of cm H_2O to mm Hg)

= 6 mm Hg - (-8 cm H_2O = -6 mm Hg)
= 6 mm Hg - (-6 mm Hg)

True RA Filling Pressure = 12 mm Hg

True LV Afterload = DBP - Pericardial Pressure
(at end inspiration)

DBP = 90 mm Hg (directly measured)
Pericardial Pressure ≅ Intrapleural Pressure = -8 cm H_2O
X cm H_2O / 1.36 = mm Hg (allows conversion of cm H_2O to mm Hg)

= 90 mm Hg - (-8 cm H_2O / 1.36 = -6 mm Hg)
= 90 mm Hg - (-6 mm Hg)

True LV Afterload = 96 mm Hg

Figure 39.4. Sample calculation of right heart filling pressure (**A**) and left heart afterload (**B**) in a spontaneously breathing patient. DBP, diastolic blood pressure.

that is associated with the negative intrapleural pressure. Figure 39.4B presents a sample calculation of the true left heart afterload calculation (1,3). LV afterload is primarily modulated by changes in systemic vascular resistance, but the relative differences between intrapericardial and intrathoracic pressures do affect this parameter as demonstrated in Figure 39.4B. Doppler changes in the transatrioventricular valvular velocities accompany these intrapericardial pressure dynamics. Transtricuspid velocities normally increase by approximately 20% during the inspiratory phase of spontaneous respiration (Fig. 39.5A). Transmitral velocities normally decrease by approximately 10% during spontaneous inspiration (Fig. 39.5B) (1). Intermittent positive pressure ventilation (IPPV) will produce opposite changes in velocities. (Fig. 39.5C and D) (4). The increase in intrathoracic pressures relative to extrathoracic systemic pressures during IPPV inspiration favors an increase in left heart output. Additionally, the increased intrathoracic pressure during IPPV inspiration expels blood from the lower compliance pulmonary veins into the LA and thus augments left heart filling and

output (1). These changes in transatrioventricular velocities have been termed *respirophasic variation*.

The absolute values of these velocities are affected by several physiologic variables that include age, heart rate, rhythm, preload, volume flow rate, ventricular systolic function, diastolic function, and atrial contractile function. The transmission of intrathoracic pressures to the intrapericardial structures appears blunted in patients with certain pericardial pathologies (e.g., pericarditis or pericardial effusions severe enough to elicit tamponade physiology) (4).

Note that under conditions of intravascular volume depletion, an alternative transmitral velocity pulse wave Doppler velocity profile has been described in an animal model. In one report using a canine model, 45% of the observed transmitral profiles revealed a slight decrease in maximal amplitude during IPPV inspiration that further decreased during expiration and eventually reached a nadir during expiration (Fig. 39.5E). The authors attributed the observation of this pattern to intravascular volume depletion which was manifest as a direct result of reduced pulmonary venous vascular reserve (4).

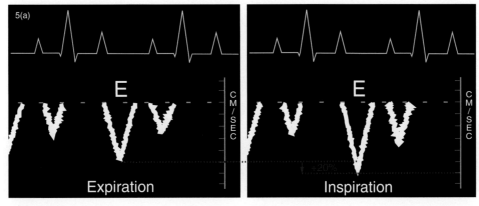

Figure 39.5. Idealized transtricuspid and transmitral valve pulse wave Doppler tracings in both spontaneously (**A, B**) breathing patients and those ventilated with IPPV. (**C–E**) illustrating respirophasic variation; effects of hypovolemia in IPPV are also presented (**E**). **A:** Transtricuspid pulse wave Doppler signals during spontaneous ventilation.

(*Continued*)

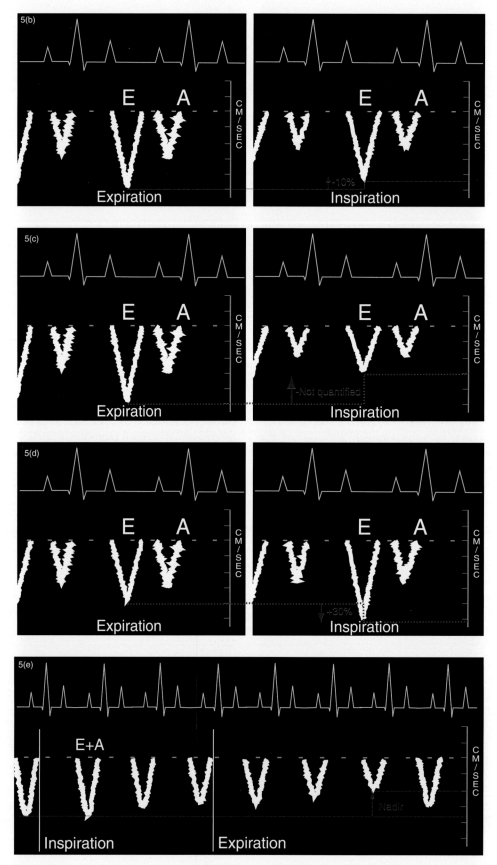

Figure 39.5. (*Continued*). **B:** Transmitral pulse wave Doppler signals during spontaneous ventilation. **C:** Transtricuspid pulse wave Doppler signals during IPPV. **D:** Transmitral pulse wave Doppler signals during IPPV. **E:** Transmitral pulse wave Doppler signals during IPPV during presumed hypovolemia. E, early diastolic filling wave; A, late diastolic filling wave related to atrial contraction.

TABLE 39.1	General Categories of Pericardial Pathology

Congenital pericardial defects

Pericarditis

Pericardial effusion

Pericardial tamponade

Pericardial masses

PERICARDIAL PATHOLOGY

Congenital Pericardial Defects

Echocardiographic evaluation of pericardial disease is performed to rule out specific pathologies that can affect myocardial function. The fact that the pericardium covers the entire myocardium and its associated structures necessitates that a multiwindow, multiplane transesophageal echocardiographic (TEE) examination be performed when assessing this structure. Table 39.1 presents the five basic categories of pericardial pathology (5).

Congenital pericardial defects are rare and consist of partial or total absence of the pericardium and mulibrey nanism, an autosomal recessive disorder, primarily found in the Finnish population, that can lead to congestive heart failure in early adult life and is partially characterized by the development of constrictive pericarditis (CP) in some affected individuals (6,7). TEE findings of CP are discussed in a later section. The significance of pericardial absence varies although appears minor in that most of these patients are clinically asymptomatic (Table 39.2). One small observational study (n = 10) reviewing this disorder found paroxysmal stabbing chest pain that mimicked coronary ischemia was the most common clinical presentation (6). Individuals with congenital absence of the pericardium are at increased risk for additional congenital abnormalities in that 30% of these patients will have other pathology (8,9).

Echocardiographically, one may observe cardiac hypermobility, paradoxical or flat systolic ventricular septal motion, an exaggerated posterior LV wall, and possibly the appearance of a dilated RV together with a reduced dimension of the right atrium (9). A small series of patients (n = 8) from a Japanese group reported more marked alterations in venous return in the right heart (measured in the superior vena cava) than in the left heart (measured in the pulmonary veins) (10). Cardiac magnetic resonance imaging (MRI), computed axial tomography (CT), and, to some extent, a plain chest film are the imaging modalities that appear to be most useful in making the definitive diagnosis of congenital absence of the pericardium. Electrocardiographic (ECG) findings in these patients may include bradycardia, right bundle branch block, poor R-wave progression in the precordial transition leads, and prominent P-waves in the mid precordial leads (9).

Pericarditis

Pericarditis is an inflammation of the pericardium and can occur as the result of multiple pathologies. Pericarditis may present as either a *chronic* or *acute* process and is often associated with the development of a variably sized pericardial effusion. Acute pericarditis can progress to chronic pericarditis that may induce severe diastolic dysfunction. This disorder is termed CP and is discussed in a later section.

Clinically, one examines the patient suspected of having pericarditis for the presence of the classic triad of chest pain, ECG evidence of pericarditis (e.g., diffuse ST segment elevations), and a pericardial rub on auscultation. The various clinical etiologies of pericarditis are listed in Table 39.3 (5).

Echocardiographically, one inspects the pericardium for evidence of thickening that appears as an increase in the brightness, or echogenicity of the ultrasound signal. Normal pericardial thickness is approximately 2 to 3 mm. M-mode analysis of a patient with pericarditis will reveal multiple parallel ultrasound reflections and can be helpful

TABLE 39.2	Pathologic Characteristics of Forms of Pericardial Absence	
Form	**Incidence**	**Clinical Significance**
Total bilateral absence	Rare	Mostly asymptomatic
Partial left absence	70%	Increased risk for aortic dissection if augmented heart mobility: possible herniation or strangulation of heart structures through the defect with chest pain, shortness of breath, syncope
Partial right absence	17%	Increased risk for aortic dissection if augmented mobility of the heart exists as a result of the defect
Overall	0.01%	

Incidence values represent a percentage of the overall incidence of 0.01%.

TABLE 39.3	Clinical Disorders Related to the Development of Pericarditis
Category	**Detailed Causes**
Immune/Inflammation related	rheumatoid arthritis, systemic lupus erythematous, acute rheumatic fever, dermatomyositis, Wegener granulomatosis, mixed collagen vascular disease, post myocardial infarction (Dressler syndrome), uremia, post cardiac surgery inflammation related
Infection related	bacterial infections (e.g., tuberculosis), post-viral
Neoplasm related	primary mesothelioma, fibrosarcoma; secondary metastatic disease (e.g., melanoma, lymphoma, leukemia, or direct extension of a pulmonic or breast tumor)
Intracardiac/Pericardial Communication Related	chest trauma, post percutaneous catheter interventional procedures (e.g., cardiac valve replacement or valvuloplasty, coronary interventions, arrhythmia-related procedures)

to discern the thickened pericardium (Fig. 39.6). Multiple echo windows should be obtained to verify the diffuse or localized nature of the pericarditis. Echocardiography lacks sufficient fidelity to consistently quantify the degree of pericarditis and thus carries an unreliable sensitivity and specificity for detecting this disorder compared to other imaging techniques (e.g., cardiac MRI or high resolution [64-slice CT]). Figure 39.7 presents an MRI image of a focally thickened pericardium.

Pericardial Effusion and Tamponade

A pericardial effusion is a collection of fluid within the pericardial sac that can either be diffusely distributed within the pericardium or localized (i.e., loculated). Depending on patient position and the amount of volume contained in the effusion, different patterns of fluid distribution can be seen assuming that the pericardial space does not contain fibrous adhesions, or a mass that may redirect accumulating fluid. Echocardiographically, a pericardial effusion appears as an echolucent signal immediately adjacent to the epicardium. General guidelines on pericardial effusion size and fluid distribution patterns are presented in Table 39.4 (5). Caution is warranted when diagnosing a pericardial effusion to rule out the presence of epicardial fat, which can appear similar to a pericardial fluid collection at first glance. Close observation of epicardial fat demonstrates a weak echogenic signal compared to the more echolucent signal of a pericardial fluid collection.

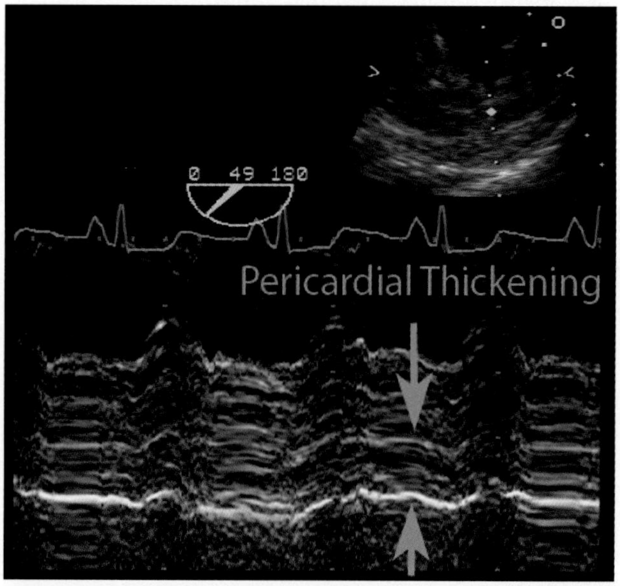

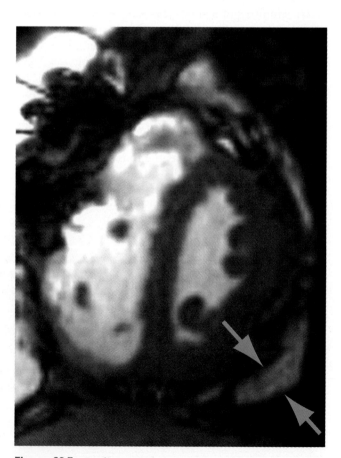

Figure 39.6. M-mode tracing of a patient with a markedly thickened parietal pericardium; the *arrows* indicate the pericardium.

Figure 39.7. Cardiac magnetic resonance image of a focally thickened pericardium denoted by the *two arrows*.

TABLE 39.4	**Pericardial Effusion Characteristics**		
Severity	**Width by Echo**	**Volume (mL)**	**Localization Region**
Small	<5 mm	<100	Behind posterior LV wall
Moderate	5–20 mm	100–150	Expand laterally and apically
Large	>20 mm	>500	Evenly distributed around the heart

Figure 39.8 presents the gross surgical image of epicardial fat (A) and its corresponding TEE appearance (B).

The clinical significance of a pericardial effusion relates to the amount of fluid present and the time course over which it accumulates. Large, chronic effusions are frequently associated with excessive antero-posterior heart motion as well as counterclockwise rotation in the horizontal plane (sometimes termed the "swinging heart"). Effusions can lead to cardiac translation within the pericardial space that can create the ECG finding termed *electrical alternans* (Fig. 39.9). Electrical alternans is the regular occurrence of alternating heights of the QRS complex that may also involve the P, T, U waves and ST segments; this finding is not specific to pericardial effusions (11).

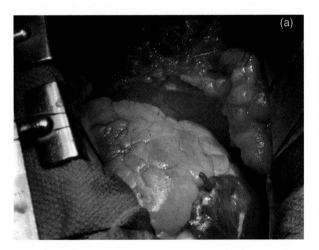
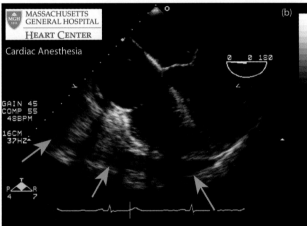

Figure 39.8. Gross surgical (**A**), and TEE image (**B**) illustrating epicardial fat. *Orange arrows* in (**B**) highlight the characteristic echogenic signal of epicardial fat.

Figure 39.9. Electrocardiogram demonstrating electrical alternans in a patient with tamponade physiology.

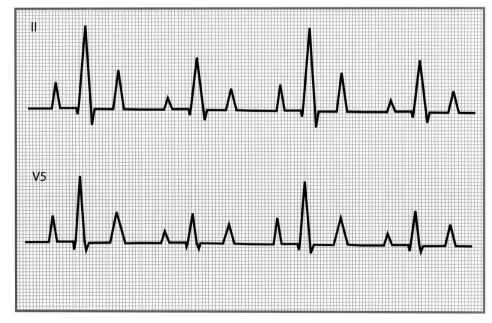

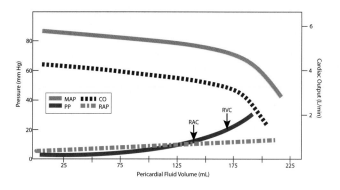

Figure 39.10. Graphic relationship of increasing pericardial fluid volume to cardiac hemodynamics. MAP, mean arterial pressure; PP, pericardial pressure; CO, cardiac output; RAP, right atrial pressure; RAC, right atrial collapse; RVC, right ventricular collapse.

Pericardial effusions are highly common in cardiac surgical patients (i.e., up to 85% will develop some extent of an effusion) and generally peak by the tenth postoperative day (12). The relevance of a pericardial effusion relates to the volume of fluid that accumulates and the chronicity with which it accumulates (Fig. 39.10) (5). Over time, the pressure in the pericardial space will increase as the effusion grows in volume and eventually intrapericardial pressure will exceed cardiac chamber pressures. When intrapericardial pressure increases to the point that cardiac chamber filling is compromised, the patient is considered to have developed tamponade physiology resulting in the clinical finding of *pericardial tamponade*. Additionally, when the amount of accumulating fluid causes a more extreme increase in pericardial pressure (i.e., the pressure-volume relationship has reached the steep point on the curve which relates these two physiologic variables), *ventricular interdependence* will be manifest (Fig. 39.3) (2,13). Note the adaptive nature of the pericardium that is observed with slowly

accumulating effusions in Figure 39.3 (2). The mesothelial cells that comprise the pericardium have the ability to reorganize and hypertrophy. This hypertrophy will allow the pericardium to accommodate greater amounts of pericardial fluid over time provided that the fluid is slowly accumulating. The importance of ventricular interdependence is manifest when one considers that as the RV fills the interventricular septum will shift toward the left and thus compromise LV filling and LV output as evidenced by a decrease in systemic blood pressure (Fig. 39.11) (14). Loss of the y-descent in the right atrial pressure tracing is also characteristic of tamponade.

Tamponade physiology occurs when the pericardial pressure exceeds cardiac chamber pressure; lower pressure chambers (e.g., RA in systole) will be affected initially followed eventually by all cardiac chambers if pericardial pressures continue to rise. In fully developed tamponade, all cardiac chambers will have elevated and equal diastolic pressures. Loculated effusions can elicit tamponade physiology with a considerably smaller volume of fluid than unloculated effusions if the fluid collection is strategically located near a low-pressure cardiac chamber (e.g., the right or left atrium). Consider that solid matter in the pericardial space (e.g., clotted blood or tumor) may also elicit tamponade physiology. Echocardiographic examination must involve a two-dimensional (2D) interrogation from multiple windows to assess for the potential presence of one or more loculated effusions. Pericardial effusions can create a host of echocardiographic findings that include

■ An echolucent signal of variable width (Table 39.3) adjacent to the pericardium (note that the echolucent signal can brighten if the pericardial space is filled with blood that has clotted as may be seen with *hemopericardium*). Figure 39.12 presents a TEE image

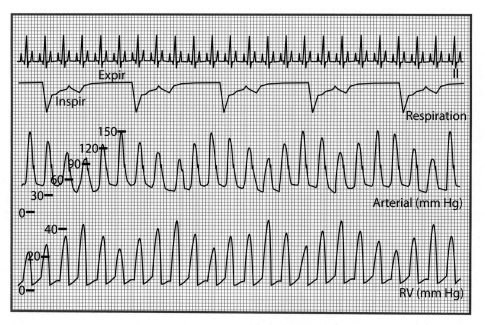

Figure 39.11. Electrocardiogram, associated left and right heart hemodynamic tracings, and respiratory cycle in a patient with pericardial tamponade demonstrating interventricular dependence (pulsus paradoxus). Expir, expiration during spontaneous breathing; Inspir, inspiration during spontaneous breathing; RV, right ventricular pressure.

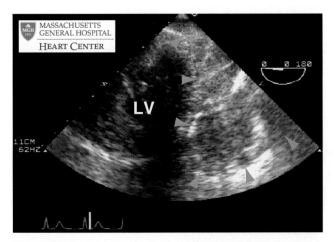

Figure 39.12. Transesophageal 2D transgastric short-axis mid-papillary echocardiographic image of a large, solid clot burden in the pericardial space lateral to the LV. *Arrowheads* outline a large clot burden.

of a postoperative cardiac surgical patient with a large collection of thrombus in the pericardial space adjacent to the LV lateral wall.

- Fibrinous stranding within the pericardial fluid may be seen in patients with long-standing pericardial disease
- Regional septal wall motion abnormalities
- Mitral valve and tricuspid valve prolapse
- Systolic anterior motion of the anterior mitral leaflet
- Early systolic closure of the aortic valve
- Midsystolic notching (partial closure) of either the aortic valve or pulmonic valve

When pericardial effusions grow to an extent that elicits pericardial tamponade, there are a host of echocardiographic findings that can be observed:

- RA systolic collapse, or inversion (inversion for > 1/3 of systole, has a 94% sensitivity and 100% specificity for tamponade) (Fig. 39.13)

- RV diastolic collapse (sensitivity 60%–90% and specificity 85%–100% for the diagnosis of tamponade) (Fig. 39.14)
- Reciprocal respiratory changes in RV and LV volumes (during spontaneous inspiration, an increase in RV volume will occur that will result in a shift of the interventricular septum toward the LV in diastole; these changes reverse during expiration and *pulsus paradoxus* [Fig. 39.11] will be observed on the arterial waveform under these physiologic conditions.)
- Inferior vena cava (IVC) plethora (dilated IVC with less than 50% inspiratory reduction in diameter near the IVC-RA junction; this a sensitive [97%] but nonspecific indicator of tamponade) (5)

Note that Doppler evaluation of tamponade physiology in spontaneously breathing patients can also provide useful information to confirm the diagnosis of pericardial tamponade. As seen during spontaneous respiration in normal transatrioventricular valve Doppler profiles, there is a decrease in transmitral velocity flow profiles during inspiration (Fig. 39.5B). In severe tamponade, this decrease can be as much as 37% (Fig. 39.15A). The transtricuspid valve velocities increase by as much as 77% with tamponade physiology during spontaneous respiration (15) (Fig. 39.15B). The magnitude of the transatrioventricular velocities will be reduced in absolute value although the respirophasic variation will be accentuated in pericardial tamponade during spontaneous respiration. The mechanism accounting for the exaggerated respirophasic variation in tamponade is an insulation of the heart from the intrathoracic pressure changes associated with the respiratory cycle.

Doppler interrogation of transmitral valve velocities during IPPV will reveal a markedly different pattern than seen with spontaneous respiration. According to work done in a canine model, the normally observed dynamics in transmitral valvular velocities seen in pericardial

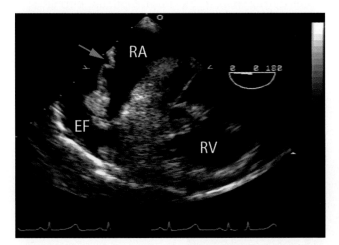

Figure 39.13. Midesophageal four-chamber view demonstrating systolic right atrial collapse/inversion in a patient with pericardial tamponade. RA, right atrium; RV, right ventricle; EF, effusion; Arrow indicates right atrial wall collapse.

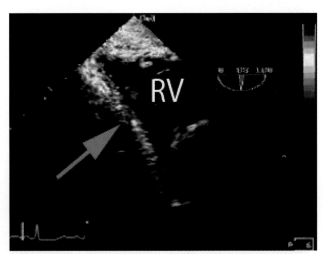

Figure 39.14. Transesophageal transgastric long-axis RV inflow view demonstrating anterior RV wall diastolic collapse in a patient with pericardial tamponade. *Arrow* indicates anterior RV wall diastolic collapse.

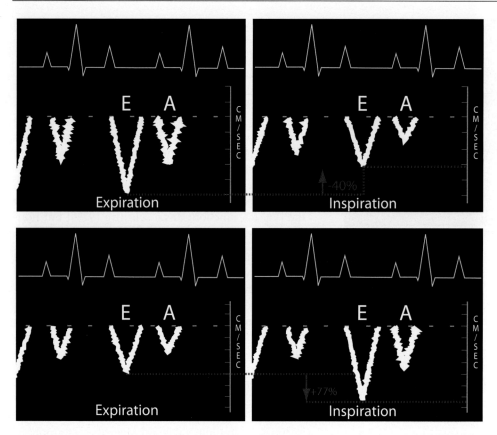

Figure 39.15. A: Transmitral pulse wave Doppler signals during spontaneous ventilation in a patient with tamponade physiology. **B:** Transtricuspid pulse wave Doppler signals during spontaneous ventilation in a patient with tamponade physiology. E, early diastolic filling wave; A, late diastolic filling wave related to atrial contraction.

tamponade will be opposite in direction (i.e., there will be an increase in transmitral flow velocity during inspiration in contrast to the decrease [Fig. 39.5B] observed in spontaneously breathing subjects) and markedly attenuated (4). Thus, the characteristic exaggerated respirophasic variation in transatrioventricular velocities seen with tamponade in spontaneously breathing patients is absent during IPPV (Fig. 39.16). However, consistent with the pattern seen in spontaneously breathing patients with tamponade, there will be an overall decrease in the amplitude of the flow velocities during mechanical ventilation compared to values obtained in individuals without tamponade (2,4).

In addition to interrogation of the transatrioventricular valve velocities, assessment of the *hepatic vein flow*

profiles can also provide useful diagnostic information in spontaneously breathing patients suspected of having tamponade physiology. Normally the pulse wave Doppler profile of the hepatic vein is bimodal with the forward flow during systole being equal to or greater than the forward flow during diastole throughout the respiratory cycle as depicted in Figure 39.17A. The systolic and diastolic forward velocities increase during spontaneous inspiration. Under conditions of tamponade physiology, the systolic and diastolic forward flow velocities also increase in magnitude during spontaneous inspiration, but during expiration, there is a marked reduction, or reversal of both the S and D waves, which is not seen in normal subjects (Fig. 39.17B) (15). Data on respirophasic changes in the

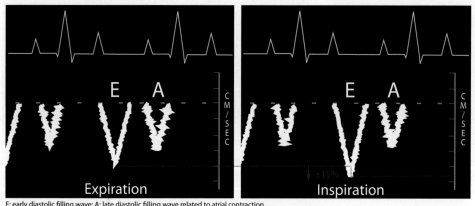

E: early diastolic filling wave; A: late diastolic filling wave related to atrial contraction

Figure 39.16. Transmitral pulse wave Doppler signals during IPPV in a patient with tamponade physiology. E, early diastolic filling wave; A, late diastolic filling wave related to atrial contraction.

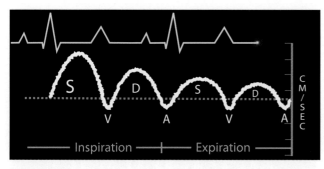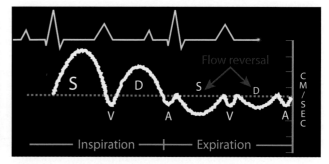

Figure 39.17. **A:** Idealized hepatic vein Doppler flow profile in a spontaneously breathing normal subject. **B:** Idealized hepatic vein Doppler flow profile in a spontaneously breathing subject with tamponade physiology. S, systolic flow; V, flow wave related to recoil of the tricuspid annulus; D, diastolic flow; A, atrial flow reversal.

hepatic veins during IPPV are not available, and thus, evaluation of the hepatic vein profiles with TEE during IPPV is not useful at present.

A final Doppler echocardiographic quantitative method that can be integrated into the assessment of a pericardial effusion and tamponade physiology is measurement of the isovolumic relaxation time (IVRT). In one transthoracic echocardiographic study that compared spontaneously breathing normal adults to individuals with tamponade as well as to individuals with an effusion, but no tamponade, a significantly prolonged IVRT was observed in patients with tamponade compared to normal individuals. Normally the IVRT is less than 100 milliseconds in most age groups (mean value of 82 msec was observed in this study), and a mean value of 104 milliseconds was observed in the tamponade group that was studied (p < 0.01) (15). Changes in the IVRT in patients with pericardial tamponade who are receiving IPPV have not been described.

Constrictive Pericarditis

The evaluation of a subtype of pericarditis termed *constrictive pericarditis* is important to be aware of when diagnosing pericardial disease. In some cases, acute pericarditis may progress to CP. CP represents a chronic and more severe form of the acute pericarditis. Clinically significant CP will affect ventricular filling in that it may mimic restrictive diastolic dysfunction. CP has been reported to occur in 0.2%–0.3% of cardiac surgical patients and has a number of pathophysiologic features that include fibrotic pericardium, inflamed pericardium, calcific thickening of the pericardium, abnormal diastolic filling, a narrow RV pulse pressure (i.e., the systolic RV pressure is normal but the diastolic RV pressure is elevated), and a prominent early diastolic RV pressure dip and later plateau termed the "square root sign" (Fig. 39.18) (12,16). Additionally, the RA pressure exhibits a pronounced systolic drop (y descent followed by an increase and then plateau) that appears as an "M-like" wave on the CVP tracing (Fig. 39.18).

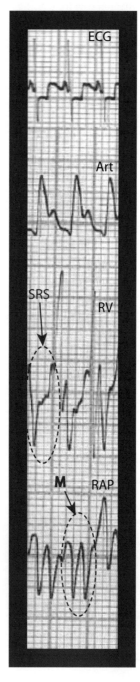

Figure 39.18. Physiologic waveforms in a patient with CP. ECG, electrocardiogram; Art, arterial waveform; RV, right ventricular waveform; SRS, square root sign; RAP, right atrial pressure tracing; M, "M" sign.

The diagnosis of CP is made by using a combination of 2D echocardiographic analysis, Doppler echocardiographic assessment, and the use of a high fidelity imaging technique. The 2D echocardiographic examination will generally reveal a thickened, highly reflective pericardium in patients with CP. TEE can detect the thickened pericardium, but computed tomography and magnetic resonance imaging are considered to provide more accurate measurements of the pericardial thickness (Figs. 39.6 and 39.7). Table 39.5 lists a number of nonspecific echocardiographic findings associated with CP (12).

Doppler assessment of patients with CP is complex in that multiple Doppler modalities are recommended to accurately diagnose this pathology. Doppler modalities used to assess CP include pulse wave Doppler transmitral tracings, pulse wave Doppler pulmonary vein tracings, tissue Doppler imaging of the mitral annulus, and color Doppler M-mode (flow propagation, V_p) of transmitral inflow. Transmitral blood flow assessment has proven to be a useful diagnostic and prognostic tool for individuals with CP. By color Doppler assessment, patients with CP may exhibit tricuspid or mitral valve incompetence. Similar to pericardial tamponade, the transmitral pulse wave Doppler profile of most spontaneously breathing patients with CP will demonstrate an exaggerated respirophasic variation (i.e., it will decrease by ~25% during inspiration). Figure 39.19 depicts a transthoracic pulse wave Doppler profile illustrating a 30% drop in the transmitral velocity during spontaneous inspiration (recall that under normal conditions there is only a 10% decrease in this parameter). Note that up to 20% of patients with CP will not exhibit this Doppler finding although the application of preload reducing maneuvers (e.g., reverse Trendelenburg position) may be useful to amplify the transmitral velocity respiratory variation that is expected in these patients (17). The thickened pericardium insulates the intrapericardial structures from the intrathoracic pressure changes associated with the respiratory cycle and produces an exaggerated respirophasic variation as a result

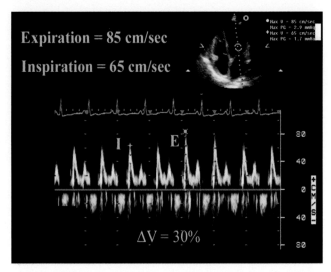

Figure 39.19. Transthoracic pulse wave transmitral Doppler profile in a patient with CP obtained during spontaneous respiration.

(as seen in tamponade). Similar respirophasic variation is observed in the pulmonary veins with CP, and the systolic:diastolic (S:D) ratios are similar to those of patients with restrictive myocardial pathology (e.g., the pulmonary vein diastolic flow velocity will be greater than the systolic flow velocity in patients with a restrictive LV filling pattern, or S:D ratio < 1) (18). Additionally, unique to CP relative to restrictive cardiomyopathy (RCM) is that the peak amplitude of the pulmonary venous D wave has been noted to exhibit pronounced respiratory variation (>18% increase upon inspiration in patients receiving IPPV) in CP (19). Figure 39.20 depicts an idealized pulmonary vein pulse wave Doppler tracing in a mechanically ventilated patient with CP (note the S:D < 1 and the exaggerated D wave velocity during inspiration).

During mechanical ventilation, the transmitral E-wave velocity will increase with early inspiration in CP and the exaggerated respirophasic variation seen with spontaneously breathing CP patients is also observed with IPPV, although the direction of change in velocity will

TABLE 39.5	2D-Echocardiographic Findings Associated with CP

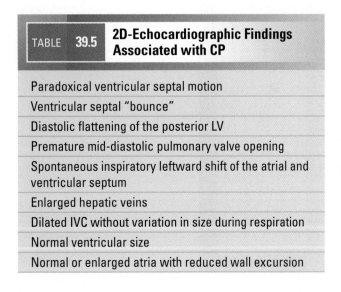

Paradoxical ventricular septal motion
Ventricular septal "bounce"
Diastolic flattening of the posterior LV
Premature mid-diastolic pulmonary valve opening
Spontaneous inspiratory leftward shift of the atrial and ventricular septum
Enlarged hepatic veins
Dilated IVC without variation in size during respiration
Normal ventricular size
Normal or enlarged atria with reduced wall excursion

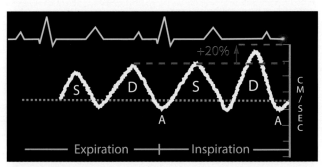

Figure 39.20. Idealized transesophageal pulmonary vein pulse wave Doppler profile in a patient with CP obtained during IPPV. S, systolic pulmonary vein wave; D, diastolic pulmonary vein wave; A, atrial pulmonary vein wave.

be opposite (16,19,20). The increase in intrathoracic pressure expels blood from the low compliance extrapericardial pulmonary veins into the left atrium, which results in an increase in transmitral flow velocity (Fig. 39.21) The mechanism for the exaggerated respirophasic variation observed in CP patients is that the thickened pericardium insulates the intracardiac chambers (the LA in this case) from the changes in intrathoracic pressure, thus increasing the gradient between the pulmonary veins and the LA during inspiration. Overall, as with pericardial tamponade, the transmitral velocities will be reduced in amplitude in CP. Given that the CP limits the volume of both cardiac chambers, the inspiratory increase in transmitral E wave velocity will be accompanied by a simultaneous decrease in transtricuspid E wave velocity for two reasons. First, the increase in intrathoracic pressure will limit right-sided filling, and second, the increased filling velocity and increased amount of blood in the LV will result in a shift of the interventricular septum to the right and thus compromises RV filling during inspiration (i.e., ventricular interdependence is demonstrated). These changes in the transmitral velocities appear to be reversible with surgical treatment (pericardial stripping or pericardiectomy) of CP although in some cases this therapy has been associated with LV dilation and transient ventricular diastolic dysfunction (21).

Perioperative echocardiographers should be aware that much has been written about making the distinction between CP and RCM. Both of these pathologies share the common pathophysiology of decreased LV compliance, but different mechanisms account for the decreased compliance in each case. In CP, the decreased compliance relates to the restrictive nature of the thickened pericardium while in RCM the restriction is related to pathology within the myocardium (e.g., infiltrative disease of the muscle or hypertrophy). Recall that severely decreased LV compliance will present a restrictive LV filling pattern (Fig. 39.22).

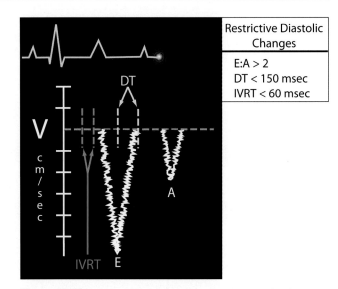

Restrictive Diastolic Changes
E:A > 2
DT < 150 msec
IVRT < 60 msec

Figure 39.22. Idealized transesophageal transmitral pulse wave Doppler profile representative of a restrictive pattern of diastolic dysfunction. V, velocity; DT, deceleration time; IVRT, isovolumic relaxation time; E, early diastolic filling; A, atrial diastolic filling.

The differentiation of CP from RCM is best approached by assessing the patient for the described exaggerated respiratory variation in the transmitral (Fig. 39.21) and pulmonary venous Doppler flow velocity profiles (i.e., S:D < 1 with a ≥18% variation in the D wave on inspiration in a mechanically ventilated patient [Fig. 39.20] and for echocardiographic or cardiac MRI/high resolution CT scan evidence of pericardial thickening [Fig. 39.7]). The exaggerated respirophasic variation has been demonstrated in anesthetized patients using TEE (19). Newer echocardiographic modalities being used to differentiate CP from RCM include color M-mode flow propagation velocities (Vp), Doppler tissue imaging (DTI) at the level of the mitral annulus, and Doppler myocardial velocity gradients (MVGs) (20,22–24). DTI has been demonstrated to provide a highly sensitive and specific means to differentiate CP from RCM in one study of a homogeneous CP patient population. Table 39.6 presents the sensitivity and specificity data for the various Doppler techniques and their ability to distinguish CP from RCM. DTI has been shown to be less sensitive to preload (a limitation of transmitral pulse wave Doppler) in differentiating CP from RCM (20). DTI at the level of the lateral mitral annulus with both TTE and TEE provides a reproducible means to align the pulse wave tissue Doppler cursor with the longitudinal axis of myocardial excursion during relaxation of the muscle. Patients with CP generally have preserved myocardial diastolic function that therefore will demonstrate normal (E_m > 8 cm/s) myocardial velocities. The converse is true for patients with RCM in that the muscle is inherently pathologic in these patients with infiltrative cardiomyopathies and thus will demonstrate an abnormality (E_m < 8 cm/s) (Fig. 39.23) (10).

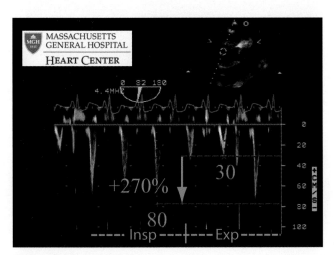

Figure 39.21. Transesophageal transmitral velocity profile in a patient with CP during positive pressure ventilation. Insp, inspiration; Exp, expiration.

TABLE 39.6	Relative Sensitivities and Specificities of Various Doppler Techniques to Distinguish Between CP and RCM		
Doppler Modality		**Sensitivity**	**Specificity**
Transmitral peak E wave PW Doppler velocity (respiratory variation ≥ 10%)		84	91
Pulmonary vein peak D wave PW Doppler velocity (respiratory variation ≥ 18%)		79	91
Transmitral color M-mode (V_p) slope ≥ 100 cm/s		74	91
Tissue Doppler imaging of the lateral mitral annulus demonstrating E_m ≥ 8 cm/s		89	100

Color M-mode, or the velocity of propagation (V_p) of transmitral flow, is also recommended to be incorporated into the assessment of patients suspected of CP. Although the results of color M-mode are not as easily reproduced as TDI, it is advantageous in that it appears to be preload independent and has the benefit of providing both excellent spatial and temporal resolution of diastolic mitral inflow. Color M-mode assessment of patients with CP will generally demonstrate high values of flow propagation toward the LV apex (i.e., ≥100 cm/s) while those with RCM will have decreased V_p values (i.e., <35 cm/s) (Fig. 39.24) Note that although these newer Doppler techniques are considered validated for use in determining diastolic dysfunction, direct validation studies for TEE and patients receiving IPPV have not been performed.

Pericardial Masses

Pericardial masses include benign pericardial cysts, pericardial neoplasms (e.g., mesothelioma, sarcoma, and teratomas are all gratefully rare), and tumors that invade the pericardium from neighboring tissue (e.g., breast or lung). Pericardial cysts are usually round and asymptomatic but can be associated with chest pain, dyspnea, cough, arrhythmias, and compression of the left atrium or pulmonary vein(s). Figure 39.25 presents an example of a pericardial cyst obtained with transthoracic echocardiography. Some pericardial cysts are not well visualized with echocardiography but will image well with cardiac

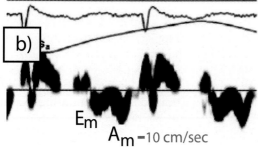

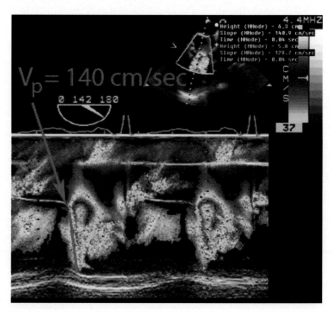

Figure 39.23. Transthoracic tissue Doppler image of the lateral mitral annulus in a patient with (**A**) CP and with (**B**) RCM. E_m, early diastolic motion of the mitral annular tissue; A_m, late diastolic motion of the mitral annular tissue.

Figure 39.24. TEE image of the LV flow propagation (V_p) in a patient with CP V_p: color M-mode, or flow propagation. The *arrow* indicates the predominant slope of the line, V_p.

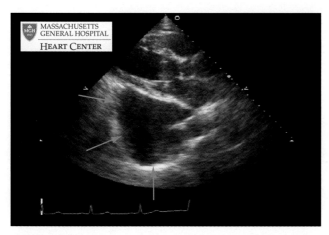

Figure 39.25. Transthoracic echocardiographic image of a pericardial cyst from the parasternal long-axis view. *Arrows* highlight the cystic structure.

MRI (Fig. 39.26). Any of these masses may inhibit cardiac chamber filling and result in hemodynamic compromise, if they grow large enough in a critical location. Pericardial thrombus formation is another pericardial mass that may precipitate hemodynamic compromise, most commonly in the postsurgical state. Hemopericardium (Fig. 39.12) may result from a number of different pathologies (e.g., aortic dissection with extravasation of blood into the transverse sinus, percutaneous catheter interventions, pacer wires or postinfarction myocardial necrosis and rupture).

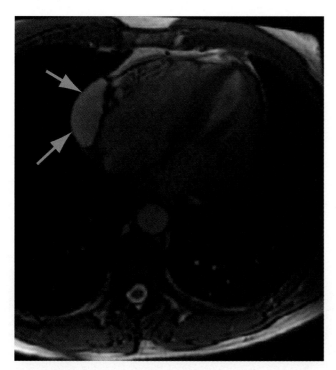

Figure 39.26. Cardiac magnetic resonance image of a pericardial cyst anterior to the right atrium that was not well imaged with cardiac ultrasound. *Arrows* highlight the cystic mass.

KEY POINTS

- Transtricuspid velocities increase by approximately 20% during the inspiratory phase of spontaneous respiration. Transmitral velocities normally decrease by approximately 10% during spontaneous inspiration. The changes in transatrioventricular valvular velocities have been termed *respirophasic variation.* IPPV will produce opposite changes in velocities. The increase in intrathoracic pressures relative to extrathoracic systemic pressures during IPPV inspiration favors an increase in left heart output. Additionally, the increased intrathoracic pressure during IPPV inspiration expels blood from the lower compliance pulmonary veins into the left atrium and thus augments left heart filling and output. The transmission of intrathoracic pressures to the intrapericardial structures appears blunted in patients with certain pericardial pathologies (e.g., pericarditis or pericardial effusions severe enough to elicit tamponade physiology).

- The characteristic respirophasic variation in transatrioventricular velocities seen with tamponade in spontaneously breathing patients is absent during IPPV. However, consistent with the pattern seen in spontaneously breathing patients with tamponade, there is an overall decrease in the amplitude of the flow velocities during mechanical ventilation compared to values obtained in individuals without tamponade.

- Systolic and diastolic forward hepatic vein velocities increase during spontaneous inspiration. However, under conditions of tamponade physiology, the systolic and diastolic forward flow velocities also increase in magnitude during inspiration, but during expiration, there is a marked reduction, or reversal of both the S and D waves, which is not seen in normal subjects.

- Similar to pericardial tamponade, the transmitral pulse wave Doppler profile of most patients with CP will demonstrate an exaggerated respirophasic variation. The thickened pericardium insulates the intrapericardial structures from the intrathoracic pressure changes associated with the respiratory cycle and produces an exaggerated respirophasic variation as a result similar to patients with tamponade. Similar respirophasic variation is also observed in the pulmonary veins with CP, and the S:D ratios observed are similar to those of patients with restrictive myocardial pathology. Additionally, unique to CP relative to RCM is that the peak amplitude of the pulmonary venous D wave has been noted to exhibit pronounced respiratory variation in CP.

- The exaggerated respirophasic variation seen with spontaneously breathing CP patients is also observed with IPPV, although the direction of change in velocity will be opposite in direction.

REFERENCES

1. Spodick DH. Macrophysiology, microphysiology, and anatomy of the pericardium: a synopsis. *Am Heart J* 1992;124:1046–1051.
2. Spodick DH. Acute cardiac tamponade. *N Engl J Med* 2003;349:684–690.
3. Shabetai R. Pericardial and cardiac pressure. *Circulation* 1988;77:1–5.
4. Faehnrich JA, Noone RB, White WD, et al. Effects of positive-pressure ventilation, pericardial effusion, and cardiac tamponade on respiratory variation in transmitral flow velocities. *J Cardiothorac Vasc Anesth* 2003;17:45–50.
5. Otto C. Pericardial disease. In: Otto C, ed. *Textbook of Clinical Echocardiography*. 3rd Ed. Philadelphia: Elsevier Saunders, 2004:259–275.
6. Gatzoulis MA, Munk MD, Merchant N, et al. Isolated congenital absence of the pericardium: clinical presentation, diagnosis, and management. *Ann Thorac Surg* 2000;69:1209–1215.
7. Kivisto S, Lipsanen-Nyman M, Kupari M, et al. Cardiac involvement in mulibrey nanism: characterization with cardiac magnetic resonance imaging. *J Cardiovasc Magn Reson* 2004; 6: 645–652.
8. Maisch B, Seferovic PM, Ristic AD, et al. Guidelines on the diagnosis and management of pericardial disease. *Eur Heart J* 2004;25:587–610.
9. Abbas AE, Appleton CP, Liu PT, et al. Congenital absence of the pericardium: case presentation and review of the literature. *Int J Cardiol* 2005;98:21–25.
10. Fukuda N, Oki T, Iuchi A, et al. Pulmonary and systemic venous flow patterns assessed by transesophageal Doppler echocardiography in congenital absence of the pericardium. *Am J Cardiol* 1995;75:1286–1288.
11. Goldschlager N, Goldman MJ. *Principles of Clinical Electrocardiography*. 13th Ed. East Norwalk: Appleton and Lange, 1989:300–302.
12. Shernan S. Echocardiographic evaluation of pericardial disease. In: Konstadt SN, Shernan S, Oka Y, eds. *Clinical Transesophageal Echocardiography: A Problem Oriented Approach*. Philadelphia: Lippincott Williams & Wilkins, 2003:203–213.
13. Hoit BD. Pericardial disease. In: Fuster VR, O'Rourke RA, Walsh RA, eds. *Hurst's The Heart*. 12th Ed. http://phstwlp1.partners.org:2270/content.aspx?aID=3079080

14. Lewinter MM, Kannani S. Pericardial diseases. In: Zipes DP, Libby P, Bonow RO, Braunwald E, eds. *Braunwald's Heart Disease*. 7th Ed. Philadelphia: Elsevier Saunders, 2005:1764.
15. Burstow DJ, Oh JK, Bailey KR, et al. Cardiac tamponade: characteristic Doppler observations. *Mayo Clin Proc* 1989;64:312–324.
16. Skubas NJ, Beardslee M, Barzilai B, et al. Constrictive pericarditis: intraoperative hemodynamic and echocardiographic evaluation of cardiac filling dynamics. *Anesth Analg* 2001;92:1424–1426.
17. Oh J, Tajik J, Appleton C, et al. Preload reduction to unmask the characteristic Doppler features of constrictive pericarditis: a new observation. *Circulation* 1997;95:796–799.
18. Klein AL, Cohen GI, Pietrolungo JF, et al. Differentiation of constrictive pericarditis from restrictive cardiomyopathy by Doppler transesophageal echocardiographic measurements of respiratory variations in pulmonary vein flow. *J Am Coll Cardiol* 1993;22:1935–1943.
19. Abdalla IA, Murray D, Awad HE, et al. Reversal of the pattern of respiratory variation of Doppler inflow velocities in constrictive pericarditis during mechanical ventilation. *J Am Soc Echocardiogr* 2000;13:827–831.
20. Rajagopalan N, Garcia M, Rodriguez L, et al. Comparison of new Doppler echocardiographic methods to differentiate constrictive pericardial heart disease and restrictive cardiomyopathy. *Am J Cardiol* 2001;87:86–94.
21. Senni M, Redfield M, Ling H, et al. Left ventricular systolic and diastolic function after pericardiectomy in patients with constrictive pericarditis: postoperative and serial Doppler echocardiographic findings. *J Am Coll Cardiol* 1999;33:1182–1188.
22. Rodriguez, Ares MA, Vandervoot PM, et al. Does color M-mode flow propagation differentiate between patients with restrictive vs. constrictive physiology? [Abstract] *J Am Coll Cardiol* 1996;27:268A.
23. Palka P, Lange A, Donnelly E, et al. Differentiation between restrictive cardiomyopathy and constrictive pericarditis by early diastolic Doppler myocardial velocity gradient at the posterior wall. *Circulation* 2000;102:655–662.
24. Garcia MJ, Thomas JD, Klein AL. New Doppler echocardiographic applications for the study of diastolic function. *J Am Coll Cardiol* 1998;32:865–875.

QUESTIONS

1. Which of the following echocardiographic signs pertaining to pericardial effusions is most correct?
   A. Echocardiographically, a pericardial effusion appears as an echodense signal immediately adjacent to the epicardium
   B. Epicardial fat demonstrates a more echolucent signal than a pericardial fluid collection.
   C. Moderate pericardial effusions have a measured width of less than 15 mm
   D. Small pericardial effusions tend to be localized behind the posterior wall of the LV

2. Which of the following echocardiographic techniques has the highest sensitivity and specificity for differentiating CP from RCM ?
   A. Pulmonary vein peak D wave pulse wave Doppler velocity
   B. Tissue Doppler imaging of the lateral mitral annulus
   C. Transmitral peak E wave pulse wave Doppler velocity
   D. Transmitral Color M-mode (Vp) slope

3. Which of the following echocardiographic signs is most consistent with a clinical diagnosis of cardiac tamponade?
   A. Diastolic rightward shift of the interventricular septum during spontaneous inspiration
   B. IVC collapse during inspiration
   C. Right atrial diastolic collapse
   D. RV diastolic collapse

4. Which of the following echocardiographic findings are least likely to be seen in patients with pericardial effusions?
   A. Early systolic closure of the aortic valve
   B. Fibrinous strands in the pericardial space
   C. Midsystolic partial closure of the pulmonic valve
   D. Regional apical wall motion abnormalities

ANSWERS

Chapter 1

1. **D.** Ultrasound propagates poorly through a gaseous medium
2. **C.** Poor TEE imaging of the ventricular apex from midesophageal depths
3. **A.** Imaging at shallower depths
4. **A.** Aligning the Doppler angle parallel to transducer beam-flow direction
5. **A.** Adjusting the system for a higher-amplitude, lower-frequency signal

Chapter 2

1. **B.** Resolution is the ability to distinguish two objects that are close to one another. The resolution of an image is no greater than 1 to 2 wavelengths. The shorter the wavelength, the more compressions and rarefractions there are per unit of time; therefore, the resolution is better. Frequency is indirectly proportional to wavelength. The shorter the wavelength, the higher the frequency and the better the resolution. Higher frequencies, however, sacrifice penetration.
2. **C.** Refraction is the deflection of ultrasound waves from a straight path and can occur as the waves pass through a medium with different acoustic impedance. When an ultrasound wave is refracted, the transducer assumes that it has returned from the original scan line and therefore places the image along the original path rather than its actual location.
3. **D.** Range ambiguity occurs because of increased pulse repetition frequency. With a high pulse repetition frequency, a second signal is sent out before the first signal is received. The transducer cannot discriminate between the returning pulses, that is, whether they represent the first, second, or even later pulses. Decreasing the depth decreases the pulse repetition frequency.
4. **A.** The Eustachian valve is an embryological remnant of the sinus venosus. It is a thin, elongated structure located at the junction of the IVC and the right atrium. While the Eustachian valve is not pathologic, it can be confused with a cardiac thrombus or mass.

Chapter 3

1. **D.** Axial resolution is the ability to distinguish two structures that are close to each other along the direction of beam propagation, as two separate structures. Axial resolution can be optimized by increasing the transducer frequency, which decreases the wavelength, and therefore shortens the PD. The pulse duration can also be shortened by using transducers with broad frequency bandwidths, which include a greater mixture of high and low frequencies compared to narrow bandwidths. Consequently, broad bandwidth transducer pulses are more likely to preserve higher frequencies as ultrasound waves penetrate through tissue, and therefore have greater sensitivity than narrow frequency bandwidths. Finally, the use of damping material in the construction of transducers minimizes piezoelectric crystal ringing and vibration, thereby producing shorter pulse duration. Thus, axial resolution can be improved by assuring a short-pulse duration using an appropriately dampened transducer with a high-frequency and broader-frequency bandwidth. (See "The Impact of Ultrasound Instrumentation on Image Generation and Display.")

2. **C.** Lateral resolution describes the ability of a transducer to resolve two objects that are adjacent to each other and perpendicular to the beam axis. Lateral resolution also refers to the ability of the beam to detect single small objects across the width of the beam. In general, lateral resolution is most optimal when the ultrasound beam width is narrow. Lateral resolution may therefore be improved by increasing the frequency (i.e., shortening the wavelength). Increasing the transducer aperture diameter may also improve lateral resolution by lengthening the near-field depth at the expense of a wider proximal near field. Increasing the ultrasound signal amplitude (i.e., POWER) increases the detection of echoes at the beam margins, thus effectively increasing beam width and decreasing lateral resolution. Lateral resolution can also be improved by focusing the transducer. Thus, lateral resolution is an important variable in determining ultrasound image quality and is ultimately influenced by transducer size, shape, frequency, and focusing. (See "The Impact of Ultrasound Instrumentation on Image Generation and Display.")

3. **A.** Temporal resolution refers to the ability to rapidly display moving structures and distinguish closely spaced events in time. Temporal resolution is related to the time required to generate one complete frame and is therefore directly related to the frame rate. Assuming preservation of scan line density and spatial resolution, the temporal resolution and frame rate can be improved only by reducing depth or sector size. Alternatively, for a given depth and sector size, using a higher-frequency transducer with decreased tissue penetration will also permit an increased frame rate and improved temporal resolution. Thus, temporal resolution is dependent upon depth, sector scan angle, scan line density, and transducer frequency. (See "The Impact of Ultrasound Instrumentation on Image Generation and Display.")

Chapter 4

1. **B.** The fibrous skeleton of the heart is formed by the U-shaped cords of the aortic annulus and their extensions forming the right trigone, left trigone, and a smaller fibrous structure from the right aortic coronary cusp to the root of the pulmonary artery (1). This "skeleton" plays a primary function of supporting the heart within the pericardium. A continuum of fibrous tissue extends from the fibrous skeleton providing attachments for the atriums, ventricles, and valve leaflets (Fig. 4.1). The right fibrous trigone extends from the base of the noncoronary cusp and is more substantial than the left fibrous trigone. The left fibrous trigone extends from the base of the left coronary cusp.

2. **C.** The mitral valve annulus assumes an ellipsoid shape of an English riding saddle during systole. This effectively reduces the size of the mitral annulus and reduces the leaflet tissue required to prevent regurgitation.

3. **D.** The annuli fibrosi of the mitral annulus becomes thinner and poorly defined as it extends posteriorly from the left and right trigones. This portion of the annulus is poorly supported and is prone to dilation in pathologic states. The posterior leaflet of the mitral valve attaches to this portion of the annulus. Dilation of the annular attachment of the posterior leaflet creates increased tension on the middle scallop of the posterior leaflet, explaining the 60% occurrence of chordal tears in the middle scallop of the posterior leaflet (2).

4. **C.** The Society of Cardiovascular Anesthesiologists and the American Society of Echocardiography has developed a 16-segment model of the LV based on the recommendations of the Subcommittee on Quantification of the ASE Standards Committee. This model divides the LV into three levels: basal, mid, and apical. The basal and mid levels are each divided circumferentially into six segments and the apical into four (Figs. 4.4 and 4.5) (5).

5. **B.** Chordae from the papillary muscles radiate upward attaching to the corresponding halves of the anterior and posterior leaflets. Chordae arising from the anterior papillary muscle attach to A1, P1, (AC), and the lateral half of P2 and A2. Chordae arising from the posterior papillary muscle attach to A3, P3, (PC), and the medial half of P2, and A2 (Figs. 4.12, 4.13, and 4.14; Table 4.2). This relation aids in defining the portion of the mitral valve that is echocardiographically visualized.

   There are two chordae attaching to the ventricular surface of the anterior leaflet that are by far the thickest and largest of the chordae to the mitral valve. They have been called strut or stay chordae. One arises from the anterior papillary muscle and attaches to the middle A1/A2 area of the anterior leaflet; the other arises from the posterior papillary muscle and attaches to the middle A2/A3 portion of the anterior leaflet (Fig. 4.14).

Chapter 5

1. **A.** The deep transgastric long-axis view allows the ultrasound beam to be aligned reasonably parallel to the flow through the LVOT and the AV for accurate Doppler measurements of these velocities. Midesophageal views of the AV provide better 2D images of the valve. The LV is usually foreshortened in the deep transgastric long-axis view. The diameter of the LVOT is usually best measured in the midesophageal AV long-axis view. The transgastric two-chamber view usually shows the mitral chordae most clearly.

2. **E.** Four-chamber views show the septal and lateral walls. Two-chamber views show the inferior and anterior walls. Transgastric short-axis views show the six segments at the basal or mid levels of the LV including the posterior segment.

3. **C.** Four- and two-chamber views cut across the mitral valve obliquely. The mitral commissural view transects the MV along the intercommissural plane and the long-axis view through the middle of the anterior and posterior leaflets.

4. **B.** Eight views are needed to provide a basic perioperative TEE exam to detect markedly abnormal ventricular filling or function, extensive myocardial ischemia or infarction, large air embolism, severe valvular dysfunction, large cardiac masses or thrombi, large pericardial effusions, and major lesions of the great vessels.

Chapter 6

1. **C.** The recommendations refer to clinical problems rather than to individual patients, who often have more than one potential reason for performing TEE. Thus, although a patient may not necessarily require perioperative TEE because of a Category III indication (e.g., cardiomyopathy), the same patient may need TEE because of coexisting hemodynamic problems (Category I). See "Practice Guidelines."

2. **B.** The AHA/ACC guidelines utilize the following classification system for indications.
   Class I: Conditions for which there is evidence and/or general agreement that a given procedure or treatment is useful and effective.
   Class II: Conditions for which there is conflicting evidence and/or a divergence of opinion about the usefulness/efficacy of a procedure or treatment.
   Class III: Conditions for which there is evidence and/or general agreement that the procedure/treatment is not useful/effective and in some cases may be harmful. See "Practice Guidelines."

3. **E.** Published reports have indicated that TEE facilitates the placement of intravascular catheters during port-access surgery, the detection of regurgitation after minimally invasive valve surgery, the diagnosis of new regional wall motion abnormalities (RWMA) during coronary artery clampings, and air embolism after ter-

mination of CPB following "open heart" procedures. (See "Indications for Specific Lesions or Procedures: Minimally Invasive Cardiac Surgery.")

4. **D.** In a recent review of 7,200 adult cardiac surgical patients, Kallmeyer et al. reported on the safety of intraoperative transesophageal echocardiography. They observed no mortality and a morbidity of only 0.2%. Most complications were related to probe insertion or manipulation that resulted in oropharyngeal, esophageal, or gastric trauma. (See "Complications.")

Chapter 7

1. **B.** There is an increased risk of esophageal perforation when a TEE probe is placed in a patient with a history of an esophageal stricture. All of the other choices are relative contraindications. (See Table 7.3. Procedures and Chemicals That Damage TEE Probes.)

2. **C.** Antibiotic prophylaxis is not required for procedures with a low risk of induced bacteremia. Therefore, endocarditis prophylaxis is not needed prior to or during TEE exams, except in patients at high risk for developing endocarditis. (See "Safety" and "Infection.")

3. **C.** The duration of the disinfecting process of the TEE probe should be at least 20 minutes to eliminate bacterial and viral contaminants. (See "Infection.")

Chapter 8

1. **E.** Essential components of basic training include independent work, supervised activities and assessment programs as well as comprehensive exam.

2. **D.** Ability to quantify normal and abnormal native and prosthetic valvular function.

3. **C.** Knowledge of congenital heart disease belong to advanced cognitive skill group.

4. **D.** Comprehensive perioperative echocardiographic exam should consist of 20 images.

5. **E.** Beside independently performing 150 studies and reviewing 300 studies, diplomat in NBE needs to pass NBE exam, fulfill requirement of passing ABA Oral Board exam, and finish 1 year of advanced clinical training (fellowship).

Chapter 9

1. **A.** Leftward bowing of the interatrial septum in midsystole is a normal echocardiographic finding. Normally, due to higher left-sided pressures, the interatrial septum bulges toward the right atrium. During passive mechanical expiration, right atrial pressure transiently exceeds left atrial pressure, and the atrial septum momentarily bows towards the left atrium. This midsystolic atrial reversal occurs when the corresponding pulmonary artery occlusion pressure (PAOP) is ≤15 mm Hg. A rightward midsystolic bowing or absence of the leftward bowing of the interatrial septum indicates PAOP

>15 mm Hg with a sensitivity of 89%, specificity of 95%, and a positive predictive value = 0.97. As a general guideline, an E/Ea >10 predicts a mean PCWP >15 mm Hg with a 92% sensitivity and 80% specificity.

2. **E.** The deep transgastric long-axis view is not normally a part of a comprehensive exam of the left ventricle. Although the left ventricle can be seen in this view, often it is foreshortened. This view allows for measurements of the flow velocities of the LVOT and the aortic valve using pulsed or continuous wave Doppler because there is good alignment of these structures to the Doppler interrogation beam.

3. **C.** Echocardiography can be used to noninvasively measure meridional and circumferential wall stress. Meridional stress acts on the long axis of the LV; the circumferential stress acts on the short axis of the LV. Meridional wall stress can be calculated using noninvasive BP and myocardial area measured with M-mode. The normal left ventricle resembles the ellipsoid model in which circumferential stress at the end of systole is 2.57 times higher than meridional stress. In a dilated failing heart, the left ventricle gradually begins to resemble a sphere, and the meridional and circumferential stress gradually equalize to a ratio of 1.

4. **D.** Sinus tachycardia may cause the systolic and diastolic waves to fuse. The peak systolic-to-diastolic filling ratio increases with sinus tachycardia because the diastolic filling period is shortened. In patients with atrial fibrillation, systolic forward flow is diminished or absent, and diastolic flow is the main contributor to left atrial filling. In the presence of low left atrial pressure, the biphasic nature of the S wave becomes more prominent because of the temporal dissociation of atrial relaxation and mitral annular motion. With TEE, the biphasic systolic wave is commonly seen. The descent of the S wave corresponds with the V wave in the left atrial pressure tracing. The second large flow velocity is the diastolic wave prompted by the antegrade flow of blood from the pulmonary veins into the left ventricle during early diastole. It coincides with the Y descent of the left atrial pressure tracing during early ventricular filling.

5. **D.** Cross-sectional area can be calculated by measuring the LVOT diameter in the midesophageal long-axis view using the equation AVA $\pi \times (D/2)^2$. The cross-sectional area can also be calculated by measuring the length of each side of the aortic valve seen in the aortic valve short-axis view using the equation AVA = $0.433 \times S^2$. The transgastric long-axis view can be used to obtain the spectral envelope for measuring the velocity time integral used in the stroke volume calculation. The spectral envelope obtained from the pulmonary artery is not equivalent to that from the aorta in the transgastric long-axis view. The cardiac output derived from measuring the spectral envelope at the pulmonary artery only correlated modestly with cardiac output measured by the thermodilution method (r = 0.65).

Chapter 10

1. **A.** With volume overload of the right ventricle, the interventricular septum is pressed to the left. This will be maximal when right ventricular volume is the largest, which occurs at end-diastole just before ejection.

2. **D.** The first three structures (Chiari network, Crista Terminalis, and the Eustachian valve) are all remnants of structures from embryonic life, which can be seen in the right atrium. The Thebesian valve is also located in the right atrium, covering the opening of the coronary sinus, and rarely seen by transesophageal echocardiography. The Moderator band is a thick muscle bundle inside the chamber of the right ventricle.

3. **D.** Systolic pulmonary artery pressure can be estimated as right atrial pressure plus the ventriculo-atrial systolic pressure gradient as the open pulmonary valve adds very little resistance during systole. Ventriculo-atrial pressure gradient can be calculated by measuring peak velocity of a tricuspid regurgitation jet, as long as the jet direction is aligned with the Doppler ultrasound beam. This can usually be achieved starting with the RV inflow-outflow view and increasing the multiplane angle.

4. **D.** Much of right ventricular contraction is contributed by shortening of longitudinal muscle fibers. This can be measured by the excursion of the tricuspid valve annulus, normally 15 to 20 mm. Smaller excursion is a sign of RV dysfunction, for example due to infarction.

5. **A.** Normal size of the right ventricle is about half to two thirds that of the left ventricle. When the right ventricle dilates, its cross-sectional area equals, and even surpasses, that of the left ventricle. Also, it lengthens so that the cardiac apex is composed of both the left and right ventricles. While tricuspid valve regurgitation commonly accompanies right ventricular dilatation, prolapse of the valve leaflets into the right atrium is very rare.

Chapter 11

1. **E.**

2. **C.** Both low-dose and high-dose dobutamine will improve function in stunned myocardium. Low-dose dobutamine will improve function in hibernating myocardium but function will worsen with high-dose dobutamine.

3. **A.** Normally the interventricular septum bulges towards the right ventricle in both systole and diastole due to higher pressures in the left ventricle. In situations of right ventricle volume overload, the interventricular septum tends to flatten in end-diastole while in situations of right ventricle pressure overload the interventricular septum tends to flatten at end-systole and early-diastole.

4. **E.** Tissue Doppler displays high-amplitude, low velocity signals coming from the myocardium. The velocities are usually lower than 15 cm/s. The velocities of the septal portion of the mitral annulus are lower than the velocities of the lateral mitral annulus.

5. **E.**

Chapter 12

1. **C.** Diastolic function evaluation is an integral part of every comprehensive TEE exam. The normal transmitral flow pattern in this patient with uncontrolled hypertension and concentric hypertrophy most likely represents a pseudonormal pattern (grade II diastolic dysfunction) which is accompanied by elevated filling pressures (S/D<1, AR duration more than 30 cm/sec) and E' less than 8 cm/sec. An E/Vp ratio more than 2.5 predicts elevated filling pressures.

2. **B.** Constrictive pericarditis is characterized by a restrictive pattern of the transmitral flow (E/A>1.5, E wave DT< 160 msec), preserved annular excursion (E'> 8 cm/sec), and normal or high Vp. Lateral E' velocity may be lower than the septal E' velocity due to the limited lateral annular excursion in diastole.

3. **B.** A decrease in preload through infusion of nitroglycerin, Valsalva maneuver, or steep reverse Trendelenburg position will result in the following changes:
   - In a healthy young adult with normal diastolic function, it will result in decreased E and A velocities, unchanged E/A ratio, and unchanged E wave DT.
   - A reversible restrictive pattern (grade IIIa) will be changed into a pseudonormal or impaired relaxation pattern.
   - An irreversible restrictive pattern (grade IIIb) will not be changed.

4. **C.** Elevation of PCWP indicating elevated left atrial pressure in the setting of LV systolic dysfunction is most likely to reveal a restrictive diastolic filling pattern. The E wave deceleration time in this scenario is most likely to be less than 150 msec.

5. **B.** With impaired relaxation, there is a decrease in peak early flow (E) velocity and a consequently higher atrial filling (A) velocity. Therefore, the E/A ratio is **decreased**. The IVRT is increased in this early stage of diastolic dysfunction as relaxation is impaired and mitral valve opening is delayed. An 'L' wave is more commonly seen in slow heart rates in advanced heart failure.

Chapter 13

1. **B.** Standard nomenclature adopted by the Society of Cardiovascular Anesthesiologists and the American Society of Echocardiography divides the anterior and posterior leaflets into three segmental regions. Indentations along the free margin of the posterior mitral leaflet give it a scalloped appearance, allowing identification of individual scallops P1, P2, and P3. The anterior mitral leaflet is also divided into three segments located opposite the corresponding segments of the posterior mitral leaflet: A1, A2, and A3. The P1 and A1 segments are adjacent to the anterolateral commis-

sure, while the P3 and A3 segments are adjacent to the posteromedial commissure (Fig. 13.2).

2. **C.** Normal pulmonary venous waveform patterns consist of a biphasic forward systolic waveform occurring during ventricular systole, a forward diastolic velocity waveform that occurs after mitral valve opening, and a retrograde atrial flow reversal waveform that occurs in response to atrial contraction. Significant degrees of mitral regurgitation increase left atrial pressure and alter forward flow through the pulmonary veins. Klein et al. investigated the relationship between the ratio of peak systolic and peak diastolic flow velocities in the pulmonary veins to varying degrees of mitral regurgitation, as measured with TEE color-flow mapping. The ratio of peak systolic to diastolic pulmonary venous waveform velocities were categorized as having a normal pattern where the ratio of peak systolic/diastolic waveform was greater than or equal to one, a blunted pattern where the ratio of peak systolic to peak diastolic waveform was between 0 and less than 1, and reversed systolic waveform represented by a peak systolic velocity value of less than 0 sensitivity and specificity for reversed systolic flow detecting four-plus mitral regurgitation was 93% and 100%, respectively. Blunted systolic flow for detecting three-plus mitral regurgitation had lower sensitivity and specificity of 61% and 97%, respectively. Pulmonary venous flow patterns may not be a reliable marker of valvular insufficiency for all grades of mitral regurgitation. A reversed pattern is highly specific marker for detecting a large regurgitant orifice area greater than 0.3 cm^2 with a sensitivity, specificity, and predictive value of 69%, 98%, and 97%, respectively, except severe MR.

3. **B.** The regurgitant orifice area is a reliable quantitative measure of the severity of mitral regurgitation. It can be measured with two-dimensional and pulsed Doppler echocardiography or with the proximal isovelocity surface area (PISA) method. The PISA method applies the continuity principle to color Doppler mapping in the region of the mitral valve orifice where flow converges toward the mitral regurgitant orifice on the left ventricular side of the mitral valve. As blood flow converges toward the mitral regurgitant orifice, it forms a series of isovelocity shells whose surface area is hemispheric in shape (Fig. 13.10). Color-flow Doppler displays a measure of velocity at a specific distance from the regurgitant orifice (Fig. 13.11). By the law of conservation of mass, flow at each layer should equal orifice flow because it must all pass through the orifice. Maximal instantaneous flow rate can be calculated. Once the maximal instantaneous flow rate is calculated, the regurgitant orifice area (ROA) can be calculated. In general, an ROA = 0.4 cm^2 is associated with severe mitral regurgitation.

4. **D.** The pressure gradient half-time (PHT) measures the rate of decline in the atrioventricular pressure gradient. It is defined as the time required for maximal diastolic pressure difference to decrease by one half of its initial value. In velocity terms, it is equivalent to the time required for the maximum transmitral velocity curve to decrease by a factor of the square root of 2. The pressure PHT can be quantitatively related to the severity of mitral stenosis. A normal mitral valve area of 4 cm^2 allows the atrioventricular flow to reduce the transmitral pressure difference to negligible values in less than 50 msec after the onset of the diastolic rise in left ventricular pressure. As the severity of mitral stenosis increases, there is a proportionately slower rate of pressure decline between the left atrium and left ventricle and the atrioventricular pressure gradient is maintained for a longer period of time. A PHT of ≥ 300 m/s is associated with severe mitral stenosis.

5. **C.** Potential sources of error should be considered when applying the PHT method in specific clinical settings. PHT is influenced by the peak transmitral pressure gradient and left atrial and left ventricular compliances. Conditions that alter left atrial or left ventricular compliance, rapid heart rates, or severe aortic insufficiency will impact the measurement accuracy. Moderate-to-severe degrees of aortic insufficiency cause a rapid rise in left ventricular diastolic pressure with a resultant shortening in the PHT and an overestimation in mitral valve area.

Chapter 14

1. **A.** Patients with left ventricular dysfunction are unable to generate the high transaortic velocities and high aortic valve gradients characteristic of aortic stenosis. For a given valve area, patients with a lower ejection fraction will generate a lower gradient and valvular velocity; that is why B and D are wrong. Reduced cusp separation is a qualitative sign of stenosis, but a determination of valve area (answer A) is required to quantify the severity of stenosis.

2. **B.** An examination of Figure 14.22 explains the answer to this question. Cath lab gradients are typically reported as peak-to-peak gradients, which are not "true" gradients, but rather the difference between peak pressures. A peak instantaneous gradient such as the one derived by using echocardiography is usually greater than the difference between peak pressures. The presence of aortic insufficiency may result in increased flow during systole because of the diastolic regurgitant volume, but this does not account for the different gradients obtained by the two techniques.

3. **D.** Color-flow, continuous wave, and pulsed wave Doppler are used to quantify the severity of aortic insufficiency. Color-flow Doppler applied to the aortic valve short-axis view is useful for identifying the location of the coaptation defect. However, two-dimensional echocardiography is the one answer that provides definitive information regarding the etiology of the valve dysfunction. Examples would include a dilated root and annulus, prolapsing leaflet, a calcific or rheumatic valve in which the leaflets do not fully open and do not completely close, and endocarditis. The diagnosis of all of these conditions is made with two-dimensional echocardiography. (See "Echocardiographic Evaluation of Aortic Insufficiency.")

4. **D.** The aortic valve regurgitant velocity deceleration slope increases with the severity of aortic regurgitation and decreased left ventricular compliance. A deceleration slope of 5 m/s indicates severe aortic insufficiency. A patient with a competent aortic valve would not be expected to have a regurgitant velocity slope. (See "Echocardiographic Evaluation of Aortic Insufficiency.")

Chapter 15

1. **C.** The PV can be viewed easily via a transgastric approach. It is embryologically derived from the same structure as the aortic valve, namely, the aortic and pulmonary trunks after partition of the bulbis cordis and the truncus arteriosus. In a similar manner to the AV, the tips of the PV leaflets may have nodules, known as the nodulus arrantii. The Ross procedure involves replacement of the aortic valve with the native PV, and subsequent placement of a PV homograft in the pulmonic position. TEE is especially useful in this setting to evaluate the relative sizes of the aortic annulus and the PV. In this way, the long-term consequences of mechanical valves are avoided.

2. **A.** Tricuspid regurgitation can be either pathologic or a normal finding. Its incidence increases with age, being found in up to 93% of patients over the age of 70. Differentiating benign TR from pathologic TR involves assessing the degree of regurgitation, the turbulence of the jet, and the peak velocity of transtricuspid flows. Likewise, the peak velocity of the regurgitant jet may be used to estimate the peak pressure in the main pulmonary artery. TR is graded by evaluation of hepatic venous flow patterns, as well as the degree of extension of the color-flow jet into the right atrium.

3. **C.** Carcinoid heart disease results from chronic exposure to vasoactive amines secreted by the primary tumors, most often from hepatic metastases of primary gastrointestinal tumors. As such, involvement primarily occurs in the right-sided cardiac structures, most specifically on the ventricular side of the TV and the arterial side of the PV. The primary tumors are slow growing, and in those with cardiac involvement death most often follows progressive cardiac failure. TEE may be used to assess results of medical therapy. The TV often develops a mixed picture of TS and TR, with fixed immobile valves.

4. **B.** Valvular stenosis often involves fusion of the leaflets along their commissures. Right atrial enlargement may result from obstruction to flow through either TS or PS. The degree of stenosis is proportional to the peak velocity of the regurgitant jet. The leaflets in both TS and PS develop doming as well as leaflet thickening and restricted motion. It is rare for rheumatic disease to involve either the TV or the PV.

Chapter 16

1. **B.** "Profile" describes the height from the base of the prosthetic valve to the top of the supporting struts. Low profile mechanical valves include tilting disk valves and bileaflet valves. Bileaflet valves have the advantage of being less obstructive to flow, with flow occurring across three orifices. (See "Low Profile Valves.")

2. **C.** Stentless porcine valves are used in the aortic position. They lack the supporting struts used with the Carpentier-Edwards and Hancock valves, thereby giving them a larger effective orifice area and lower pressure gradients. (See "Stentless Porcine Valves.")

3. **D.** Perivalvular leaks must be distinguished from the "normal" regurgitant jets seen with many of the prosthetic valve types. Perivalvular leaks can be caused by valve dehiscence, suture fracture, and endocarditis. (See "Prosthetic Valve Regurgitation.")

4. **A.** Prosthetic transvalvular gradients are affected by many factors, including size and type of prosthetic valve, time of implantation, anatomic location, flow, and cardiac function. (See "Prosthetic Valve Stenosis.")

5. **D.** TEE is considered the best modality for defining anatomic valve abnormalities seen with prosthetic valve endocarditis. TEE is five times more sensitive than transthoracic echocardiography in the detection of prosthetic valve endocarditis. (See "Prosthetic Valve Endocarditis.")

Chapter 17

1. **D.** Most secondary involvement of the heart by malignancy is pericardial (~75%).
2. **B.** Myxomas are the most common primary tumor.
3. **C.** LV apical thrombi should be visualized in systole and diastole as well as in more than one view to ensure differentiation from artifact and tangential cuts through the LV apex.

Chapter 18

1. **C.** Right ventricular hypokinesis with apical sparing
2. **A.** Atrial pacing
3. **B.** Open cholecystectomy

Chapter 19

1. **C.** Image resolution is directly related to the frequency of the transmitted ultrasound, while penetration is inversely related to the frequency. Vascular structures are generally within a few centimeters the surface, and therefore higher-frequency ultrasound is preferred because resolution is more desirable than penetration.

2. **A.** The use of short-axis image plane is easier for the novice to master in a relatively short amount of time. Short-axis imaging has the advantage of allowing the operator to visualize the vein and artery simultaneously. However, the needle is also seen on its short axis. In this situation, it is difficult to ascertain if the hyperechogenicity produced by the needle is the tip or the shaft of the needle. Overshoot, that is, double wall puncture through the anterior and posterior walls of the vein, may

occur. If the vein significantly overlaps with the artery, unintentional arterial puncture may occur. The long-axis and oblique axis imaging require greater "hand eye" coordination to master these imaging planes.

3. **False.** MRI scanning and ultrasound imaging both have illuminated that when the head is turned to the contralateral side during internal jugular vein (IJV) cannulation, the vein assumes a more anterior position in relation to the carotid artery. The anterior position predisposes toward unintentional arterial puncture (see answer 2).

4. **D.** Three-dimensional (3D) vascular ultrasonography (U/S) will be the next logical step in advancing the success rate and decreasing the complication rate of ultrasound-guided vascular access. It makes use of three imaging planes integrating the advantageous aspects of each. Furthermore, 3D U/S can provide information about the topography of the intraluminal space, for example, presence of an intimal dissection, clot or, thrombus. However, to state that 3D U/S leads to the avoidance of complications would be false because there are many other surrounding structures that may be irritated or injured despite direct vessel visualization.

Chapter 20

1. **C.** Aortic arch vessels
2. **A.** Hypotension
3. **C.** End diastolic area
4. **C.** On table TEE
5. **D.** Hypovolemia

Chapter 21

1. **B.** By utilizing the Bernoulli equation ($\Delta P = 4V^2$), Doppler-derived blood-flow velocities can be converted to pressure gradients. Velocities measured across regurgitant valves can then be used to determine the pressure difference between two cardiac chambers and, hence, intracardiac filling pressures. The Continuity equation allows estimations of valvular orifice areas, while the proximal isovelocity surface area (PISA) is most often used to assess the severity of a regurgitant valve.

2. **B.** In constriction, as opposed to restriction, the right ventricular end-diastolic pressure is often greater than 1/3 the right ventricular systolic pressure. In constriction, pulmonary pressures tend to be less than 55 mm Hg and mitral inflow variation is usually greater than 25% with respiration.

3. **C.** An elevated mitral E-wave to tissue Doppler E_A wave ratio is most suggestive of elevated left ventricular filling pressures. Findings consistent with a diagnosis of pulmonary hypertension include IVC dilatation with attenuated respiratory collapsibility, interventricular septal flattening, flow reversal in the hepatic veins, and the "flying W" sign by M-mode, among others.

4. **D.** Only visualization of thrombus-in-transit is diagnostic of pulmonary embolism (PE). All other findings can suggest right ventricular dysfunction and elevated right-sided heart pressures but are not pathognomonic for PE.

Chapter 22

1. **B.** Oscillating mass
2. **D.** Diagnosis of IE in patients with nosocomial staphylococcal bacteremia
3. **A.** Downstream of the valve
4. **D.** Mitral-pulmonic intervalvular fibrosis

Chapter 23

1. **E.** All of the above.
2. **D.** Rightward bowing of the interatrial septum
3. **A.** Atrial pacing
4. **B.** Early systolic collapse of the right ventricle

Chapter 24

1. **C.** To better visualize posterior structures
2. **A.** The examination includes the length of the ascending aorta from the sinotubular junction to the main pulmonary artery bifurcation.
3. **D.** The individual responsible for diagnostic interpretation of the epicardial and epiaortic images should be trained as an advanced echocardiographer as recommended in the ASE/SCA guidelines.

Chapter 25

1. **B.** The most common type of atrial septal defect is the secundum type. (See "Atrial Septal Defects.")
2. **D.** The degree of aortic override is best seen with the longitudinal plane. (See "Tetralogy of Fallot"; Fig. 25.7.)
3. **C.** Protein-losing enteropathy is seen after the Fontan procedure. All other answers can occur after the arterial switch operation. (See "Transposition of the Great Arteries.")

Chapter 26

1. **D.** VTI and area should be determined at the same time when calculating a Doppler-derived stoke volume. They may be measured during systole in the LVOT or at the aortic valve when determining cardiac output. However, for determination of mitral regurgitant volume, stroke volumes need to be determined during diastole at the mitral valve and during systole in the LVOT.

2. **D.** Results using the simplified proximal flow convergence method for determining mitral regurgitation severity correlate well with those obtained using the standard method.

3. **C.** The primary concern in determining aortic valve area with the continuity equation using TEE is related to the possible underestimation of time-velocity integrals (or peak velocities) in the LVOT and/or aortic valve due to inadequate beam alignment.

4. **D.** The pressure half-time method overestimates the area of normal prosthetic mitral valves.

5. **B.** Estimation of RVSP from the systemic systolic blood pressure and the peak velocity across the VSD is not valid in the presence of aortic stenosis or LVOT obstruction (systolic blood pressure will not approximate LV systolic pressure).

Chapter 27

1. **A.** Jones et al. combined data from seven studies to evaluate those recurring factors contributing to in-hospital mortality following CABG. In a clinical study of more than 172,000 patients, those variables having the strongest correlation included
   1. Patient's age
   2. Gender
   3. Previous cardiac surgery
   4. Operation urgency
   5. Ventricular ejection fraction
   6. Characterization of coronary anatomy (left main >50% stenosis, number of vessels with >70% stenosis)

   Of these variables, age, urgency of procedure, and reoperation were the ones that most strongly correlated with patient mortality following CABG surgery.

2. **B.** The diagnosis of a central mitral regurgitant jet may help guide the surgical team in the repair of the type IIIb mechanism of mitral valve dysfunction CF. However, the presence of a protruding and mobile plaque in the ascending aorta is indicative of a high risk of type I postoperative neurologic dysfunction. Such findings would direct the surgical team to consider an alternative site of cannulation (axillary or femoral) and evaluation of the cross-clamp site with epiaortic echo, and/or consideration of the use of circulatory arrest or off pump CABG. A deceleration time of less than 120 msec has been associated with a poorer long-term prognosis in patients with congestive heart failure.

3. **A.** The National Center for Health Statistics and Centers for Disease Control and Prevention estimates that the number of individuals over the age of 65 will be more than 50,000,000 by the year 2020. Eleven percent of females and 17.7% of males in the age group have clinically significant coronary artery disease. Unless there is a significant decline in the incidence or management of diabetes and hypertension, the health-care system will be confronted with this rapidly expanding patient population.

4. **A, B, and C.** Patients with coronary artery disease and significant aortic regurgitation present the surgical team with challenges for myocardial protection. Strategies may include the direct administration of cardioplegia using handheld devices that engage the coronary ostia, retrograde cardioplegia via the coronary sinus, and venting of the LV during periods when the aorta is not cross-clamped.

5. **A, B, D, and E.** Patients with ischemic heart disease may have mitral regurgitation as a result of structural abnormalities of the components of the mitral valve apparatus. This may be due to a number of mechanisms, including eccentric remodeling of the LV with bileaflet tethering (symmetric IIIb with central MR), an inferoposterior or anterolateral infarct with systolic restriction of the PMVL (asymmetrical IIIb) with an override of the AMVL and posteriorly directed MR jet, an infracted papillary muscle with focal prolapse (type II) or rupture papillary muscle (type II), and chronic enlargement of the MV annulus (type I). Transient ischemia may produce global or regional dysfunction creating either apical tethering or restriction of the PMVL. In elderly patients with extensive mitral annular calcification, the patient may even exhibit diastolic and systolic restriction of the MV leaflets producing a type IIIa mechanism. While mitral annular calcification has been associated with elevated LDL cholesterol, coronary artery disease, and significant atheroma of the aorta, MACa^{++} is not a manifestation of ischemic heart disease.

Chapter 28

1. **C.** The functional subset of annular dilatation or restrictive leaflet motion was found to have the worst 5-year survival rate (43%) compared to ruptured chordae or papillary muscle (76%). The predictor of worse long-term outcome indicated that the pathophysiology may be the major determinate of survival rather than the type of surgical intervention (12–14,34,39).

2. **A.** The blood supply to the posterior medial papillary muscle is either the right coronary artery or the obtuse marginal artery in 63% of patients and more than one vessel in 37% of patients. It has been observed and concluded that papillary muscle dysfunction paradoxically decreases ischemic MR because the inferiobasal ischemia reduces leaflet tethering and improves coaptation (21,23,28–30,40).

3. **D.** Research indicates that ring implantation reliably prevents delayed leaflet coaptation after acute ischemia, and also preserves papillary-annular distances, which invariably increase after induction of ischemia. Ring annuloplasty also preserved tethering distance and prevented disturbances in the geometry of the mitral and valve leaflets (30,31,33,40,42,48).

Chapter 29

1. **C.** In cases of mitral valve prolapse, the regurgitant jet generally travels opposite to the prolapsing leaflet. (See "Introduction: Primary Mitral Valve Disease.")

2. **D.** The most common cause of tricuspid regurgitation is functional, with no structural abnormality of the leaflets. (See "Tricuspid Valve: Functional Tricuspid Regurgitation.")

3. **E.** The mitral chordae have several functions. Third-order chordae insert into the annulus and maintain ventricular geometry. They may be important to

maintenance of ventricular function. (See "Structure and Anatomy: The Chords.")

4. **B.** Posterior leaflet prolapse is the most common finding in patients coming to surgery for degenerative mitral valve disease. It is easily and reliably repaired. (See "Pathology: Mitral Valve.")

5. **A.** SAM occurs in about 5% of patients having mitral valve repair for degenerative disease. It is associated with excess leaflet tissue and a narrow left ventricular outflow tract. It can be prevented by the use of sliding leaflet repair. (See "Pathology: Mitral Valve.")

Chapter 30

1. **D.** Systolic leaflet restriction
2. **D.** A3
3. **B.** Severe mitral annular calcification
4. **A.** Barlow's syndrome
5. **E.** Proximal isovelocity surface area
6. **D.** Commissural prolapse with a commissuroplasty
7. **C.** Should to use a different method to estimate ROA
8. **C.** Decreased line density

Chapter 31

1. **B.** The planimetric method of area determination using the *midesophageal aortic valve shor- axis* view in two and three dimensions provides good correlation with other methods used for assessment of aortic stenosis and is usually very accurate and easy to perform in patients with mild-to-moderate aortic stenosis. Three-dimensional planimetry is as reliable as two-dimensional planimetry in determining valve size. This method of determining aortic valve area is more difficult and less reliable if the valve is severely calcified. Calcium deposits, particularly if they are located along the *posterior aspect* of the valve, will shadow the anterior aspect of the valve and make it difficult to define the leaflet edges, making valve area determination with planimetry more challenging.

2. **C.** Patients *without* true anatomically severe stenosis will exhibit an increase in valve area and little change in gradient during dobutamine administration. For example, a valve area increase of 0.2 cm² or greater following dobutamine administration with little change in gradient most likely does not represent true severe anatomic stenosis. In contrast, patients with an anatomically fixed stenotic valve will exhibit an increase in their gradient but no change in their valve area as stroke volume increases during dobutamine administration. Six-year survival after aortic valve replacement among patients with contractile reserve is greater than 75%, while patient without contractile reserve is less than 50%. Systolic dysfunction due to aortic stenosis is usually reversible with valve replacement, but systolic dysfunction due to myocardial infarction, extensive coronary artery disease, or superimposed myocardial fibrosis may not improve after AVR and causes an underestimation of the severity of aortic

stenosis by gradient determination. The presence of concomitant mitral stenosis causes an *underestimation* of the severity of aortic stenosis by gradient determination because of *decreased* transaortic blood flow.

3. **C.** Stenotic valves and valves with regurgitation due to leaflet restriction (degenerative, calcific) or retraction (rheumatic) comprise the most common etiologies of aortic regurgitation, but unfortunately, these valves are not amenable to repair. Repair is a suitable option among patients with aortic regurgitation due to single-leaflet prolapse of either a tricuspid or congenitally bicuspid valve. (Figure 31.22) Although leaflet prolapse is observed in tricuspid aortic valves, this lesion most commonly affects bicuspid valves (54). TEE provides a highly accurate anatomic assessment of all types of aortic regurgitation lesions and the functional anatomy defined by TEE is an independent predictor of valve reparability and postoperative outcome.

4. **D.** All of the described approaches have been shown to be viable options during percutaneous aortic valve surgery. The antegrade transseptal approach via the femoral vein and the transapical approach to aortic valve replacement provide viable options in the setting of severe peripheral vascular disease that prohibits a femoral artery approach.

Chapter 32

1. **C.** The incidence of newly diagnosed thoracic aneurysms in the United States approximates 5.9 per 100,000 person-years with a lifetime probability of rupture of 75% to 80%. If left untreated, 5-year survival rates range from 10% to 20%. In nondissecting thoracic aortic aneurysms, absolute size is a major predictor of median time to rupture. Aneurysms, which are larger than 6 cm have a 43% risk of rupture within one year, while those larger than 8 cm have an 80% risk. Other factors, which independently predict risk of rupture include advanced age, pain, and chronic obstructive pulmonary disease.

2. **D.** The increased use of thoracic endovascular stents for the management of complicated type B aortic dissections and descending thoracic aortic aneurysms has led to a new use for intraoperative TEE. The success of a thoracic endograft depends on correct anchoring within a portion of normal-sized aorta at its proximal and distal ends (i.e., proximal and distal landing zones). Intraoperative TEE can be useful to confirm stiff-guidewire position within the aorta (usually "parked" just above the aortic valve), aid in device placement, and finally confirm the absence of endoleak. Intraoperative TEE currently serves as an adjunct to angiography.

3. **A.** Intraoperative TEE evaluation of an aortic dissection is crucial for successful operative management.[18] Specific findings on TEE will direct the surgical approach and lead to surgeon to consider different cannulation sites, root or valve replacement, bypass grafting, and arch replacement in addition to the usual repair

techniques. At the Cleveland Clinic, our minimum standard approach to a type A aortic dissection involves right axillary artery cannulation, reconstruction of the dissected layers (without the use of glue), placement of a supracoronary graft after aortic valve resuspension, and creation of an open distal anastomosis under deep hypothermic circulatory arrest. Intraoperative TEE by an experienced operator is quintessential to the success of the surgical endeavor. The goals of intraoperative TEE during a type A dissection repair include the following:

1. Confirmation of the diagnosis
2. Assessment of the aortic root, including the size of the sinus segment, the degree of aortic insufficiency, and patency of the coronary ostia;
3. Assessment of global left and right ventricular (LV and RV) functions and localization of any regional wall-motion abnormalities;
4. Monitoring for LV distension during cooling in the setting of aortic insufficiency;
5. Postrepair assessment of LV and RV functions, aortic valve competence, and coronary ostial patency.

4. **A.** The presence of thoracic aortic atheroma has been correlated with perioperative strokes in multiple studies. The ability to detect significant atheromatous or calcific burden within the portions of the ascending aorta can direct the surgical team to alternate methods of cannulation and even overall surgical strategy in order to prevent untoward events of brain embolization. From an echocardiographic perspective, the ascending aorta has been divided into six zones corresponding to sites of surgical manipulation. Zones 1 through 3 correspond to the proximal, mid, and distal ascending aorta and represent sites for aortotomies, proximal anastomoses/vent catheters, and cross-clamping, respectively. Zone 4 is the proximal aortic arch and typically the site of aortic cannulation. Zones 5 and 6, which are the distal arch and proximal descending thoracic aorta, are rarely manipulated during standard open heart surgeries. Royse demonstrated that adequate intraoperative TEE imaging of zone 3 occurred in only 58% of cases and zone 4 in only 42% of cases. Additionally, manual surgical palpation detects only 50% of important aortic disease identified by epiaortic ultrasonography. As such, TEE has an important role as a screening tool for disease of the ascending aorta and proximal aortic arch. If significant atheroma or calcification is identified in zones 1, 2, 5, or 6, then epiaortic scanning should be performed by the surgeon (Figs. 32.13 and 32.14). Finally, identification of mobile thrombi in zone 6 should alert the surgeon to the possibility of disrupting this plaque if an intraaortic balloon should need to be placed.

5. **A.** Two classifications systems are used to describe the extent of aortic dissections: the DeBakey system and the Stanford system. DeBakey classifies dissections into three types: Type I: intimal tear in the ascending aorta with extension of the dissection to the descending aorta; Type II: tear in the ascending aorta with dissection confined to the ascending aorta; and Type III: tear beginning in the descending aorta. The Stanford classification system is simpler and uses two groups: Type A dissections involve the ascending aorta, and Type B dissections do not involve the ascending aorta (Fig. 32.2) The Stanford classification not only simplifies the topographic description of the dissection but also identifies the preferred line of therapy based on risk. Type A dissections carry a mortality of 90% to 95% without surgical intervention and account for approximately 65% to 70% of all aortic dissections. Due to a 1% per hour mortality, they require urgent repair.[7] Type B dissections carry a 40% mortality, and medical management is the preferred type of therapy except for Type B dissections, which involve the aortic arch.

Chapter 33

1. **C.** Coverage of the left subclavian artery. The aneurysm involves the distal arch and likely includes the origin of the left subclavian artery that supplies the left radial artery that is being used to monitor systemic arterial pressure. Sudden vasodilation and aortic rupture are likely to change heart rate and central venous pressure, which remain unchanged in this case. Acute type A dissection involves the ascending aorta and is unlikely to result exclusively in hypotension without a change in other monitoring parameters. Acute myocardial ischemia is also likely to result in a change in all monitored parameters.

2. **D.** M-mode pattern of flap motion. The M-mode pattern of the motion of the intimal flap can be very useful for distinguishing between the true and false lumens. The flap tends to move away from the true lumen and into the false lumen during systole due to the higher pressure and flow within the true lumen. Simple identification of an intimal flap, 'smoke,' and holodiastolic flow in either lumen are all insufficient in isolation for the proper identification of lumens. Harmonic imaging is the same for both lumens and is not useful for distinguishing between them.

3. **B.** Mirror image. A mirror image artifact results from the ultrasound beam that bounces off a strong reflector—the distal aortic wall—twice. The received beam is then interpreted by the transducer as having been reflected off a structure at twice the distance from the original reflector. Hence, the appearance of a parallel aorta. This may be mistaken for a type B dissection.

4. **A.** Pulmonary artery catheter. A type A dissection involves the ascending aorta and, during intraoperative imaging, can be easily confounded by the reflection of a PA catheter in the right pulmonary artery that produces a mirror-image artifact in the ascending aorta. Pleural effusion and intraaortic balloon pump catheter may be confused for a Type B dissection during imaging of the descending aorta, while a pericar-

dial effusion is unlikely to produce an artifact in the ascending aorta.

5. **B.** Carotid dissection. A type A dissection involving the carotids should always be suspected when a patient develops deterioration of mental status. While ascending atheroma could be a potential cause, it is unlikely to lead to deterioration in this setting without aortic manipulation. Other lesions listed as options are even less likely to produce a gradual deterioration unless contributing to circulatory shock. Carotid involvement remains the most likely suspect in this scenario.

Chapter 34

1. **E.** Shorter transmitral A-wave compared to the pulmonary venous A-wave
2. **A.** Delayed closure of the aortic valve
3. **A.** Dilated cardiomyopathy
4. **A.** Increased atrial contribution to left ventricular filling
5. **D.** Interventricular septum measuring more than 18 mm in thickness
6. **C.** Persistent left ventricular outflow tract obstruction
7. **B.** Free wall

Chapter 35

1. **A.** 7%
2. **C.** 85%
3. **E.** All of the above
4. **D.** RV function
5. **E.** Correctable cardiac lesions are not absolute contraindications to LVAD implantation. Systemic infections are a contraindication to LVAD implantation related to the difficulty in effectively treating a systemic infection in the presence of a mechanical device.

Chapter 36

1. **D.** There are many 2D-echocardiographic findings of the LV, which would be considered abnormal in the general population, that are characteristic of transplant recipients, including an increase in LV wall thickness (especially the posterior and septal walls), observation of LV mass and LV mass index, paradoxical or flat interventricular septal motion, and decreased interventricular septal systolic thickening compared to normal (31% vs. 44%) (23). Because the donor heart is normal in size, it is typically smaller than the original dilated failing heart and, therefore, it is positioned more medially in the mediastinum and tends to be rotated clockwise, which usually necessitates using nonstandard transducer locations and angles for echocardiography. Residual fluid accumulations in the posterior pericardial space contribute to the common small postoperative pericardial effusions (30).

2. **D.** The echocardiographic assessment of LV diastolic function in the transplanted heart is complicated by the variability of the Doppler velocity profiles from the atrioventricular valves, which may be observed when the remnant recipient atria retain mechanical activity. This results in asynchronous atrial contractions, modifying the filling patterns of both ventricles (23–27). The beat-to-beat variations in transmitral (and tricuspid) diastolic velocities, assessed by pulsed-wave Doppler, relate to the timing of contraction of the recipient atria within the cardiac cycle. Therefore, it is important to locate the recipient P waves within the donor cardiac cycle before making the required Doppler measurements. When the recipient P waves occur during late systole to mitral valve opening, the flow signals should not be used to measure diastolic indices. Recipient P waves occurring during this period decrease isovolumic relaxation time and pressure half-time and increase the mitral inflow peak E-wave velocity. If the recipient P waves occur anywhere from late diastole through midsystole, the flow signals may be used (23,24,26).

3. **C.** The decision regarding RV assist device implantation is dependent upon a stepwise review of overall hemodynamics after the institution of maximal inotropic and vasodilator support. The assessment includes an evaluation of the size and function of both ventricles by TEE, the status of mediastinal bleeding, oxygenation, presence of arrhythmias, and urine output. This assessment usually takes place after several unsuccessful attempts to separate the patient from CPB and approximately 1 hour after removal of the aortic cross-clamp. The observation of a small hyperdynamic LV and a dilated RV by TEE, marginal urine output, arrhythmias, or coagulopathy should prompt the insertion of a RV assist device. The presence of coagulopathy will require ongoing volume resuscitation with blood products, likely resulting in a worsening of pulmonary hypertension, pulmonary edema, and RV failure with its secondary effects on cardiac output and end organ perfusion.

4. **B.** The combination of disturbed atrial hemodynamics caused by asynchronous contraction of the atria and atrial enlargement might contribute to slow blood flow within the atrial cavities and explain the relatively high incidence of spontaneous echo contrast (SEC) (25%–55%) despite normal ventricular function in heart transplant recipients (27,29,39,40). This is usually confined to the donor atrial component and characterized by multiple microechoes visible at normal gain settings slowly swirling within the enlarged atrial cavity and disappearing after passage through the mitral valve, which allows clear discrimination from noise echoes or reverberations (29). The importance of diagnosing LA SEC in the heart transplant recipients stems from its association with LA thrombi and systemic embolic events on postoperative follow-up studies (29,40,48). In most cases, the thrombi are attached to the atrial free wall underneath the protruding

suture in a niche formed after partial removal of the left atrial appendage during transplantation but can also be localized on the posterior LA wall or on the suture line (27,29,40). Therefore, the presence of LA SEC on intraoperative TEE should prompt postoperative follow-up studies to assess for the presence of atrial thrombi and the need for antiplatelet or anticoagulation therapy. The incidence of left atrial SEC and subsequent left atrial thrombi and systemic embolic events on postoperative follow-up is decreased by using the bicaval (48) or total orthotopic (27) anastomotic techniques.

5. A. Tricuspid regurgitation (TR), found in 85% of transplant recipients, occurs immediately after heart transplantation, and it is usually moderate, with an eccentric jet direction pointing toward the interatrial septum (29,55). There is no association between the incidence and severity of TR immediately after cardiac transplantation and the presence of RV dysfunction (56). Quantification of the severity of TR by color-flow Doppler is best achieved using the ratio of the maximum area of the regurgitant jet to the right atrial area (57) (<10% trivial, 10%–24% mild, 25%–49% moderate, 50% severe). The severity of posttransplant TR correlates with echocardiographic indices of atrial distortion (recipient to donor atrial area ratio) and the systolic shortening of the tricuspid annulus (55). The significantly reduced incidence of moderate and severe TR with the bicaval anastomotic technique, and both TR and MR after total orthotopic heart transplantation (38), further supports this hypothesis.

Chapter 37

1. C. Both TTE and TEE are used to confirm the preintervention diagnostic assessment, determine the potential for complications, and to guide the procedure. Along with fluoroscopy, TEE is used to position the BAV catheter for the initial balloon valvuloplasty and then to confirm proper orientation of the device prior to its deployment. Following deployment, the TEE is essential to evaluate for potential complications including assessment of the severity of AS, interruption of coronary flow, or creation of an aortic dissection.

2. E. Wilkins et al. first reported the ability of an echocardiographic score to predict the long-term course of patients undergoing percutaneous valvuloplasty. Factors, which predicted a successful valvuloplasty over

6 months included leaflet mobility, thickness, and calcification in addition to the degree of involvement of the subvalvular apparatus. Sotaria et al. subsequently demonstrated the importance of the degree of commissural calcification in predicting a successful valvuloplasty.

3. D. The MitraClip technology is based on the surgical edge-to-edge repair technique first reported by Alfieri et al. in the early 1990s as an approach to mitral repair for all etiologies of MR. At the time of the original report, Alfieri predicted the potential application of this approach for percutaneous correction of MR.

4. E. TEE guidance during percutaneous mitral valve procedure is essential for the initial diagnostic evaluation and provides the mechanism(s), location of abnormal MV, the precise coaptation gap, and width of segments requiring redress. TEE also provides guidance for the initial positioning and delivery of the MitraClip device for attachment. A thorough echocardiographic assessment is performed to confirm adequate placement with complete or near-complete elimination of mitral regurgitation.

5. C. Along with left and right atrial as well as right ventricular diastolic collapse, respiratory variation in flow and volume of hepatic vein and cardiac chambers are part of criteria used to diagnosed cardiac tamponade. Although LV wall motion abnormalities can be present in patients with tamponade, they are not useful for making the diagnosis.

Chapter 38

1. D. Strain is load dependent
2. C. DTI-strain displays deformation along a single dimension – the plane of the ultrasound beam
3. B. It is angle independent
4. E. Ideal tracking requires an optimal frame rate less than 100 frames/s
5. D.

Chapter 39

1. D. Small pericardial effusions tend to be localized behind the posterior wall of the left ventricle
2. B. Tissue Doppler imaging of the lateral mitral annulus
3. C. Right atrial diastolic collapse
4. D. Septal regional wall motion abnormalities

INDEX

Page numbers those followed by f indicate figures; those followed by t indicate tables.

Summary Tables

| TABLE A.1 | Normal and Abnormal TEE Parameters |

Left and Right Atrial Size	Women				Men			
	Reference	Mild Abnormality	Moderate Abnormality	Severe Abnormality	Reference	Mild Abnormality	Moderate Abnormality	Severe Abnormality
Atrial dimensions (ME 2 and 4 Chamber)								
LA diameter, cm	2.7–3.8	3.9–4.2	4.3–4.6	≥4.7	3.0–4.0	4.1–4.6	4.7–5.2	≥5.2
LA diameter/BSA, cm/m²	1.5–2.3	2.4–2.6	2.7–2.9	≥3.0	1.5–2.3	2.4–2.6	2.7–2.9	≥3.0
RA minor-axis dimension, cm	2.9–4.5	4.6–4.9	5.0–5.4	≥5.5	2.9–4.5	4.6–4.9	5.0–5.4	≥5.5
RA minor-axis dimension/BSA, cm /m²	1.7–2.5	2.6–2.8	2.9–3.1	≥3.2	1.7–2.5	2.6–2.8	2.9–3.1	≥3.2
Atrial area								
LA area, cm²	≤ 20	20–30	30–40	>40	≤20	20–30	30–40	>40
Atrial volumes								
LA volume, mL	22–52	53–62	63–72	≥73	18–58	59–68	69–78	≥79
LA volume/BSA, mL/m²	22 ± 6	29–33	34–39	>40	22 ± 6	29–33	34–39	>40

LV Mass and Geometry	Women				Men			
	Reference	Mild Abnormality	Moderate Abnormality	Severe Abnormality	Reference	Mild Abnormality	Moderate Abnormality	Severe Abnormality
Linear method (ME 4 and TG Mid 2 Chamber)								
LV mass, g	67–162	163–186	187–210	≥211	88–224	225–258	259–292	≥293
LV mass/BSA, g/m²	43–95	96–108	109–121	≥122	49–115	116–131	132–148	≥149
LV mass/height, g/m	41–99	100–115	116–128	≥129	52–126	127–144	145–162	≥163
LV mass/height2,7, g/m2,7	18–44	45–51	52–58	≥59	20–48	49–55	56–63	≥64
Thickness (TG Mid SAX)								
Relative wall thickness, cm	0.22–0.42	0.43–0.47	0.48–0.52	≥0.53	0.24–0.42	0.43–0.46	0.47–0.51	≥0.52
Septal thickness, cm	0.6–0.9	1.0–1.2	1.3–1.5	≥1.6	0.6–1.0	1.1–1.3	1.4–1.6	≥1.7
Posterior wall thickness, cm	0.6–0.9	1.0–1.2	1.3–1.5	≥1.6	0.6–1.0	1.1–1.3	1.4–1.6	≥1.7
2D Method (ME 4 and TG Mid 2 Chamber)								
LV mass, g	66–150	151–171	172–182	>193	96–200	201–227	228–254	>255
LV mass/BSA, g/m²	44–88	89–100	101–112	≥113	50–102	103–116	117–130	≥131

(continued)

Published in Savage RM, Solomon A, Shernan SK. *Comprehensive Textbook of Perioperative Transesophageal Echocardiography*. 2nd Edition. Philadelphia: WK Health/Lippincott Williams & Wilkins, 2011.

TABLE A.1 Normal and Abnormal TEE Parameters (Continued)	Women				Men			
LV Size	Reference	Mild Abnormality	Moderate Abnormality	Severe Abnormality	Reference	Mild Abnormality	Moderate Abnormality	Severe Abnormality
LV dimension (ME 2 and TG 2 Chamber)								
LV diastolic diameter	3.9–5.3	5.4–5.7	5.8–6.1	≥6.2	4.2–5.9	6.0–6.3	6.4–6.8	≥6.9
LV diastolic diameter/BSA, cm/m²	2.4–3.2	3.3–3.4	3.5–3.7	≥3.8	2.2–3.1	3.2–3.4	3.5–3.6	≥3.7
LV diastolic diameter/height, cm/m	2.5–3.2	3.3–3.4	3.5–3.6	≥3.7	2.4–3.3	3.4–3.5	3.6–3.7	≥3.8
LV volume (ME 4 and 2 Chamber)								
LV diastolic volume, mL	56–104	105–117	118–130	≥131	67–155	156–178	179–201	≥201
LVdiastolic volume/BSA, mL/m²	35–75	76–86	87–96	≥97	35–75	76–86	87–96	≥97
LV systolic volume, mL	19–49	50–59	60–69	≥70	22–58	59–70	71–82	≥83
LVsystolic volume/BSA, mL/m²	12–30	31–36	37–42	≥43	12–30	31–36	37–42	≥43

	Women				Men			
LV Function	Reference	Mild Abnormality	Moderate Abnormality	Severe Abnormality	Reference	Mild Abnormality	Moderate Abnormality	Severe Abnormality
Linear method (ME and TG 2 Chamber, TG Mid SAX)								
Midwall fractional shortening,%	15–23	13–14	11–12	≤10	14–22	12–13	10–11	≤10
2D method (ME 4 and 2 Chamber)								
Ejection fraction, %	≥55	45–54	30–44	≤30	≥55	45–54	30–44	≤30

Modified and reprinted from Lang RM, Bierig M, Devereux RB, et al. ASE Committee Recommendations: Recommendations for Chamber Quantification: A Report from the American Society of Echocardiography's Guidelines and Standards Committee and the Chamber Quantification Writing Group. Developed in Conjunction with the European Association of Echocardiography, a Branch of the European Society of Cardiology: J Am Soc Echocardiogr 2005; 18:1440–1463, with permission.

Published in Savage RM, Solomon A, Shernan SK. *Comprehensive Textbook of Perioperative Transesophageal Echocardiography*. 2nd Edition. Philadelphia: WK Health/Lippincott Williams & Wilkins, 2011.

TABLE A.2	Normal and Abnormal TEE Parameters

RV and PA Size	Reference	Mild Abnormality	Moderate Abnormality	Severe Abnormality
RV dimensions (ME 4 chamber)				
Basal RV diameter (RVD 1 or TV Anulus), cm	2.0–2.8	2.9–3.3	3.4–3.8	≥3.9
Mid-RV diameter (RVD 2), cm	2.7–3.3	3.4–3.7	3.8–4.1	≥4.2
Base-to-apex length (RVD 3), cm	7.1–7.9	8.0–8.5	8.6–9.1	≥9.2
RVOT diameters (ME RV inflow-outflow)				
Above aortic valve (RVOT 1), cm	2.5–2.9	3.0–3.2	3.3–3.5	≥3.6
Above pulmonic valve (RVOT 2), cm	1.7–2.3	2.4–2.7	2.8–3.1	≥3.2
PA diameter (ME RV inflow-outflow)				
Below pulmonic valve, mid RCC (PA 1), cm	1.5–2.1	2.2–2.5	2.6–2.9	≥3.0
At pulmonic valve (PA 1), cm	1.7–2.3	2.4–2.7	2.8–3.1	≥3.2

RV Size and Function (ME 4 Chamber)	Reference	Mild Abnormality	Moderate Abnormality	Severe Abnormality
RV diastolic area, cm^2	11–28	29–32	33–37	≥38
RV systolic area, cm^2	7.5–16	17–19	20–22	≥23
RV fractional area change, %	32–60	25–31	18–24	≥17
Tricuspid annular systolic excursion	1.5–2.0 cm			<1.5

Inferior Vena Cava (LAX, SAX)	Reference	Mild Abnormality	Moderate Abnormality	Severe Abnormality
	(AP < 5 mm Hg)	(RAP = 6–10 mm Hg)	(RAP = 0–15 mm Hg)	(RAP > 15 mm Hg)
IVC diameter (cm)	< 1.7	≥ 1.7	≥ 1.7	≥ 1.7
Respiratory decrease in IVC diameter (%)	50%	≥50%	<50%	0%
IVC ≤ 1.2 cm and spontaneous collapse = Vol Depletion				

Modified and reprinted from Lang RM, Bierig M, Devereux RB, et al. ASE Committee Recommendations: Recommendations for Chamber Quantification: A Report from the American Society of Echocardiography's Guidelines and Standards Committee and the Chamber Quantification Writing Group, Developed in Conjunction with the European Association of Echocardiography, a Branch of the European Society of Cardiology. J Am Soc Echocardiogr 2005;18:1440–1463, with permission.

Published in Savage RM, Solomon A, Shernan SK. *Comprehensive Textbook of Perioperative Transesophageal Echocardiography.* 2nd Edition. Philadelphia: WK Health/Lippincott Williams & Wilkins, 2011.

TABLE **A.3**	Normal and Abnormal TEE Parameters			
	Mean ± SD (mm) Not Indexed	Range (mm) Not Indexed	Mean ± SD (mm) Indexed to BSA	Range (mm) Indexed to BSA
Atria (ME 4 chamber)				
Left atrium (ME 4 chamber end-systole)				
Antero-posterior diameter	38 ± 6	20–52	21 ± 4	13–33
Medial-lateral diameter	39 ± 7	24–52	22 ± 4	13–33
Left atrial appendage				
Length	28 ± 5	15–43	16 ± 3	10–23
Diameter	16 ± 5	10–28	9 ± 3	5–17
Right atrium (ME 4 chamber end-systole)				
Antero-posterior diameter	38 ± 5	28–52	22 ± 3	16–28
Medial-lateral diameter	38 ± 6	29–53	21 ± 3	16–32
Coronary sinus diameter	6.6 ± 1.5	4–10	4 ± 1	2–6
Ventricles				
Left ventricle (TG Mid SAX)				
Antero-posterior diameter (diastole)	43 ± 7	33–55	25 ± 3	19–31
Medial-lateral diameter (diastole)	42 ± 7	23–54	24 ± 4	11–30
Antero-posterior diameter (systole)	28 ± 6	18–40	16 ± 4	10–25
Medial-lateral diameter (systole)	27 ± 6	18–42	15 ± 4	11–24
Right ventricular outflow tract diameter (ME RV Inflow-Outflow)	27 ± 4	16–36	15 ± 2	10–20
Valves (ME 4 chamber, mid-diastole)				
Tricuspid annular diameter	28 ± 5	20–40	16 ± 3	11–24
Mitral annular diameter	29 ± 4	20–38	17 ± 2	11–22
Aorta				
Aortic root diameter (ME RV inflow-outflow)	28 ± 3	21–34	16 ± 2	12–23
Descending thoracic aorta diameter				
Proximal	21 ± 4	14–30	12 ± 2	9–17
Descending	20 ± 4	13–28	11 ± 2	8–15
PA / SVC				
Pulmonary artery and vein				
Right pulmonary artery diameter (ME Asc Ao SA)	17 ± 3	12–22	10 ± 1	7–12
Left upper pulmonary vein diameter	11 ± 2	7–16	6 ± 1	5–10
Superior vena cava diameter	15 ± 3	8–20	8 ± 1	4–11

Modified and reprinted from Cohen G, White M, Sochowski R, et al. Reference values for normal adult transesophageal measurements. J Am Soc Echocardiogr 1995;8:221–230, with permission.

Published in Savage RM, Solomon A, Shernan SK. *Comprehensive Textbook of Perioperative Transesophageal Echocardiography.* 2nd Edition. Philadelphia: WK Health/Lippincott Williams & Wilkins, 2011.

TABLE A.4   Intraoperative Assessment of AR Severity

Parameter	Utility/Advantages	Limitations	Mild	Moderate	Severe
2D imaging					
LV size Nl LV minor-axis ≤ 2.8 cm/m² LVEDV ≤ 82 ml/m²	Simple LV enlarged in chronic AR Normal LV excludes severe chronic AR	LV enlarged in other conditions. Normal in acute AR	Normal in chronic	Normal or dilated	Dilated in chronic
Aortic leaflets	Simple Abnormal in severe AR Flail denotes severe AR	Nonspecific May not reflect severity	Normal or abnormal	Normal or abnormal	Abnormal, flail, or coaptation defect
Doppler					
CF doppler LVOT jet diameter Aliasing velocity 50–60 cm/s	Simple, Very sensitive Quick screen for mechanism	Eccentric jets inaccurate	Small diameter	Medium diameter	Large in central jets Eccentric jets variable
Vena contracta width (cm) Aliasing velocity 50–60 cm/s	Simple Quantitative Identifies mild or severe AR	Not useful with multiple jets Difficult to determine width in eccentric ROA	<0.3	0.3–0.60	>0.6
Jet width/LVOT width (%) Aliasing velocity 50–60 cm/s	Simple, sensitive, quick screen	Eccentric jets inaccurate	<25	25–65	>65
Jet CSA/LVOT CSA (%)	Simple Sensitive quick screen for AR	Eccentric jets inaccurate	<5	5–60	>60
PW doppler flow reversal descending aorta	Simple	Aortic stiffness dependent Brief reversal normal–mild	Brief early diastolic reversal	Prolonged	Holodiastolic reversal
CW doppler spectral density	Simple Faint/incomplete with mild AR	Qualitative Mod and Sev AR overlap	Faint	Dense	Dense
CW doppler jet pressure half time	Simple Semiquantitative	Qualitative Aortic – LV gradient dependent	Slow >500	Medium 500–200	Steep <200
Regurgitant volume (mL/beat)	Quantitative, Valid with multiple or eccentric jets Estimates severity and volume overload	Not valid combined MR and AR	<30	30–60	>60
PISA					
PISA Proximal flow convergence (PFC)	Quantitative Provides severity (ROA)	Limited by aortic Ca⁺⁺ Not valid multiple jets Eccentric jets inaccurate Max ROA Ao aneurysms underestimate	Mild	Moderate	Severe
Regurgitant volume (mL/beat)	Quantitative Provides severity (ROA)	Time consuming Non-physiologic Index (peak ROA X TVI)	<30	30–60	>60
Regurgitant fraction (%)	Quantitative Provides severity (ROA)	Time consuming	<30	30–50	>50
Peak ROA (cm²)	Quantitative Provides severity (ROA)	Not average ROA	<0.10	0.10–0.30	>0.30

Published in Savage RM, Solomon A, Shernan SK. *Comprehensive Textbook of Perioperative Transesophageal Echocardiography*. 2nd Edition. Philadelphia: WK Health/Lippincott Williams & Wilkins, 2011.

| TABLE A.5 | Intraoperative Assessment of AS Severity |

Parameter	Utility/ Advantages	Limitations	Mild	Moderate	Severe
2D imaging					
M mode Maximum cusp separation (mm)	Simple	Qualitative Cursor must be perpendicular	>20	10–20	<10
Aortic valve leaflets	Simple	Qualitative estimation	≤ 1 leaflet immobility	2 leaflet immobility	3 leaflet immobility
Planimetered valve area (cm²) Normal 3–4 cm² Systolic doming increases error risk 3D directed 2D may increase accuracy	Simple	Inaccurate with Ca++ Image plane must be perpendicular Influenced by flow	>1.5	1.0–1.5	≤1.0
Doppler					
CW doppler peak velocity (m/s)*	Simple Little inducable error	Increased with AR	<2.6–3.0	3.0–4.0	>4.0
CW doppler mean gradient (mm Hg)* Pressure Recovery may underestimate gradient when aorta D < 30mm	Simple Little inducable error	Flow dependent Low Flow-Low Gradient AS (use dobutamine if questionable)	<20[a] <30[b]	20–40[a] 30–50[b]	>40[a] >50[b]
Velocity ratio	Simple	Less quantitative	>0.50	0.25–0.50	<0.25
Continuity equation (cm²) $$AoV\ area = \frac{TVI_{LVOT} \times Area_{LVOT}}{TVI_{AoV}}$$	Accurate May be used with AR if LVOT is reference volumetric flow	Squared diameter introduces large error Not valid with Regurg non-LVOT reference valve, LVOTO, or M	>1.5	1.0–1.5	≤1.0

*assumed normal CO
[a]AHA/ACC
[b]ESC
LVOT VTI: Trace Modal Velocity Spectral Envelope
AoV VTI: Trace Outer Velocity Spectral Envelope
LVOT D: Inner Edge-Inner Edge, at af PWD Interrogation

Published in Savage RM, Solomon A, Shernan SK. *Comprehensive Textbook of Perioperative Transesophageal Echocardiography.* 2nd Edition. Philadelphia: WK Health/Lippincott Williams & Wilkins, 2011.

| TABLE A.6 | Intraoperative Assessment of MR Severity | | | | | |

Parameter	Utility/Advantages	Limitations	Mild	Moderate	Severe
2D imaging					
LA size	LAE with chronic MR Normal LA size excludes ser chronic MR	Enlargedother conditions. May be normal in acute MR	Normal	Normal or dilated	LAE
LV size	Normal LV size excludes severe chronic MR	Non-specific	Normal	Normal or dilated	Dilated Enlarged
MV apparatus	Flail or ruptured PM — severe MR	Limited to Flail and Ruptured PM	Normal or abnormal	Normal or abnormal	Flail leaflet Rupuredt Pap Muscle
Doppler			MJA 4–8		
CF doppler maximum jet area (cm²) (CFD-MJA) Aliasing velocity 50–60 cm/s	Efficinet *screen* for mild or severe MR Used for mechanism valuation PFC at aliasing velocity of 50–60 cm/s sign MR	Technical: wall filter, power, aliasing velocity, color gain, frequency Load dependent Wall impengement underestimates 60%	MJA < 4 No PFC	Variable	MJA > 8 Large PFC Wall jet
PW doppler	A-wave dominance excludes severe MR	Dependent on load, diastolic fx, MVA, a fib indirect inication	Dominant A wave	Variable	Dominant E-wave E > 1.2 m/s
PW doppler PV flow	Systolic flow reversal indicates severe MR	Increased LAP, a, fib, need R and L PV to call severe	Systolic dominance	Diastolic dominance	Systolic flow reversal
CW doppler spectral density	Easy to perform	Qualitative	Faint envelope	Dense	"v" wave cut off sign
CW doppler contour	Simple	Qualitative	Parabolic	Variable	Early peaking – triangular
Vena contracta width (cm)	Good eccentric jets Efficient	Not useful for multiple VC Diameters not additive	< 0.3 cm	0.3–0.69 cm	Vena contracta width ≥ 0.7 cm
PISA					
Regurgitant vol (mL)	Quantitative Provides severity (ROA)	Time consuming Non-physiologic index (peak ROA X TVI)	< 30	30–59	≥ 60
Regurgitant fraction (%)	Quantitative Provides severity (ROA)	Not average ROA	< 30	30–49	≥ 50
ROA (cm²)	Quantitative Provides severity (ROA)	Peak ROA, not average Reg Vol by ROA is non-physiologic	< 0.20	0.20–0.39	≥ 0.40

Published in Savage RM, Solomon A, Shernan SK. *Comprehensive Textbook of Perioperative Transesophageal Echocardiography.* 2nd Edition. Philadelphia: WK Health/Lippincott Williams & Wilkins, 2011.

TABLE A.7	Proximal Isovelocity Surface Area

Proximal Flow Convergence Radius and Severity of MR
Simplified ROA for Range of MR V_{Max}

$V_{aliasing}$ = 40 cm/s or 1/ 12th (0.8) peak V_{MR}

Grade	PISA Radius	ROA = PFC Radius^2 /2	Estimated Peak Regurgitant Vol
Mild	<6.3 mm	<0.2 cm^2	<30 mL
Moderate	6.3–8.9 mm	<0.2–0.39 cm^2	30–59 mL
Severe	>9 mm	> 0.40 cm^2	>60 mL

TABLE A.8	Mitral Stenosis Echocardiographic Splitability Index

Grade	Mobility	Leaflet Thickening (mm)	Subvalvular Thickening of Chordal Length	Leaflet Calcification
1	Tips restricted	Normal 4–5	Minimal	Single area
2	Mid and base normal	Margins thick 5–8 mm	1/3	Scattered Ca^{++} confined to margins
3	Base normal	All leaflet thick 5–8 mm	2/3	Ca^{++} to mid-leaflet
4	No movement	All leaflet thick 8–10 mm	3/3	Ca^{++} throughout >8–10 mm

Wilkins GT, Weyman AE, Abascal VM, et al. Percutaneous balloon dilatation of the mitral valve: an analysis of echocardiographic variables related to outcome and the mechanism of dilatation. Br Heart J 1988;60:299–308.

Published in Savage RM, Solomon A, Shernan SK. *Comprehensive Textbook of Perioperative Transesophageal Echocardiography.* 2nd Edition. Philadelphia: WK Health/Lippincott Williams & Wilkins, 2011.

| TABLE A.9 | **Assessment of MV Stenosis Severity** |

Parameter	Utility/ Advantages	Limitations	Mild	Moderate	Severe
2D imaging					
LA size (mm) AP diameter Exclude LAA thrombi	Simple Normal excludes chronic MS	Nonspecific	<45	45–60	>60 in Chronic MS
Spontaneous contrast	Simple **Predictive of stroke**	Nonspecific	Absent	Usually Present	Always Present
MV apparatus morphology	Simple	Inaccurate with Ca++ or previous commissurutomy	<4	4–12	>12
Planimetered valve area (cm²) Normal 3–4 cm² Measure in mid-diastole Atrial fib: average beats Locate max stenosis with TG 2 Chr CFD	Simple	Inaccurate with Ca++ Image plane must be perpendicular Not valid post-commissurotomy	1.5–2.0	1.0–1.5	<1.0
Doppler					
CF doppler prox flow convergence (Aliasing Velocity 50–60 cm/s)	Simple screening method Presence excludes normal	Nonspecific Flow related Present after MVp and MVR	Not present	Usually present	Always present
CW doppler mean gradient (mm Hg) Assumed normal CO Trace diastolic Spectral envelope edge	Simple Little inducable error	Flow rate dependent Increased with MR AR decreases	<5	5–10	>10
CW doppler estimation of PA systolic (mm Hg)	Simple	Nonspecific	<30	30–50	>50
Continuity equation(cm²) $$MV\ Area = \frac{Area_{LVOT} \times TVI_{LVOT}}{TVI_{MV}}$$	Accurate May be used with AR if LVOT is reference volumetric flow	Squared diameter introduces large error Not accurate with AR, MR, or Atrial Fib Not indexed to BSA	1.5–2.0	1.0–1.5	<1.0
Pressure half-time (ms) $$MVA = 220/PHT$$ Bimodal diastolic spectral envelope: use linear mid-portion	Fast	Inaccurate with Abnormal Compliance (LA,LV) Inaccurate with AR, post Valvuloplasty, Atrial Fib AR invalidates $PT_{1/2}$, overestimates valve area Diastolic dysfunction with LVH, AS, aging invalidates	<330 ms	330–220 ms	>220 ms
Proximal isovelocity surface area (PISA) $$MVA = 2\pi R^2 \times V_{Alising} / Peak\ V_{MS} \times \alpha° / 180°$$ $V_{Alising}$ = Aliasing Velocity of Color Doppler R = radius from orifice to PISA interface	Accurate Accurate in presence of MR	Subvalvular stenosis less accurate Funnel shaped angle Time for calculation	1.5–2.0	1.0–1.4	<0.9

Asymptomatic MVA ≥1.5 cm: Intervention not considered; MVA ≤1.5 cm: intervention directed by symptoms, atrial fib, Pulm HTN, potential for BAV. Asymptomatic MVA, ≤1.5 cm: exercise testing

Published in Savage RM, Solomon A, Shernan SK. *Comprehensive Textbook of Perioperative Transesophageal Echocardiography.* 2nd Edition. Philadelphia: WK Health/Lippincott Williams & Wilkins, 2011.

| TABLE A.10 | Intraoperative Assessment of TR Severity | | | | | |

Parameter	Utility/Advantages	Limitations	Mild	Moderate	Severe
2D imaging					
RA, RV, and IVC size *RA diameter <4.6 cm RV diameter <4.3 cm*	RAE and RVE indicates chronic TR Normal RA and RV excludes sign chronic TR.	RAE not specific RA normal in severe acute TR	Normal	Normal or dilated	Usually dilated
TV morphology	Flail and poor coaptation with significant TR	Other findings no specific for significant TR	Normal	Normal or abnormal	Flail and Incomplete coaptation
Doppler					
CF doppler max jet area (cm²) (CFD-MJA) *Nyquist limit 50–60 cm/ Not valid eccentric jets*	Efficient screen for TR	Note: tech factors and load conditions Underestimates eccentric jets	<5	5–10	>10
PW doppler hepatic vein flow	Simple	Blunting multiple causes	Systolic dominance	Systolic blunting	Systolic reversal
CW doppler spectral envelope *Jet density Contour*	Simple Readily available	Qualitative, complementary data	Soft parabolic	Dense variable contour	Dense triangular early peaking
CF doppler vena contracta width (cm)	Efficient Quantitative distinguishes |mild from severe TR	Intermediates direct need of other parameters confirmation	Not defined	<0.7	>0.7
PISA					
PISA radius (cm) *Baseline shift with Nyquist 28 cm/s*	Quantitative	Validated in only a few studies	<0.5	0.6–0.9	>0.9

Published in Savage RM, Solomon A, Shernan SK. *Comprehensive Textbook of Perioperative Transesophageal Echocardiography.* 2nd Edition. Philadelphia: WK Health/Lippincott Williams & Wilkins, 2011.

| TABLE **A.11** | **Assessment TV Stenosis Severity** |

Parameter	Utility/ Advantages	Limitations	Mild	Moderate	Severe
2D imaging					
TV morphology Thickness Ca^{++} Reduced mobility	Simple	Nonspecific	Normal valve	Variable	Abnormal
RA size					
IVC					Dilated
RV size >4.3 cm RV ED area ≥35.5 cm²			Normal RV	Variable	Dilated RV
Doppler					
CF proximal flow convergence (Nyquist 50–60 cm/s)	Simple	Nonspecific Not Quantitative			
CW jet density	Simple	Validation	Faint	Dense	Dence
CW jet deceleration	Slow decel if PR or L-R shunt	Vlidation	Steep decel	Variable decel	Delayed decel
CW doppler half-time $TVA = 190/PT_{1/2}$ Bimodal diastolic spectral envelope: use linear mid-portion	Fast	RA/RV decreased PR reduces $PT_{1/2}$ overestimates area			>190ms
Continuity equation (cm²) $Tv\ Area = \dfrac{TVI_{LVOT} \times Area\ LVOT}{TV}$	Accurate May be used with AR if LVOT is reference volumetric flow	Squared diameter introduces large error Not accurate with TR, Reference Valve Regurgittion or Atrial Fib Not indexed to BSA		>1.0	< 1.0
CW velocity (m/s)	Simple Minimizes inducible error	Flow dependent Correct alignment required	<1	1–2.5	>2.5
CW TVI (cm)	Simple Minimal inducible error	Requires Correct alignment Flow dependent			>60
CW mean gradient (mm Hg)	Simple	Flow dependent			≥5

Published in Savage RM, Solomon A, Shernan SK. *Comprehensive Textbook of Perioperative Transesophageal Echocardiography.* 2nd Edition. Philadelphia: WK Health/Lippincott Williams & Wilkins, 2011.

TABLE A.12   Intraoperative Assessment of PR Severity

Parameter	Utility/ Advantages	Limitations	Mild	Moderate	Severe
2D imaging					
Pulmonic valve morphology Cusp number, motion, structure	Simple Mechanism	Nonspecific	Normal	Normal or abnormal	Flail / no coaptation
RV size RV diameter < 4.3 cm RV ED area ≤ 35.5 cm²	Normal size excludes significant PR	RV enlargement in other conditions.	Normal*	Normal or dilated	Dilated
Paradoxical septal motion (volume overload pattern)	Simple sign of severe PR	Not specific for PR	Normal	Variable	Abnormal
Doppler					
Color flow Doppler jet length Nyquist limit 50–60 cm/s	Simple	Poor correlation with severity of PR	Thin <10 mm length	Variable	Large Wide origin
CFD vena contracta	Simple	Not Validated	Small	Variable	Large
CW doppler jet density	Simple	Qualitative	Faint	Variable	Short dense
CW doppler deceleration	Simple	Qualitative	Slow deceleration	Variable deceleration	Steep deceleration Early termination
Pulmonic systolic flow compared to systemic	Quantitative	Time consuming	Slightly increased	Intermedi- ate	Greatly increased

TABLE A.13   Intraoperative Assessment of PS Severity

Parameter	Utility/ Advantages	Limitations	Mild	Moderate	Severe
2D imaging					
RV hypertrophy Normal RV thickness = 2–3 mm	Simple	Nonspecific foreshortening	<3	3–5	> 5 mm
Doppler					
CF doppler max jet area (MJA) cm² Nyquist limit 50–60 cm/s	Simple	Qualitative	Proximal flow convergence	Variable flow convergence and turbulence	Turbulence
CW doppler peak velocity	Simple	Alignment with flow	<3	3–4	>4
CW doppler peak gradient	Simple	Alignment with flow	<36	36–64	>64

Published in Savage RM, Solomon A, Shernan SK. *Comprehensive Textbook of Perioperative Transesophageal Echocardiography.* 2nd Edition. Philadelphia: WK Health/Lippincott Williams & Wilkins, 2011.

| TABLE | **A.14** | **Estimation of Hemodynamic Pressures** |

Pressure Estimated	Required Measurement	Formula	Normal Values (mm Hg)
Estimated CVP	Respiratory IVC collapse (spontaneously breathing)	$\geq 40\% = 5$ mm Hg $< 40\%$, (nl RV) = 10 mm Hg None (RV Dysfx) = 15 mm Hg	5–10 mm Hg
RV systolic (RVSP)	Peak velocity$_{TR}$ CVP estimated or measured	$RVSP = 4(V_{TR})^2 + CVP$ (No PS)	16–30 mm Hg
RV systolic (with VSD)	Systemic systolic BP Peak $V_{LV\text{-}RV}$	$RVSP = SBP - 4(V_{LV\text{-}RV})^2$ (No AS or LVOT obstruction)	usually >50 mm Hg
PA systolic (PASP)	Peak velocity$_{TR}$ CVP estimated or measured	$PASP = 4(V_{TR})^2 + CVP$ (No PS)	16–30 mm Hg
PA diastolic (PAD)	End-diastolic Velocity$_{PR}$ CVP estimated or measured	$PAEDP = 4(V_{PR\ ED})^2 + CVP$	0–8 mm Hg
PA mean (PAM)	Acceleration time (AT) to peak V_{PA} (in m/s)	$PAM = (-0.45)\ AT + 79$	10–16 mm Hg
RV dP/dt	TR spectral envelope $T_{TR\ (2\ m/s)} - T_{TR\ (1\ m/s)}$	$RV\ dP = 4V^2_{TR(2\ m/s)} - 4V^2_{TR(2\ m/s)}$ $RV\ dP/dt = dP / T_{TR(2\ m/s)} - T_{TR(1\ m/s)}$	>150 mm Hg/ms
LA systolic (LASP)	Peak V_{MR} Systolic BP (SBP)	$LASP = SBP - 4(V_{MR})^2$ (No AS or LVOT obstruction)	3–15 mm Hg
LA (PFO)	Velocity$_{PFO}$ CVP estimated or measured	$LAP = 4(V_{PFO})^2 + CVP$	3–15 mm Hg
LV diastolic (LVEDP)	End-diastolic Velocity$_{AR}$ Diastolic BP (DBP)	$LVEDP = DBP - 4(V_{AR})^2$	3–12 mm Hg
LV dP/dt	MR spectral envelope $T_{MR\ (2\ m/s)} - T_{MR\ (1\ m/s)}$	$LV\ dP = 4V^2_{MR(3\ m/s)} - 4V^2_{MR(1\ m/s)}$ $LV\ dP/dt = dP / T_{MR\ (3\ m/s)} - T_{MR\ (1\ m/s)}$	>800 mm Hg/ms

Published in Savage RM, Solomon A, Shernan SK. *Comprehensive Textbook of Perioperative Transesophageal Echocardiography.* 2nd Edition. Philadelphia: WK Health/Lippincott Williams & Wilkins, 2011.

| TABLE | A.15 | Assessment of Diastolic Function |

Patterns of diastolic dysfunction measured by transesophageal echocardiography

| | Mitral inflow | PV flow | Tissue doppler | Color M-mode |

Labels under panels: Normal (Age <50) | Normal (Age >50) | Stage I Delayed Relaxation | Stage II Pseudo normal | Stage III Restrictive

| TABLE | A.16 | Assessment of Diastolic Function |

	Normal (age 21–49)	Normal (age > 50)	Stage I (delayed relaxation)	Stage II (pseudonormal filling)	Stage III (restrictive filling)
E/A	>1	>1	<1	1–2	>2
DT (ms)	<220	<220	>220	150–200	<150
IVRT (ms)	<100	<100	>100	60–100	<60
S/D	<1	≥1	≥1	<1	<1
AR (cm/s)	<35	<35	<35	≥35	≥25
Em (cm/s)	>10	>8	<8	<8	<8
Vp (cm/s)	>55	>45	<45	<45	<45

Unless atrial mechanical failure is present. AR, pulmonary venous peak atrial contraction reversed velocity; DT, early left ventricular filing deceleration time; E/A, early-to-atrial left ventricular filing ratio; Em, peak early diastolic myocardial velocity; IVRT, isovolumic relaxation time; S/D, systolic-to-diastolic pulmonary venous flow ratio; Vp, color M-mode flow propagation velocity. (With permission from Garcia et al. JACC 1998).

Published in Savage RM, Solomon A, Shernan SK. *Comprehensive Textbook of Perioperative Transesophageal Echocardiography.* 2nd Edition. Philadelphia: WK Health/Lippincott Williams & Wilkins, 2011.